Thieme

Minimally Invasive Spine Surgery

A Primer

Luis Manuel Tumialán, MD
Associate Professor of Neurosurgery
Barrow Neurological Institute
St. Joseph's Hospital and Medical Center
Phoenix, Arizona, USA

Director of Minimally Invasive Spine Surgery
Greenbaum Surgical Specialty Hospital
HonorHealth Neuroscience Research Institute
Scottsdale, Arizona, USA

Illustrated by Joshua Lai, MScBMC
Medical Illustrator
Neuroscience Publications
Barrow Neurological Institute
St. Joseph's Hospital and Medical Center
Phoenix, Arizona

530 illustrations

Thieme
New York • Stuttgart • Delhi • Rio de Janeiro

Library of Congress Cataloging-in-Publication Data

Names: Tumialán, Luis Manuel, author. | Lai, Joshua, illustrator.
Title: Minimally invasive spine surgery : a primer / Luis Manuel Tumialán; illustrator, Joshua Lai.
Description: New York : Thieme [2020] | Includes bibliographical references and index. | Summary: "The purpose of this work is to be a readable cohesive single-authored introductory text that discusses the principles of minimally invasive spine surgery and then explains the technique procedure by procedure. It is the goal for the reader to experience each chapter as if they are in the operating room with the author. The hope is that the words from the book become the voice inside the resident's head as they see, learn and eventually perform the procedure. This work is written as if the author were actually teaching the resident in a rotation. He begins discussing the philosophical approach to minimally invasive spinal surgery as compared to open procedures and the mindset that one should apply. He then walks the reader through the basic procedures, such as microdiscectomies and laminectomies. Principles introduced in early chapters are reinforced in the later chapters; in this manner, the earlier chapters become the building blocks for the later chapters. This is analogous to resident education, where one would teach a resident a minimally invasive microdiscectomy before going into a lumbar fusion. Each chapter has narrated video for review"– Provided by publisher.
Identifiers: LCCN 2019053438 | ISBN 9781626232181 hardcover | ISBN 9781626232198 eISBN
Subjects: MESH: Spine–surgery | Minimally Invasive Surgical Procedures–methods | Orthopedic Procedures–methods
Classification: LCC RD768 | NLM WE 725 | DDC 617.4/71–dc23
LC record available at https://lccn.loc.gov/2019053438

Thieme Publishers New York
333 Seventh Avenue, New York, NY 10001 USA
+1 800 782 3488, customerservice@thieme.com

Thieme Publishers Stuttgart
Rüdigerstrasse 14, 70469 Stuttgart, Germany
+49 [0]711 8931 421, customerservice@thieme.de

Thieme Publishers Delhi
A-12, Second Floor, Sector-2, Noida-201301
Uttar Pradesh, India
+91 120 45 566 00, customerservice@thieme.in

Thieme Revinter Publicações Ltda.
Rua do Matoso, 170 – Tijuca
Rio de Janeiro RJ 20270-135 - Brasil
+55 21 2563-9702
www.thiemerevinter.com.br

Cover art designed by Luis Manuel Tumialán and Joshua Lai; illustrated by Joshua Lai
Cover design: Thieme Publishing Group
Typesetting by Thomson Digital, India

Printed in the United States of America by
King Printing Co., Inc. 5 4 3 2 1

ISBN 978-1-62623-218-1

Also available as an e-book:
eISBN 978-1-62623-219-8

On the cover:

A posterior view of the lumbosacral spine is shown, with various minimally invasive approaches shown on the right side of the spine: A minimal access port in position for a microdiscectomy at L5-S1, an expandable minimal access port with a view of the completed osteotomy cuts for a transforaminal lumbar interbody fusion at L4-5 (pedicle screws in position at L4 and L5) and at L3-4, an access port is positioned for removal of a far lateral disc extrusion. A dilator up against the L2 lamina with the various trajectories of exposure is shown for the decompression. Kambin's prism is shown over the right L2-3 disc space. Finally, a dilator navigates the branches of the lumbar plexus for a transpsoas approach into the L2-3 disc space.

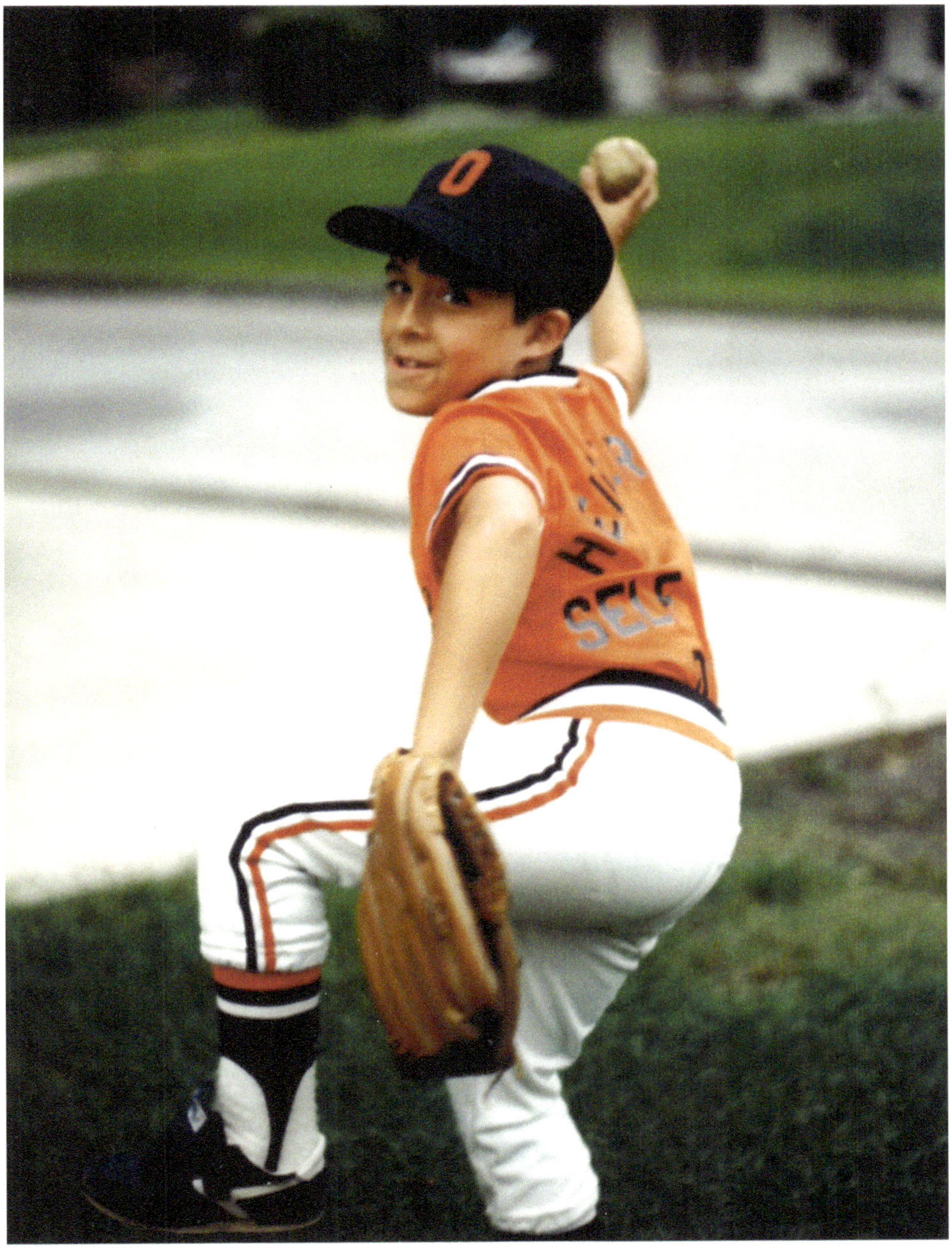

For Jorge

August 11, 1975 – October 19, 2001

Contents

Foreword

In the 10 years that I have known Luis Manuel Tumialán, he has been at the forefront of developing minimally invasive approaches to spine surgery. This Primer is a testament to his passion for improving patient outcomes and striving to advance the knowledge and understanding of the art and science of minimally invasive spine surgery.

The Primer is a comprehensive, well-written volume on minimally invasive spine surgery encompassing the cervical, thoracic and lumbar spine. It is superbly illustrated with detailed 3D illustrations, drawings and diagnostic studies. In it, Dr. Tumialán not only details the surgical techniques and nuances of minimally invasive spine surgery but also eloquently describes the evolution and historical perspectives of the techniques as they evolved into the minimally invasive procedures he uses daily. Within each chapter, he emphasizes the grounds for surgical intervention plus the advantages of using minimally invasive techniques. Each chapter meticulously details and beautifully illustrates the surgical anatomy. Throughout the book, he underscores the unique anatomy of the spine at each level. Fortunately for the reader, Dr. Tumialán applies his extensive experience with minimally invasive spine procedures to guide the reader through each technique as if they were assisting with the surgery.

Chapter 1 presents the history of the conversion from open spine surgery to minimally invasive surgery. Chapters 2 through 6 describe minimally invasive discectomy, laminectomy, transforaminal lumbar interbody fusion, lateral microdiscectomy and lateral transpsoas interbody lumbar fusion. Chapters 7 through 9 portray minimally invasive techniques in the cervical spine and describe in beautiful detail posterior cervical foraminotomy, posterior cervical laminectomy and anterior cervical discectomy with arthroplasty or fusion. Chapters 10 and 11 feature minimally invasive procedures for spinal cord decompression in metastatic spine disease along with the removal of intradural extramedullary lesions within the thoracic spine. Finally, Chapters 12 and 13 focus on the use of fluoroscopy and radiation safety in minimally invasive spine surgery.

Dr. Tumialán also scrutinizes the learning curve of becoming familiar with minimally invasive techniques, always with the aim of accomplishing the surgical task with the least disruption of the vertebral bone and musculature. Throughout the book, he emphasizes the historical aspects of each procedure and how he personally learned from the early maverick surgeons and adapted their techniques to the minimally invasive approach. He describes the pitfalls and pearls of converting to the minimally invasive approach at each level of the spine with instructive cases. For example, in Chapter 3, he describes the removal of the ligamentum flavum in patients with lumbar stenosis and reveals the conversion from piecemeal removal to en bloc removal and discusses the advantages of the latter procedure. He not only describes in detail each specific surgical procedure but also emphasizes the potential complications and their treatment. Minimally invasive spine surgery has changed tremendously over the past few decades, from rudimentary approaches to exquisitely refined minimally invasive techniques.

This extraordinary volume covering fundamental and sophisticated minimally invasive spine techniques should be on every spine and orthopedic surgeon's reading list and reference shelf, and even in the operating room. The Primer and its video accompaniments are certainly essential for the surgeon, resident or fellow who desires to learn and develop expertise in minimally invasive spine surgery.

In the spirit of advancing our craft,

Volker K.H. Sonntag, MD
Emeritus Professor, Vice Chairman, and Spine Section Chief
Department of Neurosurgery
Barrow Neurological Institute
St. Joseph's Hospital and Medical Center
Phoenix, Arizona
December 2019

Preface

We all come from the past, and children ought to know what it was that went into their making to know that life is a braided cord of humanity stretching up from time long gone, and that it cannot be defined by the span of a single journey from diaper to shroud.

Russell Baker

The practice of spine surgery is remarkable in that every spine surgeon I have ever met has been so willing to share their knowledge, teach me their tricks and talk to me about their failures as much as their successes. The entire basis of all of our professional meetings is sharing our recent experiences in the management of the spine and discussing new developments for its surgical treatment. The objective is as simple as it is noble: teach other surgeons how to help patients. Such an open-source environment can only lead to the rapid development of technology and seismic advances in a field. A fast-paced advancement has indeed been the case for modern spine surgery, which is less than 100 years old. Although it may be hard to fathom, it was only a modest 85 years ago that Mixter and Barr first reported the surgical management of radiculopathy by removing an extruded lumbar herniated disc that was compressing a nerve root. I have patients older than Mixter and Barr's operation. It has been 61 years since Cloward, Smith and Robinson described anterior cervical approaches that revolutionized the management of cervical radiculopathy and myelopathy. Most of my patients are older than that operation. Roy-Camille began routinely using lumbar pedicle screws in 1986, which makes me older than that technique.

The common denominator among all these developments is that these pioneering surgeons identified a structural problem amenable to a surgical solution. Whether a compressed nerve root in the cervical or lumbar spine or a dynamic instability, surgeons conceived and then executed a surgical intervention, analyzed their results and published their findings. Successes or failures, they hid nothing. Instead, they shared their experiences with the world. They taught generation after generation of surgeons how to perform these procedures. In turn, each generation of surgeons made their contribution to refining each procedure, or in some circumstances, they developed something entirely new. The development of minimally invasive spine surgery is part of that continuum.

Throughout the decades of development and iterations, surgeons established patterns and traditions that were inevitably passed on as well. In much the same way, my son may sputter out an adage spoken by my father's grandmother, which he has heard a thousand times come from my mouth. Similarly, we must indeed utter statements in the operating theater, the origins of which we do not necessarily know short of our mentors. But our mentors may have repeated it from their mentors, who may have, in turn, repeated the same statement from another generation. Some of those classic quotations have undoubtedly bubbled to the surface in this work. *Vox audita perit, litera scripta manet.*

This Primer is a continuation of the open-source mentality that is the specialty of spine surgery. In its simplest form, it is nothing more than a historical account of where we have been, a snapshot in time of where we currently are and a modest hint of where we have the potential to go. The material in this book came from "*a braided cord of humanity stretching up from time long gone*," which has been so well captured in our peer-reviewed literature. For each procedure, I have gathered those writings of pioneering surgeons, reviewed the more recent rigorous analyses of our peer-reviewed literature and placed them alongside the wise words of mentors and the tricks I have been taught along the way. I have attempted to lay the material out in a manner that would be beneficial to the medical student, resident, fellow or practicing spine surgeon. The goal is to understand the origins of the procedure, the anatomical basis and the nuances of the surgical technique. The hope is that the contents of this book will help surgeons help their patients, the same way the mentors, friends and the timeless voices in our spine literature have helped me help my patients. And so, to paraphrase the late Russell Baker quote that begins this preface, I leave the reader with the following thought before embarking on this Primer of minimally invasive spine surgery:

> We all come from the past, and spine surgeons ought to know what it was that went into the ability to routinely perform both the simple and complex spine operations of today. To know that our specialty is a braided cord of experiences, both successes and failures, stretching from time long gone, and that it cannot be defined by the span of a single journey from residency to retirement.

Luis Manuel Tumialán
Phoenix, Arizona
December 2019

Acknowledgments

I did not know precisely what form this book would eventually take when I blissfully and quite naïvely embarked upon writing it 4 years ago. One thing is certain: At the time, I had no concept of how to bring to life the images in my mind; how to organize an entire library of intraoperative photographs, MRIs and operative footage; or even how to appropriately assemble all the chapters. All I knew is that there was the concept of a book percolating in my mind, and I just started typing. The reality is that assembling a book such as this Primer is a veritable construction project, where an entire team of professionals is needed. I was fortunate to have such a team of experts in the Barrow Neuroscience Publications Department. Without that team, the Primer would not resemble the final, fully matured form you have before you. In fact, it would never have seen the light of day. Instead, it would be a half-baked idea still percolating in my mind.

The construction foreman of this project was Mark Schornak, who leads the Neuroscience Publications team. Mark proficiently coordinated the efforts of the animators, illustrators and video editors while Mary Ann Clifft led the early editorial process. They created method for the chaos I would bring week after week when I visited the department. Throughout the submissions of the chapters, Lynda Orescanin untethered my tangled prose and put appropriate limits on my use of metaphors. She tempered my desire to anthropomorphize surgical instruments but, at the same time, encouraged my voice to surface in the writing, which allowed me to jettison the neutral academic voice from the pages of this book. Somehow, Lynda struck a perfect balance. Time and again, Lynda's keen eye would identify opportunities to clarify a point or restructure a sentence. Thus, the neologism, to "Orescan" a chapter came into being to describe Lynda's work. As a result of the proficient "Orescanning," the Primer is a vastly improved product.

It became evident very early in this project that to communicate a concept or idea central to minimally invasive spine surgery, the artwork had to depict what a surgeon sees through an operating microscope. Artists created wonderful hand-drawn art early in this project, but those works could not capture the spatial lighting and stereovision the eyes see with the operating microscope, especially through a minimal access port. Nor do two-dimensional photographs from a microscope capture the essence of depth. An important decision was made very early in this project to invest the time needed to build a computer model that would allow for the necessary perspectives that would better communicate the images seen in minimally invasive spine surgery. Over several months, Joshua Lai brought our spine model, affectionately known as *Gilgamesh*, to life, and with it, a new perspective on artwork for minimally invasive spine surgery. While the creation of *Gilgamesh* threw off all the timelines for the completion of the book, I believe that it was a worthwhile endeavor. I am grateful for the support offered by Mark Schornak throughout that creative process and the backing by Barrow Neurological Institute to see it through. I trust the reader will find genuine benefit in the various computer-generated figures created for this work.

I am grateful to Michael Hickman, who brought to life those concepts that require animation to communicate the point superbly. Phillip Hoppes expertly breathed life into radiation physics with his illustrations and animations in Chapters 12 and 13. Phil's work positively impacts the reader's ability to comprehend and absorb what is otherwise an esoteric topic and help them decrease their radiation exposure throughout their careers in spinal surgery.

Cassandra Todd somehow organized a library of over a thousand images, sought the necessary copyright permissions for previously published images and edited countless figures, adding measurements, arrows or highlights that offered clarity. Marie Clarkson weaved my narrations to correspond with the operative video footage, Josh's spectacular artwork and the animations created by Mike and Phil to produce a seamless video for each chapter that summarizes the key points. Danielle VanBrabant and Peter Lawrence also lent their talents to the project, enhancing, modifying or creating images to fill the voids recognized at the eleventh hour.

Finally, no chapter was considered complete until processed by the scrutinizing eye of Samantha Soto. Samantha identified the glaring omissions committed by the author and systematically formatted each chapter, bringing further order and organization to each chapter and the Primer as a whole. Samantha's work is best captured with the neologism "Sotorization," which means the complete and exhaustive analysis and correction of the form, content and structure of a chapter. Samantha left no "t" uncrossed and no "i" undotted. Without this remarkable team of professionals coordinated by a thoughtful construction foreman, there would be no Primer.

I am indebted to my Minimally Invasive Ensemble at Greenbaum Surgical Specialty Hospital, where I perform the majority of the surgeries I present in this book. The unparalleled level of professionalism exhibited by that team allows me to deliver the highest level of care to my patients.

Finally, I wish to thank the patients who have entrusted me with their care. Without that trust, I never would have gained the knowledge and experience to have produced this work. The gratitude that I have for my patients' faith in me is the basis for my unfailing dedication to continuing to advance the field of spine surgery. In the end, this Primer is a meager token of appreciation for that trust and faith.

Luis Manuel Tumialán
Phoenix, Arizona
December 2019

Video Contents

Introduction

I distinctly remember the first time I gazed down into a minimal access port. I felt lost. Completely lost. Nothing more than a tuft of muscle lay within my field of view, without so much as a hint of bone to offer me a glimmer of hope. The preliminary exposure looked nothing like what I had seen in the figures from the article I had read the night before. I remember my anxiety as I studied every millimeter offered to me by that 14-mm-diameter minimally invasive access port. I wondered where and how to even begin. As I zoomed out from the microscope, I wondered how it would be possible to perform an operation through such a constrained device. As I zoomed back in, I reaffirmed that my objective was to decompress a cervical nerve root. That event would not happen if I just stared at the hole. I had to actually do something. The only problem was that I could not conceive how to possibly accomplish the task at hand while looking at an unknown landscape at the bottom of this port. With great trepidation, I took the cautery and lightly touched a tuft of muscle. With that simple step, my career in minimally invasive spinal surgery began.

As I continued to work, I was uncertain about the midline and concerned about the exposure. I did not want to venture into the canal, but at the same time, I did not want to interrupt the facet. I desperately needed to visualize the lamina, the facet, or any bony prominence to gain some element of orientation. Even as I began the exposure, I still had no idea where I was relative to the midline. With foreboding unease, I began to unveil the bony anatomy that hid underneath. I slowly began to recognize parts of the posterior cervical spine. With a countless number of anteroposterior, lateral and even owl's eye fluoroscopic images, along with hints of the partially exposed bony anatomy, I was able to assemble the structures at depth. As my confidence grew, my anxiety receded. Finally, I exposed the requisite anatomy and began to drill slowly, very slowly. The terrain was still unfamiliar, but at least the elements of the anatomy were now somewhat recognizable. No one was more surprised than I that I was ultimately able to accomplish the objectives of the operation. My first minimally invasive operation was far from efficient. In fact, it took hours. But I was genuinely surprised when I saw how well the patient did afterward, despite my struggle. Although the case I have shared with you represented the beginning of my career in minimally invasive spine surgery, I do not want it to represent the beginning of yours. For that reason, I have written this book.

Upon completion of my residency years ago, I developed a strong interest in applying minimally invasive techniques to the various spine surgeries I was performing. But what I sought did not exist: a practical introductory text that would convey the essentials of minimally invasive spine surgery. I did find several comprehensive multi-authored texts but no introductory text that could serve as a primer. There was no book that I could read from beginning to end. Nor was there a book from which I could select one chapter as a practical guide for a procedure such as a posterior cervical foraminotomy. Several wonderful surgical technique articles exist in our vast spine literature, but they are constrained by scientific writing that inhibits the friendly voice inside the reader's head from talking one through the operation. Equally important were the practical aspects of the operation, such as room set up, recommended instruments and tricks of the trade, all of which are difficult to convey in a peer-reviewed technique paper. As I surveyed the landscape of textbooks, I felt a need to fill the void of reading material that exists for residents and fellows who are interested in minimally invasive spine surgery. The current text represents my effort to do just that. But as I set about writing this Primer with the intent of filling that void, I realized that I needed to understand more about how the mind transitions from open spine surgery to minimally invasive spine surgery.

As I reflect on my own learning experience and watch the early experience of the residents and fellows with whom I am privileged to work, I ask myself: Why is it that minimally invasive surgery presents so many hurdles? After all, the anatomy of the spine does not change simply because of the selection of a minimal access port over a Williams retractor. Moreover, a minimally invasive exposure, while limited, should be no different than an open exposure. In fact, the exposure of the requisite anatomy should be exactly the same. The logical question now becomes: What is the essential difference between minimally invasive spine surgery and traditional midline open spine surgery? Perhaps embedded in the answer to that question is a path forward to learning how to perform minimally invasive surgery on the spine. The pages before you represent my attempt to answer that question. But first, I must begin by comparing minimally invasive spine surgery to traditional midline spine surgery.

The Premise of Minimally Invasive Spine Surgery

I have long marveled at how little of an open exposure I actually use to accomplish an operation on the spine. In years past, I often looked down into a wound with retractors open at the end of a single-level fusion or simple lumbar decompression, astounded by the degree of retraction of muscle and skin. Whether performing a microdiscectomy or a lumbar fusion, I have observed that the exposure was more a consequence of the midline approach than of an actual need to expose the requisite anatomy to accomplish the operation at hand. The issue was obvious. Most of the anatomy I was exposing was the consequence of starting in the midline but needing to expose lateral enough to reach the pedicle screw entry points and transverse processes for an instrumented fusion or reaching the lateral aspect of the lamina for a decompression.

As I ventured into minimally invasive spine procedures, I noticed the exact opposite: I used almost every millimeter of exposure granted to me by an access port. I had to. Little if any anatomy that I exposed was unnecessary for the operation, so I had better be in the right place. From these observations, I generated what I believe to be the three premises of minimally invasive spine surgery. The first premise is that surgeons use only a small percentage of a traditional midline open exposure to perform the actual operation. The rest of that exposure is the inevitable consequence of the midline approach. The second premise is that the same operation may be performed with a precisely focused but limited exposure, where the surgeon uses almost the entire exposure to perform the operation. One may consider the second premise to represent the efficiency of an exposure, a concept that warrants further explanation.

If one were to consider the efficiency of an exposure as the ratio of requisite anatomy needed to actually perform the operation relative to actual anatomy exposed, then minimally invasive exposures are highly efficient. Caspar first introduced the concept of a ratio between the surgical target and the surgical exposure as he reflected on the management of patients with lumbar radiculopathy. Caspar believed that the outcomes of those patients were compromised by disproportionately large exposures relative to the surgical target. In his 1977 publication on microdiscectomy, Caspar[1] advocated precise monosegmental unilateral access to the lumbar segment with minimal disruption of the paraspinal musculature. Most importantly, he emphasized the significance of minimizing the surgical exposure relative to the surgical target. To acknowledge Caspar's contributions to advancing this central principle of minimally invasive surgery, I will refer to the efficiency of a surgical exposure as the Caspar ratio throughout this Primer (i.e., the ratio of surgical target to surgical exposure).

$$\text{Efficiency of a Surgical Exposure} = \frac{\text{Surgical Target (mm}^2\text{)}}{\text{Surgical Exposure (mm}^2\text{)}} = \text{Caspar Ratio}$$

Striving for a Caspar ratio of 1 is a central theme of the Primer. After all, striving for equivalence between the surgical exposure and target is the foundation of minimally invasive surgery of the spine (▶Fig. 1).

The third and final premise is that minimally invasive operations must be indistinguishable from their open counterparts. This last premise traces its origins to Dr. Richard Fessler's thoughtful foreword to the *Neurosurgery* supplement on minimally invasive spine surgery that was published in 2002, which is a must-read for anyone beginning to learn minimally invasive spine surgery.[2]

These premises will serve as our guideposts throughout the various chapters in this Primer. They are the standards by which we will measure each minimally invasive procedure and technique.

The Organization of the Primer

The Primer is divided into four sections. The first three sections are the various minimally invasive procedures for the lumbar, cervical and thoracic spine. I have found that most minimally invasive texts begin with the cervical spine, which is the logical approach from an anatomical standpoint. However, I chose to begin with the lumbar spine in this Primer because it is the most practical place to commence the minimally invasive conversion. I would recommend against starting your minimally invasive career (as I did) with a posterior cervical foraminotomy.

Within the lumbar spine section, I predictably begin with the lumbar microdiscectomy. If there is a minimally invasive procedure to cut your teeth on, it is the microdiscectomy. For several reasons, it is the perfect gateway procedure for minimally invasive approaches. The exposure of the surgical anatomy is similar to that with an open approach and thus is familiar to the surgeon. The reconstruction of the anatomy at depth that has to occur in the surgeon's mind is limited because it is so close to the midline. The surgeon can therefore connect the lines of what is seen to what is unseen in a relatively straightforward manner. In the microdiscectomy, those lines are short because the relevant surgical anatomy is just off the midline. Perhaps the most important aspect of the minimally invasive microdiscectomy is that it offers the opportunity to become familiar with the various bayoneted instruments and to work with them within the constraints of a minimal access port. It is also an opportunity to become comfortable working with a minimally invasive drill attachment.

As your familiarity with bayonetted instruments develops and your comfort level with precisely docking the minimal access port increases, you will be able to expand your minimally invasive armamentarium. Converging the minimal access port toward the midline instead of just over the nerve root paves the way for decompression of the entire thecal sac. The minimally invasive laminectomy is the next logical step. The increased angulation will affect your capacity to remain oriented, but building on the subtle angulation that your mind has become accustomed to with the microdiscectomy will make bridging that gap less of a leap and more of an inevitable step. The acquired skill set resulting from the combination of these two procedures

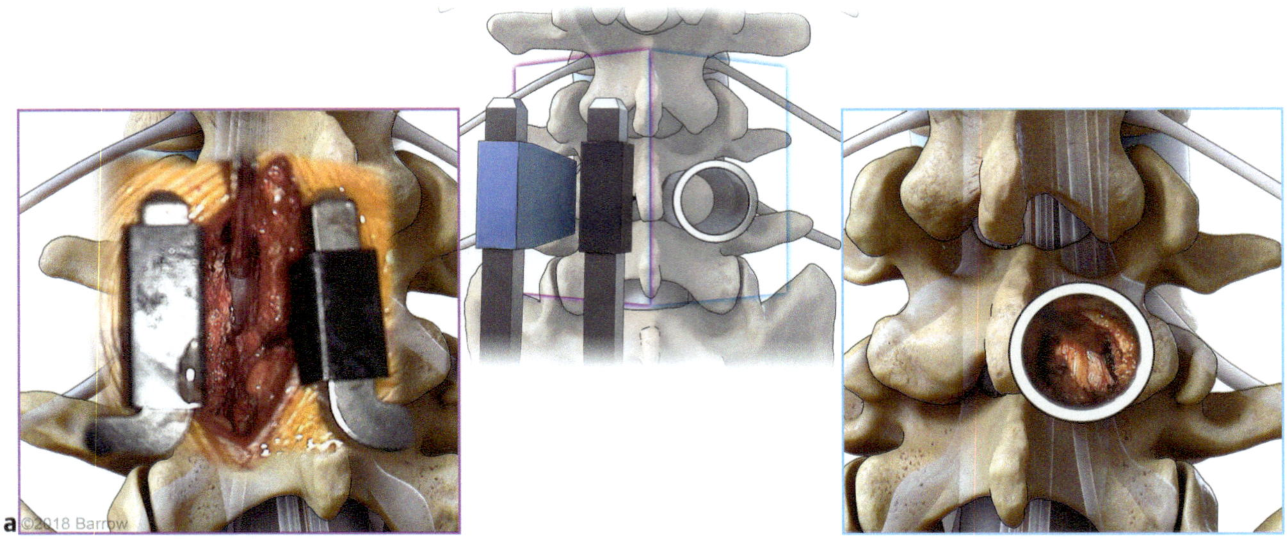

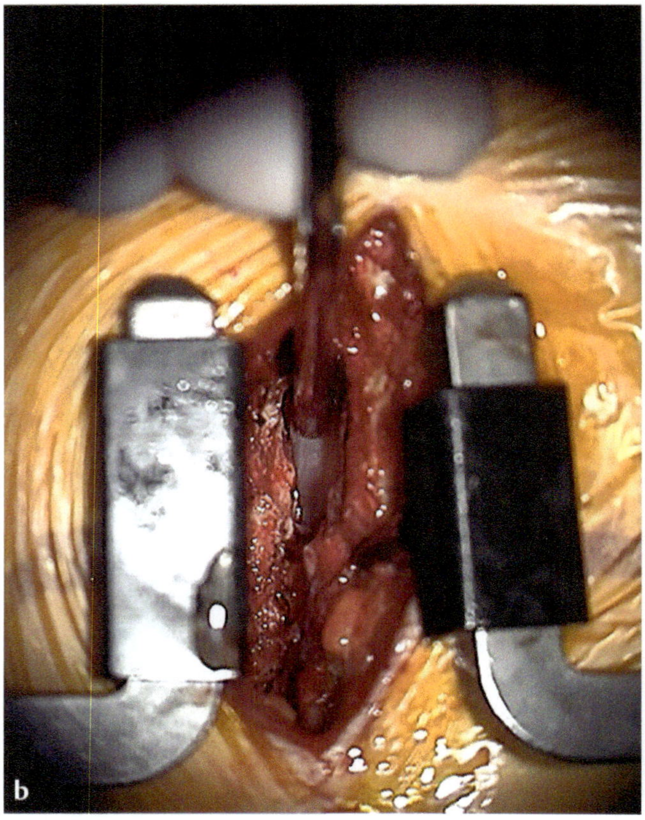

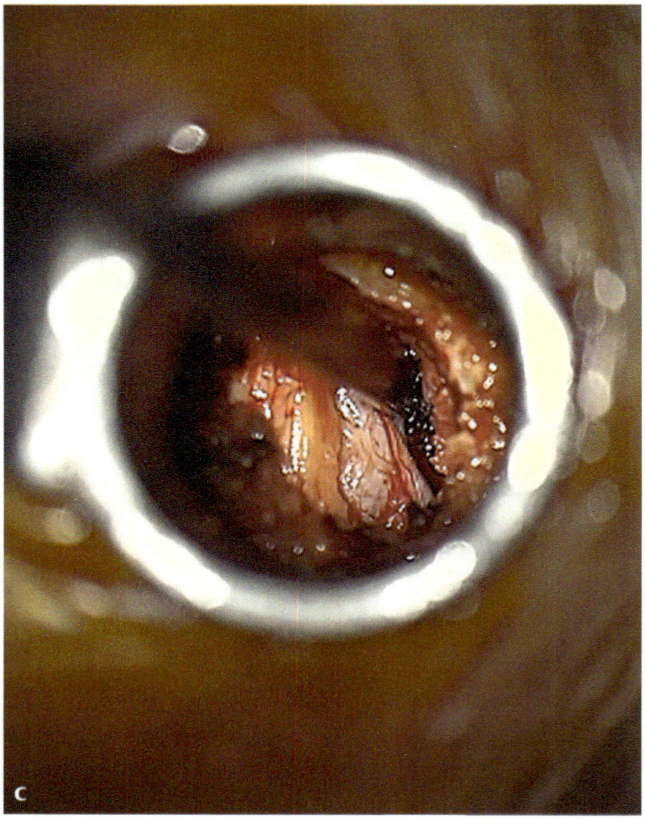

Fig. 1 Juxtaposition of two exposures for a lumbar microdiscectomy. **(a)** By its very nature, the traditional midline approach (***purple outline***) requires more exposure than the minimally invasive approach (***blue outline***), but the requisite anatomy required for the operation remains the same. **(b)** Magnified view of a traditional midline open left L4-5 microdiscectomy with use of a McCulloch retractor. To fully visualize the requisite anatomy in a midline approach, the surgeon will need to make a longer incision and expose more of the anatomy. **(c)** In this intraoperative photograph, the L4-5 segment has been exposed for a minimally invasive microdiscectomy. The nerve root suction retractor is in position, retracting the traversing nerve root of L5. The disk space can be seen lateral to the nerve root. Precise placement of a minimal access port over the requisite anatomy accomplishes the same goal through a 16-mm diameter aperture. When the efficiency of the exposure is the ratio of requisite anatomy to exposed anatomy, the minimally invasive exposure is highly efficient.

will form the basis for beginning minimally invasive transforaminal lumbar interbody fusions, the fourth chapter of this Primer.

By the same token, the expertise gained by working through the transforaminal corridor for interbody fusion translates immediately to the far lateral microdiscectomy, which I cover in Chapter 5. The far lateral microdiscectomy places the surgeon the farthest from the midline and therefore has the potential to be the most disorienting. Early in my experience, I found this procedure to be quite challenging. It is obvious to me now why that was the case. In the far-lateral approach, the lines that are seen are the farthest from those that are unseen. My mind had the greatest amount of anatomy to reconstruct at depth with this procedure, more so than for any other. Distance from the midline underscores a constant theme that will develop in your conversion: Midline is the basis of your orientation. Therefore, the farther you migrate off the midline, the greater the likelihood you will become disoriented.

The lumbar section ends with a chapter on the transpsoas approach to the lumbar spine. The lateral approach to lumbar disc spaces has caused a seismic shift in spine surgery since its introduction, especially in the management of adjacent segment degeneration, coronal imbalance and scoliosis.

I cover minimally invasive approaches to the cervical spine in the second section. The cervical section proceeds in a similar manner to the lumbar section. It begins with the posterior cervical foraminotomy then moves to the cervical laminectomy before ending with the anterior cervical discectomy. The inclusion of a chapter on the anterior cervical discectomy may mystify residents and fellows. That particular chapter may at first seem extraneous and out of place in this Primer, but I hope that after reviewing it, the reader will understand my logic for including it and find it especially relevant to the overall text.

The third section delves into the minimally invasive management of more complex clinical scenarios, such as nerve sheath tumors in the lumbar and thoracic spine and the management of metastatic disease. This section ends with a chapter on the minimally invasive management of a constellation of intradural extramedullary lesions, both vascular and neoplastic.

The fourth and final section contains two chapters on a topic important not only to patients but also to spine surgeons and their operating room staff. The material in that chapter could have been combined with that of another section or even this introduction, but I chose to place it into its own section to underscore its significance. The topic is radiation exposure in minimally invasive spinal procedures. I believe that the current generation of residents and fellows —our next generation of surgeons—is being exposed to more ionizing radiation than the generation before us. We will probably have no concrete idea of what the impact of that increased radiation exposure will be until the end of our careers. By that time, it will be too late to do anything about it. Thus, this concluding section on radiation awareness is intended not only to heighten our awareness of radiation exposure but also to discuss ways to decrease that exposure. Understanding the fundamentals of fluoroscopy, which I review in Chapter 12, is an essential component of decreasing radiation exposure. That understanding will form the basis for my discussion of a low-dose radiation protocol in Chapter 13. It is my hope that minimally invasive spine surgeons will use this understanding and some form of this protocol to decrease their radiation exposure over their lifetimes.

My concern about radiation exposure should also serve as an explanation for the noticeable absence of a chapter covering percutaneous techniques. In the absence of navigation, the radiation exposure for placement of a percutaneous screw is simply too dear in my estimation. Admittedly, computer-assisted navigation immediately neutralizes this argument, but as the reader will see in the minimally invasive transforaminal lumbar fusion chapter, there are other reasons I have shifted away from percutaneous techniques. The absence of material on percutaneous techniques should in no way be misconstrued as a criticism of that technology, which several of my colleagues use every day to improve the lives of their patients. More than anything, it represents the path I happened upon as I went through my own learning curve, exploring the various minimally invasive options for instrumentation.

The organization of each chapter in this Primer is consistent throughout the text, beginning with an overview, evolution and history of the procedure before discussing the anatomical basis for a minimally invasive approach for that particular procedure. I then discuss the technique from operating room setup to the phases of the operation and operative nuances. Each chapter ends with a review of clinical cases in which the minimally invasive procedure was applied.

Finally, a word on the references included at the end of each chapter. I have approached referencing the spine surgery literature in the Primer differently than I have any of my previous works. For a reference to find its way into this Primer, it must have met the following criteria: I must possess the actual manuscript (not just the abstract), and I must have read the entire manuscript—often more than once. If these criteria are not met, then I will assure my reader the reference will not adorn the bibliography. My hope is that this stringent approach will offer readers a meaningful bibliography that will prove worthwhile reading. In doing so, I hope to make up for the various book chapters and articles I have written in the past that contained a seemingly endless bibliography, empowered by bibliography software that makes references so readily available.

A Minimally Invasive Spine Surgery Philosophy and Disclaimer

I readily concede that the contents of this book represent one surgeon's approach to minimally invasive surgery on the spine. It is certainly not the be-all or end-all. No two procedures are ever conducted exactly the same way by any two surgeons, even those who trained in the same program under the same mentor. We all evolve our own techniques with each procedure based on our own experiences and training. My hope is simply to offer a starting point for spine surgeons interested in minimally invasive techniques. Such a framework can aid residents in preparing for a case the following day, seasoned fellows examining the anatomical basis for a minimally invasive approach and attending surgeons who are beginning to apply minimally invasive techniques in their practices. Each surgeon reading this Primer will undoubtedly develop his or her own technique, incorporating or dismissing the various elements of each chapter. Not only do I expect this reaction, but I encourage it. I have little doubt that, at some point, a reader of this work will develop a superior technique for one of the procedures mentioned in it. Perhaps a reader will even develop a new technique that was not mentioned at all or not even conceived at the time of this writing. In the years to come, I want my readers to eclipse the contents of this current work and to advance our specialty for the betterment of our patients.

More than anything, the contents of this book reflect my journey through my own learning curve. I wish to share some of that experience in the form of a stepwise approach to the common minimally invasive procedures that are routinely performed and then to proceed with more advanced techniques to address more complex clinical scenarios. I hope to eliminate the snares that entrapped me during my journey and to smooth out the terrain so that the reader may have a seamless transition into the minimally invasive precinct. No book can diminish the challenges or eliminate the complexity of learning minimally invasive surgery. But perhaps the contents of the Primer will serve as a lens through which you can view and begin to understand what your mind must unravel to become proficient.

All the procedures I discuss follow simple and consistent philosophical principles regarding minimally invasive surgery on the spine. The first and foremost principle builds on the third premise introduced earlier, which bears repeating: There should be no difference between operations performed minimally invasively and those conducted with a traditional midline approach. The incisions may vary in length and location, but the work performed at depth should be indistinguishable. The second principle is the importance of minimizing ionizing radiation. The literature is replete with manuscripts reporting increased radiation exposure in minimally invasive spine surgery. Radiation exposure is a frequent criticism of minimally invasive approaches. Some surgeons consider it a barrier to the application of minimally invasive techniques. I would like for readers to develop a mindset that there is no reason why a minimally invasive procedure cannot be done with less radiation than an open procedure. In fact, there is no reason these procedures cannot be done with less radiation than ever before.

A Historical Perspective

Before closing this chapter, I would like to invite the reader to consider the rise of minimally invasive surgery as part of a continuum that began at the dawn of our specialty. Initially, I erroneously conceived the rise of minimally invasive spine surgery as a sudden sea change in spine surgery that occurred during the early part of this century. In writing this book, I have discovered that my initial notion could not be further from the historical reality. Less invasive techniques have always been part of the spirit of innovation for surgeons challenged with various degenerative and neoplastic diseases of the spine. Over the years, surgeons undoubtedly saw the adverse consequences of extensive exposures. The disability caused by postoperative pain and, at times, instability in postoperative patients had to have prompted an "I can do more with less" mentality in these surgeons.

Modifications to procedures arose to address what surgeons obviously viewed as the unnecessary disruption of the native spine. The desire to do more with less has been part of a continuum ever since the first descriptions of lumbar disc herniations as a cause of radiculopathy. In fact, no procedure over the decades better demonstrates the desire of surgeons to disrupt less and less of the anatomy to accomplish an operation than the surgical management of lumbar disc herniations. For that reason, I end this introductory commentary with the evolution and refinement of that procedure.

Originally managed with bilateral laminectomies and transdural resection of the disc material, lumbar discectomies quickly evolved into bilateral laminectomies and extradural resection of disc material as described by Mixter and Barr. In short order, Semmes and Love described hemilaminectomy for discectomy, and soon thereafter, Love described the discectomy, working solely within the intralaminar space with no bone removal at all. That evolution occurred over the span of 11 short years after Dandy's original description of this clinical entity.[3] The ensuing decades brought forth the operating microscope by Yaşargil and Caspar, with further modifications to minimize the extent of exposure made by Williams soon thereafter.[4] The most recent step in this evolution was the migration from a subperiosteal dissection of the spinous process and lamina to a paramedian transmuscular approach precisely and directly onto the lamina facet junction with a table-mounted minimal access port as described by Foley and

Smith.[5] The migration from a subperiosteal dissection to direct access onto the spine ushered in the current modern era of minimally invasive techniques described in this Primer, but the progression toward minimally invasive approaches began decades ago. The next step in the evolution of microdiscectomy awaits unveiling by yet another innovative surgeon, who is perhaps reading this text. We would be fools to think that the treatment of the herniated lumbar discs of the future awaits no further development.

The evolution of the microdiscectomy is only one example. The evolution of the lumbar laminectomy is yet another. Even the resection of intradural extramedullary lesions follows the same pattern of surgeons venturing off the midline to achieve resections that were previously thought feasible only through midline approaches. Decompression of the lumbar spine for lumbar stenosis without sacrificing the midline elements was described as early as 1982 by Lin.[6] Yaşargil[7] described unilateral hemilaminectomy for management of intradural extramedullary lesions in 1991. As I read these manuscripts, I can almost hear the authors' voices urging me not to consider the midline an obstruction to pathology within the canal. Whether you are managing lumbar stenosis or a dural arteriovenous fistula, the canal is readily accessible without sacrifice of the midline elements when it is viewed in three dimensions. Long before the development of minimal access ports, another theme was already prevalent among the most innovative surgeons: The preservation of the midline.

From that standpoint, the spirit of minimally invasive surgery is nothing new. The contents of this Primer are another manifestation of that mentality. The "I can do more with less" mindset is part of our heritage. Defining the requisite anatomy and efficiently accessing the surgical target have long been objectives for all surgeons trying to do more with less. That is the spirit of minimally invasive spine surgery. I hope that resonating throughout this Primer, you will hear the voices of surgeons from the past urging us not to consider the midline elements as an obstruction to the central canal. They would urge us instead us to preserve the posterior tension band, the ligamentous structures, and the paraspinal muscles while encouraging us to accomplish the same operation through a more efficient and targeted exposure. In keeping with that same spirit, I begin the first chapter in the Primer, which invites you, the reader, to consider conversion to a minimally invasive mindset.

References

[1] Caspar W. *A new surgical procedure for lumbar disc herniation causing less tissue damage through a microsurgical approach.* Berlin: Springer-Verlag; 1977

[2] Fessler RG. Minimally invasive spine surgery. *Neurosurgery.* Nov 2002;51(5 Suppl):Siii-iv

[3] Dandy WE. Recent advances in the diagnosis and treatment of ruptured intervertebral disks. *Ann Surg.* Apr 1942;115(4):514-520

[4] Maroon JC. Current concepts in minimally invasive discectomy. *Neurosurgery.* Nov 2002;51(5 Suppl):S137-145

[5] Perez-Cruet MJ, Foley KT, Isaacs RE, et al. Microendoscopic lumbar discectomy: technical note. *Neurosurgery.* Nov 2002; 51(5 Suppl):S129-136

[6] Lin PM. Internal decompression for multiple levels of lumbar spinal stenosis: a technical note. *Neurosurgery.* Oct 1982;11 (4):546-549

[7] Yaşargil MG, Tranmer BI, Adamson TE, Roth P. Unilateral partial hemi-laminectomy for the removal of extra- and intramedullary tumours and AVMs. *Adv Tech Stand Neurosurg.* 1991;18: 113-132

1 A Minimally Invasive Perspective: The Conversion

Abstract
A distinct difference exists in the way the mind processes an open exposure as compared to a minimally invasive exposure. In the absence of the midline structures, the basis of orientation is different. The angles converging on the spine on a lateral to medial trajectory alter the appearance of the otherwise familiar surface anatomy. The absence of the recognizable midline structures, along with an unfamiliar perspective of the surface anatomy, has the potential to disorient the mind. This chapter analyzes the difference between these exposures and explores how the mind can become oriented in minimally invasive approaches without the midline structures. Delving into the topics of recall memory and recognition memory of the spinal anatomy furthers our understanding of the basis of orientation and disorientation. Deconstructing the origin of disorientation in minimally invasive approaches becomes the foundation upon which to build a path to a more efficient learning curve for minimally invasive spine surgery. The chapter ends with covering the essential components of minimally invasive spine surgery and reviewing the premise and principles of minimally invasive spine surgery that will be the basis of the subsequent chapters in this Primer.

Keywords: exposure, facet, lamina, learning curve, orientation, recall memory, recognition memory, spinous process, three-dimensional spinal anatomy

The mind once enlightened cannot again become dark.
Thomas Paine

1.1 Introduction

The capacity to reconstruct the spinal anatomy at depth without the midline structures to orient the mind is the very essence of minimally invasive spine surgery. In traditional open approaches, we begin in the midline and work outward. In doing so, we expose the landmarks of the spinous process, lamina, facets and transverse processes in sequential order. These landmarks orient our mind and allow us to move through the procedure confidently and efficiently. Our visualization of these midline landmarks provides us certain knowledge of the anatomy. In minimally invasive approaches, we have neither the midline nor the conventional exposure of these landmarks. Instead, we must rely on visualization of the anatomy in the mind's eye of what is not seen or even unveiled. The mind must visualize the entire facet, although only a hint of that facet may be exposed. The ability to reconstruct that anatomy with only limited exposure will prevent the mind from becoming disoriented. The capacity to maintain orientation will directly affect the proverbial learning curve in minimally invasive surgery on the spine. Therefore, the concept of what orients our minds in spine surgery is the focus of this chapter.

To borrow from nautical analogy, we should consider how, when learning to sail the ocean, we would be ill-advised to lose sight of the shore. The shoreline orients the mind of the sailor to the cardinal directions of north, south, east and west. Becoming familiar with a vessel by doing nothing more than sailing up and down the coastline provides the sailor with a foundation to venture farther and farther out to the sea. Eventually, the sailor no longer requires a view of the shoreline to remain oriented. With an understanding of the position of the sun, the stars, a sextant and even the use of computer-assisted navigation, the sailor can safely bring the ship back into a safe harbor.

In traditional midline open spine surgery, the midline structures are the shoreline that forms the basis of orientation for the surgeon. Recognizing it as such helps the surgeon to understand how the absence of the midline in minimally invasive approaches is the root cause of disorientation, the same way the loss of the shoreline is potentially disorienting for the novice sailor. The reader must always keep this key principle in mind. The limited exposure of a transverse process or the inferior aspect of a facet can become indistinguishable when viewed through a 16-mm-diameter aperture (▶ Fig. 1.1).

The mind must replace those visual reference points with its own reconstruction of the anatomy. The angle of convergence of a minimal access port onto the spine or its rostrocaudal trajectory further affects that reconstruction. Although such factors are not relevant in an open procedure, they can change the entire landscape in a minimally invasive procedure. On the one hand, the traditional midline exposures offer the visual cues of spinous processes, lamina and facets (▶ Fig. 1.2). These reference points allow you to keep your bearings during an operation. On the other hand, a minimally invasive approach does not unveil any of these midline bony landmarks. Instead, only limited portions of these landmarks in isolation are available to orient the mind. In the end, minimally invasive approaches require more from your mind than the open equivalent.

What you accomplish with a midline exposure is a complete unveiling of the spinal anatomy at depth. As a result, there is no need for the mind to reconstruct any component of that anatomy or to speculate on whether a bony prominence is a facet or a transverse process, as demonstrated in ▶ Fig. 1.1. Whether or not you realize it, your eye is constantly scanning these visual cues in an open exposure to keep your mind oriented. In a midline open approach, you never lose sight of the shore.

A minimally invasive exposure is completely different. It forces your mind to become oriented and to stay oriented without the midline and with less visualization of the spinal anatomy. Although it is a highly efficient exposure with regard to the surgical target relative to the surgical exposure, there is no midline and very little anatomy to scan as a reference point. Your mind is left to reconstruct the anatomy around the limited exposure offered by the diameter of the minimal access port. Open approaches teach us the anatomy, but reconstruction of the anatomy is unnecessary by the nature of the exposure. We can see everything. Therefore, the capacity to accurately and efficiently reconstruct this anatomy is an acquired skill unique to minimally invasive spine procedures. To confidently and expediently move through a procedure, the minimally invasive surgeon must learn how to connect the lines of the anatomy from what is seen to what is unseen. The mind must also incorporate the trigonometry of convergence and the effect it has on

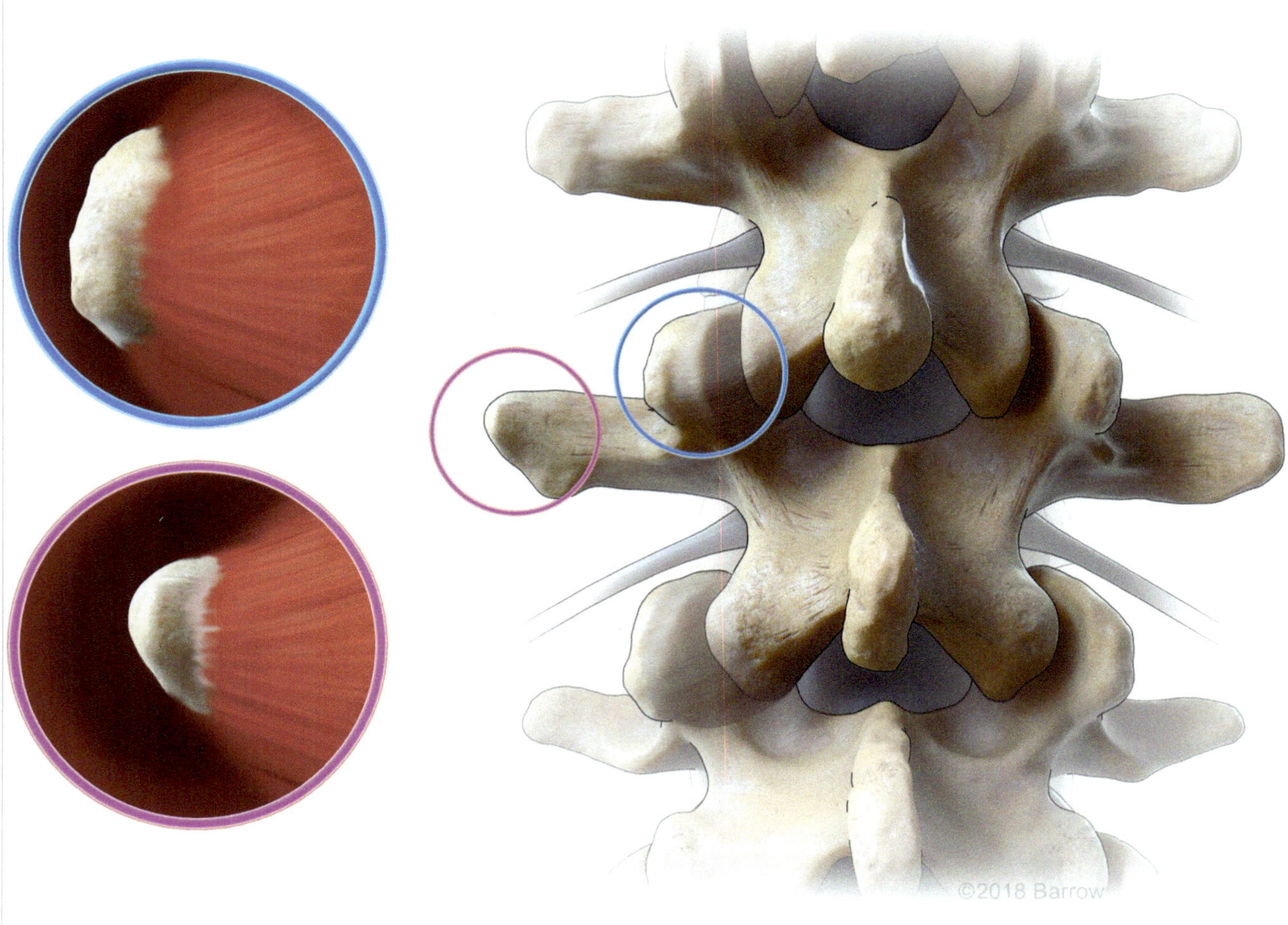

Fig. 1.1 A juxtaposition of two exposures. Two minimally invasive exposures seen through a 16-mm minimal access port. At first glance, both exposures look very similar. However, each represents a completely different part of the lateral spinal anatomy, as shown by the fully dissected exposure on the right. In the absence of the midline elements, orientation with limited exposure can be quite challenging. In the end, one exposure appears ideally suited for a transforaminal approach, whereas the other exposure is too lateral to access the foramen. The length of the access port and the starting distance from the midline collectively orient the mind by incorporating the trajectory of convergence.

the exposure at depth. ▶ Fig. 1.3 illustrates this point by demonstrating how the degree of convergence can result in two different exposures despite the same incision. You will find that as the length of the minimal access port increases, the effect of convergence plays an increasingly detrimental role in envisioning the ideal position of the exposure.

You must not think that the reconstruction of the spinal anatomy at depth depends solely on recognizing limited glimpses of the lamina or the facet or the transverse process. Several components other than direct visualization remain at your disposal. Use them all. Precise planning of the incision will place the exposure in the vicinity of familiar and relevant anatomy. Sounding the anatomy with the initial dilator will provide tactile feedback as to the location of the facet, the lamina and the interlaminar space. Lateral and anteroposterior fluoroscopic images reveal the degree of convergence and confirm the location. All these components combine to provide information that will begin the reconstruction process before you ever peer down the minimal access port. Incorporating every aspect of these components fills the void created by the absence of a wide exposure and the lack of orienting structures of the midline. When you finally do peer down the minimal access port, your eye will possess the absolute certainty of location from the integration of all these components. Again, it is the reconstruction of the spinal anatomy at depth with limited exposure and absence of the midline elements that is the essence of minimally invasive spine surgery. It is the skill that must be mastered. Having introduced the concept of orientation, I would like to examine the often-discussed learning curve in minimally invasive spine surgery from a different perspective.

1.2 The Proverbial Learning Curve

The learning curve in minimally invasive spine surgery is steep. I hear surgeons utter this statement time and time again in course after course and in lecture after lecture. Yet, I have never found this statement to be particularly helpful to the aspiring spine surgeon who wishes to embrace minimally invasive techniques. If anything, it serves instead as a potential deterrent. I

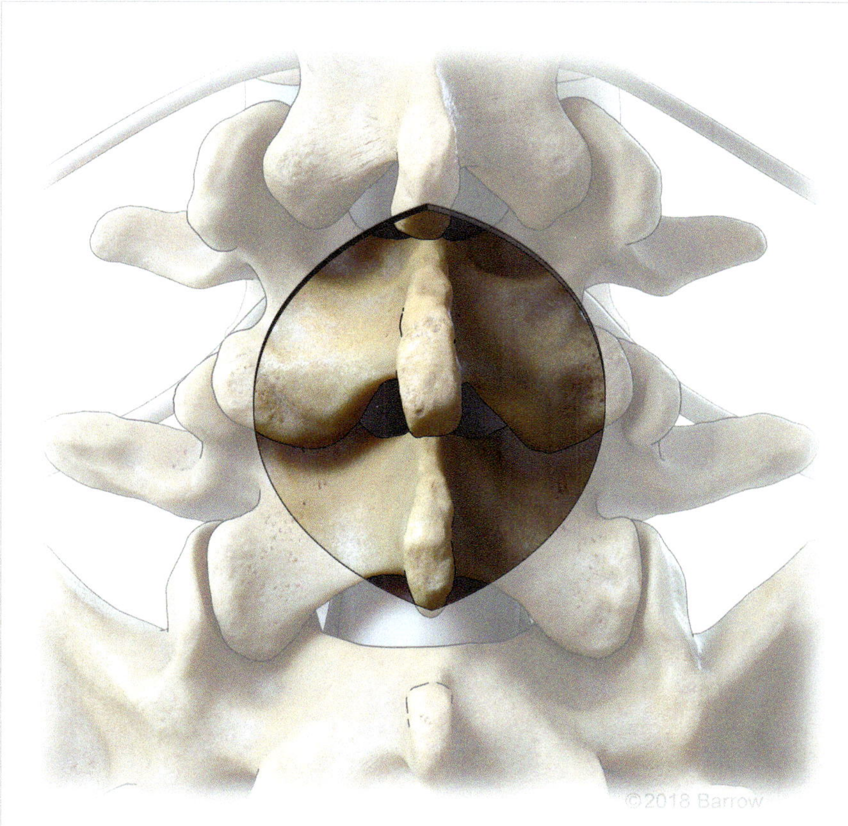

Fig. 1.2 Traditional midline open exposure for a lumbar laminectomy. Illustration demonstrates the midline elements, which remain in the surgeon's field of view. The midline keeps the mind oriented throughout the procedure. The absence of these midline elements in minimally invasive exposures can make bony prominences resemble one another, as shown in ▶ Fig. 1.1.

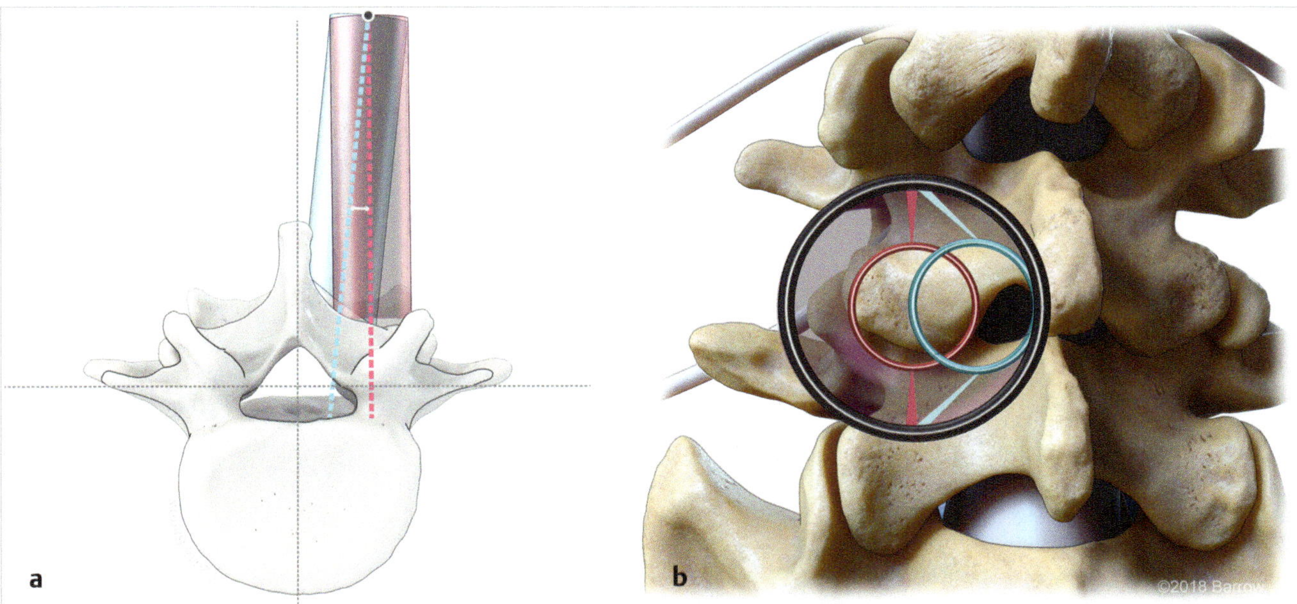

Fig. 1.3 The effect of convergence. **(a)** Illustration of a lumbar segment in the axial plane demonstrates two exposures (medial, *turquoise dashed line*; lateral, *ruby dashed line*) through the same access port (16 mm in diameter and 7 cm in length). The mind must consider several factors to reconstruct the spinal anatomy at depth. The location of the incision off the midline, the degree of convergence of the access port, and the rostrocaudal trajectory collectively affect the exposed anatomy at depth. **(b)** Posterior view of the spine of the previous axial image again demonstrates that both incisions can be placed 2 cm off the midline. A different exposure of the anatomy at depth may be the result, depending on the degree of convergence. The *large dark ring* represents the proximal aspect of the port at the level of the skin, and the smaller colored rings represent the access port at the level of the spine. The degree of convergence is the difference in these two exposures, which otherwise are identical with regard to the location of the incision and the length of the minimal access port. The medial exposure (*turquoise ring*) is ideal for a microdiscectomy, whereas the more lateral exposure (*ruby ring*) is too lateral and suboptimal for the procedure.

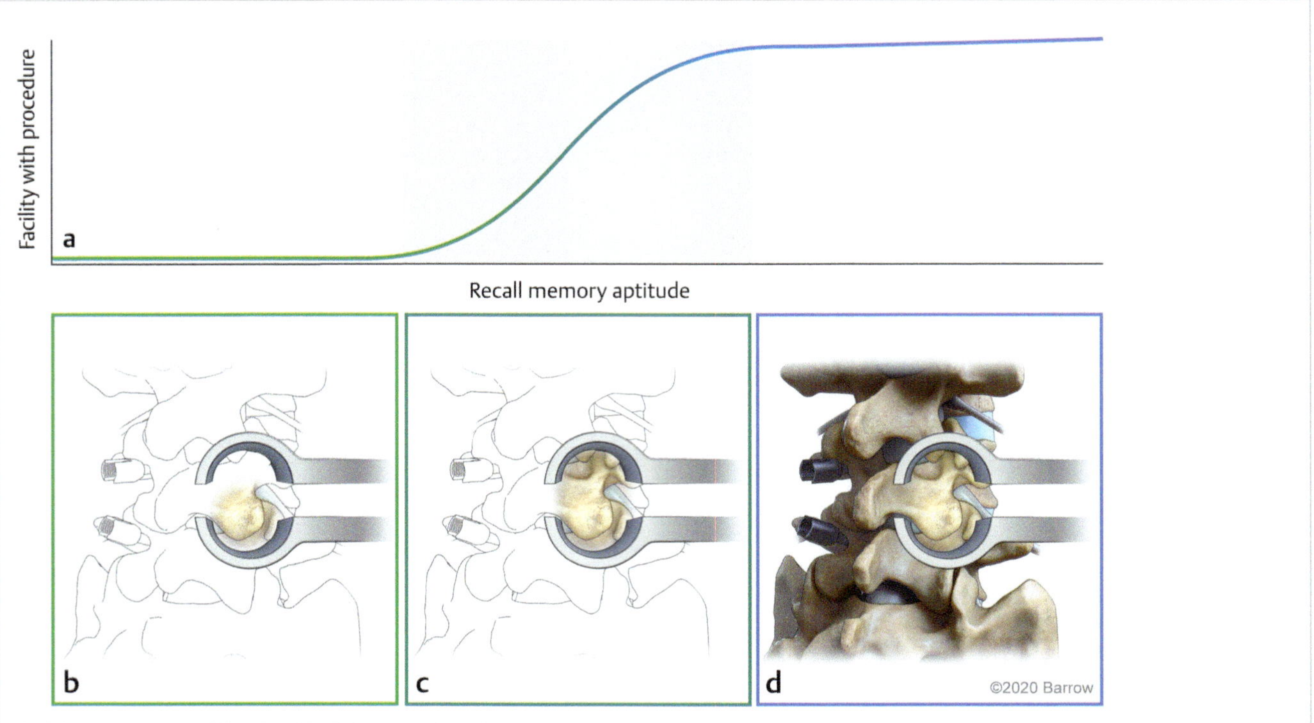

Fig. 1.4 The minimally invasive learning curve. **(a)** Learning minimally invasive surgery should require more of an emphasis on understanding what transpires in the area beneath the curve than a concern for the upward slope of the curve. The area beneath the curve represents the mind acquiring the capacity to reconstruct the spinal anatomy at depth and the surgeon being able to move through the exposure and the operation more confidently. **(b)** Initially, the surgeon's eye will see only what is directly exposed. The facility of the procedure will be lowest at this juncture because the ability to reconstruct the anatomy at depth is limited. **(c)** As recall aptitude of the spinal anatomy builds, the mind's eye can "see" more than what is visualized. **(d)** When a surgeon's recall aptitude is highest, the mind will be able to reconstruct the anatomy at depth as shown, where the mind can "see" beyond what is exposed. Proficiency with the procedure will be highest at that point because of recall memory aptitude, not necessarily because of the number of cases completed.

would suggest that such a statement, which I believe does have a kernel of truth to it, requires further examination from a different vantage point. I often tell residents and fellows to forget about the slope of the learning curve and to instead consider what is actually going on in the area beneath that curve (▶ Fig. 1.4). What happens as the cases continue to accumulate along the *x*-axis and your proficiency with the procedure increases along the *y*-axis? What is going on that explains that change?

The only adequate explanation of what transpires in the area beneath the curve is some form of conversion in the mind. As the surgeon learns minimally invasive surgery on the spine, the mind achieves a greater understanding of the relevant but limited surgical anatomy at depth and a greater appreciation of trajectories onto the spine, without all the customary visual cues. Those visual cues are the familiar and orienting midline structures mentioned previously. It bears repeating that the limited exposure challenges the mind of the surgeon to connect lines from what is exposed and therefore seen to what is not exposed and therefore unseen. Those unseen elements are what orient the mind in open approaches because they are the midline structures. Therein lies the essence of the learning curve: teaching the mind how to orient itself without direct visualization of the midline structures. From that perspective, a more appropriate label for the *x*-axis in ▶ Fig. 1.4 may be aptitude to reconstruct the spinal anatomy at depth, instead of number of cases. After all, it is only an increase in the capacity to assemble the anatomy in the mind's eye with limited visualization that will result in a rise in proficiency on the *y*-axis. It is not necessarily the number of cases, but rather the proficiency to learn the anatomy from those cases that results in altering the slope of the learning curve.

At the beginning of my learning curve, I was slow because I was uncertain. I was not yet adept at orienting my mind without conventional exposures. I could not effectively integrate the information provided by the fluoroscopic image, the tactile feel of the anatomy and the angle of convergence. So I spent more time in those early cases confirming what I thought I saw or repositioning my minimal access port, which I sometimes positioned in a suboptimal trajectory. Without the shoreline, I felt lost at sea. However, as my experience grew, my ability to reconstruct the anatomy at depth increased, and I became more skilled at becoming oriented. I recognized the anatomy with less exposure. I prevented disorientation by instantly recognizing a previous misstep and correcting it. I became more adept at integrating the indirect visual cues, such as the tactile feedback offered to me by a dilator or the subtleties of the anatomy presented by a lateral fluoroscopic image. As I began to feel more certain, I became more efficient. By extracting information from these nonvisual cues, I was able to reconstruct the anatomy at depth, which allowed me to sail by the stars.

With increasing experience, you will learn how to integrate indirect visual cues into a mental image of the spinal anatomy. Gradually, greater precision develops with the trajectory of an access port. The tactile sense of the probing dilator will feed more meaningful information to the mind. There will be subtleties identified on the fluoroscopic images that will also prompt immediate adjustment. As a nascent minimally invasive surgeon, you should focus on this growing accumulation of experience, not on the slope of the learning curve that lies ahead. By focusing intently on learning how to orient your mind without midline structures, you will begin to learn minimally invasive spine surgery. Always remember that the anatomy at depth does not change because of the use of a minimal access port. Only the visual cues are different.

1.3 Back to the Midline

This chapter began with the first principle of minimally invasive spine surgery: The midline is the basis of orientation in open spine surgery. Allow me to expand on that key concept by way of an example. Building on the concept introduced earlier, the surgeon performing an open lumbar fusion begins with an incision in the midline, which allows for immediate orientation of the mind. The surgery proceeds in a logical anatomical manner, with exposure of the spinous processes, the lamina, the facets, the pars interarticularis and the transverse processes. If at any time the anatomy is not clear, more can be exposed by lengthening the incision and widening the retractors. The eye of the surgeon may view all this anatomy simultaneously, which allows the mind to remain oriented by constantly scanning the exposed bone. Such an exposure makes it virtually impossible to misidentify a transverse process as a facet. However, the exposed anatomy is more of an inevitable consequence of a midline approach than a necessity for the operation. As mentioned in the "Introduction," this premise is a key aspect of minimally invasive spine surgery. Experienced spine surgeons will concede that only a portion of the exposed anatomy in an open surgical exposure is actually necessary to accomplish all the objectives of the operation. The remainder of the exposure is the unavoidable consequence of a midline incision (▶ Fig. 1.5).

In contradistinction to the open midline approach, a minimally invasive spine procedure uses almost all the exposure provided by a minimal access port for the procedure. Accomplishing this same procedure with minimally invasive techniques requires the precise placement of a minimal access port and limited exposure of anatomy with absolute certainty of that anatomy without the familiar midline visual reference points that would otherwise orient the mind. Thus, the mind of the minimally invasive spine surgeon has to instead recreate the unseen anatomy to confidently, efficiently and safely proceed with the operation. Without midline structures to reorient the mind, it is not always entirely clear whether a bony prominence is a portion of the inferior articular aspect of the facet or a

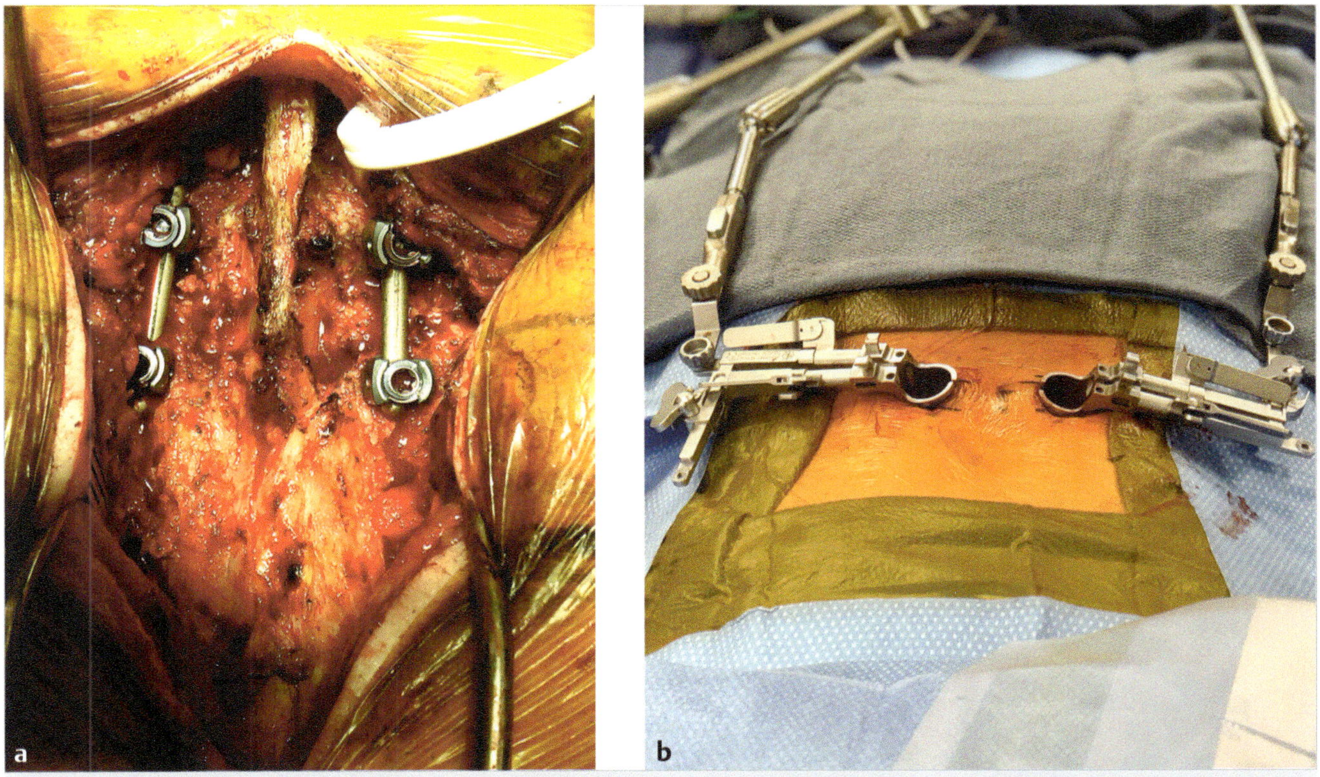

Fig. 1.5 Juxtaposition of two transforaminal lumbar interbody fusions. Intraoperative photographs show exposures for an L3–4 transforaminal lumbar interbody fusion. **(a)** The midline open approach demonstrates the amount of exposure that comes as the inevitable consequence of beginning in the midline and working laterally to the entry points and the transforaminal corridor. Only a portion of this exposure is actually needed for the procedure. **(b)** The same operation can be performed through two minimal access ports. In such an approach, almost the entire exposure is used. From that standpoint, minimally invasive exposures are highly efficient.

transverse process. As demonstrated in ▶ Fig. 1.1, these two bony prominences may look exactly alike. By the same token, the uncertainty about such bony prominences is what slows down a procedure, whereas the absolute certainty of what that bony prominence represents expedites it.

In its simplest form, what happens in the area under the learning curve is a conversion. You will develop the skill to allow your mind to connect the anatomical lines of what is seen to what is unseen. The midline will be reconstructed in your mind. Instead of an exposed spinous process, the base of a spinous process palpated with the first dilator will take its place. Instead of visualizing the entire lamina for a laminectomy, you will use anteroposterior and lateral fluoroscopic images to fill in the blanks that a minimally invasive exposure does not offer. The combination of tactile feel and fluoroscopic imaging will provide indirect visual data points. Integrating all these elements will allow you to know precisely where you are, where you need to go and—equally important—where you must not go. Orientation, efficiency, and fluidity of surgery occur, despite the smaller corridor and more limited exposure. In a nutshell, the crux of minimally invasive spine surgery is the capacity to integrate all the indirect visual components into the limited field of view to accomplish the same operation that would otherwise require a larger incision and a broader exposure.

1.4 Three-Dimensional Spinal Anatomy: Recognition versus Recall Memory

The perfect framework to further analyze how our minds learn minimally invasive spine surgery is the memory-retrieval model of recognition versus recall memory. The main difference between these two types of memory activation is the number of cues that activate the memory retrieval and the depth of knowledge required for that activation. For instance, it is one thing to simply recognize someone walking down the street; it is something entirely different to recall that person's name, where the person is from and how you know the person. The former is analogous to open spine surgery; the latter is akin to minimally invasive surgery.

In open spine surgery, the mind primarily employs recognition memory to proceed with the operation. As the anatomy is exposed, the cues accumulate until the exposure is fully recognized by the mind. The visual cues available by this open exposure spread activation from several parts of the memory. There is never a need to assemble the three-dimensional (3D) shape of a facet or a transverse process from memory alone. You need only to recognize these structures and shapes. If you do not entirely recognize something, you may further expose it until you do. The depth of knowledge required for memory activation need not exceed the recognition of the anatomy. The visual cues offered by the exposure essentially pave the way to recognition.

In contrast, minimally invasive exposures primarily employ recall memory. They provide less exposure and therefore fewer direct visual cues from the anatomy. Activation of recall memory demands a greater depth of knowledge of the 3D anatomy. As already mentioned, the mind must do more with less. Indirect visual cues, such as sounding the anatomy, examining the trajectory onto the anatomy and using fluoroscopic imaging, must supplant direct visual cues. The mind must integrate these indirect cues and the limited exposure to activate the 3D spinal anatomy within the memory. Doing so requires a depth of knowledge of the 3D anatomy far beyond what is required to activate recognition memory.

The depth of knowledge for recall of the 3D anatomy is another skill that you must hone for proficiency in minimally invasive approaches. You can do so by passively studying models and performing surgeries. Over time, that depth of knowledge will accumulate. Or you can develop this skill set more actively, which is my recommendation. Assembling your own models of the lumbar, thoracic and cervical vertebral segments from memory may be the most efficient manner to acquire the depth of knowledge of the 3D anatomy that is necessary for minimally invasive exposures.

Early in my minimally invasive experience, I attempted to construct a model of the lumbar spine vertebrae from my son's colored modeling compound (Play-Doh). I was shocked at how little my finished fuchsia-tinted creation actually resembled the anatomy. I had no true appreciation of the distance between facets or the curvature of the lamina into the spinous process. I could recognize all that anatomy, but I could not recall it well enough to create an accurate model. What I had produced at the end of my first attempt was hardly recognizable as mammalian. From that point forward, I focused on building models of the vertebral bodies with precise dimensions. I focused on the thickness of the pars interarticularis, the alignment of the facets and the shape of the transverse process. Taking a mass of a child's modeling compound and forming a 3D model of the lumbar vertebrae forced me to identify the holes in my depth of knowledge needed to activate my recall memory. Reiterating this process again and again with the lumbar, thoracic and cervical vertebral bodies filled the gaps in my knowledge. Over time, my models had greater anatomical fidelity. My spine model-making endeavors facilitated my capacity to activate my recall memory of the 3D anatomy that I needed in minimally invasive spine surgery. The value I find in this exercise is such that I continue to do it even today.

If we place recall memory and 3D spine model-building proficiency in the framework of the learning curve, the *x*-axis may be labeled the number of attempts and analyses of the models built and the *y*-axis may be labeled aptitude of recall memory of 3D spinal anatomy. With each iteration, the spinal model will become more and more accurate, provided an appropriate analysis of the model is undertaken. The results of this thought experiment are captured graphically in ▶ Fig. 1.6. When we transpose this concept to ▶ Fig. 1.4, it becomes evident that what matters is not the number of cases, but rather what the mind learned from the cases. The increased aptitude of recall memory is what allowed for a rise in proficiency. Again, when it comes to that proverbial learning curve, I want you to focus on what transpires in your mind and less on the shape of the curve itself. I want you to focus on learning the 3D anatomy and orienting your mind without the midline (Video 1.1).

1.5 Proviso

You will not be able to achieve this conversion by reading this book—or by reading any other book for that matter. As surprising as it may be to read such a caveat in a primer on minimally

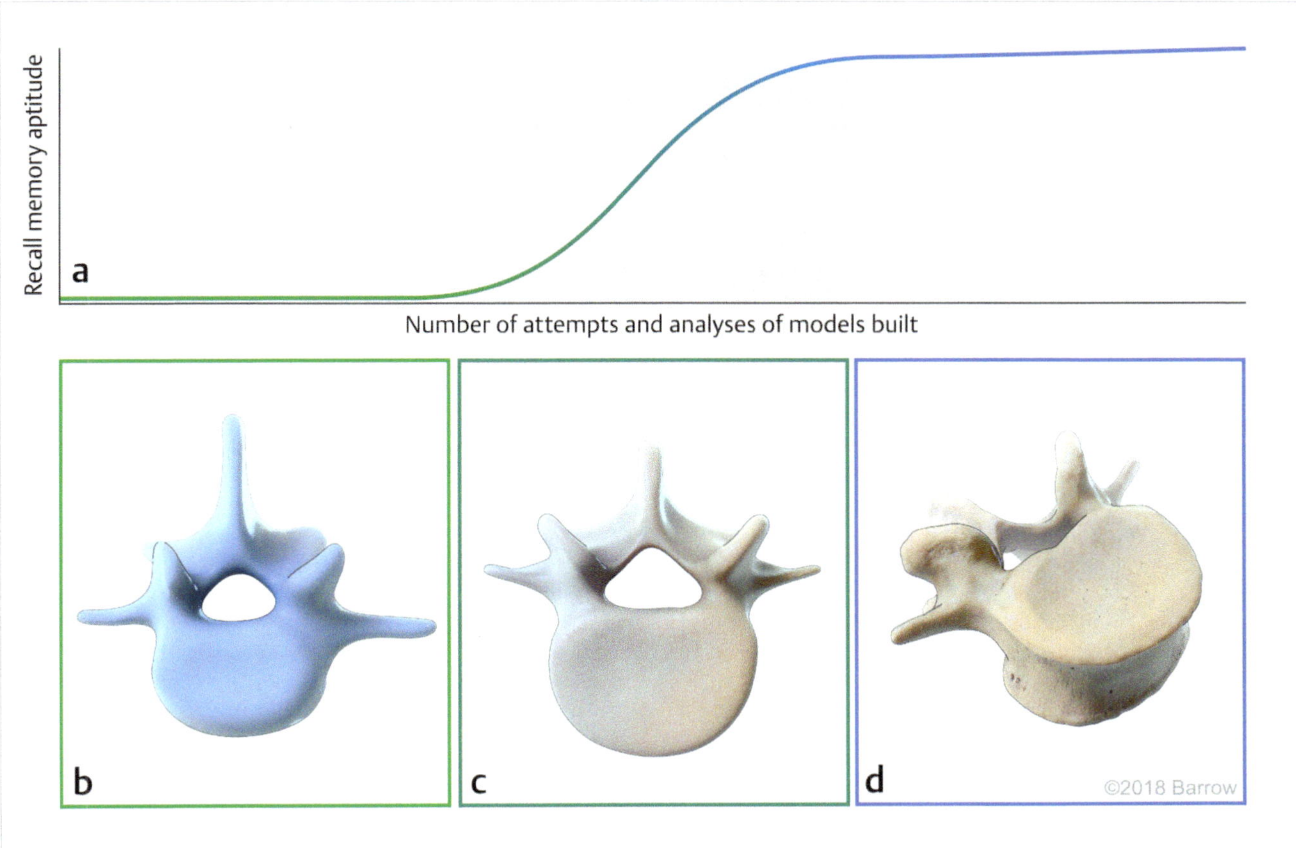

Fig. 1.6 Developing recall memory. **(a)** The graph above is identical to the graph in ▸ Fig. 1.4, but the *x*-axis and *y*-axis are labeled differently. In this graph, the *y*-axis represents the aptitude to recall the three-dimensional spinal anatomy. As this aptitude increases, the anatomical models of the spine you create become more and more accurate. When that aptitude is applied to the minimally invasive learning curve, it becomes evident that recall memory and the capacity to remain oriented are what lead to proficiency. The number of cases performed does not necessarily lead to an increase in that proficiency. **(b)** An example of an early model of the spine at a point when recall memory aptitude is low. **(c)** The model becomes more accurate as the mind advances its understanding of the anatomy. **(d)** Finally, a sophisticated understanding of the spine is achieved, and the result is a model of the spine that can be created purely from recall memory. When you can achieve this point, your proficiency with a minimally invasive procedure will be greatest.

invasive spine surgery, I believe that what happens to your mind during this minimally invasive conversion simply cannot be replicated in any text. Instead, it comes as a product of tirelessly operating, dissecting, scrutinizing radiographic studies, thoughtfully studying the spinal anatomy and increasing the depth of your anatomical knowledge so that recognition memory develops into recall memory. It even comes with making models out of Play-Doh. You may ask yourself: What, then, is the purpose of reading this Primer? The short answer is to increase your understanding of the maturation process going on in your mind. I believe that this awareness alone will help with the conversion process.

I hope that the chapters in this Primer will shift the lens through which you view the spinal anatomy. Instead of viewing the spine from the outside in, you will begin to view the spine from the inside out. During this conversion, limited exposures challenge your mind to reconstruct the anatomy at depth. Once you reach a level of proficiency reconstructing the anatomy at depth, you will confidently, efficiently and safely secure a screw within the pedicle, remove a disc herniation or even resect an intradural extramedullary lesion. Along the way, these chapters will provide a context for this conversion by reviewing the anatomical basis of a procedure, listing the anatomical measurements and emphasizing the trajectories onto the spine.

As your minimally invasive conversion occurs, you will find yourself looking at radiographs, computed tomograms and magnetic resonance imaging sequences in completely different ways. You will begin to visualize how an incision 20 mm off the midline with an angled trajectory of 30 degrees will place you perfectly within the axial plane of the compression of the neural elements. As you continue to use minimally invasive techniques, your capacity to reconstruct the spinal anatomy at depth will increase until you begin to feel as if you have X-ray vision. You will need less fluoroscopy to dock an access port, to place pedicle screws and to achieve a decompression. Exposures will become more obvious, and you will perform operations more efficiently.

The occasion will inevitably arise when you will perform an operation through a traditional midline approach, and it will be remarkable to you how little of the exposed anatomy you actually need to perform the operation. At that point, your conversion will be complete. In the words of Thomas Paine that began this chapter, "The mind once enlightened cannot again become dark." My hope is that this Primer will actively intensify the area beneath the minimally invasive learning curve for the surgeon who is beginning to learn minimally invasive techniques. I hope that the reader finds that the contents of this book will facilitate and encourage that conversion.

1.6 Essential Ingredients

1.6.1 Rotating Jackson Table

The essential tools for the minimally invasive spine surgeon warrant emphasis at this point. They include the operating table, microscope, drill, fluoroscope and operating room team. Let us begin with the table upon which the patient lies while you perform these procedures. Although any of these procedures may be performed on any table, a Jackson table that can be rotated is ideal for all lumbar and thoracic procedures (▶ Fig. 1.7). Except for the posterior cervical foraminotomy and posterior cervical laminectomy, I perform all minimally invasive operations on a Jackson table with a Wilson frame for simple decompression or without a Wilson frame for instrumented fusions. The design of the Jackson table allows the fluoroscope to readily enter and exit the operative field unencumbered because of the absence of a base in the center of the table. It also allows the fluoroscope to easily slide to the head or foot of the bed. However, not all Jackson tables can be rotated, so request one that does. As you will soon learn, the ability to rotate the bed away from the surgeon is of tremendous value for midline decompressions. The benefits of such a table are numerous, but at this point, suffice it to say that a table that rotates away from and toward the surgeon optimizes the line of sight and ergonomics for the surgeon, while facilitating entry and exit of the fluoroscope.

1.6.2 Operating Microscope

The benefits of using an operating microscope for decompressions in minimally invasive approaches cannot be overstated (▶ Fig. 1.8). The working channel in a minimally invasive exposure is already constrained, thus making the illumination and magnification of every millimeter of that exposure essential. When used in combination with a rotating Jackson table, the microscope allows the surgeon to have an ideal ergonomic position that optimizes visualization across the midline, beneath the spinous process and into the contralateral recess. The combination of visualization and trajectory allow for a complete decompression of the contralateral side. Although minimally invasive surgery is feasible with loupes and a headlight, the microscope eliminates any need to struggle.

A secondary benefit of an operating microscope is that it can record operative footage. Reviewing operative footage of your surgeries can be of tremendous value, especially early in your career. It will help you improve your technique. You will identify redundant steps, points of hesitation and areas where you may save time. When you review your operative footage, you already know what the exposure is going to look like and what adjustments you made to get to the ideal position and location. Watching yourself perform the operation again will provide you with feedback that you can immediately apply to your next operation.

1.6.3 Drill Attachments

The minimally invasive attachments to the drill represent the natural evolution of the drill for spine surgery. Having

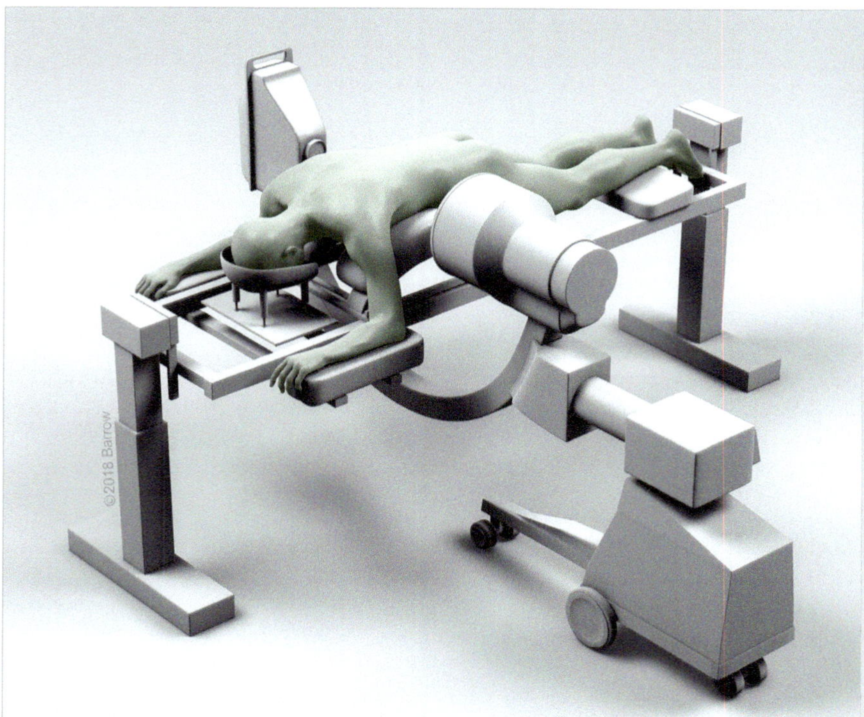

Fig. 1.7 Artist's rendition of a rotating Jackson table. The absence of a base in the center of the table allows for ready access with a fluoroscope. It also provides unencumbered access to the head and foot of the bed.

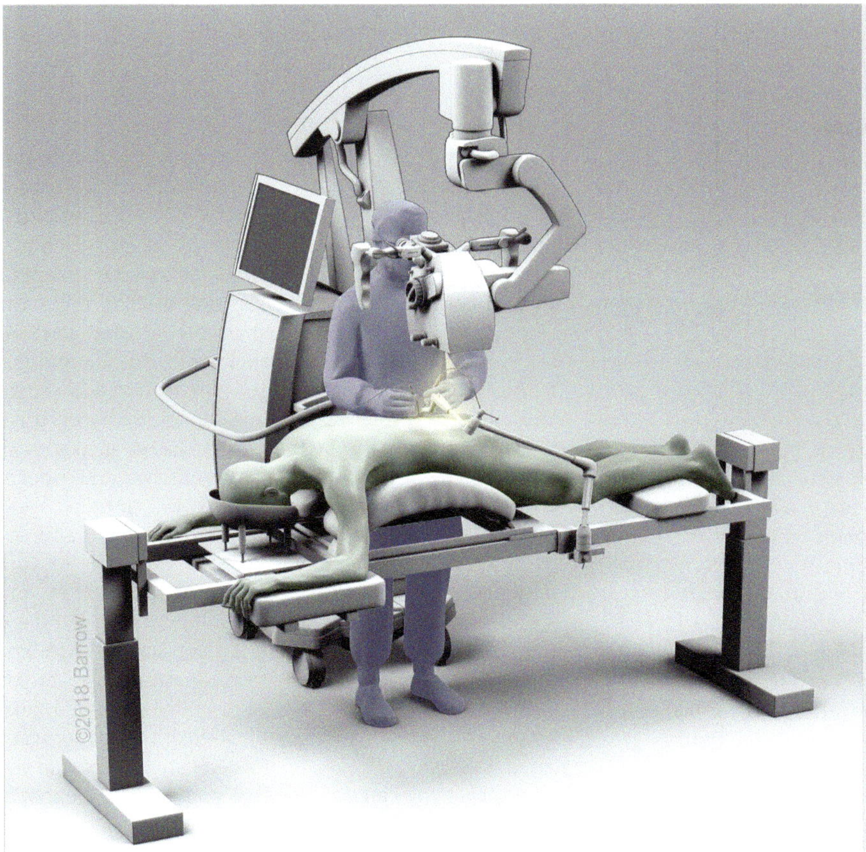

Fig. 1.8 Artist's rendition of an operating microscope. An operating microscope not only magnifies and illuminates the field but also can record operative footage. Reviewing the footage provides immediate feedback on how to improve and optimize efficiencies.

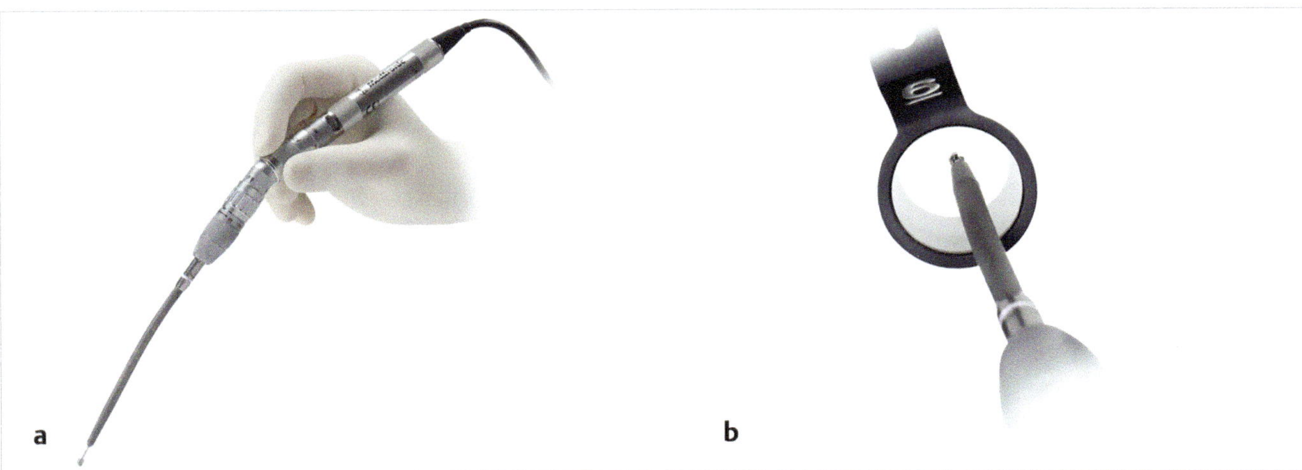

Fig. 1.9 Minimally invasive drill attachment. **(a,b)** Photographs demonstrate how the curvature of the drill attachment creates an ideal ergonomic position in the hand and optimizes visualization through **(b)** the constrained working channels of the minimal access port. (Minimally invasive Midas Rex drill, Medtronic, plc. Used with permission from Medtronic, plc.)

extensively reviewed the various writings of Dr. Ralph Cloward and his innovative approach to surgery on the spine, I would argue that if he had been shown the configuration of the minimally invasive drill attachments, he would have adopted it immediately for his surgical procedures. The gentle curve of the drill allows a line of sight to the tip of the drill bit while optimizing the stability and ergonomics within your hand (▶ Fig. 1.9). A level of comfort with using this drill arises almost immediately, and its advantages over the traditional straight and angled drill attachments are readily obvious. While there is no better drill configuration to use in a 14-mm-diameter minimal access port, I have found that this configuration is equally ideal for drilling a posterior osteophyte in an anterior cervical discectomy or for drilling a trough in a posterior cervical laminectomy. As a result, I have adopted the use of the minimally invasive drill attachments for all my spine cases, whether they are minimally invasive or open. Again, I view this as the natural evolution of the drill for spine surgery.

1.7 A Minimally Invasive Surgery Ensemble

The final and perhaps most important ingredient for a successful minimally invasive conversion is the operating room team. The operating room nurse, the scrub technician, the anesthesiologist and the fluoroscopy technologist all make up what I call the "minimally invasive ensemble." Only with the aid of your minimally invasive ensemble will you achieve efficiencies in the operating room, lower your dose of radiation exposure, minimize the time the patient is under anesthesia and successfully and effectively treat the patients who have entrusted you with their care. Making all members of the team aware of their roles in the operation optimizes the efficiency of the procedure. Spending time providing training and explaining the rationale behind the position of the microscope and the importance of securing the table-mounted arm while the scrub technician is passing the cautery and the bipolar forceps wires and the suction tubes collectively optimize the efficiency of the operation. I emphasize these elements throughout the various chapters in this Primer. Developing this ensemble pays immediate dividends regarding time spent in the operating room.

The value of a radiologic technologist who can identify a suboptimal lateral view and intuitively adjust the wag without prompting is beyond measure. When such a technologist is identified, he or she should be recognized as an invaluable member of the team. The radiologic technologist is the key to the use of less fluoroscopy and thereby less radiation. Identifying a motivated technologist and discussing methods to decrease radiation together have the potential to decrease your lifetime dose of radiation. The final two chapters in this Primer discuss the fundamentals of fluoroscopy and methods to decrease radiation. The radiologic technologist plays an essential role in reducing radiation exposure for everyone.

1.8 Complications

I hope that, in reading the pages that follow, the reader will find a clearer pathway to understanding the principles of minimally invasive spine techniques. Nothing can replace the hours under the microscope, and nothing can prevent the inevitable missteps that may lead to complications. When these occur, each situation offers a learning opportunity. Failure is always the best teacher. It is important to dissect to the very core the origin of any undesirable outcome. Reexamine everything. Review the location of the incision, the trajectory of the port, the technique used for the decompression and the entry point for the pedicle screw; any or all of these factors may have contributed to a misplaced pedicle screw, a suboptimal decompression or a dural tear.

With perseverance, you will find that, in time, the unseen spinal anatomy will become obvious despite the limited anatomy offered to you by the constrained corridor of the minimal access port. You will no longer feel disoriented. You will no longer simply recognize the anatomy, but rather you will begin to recall the subtle structures of the spine from your depth of knowledge. The lines between the seen and the unseen will effortlessly connect in your mind. Your minimally invasive conversion will be complete. After all, as Thomas Paine has said, "the mind once enlightened cannot again become dark."

The Premise of Minimally Invasive Spine Surgery

1. Only a small percentage of the exposed anatomy is needed to perform an open midline operation; the remainder of that exposure is the inevitable consequence of a midline exposure.
2. A minimally invasive exposure utilizes almost all the exposed anatomy for the operation; therefore, precise positioning of the access port is paramount.
3. The work performed at depth in a minimally invasive approach should be indistinguishable from its open equivalent.

The Principles of Learning Minimally Invasive Spine Surgery

1. The midline is the basis of orientation in spine surgery.
2. The further we venture off the midline, the more disorienting the exposure can become.
3. A minimally invasive approach asks more from your mind than its open counterpart.
4. Recall memory—not recognition memory—is needed to facilitate minimally invasive exposures.
5. Minimize ionizing radiation.

2 Minimally Invasive Microdiscectomy

Abstract
There are more similarities than differences in the exposures of a minimally invasive microdiscectomy and its open equivalent. Acknowledging these similarities allows for the mind to begin acquiring the skill of reconstructing the anatomy at depth without the orientation provided by the midline elements. Therefore, the minimally invasive microdiscectomy is the ideal procedure to embark upon as you begin to learn minimally invasive spinal surgery. You will be able to focus more of your mental energy on becoming familiar with bayoneted instruments and a minimally invasive drill attachment instead of draining yourself attempting to stay oriented. The similarities lessen the potential for disorientation and allow you to focus on building the foundation for more complex minimally invasive techniques. This chapter discusses the evolution of the minimally invasive technique for the microdiscectomy, which represents the inevitable outcome of Caspar's edict to minimize the ratio of the surgical target to the surgical exposure. From there, the chapter lays out the rationale for the diameter of the access port in the context of the requisite anatomy and thereby establishes the anatomical basis for a minimally invasive approach. Further detail regarding the nuances of positioning a minimal access port and the advantage it provides by placing the surgeon precisely in the axial plane of the compression is presented before discussing positioning, operating room setup, and the surgical technique in detail. This chapter ends with a discussion on revision microdiscectomies, complication avoidance, and a unique case illustration.

Keywords: herniated disc, lumbar spine, microdiscectomy, minimally invasive, radiculopathy, surgical technique

Knowledge is the true organ of sight.

The Panchatantra

2.1 Introduction

Minimally invasive surgery on the spine is difficult from a standing start. Navigating bayoneted instruments and operating a curved drill through a constrained working channel is always awkward at first. Even the most seasoned surgeon appears clumsy attempting to work these instruments for the first time within a cylindrical access port. Thus, as you begin to consider minimally invasive surgical procedures on the spine, your ideal approach would be to build momentum with a familiar operation that varies little whether performed open or minimally invasively. In my estimation, the microdiscectomy is the operation to do just that. It is the operation that will bridge your skill set from open surgery and allow you to translate it into the minimally invasive precinct.

As mentioned in the previous chapter, the essence of learning minimally invasive surgery is the capacity for the mind to reconstruct the anatomy at depth without visualization of the traditional landmarks. That basic principle of orientation also bears repeating as we begin this chapter on the microdiscectomy: Our orientation in spine surgery comes from the midline structures. The closer to the midline the relevant surgical anatomy lies, the more straightforward the operation becomes. As you venture away from the midline, angles begin to alter how you view the surface anatomy. The result is disorientation. Since the microdiscectomy is directly off the midline, it stands to reason that this operation is the most logical one with which to begin your minimally invasive conversion. When peering down into a 16-mm-diameter access port, you should find comfort in the fact that the distance from the orienting structures of the spinous process and lamina is limited to millimeters. Your mind may readily extrapolate those orienting midline structures from within the 16-mm diameter afforded by the exposure. The leap that you need to make from the midline exposure to the minimally invasive exposure for a microdiscectomy is not far.

2.2 Rationale

I am constantly reminded by my colleagues who routinely perform open spine surgery that there is little, if any, difference between their open incision for a microdiscectomy and my minimally invasive incision. There is truth to that statement. After all, prospective studies examining minimally invasive and open microdiscectomies have demonstrated equivalence in clinical outcomes.[1,2] That observation would suggest that the presumed benefits that I will present in this chapter may not have enough magnitude to be captured clinically. The circular argument begins again, and critics of minimally invasive surgery would question the point of investing the time and energy in developing a skill set that does not demonstrate a difference in clinical outcomes. I will not argue that the differences are in fact there and perhaps not adequately captured by the outcome measures in the current literature. Instead, I would emphasize that the microdiscectomy is the gateway procedure for the larger breadth of minimally invasive spine procedures. The gap in clinical outcomes between minimally invasive and traditional midline approaches widens considerably when the minimally invasive procedure is a lumbar fusion for a mobile grade 1 spondylolisthesis or a thoracic decompression of a metastatic lesion causing spinal cord compression.

The goal of beginning with the microdiscectomy is to develop familiarity with bayoneted instruments, which you will need to deftly maneuver through a constrained corridor. Equally important is the precise placement of the minimal access port in the ideal position and trajectory for completion of the procedure. The minimally invasive microdiscectomy begins the process of teaching the mind how to begin to reconstruct the anatomy at depth from a paraspinal approach and how to stay oriented during a minimally invasive procedure without the spinous process or the entire lamina as reference points. Thus, applying minimally invasive techniques to the microdiscectomy builds the foundation for those minimally invasive procedures that will unequivocally demonstrate clinical benefit to patients.

2.3 The Muscle–Retractor Interface: A Historical Perspective

The true benefit of minimally invasive surgery is not the length of the incision but the decreased pressure on the interface of the muscle and the retractor. In traditional midline approaches for microdiscectomies, the self-retaining retractor stays in position because of the force exerted simultaneously on the spinous process and muscle. As the retractor opens, the pressure increases on the muscle–retractor interface. Increasing the exposure and stabilizing the retractor requires pressure on the muscle to reach a certain point so that the retractor will not move. For instance, when using a McCulloch retractor, the hook engages the spinous process and allows the retractor blade to generate an asymmetrical force against the skin and paraspinal muscles. It is that anchor against the spinous process that displaces the skin and muscle, thus providing the exposure for the procedure. The inevitable consequence of that displacement is that blood flow to the paraspinal muscles plummets (▶ Fig. 2.1).[3]

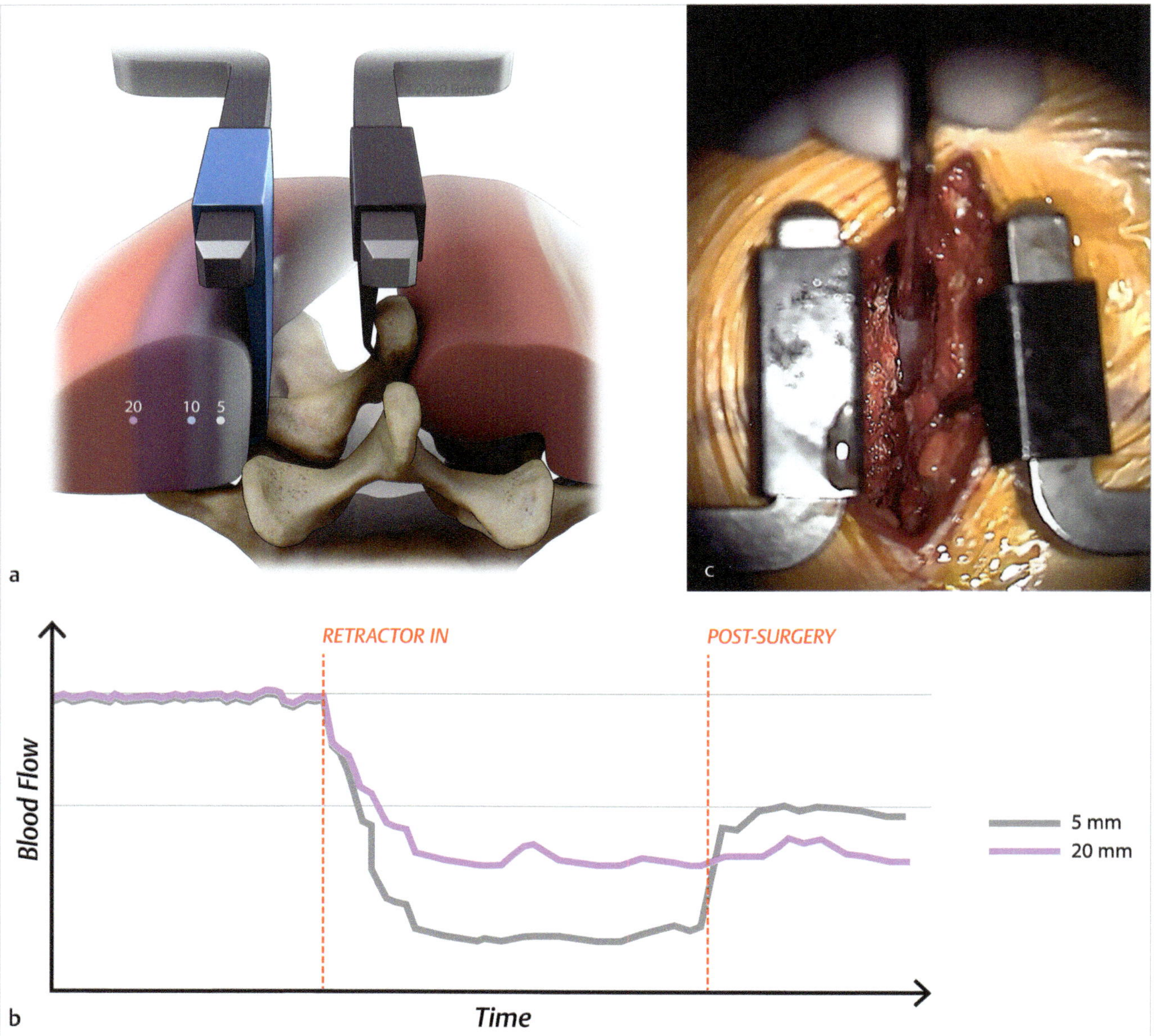

Fig. 2.1 Illustration demonstrates **(a)** the muscle–retractor interface with **(b)** corresponding blood flow graph modified from Kawaguchi et al.[3] Stability for a self-retaining retractor, such as a McCulloch retractor, is achieved when the retractor is opened and the pressure against the muscle increases. That increased pressure at the muscle–retractor interface corresponds to a decrease in blood flow. The porcine models reported by Kawaguchi and colleagues[3] showed that the greatest pressure, and thus the greatest impact on blood flow, occurs closest to the muscle–retractor interface (*gray line*). But even as far as 20 mm from the muscle–retractor interface, blood flow to the muscle is affected (*purple line*). **(c)** Intraoperative photograph of a McCulloch retractor in position for an open microdiscectomy. The blood flow to the muscle–retractor interface decreases with increased distraction. The greater distraction of the retractor translates into greater stability and lateral exposure. The consequence of the additional exposure is less blood flow to the muscle and skin.

In open midline exposures of the spine, the more the retractor is opened, the greater the exposure but the more compromised the blood flow to the skin and muscle. Exposure and blood flow are diametrically opposed to one another. The sustained compromise in blood flow from the muscle–retractor interface over time can add to the postoperative discomfort experienced by patients and may contribute to the atrophy observed on postoperative magnetic resonance imaging (MRI) years after surgery. The potential effect that sustained retraction has on the blood flow to the skin edge may also contribute to the differences in infection rates between minimally invasive approaches and their open equivalents.[4]

The muscle–retractor interface has been of interest to spine surgeons for decades. The spine surgery literature is replete with concerns about the downstream consequences of muscle retraction in spine surgery long before the rise of modern minimally invasive spine surgery. That body of literature reads almost as if it were a collective plea for a better way. Kawaguchi and colleagues[3] wrote perhaps one of the finest articles that illustrates the immediate effects of blood flow by traditional midline retractors. A carefully thought-out porcine laminectomy model elegantly demonstrated the effect of retractors on blood flow and offered the clearest explanation of the atrophy that occurs after lumbar laminectomies (▶ Fig. 2.2).[3] What is most remarkable is that their article was published well before Foley and Smith[5] described a paraspinal transmuscular approach with a table-mounted access port, which collectively addressed the blood flow at the muscle–retractor interface and the skin edge.

In the minimally invasive application, the minimal access port maintains its position not by the pressure generated at the muscle–retractor interface but instead by a table-mounted arm (▶ Fig. 2.3).[5] Herein lies the main advantage of the minimally invasive approach: The pressure is relieved from the paraspinal muscles and transferred to the table-mounted arm. Unlike an open exposure, the minimally invasive approach exerts no significant force on one side of the skin and muscle. The stability of the access port is dependent on the table-mounted arm, not on the pressure generated by the muscle–retractor interface (▶ Fig. 2.4). As a result, there is no significant decrease in blood flow to the muscle or the skin. The putative benefits are less postoperative discomfort and less paraspinal muscle atrophy. The exceptionally low infection rate reported for minimally invasive approaches further supports the optimization of blood flow at the skin and muscle–retractor interface.[4]

Equally important is a cylindrical-shaped minimal access port. Conceptually, a cylinder is the most efficient shape for distributing the forces of pressure to the entire circumference of an incision and muscle. Distribution of the forces equally to the skin and muscle prevents the asymmetric compression of one side of the incision. Thus, whatever forces exist at the muscle–retractor interface are equally distributed by the cylindrical shape of the access port (▶ Fig. 2.4).

Caspar[6] was the one who actually introduced the concept of a cylinder in lieu of a self-retaining retractor in his 1977 chapter on advancements in microdiscectomy. He had observed that the ratio of exposure to the surgical target was far too great in spine surgeries. Caspar's objective was to decrease the ratio of the requisite anatomy to the surgical exposure. To that end, he developed a speculum-type retractor that could be placed precisely over the requisite anatomy (▶ Fig. 2.5).[6]

Although Caspar[6] appears to have been the first to describe the use of a cylindrical speculum to minimize tissue trauma, the focus of his chapter was the use of the operating microscope to optimize visualization, which he and Yaşargil[7] both championed. Caspar's prescient development of a focused

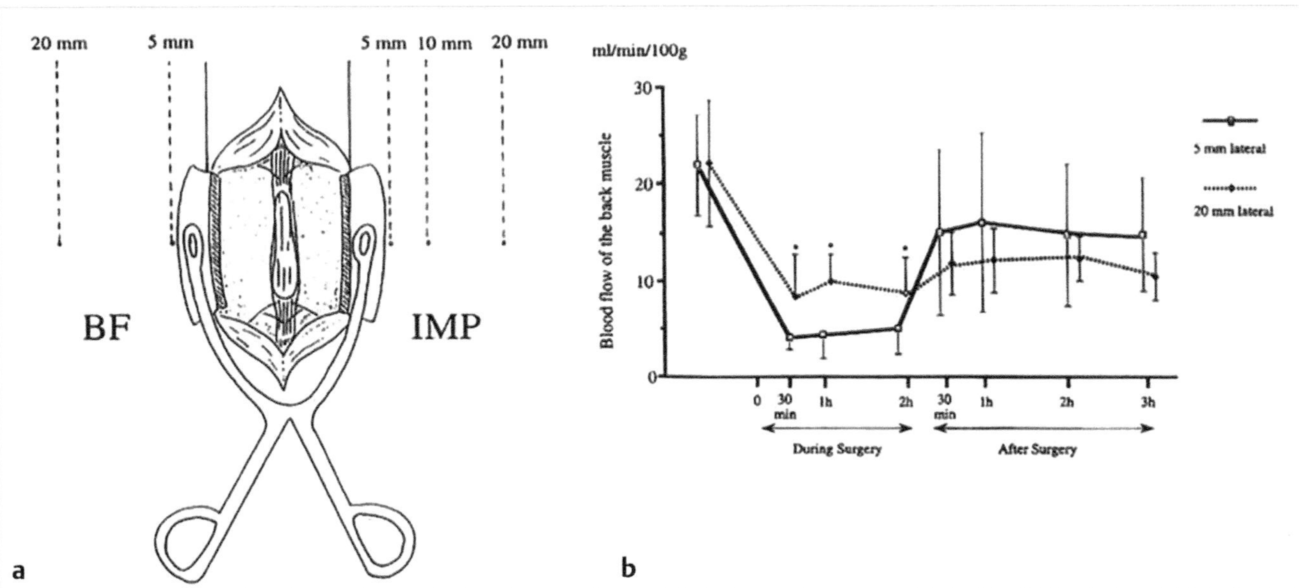

Fig. 2.2 (a) Illustration and (b) graph from Kawaguchi et al[3] demonstrate blood flow to the paraspinal muscle with a self-retaining retractor in position at various distances from the incision. Once the retractor is placed, the blood flow to the muscle plummets. Even after the retractor is removed, the blood flow does not return to preoperative levels in the hours after removal. (Reproduced with permission from Kawaguchi Y, Yabuki S, Styf J, et al. Back muscle injury after posterior lumbar spine surgery: topographic evaluation of intramuscular pressure and blood flow in the porcine back muscle during surgery. Spine [Phila Pa 1976]. 1996; 21:2683–2688.)

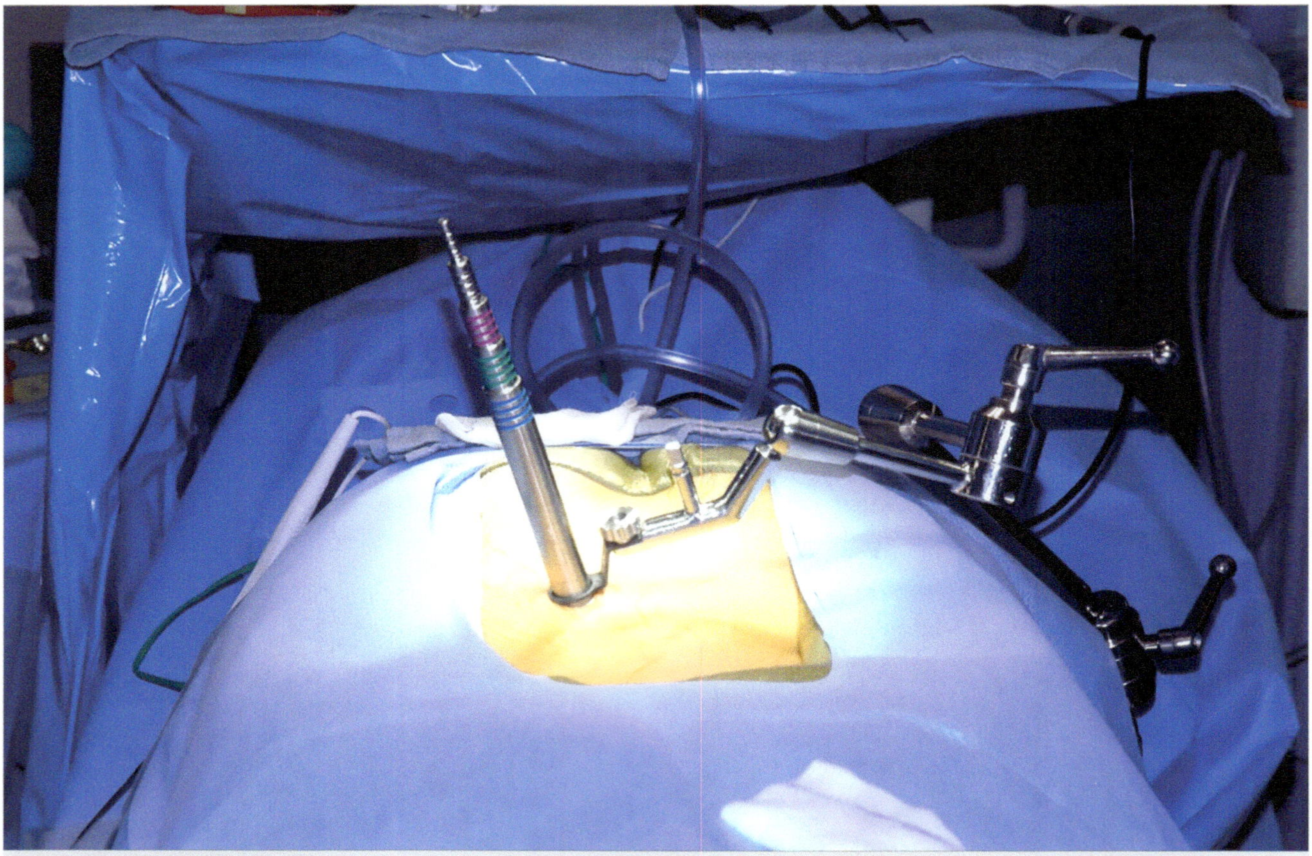

Fig. 2.3 Intraoperative photograph shows the minimal access port secured in position with the table-mounted arm as conceived by Foley and Smith.[5] Instead of all the force being translated to muscle and skin, it is translated to the table-mounted arm. The cylindrical shape of the port further distributes the forces equally to the surrounding skin and muscle.

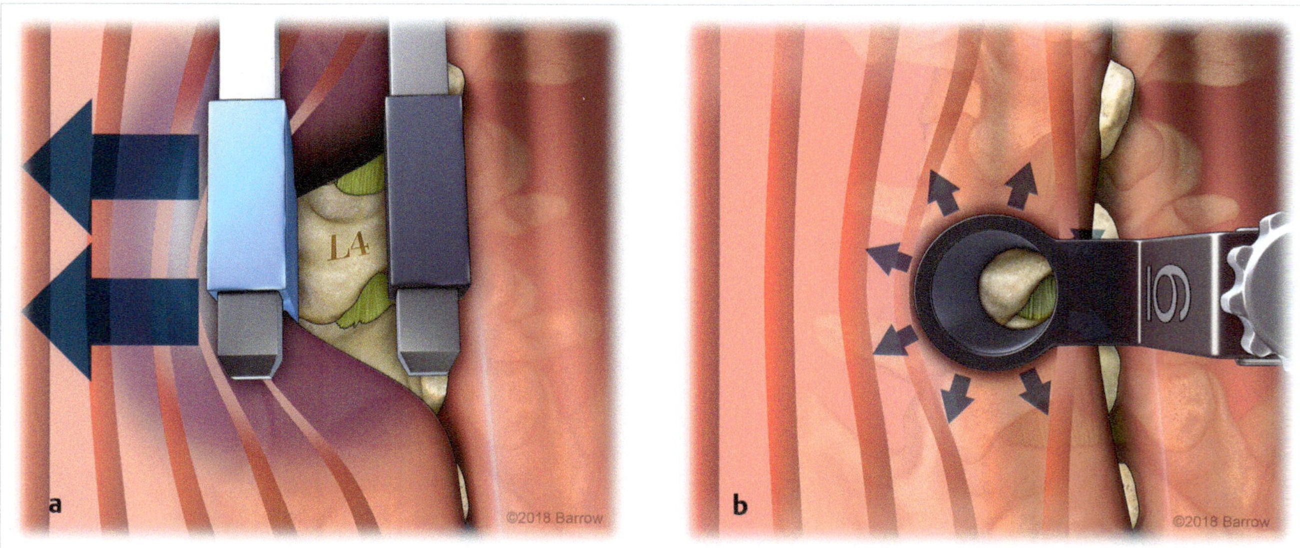

Fig. 2.4 The magnitude of forces at the muscle–retractor interface in an open exposure versus a minimally invasive exposure. **(a)** Visual rendering of the magnitude of the vector force in an exposure for an L4–5 microdiscectomy. The blood flow to the muscle is represented by vertical red lines. The directionality and magnitude of a self-retaining retractor compromise blood flow, as denoted by the darkened purple tone at the muscle–retractor interface. **(b)** The magnitude of forces is smaller, and forces are equally distributed by the cylindrical shape. Precise placement of the minimal access port immediately over the requisite anatomy precludes the need for a large vector force to expose the anatomy from the midline. The table-mounted arm holds the access port in position, instead of the forces generated by the retractor. The result is less compromise of blood flow at the interface of the minimal access port and muscle.

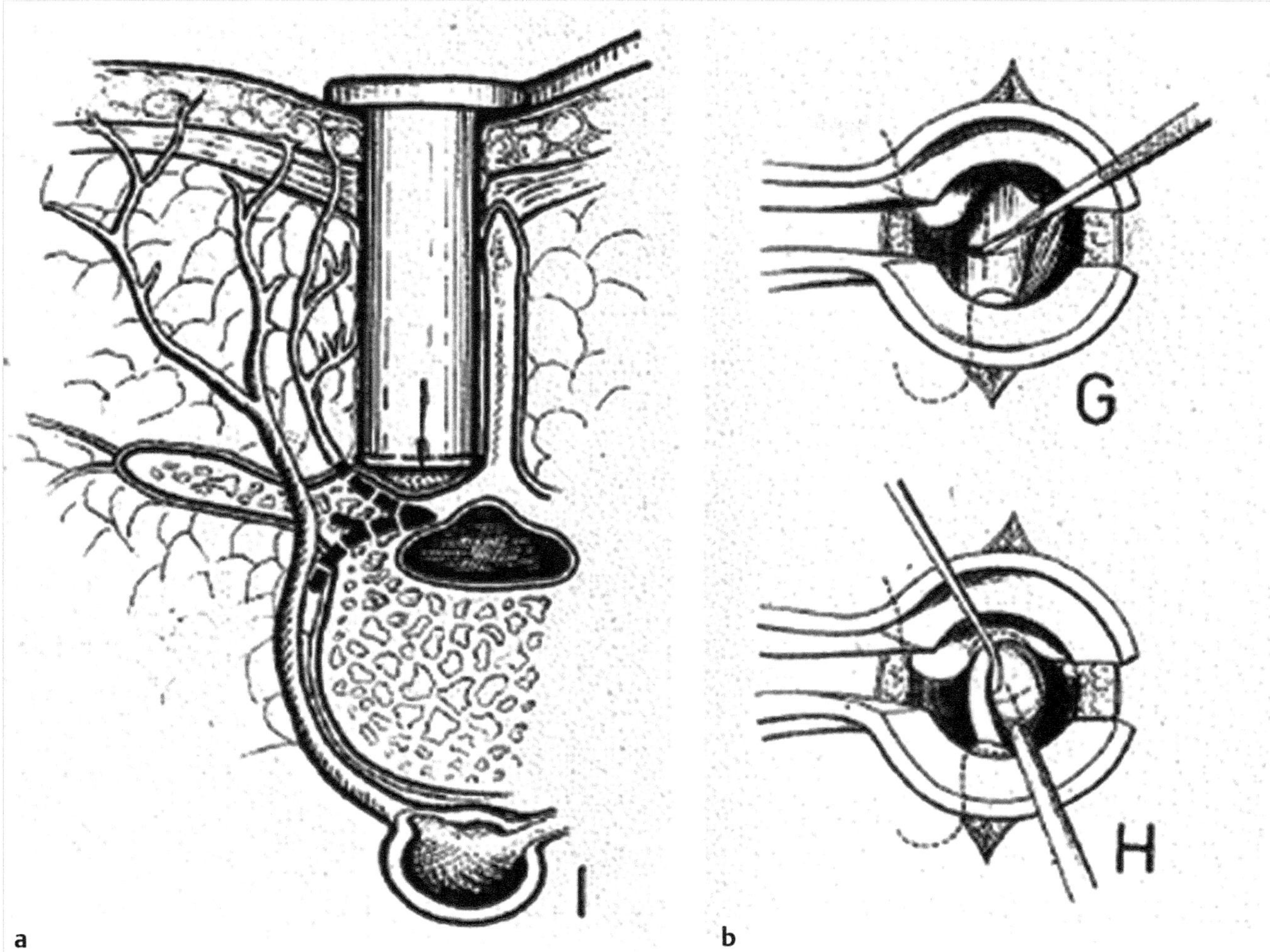

Fig. 2.5 Illustrations from Caspar's 1977 chapter[6] on microsurgical techniques for lumbar discectomy. **(a)** A cylindrical speculum that bears a striking resemblance to current minimal access ports is demonstrated in position over a lumbar segment. **(b)** Caspar recognized the liability of the muscle–retractor interface: "The smooth-walled round profile of the instrument does not cause any noteworthy pressure damage to the musculature." (Reproduced with permission from Caspar W. A new surgical procedure for lumbar disc herniation causing less tissue damage through a microsurgical approach, in: R. Wüllenweber, M. Brock, J. Hamer, et al. (Eds.), Lumbar Disc Adult Hydrocephalus. Advances in Neurosurgery, Berlin Heidelberg: Springer-Verlag. 1977.)

cylindrical port, which is strikingly like modern-day access ports, seems in large part lost to the pages of history. Caspar began his remarkably insightful manuscript with the statement:

Experience shows that there is an undesirably high incidence of substantial (unfortunately, sometimes also permanent) local back complaints after surgical treatment of lumbar disc herniation. The quality of the results of surgery is thereby reduced and sometimes indeed put in question. We believe that a considerable proportion of the complaints must be attributed to surgical trauma, in particular to muscle damage. This opinion is supported by the results of experienced surgeons such as Kuhlenedahl, Lange, Love, Youmans, and others who have long advocated an intervention which is as accurate, restricted in extent and as gentle as possible.... The hitherto practiced surgical method requires a disproportionately large access as compared to the dimensions of the surgical target area.

Caspar's observation that the exposure is disproportionately large compared to the requisite anatomy demonstrates his awareness of the need to increase the efficiency of the surgical exposure. The Caspar ratio, which I introduced in the introduction to the Primer, precisely defines the surgical efficiency as the ratio of the surgical target to the surgical exposure. Striving for a Caspar ratio of 1 is a central tenet of minimally invasive spine surgery. To remedy the perceived shortcomings of the lumbar herniation operations performed in his day, Caspar[6] set forth the following criteria:

1. Precise monosegmental access.
2. Minimal lesion in the approach to the actual area of surgery.
3. Better visual clarity (use of the operating microscope) in depth and thus more gentle manipulation of the nerve root and dural sac.

These criteria ring as true now as they did when Caspar wrote them in 1977. Collectively, adherence to these measures set a trajectory that could lead only to the current minimally invasive techniques we have today. These techniques are the inevitable outcome of fully realizing and adhering to Caspar's criteria.

Caspar's concept of a cylindrical speculum resolves several aspects of the muscle–retractor interface evenly distributing the forces to the skin and muscle. The concept was an important advancement but fell short because of the inability to maintain the stability of the speculum. My conversations with surgeons who attempted procedures through the speculum indicate that the lack of stability may have been what limited the wide adoption of the Caspar concept. Twenty years would pass before the stability of a cylindrical access port would be resolved with the introduction of the table-mounted arm by Foley and Smith.[5] Displacing the forces away from the incision and onto a table-mounted arm further minimizes the muscle–retractor interface. Foley and Smith refined the approach by shifting the incision completely off the midline, thereby eliminating the subperiosteal dissection and instead using a paraspinal transmuscular approach to the spine. Although endoscopic visualization was initially used, the microscope has become a more practical form of visualization today. The microdiscectomy performed through a paraspinal transmuscular minimal access port, secured to a table-mounted minimal access port and visualized through a microscope, is the technique I describe in this chapter.[5,8]

2.4 Requisite Anatomy

The advice I give my residents and fellows when we are performing a minimally invasive microdiscectomy together for the first time is for them to not reinvent the wheel. In other words, they should not approach a minimally invasive microdiscectomy as if it were a distinct procedure from its open counterpart. By the time residents and fellows do a rotation with me, they have already gathered some significant experience with the microdiscectomy. They have assisted in dozens of open microdiscectomies and have likely performed several virtually on their own. Their familiarity with the anatomy at depth enables them to successfully perform an open procedure—or at least to recognize how the exposure should look. These residents and fellows have reached a point in their training where reconstruction of the anatomy from memory is ripe for development. So, the first thing I emphasize to these residents is to make the exposure through the minimal access port exactly what they would expect to see if the operation was a midline open approach. It is important to recognize that the exposure in a minimally invasive operation requires, by its very nature, an element of recall memory. If you cannot see all the requisite bony landmarks that you would see in an open procedure when the minimal access port is in position, then stop and reassess. No good will come from taking a drill to anatomy about which you are uncertain.

The first logical question when considering a minimally invasive approach for a microdiscectomy is: What is the requisite anatomy for any microdiscectomy, open or minimally invasive? Compare the traditional midline microdiscectomy exposure to a minimally invasive microdiscectomy exposure with the requisite anatomy for the procedure (▶ Fig. 2.6) as defined by Williams[9] and corroborated by Maroon.[10]

In ▶ Fig. 2.6[9] the yellow highlighted area on the right of the lumbar spine represents the requisite anatomy for a microdiscectomy. Regardless of the technique you use, the lateral aspect of the thecal sac, the traversing root and the disc space must be visualized to enable you to perform the procedure. Note that the midline is not necessary for the procedure itself. ▶ Fig. 2.6c demonstrates the superimposed exposures of an open approach and a minimally invasive approach.

In an open procedure, the 1-inch or so incision is made either on the midline or slightly off the midline in the direction of the symptomatic nerve root. The medial aspect of the spinous process is exposed to allow for a subperiosteal dissection of the paraspinal muscle to unveil the lamina. The medial facet is exposed with caution so as not to interrupt the facet capsule. Typically, a Williams retractor, a McCulloch retractor or an equivalent anchors into the spinous process and is used to retract the muscle over the lamina to the medial facet after it has been exposed through the dissection.

The only difference between a minimally invasive exposure and an open exposure should be the absence of the medial aspect of the spinous process and the medial lamina, neither of which is actually required for the operation. There are no neuroanatomical structures needed for the procedures beneath the spinous process and medial lamina relevant to this procedure. Their exposure is the inevitable consequence of a midline approach. It is worth mentioning that neither the spinous process nor the medial lamina was part of the exposure in the microdiscectomy that Caspar described in 1977.[6] Other than that, the exposures should be identical. As a minimally invasive surgeon, you must adopt the mentality that a microdiscectomy with a minimal access port is simply another way to perform the same operation that otherwise would have been done with a midline incision and conventional retractors.

2.5 Efficiency of the Exposure

As demonstrated in ▶ Fig. 2.7, a magnified version of ▶ Fig. 2.6c, the minimum requisite anatomy established by Williams[9] is the inferolateral aspect of the rostral lamina, the medial facet and the superior and lateral aspects of the caudal lamina. A well-positioned 16-mm-diameter (▶ Fig. 2.7b) access port readily encompasses all the requisite anatomy. A midline approach with a conventional retractor does not expose more of the requisite anatomy; it exposes anatomy not necessary for the operation (▶ Fig. 2.7c). Remember, there is no need to try to reinvent the wheel. It is a mistake to attempt to make the operation any different from the one with which you are already familiar. The goal is to leverage the experience and skill set you have acquired from open microdiscectomies and apply them to a minimally invasive approach so that you can become familiar with the instruments and the subtleties that an altered trajectory has on the appearance of the surface anatomy.

A thoughtful examination of ▶ Fig. 2.7c demonstrates that the midline incision with a conventional lumbar spine retractor is actually outside what is necessary to perform the operation. By its very nature, this approach requires a more rostrocaudal extension of the incision to displace the muscle and skin laterally enough to expose the requisite anatomy. The exposure is more a consequence of a midline incision needing to be long enough to allow enough exposure to reach the medial facet. The result is a triangular-shaped exposure, where the rostral and caudal limbs of the triangle are a consequence of the exposure

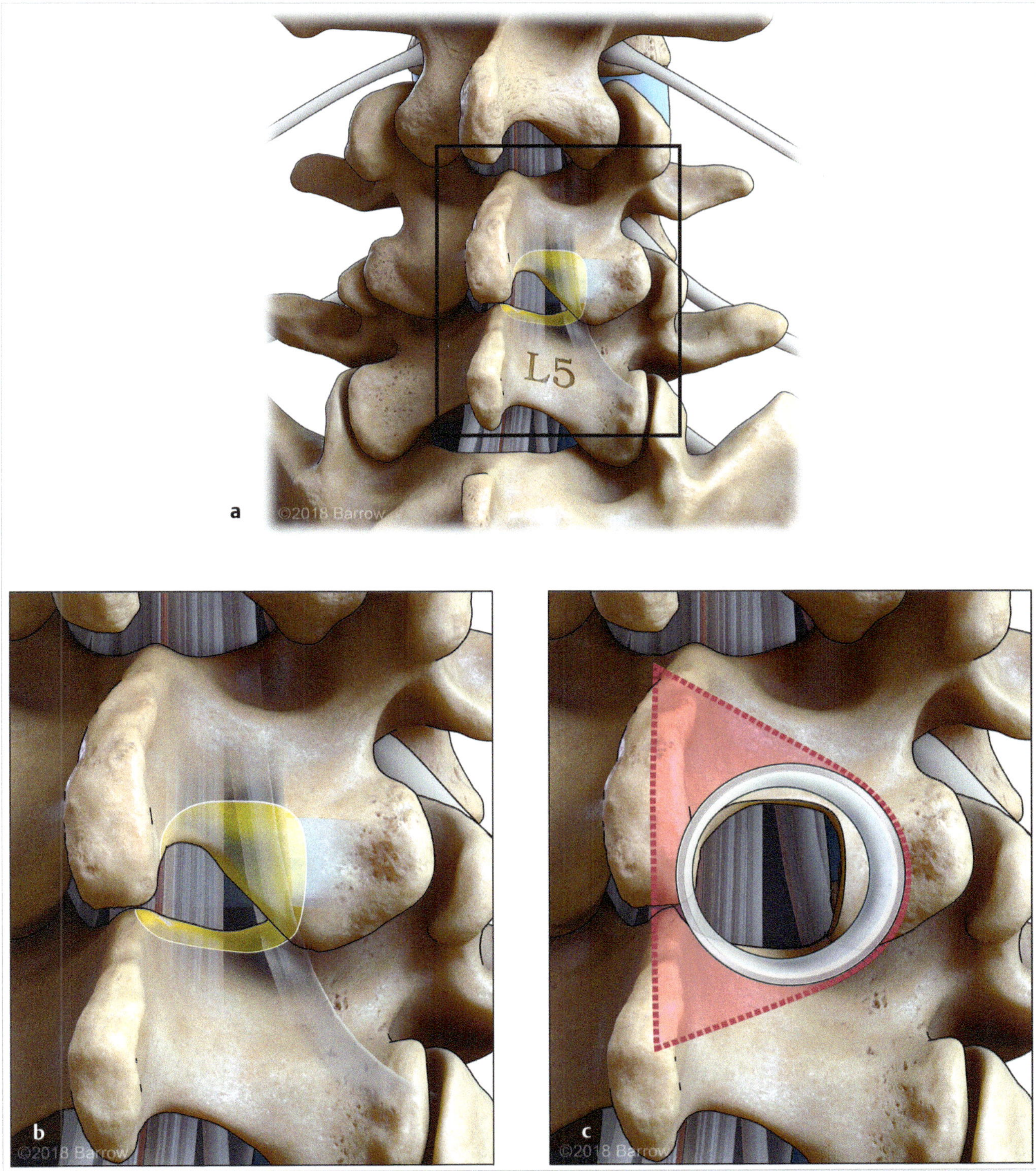

Fig. 2.6 Illustrations demonstrating the requisite anatomy exposure for a microdiscectomy as defined by Williams.[9] **(a)** The yellow highlighted area on the right of the lumbar spine represents the requisite anatomy for a microdiscectomy. Note that the midline is not necessary to perform the operation and therefore is not highlighted. The black rectangle is the area of focus for figures **b** and **c.** **(b)** Magnified view of the requisite anatomy for a microdiscectomy. The ghosted traversing root of L5 may be seen relative to the lamina and the facet along with the disc space. **(c)** Superimposed exposures of an open approach (*red shading*) and a minimally invasive approach (*encompassed by the minimal access port*). Both exposures include the requisite anatomy. However, the minimally invasive exposure is more efficient because it exposes only the requisite anatomy, whereas a midline approach exposes non-requisite anatomy (*red shading*). Exposure of non-requisite anatomy is the unavoidable consequence of beginning the exposure in the midline.

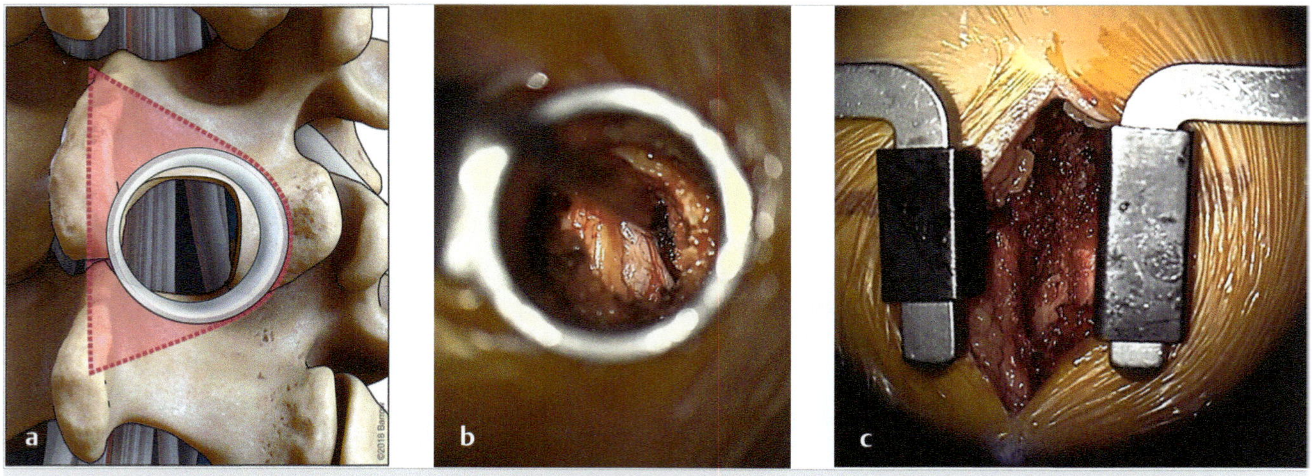

Fig. 2.7 Rationale for a minimally invasive approach. **(a)** Illustration of the requisite anatomy (magnified in ▶ Fig. 2.6c). A 16-mm-diameter access port encompasses all the requisite anatomy for the procedure. An open midline approach (*red shading*) does not offer any additional exposure of the requisite anatomy visible inside the access port (*gray circle*). **(b)** Intraoperative photograph of a minimally invasive 16-mm access port showing that it encompasses the requisite anatomy with a highly efficient exposure. **(c)** Intraoperative photograph of a McCulloch retractor exposing the lamina for a right L4–5 microdiscectomy. A midline approach does not offer more exposure of the requisite anatomy; it exposes anatomy that is not necessary for the operation.

but are not needed at all for the operation. It is important to note that a midline approach does not offer any more exposure of the requisite anatomy necessary for the operation than a well-positioned minimal access port.

The most efficient shape for exposure of the requisite anatomy is circular, as Caspar[6] championed in 1977. If the efficiency of an exposure was to be measured by the ratio of requisite anatomy to exposed anatomy, then a well-positioned cylindrical access port would demonstrate a greater efficiency than the triangular-shaped conventional midline exposure. Although the difference may be slight for a microdiscectomy, the efficiency of exposures becomes more pronounced the more lateral the requisite lies. The far lateral microdiscectomy is a perfect illustration of this concept.

2.6 Anatomical Basis

As residents and fellows begin to perform these procedures, I can sense their concern regarding the amount of exposure necessary for the procedure and whether they will be able to achieve enough exposure through the minimal access port. So, a word or two is warranted about the anatomical basis of the operation within the context of the various diameters of the access port. It is tremendously valuable to have a few anatomical measurements at your fingertips as you begin to explore minimally invasive microdiscectomies. The quote from the ancient *Panchatantra* that opened this chapter rings especially true here: "Knowledge is the true organ of sight." In this case, your knowledge of the anatomy will help orient your mind and increase your certainty of the anatomy at depth. You need not see everything to know where everything is. You do, however, need to possess the knowledge of the anatomy to have the "true organ of sight" in a minimally invasive approach. That knowledge goes beyond your recognition of the anatomy. Your goal must be complete recall of the anatomy from your memory and the aptitude to reconstruct the anatomy at depth.

Keep in mind that there are more constants than variables when it comes to the lumbar spine. While disc heights may vary even within the same patient, depending on the degree of degeneration, the diameter of the canal and the distances between the pedicles are remarkably constant. ▶ Fig. 2.8[11] and ▶ Fig. 2.9 illustrate the various measurements of canal diameter, interpedicular distance, intrapedicular distance and foraminal height.[11] Having a general sense of these measurements instills confidence when you are peering down a 16-mm-diameter access port and wondering about what is all the way down at the bottom.

As determined by Panjabi et al,[11] the intrapedicular distance (i.e., the distance between the pedicles of the same vertebral body) is on average 24 mm (range, 23–27 mm). Knowledge of this measurement indicates that the distance from the spinous process (the midline) to the pedicle is seldom more than 12 mm. The interpedicular distance (i.e., the distance between adjacent pedicles) will be inherently tied to the disc space and the level. The distance is less in patients with advanced collapse of the disc space than in healthy disc spaces. At L5–S1, where lordosis is greatest, thereby bringing the pedicles closest together, the interpedicular distance has the smallest value (typically about 28 mm), while at L3–4 where there is less segmental lordosis, the distance can increase to as much as 35 mm. The final measurement is the disc height. Although disc heights are directly related to the degree of degeneration, the height, even in a healthy disc, is seldom more than 14 mm. Collectively, these measurements point the way to the anatomical basis for a minimally invasive microdiscectomy. ▶ Fig. 2.9 demonstrates the various distances from the junction of the base of the spinous process and lamina to the medial facet and over the top of the disc space. A 16-mm diameter offers ample access to the neural elements and the bony anatomy to enable you to readily perform the operation.

At the same time, a poorly placed access port makes the operation virtually impossible. When all you have is a 16-mm-diameter view, the precise placement of that diameter is

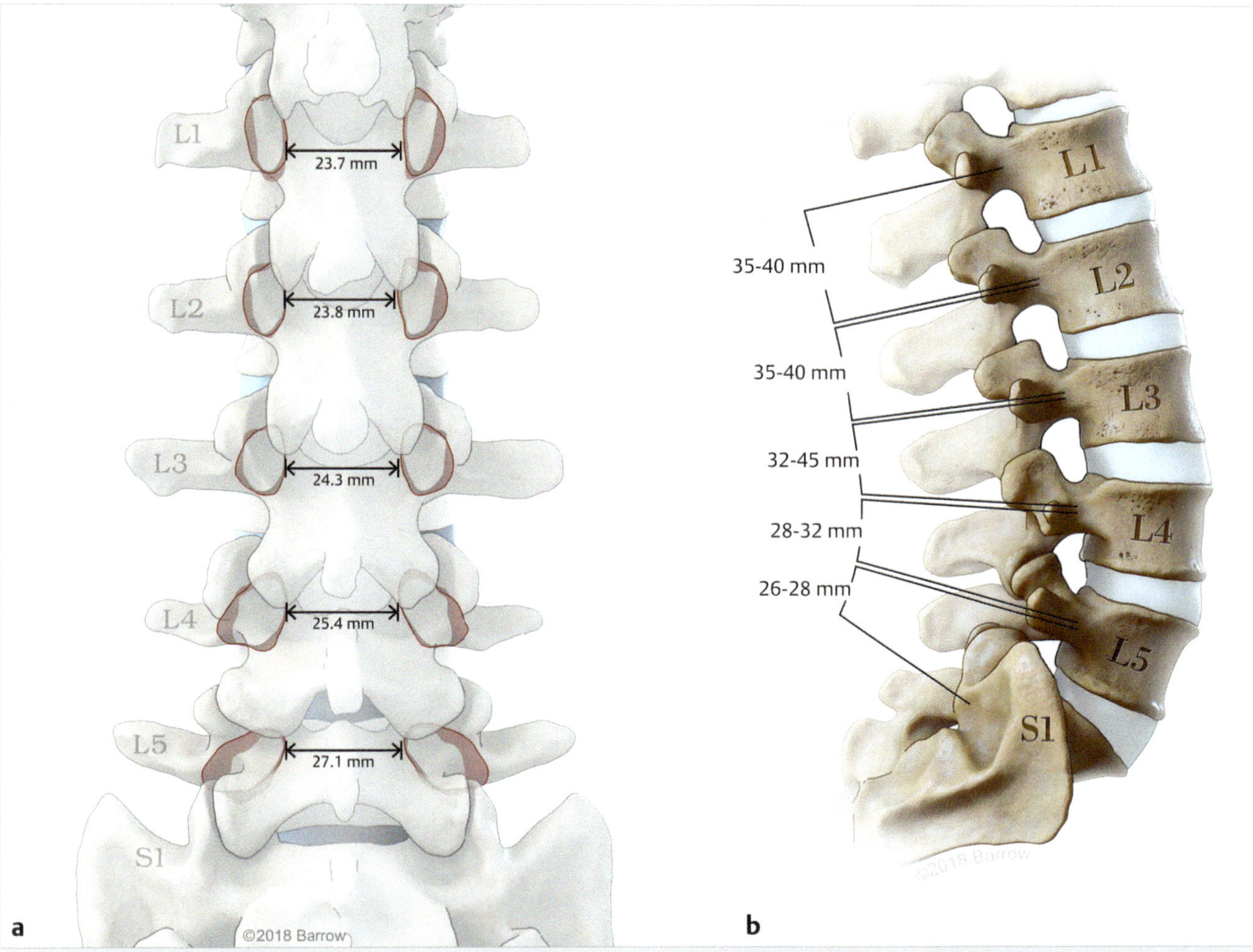

Fig. 2.8 Illustration demonstrates (a) the intrapedicular distance and (b) the interpedicular distance in the lumbar spine from L1 to S1, as reported by Panjabi et al.[11] The intrapedicular measurements define the width of the spinal canal. With a width ranging from 23 to 27 mm from L1 to L5, it becomes evident how a 16-mm-diameter access port can readily encompass the anatomy in one-half of the canal. The interpedicular distance ranges from 26 mm at L5–S1 to 40 mm at L1–2. These measurements begin to lay the foundation for a minimally invasive approach to the lumbar spine.

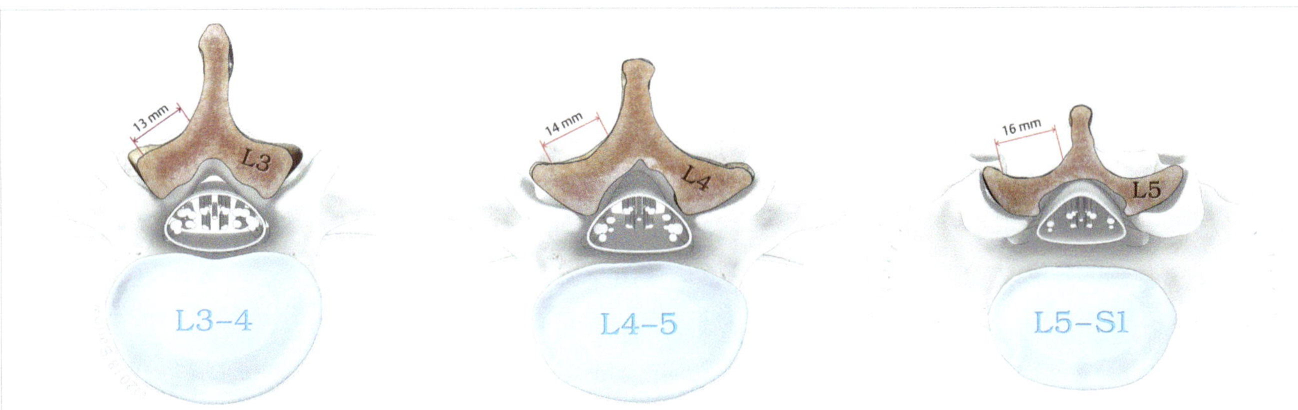

Fig. 2.9 Illustration of the axial view of the lumbar spine showing the L3, L4 and L5 laminae at the L3–4, L4–5 and L5–S1 disc space demonstrates that the distance from the base of the spinous process to the medial facet is less than 16 mm. Therefore, a well-positioned 16- to 18-mm-diameter access port will provide adequate exposure. A larger diameter would expose the facet, which is unnecessary.

imperative. How does one ensure that the requisite anatomy at depth will be there when the cautery has cleared off the soft tissue over the top of the lamina? The answer is threefold: preoperative planning, fluoroscopic guidance and sounding the anatomy.

Much in the same way we can place a ventricular catheter into the third ventricle from a point 11 cm back from the glabella and 2 cm over from the midline just as easily as we can from a point 10 cm back and 3 cm over, the incision used for a minimally invasive microdiscectomy can vary. Surgeons have recommended 1, 2 and 3 cm from the midline. Any of these distances may work because the exposed anatomy will be more a function of the trajectory. However, I prefer an incision 1.5 cm off the midline, as recommended by Foley and Smith,[5] for reasons I will expound on later. Some surgeons advocate the benefits of a transverse incision, while others see no reason not to start directly over the relevant anatomy. Again, it is not so much the incision or the location; it is what you do with that incision to accomplish the requisite exposure.

2.6.1 Anatomical Basis for Minimal Access Diameters

At this point, it is germane to discuss the diameter of the minimal access port. Of the various diameters available, 18 mm is an ideal one with which to start. Although diameters up to 22 mm are available, the measurements on ▶ Fig. 2.9 demonstrate that there is no anatomical basis for such a large diameter for a microdiscectomy. If anything, diameters larger than 18 mm may be more of a liability than an asset. Such a diameter can disrupt structures that lay outside the requisite anatomy for the operation. The illustration of the lumbar spine in an axial view shown in ▶ Fig. 2.9 demonstrates that the distance from the lateral aspect of the spinous process to the medial facet at the L3, L4, and L5 levels is no more than 16 mm.

The distance from the center of the disc space to the medial aspect of the pedicle is no more than 18 mm at L3, L4, and L5, as demonstrated in ▶ Fig. 2.10.

The measurements listed in ▶ Fig. 2.9 and ▶ Fig. 2.10 show how the necessary exposure for a microdiscectomy—open or minimally invasive—need not expose more than 18 mm lateral to the spinous process. In fact, more than 18 mm may actually be a liability, because it may expose the facet capsule. Furthermore, with these measurements in mind, one can argue that a well-positioned 16-mm, or even a 14-mm, minimal access port provides ample exposure of the requisite anatomy from a mediolateral standpoint. Ideal placement and trajectory are paramount for these diameters, as every millimeter of exposure will be indispensable for the operation.

From a rostrocaudal standpoint, the distance from just above the disc space into the foramen measures approximately 16 mm. The illustration of the lumbar spine in the coronal projection in ▶ Fig. 2.11 demonstrates that 16 mm allows the lateral aspect of the nerve root at S1 to be followed from the medial facet into the foramen.

These rostrocaudal and mediolateral measurements establish the anatomical basis for the diameters used in minimally invasive microdiscectomies. It quickly becomes evident from these measurements that an 18-mm-diameter port offers a generous exposure. With experience, a 16-mm-diameter port or even a 14-mm-diameter port will become a feasible option (▶ Fig. 2.12).

2.7 Operating Room Setup

Always set up your operating room in a manner that will optimize the flow of the operation and minimize idle time when the patient is under anesthesia. Idle time can occur at transition points, such as while waiting for the microscope or securing the table-mounted arm. To prevent delays, the scrub technician, operating room nurse and radiology technologist should all know their roles to efficiently get you to the point of making an incision, docking the access port and working under the operating microscope.

For the operating room setup, I position the microscope on the side of the prone patient's symptoms and the fluoroscope opposite the side of the radiculopathy. The scrub technician begins to drape the microscope as the patient is being anesthetized. Consequently, by the time the minimal access port is in position, there is no delay in transitioning to the microscope in the surgical field (▶ Fig. 2.13).

The operating room nurse secures the table mount and the clamp that anchors the table-mounted arm to the bed. These steps are taken before draping but immediately after positioning the patient (▶ Fig. 2.14).

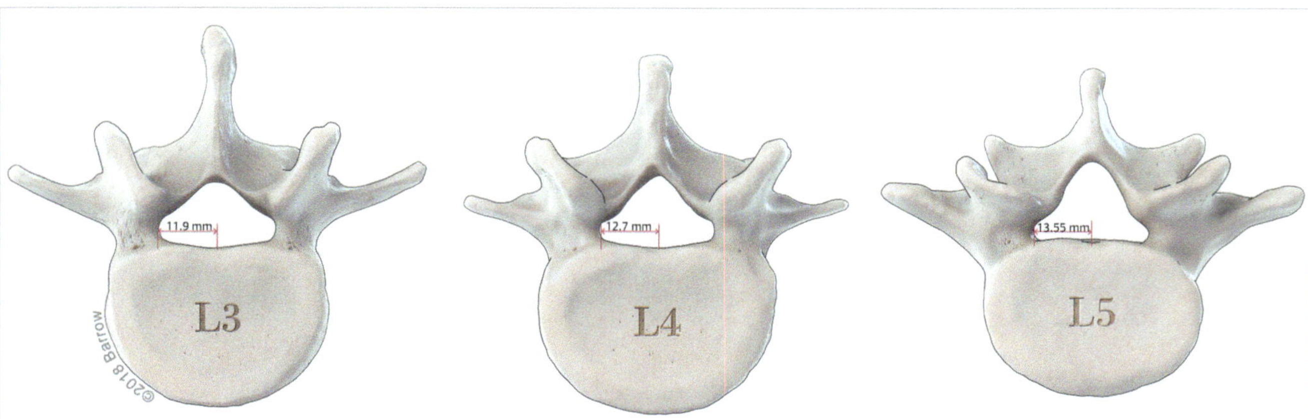

Fig. 2.10 Illustration of L3, L4 and L5 vertebrae demonstrates that the distance from the midline to the pedicle is less than 18 mm. Therefore, a 16-mm-diameter port would offer exposure from the base of the spinous process to the pedicle. The requisite anatomy for a microdiscectomy is well within that diameter.

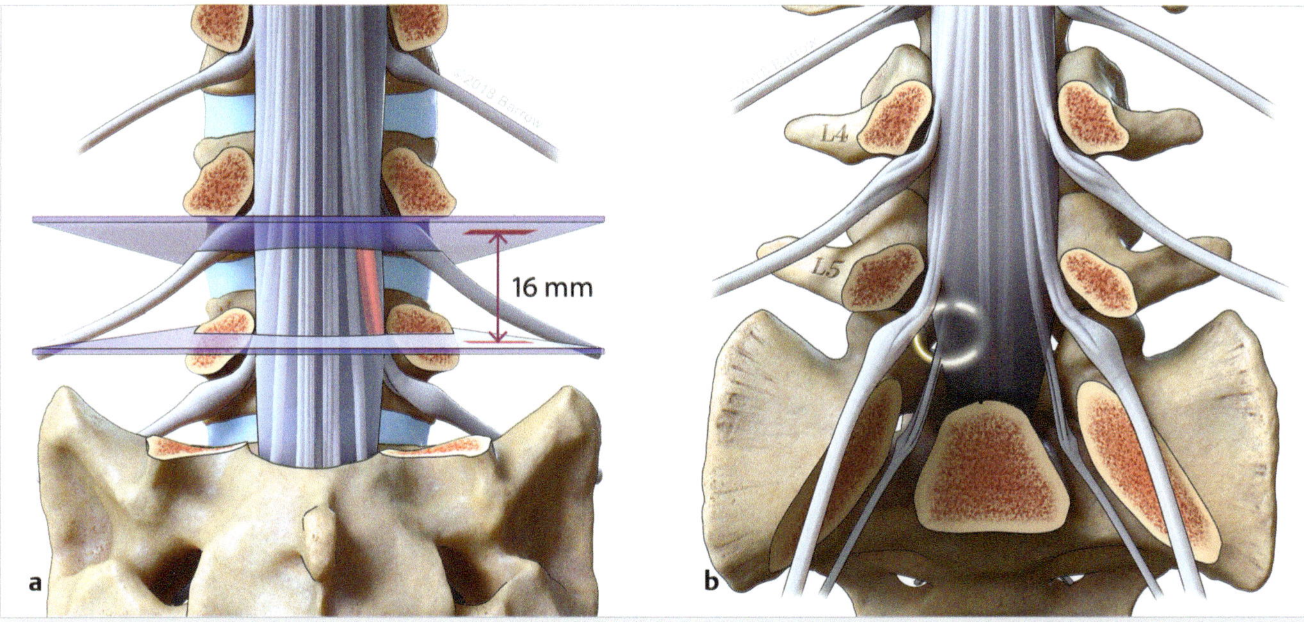

Fig. 2.11 Illustration demonstrates the lumbar spine in the coronal projection. **(a)** Posterior view with the posterior elements removed. The plane from the top of the L4–5 disc space to the plane through the mid-pedicle of L5 measures approximately 16 mm. **(b)** Anterior view with the vertebral bodies removed shows a well-positioned 16-mm-diameter minimal access port (*light ring*) over the top of the nerve root of S1 for an L5–S1 microdiscectomy. The view from inside the canal demonstrates that such a diameter offers all the exposure necessary to accomplish all the goals of the surgery.

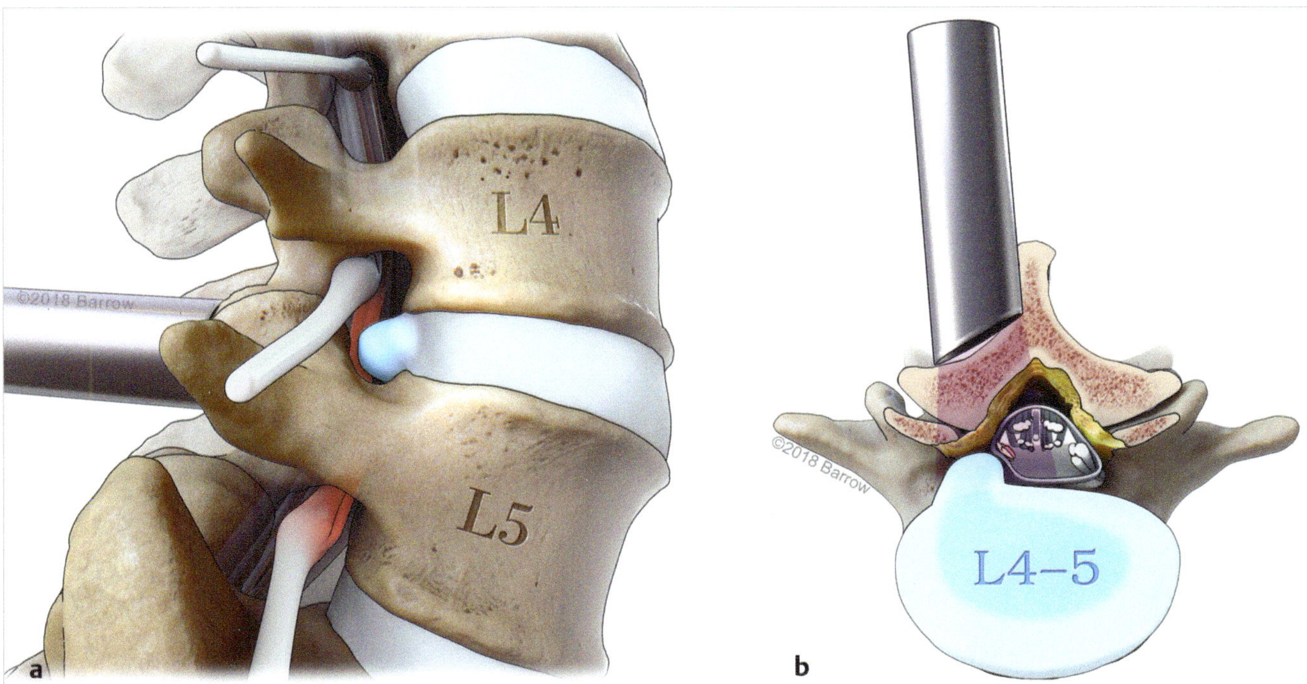

Fig. 2.12 Illustration of the lumbar spine demonstrates an L4–5 rightward disc herniation and a 16-mm-diameter access port in position. **(a)** Lateral oblique projection demonstrates the trajectory of the minimal access port in the precise axial plane of the nerve root compression and, **(b)** axial projection shows the access port in the axial plane of compression. It is clear that a 16-mm-diameter access port provides exposure of the requisite anatomy, as demonstrated by the field of view (*light purple shading*).

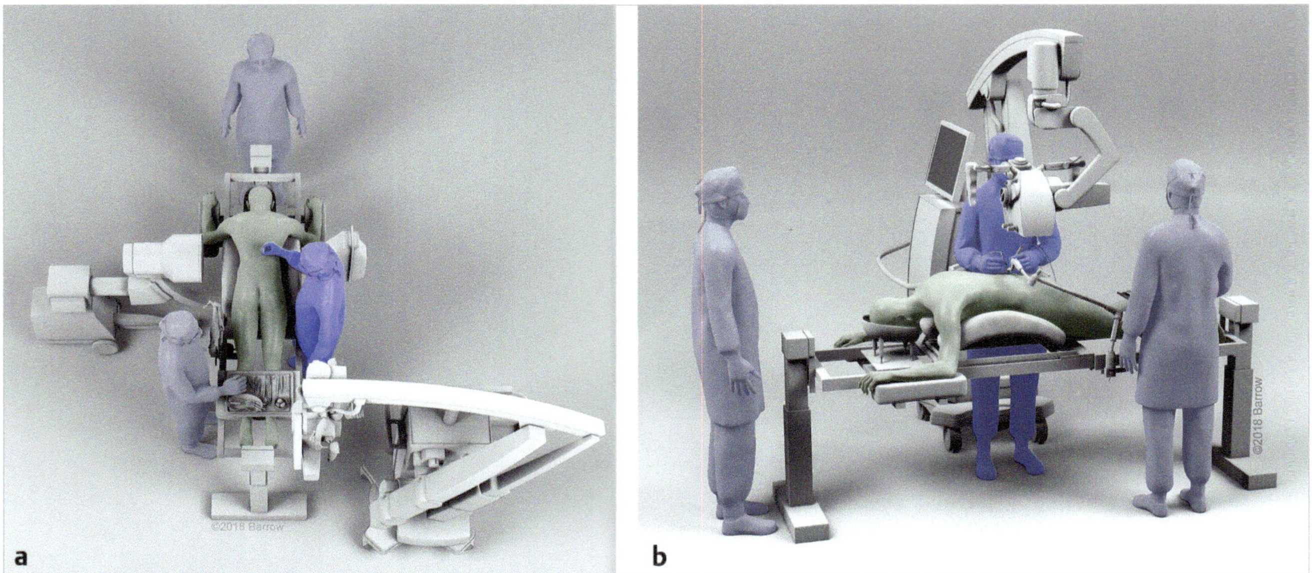

Fig. 2.13 Three-dimensional model demonstrates operating room personnel and equipment setup. **(a)** A bird's-eye view of the patient positioned prone on a Jackson table atop a Wilson frame for a right-sided microdiscectomy. The surgeon stands on the symptomatic side. The clamp that will hold the table-mounted arm is in position opposite the side of the symptoms. The image intensifier of the fluoroscope is opposite the side of the symptoms and the X-ray tube is on the symptomatic side. As shown in this illustration, the fluoroscope is in position at the start of the operation, and the microscope is draped and ready. The table-mounted arm is in position and ready to be secured once the minimal access port is in position. Such a configuration allows for the fluoroscope to be readily wheeled out and the microscope to be wheeled in with no delay in transition. **(b)** View from the front corner of the operating room demonstrates the surgeon now operating under the microscope. The fluoroscope was rolled out as the microscope was rolled in, and the minimal access port has been secured to the table-mounted arm.

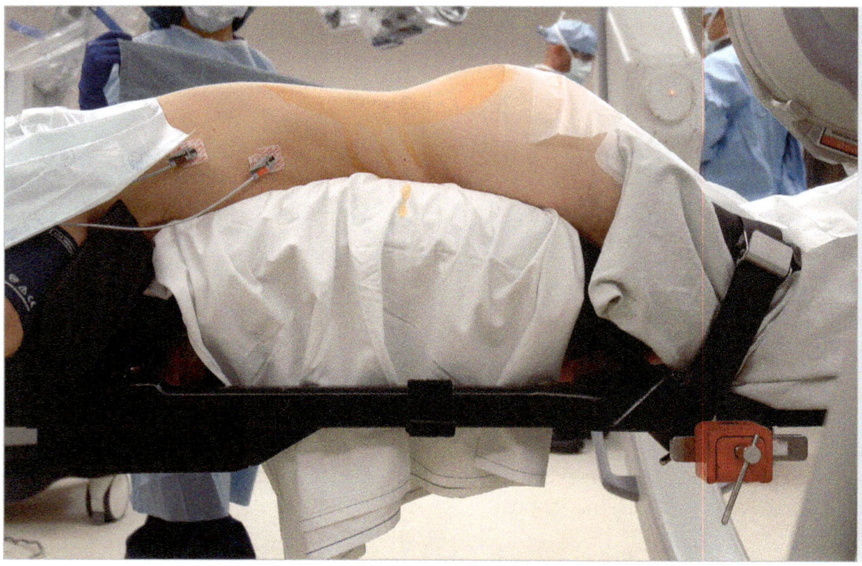

Fig. 2.14 Preoperative photograph shows patient positioning for a right L4–5 microdiscectomy. The patient rests prone on a fully expanded Wilson frame atop a Jackson table. The clamp is already in position before the patient is draped, which prevents any idle time waiting for the operating room staff to secure a clamp under the drape. The operating microscope is already draped and on the symptomatic side of the prone patient, and the clamp is already positioned opposite the side of the symptoms.

The radiology technologist brings in the fluoroscopy unit and places it at the level of the patient's knees to facilitate draping (▶ Fig. 2.15). The smaller X-ray tube is on the side of the surgeon, whereas the bulky image intensifier is on the asymptomatic side opposite the surgeon. Such a configuration facilitates draping the fluoroscope into the surgical field and eventually allows for efficient removal of the fluoroscope and transition to the operating microscope. There is no need for preoperative fluoroscopic images, consistent with the focus on minimizing radiation exposure. Preoperative fluoroscopy will not eliminate the need to obtain images as you dock the access port; so, it is best to reserve those images for the actual procedure.

After placing the sterile drapes on the patient and the fluoroscope, the scrub technician, with the assistance of the operating room nurse, secures the sterile arm to the table-mounted bracket before bringing in the Mayo stand. That proactive maneuver eliminates delays once dilatation of the incision is complete and the minimal access port is ready to be secured.

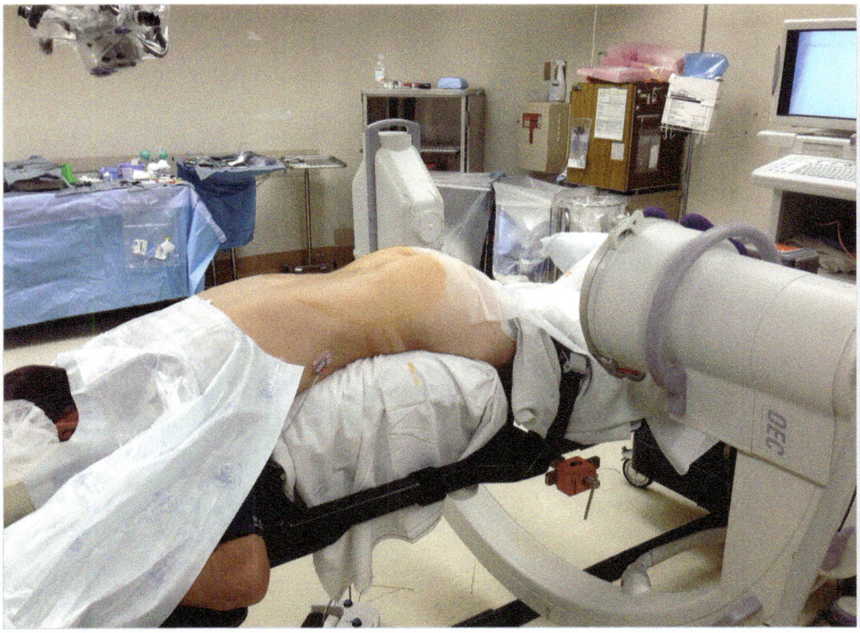

Fig. 2.15 Preoperative photograph shows operating room setup for a right L4–5 microdiscectomy. The fluoroscopic unit is positioned before the patient is draped. Placing the fluoroscope at the bend of the patient's knees facilitates draping the unit in a sterile manner. The X-ray tube is placed on the side where the surgeon will stand. The bulky image intensifier is placed opposite the surgeon. The microscope is visible in the top left of the photograph, already draped and ready to be rolled into position once the minimal access port is secured.

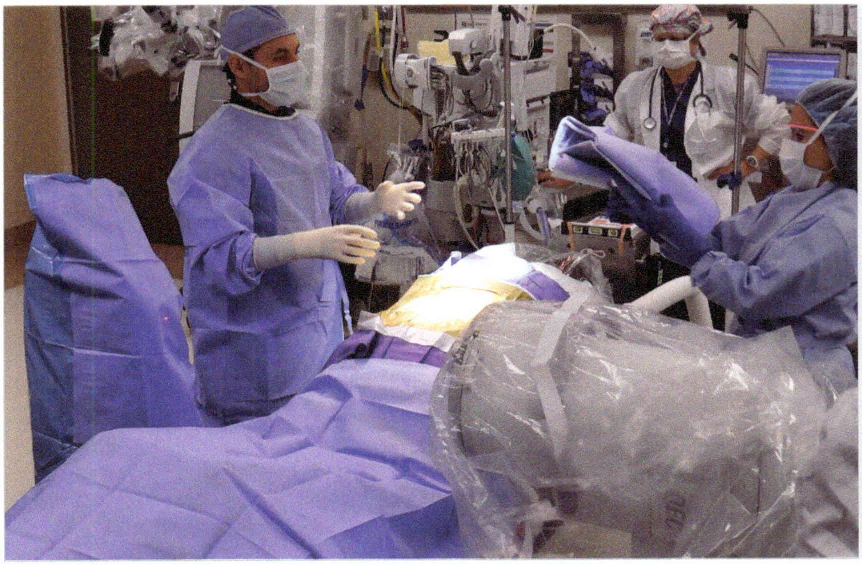

Fig. 2.16 Operating room setup for a left L4–5 microdiscectomy. A draped microscope stands ready to be used, and a draped fluoroscope can be rolled into position for imaging after the draping of the patient is completed. Localization may begin as the scrub technician passes off the cords for the drill and cautery and the tubing for the suction.

All these steps are part of the unspoken routine for the minimally invasive ensemble, which emphasizes the importance of assembling such a team (▶ Fig. 2.16).

2.8 Patient Positioning

I prefer to use a Wilson frame atop a flattop Jackson table for minimally invasive microdiscectomy operations. The Jackson table allows for unencumbered passage of the fluoroscope up and down the underside of the table. With the patient in position, I crank open the Wilson frame to its fully expanded curvature. The arc created by a fully expanded Wilson frame opens the interlaminar space and thereby limits the bone work necessary to access the lateral aspect of the canal, mobilize the nerve root, and remove the herniated disc. The Wilson frame also indicates the ideal position for the clamp that will secure the table-mounted arm. I place this clamp at the base of the Wilson frame opposite the side of the symptoms (▶ Fig. 2.13 and ▶ Fig. 2.15). This particular position of the clamp creates an ideal configuration for the table-mounted arm to readily secure the minimal access port in a low-profile manner. For disc herniations at L2–3 and L1–2, this clamp should be moved up to the midportion of the Wilson frame. As mentioned previously, securing the clamp should be part of the unspoken ritual of the smoothly functioning minimally invasive ensemble.

A Jackson table is not absolutely necessary, but it is preferable because it facilitates positioning of the fluoroscopic unit and allows its movement to the foot or the head of the bed. Attempting to navigate around the base of a standard operating room table can be more challenging and disruptive to the flow of the operation.

2.9 Surgical Technique

2.9.1 Conceptualizing the Position of the Minimal Access Port

A well-placed minimal access port will allow the surgeon to begin operating immediately after bringing in the microscope, without concern that the port is not ideally positioned over the requisite anatomy. Ensuring that the exposure at the bottom of the port will be identical to what could be accomplished with a midline approach before peering down the operating microscope requires adherence to certain principles. The first principle is to ensure that the operating corridor is precisely in the axial plane of the disc herniation. Such positioning is achieved by maintaining the minimal access port completely parallel to the disc space. The first step in achieving that position entails precisely planning the incision (▶ Fig. 2.17).

Preoperative fluoroscopy has little utility because the minimal access port needs to be anchored onto the table-mounted frame with fluoroscopy during the operation. Preoperative fluoroscopy therefore becomes redundant. As emphasized in the introduction to the Primer, the minimally invasive spine surgeon must make every attempt to minimize exposure to ionizing radiation.

2.9.2 Planning the Incision

To plan the incision, I begin by palpating the bony landmarks through the skin as classically described by Williams.[9] I palpate the anterior superior iliac spine with my index finger and approximate the L4–5 level with my thumb (Video 2.1). I then mark the level that I intend to operate on in the midline in between the spinous processes. If I am operating on the L5–S1 level, I mark the interspinous space one down from my presumptive L4–5 level; if I am operating on L3–4, then I move up one interspace, and so on (▶ Fig. 2.18). A prominent line will mark the midline of the spine. Firmly establishing and marking the midline are essential components for orientation. Although you may not be able to look directly at the spinous process or lamina, you still know where it resides. The reconstruction of the anatomy at depth for the operation begins at this point.

The guiding principle for bone work performed in microdiscectomies was set forth by Caspar,[6] Yaşargil,[7] Williams[9] and Love.[12] It is a worthwhile endeavor to read these classic articles. I have found that each one of them establishes the timeless principles and provides valuable insight into the lumbar microdiscectomy operation. Whether the microdiscectomy is performed in the open or minimally invasive manner, its focus should always be to remove the least amount of bone that will allow for safe mobilization of the nerve root and removal of the disc herniation. Every effort must be made to prevent disruption of the facet capsule or significant removal of the medial facet as shown in ▶ Fig. 2.7a. With this in mind, I measure 1.5 cm off the midline and mark my proposed incision (▶ Fig. 2.19). My rationale for this distance is twofold. First, I know from the anatomical measurements discussed previously that the distance from the midline to the pedicle throughout the lumbar spine is approximately 12 to 14 mm. The anatomy before us dictates the parameters of the exposure, and there is little utility in exceeding what that anatomy dictates. Second, I want to minimize my angle onto the spine. An incision of any greater distance off the midline may increase the angle and limit visualization of the lateral recess. Increased angles onto the spine in a microdiscectomy will require more bone removal to visualize the lateral recess and mobilize the traversing nerve root.

Regarding the length of the incision, I typically add 2 mm to the diameter of the minimal access port that I intend to use. For instance, if I intend to use a 16-mm-diameter port, then I will mark an 18-mm incision, which allows for easier passage of the access port and minimizes any stretching of the skin. I make a preliminary mark for the incision based only on my palpation of the bony landmarks. Again, I do not obtain any preoperative fluoroscopic images for two reasons: first to minimize radiation exposure to the operating room team as well as myself and second, because a preoperative fluoroscopic image does not

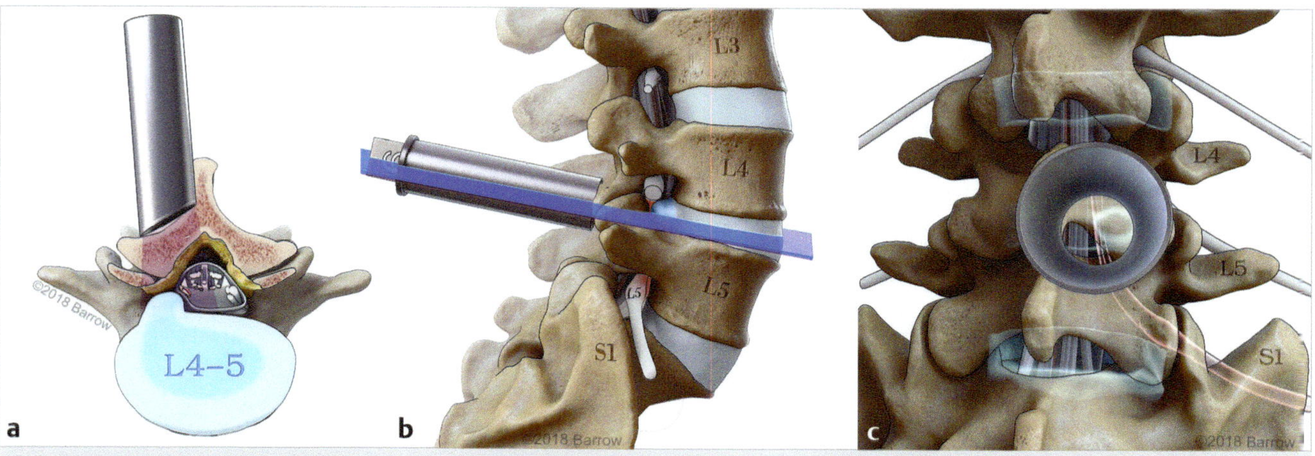

Fig. 2.17 Illustration demonstrates the axial plane of the compression in an L4–5 rightward disc herniation. **(a)** Axial plane with the minimal access port docked onto the lamina in the precise axial plane of the nerve root compression. **(b)** Lateral view of the same access port parallel to the disc space, with the trajectory of the access port in the precise axial plane of the disc herniation. Such precise positioning is necessary to optimize exposure of the requisite anatomy. **(c)** Posterior view (surgical view) of a 16-mm-diameter minimal access port position with an optimal trajectory to the spine in the precise axial plane of the compressed nerve root.

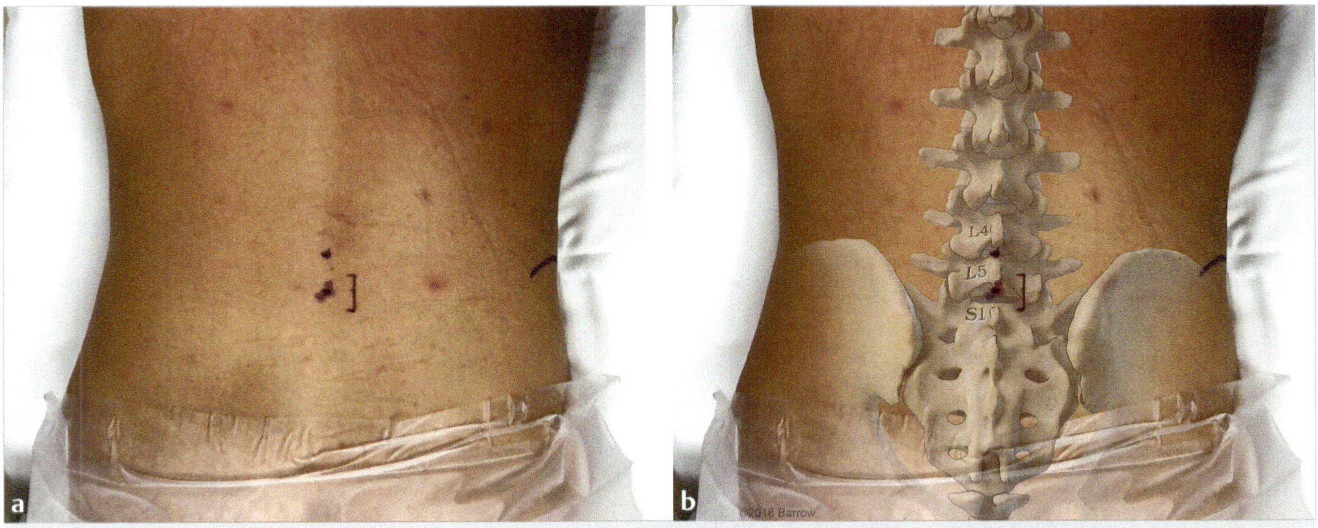

Fig. 2.18 Planning the incision for an L5–S1 right-sided microdiscectomy. **(a)** Palpate the anterior superior iliac spine (marked on the right flank with a *curved line*); approximate and mark the L4–5 interspinous process space (*upper dot*). Locate L5–S1 (*lower dot*) as the next interspace below L4–5. From the lower interspace, an incision is planned 1.5 cm from the midline (*line*). **(b)** The spinal anatomy ghosted onto the image in panel (a), which reveals the palpated anatomy relative to the planned incision.

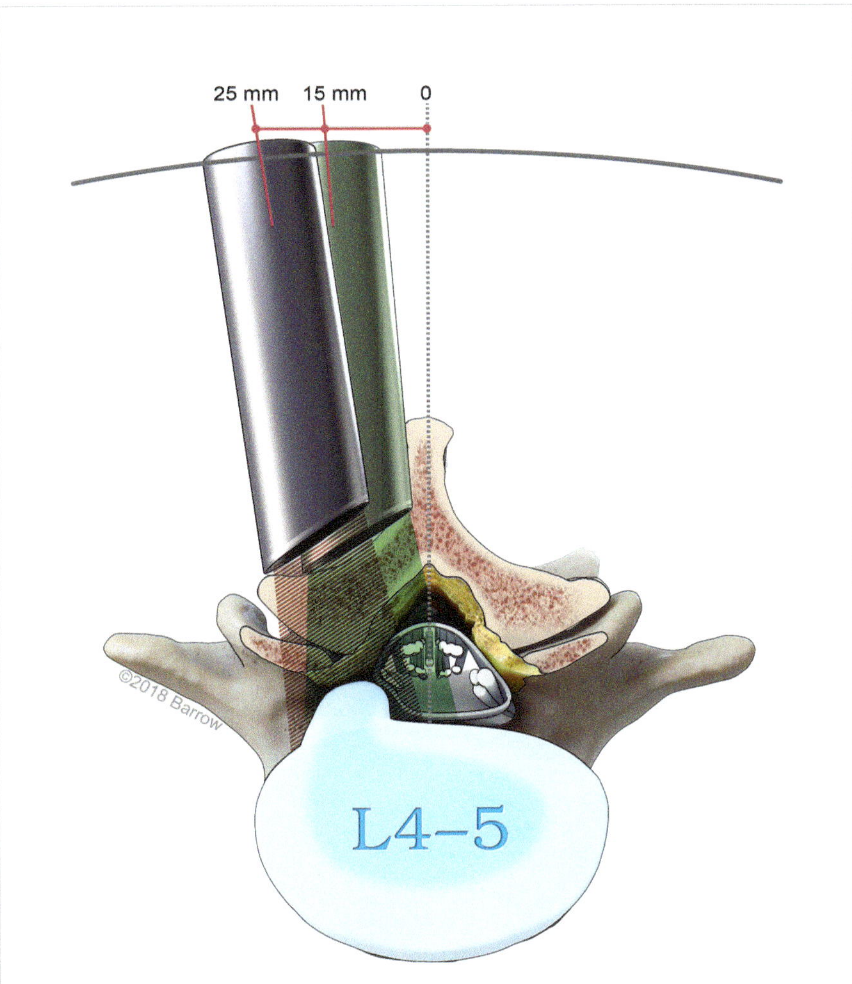

Fig. 2.19 The rationale for an incision 1.5 cm from the midline. Illustration demonstrates the angles created by an incision at 1.5 and 2.5 cm from the midline. The angle at an incision 2.5 cm from the midline creates a suboptimal trajectory onto the nerve root with more of the facet covering the nerve root, whereas an incision 1.5 cm from the midline creates a trajectory for the access port immediately over the nerve root.

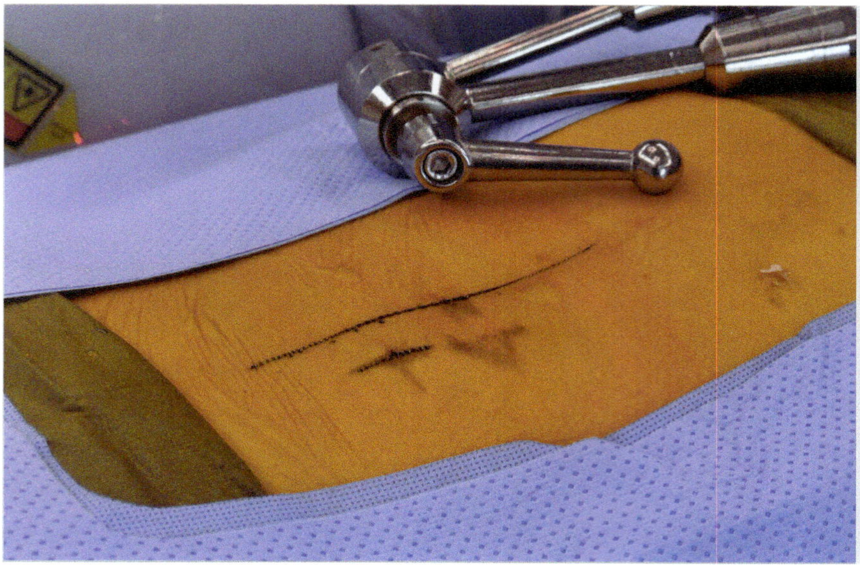

Fig. 2.20 Intraoperative photograph shows marking for an incision. The long vertical line marks the midline. The incision is planned 1.5 cm off the midline and then marked. The first fluoroscopic image is obtained after passage of the spinal needle onto the lamina to confirm the level. Any necessary adjustment is then made, and the proposed incision site is filtrated with a local anesthetic.

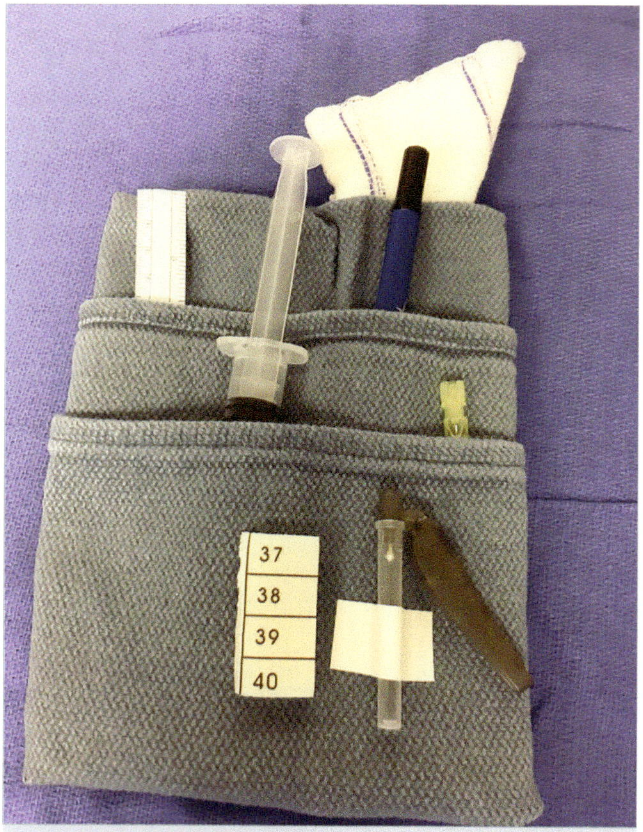

Fig. 2.21 Photograph of the infiltration and incision planning set. At the beginning of the operation, the surgeon can be given a spinal needle, a syringe filled with local anesthetic, a hypodermic needle, a marking pen and a ruler to confirm the segment and optimize the incision while the scrub technician prepares for surgery. Being able to simultaneously confirm, re-mark and infiltrate the incision while the scrub technician prepares the Mayo stand and passes off the cautery wires and suction tubing further adds to the efficiency of the procedure.

preclude the need to obtain an image later. In short, it saves time and decreases radiation exposure (▶ Fig. 2.20).

After I have marked the midline and my proposed incision, I prep and drape the patient widely in case I need to adjust the incision in either the rostral or caudal direction. The radiologic technologist rolls the previously draped fluoroscopic unit into position for a lateral image at the level of interest.

The work flow of the operation can be optimized by having the scrub technician set out a spinal needle, a syringe with local anesthetic, a ruler and a marking pen in a surgical towel before passing off wires and suction tubes and before positioning and preparing the Mayo stand for the operation (▶ Fig. 2.21). In this manner, I confirm the level and optimize the location of the incision while the scrub technician simultaneously prepares for the operation. By the time I am ready to make the incision, the scrub technician has their Mayo stand, suction and cautery instruments ready as well.

I pass a 20-gauge spinal needle through the marked incision and onto the lamina (▶ Fig. 2.22). I angle it away from midline to prevent the possibility of the tip of the needle passing interlaminar and puncturing the dura. Dural puncture with localization has happened to me on one occasion, and I will never forget it. Since that singular incident, I take every measure possible to ensure that it never happens again. When the needle encounters the lamina–facet junction, I wander as far away from the X-ray tube as sterility will allow and then request the first fluoroscopic image. The needle should be completely parallel to the disc space in the axial plane of the disc herniation. ▶ Fig. 2.17b illustrates the concept of the ideal trajectory, whereas ▶ Fig. 2.23 demonstrates the potential pitfalls of a suboptimal trajectory. I will reposition the needle to achieve the perfect position and trajectory that will ensure the ideal placement of the incision for the ideal trajectory of the minimal access port.

It is important to recognize that the trajectory of the needle in the sagittal plane determines the trajectory of the minimal access port onto the segment. The entry point of the needle at the level of the skin will define the incision. Any adjustment of

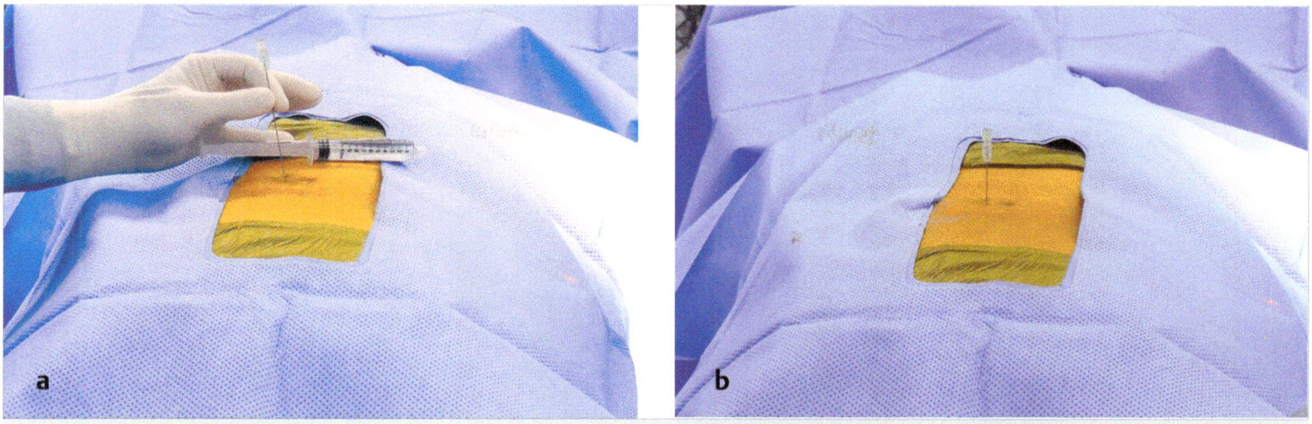

Fig. 2.22 Intraoperative photograph demonstrates placement of the spinal needle. (a) Passage of the spinal needle to the lamina facet junction. (b) After the spinal needle is in position, the first fluoroscopic image can be taken.

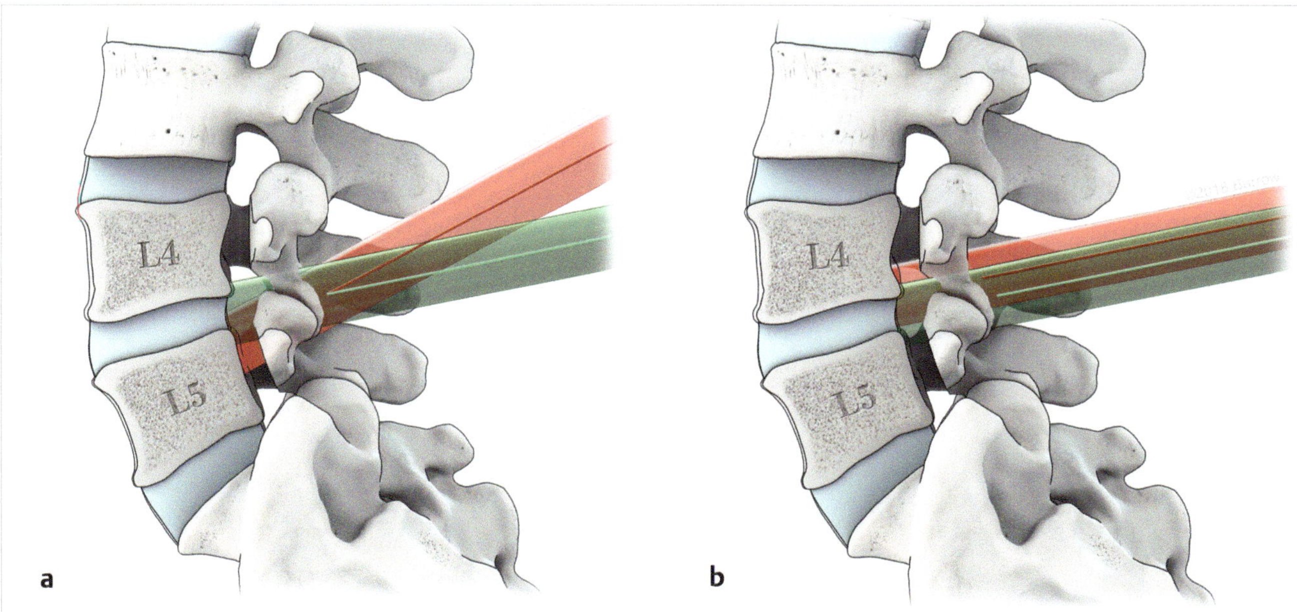

Fig. 2.23 Potential pitfalls of a suboptimal trajectory or starting point for an L4–5 microdiscectomy. Lateral projection of the spine demonstrates two distinct starting points for the incision. The line within each column represents the spinal needle. (a) The *red projection* onto the spine is not parallel to the disc space. The starting point is too high. An incision planned from this point is at the correct level but will not allow for an optimal trajectory onto the disc space and nerve root. As demonstrated in the image, the line of sight will be below the disc space. (b) In this circumstance, the *red projection* is parallel to the disc space, but the starting point is too high. While an incision planned from this point is at the correct level, the plane selected will result in exposure of the posterior aspect of the L4 vertebral body instead of the disc space. (a,b) The *green projections* in both images are precisely in the axial plane of the disc space and will provide an optimal trajectory for an operation at L4–5.

the needle prompts a remarking of the incision. With a 16-mm-diameter working channel, precise planning of the incision is imperative. It is possible to be at the correct operative level but to have a suboptimal trajectory because of poor incision planning. A trajectory that diverges from the disc space may not optimize the line of sight for adequate visualization of the nerve root and removal of the disc herniation. However, a parallel trajectory places the working channel precisely in the axial plane of the compression of the nerve root (▶ Fig. 2.23).

Once a fluoroscopic image demonstrates the spinal needle at the correct level, in the ideal position and trajectory, I remove the stylet from the spinal needle, pull back the spinal needle from the lamina 1 or 2 mm, and infiltrate a lidocaine with epinephrine and bupivacaine mixture into the future tract of the minimal access port. That mixture not only helps control bleeding from the muscle with vasoconstriction from the epinephrine but also helps control postoperative pain. The goal is for the patient to not feel the incision for the first several hours after the operation. After I inject the lidocaine–epinephrine–bupivacaine, I remove the spinal needle in its entirety and then use a hypodermic needle to infiltrate the four quadrants of the incision (▶ Fig. 2.24).

I make the incision with a No. 15 blade and obtain hemostasis with cautery. Dissection proceeds down to the lumbosacral fascia. As mentioned previously in the introduction to the Primer and in Chapter 1, it is the midline structures that maintain your orientation and their absence can be potentially disorienting. So before opening the lumbosacral fascia, I reorient my mind to the midline by palpating the spinous processes within the incision. Doing so provides my mind with another data point to help reconstruct the anatomy at depth. At times, the incision may seem to be in an ideal place but palpating the spinous process reveals that I am right over the midline—or that the spinous process is a full 2 cm away. Such a circumstance can happen especially in patients with a high body mass index. Palpating the spinous process reorients my mind when direct visualization of the midline structures is not possible. Having a confident sense of the midline allows me to use cautery to make the fascial incision approximately 1 cm away from the spinous process. Although the skin incision was 2 mm larger than the minimal access port, the fascial opening should be precisely the size of the minimal access port, which will further stabilize it (▶ Fig. 2.25).

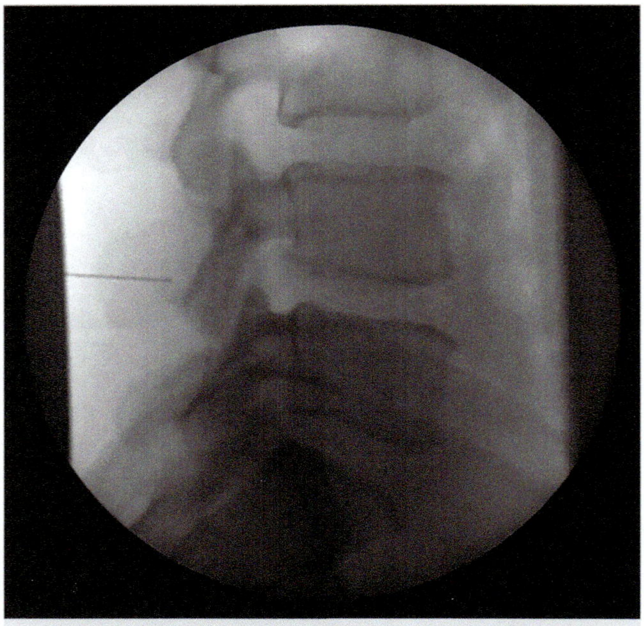

Fig. 2.24 Lateral fluoroscopic image demonstrating a spinal needle parallel to the disc space, confirming level L4–5. The incision is remarked, if necessary. The trajectory of the needle onto the spine will determine the trajectory of the minimal access port. In this circumstance, the entry point of the needle at the level of the skin is completely parallel to the disc space, assuring an optimal trajectory for the minimal access port.

2.9.3 Docking the Minimal Access Port

I optimize the efficiency of the operation by having the scrub technician and the operating room nurse secure the table-mounted arm into the clamp on the side of the bed as I make the incision. Before the patient is even draped, the clamp that will hold the arm had been secured opposite the side of the incision at the level of the base of the Wilson frame, so that the table-mounted arm will have a minimal profile during surgery. With everything ready, I place the first dilator into the incision, past the divided fascia and onto the spine with the target being the junction of the spinous process and lamina. It is important to note that several operative techniques have described the passage of a Kirschner wire onto the lamina as the first step. In fact, the first dilator has a hole designed to pass over a Kirschner wire. However, I have taken the counsel of several of my mentors not to use this technique and therefore have not described it in this chapter or in any other chapter. After the first dilator is on the lamina, I obtain the second fluoroscopic image to confirm the level (▶ Fig. 2.26 and ▶ Fig. 2.27).

Confirming the level with the first dilator presents another opportunity for me to begin reconstructing the anatomy at depth. In an open procedure, descending the plane of the spinous process onto the lamina with a subperiosteal dissection establishes the surgeon's bearings. Although that visual cue is lost in a minimally invasive approach, a tactile sense with use of the first dilator can fill that void. I sound the bony anatomy

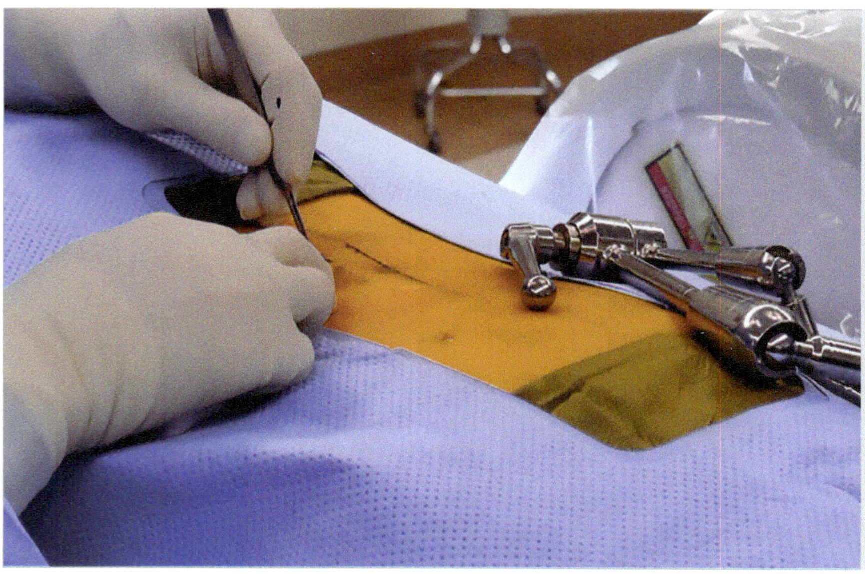

Fig. 2.25 Intraoperative photograph of the beginning of the operation. The photograph demonstrates the table-mounted arm already in position as the incision is made. The fluoroscope remains in the same position used when the localizing image was taken. Keeping the fluoroscope in position prevents delay in acquiring the same image again for localization. It also prevents any interruption in securing the access port. Collectively, these steps optimize the efficiency of the operation.

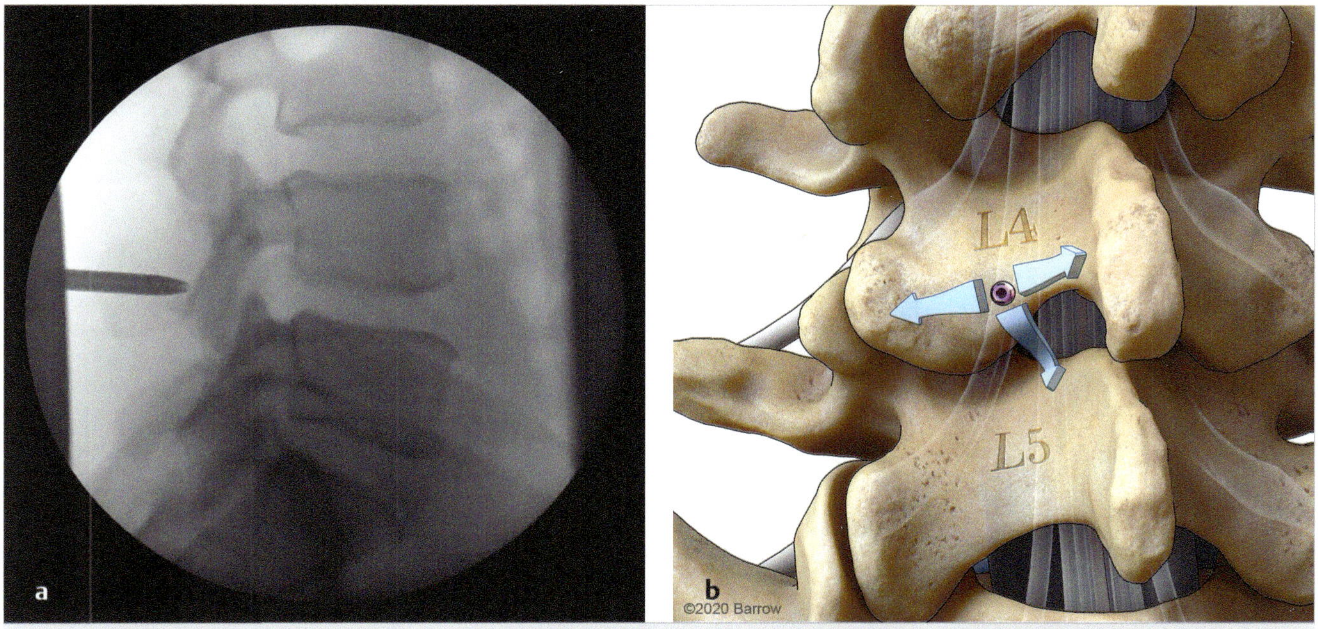

Fig. 2.26 **(a)** Lateral fluoroscopic image demonstrating the initial dilator pointing to the L4–5 segment. Note that the dilator is in the precise axial plane of the disc and parallel to the disc space. **(b)** Illustration demonstrates the location of the tip of the initial dilator. The initial dilator can be used to sound the anatomy. By probing medially and wanding the dilator, you can confirm the confluence of the lamina and spinous process. Probing laterally provides a tactile sense of the medial facet. Probing inferiorly identifies the interlaminar space. The tactile information provided by the first dilator enables the mind to reconstruct the anatomy at depth without direct visualization of the anatomy. Once these boundaries are probed, and the initial dilator is optimally placed and secured, you can perform subsequent dilatation.

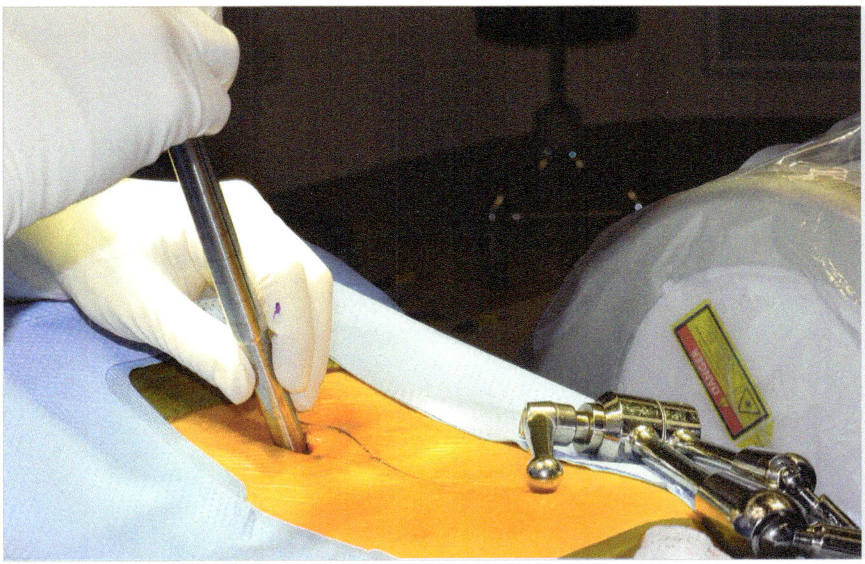

Fig. 2.27 Intraoperative photograph demonstrates dilatation of the paraspinal muscles. No additional fluoroscopy is performed after the initial dilator until the access port is in position and ready to be secured to the table-mounted arm.

with the dilators to substitute the spinous process as a visual cue. I use the first dilator to probe the junction of the spinous process and the lamina. By sliding the tip of the dilator a few millimeters up the spinous process and then over the lamina, I replace the visual cues of an open approach with the feel of the anatomy. I routinely get a sense of the interlaminar space by sliding off the inferior aspect of the lamina (▶ Fig. 2.26b). After I have mentally reconstructed the medial anatomy this way, I proceed laterally and get a sense of the inferior aspect of the lamina and the medial facet. The junction of the lamina and the medial facet is the target of the exposure (▶ Fig. 2.28).

With the anatomy reconstructed at depth in my mind's eye, I can now confidently secure the first dilator at the facet–lamina junction just above the interlaminar space and begin dilating. There will be no need for subsequent fluoroscopic images as I dilate if I firmly maintain the trajectory and position of my first dilator. I will obtain additional fluoroscopic images only if I lose my position on the lamina. After I have dilated to the appropriate diameter, I determine the necessary length of the access port by looking at the measurements on the side of the final dilator and slip the appropriate minimal access port over the dilators. With the help of the scrub technician or my surgical

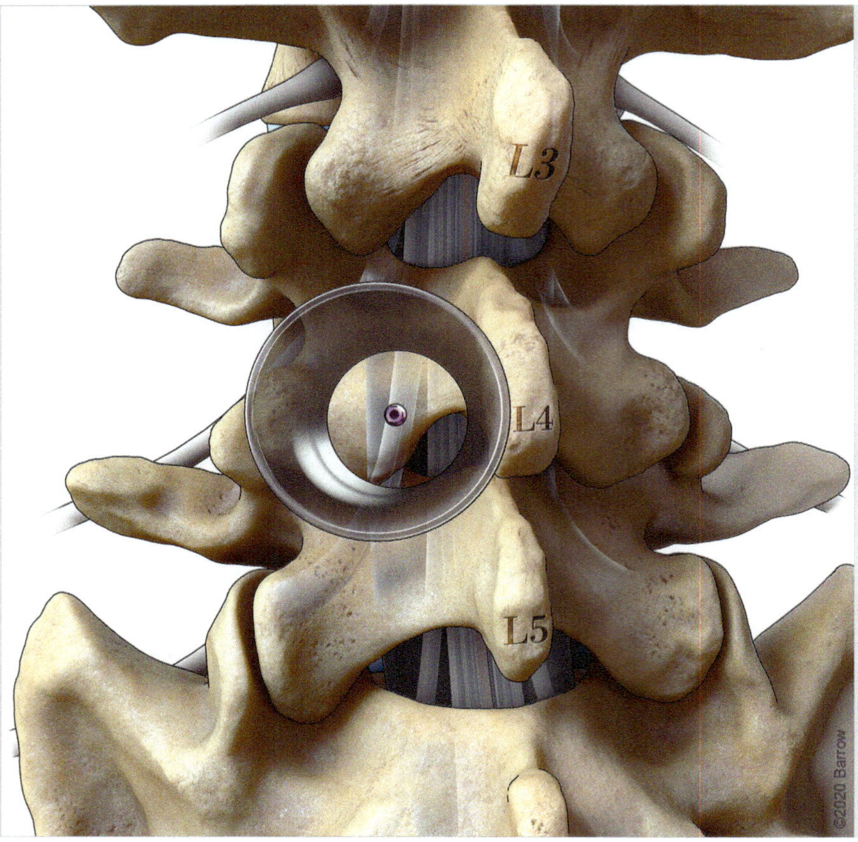

Fig. 2.28 Illustration demonstrates the junction of the medial facet and lamina as the ideal target for dilatation onto the lumbar spine for placement of a minimal access port for a microdiscectomy. The ghosted thecal sac and traversing root beneath the target demonstrate how this position offers the capacity to identify the neural elements, mobilize them and retrieve a disc herniation once the dilatation is complete over this initial position.

assistant, I secure the table-mounted arm into the stem of the access port and then obtain the third of the four fluoroscopic images to confirm the trajectory. I emphasize being completely parallel to the disc space, with the entire access port encompassing it. Even a healthy disc space is seldom more than 14 mm in height, which establishes the anatomical basis for a 16-mm-diameter port for a microdiscectomy. A parallel trajectory ensures that I will be in the axial plane of the disc herniation, causing the compression of the nerve root. The 16-mm diameter ensures access to both the rostral and caudal aspects of the disc space, provided that the access port is perfectly parallel to the disc space. By convention, I place the stem of the minimal access port pointing directly to the interlaminar space and label this the 12 o'clock position. The stem of the minimal access port becomes yet another reference point to help maintain orientation (▶ Fig. 2.29).

With the access port in position and at the ideal trajectory, I tighten the joints of the table-mounted arm to capture the position of the minimal access port. It is vital to maintain downward pressure on the stem of the access port while tightening the table-mounted arm. Downward pressure will minimize any muscle creep between the lamina and access port (▶ Fig. 2.30).

Although the lateral fluoroscopic image can help determine the optimal rostrocaudal trajectory, it does not help with the mediolateral angulation. For the most part, setting this trajectory comes with experience. Setting the medial-lateral angulation for a minimally invasive microdiscectomy is a mental game of trigonometry that requires the surgeon to incorporate the distance of the incision from the midline, based on what the sounding of the anatomy revealed and the depth of the anatomy. In doing so, the mind envisions how a subtle medial trajectory will place the diameter of the port ideally over the requisite anatomy for the operation. Too much of a medial angle will compromise the ability to get lateral to the traversing root, whereas too little of a medial angle will expose more of the facet capsule than would otherwise be necessary for the operation (▶ Fig. 2.31). An incision 1.5 cm from the midline requires only a subtle converging angle. The greater depth to the target has obvious implications for the angle. The same angle in a 9-cm access port (*red* in ▶ Fig. 2.31) and a 4-cm access port (*turquoise* in ▶ Fig. 2.31) will have two separate targets at depth, with the first being considerably more medial than the second. The angle of convergence is something to keep in mind, especially when the patient has a high body mass index.

After securing the access port to the table-mounted arm, I leave all the dilators in position and take another look at the angle. I may make minor adjustments if the angle seems suboptimal. As I look at the access port with the dilators in position, my mind processes the length of the access port and the angle. I am ensuring that there will be no surprises when I peer down the access port. Although I can confirm the angle using only the minimal access port, seeing all the dilators in position makes the angle more evident.

With the optimal trajectory determined on a lateral fluoroscopic image, I rotate the fluoroscope for an anteroposterior image. I retreat a safe distance from the X-ray source and obtain the fourth and final fluoroscopic image. I recently only incorporated this final anteroposterior image into my routine at the

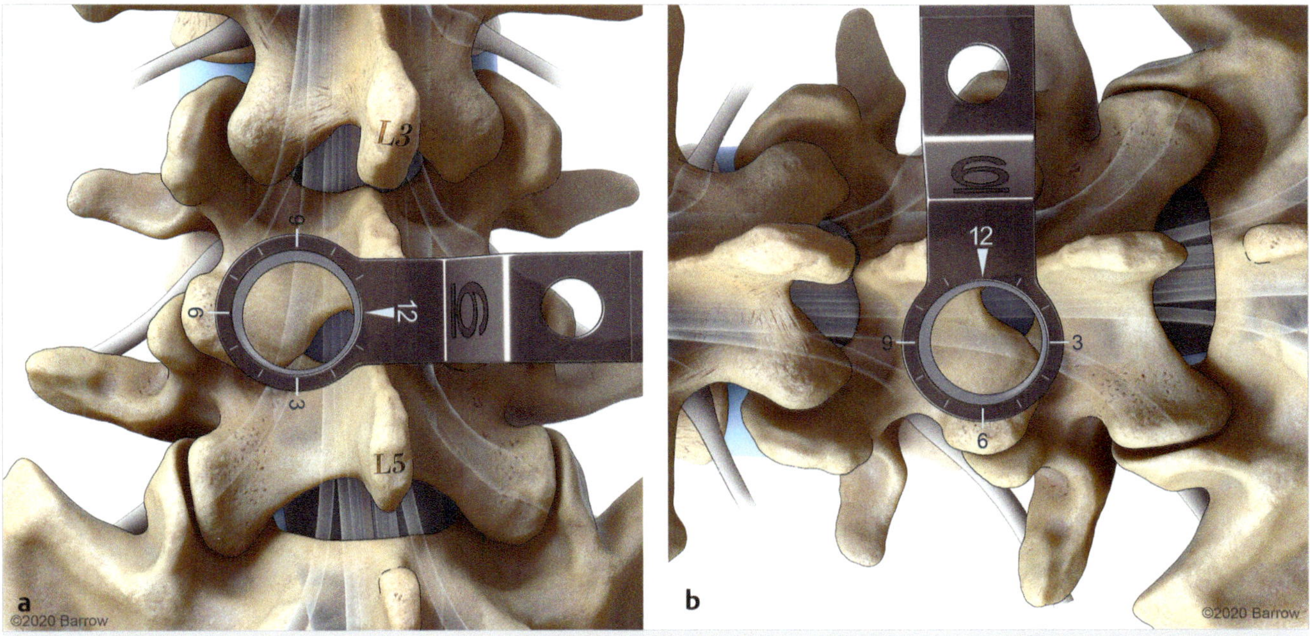

Fig. 2.29 The stem of the minimal access port used to maintain orientation. Illustration demonstrates the minimal access port in position in **(a)** a posterior view and **(b)** a surgical view with the surgeon standing on the symptomatic side of the patient. Assigning the stem of the access port a 12 o'clock position and pointing it to the interlaminar space creates an additional reference point for orientation. Under the operating microscope, the clock face becomes a useful method for maintaining one's bearings.

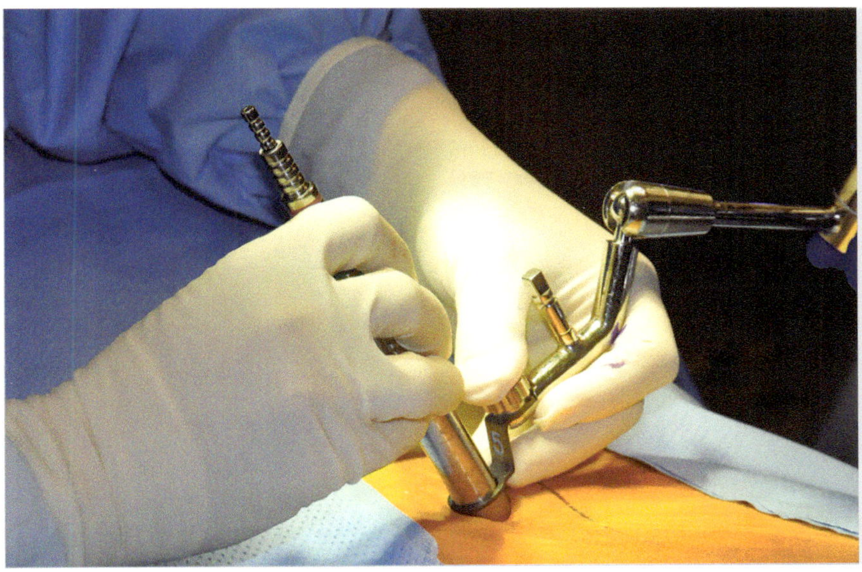

Fig. 2.30 Intraoperative photograph demonstrates the securing of the minimal access port. Downward pressure exerted by optimizing the interface of the access port against the lamina is imperative while tightening the table-mounted arm to minimize the creep of the paraspinal muscles.

request of a resident, who found it helpful to orient his mind to the anatomy at depth. Previously, I obtained an anteroposterior image only if I felt uncertain about the anatomy. Such an image is not essential, but it can help orient surgeons new to a minimally invasive approach. I use that image to look for the position of the minimal access port relative to the pedicle of the nerve root to be decompressed. The aperture of the access port should encompass a diameter just medial to the pedicle on the anteroposterior image (▶ Fig. 2.32).

The combination of sounding the anatomy, positioning the access port parallel to the disc space, and converging the trajectory onto the lamina facet interface optimizes the aperture of the access port at depth over the requisite anatomy. All this positioning is done before the operating microscope rolls into position. The fluoroscopic imaging for localization includes a total of four images, two of which place the surgeon more than 10 feet away from the X-ray source. In the anteroposterior position, the fluoroscope effortlessly pulls away from the operative site as the microscope simultaneously rolls in. I keep the final anteroposterior and lateral fluoroscopic images up on the screen throughout the operation so that I can glance at them from time to time to maintain my bearings. In my mind's eye, I

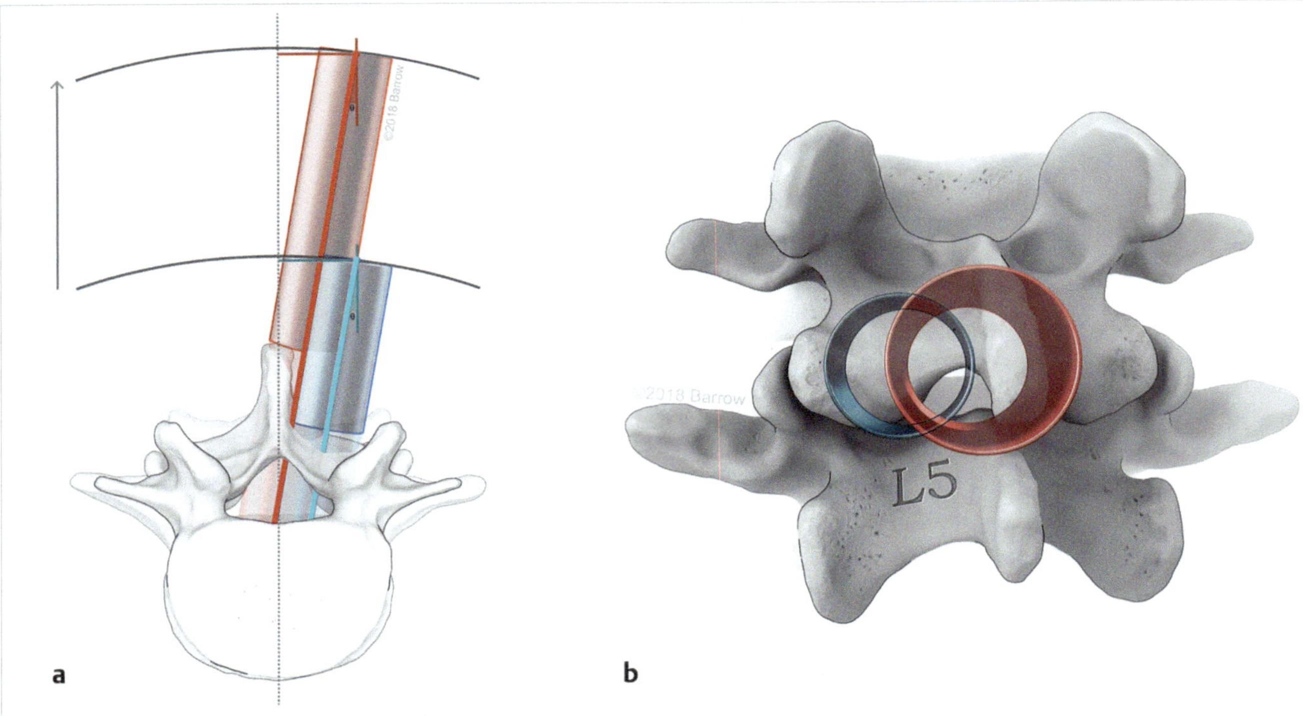

Fig. 2.31 Illustration demonstrates two anatomical scenarios based on the distance from the skin to the spine. In each circumstance, the same incision planned the same distance from the midline with the same angle for both would result in two different targets, one more medial (*red*) and the other more lateral (*turquoise*). **(a)** Axial view demonstrates that a straighter trajectory is required when using a longer access port (*red*) and **(b)** surgeon's view showing the area encompassed on the lamina by the positions of the access ports. Both targets are achieved with an incision 1.5 cm lateral to the midline with the same exact angle of convergence, but the results are two very different exposures. The impact that the angle of convergence has on these two exposures emphasizes the importance of making the necessary adjustments for a greater distance from the skin surface to the depth of the spine.

have already reconstructed the anatomy at the depth of the access port. The sounding of the lamina and facet, the fluoroscopic images and, most importantly, my knowledge of the anatomy, have me viewing the traversing nerve root, thecal sac, and disc herniation just as shown in ▶ Fig. 2.32c, c1. I focus the microscope down the access port with a suction in one hand and cautery in the other and begin the next phase of the operation (▶ Fig. 2.33).

2.9.4 Exposure

On a good day, I will peer down into the minimal access port and see nothing more than a thin veil of muscle overlying the lamina facet junction. The unmistakable ivory whiteness of the lamina should be immediately evident, without any dissection whatsoever. At times, the interface of the access port with the lamina facet junction will be suboptimal, and muscle will obscure more of the operative field of view than I would like. With the suction in my nondominant hand, I curiously, cautiously, and continuously probe the anatomy to confirm the lamina and facet before using the tip of the cautery in my dominant hand to discharge the first pulse of electricity and begin to reveal the anatomy. Once I have confirmed the lamina below, I use a bayoneted cautery tip to paint away what remains of the muscle. The bony anatomy reveals itself almost immediately. I approach the exposure in quadrants (▶ Fig. 2.34). It is always safest to start in the superior lateral quadrant, which corresponds to the 6 to 9 o'clock position (quadrant I) of the minimal access port. That quadrant will reliably have lamina below and will be an ideal location to begin establishing your bearings. Cautery in this quadrant presents little, if any, risk to the neural elements or the facet capsule. I consider the inferomedial aspect of the exposure, which corresponds to the 12 to 3 o'clock position (quadrant IV) a "no-fly zone" for cautery until I have clearly exposed the anatomy and know with certainty the location of the inferior aspect of the lamina. I continue the process of exposing the anatomy that I have already reconstructed in my mind.

My preferred method of exposure is to have a suction device in one hand to gently probe and confirm the presence of bone before ever discharging a pulse of cautery that will expose that bone. After exposure of the first quadrant, I proceed medially to quadrant II (9–12 o'clock). Within this field of view, the junction of the spinous process and the lamina should be clearly seen. Exposure of the base of the spinous process now provides my mind with a visual cue of where the midline resides. I cannot directly see the midline, but I can reconstruct it in my mind by seeing the confluence of the lamina and spinous process. My knowledge of the anatomy tells me that it is only millimeters away. Looking at this exposure gives me a sense of where the traversing root will lie, approximately 12 to 14 mm from the midline and well within my field of view using a 16-mm-diam-

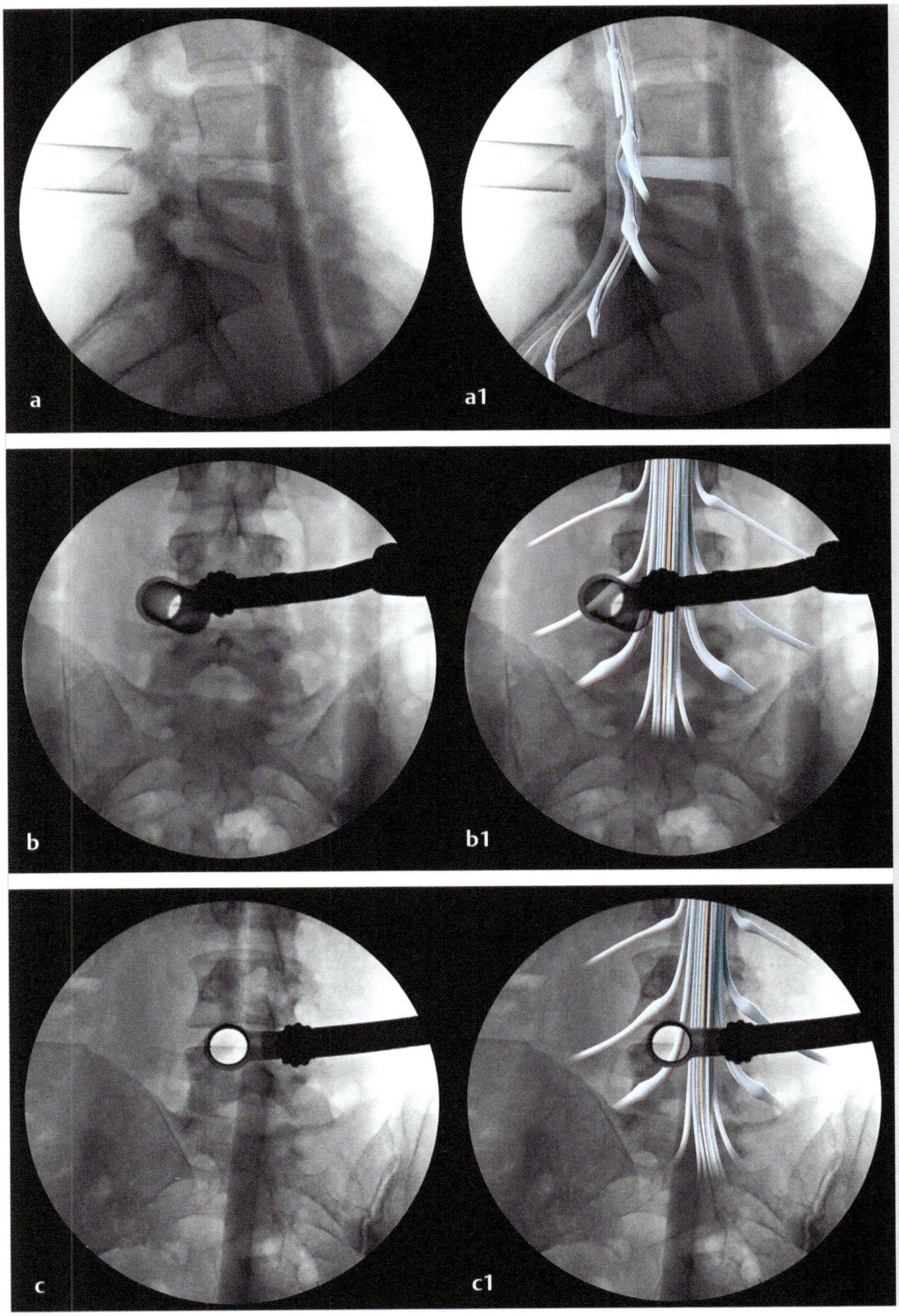

Fig. 2.32 Reconstruction of the anatomy at depth. Lateral, anteroposterior (AP) and oblique paired fluoroscopic images demonstrate the ideal placement of the 16-mm-diameter minimal access port for an L4–5 microdiscectomy, superimposed with the artist's rendition of the neural structures. **(a)** The lateral image demonstrates the access port is parallel to the disc space. **(a1)** Ghosted, superimposed neural structures. The mind should become proficient with reconstructing this view by looking at a fluoroscopic image. **(b)** The AP image demonstrates the access port just medial to the L5 pedicle with **(b1)** the superimposed neural structures shown to demonstrate their position relative to the bony structures. **(c)** The oblique view. **(c1)** Image with the superimposed neural structures demonstrates the traversing nerve root and thecal sac relative to the disc space. This view demonstrates a well-positioned access port over the top of the nerve root and disc space.

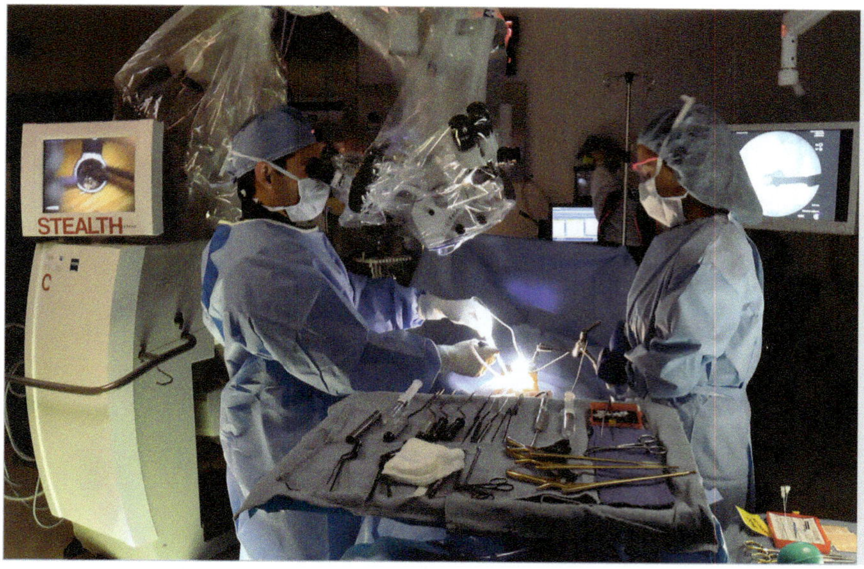

Fig. 2.33 Intraoperative photograph of a microdiscectomy. The scrub technician stands opposite the surgeon with a line of sight to the video feed of the microscope to follow the progress of the surgery and to anticipate the need for instruments. The microscope, which was draped before the incision was made, is positioned behind the surgeon. The fluoroscope has been removed from the field, but the final anteroposterior and lateral images remain available as a reference.

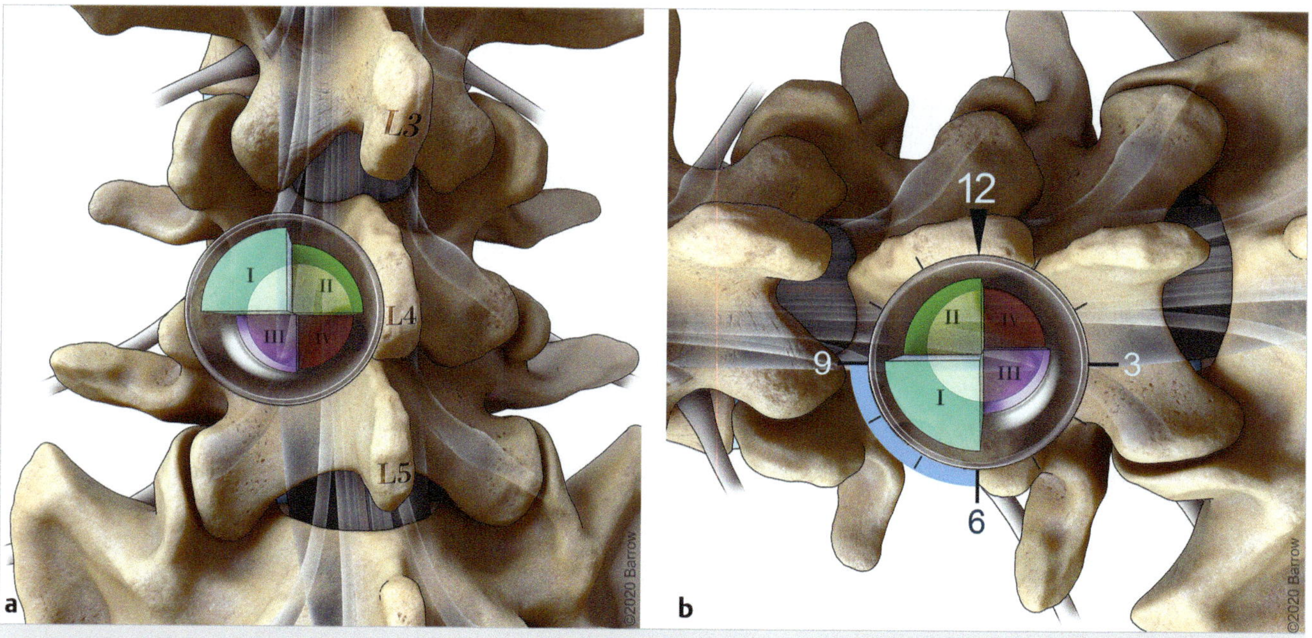

Fig. 2.34 The quadrants of exposure for a minimally invasive microdiscectomy. Illustration demonstrates that exposure begins in the safe zone of quadrant I. With direct visualization of the lamina, you can proceed to quadrant II to obtain the necessary medial exposure. Quadrant III provides access for a foraminotomy, and quadrant IV represents the inferomedial limit of the exposure where the intralaminar space resides. **(a)** Posterior anatomical view. **(b)** Surgical view with surgeon standing on symptomatic side of patient. The clock face is superimposed on the access port for orientation.

eter access port. In my mind's eye, I am viewing ▶ Fig. 2.32c1. From here, I proceed inferolaterally into quadrant III (i.e., the medial facet). The best way to avoid entering the facet capsule or the facet joint with the cautery is by proceeding from medial to lateral.

The goal of this exposure is to visualize all the components of the anatomy that would be seen in an open exposure, specifically the inferior aspect of the rostral lamina, the medial facet and the superior aspect of the caudal lamina. Except for the medial exposure consisting of the entire lateral aspect of the spinous process, there should be no difference between an open and a minimally invasive exposure.

2.9.5 Bone Work

As I begin the bone work, I keep in mind the guiding principle of the microdiscectomy: to remove the least amount of bone that will allow the safe mobilization of the traversing nerve root and thecal sac for removal of the disc herniation. That amount of bone varies slightly for every level (▶ Fig. 2.35). The characteristics of the disc extrusions also play a part in the amount of bone that must be removed. A small extrusion with caudal migration at L5–S1 requires less bone removal than a large central extrusion at L3–4, which is distinct from an L2–3 disc extrusion with rostral migration (▶ Fig. 2.35).

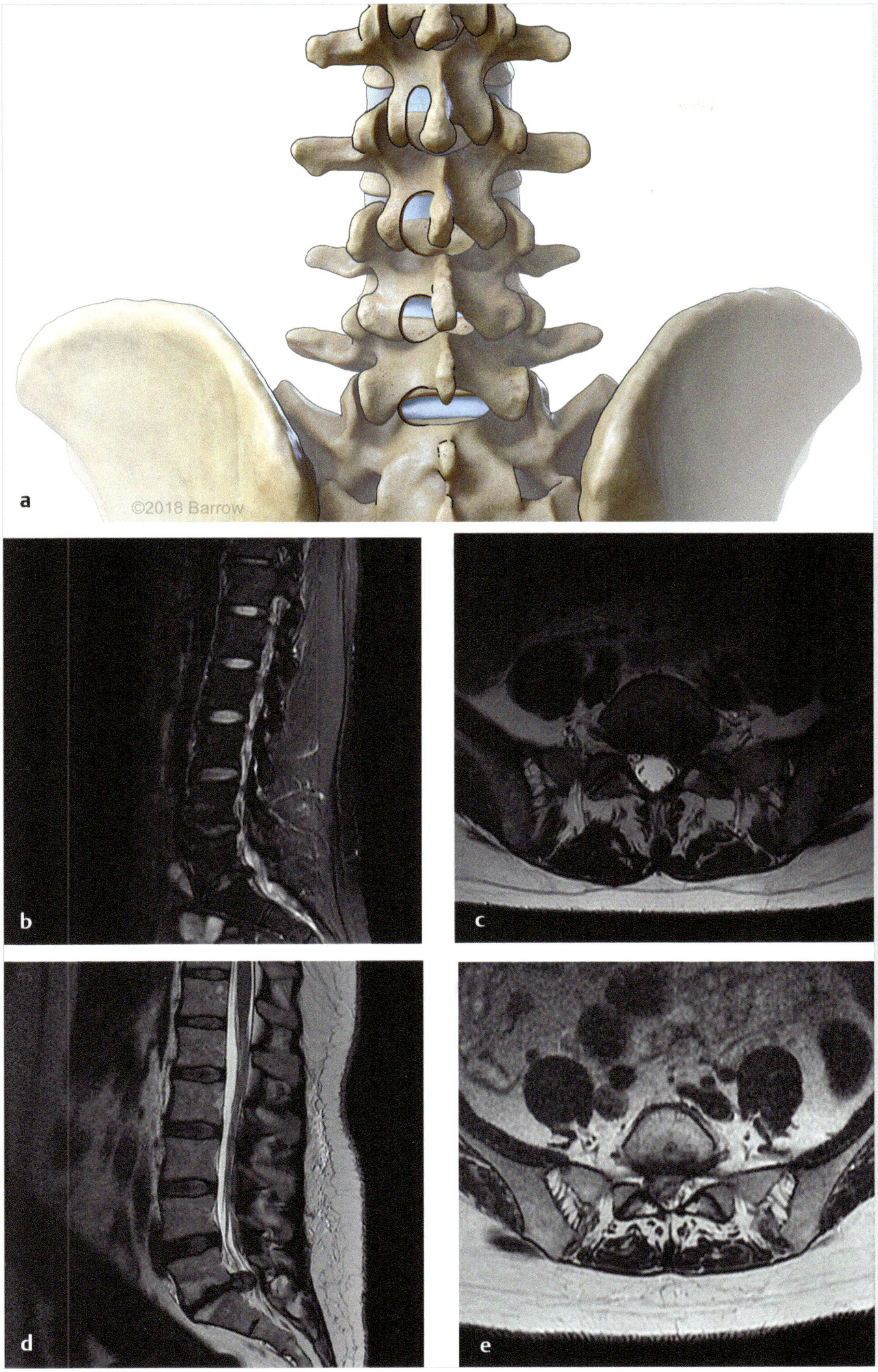

Fig. 2.35 Tailoring the bone work to the level and the size of the disc extrusion. **(a)** Illustration demonstrating the extent of bone work required at each level to access the disc space. At L5–S1 almost no bone work is required, whereas at L2–3 a considerable amount of the lamina must be removed to access the disc space. **(b-e)** Juxtaposition of two different herniations at L5–S1. **(b)** Sagittal T2-weighted magnetic resonance imaging (MRI) of the lumbar spine demonstrating a small focal disc extrusion at L5–S1 causing a left S1 radiculopathy. **(c)** The axial T2-weighted MRI demonstrates a focal disc extrusion. In this case, a small laminotomy with a medial facetectomy will be more than adequate for mobilization of the nerve root and removal of the focal disc extrusion. **(d)** Sagittal T2-weighted MRI of the lumbar spine demonstrating a large disc extrusion causing early cauda equina syndrome. **(e)** Axial T2-weighted MRI of lumbar spine demonstrating the disc extrusion occupying nearly two-thirds of the canal. A generous laminotomy, if not hemilaminectomy would be needed to safely mobilize the neural elements and remove the disc extrusion.

After exposure of the lamina and the medial facet, a small forward-angled curet can help establish the inferior aspect of the rostral lamina and unveil the interlaminar space. With the caudal border of the inferior lamina confirmed, I use a drill with a minimally invasive attachment to complete the laminotomy and medial facetectomy. The amount of bone work is determined by the compression at hand. The larger the disc herniation, the more bone work is typically required to facilitate removal of the herniation with minimal risk of injury to the neural elements. The bone work ranges from a complete hemilaminectomy for large disc herniations that completely obliterate the canal to a small laminotomy for small focal extrusions (▶ Fig. 2.35). Every effort should be made to minimize the extent of the medial facetectomy. However, enough of the medial facet must be removed to safely identify and then mobilize the traversing nerve root. At times, disc herniations may displace the nerve root into the lateral recess to such an extent that an extensive medial facetectomy will be necessary to safely reach the lateral aspect of the traversing nerve root for safe mobilization. I do not try to predict this scenario, but instead, I do the same amount of initial bone work to expose the neural elements. I prefer to remove more bone after assessing the neural elements than to have removed more of the medial facet than necessary to perform the operation.

The level of the disc herniation also affects the amount of bone work. The interlaminar space is greatest at L5–S1, where at times no bone removal is required for access to the nerve root (▶ Fig. 2.35). However, L1–2 and L2–3 have considerably less interlaminar space, prompting a need to remove more bone to safely mobilize the nerve root and retrieve the disc.

2.9.6 Exposure of the Ligamentum Flavum

After I complete the preliminary bone work, the unmistakable yellow carpet of the ligamentum flavum becomes evident. Whatever muscle tissue remains over the top of the interlaminar space can now be swept downward with a large straight curet and resected with a Kerrison rongeur. Doing so expands the amount of the exposed ligament. It also reveals the unmistakable appearance of the lateral aspect of the ligamentum flavum just beneath the facet. A few bites with a Kerrison rongeur to undercut the facet reveal the curvature of the ligamentum flavum as it forms the lateral aspect of the canal. The change from rough to smooth ligamentum represents the lateral aspect of the canal where the ligamentum flavum wraps around the thecal sac. The sublaminar ligamentum flavum has an unmistakably coarse appearance, whereas the subarticular ligamentum flavum has a characteristically smooth appearance. The traversing root is typically accessible at the interface of the sublaminar and subarticular ligamentum flavum. When I see this transition in the ligamentum flavum occur, I refrain from any further bone work for the time being. After this vast expanse of ligamentum flavum can be visualized from just off the midline to the medial facet, the exposure is complete. I may now begin division of the ligamentum flavum and expose the neural elements.

2.9.7 Division and Resection of the Ligamentum Flavum

The complications that I witnessed throughout my residency and have since encountered in my practice have been during this phase of the operation. In my estimation, it is a worthwhile investment of time to be meticulously cautious at this point. It is also surprising that no technique papers I reviewed in the literature describe the details of this component of the procedure. The task at hand is to bluntly divide a thick ligament with a precious and vulnerable water balloon (i.e., the thecal sac) directly on the other side. In some circumstances, that water balloon can be under pressure from a large disc herniation pushing in the direction of the surgeon working directly above it.

There are two approaches to reach the other side of the ligamentum flavum: direct dissection through the ligamentum or release of the ligamentum from its insertion on the underside of the lamina. The latter technique involves reaching outside the exposure, blindly sweeping for the insertion of the ligamentum flavum on the underside of the lamina and then bringing it into the field of view. While I have concerns with reaching outside my direct field of view with any instrument, my main reservation with this technique is that more ligamentum is interrupted than would otherwise be necessary to perform the operation. Instead, the technique that is more in keeping with the minimally invasive principle of disrupting the least amount of anatomy as possible is the direct dissection of the ligamentum immediately over the top of the traversing root. Therefore, I prefer to meticulously dissect the ligamentum through its various layers using a combination of curets and Penfield dissectors.

The ligamentum flavum can be divided into three distinct layers. I sequentially divide the fibers of the ligamentum at each layer to minimize the risk of injury to the contents below. After all, I intend to keep that water balloon directly beneath the ligamentum flavum intact. There are various histologic analyses of the ligamentum flavum in the literature but no formal descriptions of the distinct layers that I will describe in the next few paragraphs.[13] Regardless of whether or not the following description of the three layers of the ligamentum flavum has a histologic basis, they do have a functional basis for safe entry to the canal.

The outer sublaminar layer of the ligamentum flavum is the coarse layer or what I refer to as the *ligamentum flavum crassum*. With some limited downward pressure and using a small straight curet to scrape back and forth, I can readily establish a plane of dissection. Once I have established this plane, I use a No. 2 Kerrison rongeur to remove the remainder of the coarse layer and expose a swath of smooth ligamentum, which I refer to as the *ligamentum flavum levis* or the second layer.

The more lateral you are in the canal, the thicker the ligamentum flavum; and the more medial you are, the thinner the ligamentum flavum (▶ Fig. 2.36). Therefore, after clearing away the coarse layer of ligamentum flavum, I begin to work as medially as possible so that I can traverse the thinnest part of the ligament. With either a straight curet or a fine Penfield dissector, I use broad sweeping motions to divide the fibers of the smooth ligamentum. As the ligament divides, the final layer is revealed. The final layer of the ligament is thin enough to be diaphanous, giving it the whiter appearance of the dura below. Since it is the

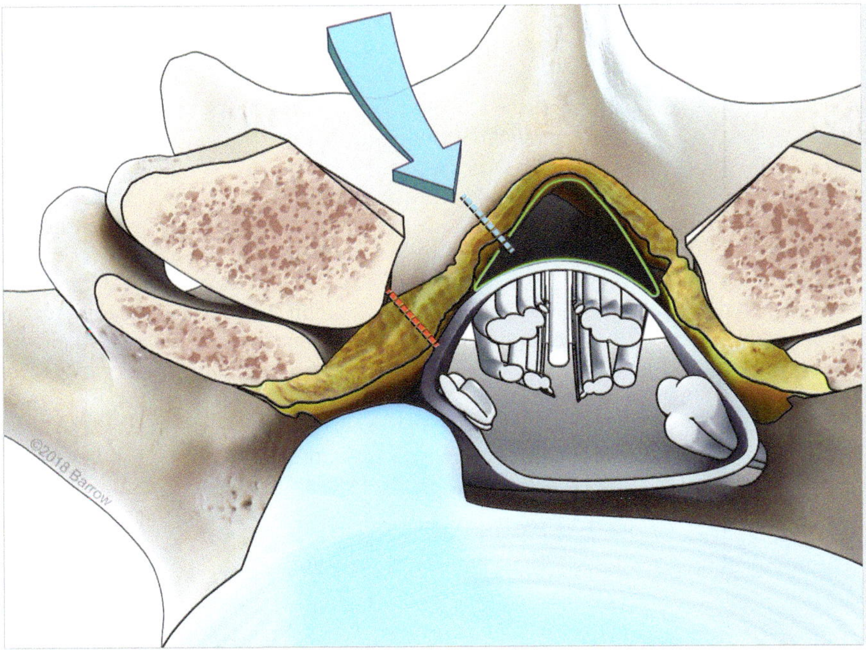

Fig. 2.36 Illustration demonstrates the potential triangular space superior to the thecal sac medially. This area is also where the ligamentum flavum is thinnest. In the lateral recess, the ligamentum flavum is thicker and traversing it places the instrument immediately over the thecal sac. Exposing the neural elements in the triangular space greatly facilitates revision microdiscectomies.

innermost layer, I refer to this final layer as *the ligamentum flavum intima*, the layer most intimately related to the dura. Once I appreciate this distinct layer, I establish a plane superficial to the smooth layer with either a forward-angled curet or a nerve hook. I then clear the exposed surface area with a Kerrison punch to reach the edges of exposed bone. Finally, I carefully divide the last diaphanous layer of ligamentum flavum with a small Penfield dissector, gently sweeping back and forth with a slight amount of downward pressure until the fibers yield and an opening appears. Epidural fat or neural elements or both will quickly come into view through a longitudinal division of the ligament. I now have a safe entry to the canal.

Next, I use a Kerrison rongeur to resect the ligamentum flavum to the perimeter of the bone work. During this resection, it is vital to ensure a clear plane between the underside of the ligament and the dura. Before resecting the remaining ligament, I pass a right-angled ball-tipped probe superficial to the dura, to ensure the safe passage of the footplate of the rongeur. I then resect the ligamentum flavum in all directions to the edge of the bone work. My goal is to resect the ligamentum flavum over the affected nerve root while leaving as much as possible of the ligamentum flavum overlaying the thecal sac.

When the thecal sac comes into clear view, I determine whether I have enough lateral exposure to mobilize the nerve root. With a medium Penfield dissector, I sweep the lateral aspect of the dura and the traversing nerve root medially until I can clearly see the disc space. A clear view of the nerve root and the disc space ensures adequate lateral exposure. I continue to develop the plane between the nerve root and the disc before introducing a suction retractor to hold the nerve root out of harm's way as I begin the disc work.

If I am unable to work lateral to the traversing root, then I have not done an adequate amount of bone work and ligamentum flavum resection. Doing too little is not a problem, for it avoids having done too much at the outset and potentially destabilizing the facet joint. Before I begin drilling again, I place a piece of thrombin-soaked Gelfoam of the size of the bony exposure to ensure coverage of the neural elements. The Gelfoam not only protects the neural elements but also collects the bone debris from the drill. I typically drill out another 2 mm of bone (the thickness of the drill bit) from the medial facet, leaving an edge of bone between the tip of the drill and the lateral recess of the canal. Doing so prevents the tip of the drill from consuming and spinning the Gelfoam. I use a Kerrison rongeur to remove this edge of bone and to further resect the ligamentum flavum. Epidural fat surrounding the traversing root may then become evident, indicating that I have advanced lateral enough with the bone work. I then use the medium Penfield dissector to sweep the thecal sac and nerve root laterally. If I am still unable to get around the thecal sac and nerve root, I will repeat the steps delineated earlier until I can. I do not begin the disc work until I am unequivocally certain of the location of the traversing root. As mentioned previously, a disc herniation may at times displace the nerve root so far out of the lateral recess that an inordinate amount of bone work must be done to reach the lateral edge of the nerve root.

Take your time with this phase of the operation. It is essential to do the necessary bone work to unequivocally identify the lateral edge of the nerve root. In some cases, you may think you have done the necessary bone work for the operation but still cannot mobilize the traversing root. At these times, glancing at the axial MRIs reaffirms the situation in your mind's eye. Time and again, I find myself recognizing subtleties in an MRI, specifically the axial view, only after having completed the exposure. In the end, you should have no doubt about what represents the lateral aspect of the traversing root. The fail-safe method is to palpate the pedicle with a right-angled ball-tipped probe and then sweep the contents of the canal medially.

2.9.8 Disc Removal

Regardless of whether the compressive pathology is a large free fragment of herniated disc or a broad-based contained disc bulge, a systematic approach to the operation ensures adequate decompression of the thecal sac and nerve root. I place the suction retractor in my nondominant hand and pass a medium Penfield dissector in my dominant hand lateral to the nerve root to mobilize it. I then use the Penfield dissector to shoehorn the suction retractor past the nerve root and into position to retract the traversing nerve root. My nondominant hand will be positioned at 12 o'clock (▶ Fig. 2.37). Then, I may begin removing the disc herniation with a pituitary rongeur in my dominant hand. At times, it is necessary to pull up on the nerve root and then retract the root over the disc herniation, lest you retract the disc herniation along with the nerve root. Retracting the disc herniation with the nerve root, which I have done, can obviously make the disc herniation very difficult to find. The large extruded fragment that you saw only moments ago on the MRI now lays hidden behind the suction retractor and the nerve root well outside your line of sight and reach (▶ Fig. 2.38). You can stare in complete astonishment at the field of view for quite some time if you do not recognize the true nature of the situation. Thoughts begin to enter your mind about whether you have exposed the correct level. Perhaps you will begin speculating that the disc has resorbed and there is nothing causing compression of the nerve root. To avoid such thoughts, astonishment, and speculation, you must recognize the possibility of retracting an extruded fragment along with the nerve root. Employing a small right-angled nerve hook to establish and develop a plane between the disc and the nerve root is the first essential step. If the nerve root is tethered and I am unable to retract it to visualize the disc, meticulous dissection of the nerve root–disc interface allows safe mobilization of the nerve root and provides the necessary exposure.

After the retrieval of a large free fragment of disc, the operation is over almost as soon as the nerve is retracted. I use a right-angled ball-tipped probe to free the disc fragment, which I then remove with a straight micropituitary rongeur. Typically, a satisfyingly large fragment of disc makes its way out within the pincers of the pituitary rongeur, and the thecal sac and nerve root fall cleanly back into their anatomical positions. Retracting the root once more to explore the annulotomy created by the disc herniation enables me to check for other free fragments of disc material. It is also helpful to explore the axilla of the nerve root and to sweep a right-angled nerve hook behind the thecal sac to clear away any other fragments that have migrated into these areas. I ask the scrub technician to collect all the disc material that I remove and place the pieces on a small sheet of Telfa (Medtronic, plc) so that I can assess the volume of the disc removed and compare it to the MRI. Doing so allows me to determine whether I have removed an adequate amount of disc material.

When the disc herniation is a broad-based disc bulge without a focal or distinct disc herniation that remains contained within the annulus, it is more of a segmental degenerative entity than an isolated disc herniation. The disc complex has begun to fail. In my experience, adequately decompressing the traversing root and thecal sac requires the removal of a larger segment of disc. In these circumstances, I mobilize the nerve root medially and then use a No. 11 blade on a bayoneted handle to make a linear incision into the disc space. In a tall disc space, I make a vertical incision in the annulus. In a collapsed disc space, a horizontal incision is the only feasible manner to enter the disc space. I try to keep this annulotomy as lateral as possible so that if reherniation should occur, the disc material will extrude laterally and may not compress the thecal sac or nerve root. I then pass a reverse-angled Epstein curet into the annulotomy and push the disc protrusion down into the disc space away from the thecal sac and traversing nerve root. A few downward strokes make the disc herniation ready for retrieval with a pituitary rongeur. Simultaneous downward pressure on the suction retractor helps deliver the disc material. I pass a right-angled ball-tipped probe into the annulotomy defect to probe for loose fragments of disc material. I also pass the right-angled ball-tipped probe beneath the thecal sac and over the top of the annulus to ensure that disc material has not migrated into these areas. Downward pressure atop the annulus dislodges subannular disc material that can then be retrieved with a pituitary rongeur. Once again, I collect the disc material, assess its volume, and compare it to what I might expect on the basis of the MRI. Any discrepancy in the expected volume of disc material will prompt me to continue exploring the disc space (Video 2.1).

2.9.9 Final Systems Check

When I believe that I have completed the operation, I zoom out with the microscope and take another look at the fluoroscopic image, the preoperative MRI and the collection of excised disc material. I then begin the final systems check before removing the access port and closing the incision. Over the years, I have recognized the tunnel vision that invariably arises from intensely focusing on a disc herniation at high magnification through the operating microscope. At the end of the case, it is crucial to step away, leave the tunnel, and view the entire landscape of the operative field once again. Viewing the operative field through low magnification allows me to reengage with a curious mind to assess my work. The final systems check keeps every operation as standardized as possible. I am always surprised when a hidden clump of disc appears that I may have left behind had I not pulled back, taken a deep breath and reassessed the operative field.

The final check ensures an adequate decompression of the thecal sac and nerve root and elimination of the hiding places where disc material can migrate. The main instrument that I use for the final systems check is the bayoneted right-angled ball-tipped probe. That instrument is ideal for providing the tactile feedback the surgeon requires to assess the surgical corridors. I also continue to use the suction retractor in my nondominant hand as I slip the probe lateral to the traversing root. I shoehorn the suction retractor into position to retract the nerve root. Then, I use the probe to pass lateral to the nerve root and curiously explore the lateral recess for any residual disc. The probe should pass freely through this corridor. Any resistance should prompt concern and further exploration. Rotating the probe clockwise or counterclockwise (depending on the side of the patient I am operating on) allows its tip to encounter the pedicle. Palpating the pedicle completes the first element of the systems check.

A quick review of the axial and sagittal MRIs helps guide this final review. For instance, if the axial MRI demonstrates caudal migration of the disc herniation against the pedicle, then more attention should be focused on this region. The rotation of the probe may mobilize a wayward fragment of disc which then comes into view and becomes accessible to the pincers of the pituitary rongeur. At the same time, this same motion may also interrupt the veins of the pedicle and cause considerable bleeding, which can be addressed using right-angled bipolar forceps,

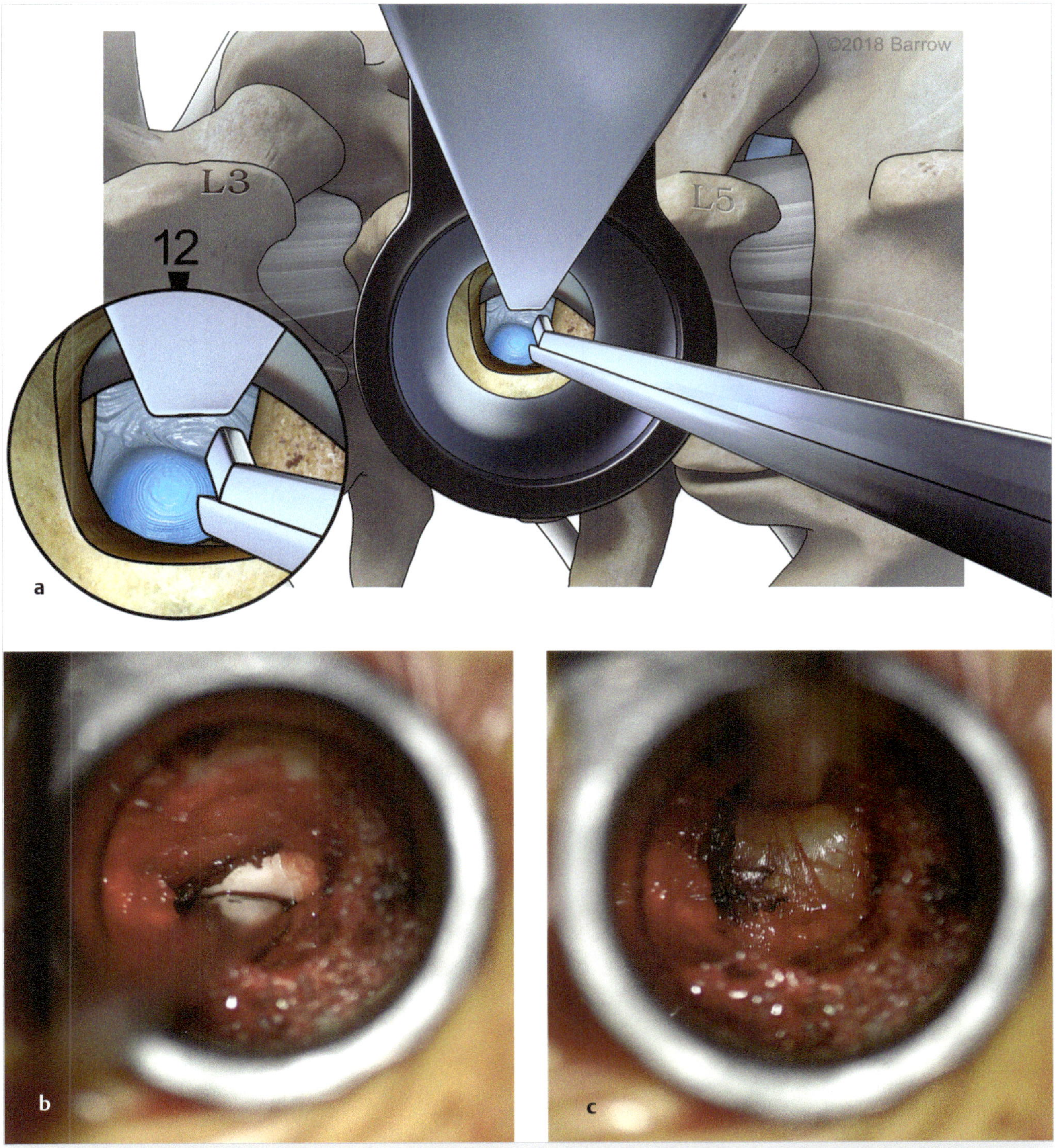

Fig. 2.37 L4–5 minimally invasive microdiscectomy, left sided. **(a)** Illustration demonstrates the surgical view of an L4–5 left-sided minimally invasive microdiscectomy performed through a 16-mm-diameter access port. In this illustration, the bone work has been completed with removal of the medial facet to the extent necessary to allow for safe mobilization of the nerve root. The ligamentum flavum has been divided and resected to allow visualization of the lateral aspect of the thecal sac and the lateral aspect of the nerve root. A suction retractor is placed in the 12 o'clock position (inset), and the nerve root is retracted. With the nerve root retracted, the disc herniation now comes clearly into view and can be removed with a pituitary rongeur. **(b)** Intraoperative photograph demonstrating the ligamentum flavum resected only over the top of the nerve root. The lateral aspect of the nerve root has been identified and a suction retractor is in position for retraction. **(c)** Retraction of the left L5 nerve root revealing the disc herniation.

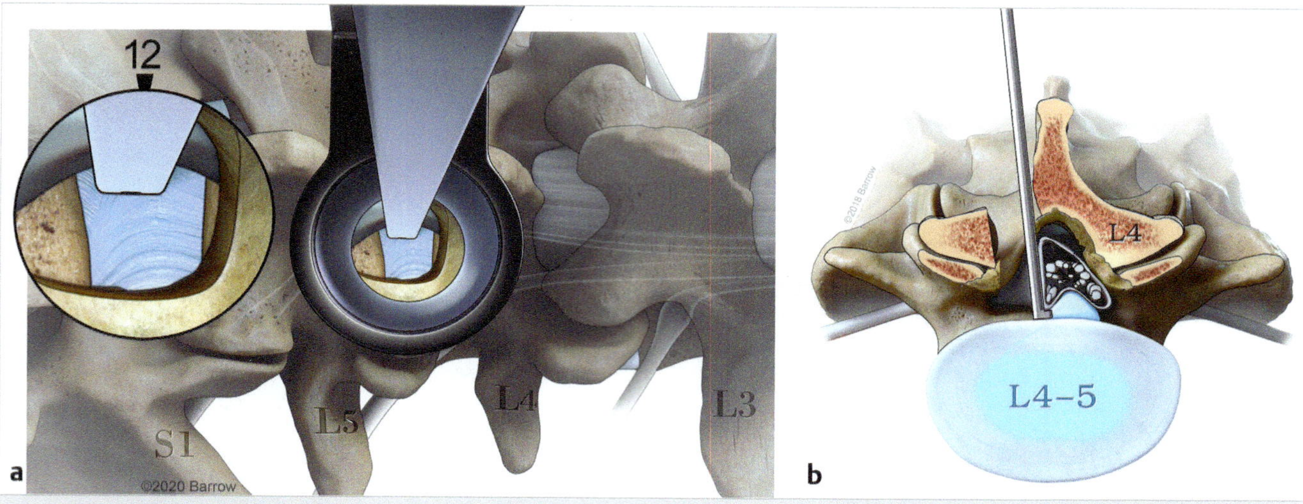

Fig. 2.38 Illustration of a right-sided L4–5 microdiscectomy with the traversing nerve root and thecal sac retracted. **(a)** Surgical view of the minimal access port in position. The view through the port under the operating microscope reveals no disc extrusion. **(b)** The axial view reveals why the disc extrusion cannot be identified. As the nerve root was retracted, the disc material was carried along with it. A right-angled ball-tipped probe placed into the field without the suction retractor will encounter stiff resistance. Without dissecting a plane between the nerve root and the disc extrusion and then retracting the nerve up and over the disc extrusion, the disc material will lay hidden. Using a combination of a right-angled nerve hook and a right-angled ball tipped probe to accomplish the task of separating the nerve root from the disc extrusion will allow for separation of the nerve root from the disc extrusion. Pulling the nerve root upwards with the suction retractor will now unveil the disc extrusion and make it ripe for retrieval.

Floseal Hemostatic Matrix (Baxter Healthcare Corp.) and a half-by-half cottonoid. After the corridor has been explored and the bleeding has been contained, there is no reason to venture farther into the lateral recess.

Once I am satisfied with the decompression of the lateral recess, I ensure that there is nothing in the midline to cause central stenosis or compression of the shoulder of the nerve root. I slide the ball-tipped probe behind the dura and gently lift and retract it to reveal whether any disc material has been retracted along with the thecal sac. I have encountered some circumstances where the large disc extrusion I was searching for eluded me until this final systems check. In one case, I distinctly remember gazing at the MRI and clearly seeing a large free fragment of disc severely compressing the thecal sac and traversing root. However, as I studied the disc material resting on the Telfa, I saw nothing but tiny fragments of the size of a grain of rice. I went to review the date of the MRI and began to wonder whether the disc had resorbed. Then, I wondered whether the decompression was inadequate. The reality was that I had been retracting the thecal sac along with the central disc herniation while performing the discectomy as illustrated in ▶ Fig. 2.38. When I passed the right-angled ball-tipped probe beneath the thecal sac, I encountered stiff resistance. I then worked the probe above the disc space and behind the thecal sac. Rotating the probe revealed a disc herniation that was as large, if not larger, than what was demonstrated on the MRI. Such cases underscore the importance of being able to pass the ball-tipped probe posterior to the thecal sac up and down the span of the disc space. The systems check is the final element of the operation. After completing it, I irrigate the surgical site and begin the closure.

2.9.10 Closure

With the microscope still in position, I place the bipolar cautery in one hand and hold the stem of the minimal access port in the other. My assistant or the surgical scrub technician holds the suction over the top of the minimal access port to draw off the smoke created by the cautery. I slowly pull out the access port, cauterizing any bleeding in the muscle. At times, I will encounter a vein that the access port was able to tamponade when it was in position, but that begins to bleed as I remove the port. Bleeding may occur with variable degrees of intensity, requiring a suction in one hand and the cautery or a bipolar forceps in the other hand. Once I have controlled the bleeding, I irrigate the incision to flush away any blood that may have made its way down to the nerve root. Minimizing the blood by the nerve root will decrease the inflammatory reaction caused by the breakdown of blood products during recovery. Under ideal circumstances, I like to see the whiteness of the nerve root and the thecal sac as I remove the access port and cauterize any superficial bleeding.

I again infiltrate the muscle layer and the subcutaneous layer with a lidocaine–epinephrine–bupivacaine mixture to minimize postoperative discomfort. My goal is for the patient to not be able to feel the incision for the first 8 to 12 hours after the operation. I close the fascia with a zero Vicryl (Ethicon, Inc.) suture on a UR6 needle, the subcutaneous layer with 2.0 Vicryl on an X-1 needle, and the skin edges with 4.0 Vicryl on an RB-1 needle, if necessary.

The design of the UR-6 needle allows for rotation within narrow corridors. Designed for the closure of laparoscopic incisions, the UR-6 is configured in a 5/8-inch circle, which is ideal for working deep within small incisions and grabbing either side of the fascia. I routinely use the UR-6 to close the fascia in all minimally invasive approaches. The X-1 needle has a half-circle configuration that facilitates rotating the needle in the subcutaneous tissue. Finally, I apply benzoin or Mastisol Liquid Adhesive (Ferndale Laboratories, Inc.) to the surrounding skin, and I apply half-inch Steri-Strips (3M) over the incision. A piece of Telfa covers the Steri-Strips, and a lidocaine 5% patch covers the entire incision. The operating room team places the patient in the supine position, signaling the completion of the minimally invasive microdiscectomy.

2.10 Operative Time

In a report on 530 consecutive microdiscectomies, Williams[9] reported a mean operative time of 37 minutes. Such a concise operative time reflects a surgeon at the acme of their skill. The surgeon achieves such an operative time only with certainty about the anatomy, comfort with the exposure, years of experience and an efficient operating room team. However, an operative time of less than 40 minutes is not a standard to which you should hold yourself from the outset. No operation should ever be rushed to completion. How much time it takes to conduct a procedure is never as important as the complete achievement of the goals of the operation itself. I would prefer a 1-hour procedure with complete decompression and alleviation of symptoms to a 30-minute procedure with incomplete decompression and persistent symptoms. Nevertheless, there is value in a shorter duration of procedure for the patient and the clinical outcomes; so, it is worthwhile to monitor procedure time as you progress through your learning curve. The advantage of the minimally invasive approach is the capacity to begin operating under the microscope almost immediately after making the incision. If the operation was divided into three phases, the first phase of the operation, which includes the incision and docking the minimal access port, is going to be the fastest. The first phase can take as little as 5 minutes after making the incision. For this reason, the microscope should be draped and ready, the fluoroscope should be in position, and the table-mounted arm should be on standby. A well-trained operating room staff is an essential component of accomplishing such efficiency. The second phase under the microscope is where most of the operating time (roughly 30–45 minutes) is spent. The final phase of closure can require as little as 5 minutes. These time approximations assume ideal placement of the minimal access port, which is seldom perfect in the first few procedures. Over time, however, your operating times will trend toward these approximations. You will be able to tell your patients that the operation can be safely completed in 45 to 60 minutes. I have performed operations that required as little as 36 minutes and others that have taken as long as 122 minutes. The overall goal is effective efficiency in accomplishing the operation step by step, not rushing through the procedure for the sake of time.

2.11 Postoperative Management

I perform most lumbar microdiscectomies as an outpatient procedure. Thus, infiltration of local anesthetic before closure is of great value for same-day discharge. After a period of observation in the recovery room, patients are typically discharged home 60 to 90 minutes after surgery. For pain control, all discharged patients are prescribed a muscle relaxant, an acetaminophen–narcotic combination, and a methylprednisolone dose pack based on the historic experience in the literature.[14] I encourage all patients to ambulate every day, restrict them from carrying anything heavier than 5 pounds, and ask them to limit any bending or twisting at the waist for 1 month. Patients begin physical therapy at 1 month postoperatively but should refrain from impact training for another 2 months. At 3 months, patients can return to unrestricted activity.

2.12 Revision Microdiscectomies

I have intentionally separated the final part of this chapter into a different section for what I believe to be a completely distinct operation. I approach minimally invasive revision microdiscectomies with an entirely different mindset and a different technique. Whether conducted as a minimally invasive or open procedure, the revision microdiscectomy is more challenging, with a greater risk to the nerve root and a greater risk of cerebrospinal fluid (CSF) leak. These operations require patience and even more thoughtful analysis of the anatomy as the surgery proceeds. Scar tissue may resemble nerve root, and nerve root may resemble scar tissue. I never hesitate to tell the residents and fellows who operate with me that two of the top-three most difficult cases I have ever performed were revision microdiscectomies.

Minimally invasive revision microdiscectomies should be undertaken only after acquiring facility with de novo minimally invasive microdiscectomies. This operation is not an operation I would advise taking on early in your minimally invasive surgical career. When I began performing revision procedures, I started by revising my own microdiscectomies. These patients are ideal candidates early on because of your familiarity with the bone work that was done. As my experience grew, I began to revise all reherniations using a minimally invasive technique. I found several advantages to revising reherniations that were initially managed with a midline approach. The first is that it avoided opening a previous incision and working through the scar. Instead, I found myself traversing a virgin plane to the spine. The second was that I was able to safely approach the laminotomy defect, docking firmly on bone and proceeding laterally to medially. My initial concern was whether a second incision lateral to the initial midline incision would prove problematic in healing, but over the years, a problem from that second incision off the midline has never materialized. If anything, patients are often pleased with the size of their revision incision, which they readily compare to their initial surgery incision.

Revising a previous minimally invasive microdiscectomy does not provide a virgin plane of dissection. Thus, these procedures can be potentially challenging because of having to navigate the scar and dock onto the spine. Their main advantage is that they allow the use of the same small incision.

2.12.1 Planning the Incision

Whether the previous operation was performed through a midline microdiscectomy or a minimally invasive microdiscectomy, a patient with a recurrent disc herniation is a candidate for a minimally invasive revision. Even if I was the surgeon who performed the initial procedure, I spend a great deal of time before the operation studying the MRIs, especially the axial T1-weighted view, so that I can review the amount of bone work that was done as part of the laminotomy and medial facetectomy. There is obviously no difference in the positioning of the patient or in the operating room setup. The key difference and the greatest risk of the procedure are with dilatation and docking of the minimal access port, both of which can be safely performed in a systematic fashion.

For the patient with a previous midline incision, I plan the new incision independent of the previous midline incision. For whatever reason, a previous midline incision and a proposed minimally invasive incision seldom coincide. Open incisions often tend to be lower than the optimal minimally invasive trajectory. As with a de novo microdiscectomy, I will palpate the bony landmarks and approximate the level. I measure a distance 1.5 cm from the midline and mark the area for a 20-mm incision. In patients who have had a previous minimally invasive microdiscectomy, I mark the previous incision but still confirm it with a lateral image and a spinal needle, especially if years have passed since the initial operation. The incision itself can be equally deceiving. If the previous surgery was conducted only months earlier, I am more confident that the incision is on the mark.

After the patient is prepped and draped, I pass a spinal needle only one-half the distance to the spine, even with a lateral trajectory, because of the laminotomy defect. Doing so reduces the likelihood of an inadvertent lumbar puncture. My goal is only to confirm the operative level and establish the ideal trajectory, not to dock the spinal needle onto the spine. Once I have confirmed the level with the needle halfway to the spine, I will adjust it for an optimal trajectory or, if it is in an ideal position, I will infiltrate it with the local anesthetic mixture. I re-mark the site for the incision and begin the revision.

2.12.2 Docking the Minimal Access Port

For all revision microdiscectomies, I use an 18-mm-diameter access port, which reliably encompasses the previous laminotomy defect and untouched lamina. Unlike the target in a de novo minimally invasive microdiscectomy, my target is away from the interlaminar space and closer to the pars interarticularis, where I have confirmed the presence of bone on the axial T1-weighted MRIs. At the forefront of my mind when docking the access port for a revision microdiscectomy is the risk of passing one of the early dilators into the canal through the laminotomy defect. After all, that laminotomy defect is already present from the initial operation. For this reason, the target of the first dilator is different for a revision microdiscectomy.

After making the incision and opening the fascia, I pass the first dilator with the intent of docking much higher on the spine than I otherwise would in a de novo microdiscectomy. At first, my target is intentionally high, specifically at the junction of the lamina and the pars interarticularis (▶ Fig. 2.39). Once I contact the bone with the initial dilator, I will wand my way through any scar tissue and then dock the first dilator firmly onto the pars interarticularis. I confirm the position of the dilator with fluoroscopy. Herein lies another key difference between a de novo minimally invasive microdiscectomy and a revision microdiscectomy. In the case of the former, the initial trajectory of the first dilator will be the position and trajectory for the whole operation, and subsequent dilators will act only to increase the diameter of the working channel over that position. In the case of the latter, the initial trajectory onto the pars interarticularis merely offers a safe passage onto an area of the spine where bone is unequivocally present. Establishing that solid footing is the first and perhaps the most essential step in minimally invasive revisions. Each subsequent dilator acts to safely close in on the trajectory that will be used for the operation. So, while the first dilator is high and lateral relative to the disc space, I wand each subsequent dilator more inferiorly and

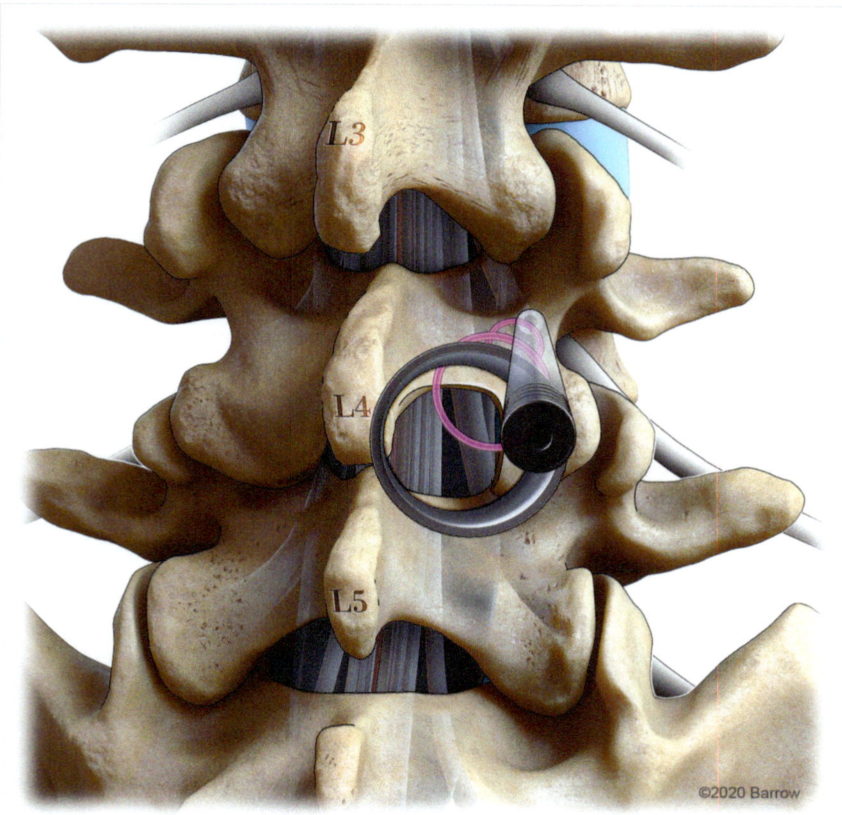

Fig. 2.39 Illustration demonstrates sequential positioning of dilators for a revision microdiscectomy. Posterior view of the lumbar spine shows the sequence in which the dilators are secured to the lumbar spine to minimize the risk of translaminar passage. The beginning dilator docks safely onto the pars interarticularis–laminar junction. With each increasing diameter size, the limits of the previous bone work become encompassed by the final diameter of dilator.

more medially, thereby closing in on the previous laminotomy defect. As the diameter of each dilator increases, the risk of translaminar passage decreases. By the time I reach my last dilator, I will be completely parallel to the disc space and converging medially. I will confirm the trajectory with anteroposterior and lateral fluoroscopic images before bringing in the microscope (▶ Fig. 2.39).

2.12.3 Exposure

The scar tissue from the previous surgery will preclude a clean plane onto the spine. As with a de novo case, I begin my dissection in the safe zone, which is rostral and lateral. Before applying cautery, I curiously but cautiously prod the area that I intend to expose with a suction device to determine whether bone resides underneath it. The higher and more lateral I go, the more confident I become that lamina is present below. I begin to use cautery to sweep away the scar tissue. My primary objective is to expose the perimeter of the bone work previously performed in the initial operation. Upon completion of this task, I should be able to visualize the entire edge of bone with the scar in the middle.

My secondary objective is to identify the virgin anatomy above and below the previous surgical site. To accomplish this, I need to enlarge the laminotomy defect by about 25% (▶ Fig. 2.40). The focus of this increase should be at the rostral and caudal poles. Equally important is my focus on removing the least amount of bone possible from the medial facet to prevent destabilization of the segment. I routinely begin drilling the lamina immediately above the previous laminotomy defect. My focus is equal parts of rostral and medial until I have exposed a small swath of untouched and previously unexposed ligamentum flavum. I then divide the ligament in the manner described in Section 2.9.6, Exposure of the Ligamentum Flavum, and Section 2.9.7, Division and Resection of the Ligamentum Flavum, above to expose the thecal sac. I resect the ligament until I reach the scar and then stop there. I have never found any value in tangling directly with the scar. I ensure that I have exposure lateral to the thecal sac above the scar tissue.

The next step is the caudal exposure. I generously expose the lamina of the caudal level, again sweeping away the scar tissue until I can visualize the unmistakable ivory whiteness of the bone. I drill this bone down to the insertion of the ligamentum flavum. A small forward-angled curet will safely cleave a plane superior to the thecal sac and nerve root just beneath the lamina. Once I have established this plane, I use a No. 2 Kerrison rongeur to complete the removal of bone and ligament, typically revealing the epidural fat from the lateral recess. Minimal dissection using a Penfield dissector and applying some light suction to the epidural fat allows the unveiling of the nerve or the thecal sac. With these neural elements in plain sight, I can identify the pedicle of the traversing nerve root with a right-angled ball-tipped probe. When I am unequivocally convinced that I have palpated the medial aspect of the pedicle, I will have almost secured a perimeter around the nerve root and the disc herniation. What remains is only the scar over the medial facet.

2.12.4 Medial Facetectomy

At this point in the operation, the thecal sac is exposed above the scar tissue of the previous surgery and the thecal sac and

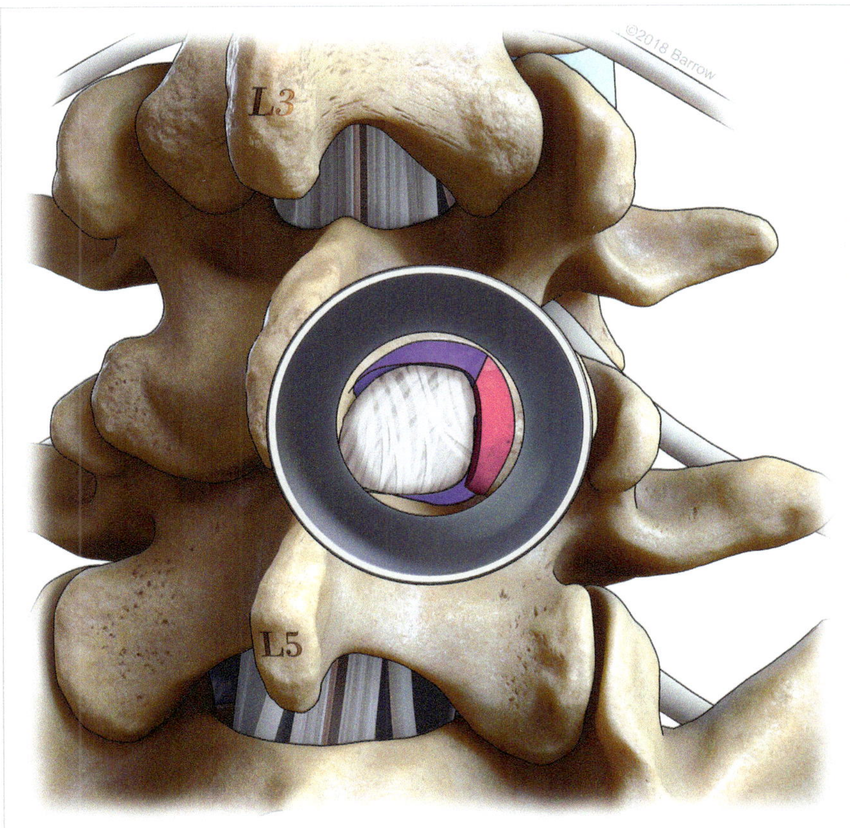

Fig. 2.40 Illustration demonstrates the extension of bone work for revision microdiscectomy through an 18-mm-diameter access port. The first step in a revision minimally invasive microdiscectomy is exposure of the boundaries of the previous bone work. The second step is extension of the laminotomy above and below (*purple shading*) so that the nerve root and thecal sac may be exposed without directly working within the scar tissue (*white shading*). Every effort must be taken to avoid direct dissection through the scar. Once the thecal sac becomes evident with extension of the rostral laminotomy and the nerve root becomes evident with the caudal laminotomy, the medial facet is drilled until virgin ligamentum flavum becomes evident (*magenta shading*). In this manner, access to the disc lateral to the nerve root becomes feasible.

nerve root are exposed below the scar tissue. I now palpate the pedicle and sweep all contents medially. However, I have not yet exposed the disc space or the area where the disc is compressing the nerve root. The final phase of the exposure—extension of the medial facetectomy—will allow me to safely perform the operation. I make every attempt to minimize the amount of bone I remove from the medial facet. At the same time, I balance this conservative approach with the need to obtain the necessary exposure to safely decompress the nerve.

I begin from the caudal aspect of the exposure, where I can see the nerve root, and I then work rostrally to where the scar envelops and conceals the nerve root. With the traversing nerve root in view at the caudal aspect of the exposure, I use a forward-angled curet to mobilize the scar tissue adherent to the medial facet. That particular area is where the medial facetectomy was performed during the initial operation. After I establish this plane, I assess whether a Kerrison rongeur will allow for extension of the bone work or whether additional drilling is required first. The key element to this component of the procedure is to ensure an adequate exposure between the bone and the scar before using the Kerrison rongeur. The goal is to expose the lateral edge of the ligamentum flavum that was resected during the initial operation. Whether it is accomplished with a drill or a Kerrison rongeur, the exposure of virgin ligamentum flavum laterally beneath the extended medial facetectomy signals that I can safely begin the discectomy.

2.12.5 Microdiscectomy

When I have exposed the ligamentum flavum lateral to previous medial facet, the procedure becomes a matter of connecting the exposures. I always attempt to stay lateral to the scar tissue as I proceed with the dissection. The goal is to safely mobilize the nerve root, which remains enveloped within the scar tissue from the initial procedure, and to expose the lateral aspect of the disc. I work above and below the scar tissue until I can mobilize the traversing nerve root within the scar tissue over the disc space. It is tremendously helpful to be able to directly visualize the traversing root in the caudal exposure while conducting this dissection. In my mind's eye, I can envision the path of the nerve root by looking simultaneously at the exposures of the nerve root below the scar and the thecal sac above it. I work lateral to the path of the nerve root with either a right-angled ball-tipped probe or a Penfield dissector. I palpate the pedicle and sweep the contents medially to develop a plane lateral to the root. I can then work above the root both within the rostral exposure and lateral to the thecal sac. Working back and forth between the two exposures eventually mobilizes the traversing root adequately to provide access to the disc space. Unlike in a de novo microdiscectomy, in which I look for the lateral aspect of the traversing root to mobilize it, in a revision microdiscectomy, I am trying to identify the disc space lateral to the previous annulotomy defect. That lateral exposure allows me to enter the disc space without first identifying and retracting the nerve root.

We are all familiar with the unmistakable white sheen of the disc space once it is amply exposed. A revision microdiscectomy makes this exposure more challenging. When I feel as if I am on the lateral aspect of the disc space but that unmistakable sheen has eluded me, I will use a micro-cottonoid (quarter-by-quarter inch) with a bayonet or a Penfield dissector as I would use a Kittner dissector in the cervical spine to expose the precervical fascia. Bluntly sweeping the cottonoid up against the disc space helps mobilize the scar and the traversing root over the disc. On occasion, this action alone begins to deliver the disc material, enabling the safe decompression of the nerve root. Most of the time, I have found it necessary to incise the disc space in the lateral aspect of the exposure. In my estimation, doing so is the most perilous part of a revision microdiscectomy. Before applying a No. 11 blade to the disc, I reassess the exposure and the anatomy. I examine what I perceive to be the disc space, I palpate the pedicle and I envision the course of the traversing root. If I have any concerns, then I refrain from plunging into an uncertain disc space and instead expose more laterally into virgin anatomy until the disc space becomes obvious.

A lateral entry into the disc allows for a safe corridor past the nerve root but does not allow for exposure of the nerve root–disc interface (▶ Fig. 2.41). Thus, I make a conscientious effort to work beneath the scar-shrouded nerve root to mobilize the disc material causing the nerve root compression. The extent of visibility of the anatomy varies widely from patient to patient. At times, I am genuinely surprised at how well the thecal sac and traversing nerve and disc can be visualized, whereas at other times, I despair at the obscurity of the anatomy. However, adhering to the anatomical landmarks, specifically the pedicle, is the surest way to avoid complications and successfully decompress the nerve root.

2.13 Complication Avoidance

To paraphrase the words of Benjamin Franklin, an ounce of prevention is worth the weight of the surgeon. Whether you are performing a minimally invasive or a traditional midline microdiscectomy, you must take every measure possible to prevent the complication of a CSF leak. The thecal sac is most vulnerable to inadvertent disruption in two phases of the operation. The first phase is during division of the ligamentum flavum, and the second is during mobilization of the nerve root. I cannot overemphasize the importance of dividing the ligamentum flavum as medially as the exposure will allow. The ligament is considerably thinner in this area, and it is therefore easier to traverse than in a lateral exposure. Furthermore, because the configuration of the thecal sac within the canal is essentially a circle within a triangle, a potential space above the dura exists where an instrument can safely enter without contacting the thecal sac (▶ Fig. 2.40). A medial opening in the ligamentum flavum is an especially valuable technique in a revision microdiscectomy because every effort should be made to avoid epidural scarring.

Completing the division of the ligamentum flavum without difficulty, however, does not offer an immediate safe harbor. It is always essential to ensure a free plane of passage for an instrument between the underside of the ligamentum flavum and the thecal sac, which is especially true for recurrent disc herniations. Forward-angled curets, right-angled ball-tipped probes and right-angled nerve hooks are all reliable instruments to sweep within the plane between the ligamentum flavum and the thecal sac to confirm safe passage of a Kerrison rongeur before taking a bite. The dura may adhere to the ligamentum flavum in patients who have had a number of epidural injections. In this circumstance, the right-angled ball-tipped

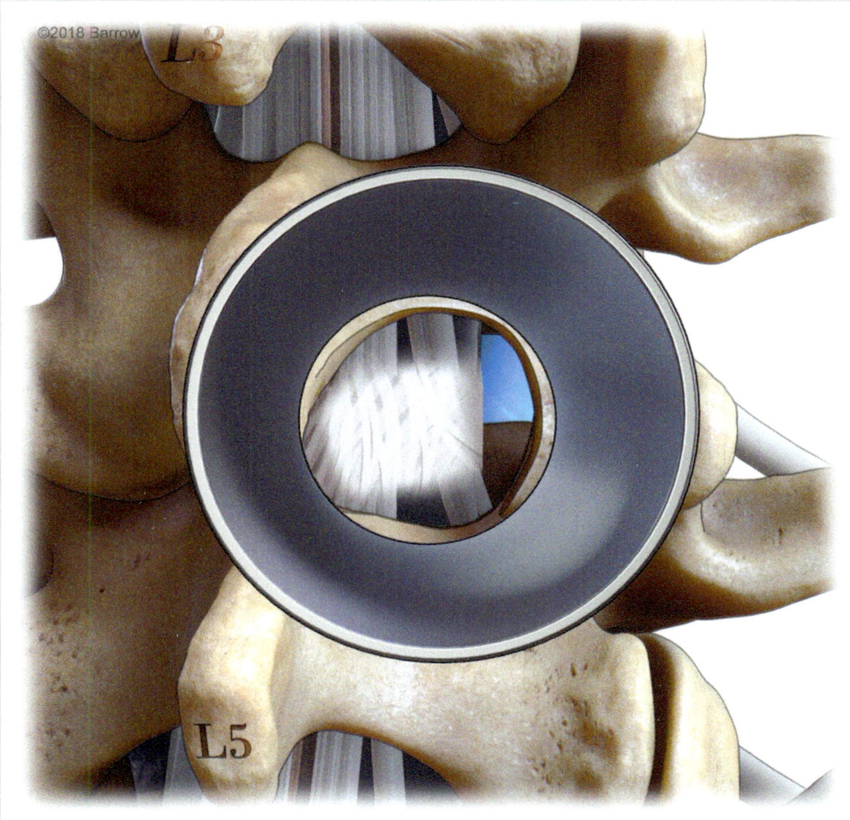

Fig. 2.41 Illustration demonstrates the exposure for a revision microdiscectomy. With the bone work extended and the nerve root and thecal sac identified in virgin planes, the disc space is accessed lateral to the line drawn between the newly exposed lateral thecal sac and the traversing root. The pedicle is also a valuable landmark in revision microdiscectomies. Entry into the disc space lateral to the nerve root is the safest corridor to begin the decompression when the nerve root is shrouded by scar tissue.

probe is my preferred instrument. If the dura moves in line with the instrument as I attempt to pass it beneath the ligamentum flavum, then further dissection with a nerve hook or a forward-angled curet will mitigate interruption of the dura.

2.14 Repair of Cerebrospinal Fluid Leaks

As mentioned in the beginning of this chapter, I have caused an inadvertent puncture of the dura with a spinal needle during the localization phase because of a medial trajectory, and I will never forget it. After taking down the ligamentum flavum, I noticed the unmistakable egress of CSF. The sight of clear fluid trickling into the field paralyzed me the first time I saw it. I quickly found the source, which was a puncture of the dura with a 20-gauge needle. The most important step to take when a CSF leak occurs, regardless of its source, is to focus on the primary objective, which is to decompress the nerve root by removing the disc herniation. Place a piece of Gelfoam and a half-by-half cottonoid over the puncture site to tamponade the leak, and then focus your attention on completing the decompression. Of course, this is easier said than done. Retraction of the thecal sac and nerve root will exacerbate the leak, which can be abated somewhat by placing the patient in the Trendelenburg position. In this particular circumstance, after I completed the decompression, I placed a quarter-inch by quarter-inch piece of dural matrix substitute over the top of the puncture site and covered it with a thin layer of fibrin glue to hold it in place. Remarkably, the patient experienced no untoward effects from the puncture. Since then, I have made certain that the spinal needle I use for localization never converges toward the midline.

A larger rent in the dura is a more difficult situation to address through a 16- or 18-mm-diameter access port. Although many reports in the literature suggest that there are minimal consequences because the transmuscular approach forgoes the need for direct repair,[15] I believe that larger defects in the dura require more than a piece of dural matrix and fibrin glue. A primary repair is the most comprehensive solution for addressing this situation. However, efficiently navigating a needle driver in a constrained working channel is a tall order. For a CSF leak in need of direct repair, the best path forward is to transition to a larger access port or to an expandable minimally invasive access port that will allow the necessary exposure and enough room to perform the repair. Reverting to an open incision is ill advised and should be avoided at all costs.

The first step in changing to a larger access port is to secure the final dilator back into the access port currently in position under direct visualization. Use one hand to ensure that the dilator is firmly secured against the lamina and then ask the assistant to loosen the table-mounted arm before you remove the access port with your other hand. Temporarily remove the operating microscope from the operative field, being careful to maintain downward pressure with the final dilator to keep the area of exposure unchanged. To lengthen the incision 2 mm in either direction, I pass a No. 15 blade down the side of the dilator to extend the skin and fascia incision. Then I may use the subsequent dilators to continue to enlarge the diameter of the exposure to 22 mm. I prefer to use an expandable minimal access port to allow for angulation of the blades and achieve greater exposure at depth. After the expandable access port is in position, I bring the microscope back into the operative field and assess the exposure.

For a primary repair, I prefer an exposure several millimeters above and below the defect. This exposure will require more bone work and resection of the ligamentum flavum, and therefore more time, but it is a worthwhile investment before attempting the repair. A minimally invasive CSF leak repair kit should always be available (Appendix). It is ideal to assemble and pack a sterile CSF repair kit in advance for ready retrieval by your operating room staff in the event the need arises. When attempting to deal with a dural tear, the last thing you need is your operating room personnel rummaging through microsets and trays attempting to find the instruments and sutures you need.

I use a bayoneted curved microsurgical needle driver and bayoneted fine Rhoton microsurgical forceps to deliver a 6.0 polypropylene suture on a PS-2 needle. Depending on the size of the defect, two or three interrupted sutures will provide a watertight closure for an adequate repair. A small muscle patch harvested from within the incision can be included in one of the sutures and a thin layer of fibrin glue can be applied over the repair.

Other criticisms of minimally invasive surgery are the perceived increased vulnerability of the patient to CSF leaks. In actuality, the risk of a CSF leak with either minimally invasive or open surgery is commensurate with the experience of the surgeon. Yet another criticism of minimally invasive techniques is that repair of a CSF leak is unduly difficult through a minimal access port. The reality is that I have never found closure of any dural defect to be an easy task—whether performed through an open or minimally invasive exposure. Regardless of the approach, the surgeon should use every measure feasible to prevent a CSF leak, which prevents the need to repair one.

2.15 Case Illustration: A Unique Circumstance

In the context of simultaneous L4–5 and L5–S1 disc herniations, a trajectory-dependent approach such as the minimally invasive microdiscectomy capitalizes on the angles to the disc space that originate from the same point. This unique circumstance is caused by the lumbar lordosis at the lumbosacral junction. Although this situation is not exceedingly common, it is one in which the minimally invasive approach offers a superior surgical option to the traditional midline open approach. This procedure requires only one 16-mm or 18-mm skin incision and two fascial openings.

This scenario is illustrated by the case of a 26-year-old woman with a rightward disc herniation at both L4–5 and L5–S1 (▶ Fig. 2.42). Trajectories through the L4–5 and L5–S1 disc spaces originate from the same point as the anatomical consequence of the lumbar lordosis. The fluoroscopic images (▶ Fig. 2.43) demonstrate two distinct trajectories originating from the same point and diverging to each respective disc space.

Thus, one incision is all that is required (▶ Fig. 2.44). I begin by planning the incision at L4–5. I infiltrate the proposed trajectory, make the incision, and then I perform the operation with the standard fascial opening as if it were a single-level operation. Upon completion of the L4–5 level, I remove the access port in its entirety and close the fascia. Next, I bring the fluoroscope back into the field and pass a spinal needle onto the lamina of L5. The trajectory is steeper than that for L4–5, which should be kept in mind when passing the spinal needle to avoid an inadvertent dural puncture at the L4–5 level. After I confirm the trajectory, I again infiltrate with local anesthetic and make a separate fascial opening. This fascial opening tends to be well below the L4–5 opening. I carefully proceed with sequential dilatation to 16 mm fully aware of the potential for passage of the early dilators into the canal through my recent bone work. I anchor the minimal access port into its optimal position and begin the second level, all through the initial 18-mm incision (▶ Fig. 2.44).

2.16 Conclusion

I end this chapter with the comment that began it: Minimally invasive spine surgery is difficult from a standing start. Many surgeons I have trained with and worked with over the years have abandoned minimally invasive techniques in favor of traditional midline techniques. Their reasons are always the same:

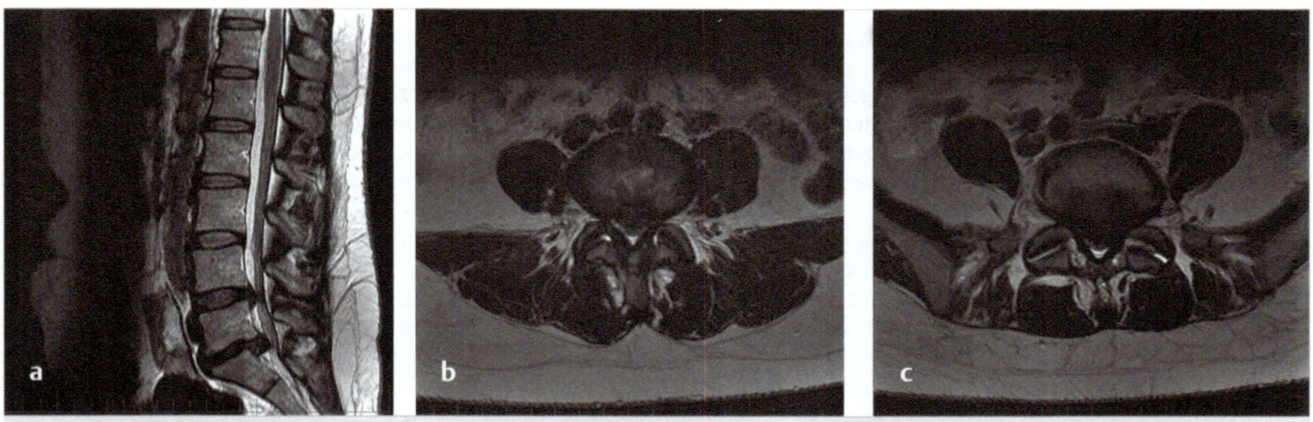

Fig. 2.42 A unique clinical circumstance: L4–5 and L5–S1 disc herniations. **(a)** Sagittal T2-weighted magnetic resonance imaging (MRI) demonstrates disc herniations at L4–5 and L5–S1. **(b)** Axial T2-weighted MRI through L4–5. **(c)** Axial T2-weighted MRI through L5–S1.

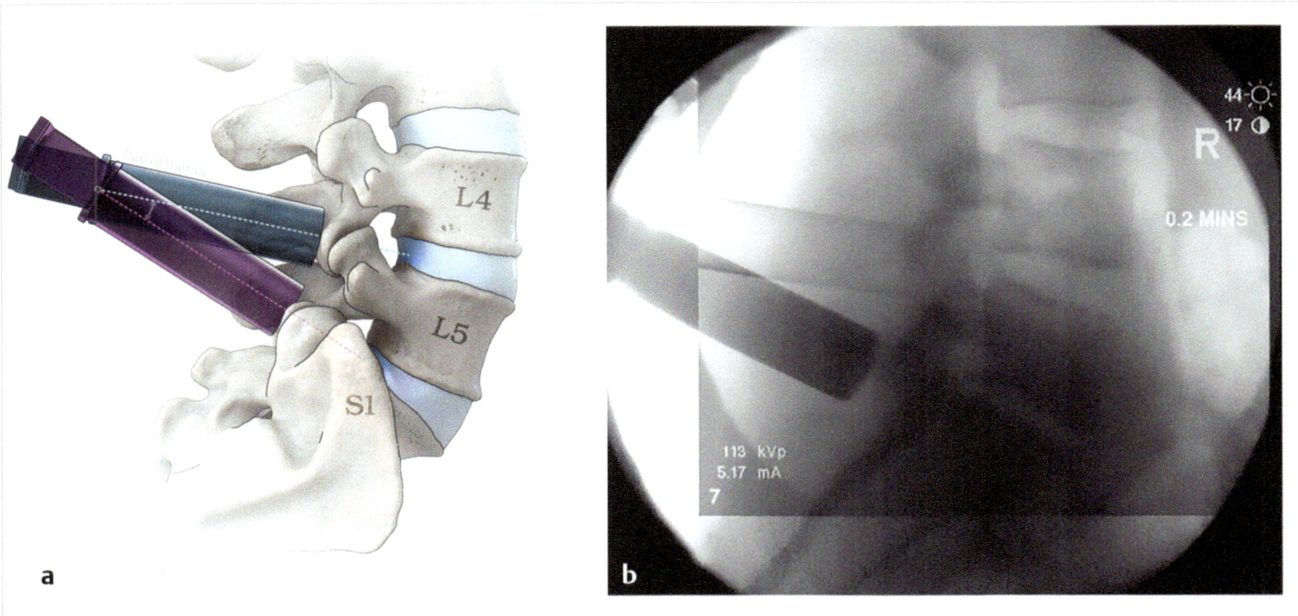

Fig. 2.43 A unique anatomical circumstance: lumbar lordosis at the lumbosacral junction. **(a)** Illustration of the lateral lumbar spine demonstrates the ability to access L4–5 and L5–S1 disc spaces with a minimal access port beginning from the same point (i.e., the incision). **(b)** Two lateral fluoroscopic images superimposed on one another show two distinct trajectories originating from the same point. There is a vast difference in performing a two-level minimally invasive microdiscectomy compared to an open microdiscectomy at L4–5 and L5–S1.

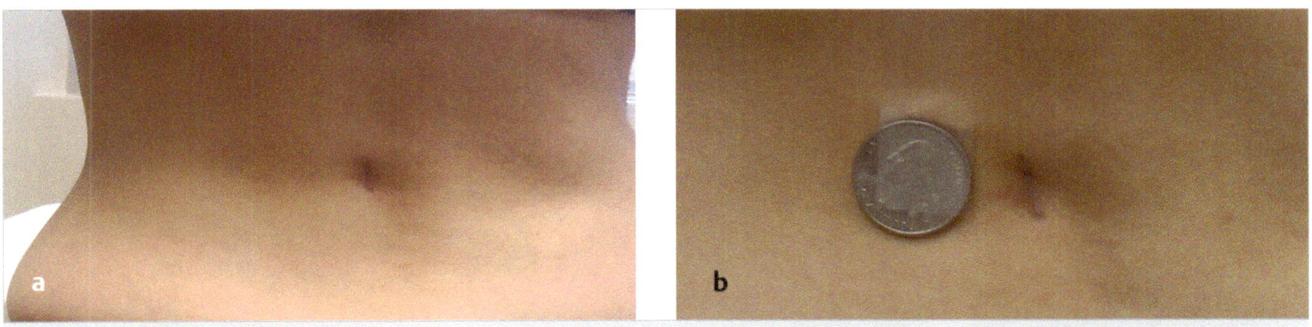

Fig. 2.44 Postoperative photographs of a patient who underwent simultaneous L4–5 and L5–S1 microdiscectomies with a minimally invasive approach. The patient was discharged home 2 hours after surgery and returned to work 20 days after the operation. **(a)** Healed scar. **(b)** Relative size of scar.

The minimally invasive procedure takes longer, it requires more radiation than open procedures, and it produces clinical results inferior to those of the open equivalents. I suspect that these surgeons attempted to gallop from the proverbial standing start instead of slowly building up momentum.

Instead, I believe that the way to build momentum is to gradually become familiar with the microsurgical instruments within the constraints of the minimal access port. Perhaps even more important is to develop the ability to reconstruct the anatomy at depth without the midline structures. Among the minimally invasive and open procedures, the bridge that spans the difference between a minimally invasive microdiscectomy and an open microdiscectomy is the shortest. It is therefore the bridge to cross first. In contrast, the bridge is far longer that spans the open transforaminal lumbar interbody fusion and the minimally invasive transforaminal lumbar interbody fusion. But for whatever reason, that procedure is where many surgeons begin—and sometimes end—in frustration, perspiration, and profanity. It is my hope that this chapter has offered the reader the fundamentals to begin the conversion to minimally invasive spine surgery through what I perceive to be the ideal gateway procedure. The minimally invasive microdiscectomy lays the foundation of the knowledge that will be the true organ of sight for those learning minimally invasive procedures. With mastery of this procedure, the reader can harness that forward momentum, turn the minimal access port inward, and apply these techniques to the minimally invasive lumbar laminectomy.

Appendix: Minimally Invasive Cerebrospinal Fluid Leak Repair Kit

1. Aesculap FD097 R Bayonet Micro Needle Holder, Curved 225 mm (× 1)
2. Codman/Symmetry 80–1512 Bayonet Micro Needle Holder, Straight, Titanium 225 mm (× 1)
3. Codman/Symmetry 80–1702 Bayonet Fine 0.5-mm Rhoton Forceps Titanium (× 2)
4. PMT 5-Fr. Barrel Tip "Inside" suction 3201–05M-06-SF (× 1)
5. PMT 7-Fr. Barrel Tip "Inside" suction 3201–07M-06-SF (× 1)

References

[1] Franke J, Greiner-Perth R, Boehm H, et al. Comparison of a minimally invasive procedure versus standard microscopic discotomy: a prospective randomised controlled clinical trial. Eur Spine J. 2009; 18(7):992–1000

[2] Arts MP, Brand R, van den Akker ME, Koes BW, Bartels RH, Peul WC, Leiden-The Hague Spine Intervention Prognostic Study Group (SIPS). Tubular diskectomy vs conventional microdiskectomy for sciatica: a randomized controlled trial. JAMA. 2009; 302(2):149–158

[3] Kawaguchi Y, Yabuki S, Styf J, et al. Back muscle injury after posterior lumbar spine surgery. Topographic evaluation of intramuscular pressure and blood flow in the porcine back muscle during surgery. Spine. 1996; 21(22):2683–2688

[4] O'Toole JE, Eichholz KM, Fessler RG. Surgical site infection rates after minimally invasive spinal surgery. J Neurosurg Spine. 2009; 11(4):471–476

[5] Foley K, Smith M. Microendoscopic discectomy. Tech Neurosurg. 1997; 3: 301–307

[6] Caspar W. A new surgical procedure for lumbar disc herniation causing less tissue damage through a microsurgical approach. In: Wüllenweber R, Brock M, Hamer J, Kinger M, Spoerri O, eds. Lumbar Disc Adult Hydrocephalus. Advances in Neurosurgery. Vol 4. Berlin Heidelberg: Springer-Verlag; 1977

[7] Yaşargil MG. Microsurgical Operation for Herniated Disc. Berlin: Springer-Verlag; 1977

[8] Perez-Cruet MJ, Foley KT, Isaacs RE, et al. Microendoscopic lumbar discectomy: technical note. Neurosurgery. 2002; 51(5) Suppl:S129–S136

[9] Williams RW. Microlumbar discectomy: a conservative surgical approach to the virgin herniated lumbar disc. Spine. 1978; 3(2):175–182

[10] Maroon JC. Current concepts in minimally invasive discectomy. Neurosurgery. 2002; 51(5) Suppl:S137–S145

[11] Panjabi MM, Goel V, Oxland T, et al. Human lumbar vertebrae. Quantitative three-dimensional anatomy. Spine. 1992; 17(3):299–306

[12] Love J. Removal of protruded intervertebral disks without laminectomy. Proc R Soc Med. 1939; 32:97–121

[13] Yong-Hing K, Reilly J, Kirkaldy-Willis WH. The ligamentum flavum. Spine. 1976; 1(4):226–234

[14] King JS. Dexamethasone–a helpful adjunct in management after lumbar discectomy. Neurosurgery. 1984; 14(6):697–700

[15] Kogias E, Klingler JH, Franco Jimenez P, et al. Incidental durotomy in open versus tubular revision microdiscectomy: a retrospective controlled study on incidence, management, and outcome. Clin Spine Surg. 2017; 30(10):E1333–E1337

3 Minimally Invasive Lumbar Laminectomy

Abstract
The difference in the exposure and approach between a minimally invasive and open lumbar microdiscectomy is slight. The difference between a minimally invasive and open lumbar laminectomy, however, is considerable. While the goals to completely decompress the thecal sac and nerve roots at a particular lumbar segment remain the same, the technical approach changes from outside in, applied in the open technique, to inside out in the minimally invasive one. This chapter focuses on the departure from a midline bilateral exposure of the lamina for decompression of a segment to a paramedian unilateral transmuscular approach for bilateral decompression of a segment. The consequence of beginning off the midline and converging onto the spine has the capacity to disorient. However, the mind prepared with the experience of minimally invasive microdiscectomies will overcome such disorientation. A historical perspective at the beginning of the chapter offers context for the inevitability of the minimally invasive approach for laminectomy. From there, review of the anatomy establishes the rationale for a minimally invasive approach. A detailed description of the surgical technique and case illustrations completes the chapter. The experience with the minimally invasive lumbar laminectomy becomes yet another building block that will be essential for the next logical step: minimally invasive lumbar fusions.

Keywords: facetectomy, laminectomy, ligamentum flavum, lumbar stenosis, minimally invasive

Based on over 45 years' experience in the surgical treatment of lumbar disc disease, it is recommended that the following operations be eliminated: the simple discectomy, which may cure the sciatica but not the back pain; the decompressive laminectomy, which leaves the patient with painful instability and nerve-root scarring; and chemonucleolysis, which does not provide permanent relief of either low-back or leg pain. The PLIF [posterior lumbar interbody fusion] technique is the answer to treatment of diseases of the lumbar spine and may be the operation of the future.

Dr. Ralph Bingham Cloward[1]

3.1 Introduction

Ralph Bingham Cloward certainly maintained a passionate and absolute opinion regarding the lumbar laminectomy. These words come from a surgeon who, over the course of a brilliant career, saw patients come in and out of his clinic after microdiscectomies, laminectomies, and posterior lumbar interbody fusions (PLIFs). Since Cloward spent his career on the island of Hawaii, his patients had few other places to go, and Cloward had no place to hide. As extreme as Cloward's position may seem in our modern era of spine surgery, given his decades of experience and the historical context of the time, it is difficult to discount his statement altogether. Perhaps we can even find some kernel of truth in his conclusion.

I can envision Dr. Cloward walking into that clinic room to examine a postoperative laminectomy patient wearing an expression of pain, anxiety, and dissatisfaction that we surgeons have all seen. He would stand there shaking his head while biting his lip as the patient described their painful instability originating only from their back without symptoms into the legs. "I should have fused this patient," he would likely have whispered beneath his breath. (How many times have I thought and mumbled the same?) I can also see Cloward knock on that same clinic door before peeking in to see a smiling patient who had undergone his PLIF procedure. As the PLIF patient thanked him and praised him, he would sigh with the satisfaction that only a spine surgeon knows. After years of this pattern repeating itself, the origins of the statement that begins this chapter become obvious.

One of the first spine surgeries I saw as a medical student at Georgetown University was a lumbar laminectomy. I was aghast. Looking at the immensity of the retractors, the length of the incision and the amount of blood loss, I wondered how this surgery could be of benefit to any patient. I remember the first step performed by the chief resident was using the Horsley Stille bone cutter to remove a pair of spinous processes. After interruption of the posterior tension band, the laminae were removed bilaterally to the edge of the facets. With each phase of the operation, the chief resident deepened the retractors and clicked them open wider and wider. I could not register in my mind that such an extensive wide-open approach was the best approach. After the case concluded, I distinctly remember asking the chief resident how a patient could possibly improve after such a procedure. I received a shrug and a muted response. I had not yet read Cloward's statement on the lumbar laminectomy, but if I had, I likely would have agreed with him.

In 1966, Love described the technique for the "decompressive laminectomy" as the removal of the spinous process and bilateral laminae.[2] In more specific terms, it can be defined by a midline approach to the spine, subperiosteal dissection of the paraspinous muscles and multifidus off the spinous process, laminae, and facets. The exposure is followed by complete resection of the spinous process, bilateral lamina, and medial facets. The very nature of this procedure interrupts the posterior intraspinous process ligament. That posterior tension band assists the body in maintaining lumbar lordosis and its loss has the potential to contribute to the flattening of our backs. With such a procedure, we lose the band that strings the bow.[3] When Cloward made his statement regarding the laminectomy, Love's description of the operation is likely what he had in mind. Since context is everything, it is important to note that Love's description of the laminectomy occurred at a time when localization in the operating room was accomplished at times by counting up from the sacrum and preoperative imaging was a rudimentary form of myelography.

Despite the preservation of the majority of the facet joint, the elimination of the posterior tension band explains how such a procedure has the potential to be destabilizing. Cloward was not alone in his opinion of the lumbar laminectomy. Over the years, spine surgeons have made the same intuitive observation about their patients regarding the lumbar laminectomy.[4,5] Few would argue that interruption of the posterior tension band, the devascularization of the paraspinous muscles along with the complete removal of the bony anatomy, does not have the capacity to affect the stability of the decompressed segment. More recent biomechanical studies have validated these intuitive concerns.[3,6]

Over the decades, surgeons must have looked at the task at hand, the anatomy they were dealing with alongside the consequences of the current techniques and thought to themselves, "There must be a better way." For Cloward, it was decompression with stabilization of the spine. Admittedly, this technique was developed in an era without full appreciation of either the impact of adjacent segment degeneration or the importance of segmental lumbar lordosis. But it certainly addressed the issue of stability.

Another approach arose that offered the same extent of decompression with minimal disruption of the native spine. Surgeons began to look at a lumbar segment in three dimensions instead of two. With this perspective, suddenly the spinous process and the lamina were no longer obstacles to the central canal (▶ Fig. 3.1). A common theme arose among the innovative surgeons who developed an approach that allowed for the preservation of the midline elements. That theme resonates in perfect pitch with modern-day minimally invasive principles. It was this rational approach to decompress without sacrifice of the midline ligamentous or bony anatomy that became the foundation of what has become the minimally invasive laminectomy.

3.2 Historical Perspective

Long before the development of modern minimally invasive techniques, surgeons sought a method to decompress the lumbar spine without sacrificing the midline elements. It was those lumbar laminectomy patients who experienced successful relief of neurogenic claudication and radiculopathy but developed new-onset back pain and radiographic evidence of instability that undoubtedly weighed heavily on the minds of those surgeons. The question was whether a successful decompression of the neural elements could be accomplished any other way?

Surgeons had made the astute observation that it is seldom the bony elements that result in central canal stenosis, but rather, the hypertrophied ligamentum flavum and facet arthropathy that cause compression of the neural elements. One thing was certain, the spinous processes and interspinous ligaments were completely innocent. Nevertheless, they became the collateral casualties of the classic wide midline decompression. Comments such as "the removal of bone is extensive for what is essentially a segmental disease confined largely to the posterolateral elements" began to surface in the literature regarding the traditional midline laminectomy.[7] Surgeons began asking why a satisfactory decompression could not be accomplished if the midline structures were not considered obstacles to the central canal.

Paul Lin[8] was one of the first surgeons to attempt to answer this question when he published his 1982 technical note on the internal decompression of the canal for the treatment of

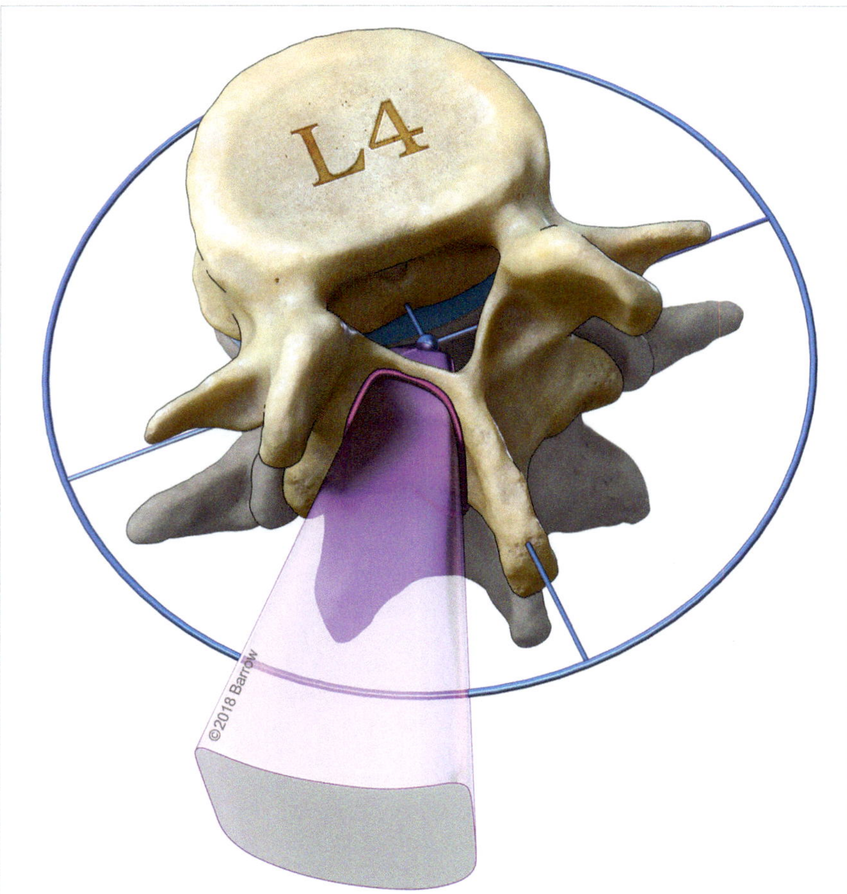

Fig. 3.1 The lumbar spine in three dimensions. Illustration of the true target of a lumbar laminectomy: the geometric center of the lumbar canal. There are several corridors that allow access to the central canal. A direct posterior approach will mandate complete resection of the spinous process and subsequently the lamina in order to decompress the neural elements. By beginning off the midline and angling onto the spine with a trajectory of 15 to 25 degrees, as illustrated in this figure, the same target may be reached without having to sacrifice the spinous process and both laminae.

lumbar stenosis. Removal of the medial aspect of the inferior and superior articular processes, the inferior aspect of the rostral lamina, and the superior aspect of the caudal lamina made possible the decompression of the neural elements with preservation of the lamina, spinous processes, and posterior tension band (▶ Fig. 3.2).[8] In 1988, Young and colleagues[7] published a similar technique of "multilevel subarticular fenestrations as an alternative to wide laminectomy" that confirmed the efficacy of Lin's technique in a series of 32 patients with up to 5 years of follow-up. In 1990, Aryanpur and Ducker[9] published another series of 32 patients using the same technique adding further evidence to the efficacy of this technique (▶ Fig. 3.3).[9]

Lin[8] made the following astute and prescient observation in his commentary on Aryanpur and Ducker's paper: "It is our experience when only the angled rongeur is being used, that adequate bony decompression of the foramen can only be accomplished if the operating surgeon stands on the opposite side of the lesion." That simple statement was prophetic. It captured the essence of the contralateral decompression achieved in current minimally invasive techniques. In 1995, Poletti[10] advanced this concept further with what appears to be the first formal description of a unilateral laminotomy with bilateral "ligamentectomy" to decompress the central canal (▶ Fig. 3.4).[10] In his patients, Poletti maintained the integrity of the posterior tension band, spinous process, and contralateral lamina. He rationalized that doing so would minimize any instability and muscle devascularization that would occur with a traditional midline approach. Through this unilateral approach, Poletti was able to completely resect the ligamentum flavum that was causing the compression by undercutting the spinous process and the contralateral lamina.

Despite the efficacy of the unilateral approach that was demonstrated through the middle and late 1990s, the midline laminectomy remained the mainstay in treatment for lumbar stenosis. It was the approach I was taught in my residency and to a large part, it continues to be taught to this day.

Parallel with the desire to maintain the native structures of the spine in the treatment of lumbar stenosis, there has been an increasing interest in minimally invasive approaches to the spine. The paramedian transmuscular approaches developed by surgeons seeking a minimally invasive procedure to access the spine would find a perfect marriage with a technique that intended to preserve the posterior tension band and as much of the midline bony elements as possible. The synthesis of these two techniques popularized by Foley and Fessler and written about by Khoo and Fessler[11] would eventually lead us to the minimally invasive laminectomy.

3.3 The Minimally Invasive Conversion

I emphasized in Chapter 2, Minimally Invasive Microdiscectomy, that there are more similarities than differences between the open and minimally invasive microdiscectomy. The approach, the bone work and the procedure are virtually identical between the two; it is the access to the requisite anatomy that is the only real difference between these two techniques. It is those very similarities that make that operation the ideal starting point for minimally invasive surgery on the spine. In this chapter, I acknowledge that the minimally invasive laminectomy is more of a departure from the midline laminectomy. The bone work is different, the exposure is different and the incision is different. Nevertheless, the decompression is the same. The advantage that you have in developing a skill set with the minimally invasive microdiscectomy is that those same skills readily translate to the minimally invasive laminectomy. From that standpoint, the minimally invasive laminectomy is the logical next chapter in this Primer.

There are key differences between the microdiscectomy and laminectomy that are worthwhile to highlight. Unlike the incision for the minimally invasive microdiscectomy, the incision for a minimally invasive laminectomy is slightly more off the midline and has a greater angle of convergence onto the spine as seen in ▶ Fig. 3.1 at the beginning of this chapter. The combination of increased angle and greater distance from the midline has the potential to disorient the surgeon's mind. After all, the midline is the basis of our orientation. A return to the basic principles of sounding the lamina, spinous process and facet that I introduced in Chapter 2 will help you reconstruct the anatomy at depth. These components will keep your mind oriented. In turn, the minimally invasive laminectomy becomes yet another building block that will become the foundation for minimally invasive lumbar fusions.

3.4 Patient Selection

The focus of this Primer is the surgical technique. However, it would be difficult not to make a comment regarding patient selection for the minimally invasive laminectomy, given some of the unique elements of this procedure. Neurogenic claudication caused by single-level lumbar stenosis is perhaps the most common condition that I treat in my practice. Over the years, I have observed that this entity seldom occurs at L5–S1 or higher than L2–3 in the absence of previous surgery. A review of my last 100 or so cases demonstrates that the vast majority of the surgeries I have performed have been at L4–5 or L3–4, or both. Remarkably, the vast majority have been single-level procedures.

The ideal candidate for a minimally invasive lumbar laminectomy has single-level stenosis, typically at L3–4 or L4–5. The subjective complaints of the patient may have a unilateral radicular component, but their history is primarily one of neurogenic claudication. A back pain component may be present, but without advanced disc degeneration, the goal of surgery is to decompress the neural elements and alleviate symptoms of neurogenic claudication. Back pain that resolves after the operation, I attribute to the inability to adequately distinguish the back pain from symptoms of neurogenic claudication.

Magnetic resonance imaging (MRI) should demonstrate the predominance of thickening in the ligamentum flavum over any disc protrusion or bony encroachment of the canal on the axial images. The amount of facet arthropathy and disc degeneration is relevant especially in the context of spondylolisthesis. Several aspects shown on the MRI in ▶ Fig. 3.5 make this patient an ideal candidate for a minimally invasive lumbar laminectomy.

First, the patient has single-level compression at L4–5 with no evidence of spondylolisthesis at that segment. The flexion-extension studies (not shown) do not demonstrate abnormal motion. The MRI demonstrates relative preservation of lumbar lordosis. There is no significant mismatch between the pelvic incidence and the lumbar lordosis.

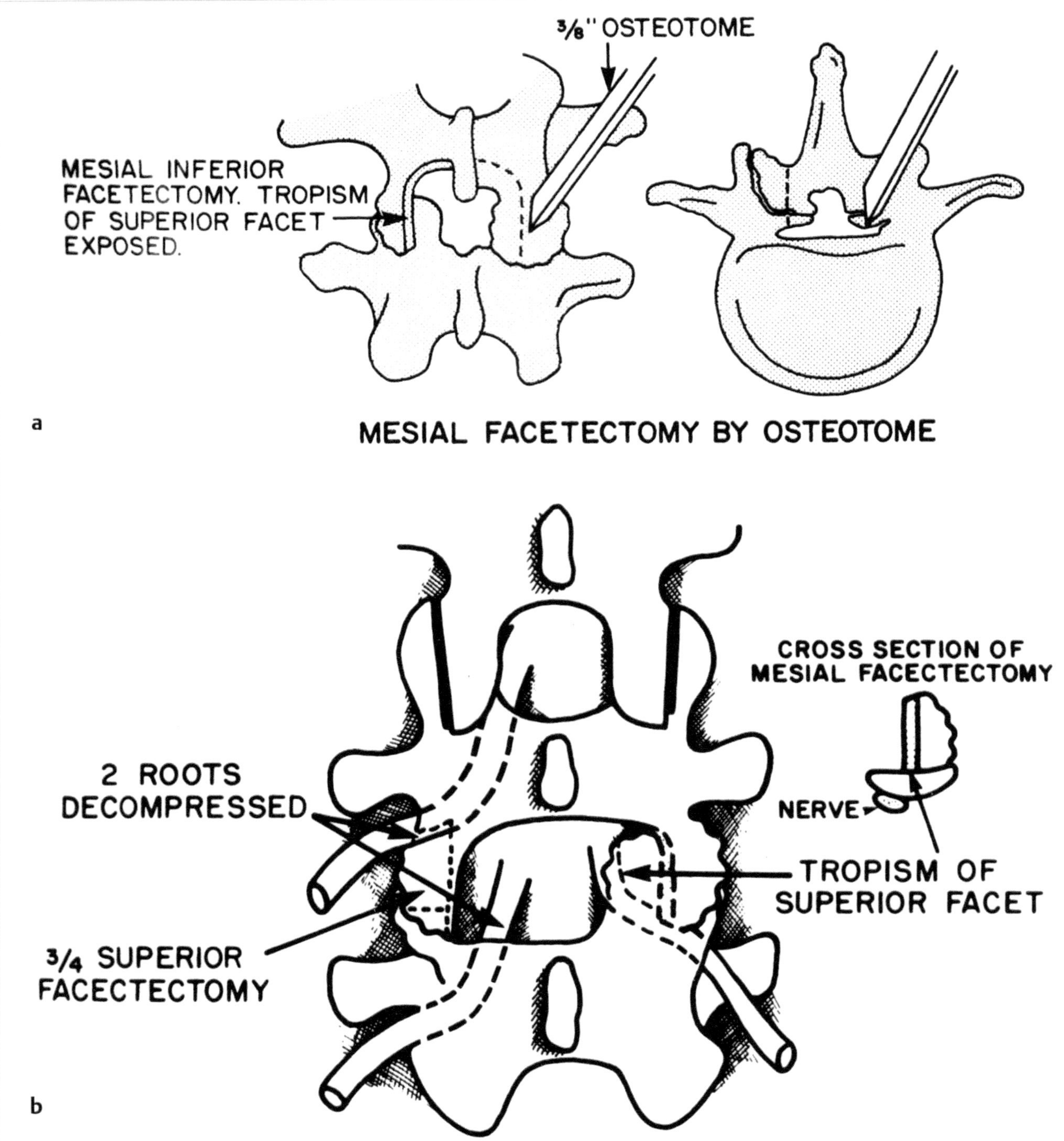

Fig. 3.2 Decompression of the central canal without sacrifice of the midline elements. Illustrations from Lin's[8] description of internal decompression of the central canal for management of lumbar stenosis. **(a)** Mesial facetectomy. **(b)** Superior facetectomy. (Reproduced with permission from Lin PM. Internal decompression for multiple levels of lumbar spinal stenosis: a technical note. Neurosurgery. 1982; 11(4):546–549.)

Second, despite the advanced disc degeneration present at L5–S1, there is no significant degeneration of the disc space at L4–5. In fact, the disc height is well preserved at L4–5. From a clinical standpoint, this patient reports a history of primarily neurogenic claudication symptoms in the legs and mild left-sided L5 radiculopathy.

Finally, the axial MRI demonstrates a mild degree of facet arthropathy with most of the compression due to the thickened ligamentum flavum. Once the ligamentum flavum has been cleared and a medial facetectomy has been performed, the canal and the lateral recess will be well decompressed. Collectively, these clinical and radiographic aspects make this

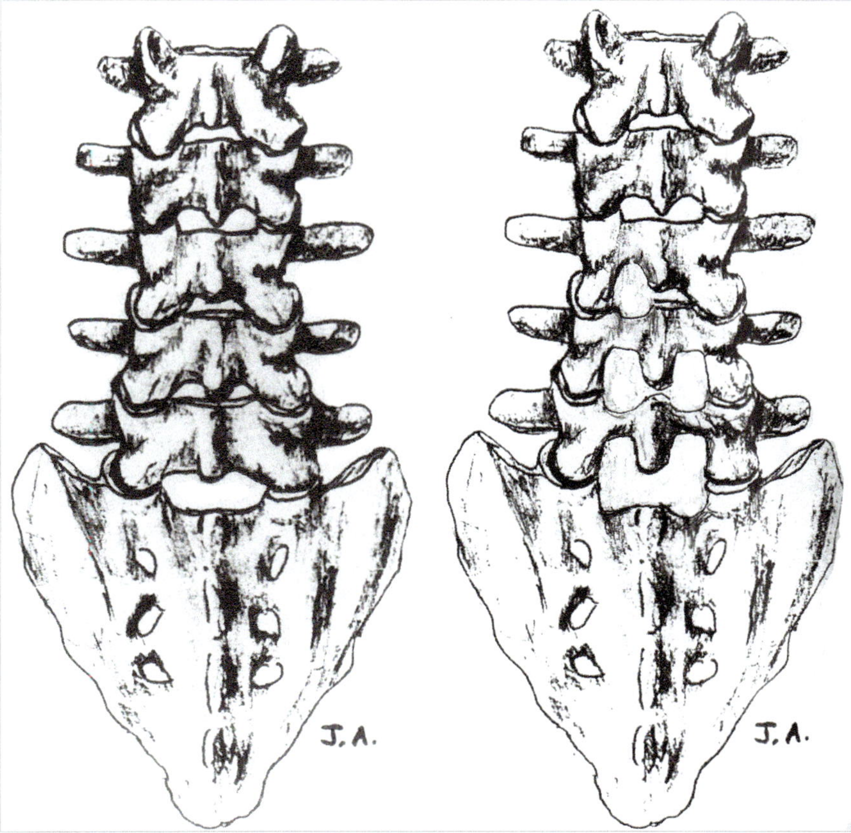

Fig. 3.3 Illustration from Aryanpur and Ducker[9] demonstrating the technique of multilevel medial facetectomies with preservation of the midline elements. (Reproduced with permission from Aryanpur J, Ducker T. Multilevel lumbar laminotomies: an alternative to laminectomy in the treatment of lumbar stenosis. Neurosurgery. 1990; 26(3):429–432; discussion 433.)

patient an ideal candidate for a minimally invasive lumbar decompression.

Characteristics in the imaging that would make the patient a less-than-ideal candidate for a minimally invasive laminectomy would include advanced degeneration, loss of lumbar lordosis and disc collapse causing neuroforaminal compromise of the L4 nerve root. In those circumstances, the restoration of the disc height and restoration of lumbar lordosis may be as important as the decompression of the neural elements.

Next, consider a patient with lumbar stenosis secondary to a grade I spondylolisthesis at L4–5 and advanced facet arthropathy (▶ Fig. 3.6). The decision-making process is slightly different for a minimally invasive approach than for a traditional midline open approach. In this patient, the absence of motion on flexion-extension studies and the preservation of the posterior tension band and the lamina with a minimally invasive approach allows for more stability than with a traditional midline approach, in which the posterior tension band and the lamina would be removed.[3,12] Furthermore, the disc height is well maintained, thus precluding the need to restore foraminal height. The extensive facet arthropathy requires removal of a substantial portion of the facet to achieve an adequate decompression. In this case, a minimally invasive decompression may be considered, with the patient monitored over time to check for any progressive instability.

Finally, consider a patient with multiple levels of stenosis. ▶ Fig. 3.7 represents the inherent limitation of a minimally invasive laminectomy. The patient has four levels of stenosis. Working through a minimal access port at four different levels is possible, but far from efficient. At some point, simultaneous exposure of all the levels that require decompression will offer greater efficiency than securing a minimal access port at four different levels. I believe that crossover in efficiency occurs after more than two levels are involved. Although attempting to decompress the worst segment or perhaps the two worst segments is an option, such extensive lumbar stenosis argues for a more comprehensive solution as perhaps the best course of action. However, a traditional midline exposure does not mandate sacrifice of the spinous process and the posterior tension band. Applying the techniques described by Lin,[8] Aryanpur and Ducker,[9] and Poletti[10] remains a viable alternative even in the setting of a midline approach for multilevel stenosis.

3.5 Anatomical Basis

From a conceptual standpoint, the operative anatomy in the axial plane may be considered a triangle formed by the two arms of the lamina and the disc space (▶ Fig. 3.8).[2] The main goal of the laminectomy, whether open or minimally invasive, is to decompress the thecal sac and the traversing nerve roots by removing the thickened ligamentum flavum and the compressive components of the hypertrophied facets. In a traditional midline laminectomy, these goals are accomplished by approaching and removing the apex of the triangle (the spinous process) along with the two limbs of the triangle (bilateral laminectomies and medial facets). In such an approach, the decompression is accomplished from the outside in (▶ Fig. 3.9).

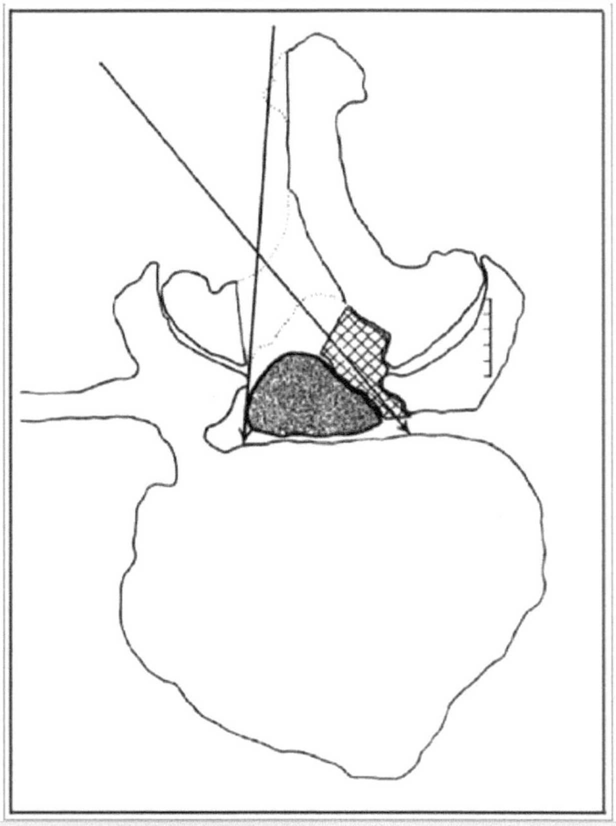

Fig. 3.4 Illustration from Dr. Poletti's 1995 publication[10] before the advent of minimally invasive spine techniques. Remarkably, this illustration augurs the technique that minimally invasive surgeons would eventually use to perform minimally invasive lumbar laminectomies through minimal access ports. (Reproduced with permission from Poletti CE. Central lumbar stenosis caused by ligamentum flavum: unilateral laminotomy for bilateral ligamentectomy. Neurosurgery. 1995; 37(2):343-347.)

With the minimally invasive technique, the surgeon approaches one face of the triangle and removes most of that side to gain access to the inside of the triangle. Since most of the compression is due to the ligamentum flavum, the surgeon may accomplish the majority of the decompression by essentially excavating the ligamentum flavum from within this triangle. Thus, in the minimally invasive approach, the decompression of the thecal sac is accomplished from the inside out (▶ Fig. 3.10).[10]

Effectively accomplishing a minimally invasive decompression requires access to the entire swath of ligamentum flavum within the canal. Thus, exposure of the rostral and caudal insertion points of the ligamentum flavum is necessary. Such access allows for the detachment and removal of the entire ligamentum flavum, thereby decompressing the whole segment. Accordingly, the operative exposure should include the insertion points of the ligamentum flavum, which are at the rostral aspects of the superior lamina and the inferior lamina of the segment. Since the theme of a minimally invasive decompression is from the inside out and the focus is the ligamentum flavum, you would do well to study the anatomy of the ligamentum flavum from the inside out. Reviewing an anatomical illustration with a perspective from the underside of the ligamentum flavum is a useful exercise. It can help you consider the anatomy as if you were lying down on the floor of the spinal canal looking outward at the targets you need for a minimally invasive decompression. Carefully studying the anatomy from this perspective provides your mind with the unique insight to achieve the goals of excavating the segment from the inside out (▶ Fig. 3.11).

Exposure to the insertion points of the ligamentum flavum in and of itself allows the piecemeal resection of the ligamentum flavum with Kerrison rongeurs and pituitary rongeurs; but this type of exposure also lends itself to a more simplified method of decompression. Conceptually, the release of the rostral and caudal insertion points of the ligamentum flavum makes possible the en bloc removal of the ligamentum flavum. A study of the precise anatomical distance from the insertions will facilitate this technique. As noted in Chapter 2, Minimally Invasive Microdiscectomy, there is great value in knowing with certainty the specific anatomical measurements relevant to the procedure. For the minimally invasive lumbar laminectomy, the distance from the insertion point to the insertion point of the ligamentum flavum is perhaps the most valuable anatomical measurement. The MRI shown in ▶ Fig. 3.12 demonstrates the insertion points of the ligamentum flavum at L4–5. Depending on the disc height, that distance is typically around 25 mm. That is the approximate distance you must cover in a minimally invasive exposure to achieve a segmental decompression. Reulen et al further corroborate the 25-mm approximation in their analysis of laminar height.[13] The analysis of 31 cadaveric lumbar spines found that the range of laminar heights for L3, L4, and L5 were 23 mm (20–32 mm), 21 mm (16–29 mm), and 17 mm (14–22 mm), respectively (▶ Fig. 3.12d–f). Laminar height in the lumbar spine is yet another valuable measurement to keep in mind as a minimally invasive spine surgeon.

It is equally valuable to appreciate the dimensions of the lumbar canal to further establish the rationale for a minimally invasive approach for a lumbar laminectomy. ▶ Fig. 3.13[14] demonstrates the dimensions of the canal as determined by Panjabi et al[14] at the various levels of L1 to L5. Recognizing that the width of the lumbar canal ranges from 23 to 27 mm provides the context for a minimal access port measuring 16 to 18 mm in diameter. Such an access port can readily cover that dimension when repositioned at the various angles.

An analysis of the axial MRIs alongside the measurements in ▶ Fig. 3.13 demonstrates the extent of the medial to lateral exposure required to accomplish the goals of the operation. It is helpful to keep in mind that the intrapedicular distance is approximately 2 cm and that the length of the lamina (one side of the triangle) is approximately 18 mm (▶ Fig. 3.14).

Looking at these various measurements collectively, the anatomical basis of the minimally invasive laminectomy begins to unveil itself. We have defined the rostrocaudal and lateral dimensions of exposures to be approximately 25 mm. It becomes conceivable how a minimal access port secured onto one of the laminae at an angle parallel to the adjacent side can provide adequate access to the entire central canal to accomplish the decompression (▶ Fig. 3.15). A diameter of 16 to 18 mm provides adequate exposure of the lamina for decompression in the axial plane of compression. However, a 16- or 18-mm aperture will not provide the necessary rostrocaudal exposure to reach the insertion points of the ligamentum

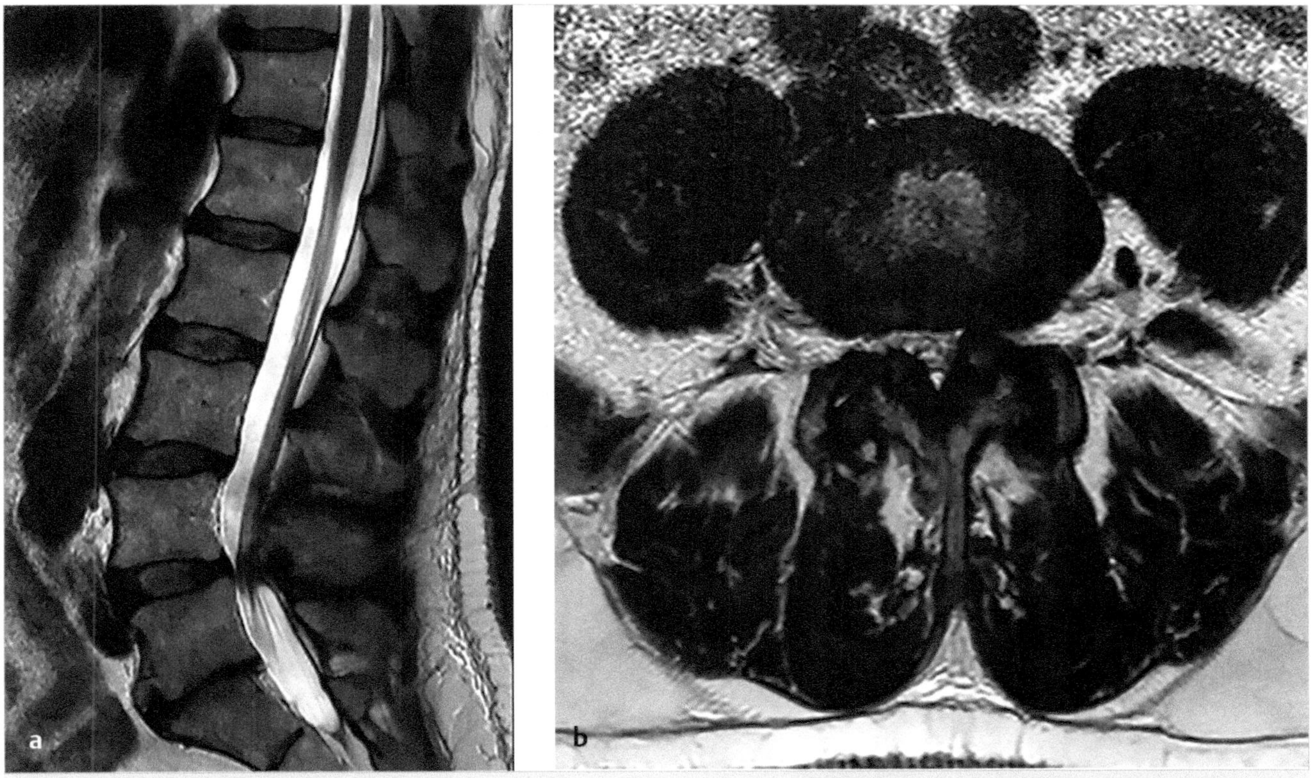

Fig. 3.5 Lumbar stenosis in a patient with neurogenic claudication. T2-weighted magnetic resonance imaging of the lumbar spine. (a) Sagittal view demonstrates single-level lumbar stenosis at L4–5. Note the preservation of the disc height at L4–5 and the relative preservation of lumbar lordosis. (b) Axial view demonstrates primarily ligamentum flavum hypertrophy with a mild facet arthropathy.

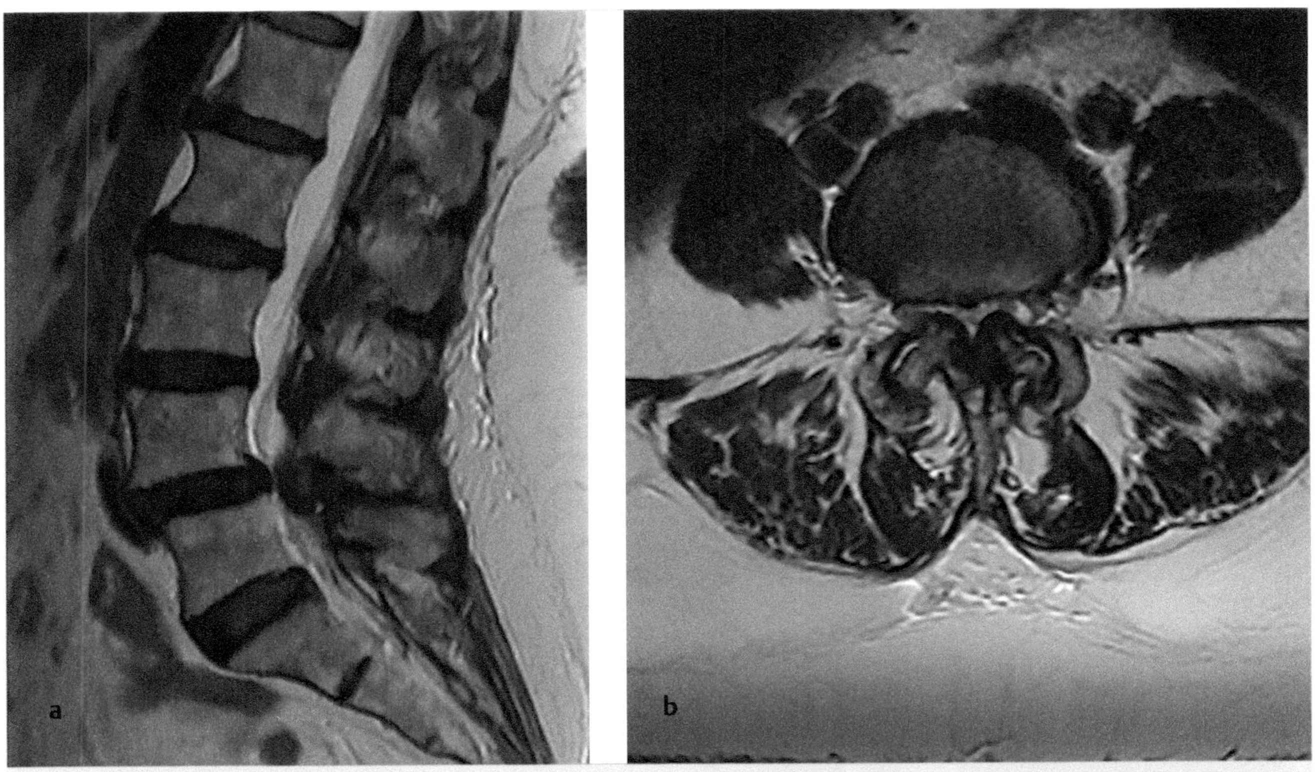

Fig. 3.6 Magnetic resonance imaging (MRI) of the lumbar spine of a patient with spondylolisthesis. (a) Sagittal T2-weighted MRI demonstrates grade I spondylolisthesis at L4–5 with well-preserved disc height. (b) Axial T2-weighted MRI demonstrates severe central canal stenosis secondary to facet arthropathy. There was no evidence of instability on flexion-extension radiographs (not shown).

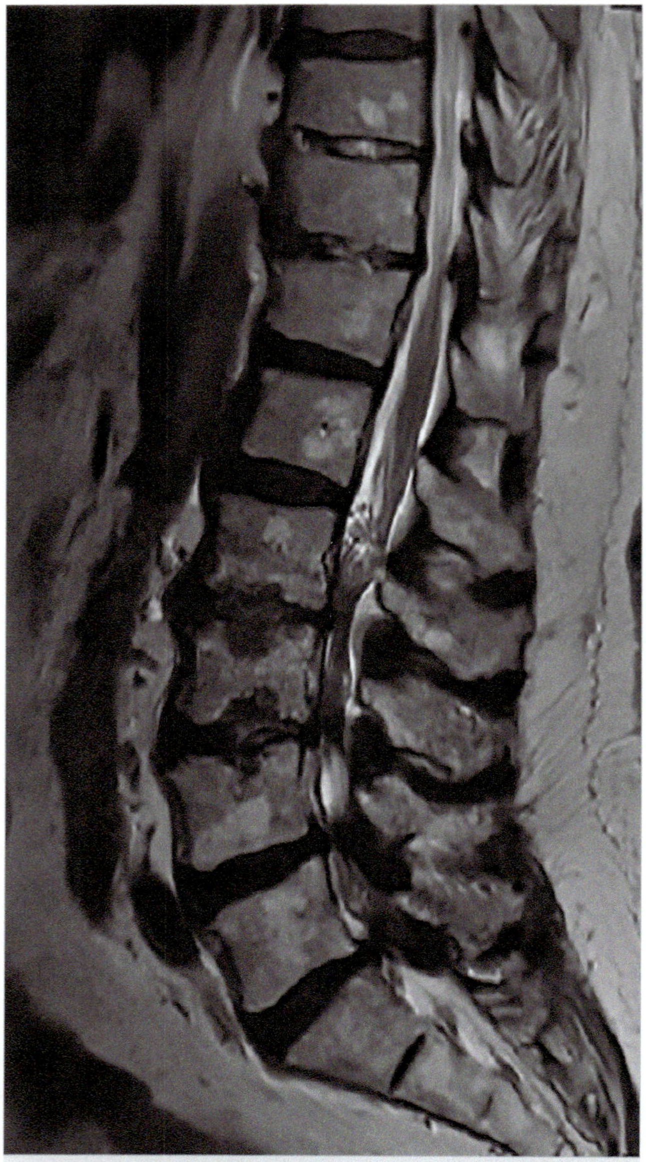

Fig. 3.7 Multiple levels of lumbar stenosis. Sagittal T2-weighted magnetic resonance image of the lumbar spine demonstrating four levels of lumbar stenosis. This patient would be a poor candidate for a minimally invasive decompression.

flavum on the lamina. As demonstrated in ▶ Fig. 3.12, up to 25 mm of exposure may be necessary. Expandable minimal access ports can simultaneously encompass all the requisite anatomy within a single field of view but will result in greater disruption to the paraspinal musculature and will bring more muscle tissue into the operative field. Furthermore, the wide exposure offered by expandable minimal access ports shifts the Caspar ratio disadvantageously. Another viable option is simply to change the trajectory of the minimal access port to reach the limits of the exposure (▶ Fig. 3.16). Such a technique allows for an expansive exposure with no further disruption of the paraspinal musculature. I prefer using this technique to cover the 25 mm required to reach the insertions of the ligamentum flavum. Returning to the concept of the Caspar ratio, where the goal is to achieve a ratio of surgical target to surgical exposure as close to 1 as possible, we find that the minimally invasive laminectomy is the one circumstance where the ratio actually exceeds 1: A surgical target of 25 mm is accomplished through an incision 18 mm in length using an access port 16 mm in diameter (▶ Fig. 3.16).

As you proceed with the operation and reposition the minimal access port, there will be overlap with the initial field of view. That overlap allows for both a continuous exposure of the initial field of view and for completion of the remaining 7 to 10 mm of exposure. With these anatomical measurements as our guide, we have established the anatomical basis for the use of a 16- to 18-mm fixed-diameter minimal access port.

3.6 Operating Room Setup

As with a microdiscectomy, I prefer patients to be positioned on a Jackson table with a Wilson frame. The Jackson table facilitates insertion and extraction of fluoroscopy. Jackson tables that have the capacity to rotate are ideal, as they optimize the ergonomics for the surgeon. Standard operating tables with a Wilson frame will work as well but will require some complex navigation of the fluoroscopic unit around the base of the table.

I always place the fluoroscopic unit into position before prepping and draping the patient so as not to interrupt the flow of the operation after it begins. The scrub technician drapes the microscope and positions it opposite the image intensifier of the fluoroscope (▶ Fig. 3.17). Patients typically have symptoms that are more prominent in one leg. By convention, I will dock the access port on the lamina of the more symptomatic side indicating to my team where to position the microscope within the operating room (▶ Fig. 3.18). In patients who have purely neurogenic claudication, the laterality of approach is by surgeon preference. Regardless of the side of the approach, the decompression is bilateral. The objective is to decompress the entire central canal.

I position the patient prone atop the Wilson frame, which is then fully expanded and then palpate the bony landmarks of the anterior superior iliac spine and the intraspinous process space. The L4–5 level is approximated in this manner and marked. That mark now becomes my reference point. I then mark the incision relative to my presumptive L4–5 mark. If I am to operate on L3–4, then I mark one interspinous process space up. If I am to operate on L5–S1, then I mark one level down and so on. After I have approximated the level, I palpate the spinous processes and mark them to establish the midline. I plan the incision to be 18 to 20 mm in length and 20 to 25 mm lateral to midline, which translates to a finger breadth lateral to the spinous process. That distance is slightly more lateral than the distance for a microdiscectomy. A slightly more lateral starting point will allow for the necessary angle of convergence to accomplish a midline and contralateral decompression. By contradistinction, in a microdiscectomy, only the ipsilateral aspect

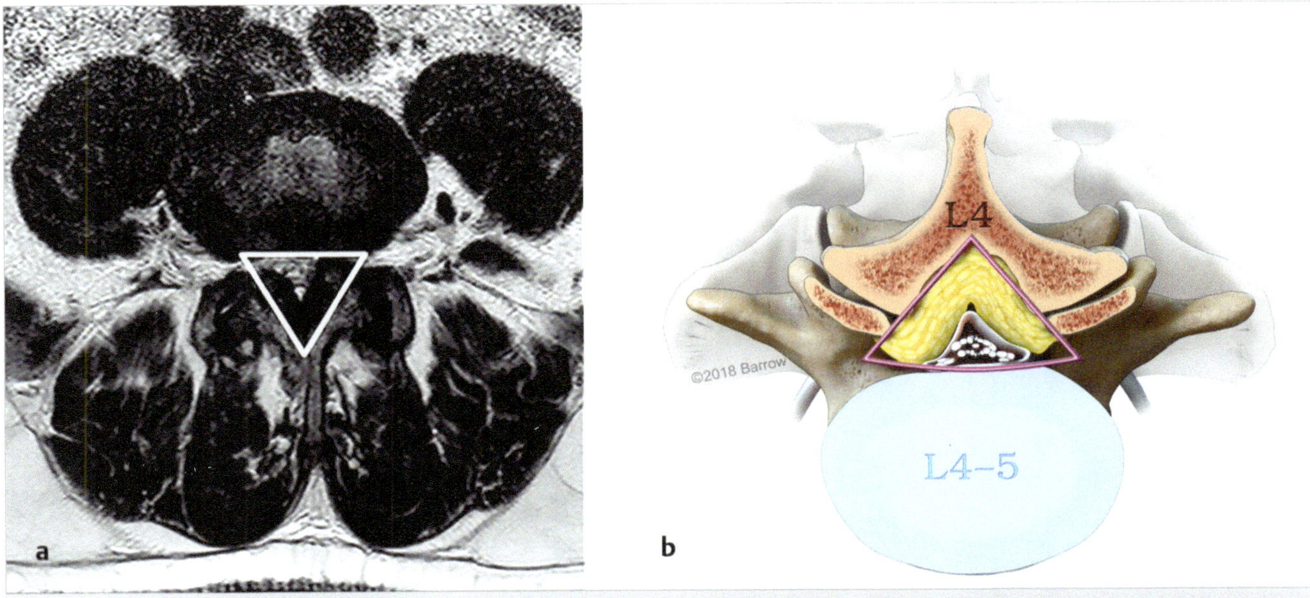

Fig. 3.8 **(a)** Axial T2-weighted magnetic resonance imaging of the lumbar spine demonstrating severe central canal stenosis at the L4–5 segment. The limbs of the lamina and the disc space form a triangle in the axial plane of the compression of the thecal sac. In a traditional midline approach, both limbs of the triangle would be removed, as described by Love,[2] thereby achieving decompression from the outside in. The minimally invasive technique approaches one side of this triangle and decompresses from the inside out. **(b)** Illustration of the thickened ligamentum flavum resulting in the compression of the thecal sac. The magenta triangle demarcates the borders of the canal: the lamina, medial facets and disc space. The spinous process clearly does not result in compression of the neural elements. Despite this, it is the first structure surgeons remove in a traditional midline lumbar laminectomy.

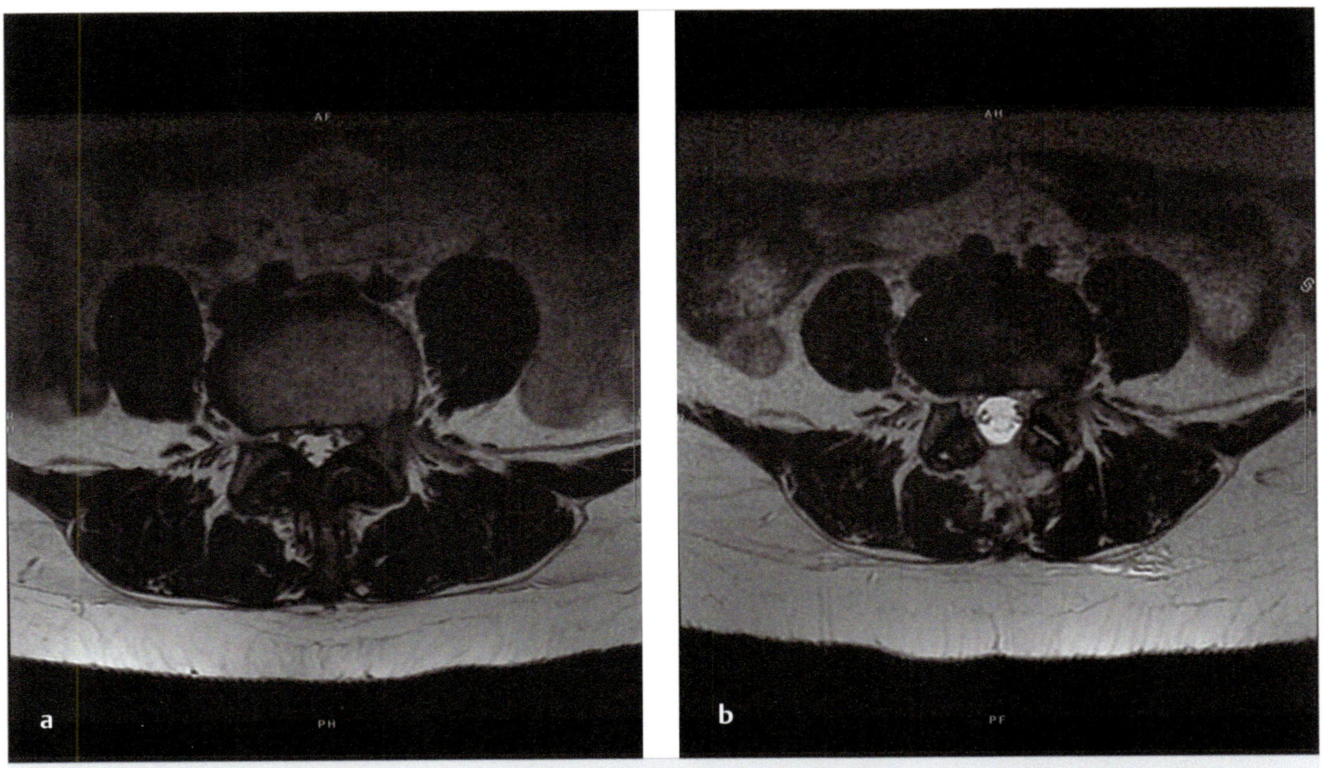

Fig. 3.9 Postoperative image of a traditional midline laminectomy. **(a)** Preoperative axial T2-weighted magnetic resonance imaging (MRI) demonstrating mild compression of the neural elements by the ligamentum flavum. **(b)** Postoperative axial T2-weighted MRI in a patient who underwent a traditional midline laminectomy. Note the removal of the spinous process, the lamina and the medial facets.

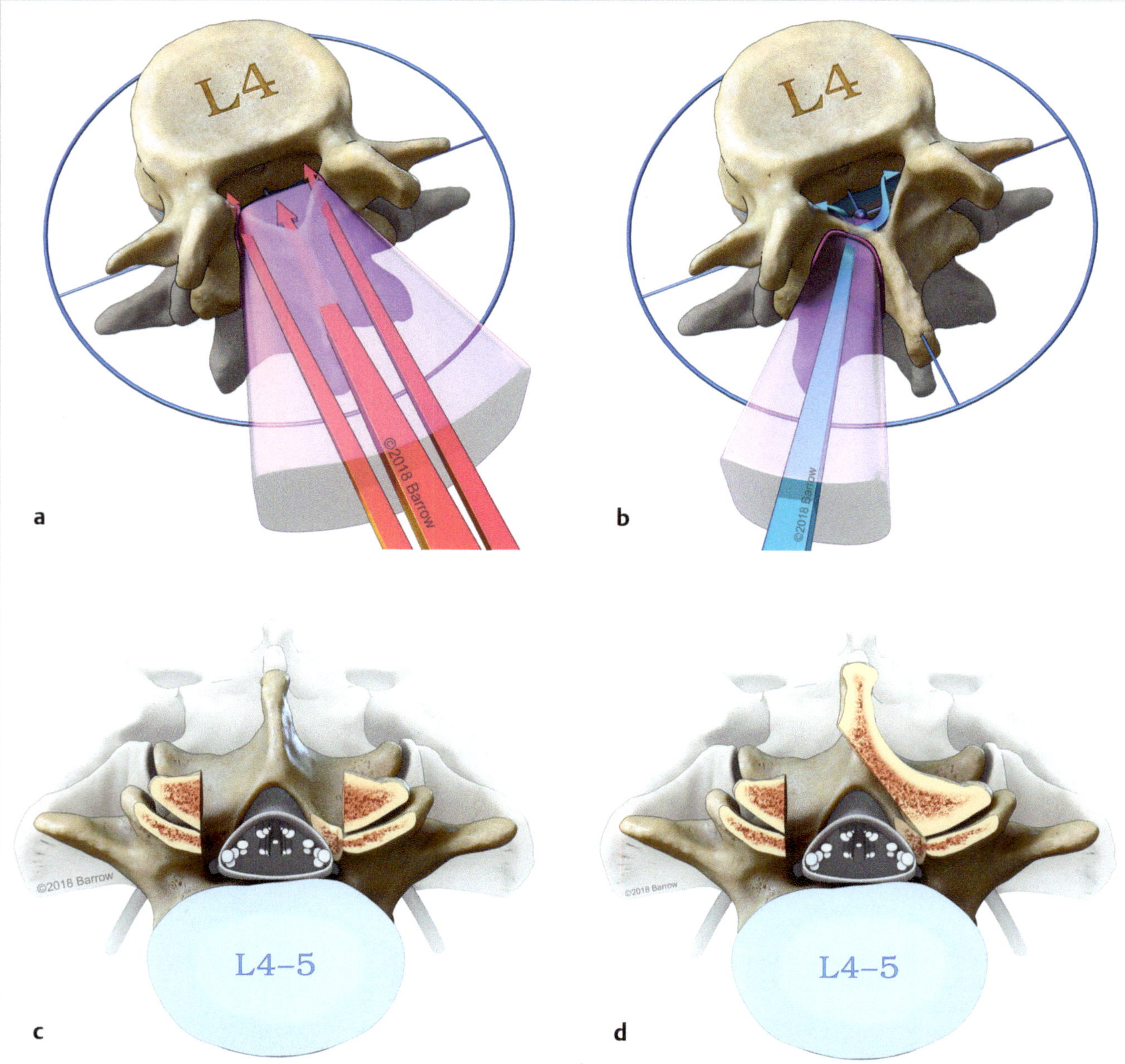

Fig. 3.10 A traditional midline open versus minimally invasive lumbar laminectomy. **(a)** Illustration demonstrating the approach for a midline lumbar laminectomy. The first structure encountered is the spinous process. After removal of the spinous process, the laminae are removed bilaterally followed by the medial facets. With access to the central canal, the ligamentum flavum is resected and the neural elements decompressed. In this circumstance the decompression would be performed from the outside in. **(b)** Illustration of a minimally invasive approach for a lumbar laminectomy. A unilateral approach to the lamina, similar to what was described by Poletti[10] in 1995. In this approach, the spinous process would be undercut, the medial facet removed and one side of the lamina removed. Access to the central canal in this manner allows for resection of the ligamentum flavum. In this circumstance, the operation would be performed from the inside out. **(c)** Illustration of a postoperative laminectomy performed through a traditional midline approach. The neural elements have been decompressed from the outside in. **(d)** Illustration of a postoperative minimally invasive laminectomy with preservation of the posterior midline structures. The decompression achieved is the same.

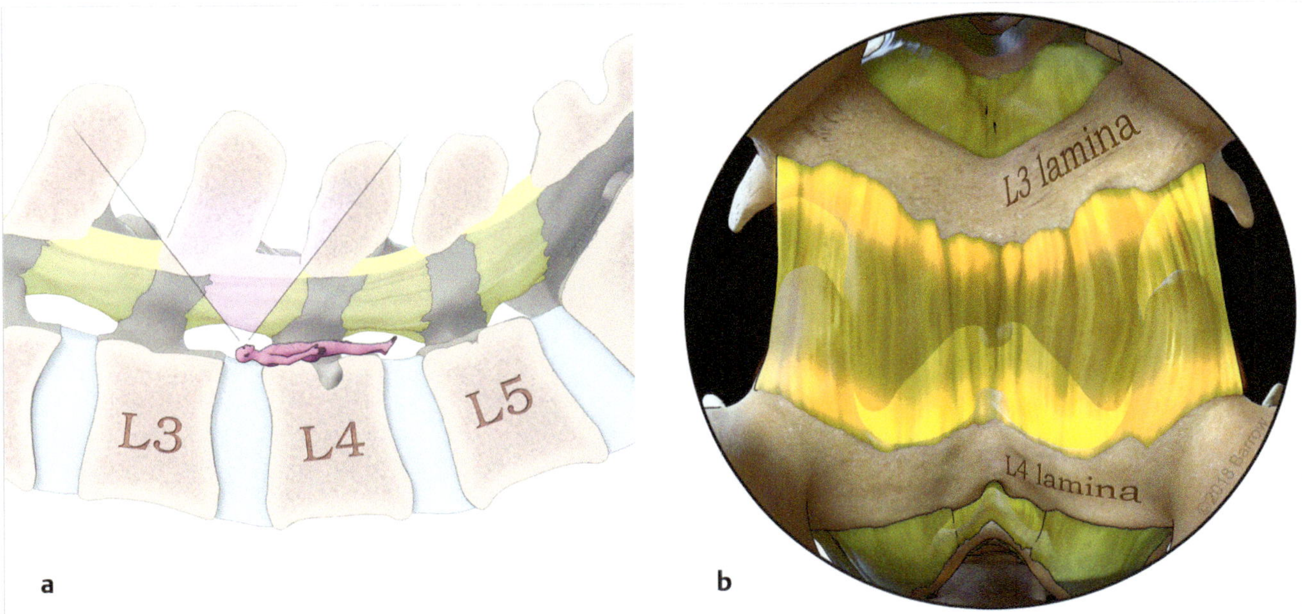

Fig. 3.11 **(a)** Illustration of viewing the ligamentum flavum from within the canal. **(b)** If you were to consider lying down in the canal looking up at the ligamentum flavum then your field of view would encompass viewing the ligamentum flavum from the underside of the laminae. The insertion points of the ligamentum flavum are clearly evident on the underside of the rostral and caudal laminae. These insertion points (highlighted in the illustration) are the targets for the exposure needed to accomplish complete decompression of the segment. Note the shadow of the facets bilaterally behind the curtain of ligamentum flavum. Ipsilateral and contralateral medial facetectomies may still be performed from a unilateral approach.

of the thecal sac and traversing nerve root need to be visualized. A more medially based incision allows for that straighter trajectory (▸ Fig. 3.19).

3.7 Localization

After the incision has been prepped and draped with the fluoroscopic unit in position at the operative level, I pass a 20-gauge spinal needle onto the lamina. Similar to localization in a microdiscectomy, care should be taken to ensure that the trajectory onto the spine is divergent from the interlaminar space, so as to minimize, if not eliminate, the risk of dural puncture. As the needle descends down its path, the tip should make contact with the lamina or facet almost immediately. If the passage of the needle seems inordinately long, then I reassess my trajectory and even obtain a fluoroscopic image. Because of the divergent trajectory, it is conceivable, although highly unlikely, that with an extreme angle the needle may pass lateral to the spine altogether. At times, securing the needle onto the spine will require what seems to be an excessively deep placement in patients with an elevated body mass index. Additional fluoroscopy can make such needle placement a more tolerable experience for the surgeon.

After I have confirmed the level, I adjust the position of the spinal needle in the rostral or caudal direction so that it is pointed to the rostral insertion of the ligamentum flavum (▸ Fig. 3.20). I infiltrate the incision with a combination of bupivacaine and lidocaine with epinephrine as I withdraw the spinal needle and then infiltrate more local anesthetic into the superficial incision with a hypodermic needle. When I have remarked the optimal location for the incision, the operation is ready to begin. Throughout the entire incision planning process, I maintain the fluoroscope in position to optimize the flow of the surgery. After all, securing the minimal access port is only moments away and moving the fluoroscopy unit back and forth only results in inefficiency.

3.8 Surgical Technique

After making an 18-mm incision with a No. 15 blade, I use cautery to dissect down to the fascia. Understandably, I cannot directly see the spinous process since the incision is off the midline, but I still recognize the importance of that structure to establish my bearings. So, in place of visual input, I use tactile input. Direct palpation of the tip of the spinous process with an index finger confirms the midline and allows me to reconstruct the anatomy at depth in my mind's eye. The additional tactile information provides me with the certainty needed to select the location of my fascial opening. To ensure that I can angulate appropriately onto the lamina, I use the cautery to make a fascial opening approximately 2 cm lateral to the midline based on my palpation of the spinous process. The fascial opening needs to be only slightly larger than the skin incision, which facilitates the rostral–caudal adjustments for the 25-mm exposure.

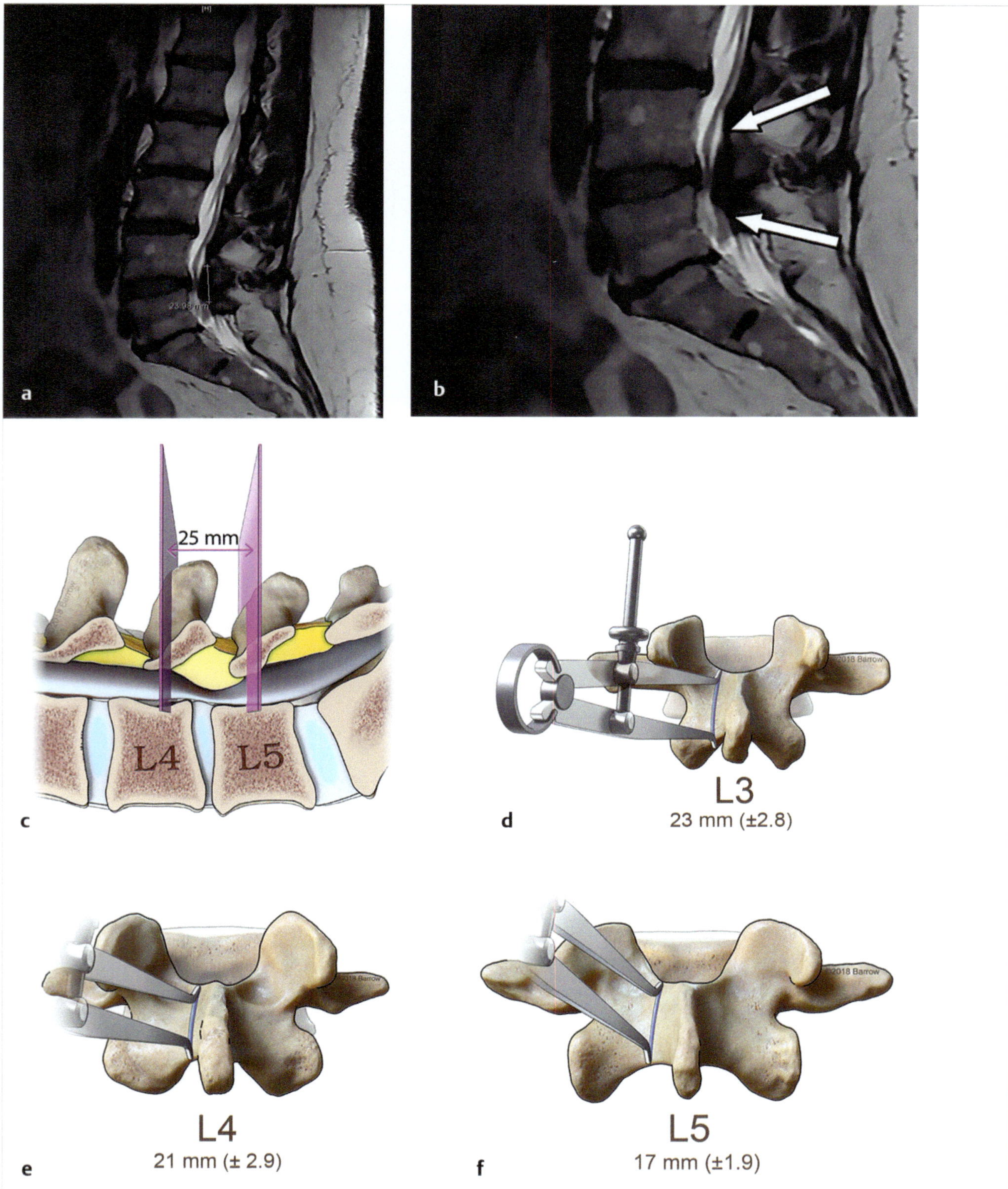

Fig. 3.12 Sagittal T2-weighted magnetic resonance imaging (MRI) demonstrating that **(a)** the distance from the rostral insertion point of the ligamentum flavum to the caudal insertion point is a distance of approximately 25 mm. **(b)** Sagittal T2-weighted MRI demonstrates the insertion points (*arrows*) that are the target for resection in a minimally invasive lumbar laminectomy. **(c)** An illustration of the distance from rostral insertion to caudal insertion of the ligamentum flavum into the lamina of a segment. The distance from insertion point to insertion point is seldom more than 25 mm. Posterior view of **(d)** L3, **(e)** L4 and **(f)** L5 laminae showing laminar measurements that further demonstrate the anatomic basis for a minimally invasive approach.

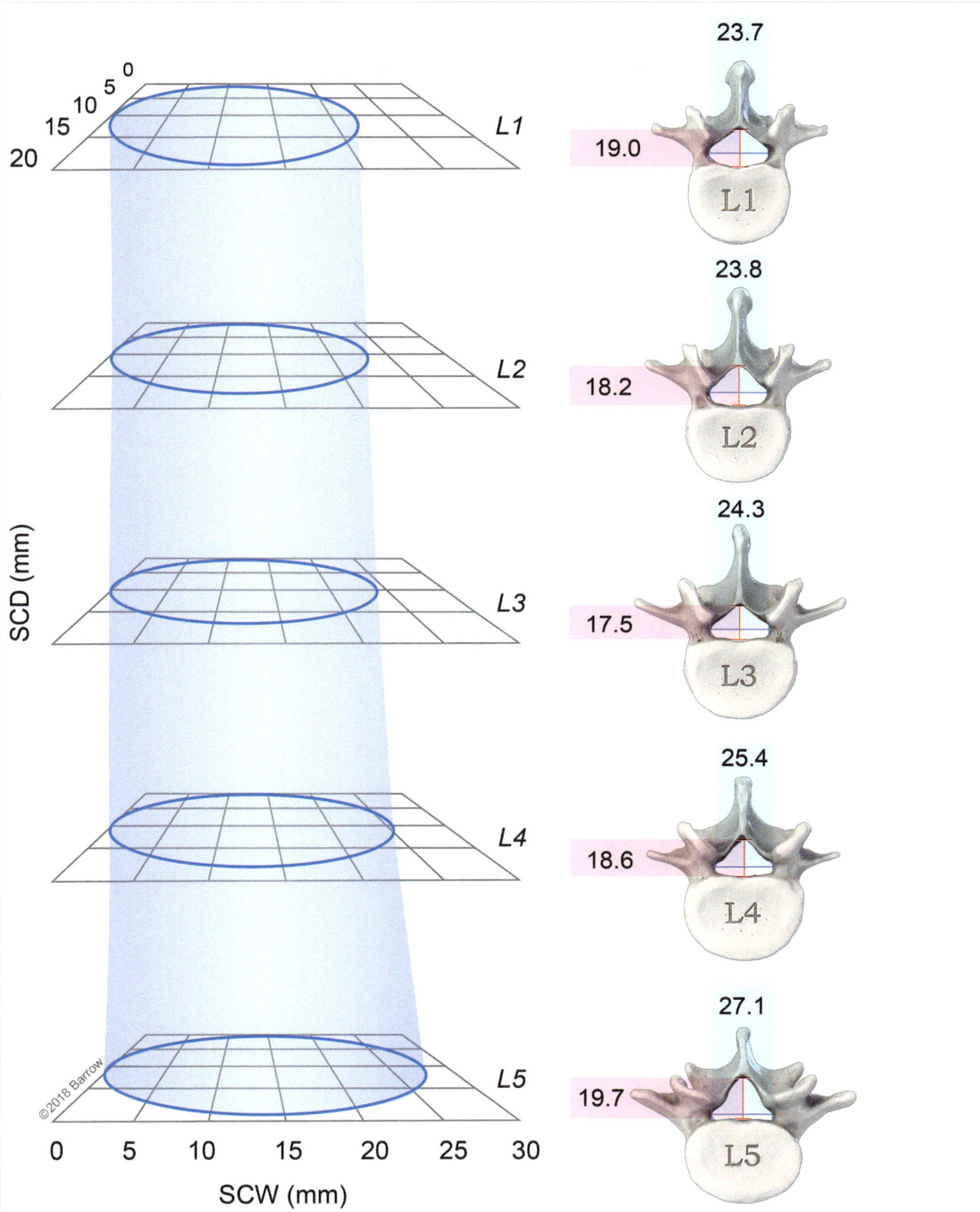

Fig. 3.13 An illustration demonstrating the varying depths and widths of the lumbar canal. The canal is widest at L5 with a measurement of 27.1 mm as reported by Panjabi and colleagues.[14] Access to the central canal through a unilateral hemilaminectomy measuring 16–18 mm will reliably provide access to the entire central canal. Abbreviations: SCD, spinal canal diameter; SCW, spinal canal width.

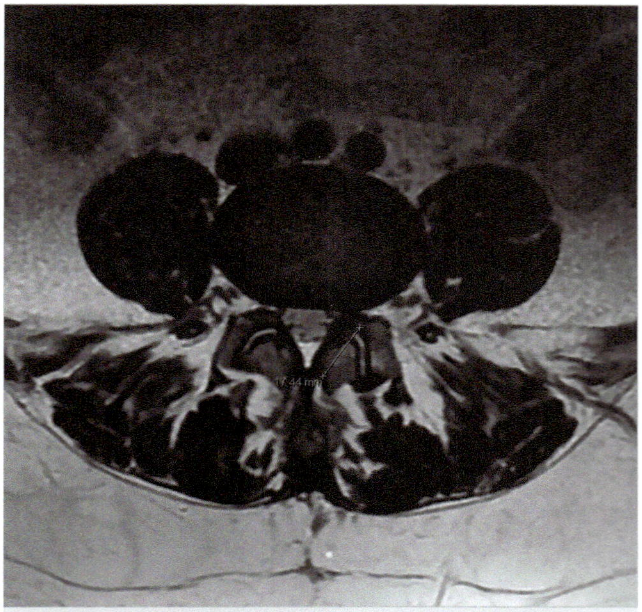

Fig. 3.14 Axial T2-weighted magnetic resonance imaging of the lumbar spine demonstrating that one limb of the triangle measures approximately 18 mm.

3.9 Dilating and Docking the Retractor

I insert the first dilator through the fascial opening at an angle of approximately 15 to 25 degrees (▶ Fig. 3.21). As I pass the first dilator, I am anticipating the unmistakable tactile feedback of a metallic tip encountering bone. Once I encounter the lamina, I firmly anchor the dilator onto lamina and begin to probe the anatomy to establish the boundaries of my exposure (▶ Fig. 3.21). The goal is to confirm my ability to reach the limits of the spinal canal. The term "wanding" has entered the minimally invasive spinal vernacular to describe this technique. Wanding encompasses the following: sounding the anatomy; confirming structures, such as the confluence of the lamina and the spinous process; and sweeping over the top of the anatomy with the dilator to establish a plane of dissection. Wanding allows for accessing different regions of the spinal segment at various trajectories to reach all aspects of the spinal canal: rostral, caudal, medial, and lateral.

In the lower lumbar levels (L4–5 and L5–S1), the diameter of the first dilator is small enough to pass through the interlaminar space and into the canal, especially when the patient is positioned on a fully expanded Wilson frame, which, by design, opens the interlaminar space. A slight upward trajectory away

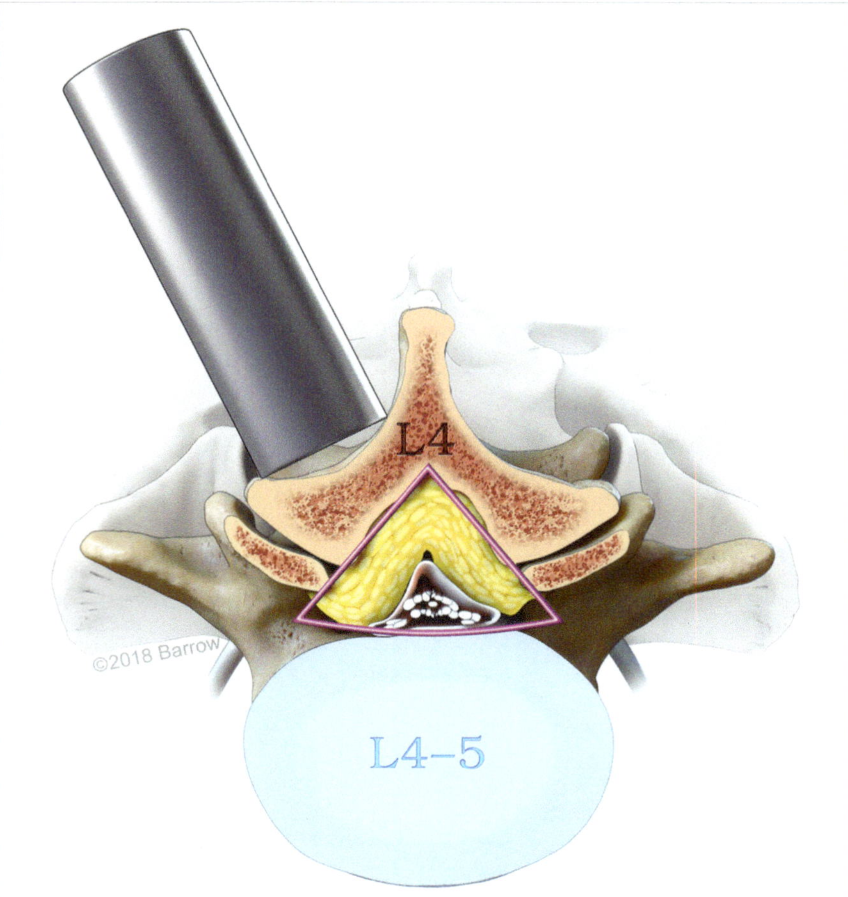

Fig. 3.15 A conceptual drawing of a minimal access port anchored onto one limb of the triangle. The trajectory of the access port in the axial plane should be parallel to the adjacent side of the lamina.

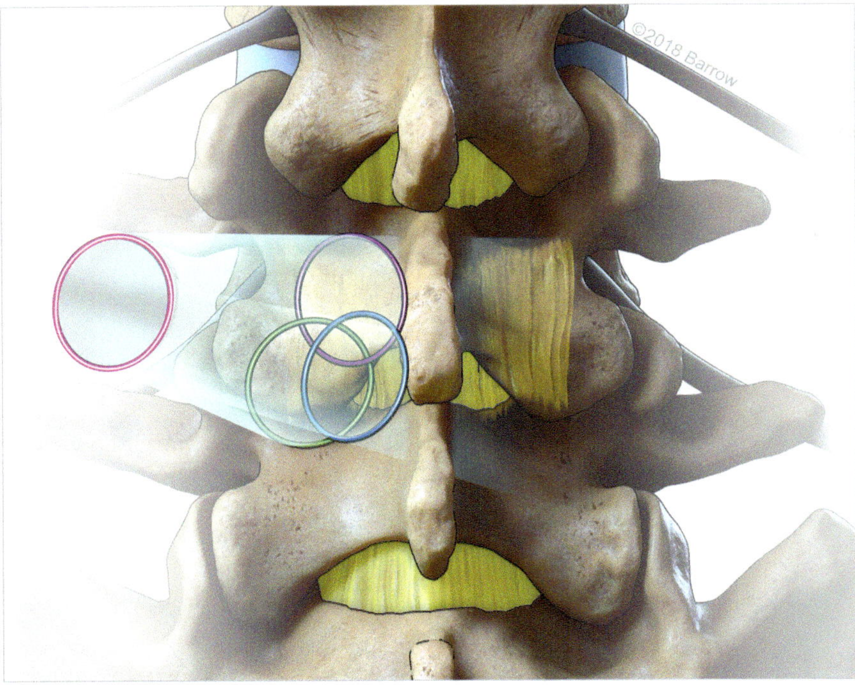

Fig. 3.16 Artist's illustration showing three concentric circles of exposure that indicate how subtle repositioning of the minimal access port allows sequential access to the insertion points of the ligamentum flavum along with the contralateral and ipsilateral canal.

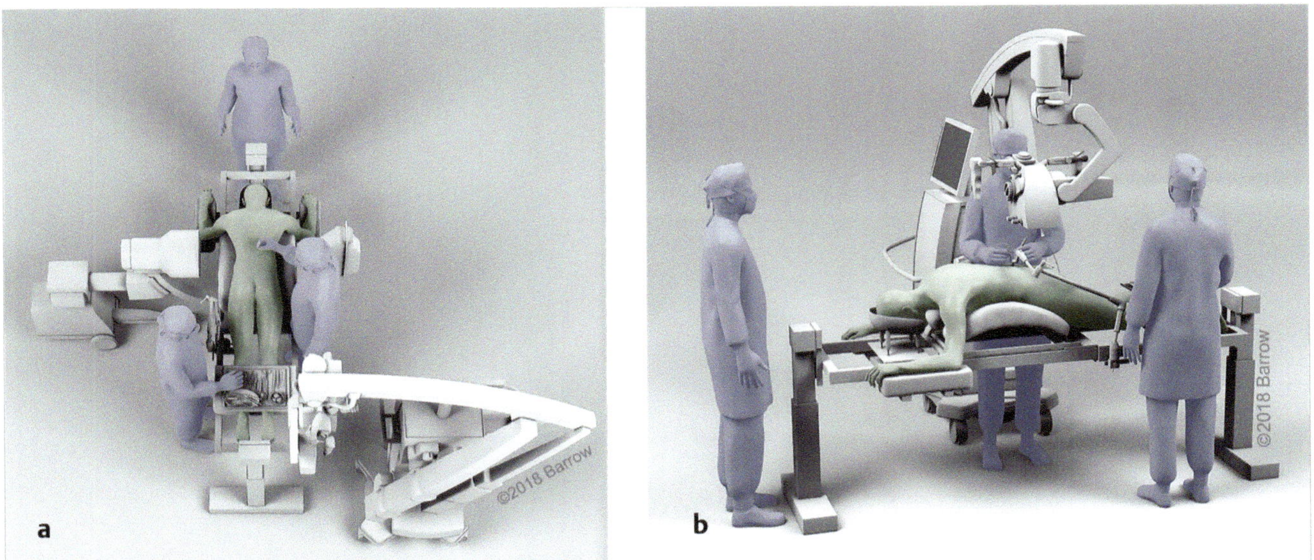

Fig. 3.17 Illustration of the operating room setup, which is identical to the setup for a minimally invasive microdiscectomy. **(a)** Bird's-eye view of a patient undergoing an L4–5 laminectomy with a right-sided approach. In this image, the surgeon is confirming the level and planning the incision. The patient is positioned on a Jackson table atop a Wilson frame. The fluoroscope is in position at the start of case with the image intensifier on the opposite side of the surgeon and the microscope at the ready on the same side as the surgeon. Having all components in position optimizes the efficiency of the operation. **(b)** Lateral view of the operating room once the minimal access port has been secured. The fluoroscope transitions out as the microscope rolls into position.

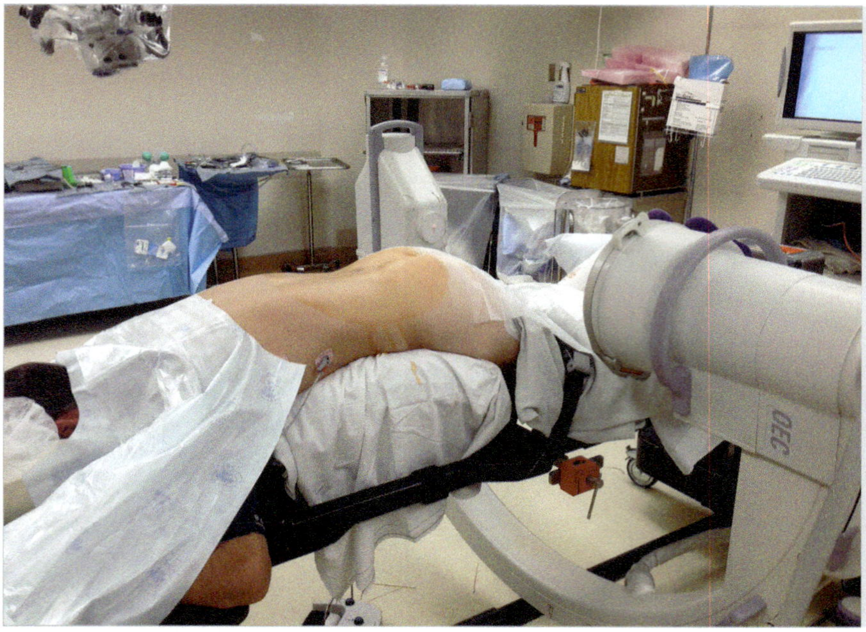

Fig. 3.18 Intraoperative photograph demonstrating operating room setup. This patient has predominantly left-sided symptoms. The draped microscope stands on the symptomatic side. The image intensifier component of the fluoroscope remains opposite the microscope. The microscope also stands at the ready on the side of the approach draped to optimize the flow of the operation.

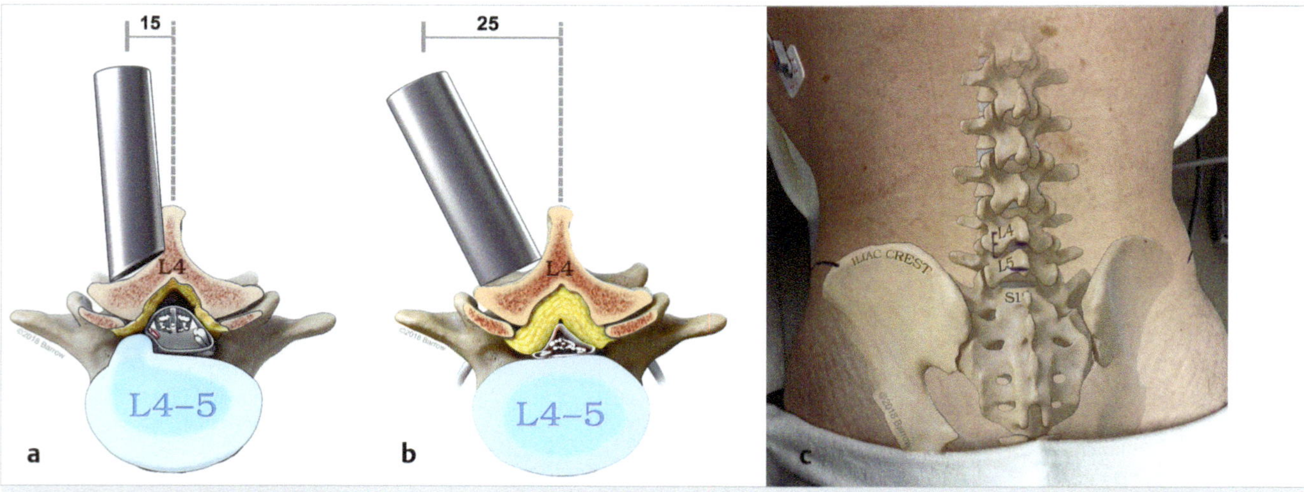

Fig. 3.19 Trajectories for microdiscectomy and laminectomy. **(a)** Illustration of the straighter trajectory for microdiscectomy to be immediately over the traversing root and lateral aspect of the thecal sac. For such a trajectory, an incision 1.5 cm from the midline is optimal. **(b)** Illustration demonstrating a greater angle of convergence onto the lamina to access the entire canal. Planning an incision 20–25 mm lateral to the spinous process will optimize that trajectory. **(c)** Intraoperative photo of a planned incision for an L4–5 laminectomy, with superimposition of the spinal anatomy on the patient.

from the interlaminar space will therefore reliably land the tip of the first dilator onto the lamina. At that point, wanding with a medial trajectory allows the tip of the dilator to encounter the base of the spinous process (▶ Fig. 3.22). The docking point is the key difference between wanding in minimally invasive microdiscectomy and minimally invasive laminectomy. Although I dock the first dilator in a microdiscectomy at the lamina facet junction and immediately over the nerve root and lateral thecal sac, in a laminectomy, I dock the first dilator at the junction of the spinous process and lamina. Doing so allows the trajectory necessary to decompress the entire thecal sac (▶ Fig. 3.23).

When the first dilator encounters the junction of the lamina and the spinous process, I obtain the first lateral fluoroscopic image (▶ Fig. 3.21b). I maintain a trajectory parallel to the disc space similar to that for a microdiscectomy but in a higher axial plane. The higher axial plane allows the access port to encompass the rostral insertion of the ligamentum flavum. I then dilate the incision up to 16 to 18 mm, depending on the diameter of the access port selected, and I pass the appropriate length minimal access port over the dilators and firmly anchor it onto the spinous process lamina junction with a medial convergence as illustrated in ▶ Fig. 3.24 and ▶ Fig. 3.25. I can minimize muscle creeping in from around the perimeter of the access port by placing downward pressure as my assistant secures the table-mounted arm into the stem of the access port. The goal is to optimize the interface of the lamina spinous process and the base of the access port.

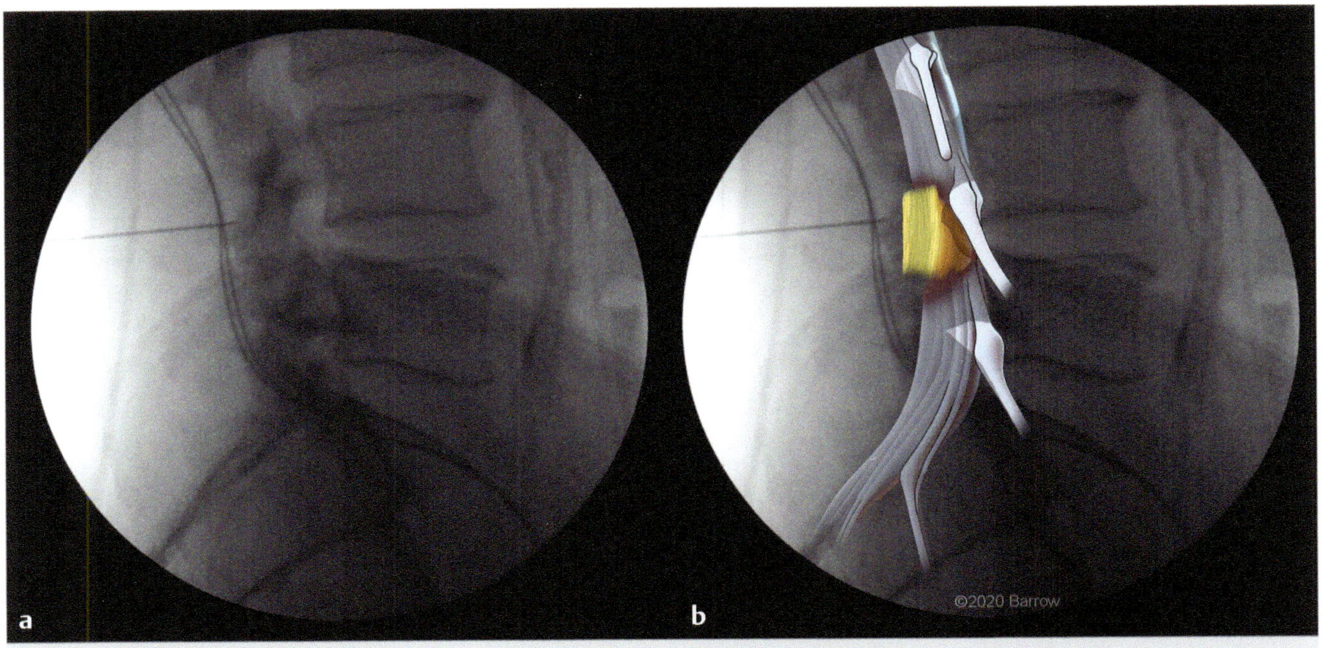

Fig. 3.20 Lateral fluoroscopic images showing localization of the level and planning the incision. **(a)** Confirmation of the L4–5 segment with a 20-gauge spinal needle. Note that the needle is pointing higher than the disc space and more to the rostral insertion of the ligamentum flavum. Planning the incision in the axial plane of the rostral insertion of the ligamentum flavum will allow immediate identification and release of that insertion once the lamina has been removed. With the level confirmed, the stylet is removed and the incision track infiltrated with local anesthetic. **(b)** A mental reconstruction of the anatomy at L4–5. Superimposed on the fluoroscopy image is the neural anatomical structures and the ligamentum flavum from rostral insertion to caudal insertion. The spinal needle points to the rostral insertion. In this image, it becomes readily evident that a 16- or 18-mm access point will encompass the rostral insertion.

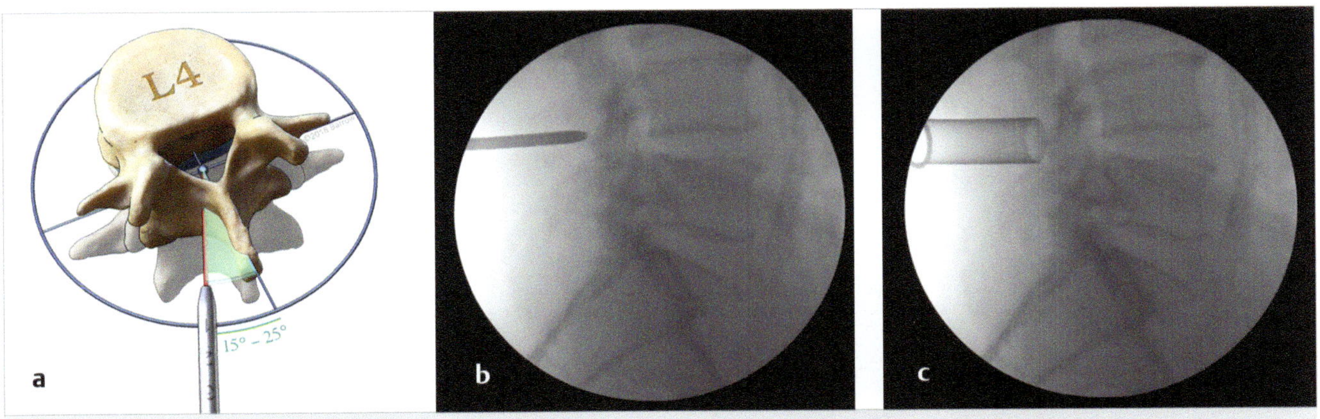

Fig. 3.21 Dilatation and securing the minimal access port for an L4–5 laminectomy. **(a)** Illustration demonstrating the trajectory onto the lamina to access the central canal. Beginning 20–25 mm off the midline and converging 15 to 25 degrees onto the lamina points the dilator at the geometric center of the canal. **(b)** Lateral fluoroscopic image demonstrating the first dilator docked onto the lamina. The first dilator is slightly rostral on the superior lamina. The goal is to have the first dilator pointing to the rostral insertion of the ligamentum flavum in the same axial plane that the spinal needle was moments ago. **(c)** Lateral fluoroscopic image with a 16-mm minimal access port in position completely parallel to the disc space but in a higher axial plane for access to the rostral insertion of the ligamentum flavum.

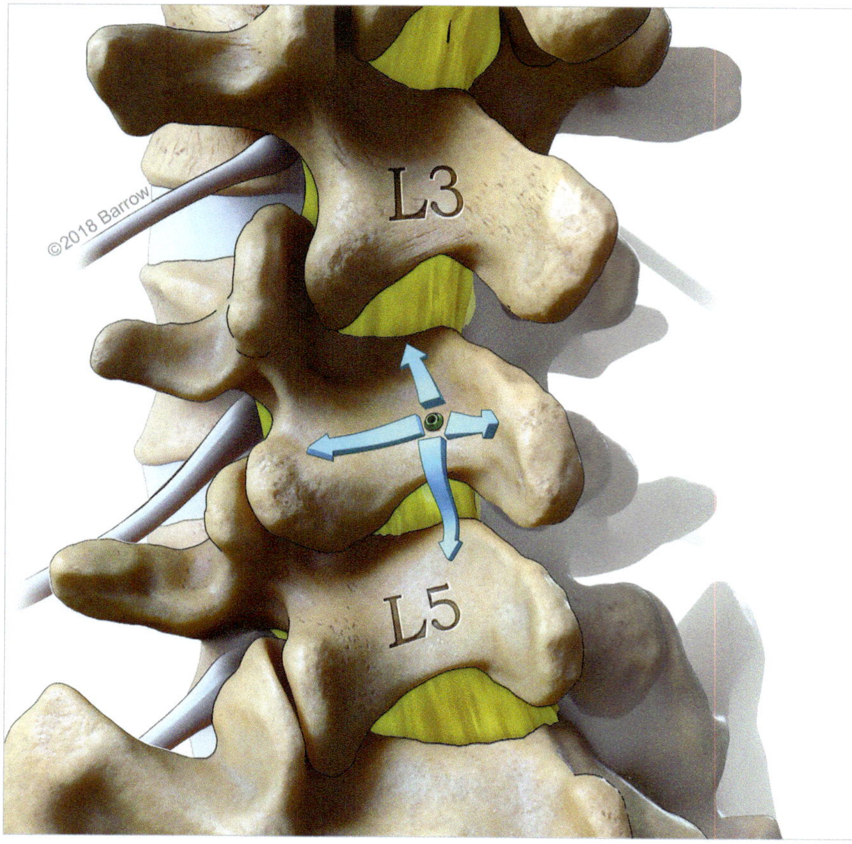

Fig. 3.22 Illustration for wanding of an L4–5 minimally invasive laminectomy. The first dilator is used to provide tactile feedback to the surgeon regarding the location of the spinous process–lamina junction and the lamina–facet junction. The intended target for securing the minimal access port is indicated by the *green fiducial* marker. By probing in the direction demonstrated by the *blue arrows*, the surgeon can begin to reconstruct the anatomy at depth. It is important to have an appreciation of the interlaminar space in order to access the caudal insertion of the ligamentum flavum.

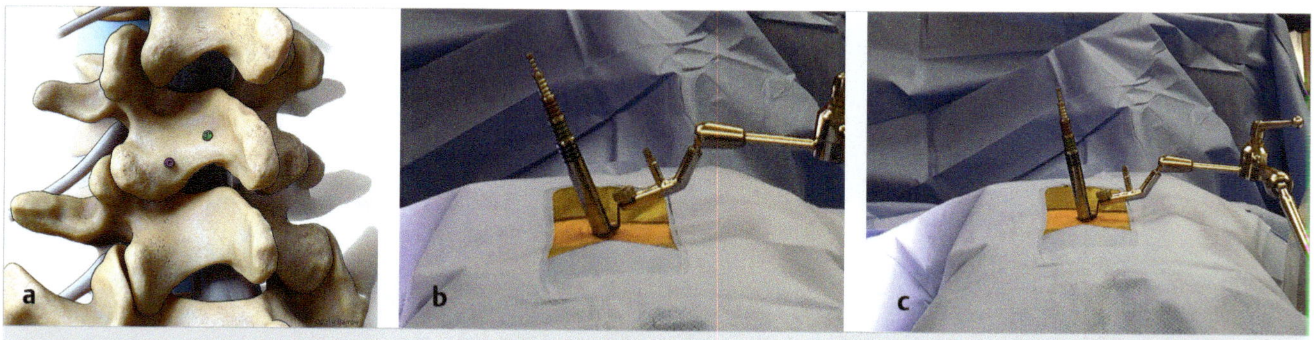

Fig. 3.23 Docking target for the minimally invasive laminectomy versus microdiscectomy. **(a)** Illustration demonstrating the two distinct targets for the first dilator in a lumbar microdiscectomy and a lumbar laminectomy. In a microdiscectomy, the first dilator is essentially pointing to the affected nerve root. Therefore, the target for the dilator and eventual minimal access port is more lateral. In this image, the microdiscectomy target is denoted by a *magenta fiducial*. For a laminectomy, the target is the rostral insertion point of the ligamentum flavum in the geometric center of the canal. The result is a more rostral and medial position as denoted by the *emerald fiducial*. **(b)** Intraoperative photograph demonstrating a minimal access port in position for a laminectomy. The angle of convergence is approximately 20 to 25 degrees. **(c)** Intraoperative photograph of a minimal access port in position for a microdiscectomy. The angle of convergence is significantly less at 10 to 15 degrees.

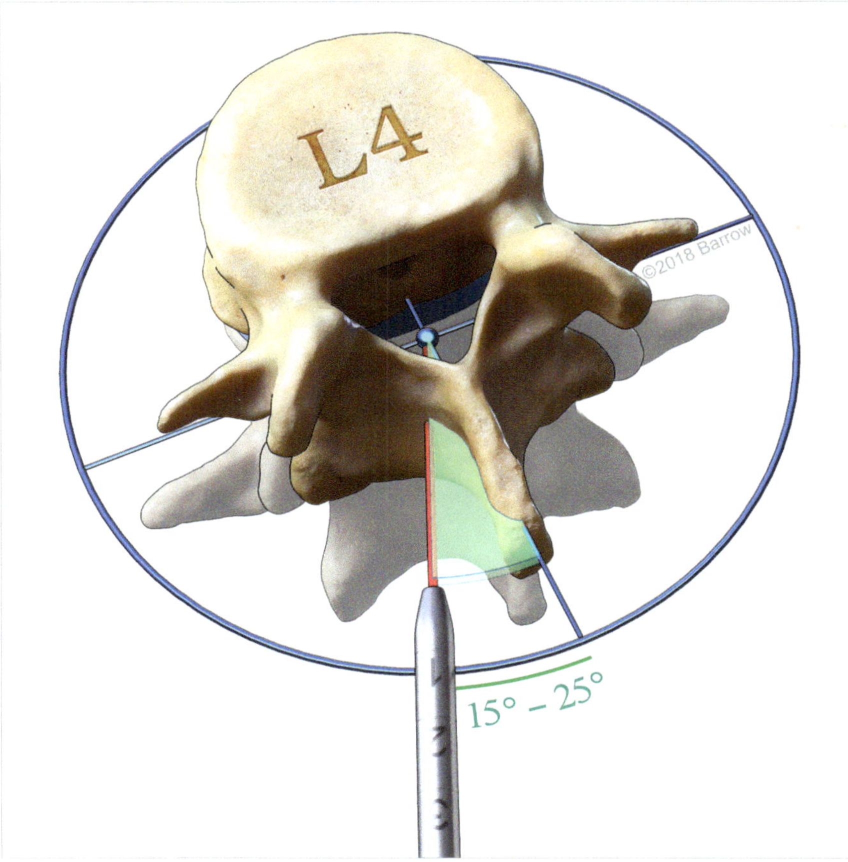

Fig. 3.24 Illustration demonstrating the trajectory onto the lamina to access the central canal. Beginning 20 to 25 mm off of the midline and converging 15 to 25 degrees onto the lamina points the dilator at the geometric center of the canal.

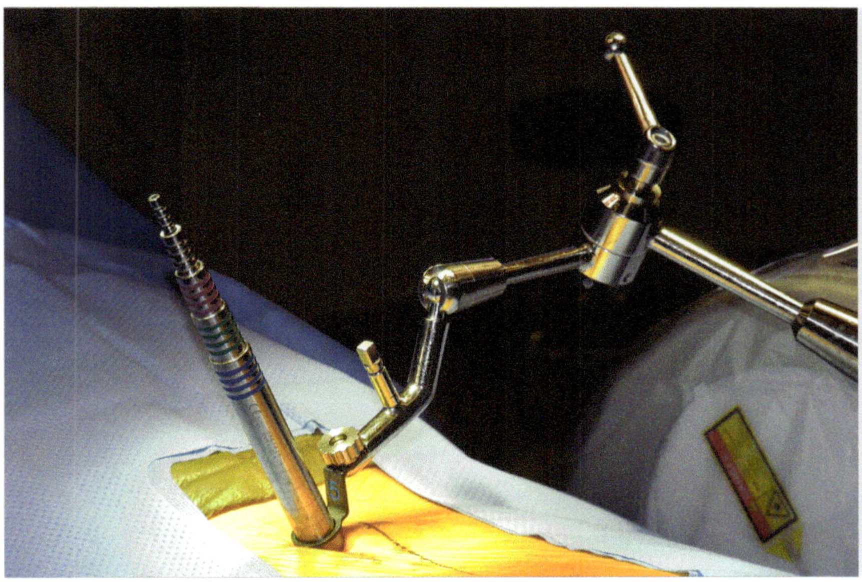

Fig. 3.25 Intraoperative photograph demonstrating the minimal access port in position with the dilators still in place. Keeping the entire series of dilators allows a better determination of the degree of convergence.

To ensure the appropriate trajectory, I anchor the port onto the table-mounted frame while the radiology technician takes the third fluoroscopic image. After I anchor the port into position, I ensure that there is a medial trajectory of at least 15 to 25 degrees. The radiology technician then rotates the fluoroscope for an anteroposterior (AP) image, which is the fourth and final fluoroscopic image. The AP image confirms that the most distal and medial aspect of the port is docked against the junction of the base of the spinous process and lamina. The AP image also provides additional cues to the anatomy that will help your mind reconstruct the anatomy at depth (▶ Fig. 3.26).

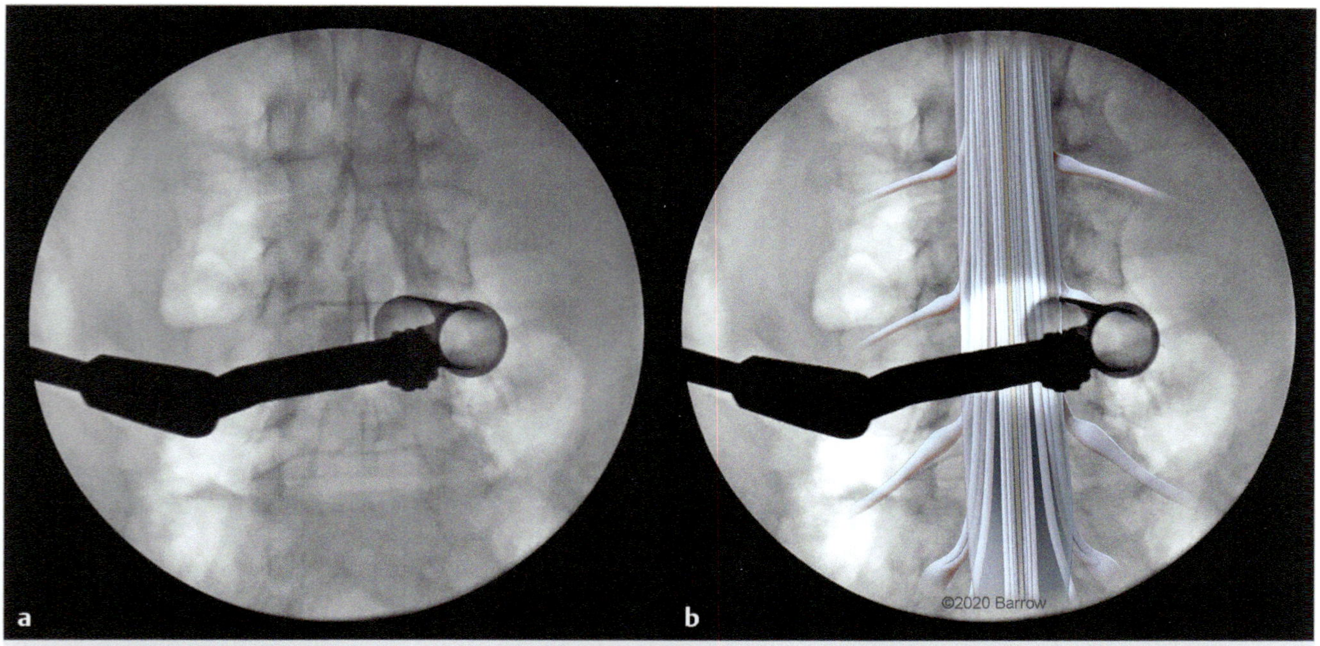

Fig. 3.26 Positioning the minimal access port for a laminectomy. **(a)** Anteroposterior fluoroscopic image demonstrating the medial aspect of the minimal access port abutting the base of the spinous process and converging toward the midline. The angulation places the center of the access port over the thecal sac, which is distinct from the position used for a microdiscectomy. **(b)** Anteroposterior fluoroscopic image with thecal sac and nerve roots superimposed onto the image. Reconstruction of the anatomy at depth in the mind's eye begins with positioning of the access port. The light shining on the thecal sac represents the extent of decompression that will be accomplished from the inside out.

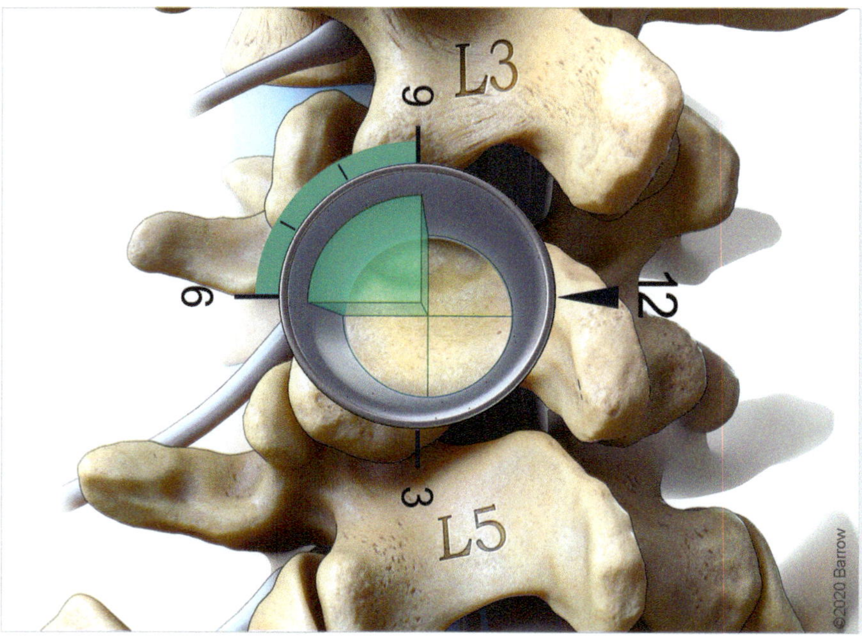

Fig. 3.27 Sequence of exposure for laminectomy. Illustration of the L4–5 with a minimal access port in the initial position for a laminectomy. The safe zone to begin the exposure is in the outer quadrant (6 to 9 o'clock) of the minimal access port. Once the lamina is exposed in that quadrant, exposure proceeds medially to the 9 to 12 o'clock and then inferomedial to the 12 to 3 o'clock quadrant. Care is taken in exposing the 3 to 6 o'clock quadrant to avoid encountering the facet capsule. The interlaminar space is not always seen in the initial position of the access port.

On a good day, when the microscope is brought in and focused through the port, you will be looking at more bone of the lamina than muscle. The thin cuff of muscle that remains readily peels away with cautery. I prefer to begin exposing the upper outer quadrant (6 to 9 o'clock) within the access port, where lamina most assuredly resides at the bottom (▶ Fig. 3.27). When I have unequivocally encountered the lamina, I brush away the veil of muscle in a lateral to medial direction. In doing so, I have exposed the base of the spinous process in the 9 to 12 o'clock position of the access port. Visualization of the base of the spinous process and the lamina in these quadrants allows for the dissection to proceed confidently in the caudal direction. After all, I now know my position relative to the midline. I complete the exposure of the entire 16- to 18-mm circumference (6 to 12 o'clock). A well-positioned port allows for exposure of the base of the spinous process, the

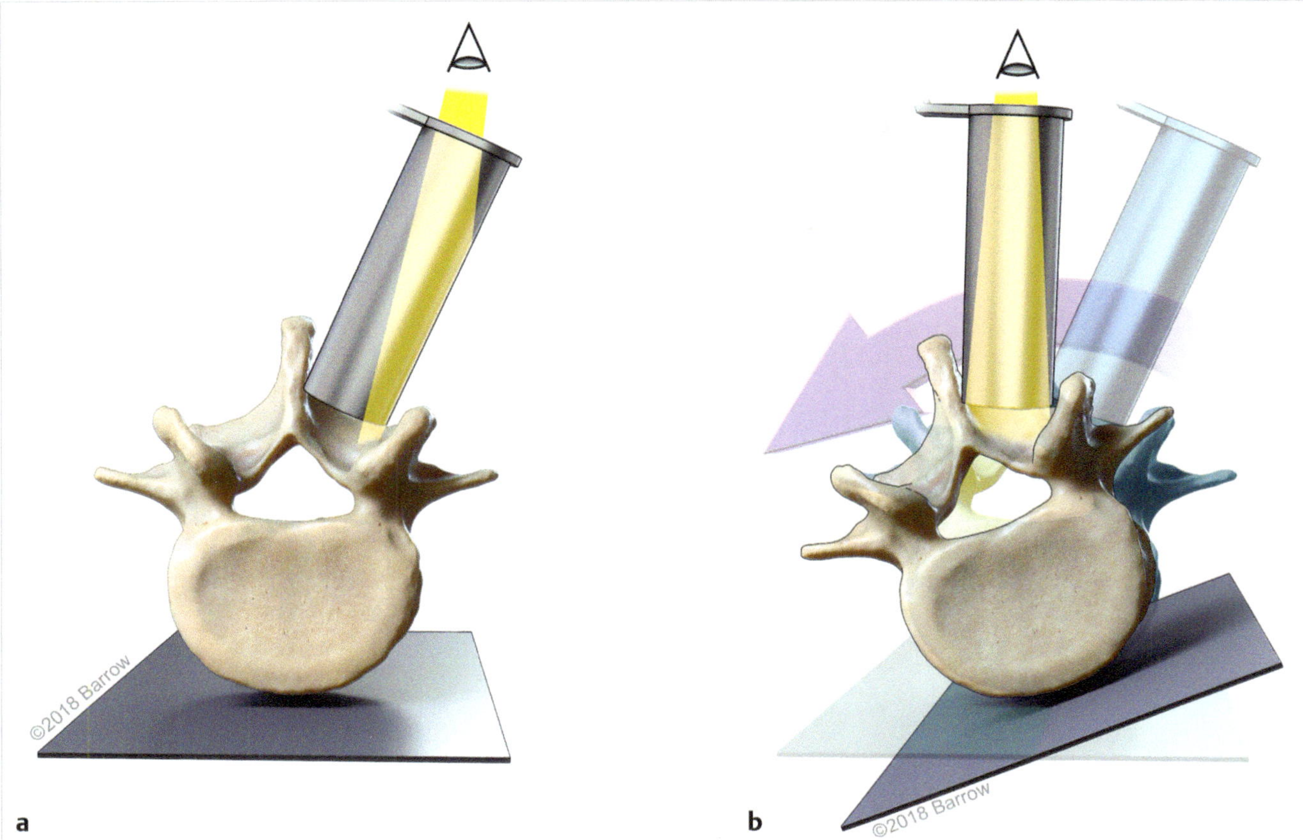

Fig. 3.28 Rotation of the bed for optimal working trajectory. Illustration of the axial perspective of the lumbar spine. **(a)** Without rotation, the angle of convergence onto the spine makes it challenging to visualize and access the contralateral recess. The line of sight onto the lamina in the unrotated bed, as demonstrated by the beam of light onto the lamina, places the surgeon in a suboptimal working angle. **(b)** Rotation of the bed, as indicated by the purple arrow, optimizes a working trajectory through the minimal access port onto the lamina and the contralateral recess. As demonstrated by the beam of light, the line of sight is directly onto the confluence of the lamina and base of the spinous process providing an ideal ergonomic working angle for the contralateral recess. The bed will be rotated back to its initial position and the access port straightened for decompression of the ipsilateral nerve root.

lamina and the medial facet as seen in ▶ Fig. 3.19. The interlaminar space will be at the caudal-most aspect of the exposure but may not be readily visible with the initial position of the access port.

3.10 Drilling

Before taking a drill to the lamina, I have the anesthesiologist rotate the bed away from me as I peer down through the microscope. I watch as the distal diameter of the access port comes into full view, stopping the rotation when I have an optimal line of sight and working angle. That maneuver will provide an ideal trajectory to the contralateral side (▶ Fig. 3.28). Rotation of the bed also allows the trajectory to become more vertical and therefore offer a more ergonomic position for the surgeon (Video 3.1). A drill with a minimally invasive attachment will maximize visibility at depth within the minimal access port and is essential for this procedure.

Identifying the base of the spinous process is the essential first step. Not only is it the initial target for the drill, but it is an important landmark that will establish your bearings and keep you oriented in what can be an unfamiliar perspective and working angle. It is imperative to unequivocally identify the confluence of the lamina blending into the spinous process prior to ever stepping on the drill pedal. Locking onto this target with an appropriate trajectory allows you to undercut the spinous process and drill into the underside of the contralateral lamina to access the contralateral recess (▶ Fig. 3.29).

There are three preliminary objectives that I keep in mind as I begin drilling. The first objective is to identify the rostral insertion of the ligamentum flavum. The second objective is to reach the contralateral recess of the canal, and the third objective is to reach the caudal insertion of the ligamentum flavum.

I begin drilling at the base of the spinous process in a rostral caudal sequence as if I were mowing a lawn. As the drill removes the outer cortex of the lamina, the cancellous bone beneath will quickly become evident. After I expose the cancellous bone at the base of the spinous process, I continue to drill beneath the spinous process until the tip of the drill begins to remove the underside of the contralateral lamina. It is that component of the bone work that will eventually grant me

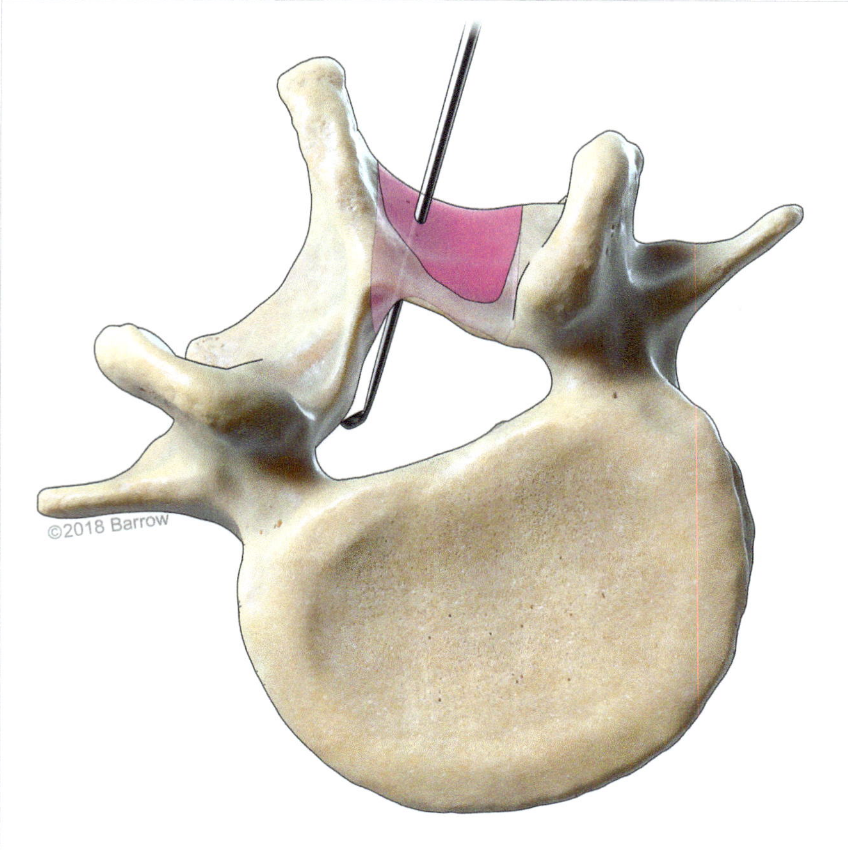

Fig. 3.29 Access to the contralateral recess. Illustration demonstrating how rotation of the bed away from the surgeon allows a more optimal trajectory through the access port and more ergonomic position for the surgeon to reach the midline and contralateral recess.

access to the contralateral recess for decompression. From undercutting the spinous process, I shift my focus to the lateral aspect of the exposure. I widen the drilling area laterally from the midline toward the pars interarticularis encompassing the area demonstrated in ▶ Fig. 3.30. As with an open laminectomy, a full 10 mm of the lateral aspect of the pars interarticularis should be preserved to minimize the risk of instability. It is always important to consider the three-dimensional anatomy while drilling because the topography and depth of the lamina can vary.

After undercutting the spinous process and drilling the underside of the contralateral lamina, my focus turns to thinning the lamina over the remaining area of the planned bone work. I feel most comfortable drilling on the caudal aspect of the lamina where I know a thick carpet of ligamentum flavum covers the thecal sac. There, the tip of the drill may breach the inner lamina and safely encounter the thickened ligamentum flavum. I continue to thin the remaining lamina in all directions from that initial breach. I keep in perspective the valuable reference point provided to me by the laminar breach, which tells me the depth of the ligamentum flavum as I thin the lamina toward its rostral insertion point. I ensure a substantial layer of ligamentum between the tip of the drill and the thecal sac until I am certain about where the insertion of the ligamentum flavum resides (▶ Fig. 3.31a).

After the ligamentum becomes evident from the laminar breach and the remaining lamina has the thickness of a shrimp shell, I develop a plane over the top of the ligamentum flavum with a small forward-angled curet. The footplate of a Kerrison can now enter the plane beneath the thinned laminar bone and the ligamentum flavum and remove what remains of the lamina (▶ Fig. 3.31b). I use the Kerrison to continue working in the rostral direction until I have removed the lamina above the rostral ligamentum flavum insertion. As I work rostrally, the tapering strands of the ligamentum flavum that give way to epidural fat are the telltale signs that I have accomplished my first objective: I am above the insertion of the ligamentum flavum at that segment (▶ Fig. 3.32).

As the ligamentum flavum inserts into its rostral insertion point, it tapers considerably. I look for that tapered insertion point at the rostral component of my laminotomy. I continue to work only with the Kerrison until I am above the entire rostral insertion of the ligamentum flavum for the segment. I emphasize once again that I attempt only to thin the bone to a shrimp shell thickness with the drill at the rostral aspect of my laminotomy where the ligamentum flavum beneath the lamina is thinnest if not altogether absent. The rostral-most aspect of the laminotomy defect should be beyond the level of the insertion of the ligamentum flavum, and accordingly, there will be no ligamentum flavum protecting the tip of the drill from the thecal sac. That is the area where the thecal sac is most susceptible to injury. So, once I establish an opening in the lamina over the top of the ligamentum at the more rostral part of the laminotomy, I use only the Kerrison to remove the remaining bone. Using the drill in this area of the lamina is ill-advised. The dura lies vulnerably underneath that part of the lamina, and the tip

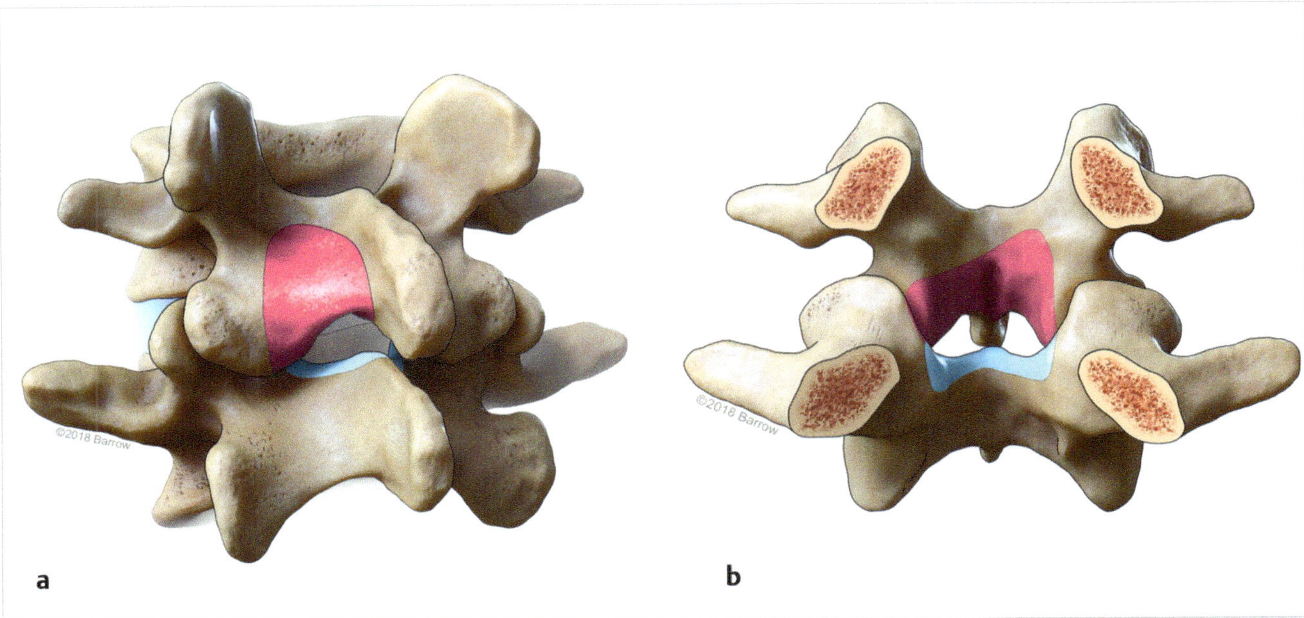

Fig. 3.30 The area of bone work for a minimally invasive laminectomy. **(a)** Artist's illustration showing the posterior lateral view of the spine. The shaded areas represent the bone removal. The *magenta shaded area* represents the bone work performed on the rostral lamina and facet, whereas the *sky blue shaded area* is the bone removal for the caudal lamina. **(b)** A view from within the canal looking outward onto the underside of the lamina. Conceptualizing the bone work from this perspective furthers the three-dimensional understanding of the spine that facilitates the learning curve. Removing the bone from these areas will encompass the insertion points of the ligamentum flavum.

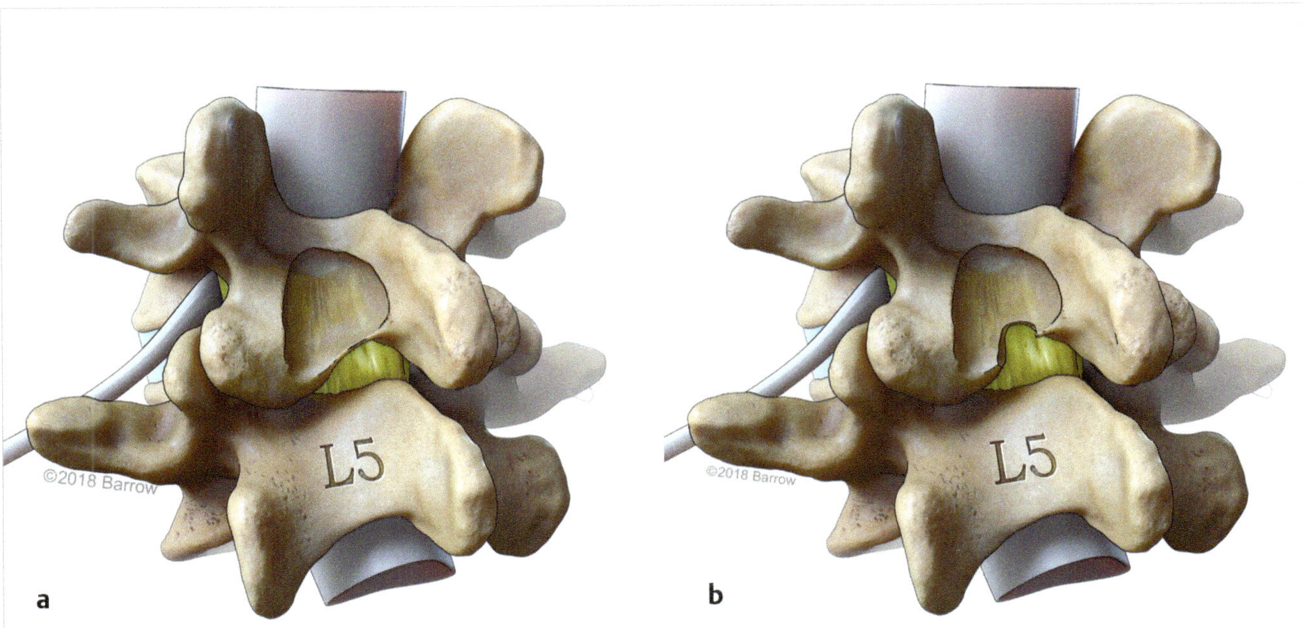

Fig. 3.31 Exposure of the ligamentum flavum. **(a)** Illustration of the preliminary bone work performed at the L4 lamina for an L4–5 decompression. In this illustration, the lamina has been thinned by drilling up to the rostral insertion of the ligamentum flavum. The base of the spinous process of L4 has been undercut and the contralateral lamina has been drilled. The ligamentum flavum becomes evident behind the thinning bone of the lamina. **(b)** A forward-angled curet establishes a plane of dissection beneath the lamina and above the ligamentum flavum. A Kerrison rongeur is then used to remove what remains of the lamina working beyond the rostral insertion of the ligamentum flavum.

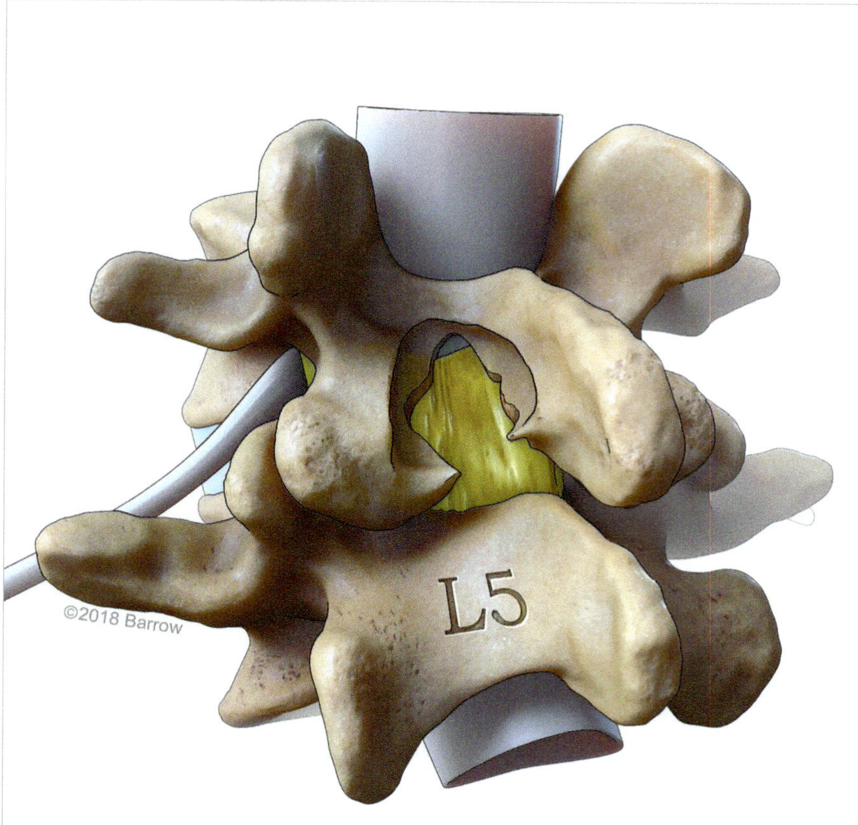

Fig. 3.32 Identification of the insertion of the ligamentum flavum. Illustration demonstrates removal of the L4 lamina up to the insertion of the ligamentum flavum. There is an unmistakable appearance of epidural fat that resides above the insertion of the ligamentum flavum. Once the rostral insertion of the ligamentum flavum is reached, I have accomplished the first objective.

of the drill has the uncanny ability to find it. I see no point in exposing the patient to such a risk once you have identified the limits of the ligamentum flavum insertion.

As soon as I reach the level of the ligamentum flavum insertion, I turn my attention caudal and contralateral, where there is an abundance of thickened ligamentum flavum protecting the thecal sac. I use the drill to continually thin the lamina on the underside of where the spinous process was undercut (▶ Fig. 3.33 and ▶ Fig. 3.34). The importance of keeping the ligamentum flavum intact for drilling the underside of the lamina cannot be emphasized enough. The thickened ligamentum is the most reliable protector of the dura. Continuing to work on the underside of the contralateral lamina facilitates the bilateral decompression as described by Härtl and colleagues.[12,15,16] My focus now shifts to the contralateral side, which will be out of reach once the access port is repositioned for the exposure of the ipsilateral nerve root.

I use a forward-angled curet to establish a plane of dissection between the thinned contralateral lamina and the ligamentum flavum. Then, I use a Kerrison punch to complete the laminectomy on the contralateral side, the midline and what I have access to on the ipsilateral side. Upon completion of this task, I have removed all the bone within my current exposure.

When I peer at the field of view at this point in the operation, I will be looking at the epidural fat and the thecal sac above the rostral insertion of the ligamentum flavum, along with a vast carpet of ligamentum flavum that extends in the caudal direction. In the rostral-most aspect of the exposure, I pass a right-angled ball-tipped probe between the ligamentum flavum and the thecal sac. The tip of that instrument will end up in a collection of epidural fat, a clear indication that I have removed the lamina into which the ligamentum flavum was once inserted. The probe encounters little if any resistance in this area. If only the thickened ligamentum flavum is visible, then the exposure is not rostral enough. The probe will not pass freely. Instead, the tip of the probe will find the insertion of the ligamentum flavum which remains firmly adhered to the underside of the lamina that still needs to be thinned and removed. Unlike in the microdiscectomy, there should be no need to divide the ligamentum flavum in a minimally invasive laminectomy. Instead, you need to identify the insertion and work above it.

If you do not see epidural fat, then it will be necessary to continue the bone work in a rostral direction until the epidural fat or the thecal sac is unequivocally visible. Otherwise, an incomplete decompression of the segment may result. Once the probe is beneath the ligamentum flavum, upward force on that probe or a forward-angled curet helps further establish a plane and ensure safe passage of the footplate of a Kerrison. Sometimes, the passage of the right-angled ball-tipped probe alone begins to separate the ligamentum from the insertion. Other times a small forward-angled curet will be needed to separate the ligamentum from the insertion.

Upon separating the ligamentum flavum from its rostral insertion, I continue to establish a plane of dissection between the ligamentum and the dura. I have two options: I can either begin with a direct resection of the ligamentum flavum with a Kerrison or identify the caudal insertion point of the ligamentum flavum for an en bloc resection of the ligament. Early in

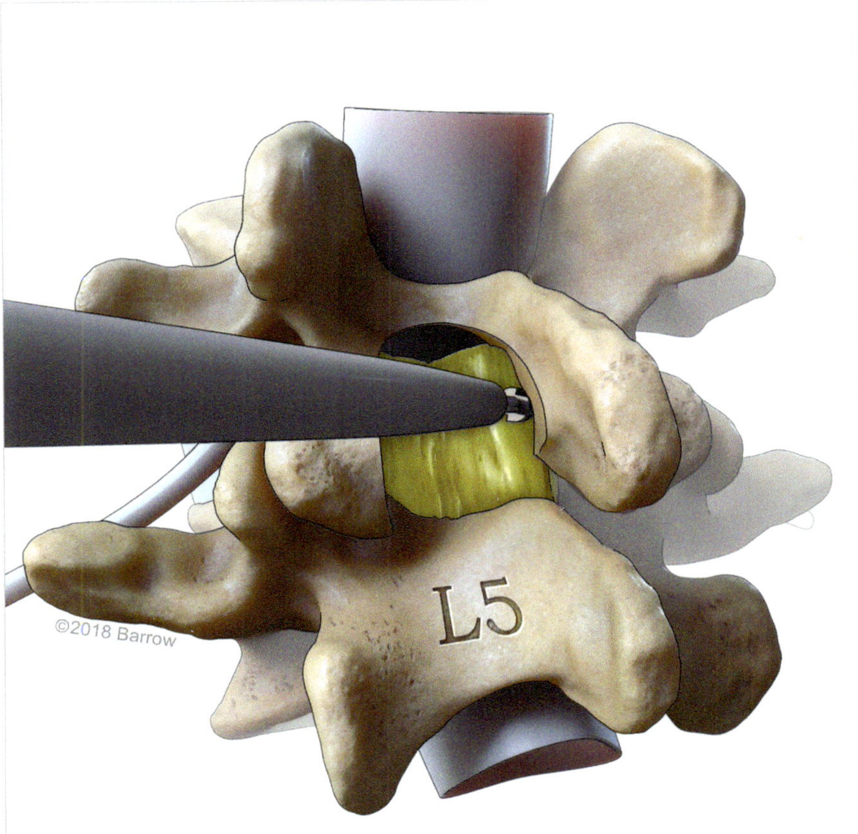

Fig. 3.33 Drilling the contralateral lamina. Illustration demonstrating the technique for drilling the contralateral lamina. To safely accomplish this task, the surgeon should keep the ligamentum flavum intact. The tip of the drill will pass over the top of the ligamentum flavum and into the contralateral recess. All the while, the thecal sac is safe from the tip of drill protected by the thickened ligamentum flavum.

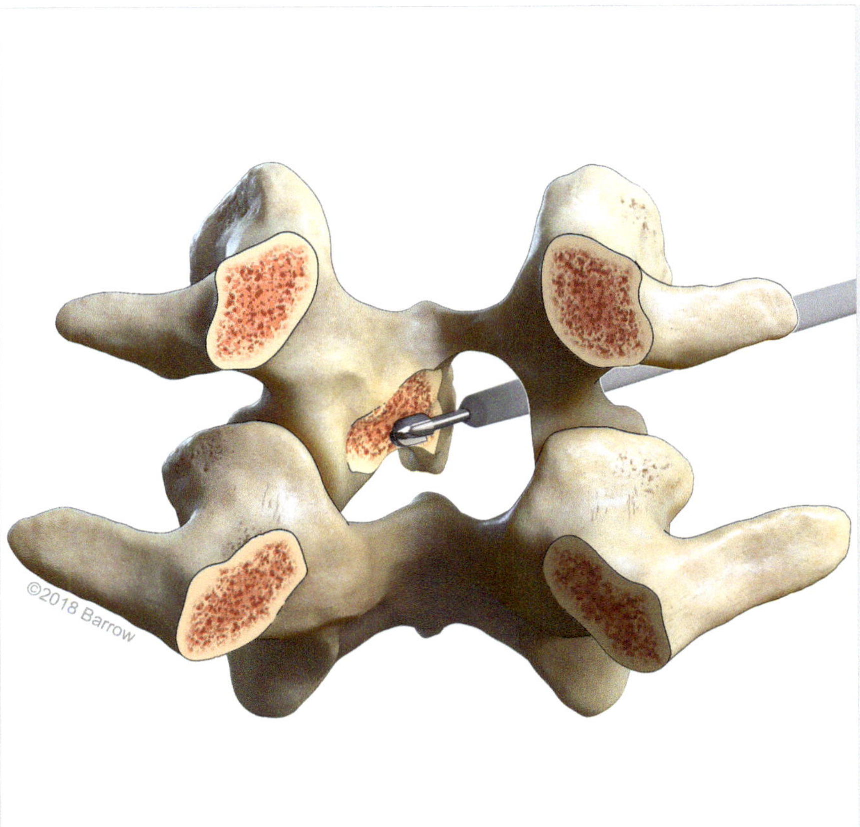

Fig. 3.34 Drilling the contralateral lamina. An illustration with a perspective from within the central canal. The illustration demonstrates the over-the-top removal of the contralateral lamina. As the drill removes the underside of the contralateral lamina, the thickened ligamentum flavum protects the thecal sac.

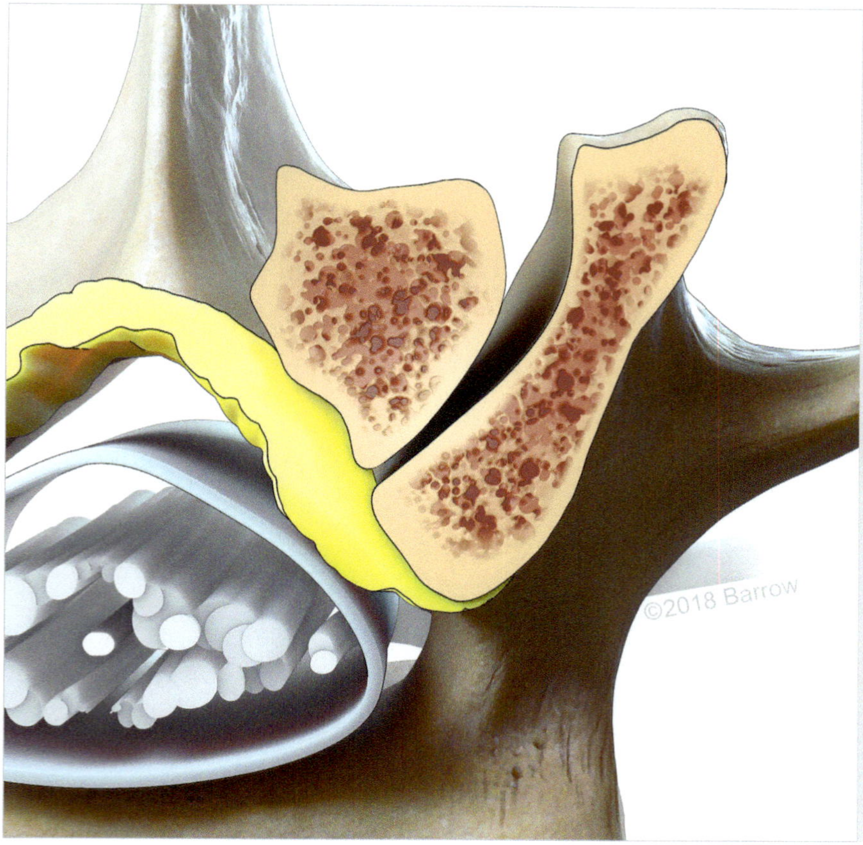

Fig. 3.35 Insertion of the ligamentum flavum in the medial facet. This illustration, adapted from an anatomical study of the ligamentum flavum performed by Yong-Hing and colleagues,[17] demonstrates the insertion of the ligamentum flavum on the underside of the medial facet.

your experience, a direct piecemeal resection of the ligament is advisable. As your experience with manipulation of the minimal access port develops, an en bloc resection of the ligamentum flavum will mitigate your risk of experiencing Kerrison-induced lateral epicondylitis.

3.11 Direct Resection

Direct resection of the ligamentum flavum involves its piecemeal removal with Kerrison rongeurs, pituitary forceps and curets until the segment is decompressed. I begin by using either a No. 2 or No. 3 Kerrison punch. I can safely resect large swaths of ligament in the midline, which affords me better visualization of the thecal sac. After performing a preliminary midline decompression, I focus the decompression on undercutting the ligamentum flavum on the contralateral side because the trajectory of the access port is optimized at this phase of the procedure.

I prefer a right-angled ball-tipped probe to ensure a safe plane between the dura and the ligamentum flavum. I also place a micro-cottonoid (0.25 × 0.25-inch patty) on the thecal sac to create a safe plane for the foot of the Kerrison to pass. With the patty in place, I can safely accomplish a contralateral resection of the ligamentum flavum with either a Kerrison punch or a forward-angled curet. A larger curet may be the more efficient instrument, as it can be safely passed over the top of the thecal sac and into the contralateral recess. The ligamentum flavum inserts on the underside of the medial facet, making it the target for the release of the ligamentum in the contralateral recess (▶ Fig. 3.35).[17]

With a forward-angled curet slipped into position between the facet and the thecal sac, you can exert upward force with the curet against the medial facet and safely begin to release the ligament from the lateral recess. Sometimes the ligament can be mobilized enough to remove it with pituitary forceps. Other times, a Kerrison punch is needed. The preliminary contralateral decompression is complete when the epidural fat in the contralateral recess becomes visible and the curvature of the thecal sac begins to fall away. I have reached the limit of what I can accomplish with the minimal access port in its current position. I have decompressed 16 mm of the segment, but my next target is out of reach. Once I have decompressed everything within the 16 mm of exposure offered by the minimal access port, it is time to reposition it over my next target: the caudal insertion of the ligamentum flavum (▶ Fig. 3.36).

I prefer to reposition the access port under direct visualization. To do so, I first place Gelfoam (Pfizer, Inc.) over the top of the decompressed thecal sac, zoom out the microscope, place the final dilator in the access port and have either the scrub technician or my assistant loosen the table-mounted arm most proximal to the port. I then redirect the port while maintaining the medial trajectory and downward angle. The new position and trajectory will allow me to reach the rostral aspect of the caudal lamina, where the inferior ligamentum flavum inserts. That is my next target. The new position will also allow me to complete the contralateral and caudal decompressions.

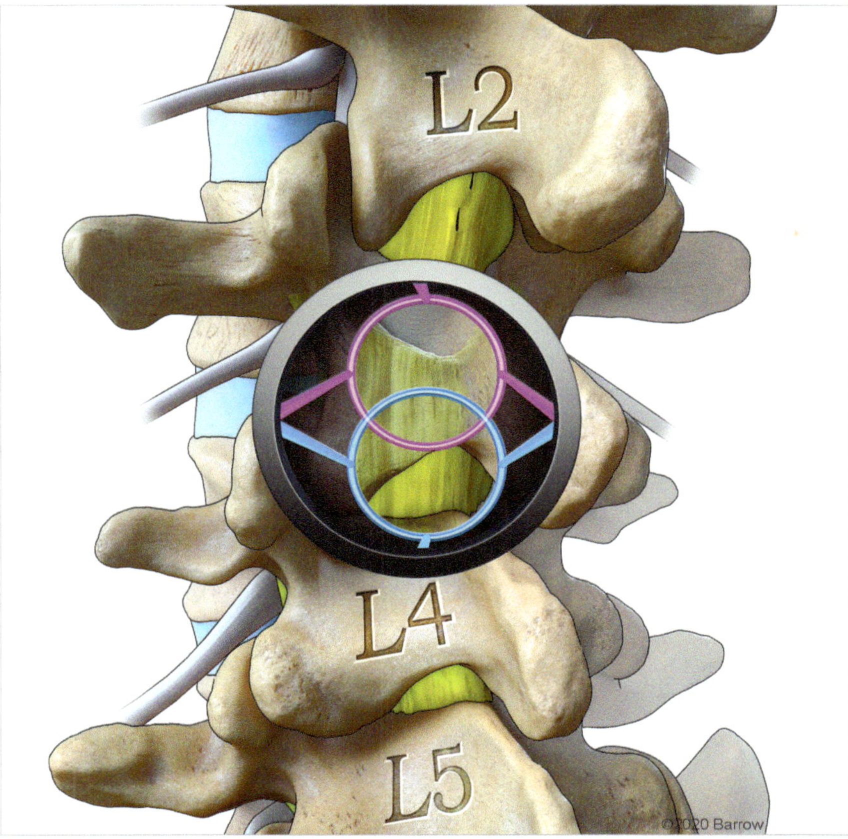

Fig. 3.36 Posterolateral perspective of the spine demonstrating the shift in trajectory of the minimal access port to incorporate first the rostral insertion point of the ligamentum flavum (*magenta ring*) and then the caudal insertion point of the ligamentum flavum *(turquoise ring)*. This transition allows a 25-mm exposure through a 16-mm access port.

With the minimal access port repositioned, I remove the final dilator and the Gelfoam and refocus the microscope. Within my field of view, I should be able to see at least 50% of my previous exposure of the dura and the remaining 50% of untouched anatomy. I simply continue along the plane of dissection over the top of the dura to decompress the thecal sac centrally before proceeding into the contralateral lateral recess to continue decompressing the contralateral thecal sac and contralateral nerve root. The goal is to pass a right-angled ball-tipped probe out of the contralateral neural foramen. Accomplishing this task requires the undercutting of an extensive amount of the ligamentum flavum. Drilling the underside of the contralateral lamina that I performed at the outset pays immediate dividends at this phase of the operation. The removal of that lamina affords a view of the contralateral ligamentum flavum from the inside out. As I continue to resect ligament, I find myself "falling off" the thecal sac and into the foramen. Creation of that corridor allows a Kerrison to slip under the contralateral facet to undercut the medial facet. That maneuver will release the ligamentum flavum from its lateral insertion point.

Finally, I complete the caudal-most aspect of the decompression by resecting the ligamentum flavum at its caudal insertion point on the lamina below. Before I resect this part of the ligamentum flavum and the caudal lamina, I can appreciate that the thecal sac has a distinct appearance of compression. The flattened appearance of the neural elements is a clear indication that my work is not yet done. The thecal sac simply does not look like a well-decompressed tube. Instead, it looks as if it had a napkin ring surrounding it. The combination of the ligamentum flavum and the caudal lamina are the source of that compression, which makes them my next target. Only after the resection of the caudal insertion point of the ligamentum and the superior aspect of the caudal lamina does the dura appear to lose that napkin-ring–like compression (▶ Fig. 3.37).

I pass a forward-angled curet or a right-angled ball-tipped probe over the top of the dura to ensure there is a safe passage for the footplate of the Kerrison rongeur. Next, I pass the footplate of the Kerrison under direct visualization above the dura and beneath the caudal lamina to complete the resection of the ligamentum. In my experience, it is this part of the surgery that has the greatest potential for a cerebrospinal fluid (CSF) leak. Using large Kerrison rongeurs may actually be safer in that the larger footplate displaces the dura away from the action of the chomping rongeur; but nothing changes the fact that I am attempting to pass instruments at the tightest point between the lamina and thecal sac with the ligamentum flavum in the way.

I continue removing lamina and ligamentum flavum until the napkin-ring appearance compression of the dura disappears, and a well-decompressed thecal sac is all that remains. Again, each action of the Kerrison in this region is fraught with the risk of a CSF leak. That risk is understandable when you consider the downward slope of the lamina into the dura at the superior aspect of that lamina (▶ Fig. 3.38). We are maneuvering a Kerrison beneath the lamina at its steepest and deepest point in the canal with a mouth already full of ligamentum flavum and grabbing only the lamina while avoiding the dura, which is innocently compressed right beside it. Nothing would be safer

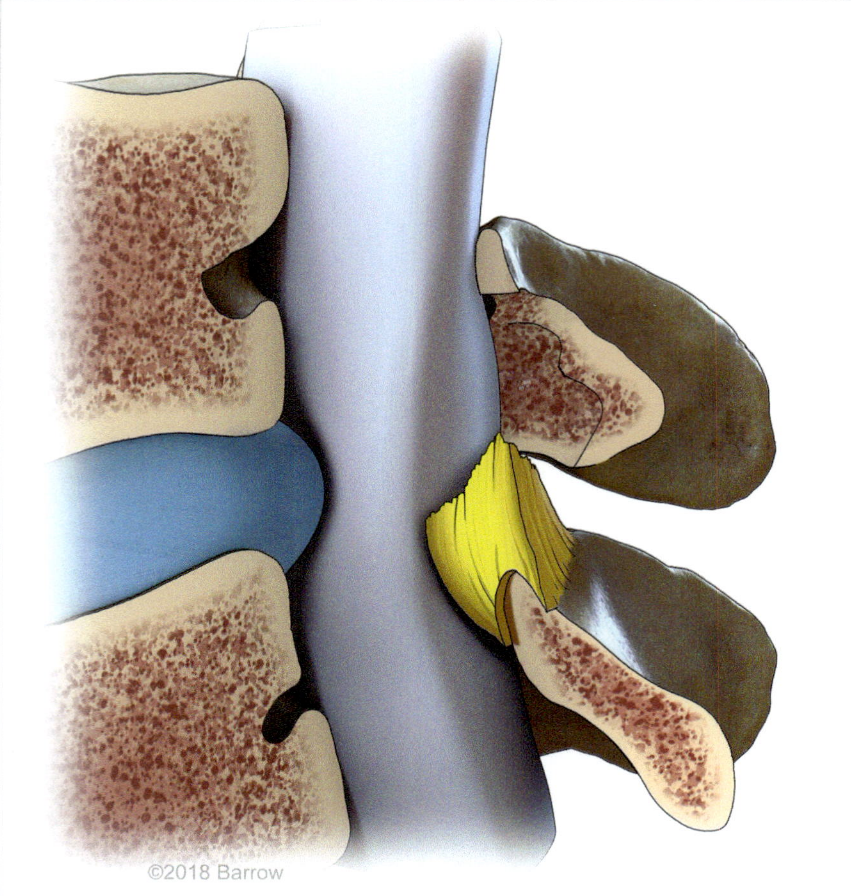

Fig. 3.37 Napkin-ring–like compression from a combination of the ligamentum flavum and the superior aspect of the caudal lamina (in this circumstance L5). After preliminary resection of the ligamentum flavum, the thecal sac expands at the level of resection, further exacerbating the napkin-ring effect.

than avoiding the passage of a Kerrison rongeur beneath the lamina altogether. An alternative to this technique, and my current preference, is the en bloc resection of the ligamentum flavum that I describe later. Working beyond the steepest and deepest point of the canal further down on the caudal lamina where it slopes upward is an alternative and potentially safer technique for handling the caudal insertion.

After I complete the work in this trajectory, the only step that remains is decompression of the ipsilateral traversing nerve root. In the current position of the minimal access port, the ipsilateral nerve root is out of the field of view. To include that nerve root into the field of view for decompression, I will reposition the access port for the third and final time laterally over the medial facet and the ipsilateral lateral recess (▶ Fig. 3.39). The access port is in the position it would be for a microdiscectomy, where the focus is the lateral aspect of the traversing root.

As with any reposition of the access port, I position a piece of Gelfoam over the top of the exposed dura and place the last dilator into the access port. I will zoom out the microscope as my assistant loosens the table-mounted arm. Peering down the diameter of the minimal access port, I will straighten out the converging trajectory (▶ Fig. 3.39). The diameter of the minimal access port will now be immediately over the medial facet. The nerve root awaiting decompression beneath that facet is now within reach. Keep in mind that the bed is still rotated away from me, and the trajectory is not optimal. As I peer down onto my field of view through the microscope, I will have the anesthesiologist rotate the bed back into the neutral position. Decompression of the ipsilateral thecal sac and ipsilateral nerve root is now possible. The access port is in the same trajectory as it would be if I were performing a microdiscectomy, where the focus is also the lateral thecal sac and nerve root.

After I remove the dilator and refocus the microscope, I should be able to visualize at least 50% of the previous exposure. The medial facet will be the majority of the field of view and will require more drilling. I cover any exposed dura with Gelfoam and complete the medial facetectomy with the drill. The Gelfoam not only protects the dura from an errant jump of the drill but also collects the bone dust. When the Gelfoam is suctioned away, the bone dust it has collected goes right along with it.

After I have adequately thinned the medial facet with the drill, I use Kerrison rongeurs to finish the decompression. I establish a plane of dissection with a right-angled ball-tipped probe over the top of the dura. The footplate of a Kerrison can now safely find its way into this plane of dissection and resect the ligamentum flavum in the lateral recess. I continue out laterally until I can clearly visualize the lateral aspect of the dura and mobilize the nerve root. If I am unable to see the traversing nerve root, I reposition the access port more laterally and remove more bone. I will continue with resection of the ligamentum flavum until the lateral aspect of the nerve root comes into view. Upon directly visualizing the nerve root, I mobilize it

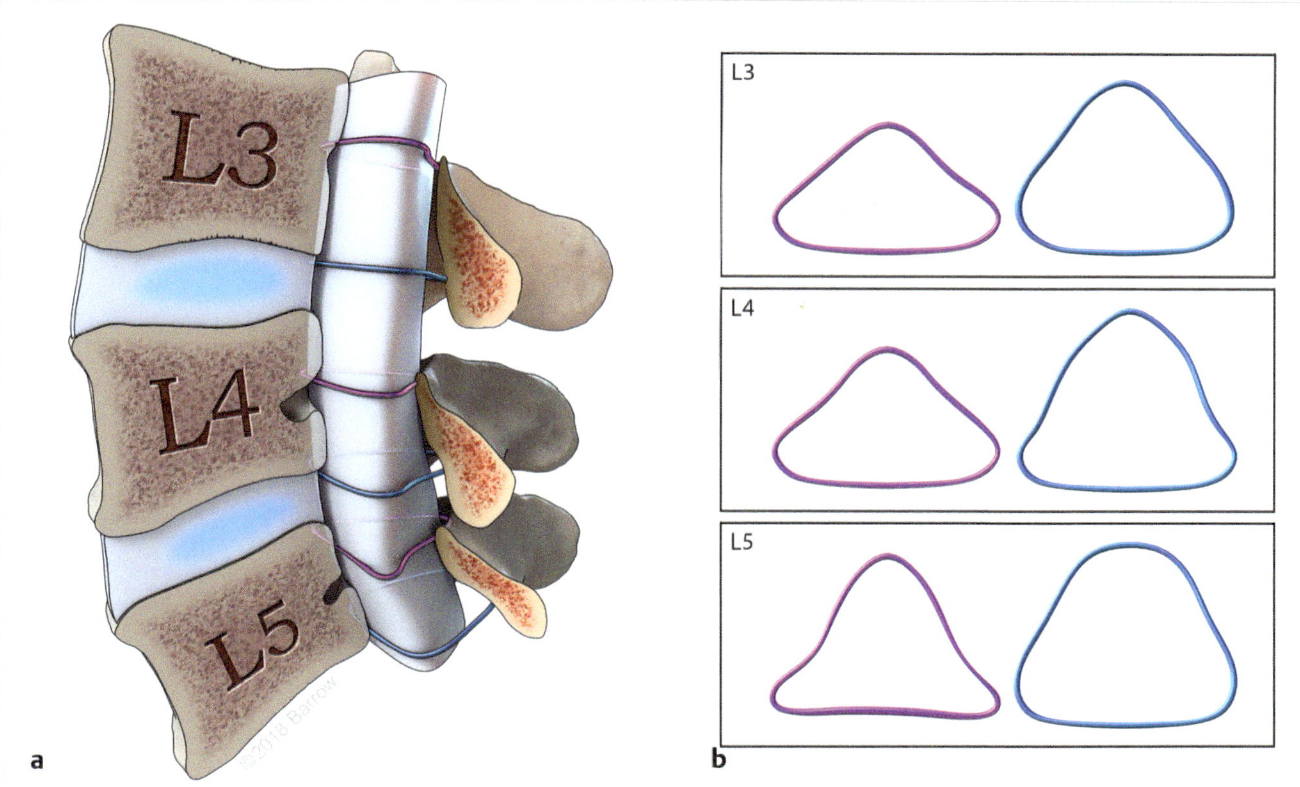

Fig. 3.38 The varying diameters within the canal. **(a)** A conceptualized illustration of the sloping lamina within the lumbar canal. Because of the slope of the lamina at each level, the rostral aspect of each lamina *(magenta ring)* is the deepest and tightest point in the canal, whereas the caudal aspect *(turquoise ring)* becomes the largest diameter. This figure illustrates how as the lamina slopes upward, the diameter enlarges. Working distal to the narrowest point in the canal for each segment has the potential to offer a greater working distance between the lamina and the thecal sac. **(b)** A side-by-side axial comparison of the diameter of the canal. In the axial plane, the difference in diameter of the canal at the rostral and caudal aspects of the lamina becomes obvious. It would be preferable to work within the turquoise ring rather than the magenta ring. Furthermore, the magenta ring has thickened ligamentum flavum further compounding the narrowing of the canal at this juncture.

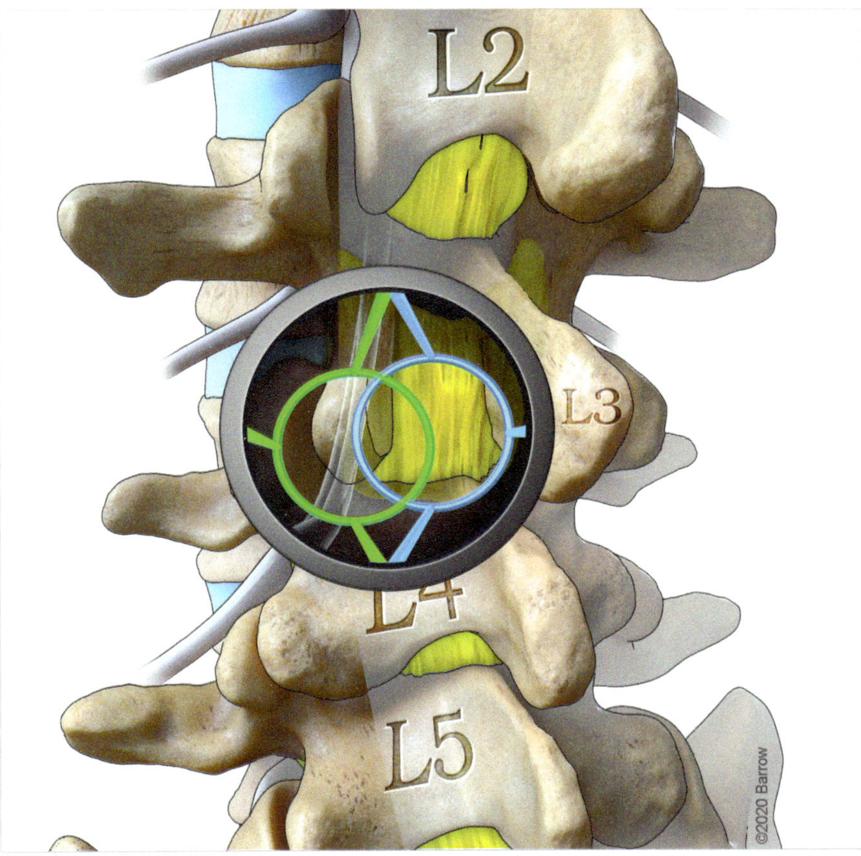

Fig. 3.39 Posterolateral perspective of the spine demonstrating the third and final transition of the minimal access port. After the contralateral and caudal decompressions are complete, the access port is shifted from the caudal contralateral exposure (*turquoise ring*) to an exposure over the ipsilateral traversing nerve root (*emerald ring*). The final position over the ipsilateral nerve root is identical to the position for a microdiscectomy. At this point, the operating table is rotated back into the neutral position.

using a suction retractor. I then pass the right-angled ball-tipped probe into the foramen to ensure safe passage of a Kerrison rongeur. The remaining ligamentum flavum in the lateral recess is now ripe for a larger mouthed Kerrison to resect it. As these final bites enlarge the foramen, the traversing nerve root hides safely away from the action behind a suction retractor.

For the final systems check, I pass a right-angled ball-tipped probe into the foramen and palpate the pedicle to confirm that I have gone lateral enough with the decompression. I will also pass that instrument over the top of the thecal sac to ensure an adequate caudal decompression.

With the foraminotomy complete, I release the nerve root from the protection of the suction retractor and pass the ball-tipped probe over the nerve root to again ensure safe passage. I take a final set of bites with the Kerrison punch over the top of the nerve root to ensure that the ipsilateral space has been adequately decompressed. As I survey the operative field, I confirm that the contralateral space has been decompressed, the central stenosis has been removed and the ipsilateral nerve root decompressed from insertion point to insertion point of the ligamentum flavum. The operation is now complete (▶ Fig. 3.40).

I fill the void with thrombin Gelfoam to obtain hemostasis, trickle in some preservative-free 0.25% bupivacaine (the same concoction approved for epidurals) and place a ½ × 1-inch patty onto the surgical field. I leave the patty in place for 1 minute, then remove it along with the Gelfoam and irrigate the field with a bacitracin solution. I have my anesthesia colleague perform a Valsalva maneuver as I take a final survey of the landscape to ensure I have achieved adequate hemostasis. I slowly remove the access port, obtain hemostasis within the muscle along the path of the port, and close the incision.

3.12 En Bloc Resection of the Ligamentum Flavum

In the previous section, I detailed the technique for piecemeal resection of the ligamentum flavum. Within that section, I mentioned my concern regarding the caudal insertion of the ligamentum flavum and the constrained corridor for instruments to pass beneath the lamina to decompress the thecal sac. I believe that concern was palpable for my reader as I began to present the case to look at alternative strategies to decompress the caudal aspect of the segment. As mentioned, the complications that I have encountered, specifically CSF leaks, have occurred as I was addressing the most compressed component of the thecal sac, which is at the superior aspect of the caudal lamina: the napkin ring. In an effort to avoid future complications, I began to explore a variety of surgical strategies that would avoid working in the deepest and most constrained part of the canal. I have settled on the en bloc resection of the ligamentum flavum that incorporates working beyond the caudal insertion of the ligamentum flavum. The strategy is to release the insertion points of the ligamentum flavum within the canal and remove the entire swath of ligamentum flavum only after I have released every insertion point (▶ Fig. 3.41).

In the en bloc technique, there is a particular focus on the caudal insertion of the ligamentum flavum into the superior aspect of the caudal lamina. Harnessing the anatomic advantages of canal diameters and laminar slope minimizes risk of interruption of the dura. It is that technique that I currently use for all minimally invasive laminectomies. The next section describes the rationale and the surgical technique of an en bloc resection that avoids the napkin ring created by the superior aspect of the caudal lamina. I focus on presenting the rationale and technique for addressing the caudal insertion of the

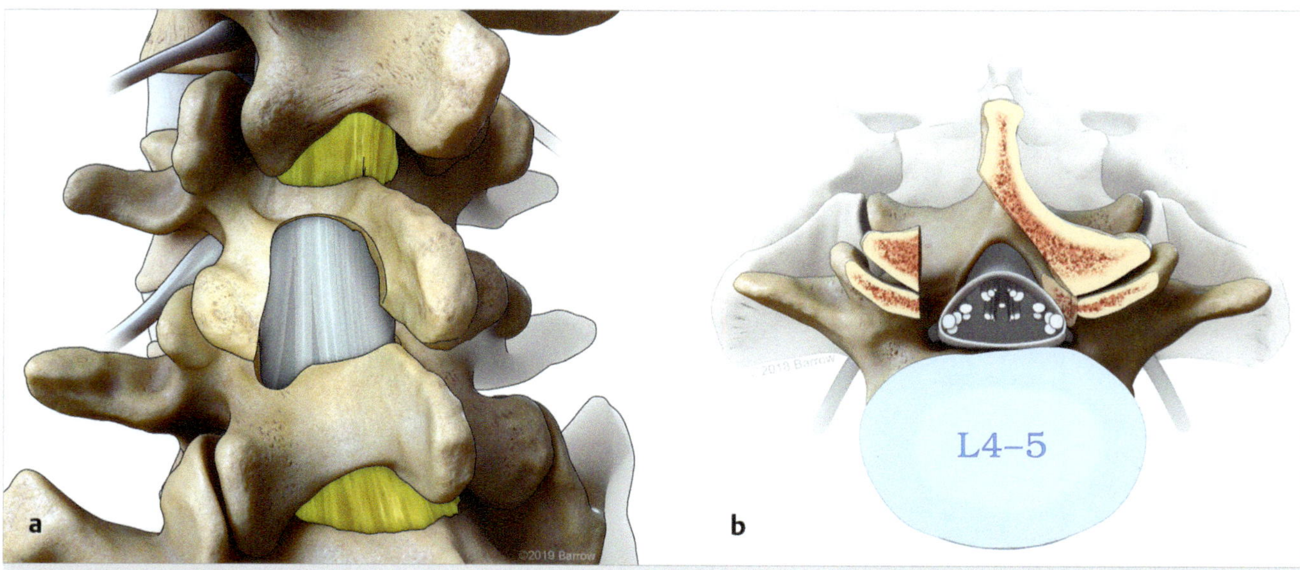

Fig. 3.40 A completed minimally invasive laminectomy. **(a)** Illustration demonstrating a postoperative view of a completed minimally invasive lumbar laminectomy. In this illustration the previously highlighted bone work has been removed and the entire ligamentum flavum for the L4–5 segment has been resected from insertion point to insertion point. The entire thecal sac appears well decompressed, along with the traversing nerve roots. Note the foraminotomy over the top of the L5 nerve root. **(b)** Illustration of an axial perspective of a minimally invasive lumbar laminectomy clearly demonstrating the undercutting of the contralateral lamina to decompress the contralateral recess.

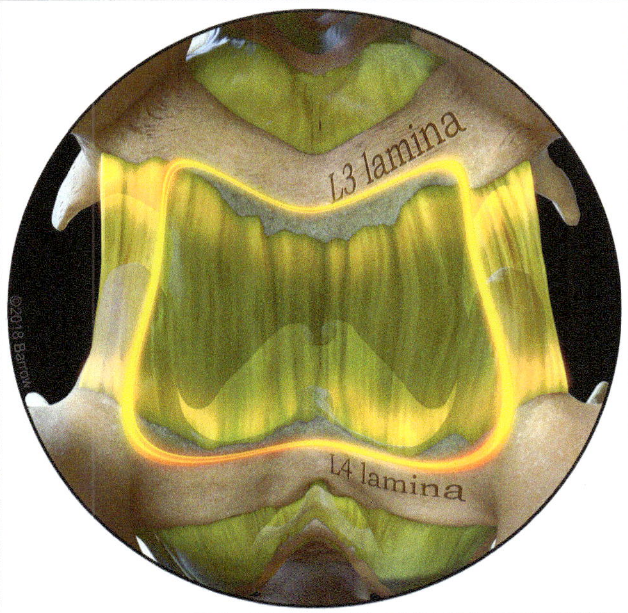

Fig. 3.41 Sequential release of the ligamentum flavum for en bloc resection. In this illustration, the insertion points of the ligamentum flavum are demarcated. The majority of the ligamentum flavum is maintained in position until the entire perimeter is released. Only the insertion points are resected. A particular focus of this technique is in the caudal insertion point of the ligamentum flavum into the superior aspect of the caudal lamina. That is the most constrained area of the canal for the segment.

ligamentum flavum first, before bringing all the component parts of the surgical technique together in the final section.

3.12.1 A Constrained Corridor: Canal Diameter and Canal Depth

The area beneath the superior aspect of the caudal lamina is the tightest diameter of the lumbar segment. The compressed thecal sac and the insertion of the caudal aspect of the ligamentum flavum both share that constrained corridor. The cross-sectional analysis of the diameter of the canal at that point measures significantly less than a measurement further down the upward sloping lamina. The importance of this principle has prompted me to repeat ▶ Fig. 3.38 in this part of the chapter to reemphasize that anatomical characteristic, which is especially relevant to this section (▶ Fig. 3.42). The result is a napkin ring enveloping the thecal sac precisely where a Kerrison needs to perform its most delicate work. Over the years, I have come to realize that the action of the Kerrison in that area is a hopeful and blind one. Hopeful in the sense that the jaws of the Kerrison come together in the tightest space within the canal having a mouth already full of thickened ligamentum flavum. Blind in the sense that the foot of the Kerrison passes beneath the lamina and outside of your direct line of sight of the thecal sac. We are asking the Kerrison to simultaneously bite the lamina and the thickened ligamentum flavum in the narrowest section of the segment while excluding a dural edge from its chops.

It is also important to recognize the working depth at various points within the same segment. The working depth to remove the lamina is deeper at the superior aspect of the caudal lamina than the working depth at the midpoint of the rostral lamina (▶ Fig. 3.43). That deeper working depth forces instruments to displace the thecal sac downward to secure a plane above the dura but below the lamina. The combination of downward displacement of the thecal sac and compression from ligamentum flavum along with bone cutting instruments is a recipe for potential disruption of the dura.

Independently, the working depth or the napkin ring alone creates a challenging scenario for the task at hand. Combine these two anatomical circumstances and it becomes evident how the decompression of the thecal sac by releasing the ligamentum flavum from its caudal insertion with a well-intended Kerrison working at a greater depth and in the most constrained corridor increases the potential for disruption of the thecal sac. It is for these various reasons that I avoid the blind and hopeful bite of a Kerrison in this area altogether. Instead, I work beyond it.

A Larger Working Zone

Working further caudal on the laminar slope and beyond the insertion of the ligamentum flavum avoids the tightest working space altogether (▶ Fig. 3.44). The diameter of the canal widens considerably in a lumbar segment caudal to the insertion of the ligamentum flavum. I will drill at a point in the lamina where it slopes up away from the thecal sac. I will continue that drilling until I make a small breach in the lamina. Instruments that I pass through the breach are further away from the thecal sac so that I can widen the breach safely while I directly visualize the thecal sac beyond the caudal insertion. All issues with line of sight vanish because once the bone work is expanded through the initial breach, the thecal sac will be in plain view. There will be nothing blind and hopeful now about the actions of the Kerrison.

And so, my strategy in the en bloc resection is to release the caudal insertion of the ligamentum flavum after release of the rostral and contralateral insertions. That caudal release requires making a breach in the lamina beyond the napkin ring (▶ Fig. 3.44). A laminar breach at the midpoint of the lamina is at a shallower working depth further away from the thecal sac than working at the superior aspect of the lamina. After all, it is an area on the upward slope of the lamina where the diameter of the canal widens.

In the end, I am looking to breach the canal beyond the insertion of the ligamentum flavum, identify the dura, and then work my way back to the ligamentum flavum insertion and ultimately the napkin ring. The goal is to mobilize the ligamentum flavum from below and work in a rostral direction while looking at the thecal sac the whole time, instead of blindly working from above hoping not to disrupt the dura of the thecal sac. Once I identify the inferior aspect of the ligamentum flavum insertion, my strategy then turns to releasing the contralateral and ipsilateral insertion points. From there I would work toward where I left off when the access port was in the first position. I want to encounter the untethered ligamentum flavum that I released moments ago when I was working in the rostral to caudal direction. The hope would be that as I work in

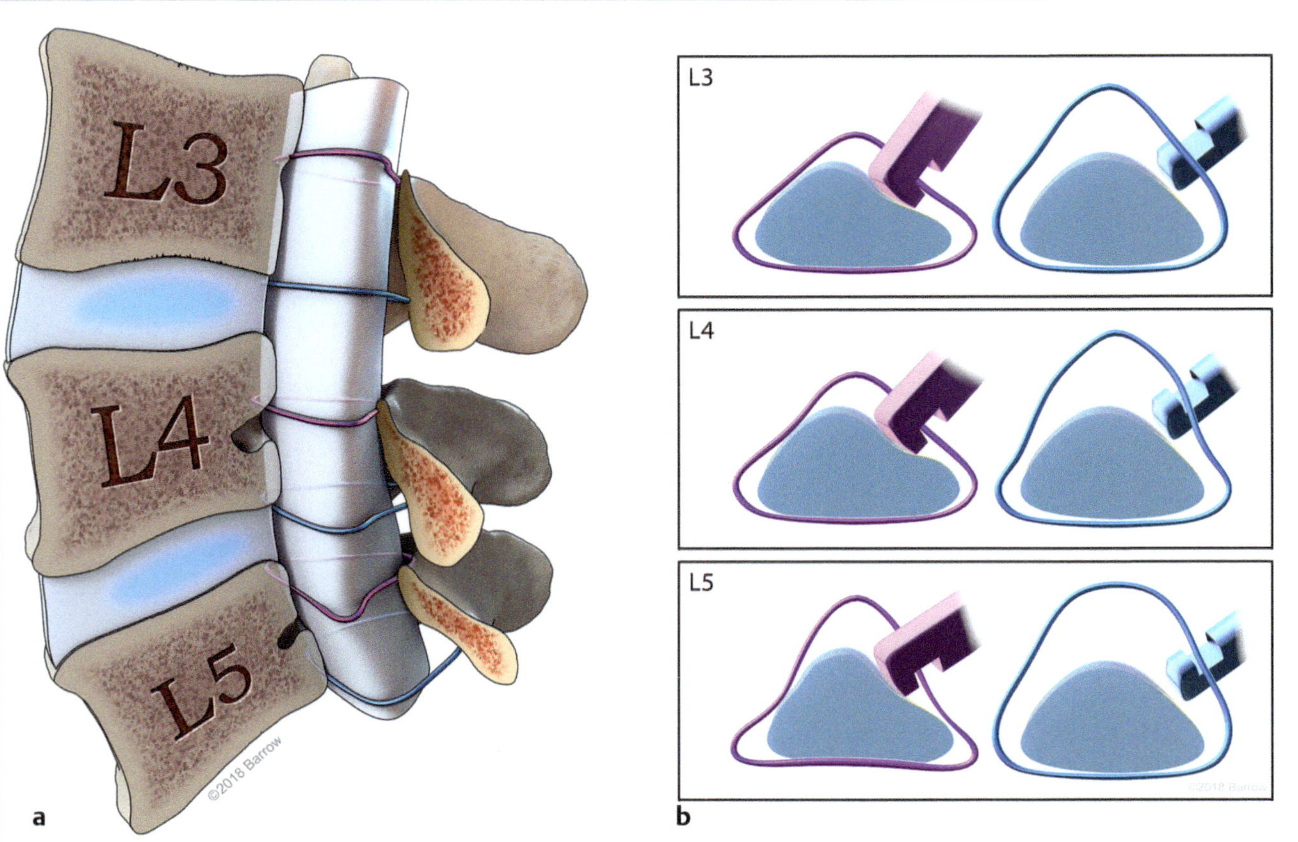

Fig. 3.42 Rationale behind working beyond the caudal insertion of the ligamentum flavum. **(a)** Illustration that demonstrates the relationship between the slope of the lamina and diameter of the canal. L3, L4 and L5 are the most common levels to demonstrate lumbar stenosis. The most superior aspect of the lamina is the narrowest aspect of the canal for that segment as demonstrated by the *magenta ring*. In comparison, the diameter widens considerably further down on the lamina as it slopes upward. The increased diameter is demonstrated by the *turquoise ring*. The combination of a larger diameter and absence of the ligamentum flavum results in a safer working zone. **(b)** Cross sectional analysis demonstrating the increased diameters as the lamina slopes away from the thecal sac.

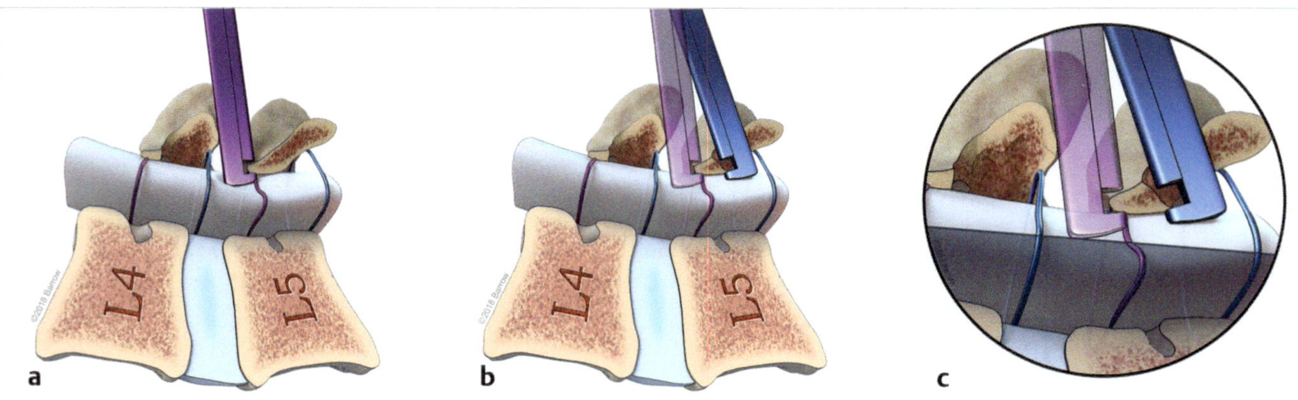

Fig. 3.43 Working beyond the caudal insertion of the ligamentum flavum. Illustration of the relative depth of the superior aspect of the caudal lamina in an L4–5 decompression. **(a)** Removing the superior aspect of the rostral lamina (L5 in this case) requires the instrument to work at a greater depth in a more constrained working channel. Further adding to the compression is the ligamentum flavum (not shown). In this figure, the *magenta-colored* Kerrison needs to displace the thecal sac downward and work a plane beneath the superior aspect of the caudal lamina. **(b)** Working as the lamina slopes upward offers a larger working channel at less depth. **(c)** A magnified and focused view of **b**. In this illustration, the *azure-colored* Kerrison clearly demonstrates the difference in working depth at these two distinct areas within the segment. The line demarcates the depth of the *magenta-colored* Kerrison footplate. The *azure-colored* Kerrison is at a shallower depth in an area where there is no ligamentum flavum.

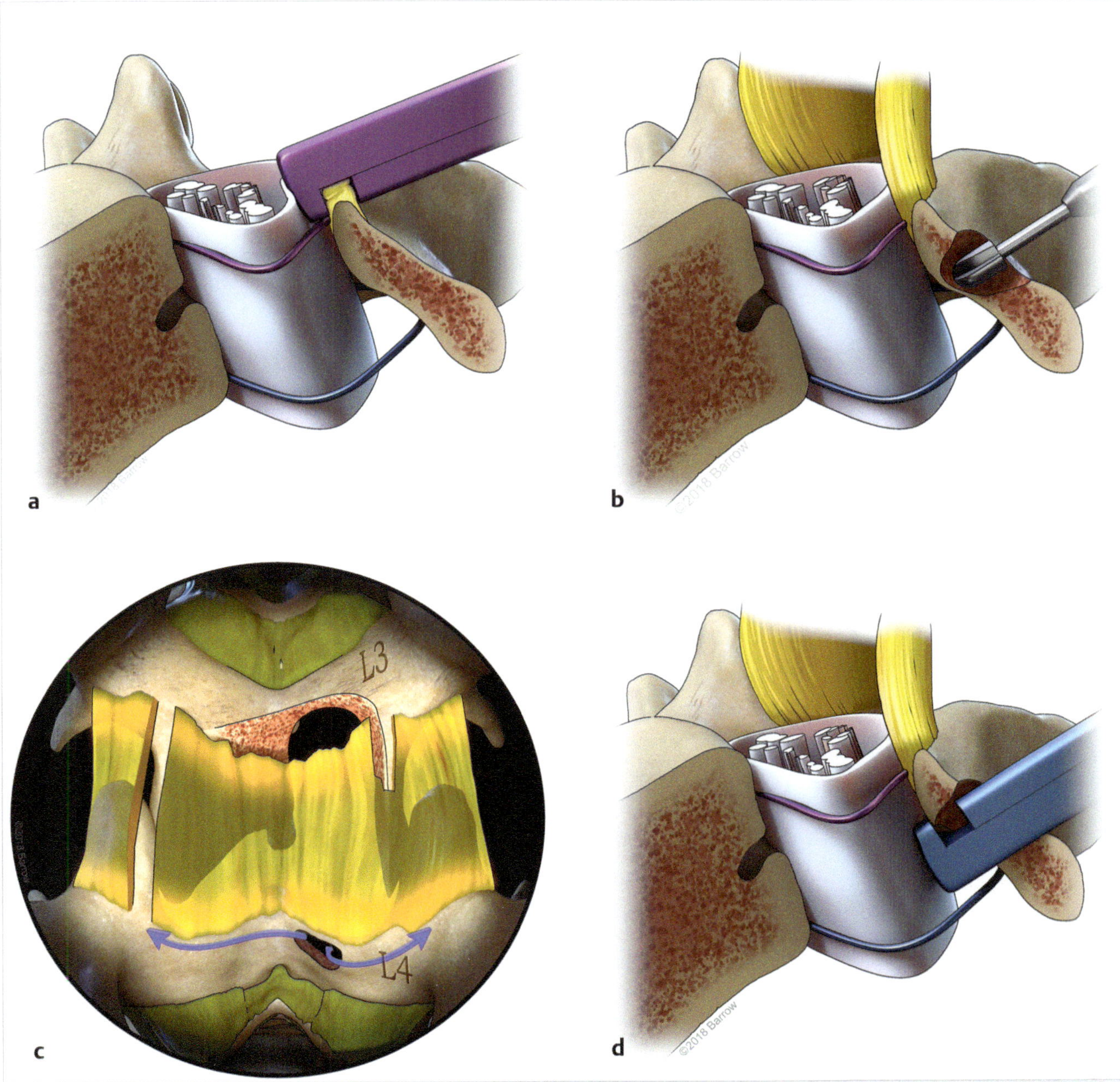

Fig. 3.44 A larger working zone. An illustration demonstrating the additional working area when working further down the caudal lamina. **(a)** Illustration demonstrating a Kerrison passing through the narrowest corridor to resect the caudal insertion of the ligamentum flavum. Action of a Kerrison at the superior aspect of the caudal lamina is fraught with the risk of a cerebrospinal fluid leak. **(b)** Illustration demonstrating the drilling of the caudal lamina to create a breach as the lamina slopes upward away from the thecal sac. **(c)** A view of the ligamentum flavum insertions with a perspective from within the canal. The site intended for the breach is below the caudal insertion of the ligamentum flavum. Once the drill creates a breach, the bone work may be extended (*arrows*) and the thecal sac visualized beyond the insertion of the ligamentum flavum. The upward slope of the lamina places instruments at a shallower working depth. **(d)** The larger diameter allows for greater distance between the dural edge of the thecal sac and actions of the Kerrison.

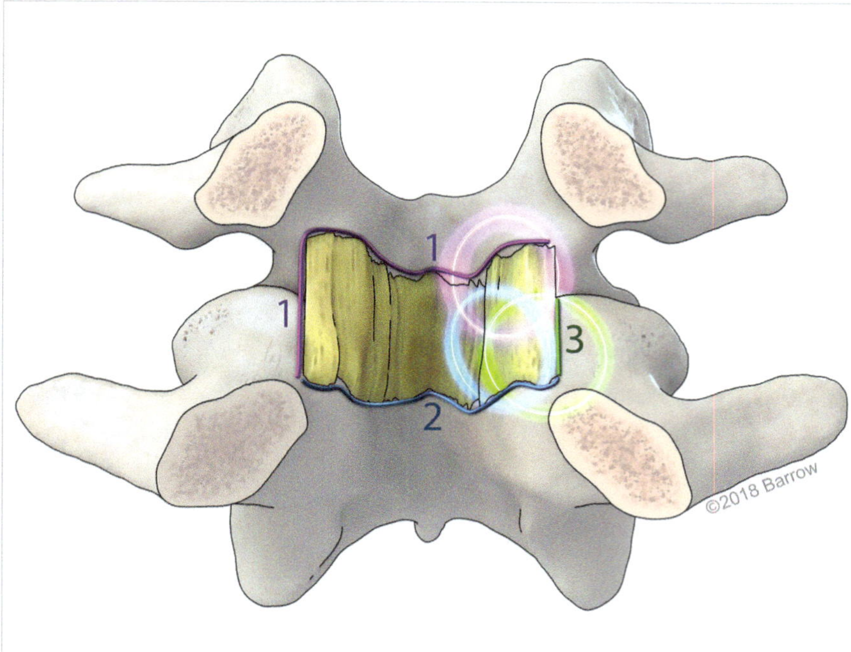

Fig. 3.45 Artist's illustration demonstrating sequential release of the insertion points of the ligamentum flavum in an L4–5 laminectomy with a left-sided approach. Initially, the bone work remains the same as piecemeal resection of the ligamentum flavum. The rostral insertion point (1, top) of the ligamentum flavum is identified and released, and then the contralateral (1, left), caudal (2) and ipsilateral (3) insertions of the ligamentum flavum are identified and released sequentially. Doing so involves shifting the minimal access port (*colored rings*) to be over the top of the caudal lamina and thinning the rostral component of the caudal lamina with the drill.

the caudal to rostral direction, I can free up the entire ligamentum and eventually remove it en bloc while never losing sight of the dura.

The last few paragraphs above have laid out the concepts, principles, and rationale for the en bloc resection. The next component is putting all these elements together in a cogent and methodical surgical technique.

3.12.2 Surgical Technique

The initial approach to the rostral insertion point of the ligamentum flavum for an enbloc resection does not differ from that of a piecemeal resection. The difference is in the sequence of the resection. I dock the minimal access port in the same initial position that I described earlier in Section 3.11, Direct Resection. There are four sides of attachments: the insertion points in the rostral and caudal lamina and the insertion points in the ipsilateral and contralateral recesses. Sequential resection and release of the ligamentum flavum around the entire perimeter allows for complete and simultaneous removal of the compressive elements of the thecal sac (▶ Fig. 3.45). Most importantly, release of the ligamentum flavum at its caudal insertion from below by removal of the lamina distal to the insertion eliminates the need to apply a Kerrison at the tightest part of the napkin ring. I believe this maneuver alone may decrease the risk of CSF leak for this operation.

My first objective remains the rostral insertion. As described earlier, I extend my laminotomy window just above the rostral insertion point of the ligamentum flavum for the segment. I will have a large swath of thickened yellow ligament lying before me with the rostral insertion point completely untethered. I will also release what I can of the ipsilateral insertion, but the current position of the access port does currently provide access to the ipsilateral medial facet. The important point at this phase of the operation is that instead of resecting the ligamentum flavum piecemeal, I focus on releasing the insertions circumferentially. ▶ Fig. 3.46 illustrates the resection of the rostral insertion from within the canal.

Once I have completely released the rostral insertion of the ligamentum flavum, the attachment in the contralateral recess becomes my next focus. I am meticulous in only removing the amount of ligament necessary to release the ligamentum flavum from its lateral insertion within the contralateral facet (▶ Fig. 3.47). The goal is actually to preserve as much ligamentum flavum as possible throughout this entire process. With the spinous process undercut and the contralateral recess in view, I continue the sequential release of the ligamentum flavum. As with a piecemeal resection, I use a combination of Kerrison rongeurs and forward-angled curets within the contralateral recess but work to release only the insertions of the ligamentum flavum. Throughout the resection of the contralateral attachments, I meticulously keep the central component of the ligamentum flavum intact. Having that thickened ligamentum flavum in place will continue to protect the thecal sac and prevent expansion of the thecal sac into my surgical field.

After completing the contralateral release, I leave the ligamentum flavum in place and shift the access port over the caudal insertion point of the ligamentum flavum as previously described. It is the approach to the caudal lamina where there is a significant departure from the direct piecemeal resection that I described earlier.

The first step is to expose the superior aspect of the caudal lamina. Understanding that the ligamentum flavum actually straddles the lamina is helpful for this phase of the operation. There are attachments on the dorsal and ventral surfaces of the lamina (▶ Fig. 3.48). I approach each attachment sequentially.

Using a small straight curet, I sweep away the ligamentum flavum over the top of the caudal lamina until I can unequivocally visualize the lamina. I focus on exposing the aspect of the lamina where the upward slope takes me the farthest away

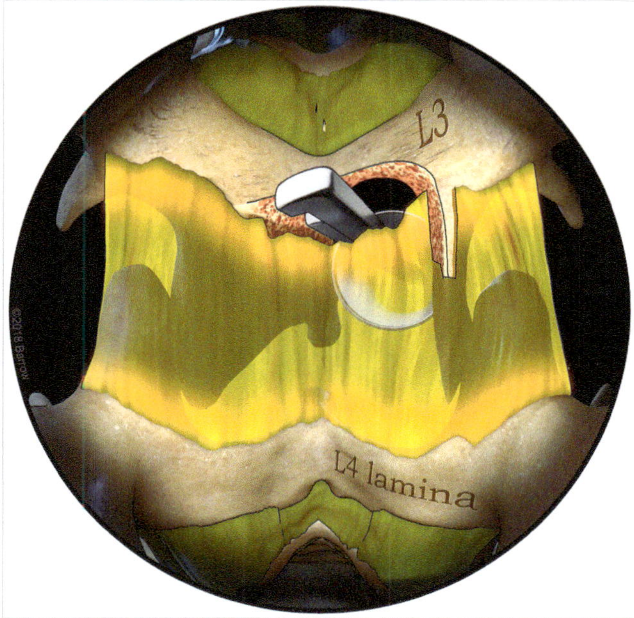

Fig. 3.46 Release of the rostral insertion of the ligamentum flavum. An illustration with a perspective from within the canal looking at the ligamentum flavum. The first step in the en bloc technique is release of the rostral insertion of the ligamentum flavum and partial release of the ipsilateral insertion as demonstrated in this image.

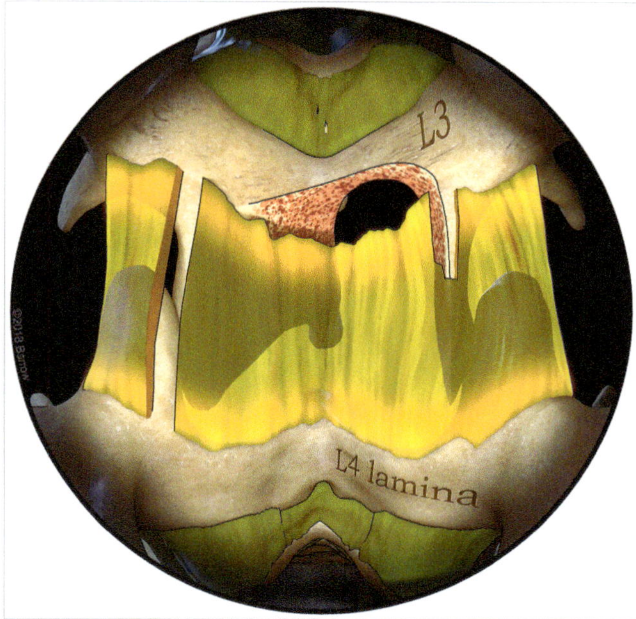

Fig. 3.47 Release of the contralateral insertion of the ligamentum flavum. The second step in the en bloc technique is release of the contralateral insertion of the ligamentum flavum. This illustration demonstrates the contralateral insertion of the ligamentum flavum released by a Kerrison.

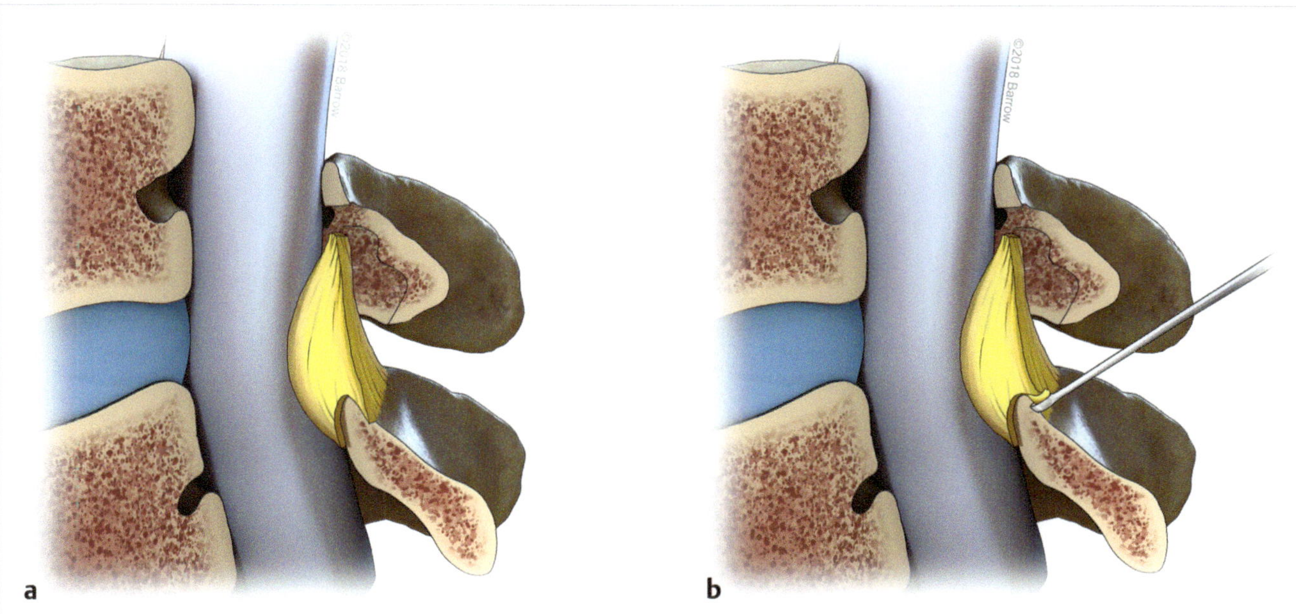

Fig. 3.48 The lamina and the ligamentum flavum. **(a)** Illustration demonstrating how the ligamentum flavum straddles the lamina on either side. **(b)** Peeling away the ligamentum on the dorsal aspect of the lamina allows for clear visualization of the laminar bone. Working farther caudal on the exposed lamina, which is beyond the caudal insertion of the ligamentum flavum and where the lamina slopes upward away from the thecal sac, provides a working corridor to create a breach distal to the "napkin ring." Working in the rostral direction from that breach, the ligamentum flavum may be safely released.

from the deepest and narrowest diameter of the canal. After all, my goal is to avoid the napkin ring. When I have exposed a wide enough surface area, I will drill the lamina down to the thickness of a shrimp shell. Again, the focus is to drill the lamina beyond the level of the caudal insertion of the ligamentum flavum, similar to what was accomplished at the rostral insertion. But in this instance, I am trying to get below the insertion, not above it. Drilling this area places me well beyond the tightest area of compression, the napkin ring. With a breach in the lamina made, a forward-angled curet can now enter the space below the insertion point of the ligamentum flavum. Familiar epidural fat and the unmistakable sheen of the dura should be obvious, analogous to the release of the rostral insertion point. Because I am working in an area further down the lamina, I will have a larger diameter to wield my instruments. I will also have direct visualization of the thecal sac.

I create an opening with the drill adequate for a modest sized Kerrison rongeur and then remove bone as far laterally and medially as the exposure will allow (▶ Fig. 3.49). Working below the insertion point of the ligamentum flavum virtually eliminates the risk of a CSF leak that can occur with a blind and hopeful passage of an instrument from above the insertion plunging beneath the lamina. As seen in ▶ Fig. 3.43, there is considerably more working space between the thecal sac and the lamina in this region, virtually eliminating the anxiety caused by attempting to bite the lamina and ligament without capturing the dura within the metallic chomps of the Kerrison. The rostral, contralateral, and caudal insertions of the ligamentum flavum are detached. One insertion remains.

The final shift of the minimal access port involves placing it immediately over the ipsilateral nerve root for the foraminotomy. I drill the medial facet, release the ligamentum flavum from its insertion on the ipsilateral facet, and then the decompression for the entire segment is complete. The entire swath of the ligamentum flavum for the segment is now free (▶ Fig. 3.50). I remove it effortlessly with nothing more than a pituitary rongeur and look at the nerve root and entire thecal sac appearing widely decompressed. The en bloc technique completes the decompression of the segment with the least number of actions of the Kerrison rongeur and, in my opinion, with less risk to the thecal sac at the caudal insertion of the ligamentum flavum.

The en bloc technique has several advantages. The first advantage is preservation of the ligamentum flavum over the top of the dura for nearly the entire decompression. Having that thick yellow carpet protecting the thecal sac as instruments pass in and out of the operative field alone mitigates the risk of a CSF leak. The second advantage is efficiency. Resecting the attachment points around the perimeter instead of piecemeal resection is a more efficient procedure, with substantially fewer actions with the Kerrison rongeur. In my experience, a considerably shorter operating time is the inevitable result.

3.13 Closure

With the microscope still in position, I loosen the table-mounted retractor arm and the surgical assistant or scrub technician slowly pulls it back. I hold the suction in one hand and the cautery in the other; I can address any bleeding that the access port had compressed. The bleeding is seldom troublesome and can readily be controlled with cautery. The various muscle and skin layers are infiltrated again with a mixture of 1% lidocaine with epinephrine and 0.25% Marcaine. Approximately 12 mL is injected into either side of the incision. The goal is for the patient to not even be aware of the incision for several hours after the operation.

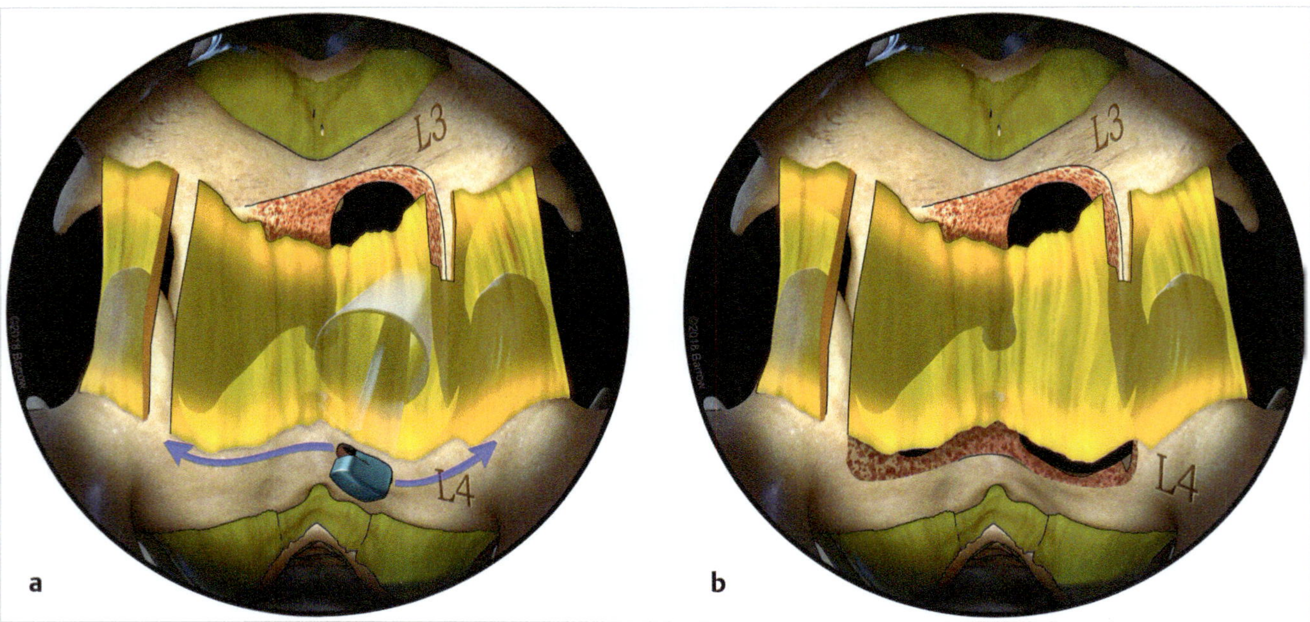

Fig. 3.49 Working beyond the caudal insertion and in the larger diameter of the canal. **(a)** Illustration demonstrating the location of the breach in the caudal lamina beyond the insertion and at a point (*arrows*) where the diameter of the canal is larger allowing for greater room to maneuver instruments. **(b)** The bone work and release of the caudal insertion is extended in both directions. In this manner, the caudal insertion of the ligamentum flavum is released with direct visualization of the thecal sac.

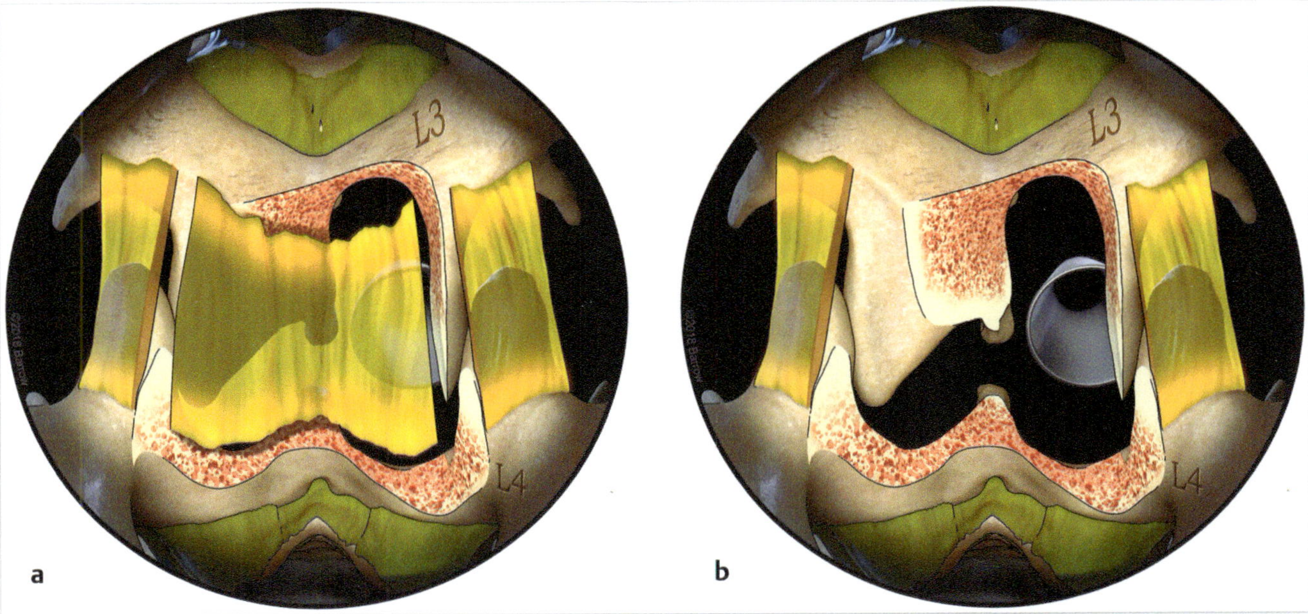

Fig. 3.50 Completion of the en bloc resection. **(a)** Illustration demonstrating the release of the ipsilateral ligamentum flavum. With the access port repositioned the final remaining attachment of the ligamentum flavum may be released. When the insertion points have been connected, the ligamentum flavum may be removed en bloc. **(b)** Illustration demonstrating completion of the decompression.

After removal of the access port, I close the wound in a multilayered fashion. The fascia is reapproximated with 0 Vicryl (Ethicon, Inc.) sutures on a UR-6 needle, the subcutaneous tissue is closed with 2.0 Vicryl on an X-1 needle, and the skin edges come together with 4.0 Vicryl on an RB-1 needle. I will apply Mastisol (Eloquest Healthcare, Inc.) or benzoin liquid adhesive to the periphery of the incision and Steri-Strips (3M) to eliminate any tension across the incision. I place a small Telfa dressing over the top of the Steri-Strips followed by a 5% lidocaine patch to continue to douse any incisional discomfort.

3.14 Postoperative Care

Healthy patients with no significant comorbidities may typically be discharged from the postanesthesia care unit after an hour or so. Patients should be able to void, should feel comfortable transitioning from a seated to a standing position, and should be able to walk 25 feet. In the presence of comorbidities or advanced age, a 23-hour admission is advisable. On occasion, I have discharged older male patients who later found that they could not urinate around midnight on the evening of the operation. Any patient who has a prostate issue or who is at risk for urinary difficulties should be observed until they have demonstrated normal urinary function.

I ask patients to leave the lidocaine patch in place overnight and then remove it the morning after surgery. Patients may shower the first postoperative day but may not submerge the incision until completely healed. To minimize epidural scarring, I prescribe a methylprednisolone dose pack and have the patient begin the pack the day after the surgery. Patients are seen at a 1-month follow-up visit and tend to be the happiest patients in my clinic. If anything, I find it challenging to bring them back for subsequent follow-ups.

3.15 Case Illustration

3.15.1 Clinical History and Neurological Examination

A 73-year-old man presented with a 12-month history of neurogenic claudication. The patient reported intermittent bouts of sciatica successfully treated with epidural injections throughout the years; however, over the past year he has found no relief with these injections. The patient reported that 1 year earlier he was walking 2 to 3 miles a day and playing nine holes of golf two to three times a week but in the past few months, he could walk no further than 100 yards without a heaviness and discomfort in both legs. While he found complete relief by sitting or leaning over, the symptoms reached a point where he had to stop both his walks and golf outings altogether.

The patient's neurological examination was notable only for blunted reflexes in the Achilles and patellar tendons bilaterally. He demonstrated nondermatomal sensory loss in the lower extremities, but on examination by confrontation exhibited 5/5 strength in all muscle groups of the lower extremities bilaterally. The Oswestry Disability Index (ODI) was 38, and the Visual Analog Score (VAS) was 40 and 60 mm for his back and legs, respectively.

3.15.2 Radiographic Studies

MRI demonstrated multiple levels of degenerative disc disease and multiple levels with varying degrees of stenosis. However, of all the segments, L3–4 demonstrated the greatest degree of ligamentum flavum hypertrophy and as a result the greatest degree of lumbar stenosis as seen on both the axial and sagittal images (▶ Fig. 3.51).

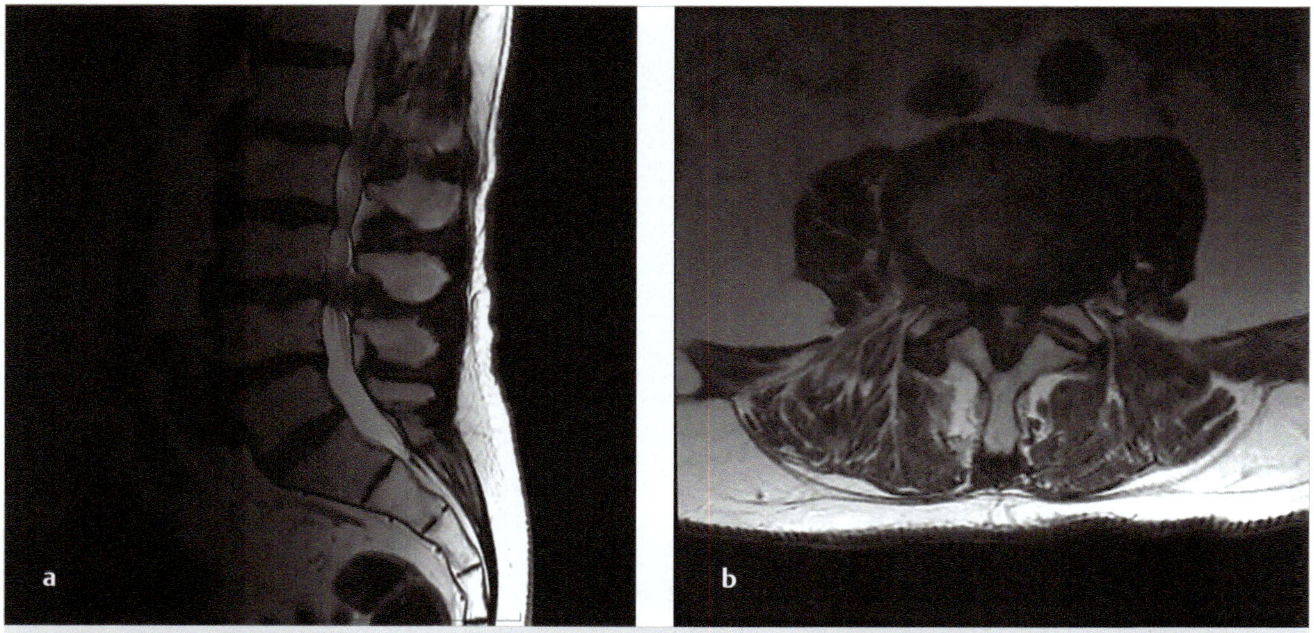

Fig. 3.51 L3–4 stenosis with neurogenic claudication. **(a)** Sagittal T2-weighted magnetic resonance imaging (MRI) demonstrating single-level stenosis at the L3–4 segment. There is no evidence of malalignment, and the L3–4 disc height is well preserved as is lumbar lordosis. Those characteristics make the patient an ideal candidate for a minimally invasive lumbar laminectomy. **(b)** Axial T2-weighted MRI demonstrating ligamentum flavum hypertrophy as the leading cause of the stenosis.

3.15.3 Operative Intervention

I recommended a minimally invasive L3–4 lumbar laminectomy with a right-sided approach. The approach was based purely on surgeon preference because in this case, the patient had symptoms that were equal in both lower extremities. I positioned the patient on a Wilson frame atop a Jackson table. After I fully expanded the Wilson frame, I approximated the L4–5 level based on the anterior superior iliac spine and the interspinous process space. I then shifted up one segment to the intended target of L3–4 and planned an incision 2 cm lateral to the midline.

By the time I have prepped and draped the patient, the microscope is draped and at the ready on the side of the approach and the fluoroscope is in position opposite the microscope. I pass a spinal needle onto the lamina and confirm the level with the first fluoroscopic image. I make any adjustment to the insertion point and trajectory of the needle that optimizes access to the segment and then infiltrate the proposed tract with the lidocaine/Marcaine mixture. I make an 18-mm incision in preparation for the 16-mm access port. Palpation of the spinous process through the incision confirms the midline in my mind's eye. I confidently divide the fascia 18 to 20 mm off the midline with cautery in preparation for the dilators. The first dilator passes through the fascial opening with an angle of convergence of 15 to 20 degrees and stops upon encountering the lamina of L3 (▶ Fig. 3.52a). The tip of the dilator wands up and down at the confluence of the spinous process and lamina.

A second fluoroscopic image confirms that I am positioned parallel to the L3–4 disc space, and I dilate sequentially up to 16 mm and then secure a 6 cm × 16 mm minimal access port (▶ Fig. 3.52b). A final lateral and AP image completes the reconstruction of the anatomy at depth in my mind's eye and the operating microscope rolls in as the fluoroscope rolls out (▶ Fig. 3.52c). My anesthetist rotates the patient away from me as I peer through the microscope. I ask them to stop the rotation when the line of sight through the microscope is directly down the minimal access port.

I zoom in and focus the microscope on the diameter at the bottom of the access port. Only a few strands of muscle remain at the confluence of the spinous process and the lamina, which I paint away with cautery. As I complete the exposure, I appreciate the confluence of the lamina and spinous process and get a sense of the beginning of the pars interarticularis. Before I begin drilling I ensure that my mind has accurately reconciled my exposure with the fluoroscopic images. I should have the entire three-dimensional anatomy reconstructed in my mind's eye.

The 16 mm of exposure allows me to drill all the lamina in my field of view and the base of the spinous process into the contralateral lamina (Video 3.1). The goal is to thin the lamina and then create a breach within the inferior aspect of the rostral lamina, where the ligamentum flavum is thickest. When I encounter the ligamentum flavum, I continue to thin the lamina and then work in the rostral direction until there is no evidence of the ligamentum flavum. My intention for this operation was an en bloc resection of the ligamentum flavum, and so my focus was the insertion points.

A forward-angled curet develops the plane between the dura and the ligamentum flavum and begins releasing the rostral insertion. From there, I undercut the spinous process and contralateral lamina which enabled me to release the ligamentum flavum from its contralateral insertion. I confirm a contralateral release with a right-angled ball-tipped probe into the contrala-

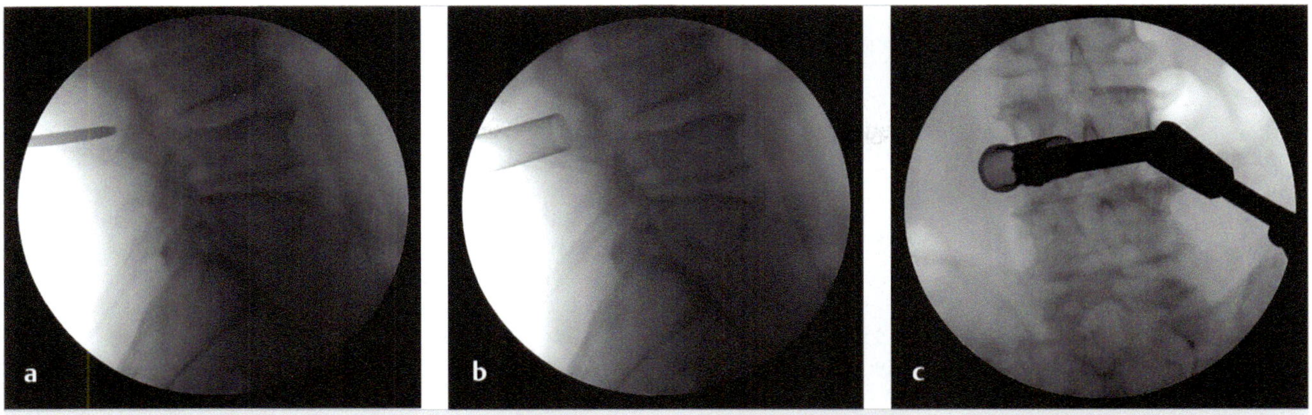

Fig. 3.52 Securing the access port for an L3–4 laminectomy. **(a)** Lateral fluoroscopic image confirming the operative segment with the first dilator and then wanding the tip of the dilator over the intended surface area for surgery. **(b)** Fluoroscopic image confirming the position of the access port with a trajectory onto the rostral insertion of the ligamentum flavum. **(c)** Final anteroposterior image confirming a converging trajectory onto the base of the spinous process.

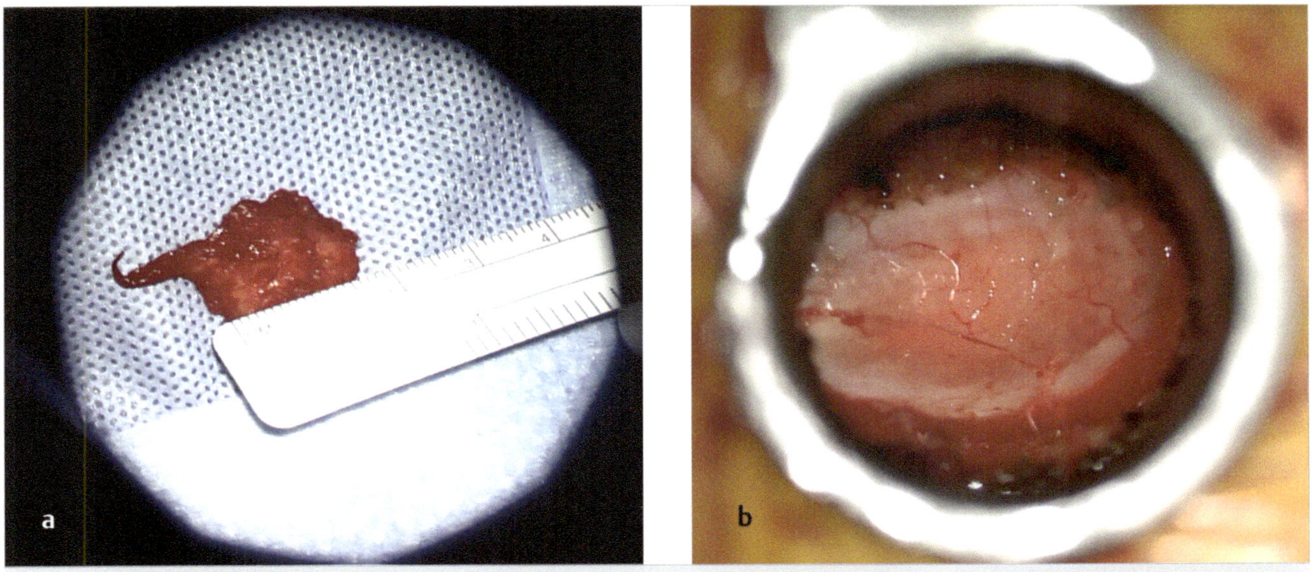

Fig. 3.53 Minimally invasive L3–4 laminectomy. **(a)** Intraoperative photo of the ligamentum flavum resected in an en bloc manner. **(b)** Intraoperative view through the minimal access port at the completion of the procedure. Although only 16 mm is visible through this view, the access port was in two different trajectories prior to the current position. Approximately 25 mm of rostral-caudal decompression was achieved.

teral foramen. With the first objective met, I placed the final dilator into the minimal access port and wand the minimal access port down to the superior aspect of the L4 lamina.

With a small straight curet in hand, I sweep away the fibers of the ligamentum flavum over the top of the lamina of L4 and expose the unmistakable white ivory appearance of the lamina. I drill the superior aspect of the lamina of L4 until it has a shrimp shell thickness. A forward-angled curet finds its way through what remains of the lamina and into the canal. I am now past the caudal insertion of the ligamentum flavum and I can clearly visualize the epidural fat and the unmistakable sheen of the dura. Any bite of the Kerrison rongeur will be neither blind nor hopeful. I will have the nerve root and the thecal sac in plain view with every action of the Kerrison. I continue to develop the exposure into the contralateral and ipsilateral recess which further releases the ligamentum from its caudal insertion. Once I have connected the caudal release to the contralateral release, I reposition the minimal access port into the final position: over the top of the ipsilateral nerve root.

The medial facetectomy exposes the remaining ligamentum flavum, which lies on top of the nerve root. The entire swath of ligamentum flavum remains over top of the neural elements as I complete the drilling of the medial facet. Once I expose the ligamentum flavum at the top of the lateral recess, I am able to complete the release from the insertion beneath the medial facet. A pituitary rongeur removes the entire ligamentum flavum from insertion to insertion and the entire segment is decompressed (▶ Fig. 3.53).

I performed a final system check before removing the access port and closing the incision. I mobilize the traversing root and perform a generous foraminotomy. I pass a right-angled ball-tipped probe over top of the thecal sac in the caudal and rostral directions and then out the foramen on the ipsilateral and contralateral sides. I obtained hemostasis as I remove the minimal access port, infiltrated the incision with a lidocaine and bupivacaine mixture, and closed the fascia, subcutaneous layer, and skin edges.

3.15.4 Postoperative Course

After a period of observation in the recovery room, the patient was discharged home, walking independently. At the 1-month follow-up, he had returned to walking 2 to 3 miles per day. By 3 months, he had returned to nine holes of golf two to three times a week. The postoperative ODI was 9, and the VAS for the back and legs were 20 and 0 mm, respectively.

3.16 Long-Term Outcomes

When it comes to counseling a patient regarding surgical intervention, offering some insight into what the future may bring has tremendous value. The most comprehensive data regarding long-term outcomes for the surgical management of lumbar stenosis come from the Spine Outcomes Research Trial (SPORT). However, it is important to note that the surgical technique used in the SPORT was not a minimally invasive approach. The impact of removing the posterior tension band has been examined in cadaveric models, but the impact on clinical outcomes is not well studied.[3] In the SPORT, both the 4-year and 8-year follow-up data demonstrated that the patients treated surgically had significantly greater improvement in outcome measures than the patients treated nonoperatively.[18,19] The 4-year rate of reoperation for recurrent stenosis was 6%, which increased to 10% by 8 years. Such robust long-term data demonstrate the sustainability of this operation. I have had a similar experience in the management of lumbar stenosis. The patient featured in ▶ Fig. 3.54 underwent a minimally invasive lumbar laminectomy and was reevaluated 7 years later at the request of an orthopaedic surgeon to rule out a spinal cause for her hip pain. The patient showed no restenosis upon long-term reevaluation.

3.17 Complication Avoidance

Cerebrospinal fluid leak, iatrogenic instability, and incomplete decompression are the three main complications that can arise from any lumbar laminectomy whether performed minimally invasive or through a traditional open midline incision. In each of these complications that I have weathered alongside my patients, I have reaffirmed the adage that failure is the best teacher. Any complication that occurs warrants a thoughtful analysis of what measures could have been taken to avoid the complication. In the end, there is no worse fate for the surgeon than not to learn from a complication that has transpired.

3.17.1 Cerebrospinal Fluid Leaks

When I think of CSF leaks in the lumbar laminectomy, I envision nearing the end of the procedure, passing the Kerrison beneath the superior aspect of the caudal lamina, and chomping. The egress of cerebral spinal fluid floods not only the surgical field, but the mind of the surgeon with thoughts of pseudomeningoceles, wound healing issues and positional headaches. My experience has been consistent with the reports in the literature that a direct repair is seldom necessary. Instead a dural patch and a dural sealant over the top of the dural interruption is all that is needed. The most important aspect to consider is completion of the decompression. Placing a cottonoid pad over the defect and continuing the decompression are the most important steps that a surgeon can take in the face of a CSF leak. Larger rents in the dura may require primary repair, which is untenable in a 16-mm access port. If after assessment of the defect in the dura, the need for primary repair becomes obvious, it would be advisable to exchange the minimal access port for a larger port, if not an expandable port as described in Chapter 2. A dedicated minimally invasive CSF leak repair kit (Appendix, Chapter 2) is necessary to have prepared and readily retrievable should the occasion arise.

I cannot recall a CSF leak that did not occur at the caudal insertion of the ligamentum flavum. It was those complications early in my experience that prompted an analysis of the lumbar diameter of the canal. Working beyond the "napkin ring" and in a larger diameter of the canal, as described in this chapter, has virtually eliminated CSF leaks in lumbar laminectomies. The en bloc resection of the ligamentum flavum is another measure that mitigates the risk of interruption of the dura. Having the ligamentum flavum in position over the dura for nearly the entire case is protective in and of itself.

3.17.2 Instability

It would be unrealistic to expect an individual with preoperative instability to become any more stable from a minimally invasive laminectomy. To that end, all patients with spondylolisthesis should have flexion and extension radiographs. If the symptomatic segment is unstable, considering a decompression and fusion may be the best course of action.

Instability of a previous stable segment may occur by removing too much of the medial facet. Similar to a microdiscectomy, only that part of the facet should be removed that is necessary to reach the lateral aspect of the traversing nerve root.

Early in your experience, an additional AP fluoroscopic image may be of value to ensure adequate medial convergence onto the lamina and facet complex. In my experience, instability is more likely to occur in the upper lumbar segments, specifically L1–2 and L2–3. At those segments the facets and the lamina have a narrow window of transition.

3.17.3 Inadequate Decompression

Suboptimal placement of the minimal access port invariably leads to inadequate decompression. It is important to reconstruct the anatomy at depth by sounding the anatomy. Reconstruction of the anatomy in your mind's eye will ensure optimal placement of the access port. Undercutting the spinous process and contralateral lamina is essential to decompress the side contralateral to the approach. Palpating the foramen on both sides with a right-angled ball-tipped probe should offer an unmistakable tactile feel of a freed nerve root. At the end of the procedure, the thecal sac should also have the unmistakable appearance of a well-decompressed segment.

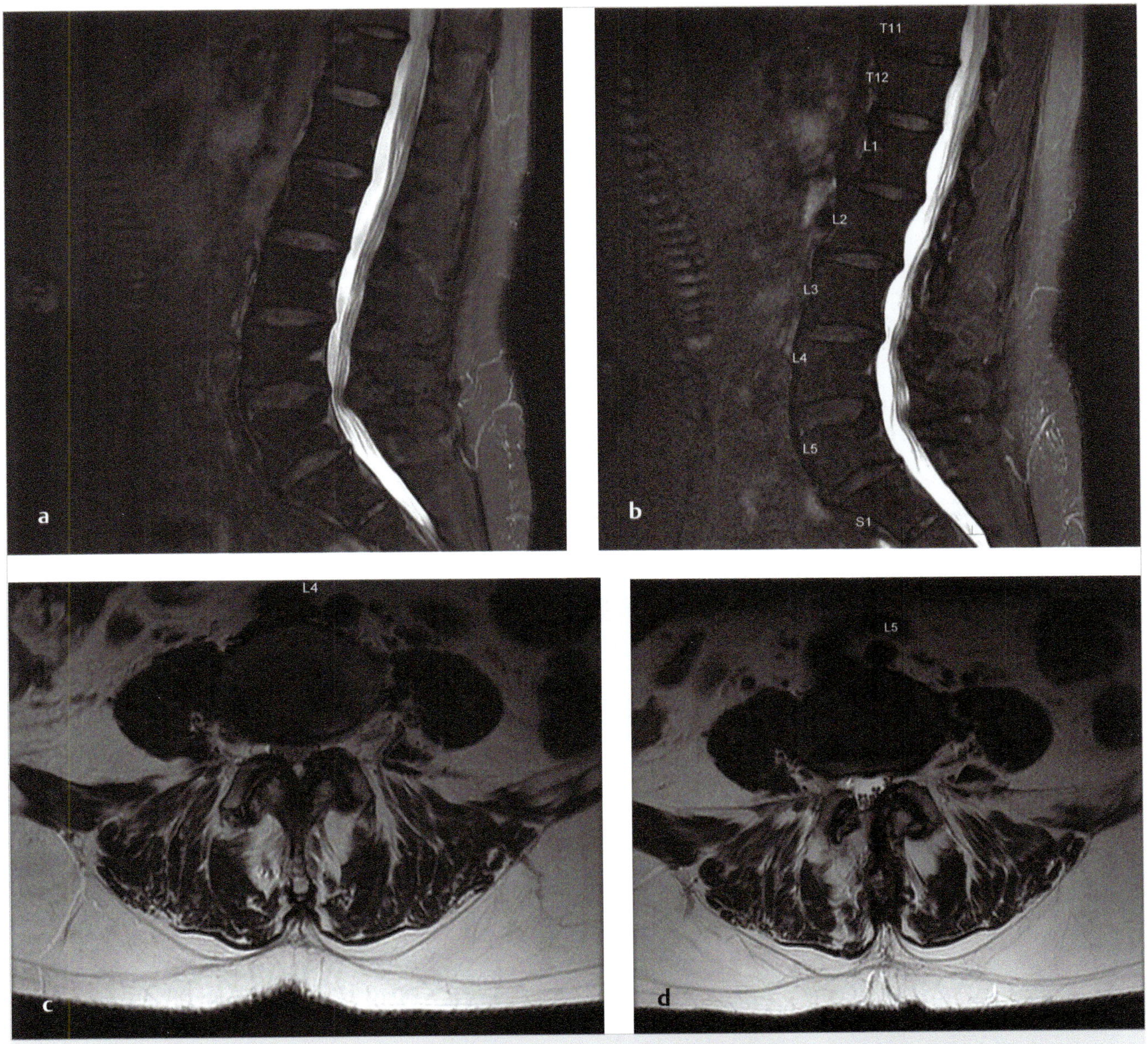

Fig. 3.54 Long-term radiographic follow-up. **(a)** Sagittal T2-weighted magnetic resonance imaging (MRI) of a then 64-year-old woman who presented with lumbar stenosis and neurogenic claudication. **(b)** Axial T2-weighted MRI through the L4–5 segment. **(c)** Sagittal T2-weighted MRI of the same patient 7 years later demonstrating a well-decompressed central canal at L4–5. The patient presented with right groin pain and was referred by her orthopedic surgeon to rule out the lumbar spine as a possible etiology. **(d)** Axial T2-weighted MRI through the L4–5 segment demonstrating a well decompressed segment. The patient at 71 years of age would go on to have a right hip replacement with complete resolution of her symptoms.

3.18 Conclusion

As a minimally invasive spine surgeon, you will readily translate the familiarity of working through a minimal access port with bayoneted instruments gained by performing minimally invasive microdiscectomies to the minimally invasive laminectomy. However, to gain further proficiency, you must first recognize the difference between these two procedures. Unlike the minimally invasive microdiscectomy, the minimally invasive lumbar laminectomy is more of a departure from its open counterpart. Although the bone work should be almost identical in a minimally invasive or open microdiscectomy, the bone work for a minimal invasive laminectomy is quite distinct. Instead of a complete laminectomy with removal of the spinous process and interruption of the posterior tension band, the minimally invasive laminectomy is more of an excavation of the lamina on top of the ligamentum flavum and a release from its insertions. Comfort will develop as you work beneath the spinous process into the contralateral aspect of the canal through a unilateral laminar approach.

The principle that “the more off the midline the starting point, the more unfamiliar the anatomy may become” begins to surface with this procedure. The angles may be more disorienting and the concept of excavating beneath the spinous process and contralateral lamina more technically demanding. However, understanding that principle allows the surgeon to better comprehend the area beneath the learning curve and to better prepare the mind for the reconstruction of the anatomy at depth.

Nevertheless, the bridge that must be spanned in the surgeon's mind does not begin from the perspective of an open laminectomy but rather from the experience of a minimally invasive microdiscectomy. That distance is shorter. Familiarity with recognizing limited fields of view while understanding the extent of bone work necessary becomes readily apparent after a thoughtful evaluation of the anatomy from a minimally invasive perspective. With those elements in mind, the area under the learning curve for this procedure will intensify and your efficiency performing the procedure will reflect that wherewithal. The experience with the microdiscectomy and laminectomy collectively forms the basis for the next step in the progression of minimally invasive surgery, the lumbar decompression, and fusion. Logically, that is the next chapter in this Primer.

This chapter began with a quotation from Dr. Cloward recommending that the lumbar laminectomy be eliminated from the spine surgeon's armamentarium. The basis for his recommendation was that the procedure "leaves the patient with painful instability and nerve-root scarring." Over three decades later, Dr. Cloward's 1985 prediction has not come to pass. The minimally invasive lumbar laminectomy is a reliable and effective treatment for neurogenic claudication for those patients with symptomatic lumbar stenosis. I cannot help but wonder what his opinion would be if he had the opportunity to scrutinize the minimally invasive lumbar laminectomy. The preservation of the musculature and the posterior tension band prevents the instability Dr. Cloward feared, and the unilateral laminar approach mitigates the "nerve root scarring" that worried him. After a thoughtful review of this procedure, would Dr. Cloward maintain the same position he so zealously stated, or would he have found a role for it in the practice of spine surgery? We are left only to wonder about his response, but I believe that in well-selected patients, he just might have become an advocate of it.

Regardless, the minimally invasive laminectomy serves as the stepping-stone upon which to embark on the operation that Dr. Cloward believed was the answer for treating degenerative disease of the spine. The eyes of the surgeon experienced in minimally invasive microdiscectomies and laminectomies will see more in the narrow corridors than will those of the unprepared mind, allowing the procedure Cloward hailed as the operation of the future to be performed minimally invasively.

References

[1] Cloward RB. Posterior lumbar interbody fusion updated. Clin Orthop Relat Res. 1985; 193:16–19

[2] Love JG. Laminectomy for the removal of spinal cord tumors. J Neurosurg 1966; 25(1):116–121

[3] Bresnahan L, Ogden AT, Natarajan RN, Fessler RG. A biomechanical evaluation of graded posterior element removal for treatment of lumbar stenosis: comparison of a minimally invasive approach with two standard laminectomy techniques. Spine. 2009; 34(1):17–23

[4] Johnsson KE, Willner S, Johnsson K. Postoperative instability after decompression for lumbar spinal stenosis. Spine. 1986; 11(2):107–110

[5] Papagelopoulos PJ, Peterson HA, Ebersold MJ, Emmanuel PR, Choudhury SN, Quast LM. Spinal column deformity and instability after lumbar or thoracolumbar laminectomy for intraspinal tumors in children and young adults. Spine. 1997; 22(4):442–451

[6] Lee MJ, Bransford RJ, Bellabarba C, et al. The effect of bilateral laminotomy versus laminectomy on the motion and stiffness of the human lumbar spine: a biomechanical comparison. Spine. 2010; 35(19):1789–1793

[7] Young S, Veerapen R, O'Laoire SA. Relief of lumbar canal stenosis using multilevel subarticular fenestrations as an alternative to wide laminectomy: preliminary report. Neurosurgery. 1988; 23(5):628–633

[8] Lin PM. Internal decompression for multiple levels of lumbar spinal stenosis: a technical note. Neurosurgery. 1982; 11(4):546–549

[9] Aryanpur J, Ducker T. Multilevel lumbar laminotomies: an alternative to laminectomy in the treatment of lumbar stenosis. Neurosurgery. 1990; 26(3): 429–432, discussion 433

[10] Poletti CE. Central lumbar stenosis caused by ligamentum flavum: unilateral laminotomy for bilateral ligamentectomy: preliminary report of two cases. Neurosurgery. 1995; 37(2):343–347

[11] Khoo LT, Fessler RG. Microendoscopic decompressive laminotomy for the treatment of lumbar stenosis. Neurosurgery. 2002; 51(5) Suppl:S146–S154

[12] Alimi M, Hofstetter CP, Pyo SY, Paulo D, Härtl R. Minimally invasive laminectomy for lumbar spinal stenosis in patients with and without preoperative spondylolisthesis: clinical outcome and reoperation rates. J Neurosurg Spine. 2015; 22(4):339–352

[13] Reulen HJ, Müller A, Ebeling U. Microsurgical anatomy of the lateral approach to extraforaminal lumbar disc herniations. Neurosurgery. 1996; 39(2):345–350, discussion 350–351

[14] Panjabi MM, Goel V, Oxland T, et al. Human lumbar vertebrae. Quantitative three-dimensional anatomy. Spine. 1992; 17(3):299–306

[15] Boukebir MA, Berlin CD, Navarro-Ramirez R, et al. Ten-step minimally invasive spine lumbar decompression and dural repair through tubular retractors. Oper Neurosurg (Hagerstown). 2017; 13(2):232–245

[16] Schöller K, Alimi M, Cong GT, Christos P, Härtl R. Lumbar spinal stenosis associated with degenerative lumbar spondylolisthesis: a systematic review and meta-analysis of secondary fusion rates following open vs minimally invasive decompression. Neurosurgery. 2017; 80(3):355–367

[17] Yong-Hing K, Reilly J, Kirkaldy-Willis WH. The ligamentum flavum. Spine. 1976; 1(4):226–234

[18] Weinstein JN, Tosteson TD, Lurie JD, et al. Surgical versus nonoperative treatment for lumbar spinal stenosis four-year results of the Spine Patient Outcomes Research Trial. Spine. 2010; 35(14):1329–1338

[19] Lurie JD, Tosteson TD, Tosteson A, et al. Long-term outcomes of lumbar spinal stenosis: eight-year results of the Spine Patient Outcomes Research Trial (SPORT). Spine. 2015; 40(2):63–76

4 Minimally Invasive Transforaminal Lumbar Interbody Fusion

Abstract
The transforaminal lumbar interbody fusion (TLIF) has become one of the most dependable procedures for decompression and stabilization of the lumbar spine since its introduction by Harms in 1998. The TLIF can be reliably used to treat a variety of conditions from recurrent disc herniations to advanced degenerative disc disease, such as radiculopathy to spondylolisthesis with instability. The introduction of minimally invasive techniques offers a natural opportunity to capitalize on the transforaminal approach, which, by its very nature, is a paramedian trajectory into the disc space. Beginning off the midline and making the facet the center of the exposure place the surgeon in the immediate vicinity of the pedicles and directly over the top of the neural elements through a focused and limited corridor. All the while, the midline structures are preserved, and the exposure is considerably less than what is needed when beginning from the midline. A minimally invasive approach with bilateral direct visualization of the facets, pars interarticularis, and laminae optimizes the Caspar ratio and preserves the midline while accomplishing the same objectives as its open counterpart. This chapter details the anatomical basis for the minimally invasive TLIF and reviews patient positioning and the operating room setup before presenting the operative technique. Finally, a review of pertinent cases illustrates the minimally invasive techniques applied in the management of a variety of diagnoses.

Keywords: facet, interbody fusion, Kambin triangle, pars interarticularis, pedicle screw, spondylolisthesis, transforaminal corridor, transverse process

The eyes will see only what the mind is prepared to comprehend.
Henri Bergson

4.1 Introduction

The previous two chapters focused on the decompression of the neural elements with minimally invasive techniques. This chapter continues to build on that skillset and introduces instrumentation of the spine through minimally invasive approaches. It is the experience of minimally invasive microdiscectomies and laminectomies that creates a natural transition from decompression to instrumentation of the spine through a paramedian approach beginning off the midline. The familiarity of the anatomy that you have acquired through a minimally invasive perspective has laid a foundation for the techniques that I describe in this chapter. It is important to recognize that the transforaminal approach is more lateral, and the angles involved are more acute than those in the microdiscectomy or laminectomy (▶ Fig. 4.1). For that reason, I will once again invoke the principle that the farther off the midline the working channel resides, the more potential there is for disorientation with the anatomy at depth. If you are cognizant of the potential cause of disorientation, you will be able to work to eliminate it. As the distance from the midline and the angles of convergence continues to increase, you must use the most recognizable and familiar structure that is off the midline as a beacon for orientation: the facet joint.

In the minimally invasive transforaminal lumbar interbody fusion (TLIF), the facet joint is the North Star that will establish your bearings (▶ Fig. 4.2). The facet guides you to the entry points for your pedicle screws, helps establish the boundaries for decompression, and offers transforaminal access to the disc space. When the exposure at depth is complete, the anatomy should be as equally obvious as it is if the approach were through a traditional midline approach. It has been the minimally invasive decompressions, both microdiscectomies and laminectomies, that have prepared your mind to comprehend the anatomy from this lateral and angled vantage point. The three-dimensional anatomical knowledge of the spine that your mind can now re-create at depth is what will allow you to do more through 28 mm of exposure than you otherwise would through an open exposure twice that size. As Henri Bergson eloquently stated, "the eyes will see only what the mind is prepared to comprehend."

4.2 Minimally Invasive TLIF: A Heterogeneous Entity

Before describing the minimally invasive TLIF in this chapter, it is important to acknowledge that there is no universally accepted minimally invasive transforaminal approach. Over the years of its development, surgeons have combined several existing technologies that include percutaneous placement of pedicle screws with minimal access approaches, unilateral fixation, facet fixation, and combinations thereof. Fluoroscopy and a variety of forms of image guidance systems have been the mainstay of imaging for the procedure. A PubMed search including the terms "minimally invasive transforaminal lumbar interbody fusion" and "technique" since 2005 generated over 100 references. However, despite the multiple permutations of this procedure, when one distills the various forms of the minimally invasive TLIF from these references, three main techniques arise:

1. Percutaneous placement of pedicle screws and decompression with interbody placement through a fixed tubular retractor as described by Fessler and Foley.[1,2]
2. Use of expandable minimal access retractors for bilateral direct exposure of the bony anatomy and placement of pedicle screws, decompression and interbody placement as described by Mummaneni and Rodts.[3]
3. A hybrid technique of 1 and 2: Percutaneous pedicle screw placement on one side of the anatomy and use of an expandable minimal access port for pedicle screw placement decompression and interbody placement on the other.

Over the years, I have employed all the above-mentioned TLIF permutations and have settled on one approach. My journey to

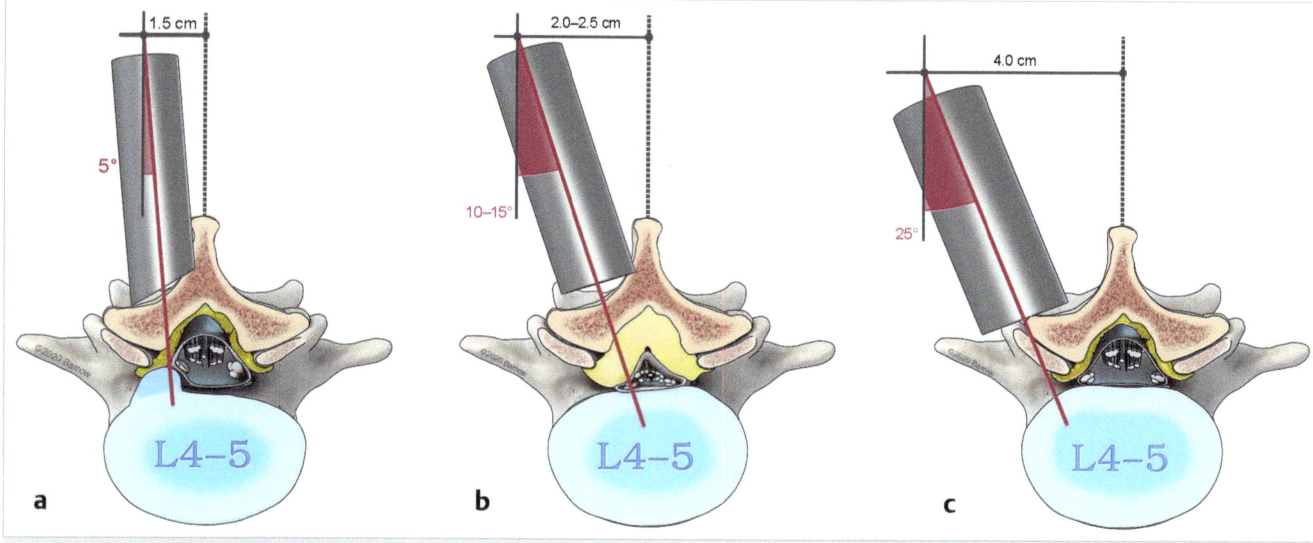

Fig. 4.1 Illustration demonstrating the distance off the midline and the angle of convergence at L4–5 for a microdiscectomy, laminectomy and transforaminal lumbar interbody fusion. **(a)** The position of a minimal access port for a microdiscectomy at 1.5 cm off the midline with an angle of convergence of 5 degrees. **(b)** The position of a minimal access port for a laminectomy at 2.0-2.5 cm off the midline with an angle of convergence of 10 to 15 degrees. **(c)** The position of an expandable minimal access port 4.0 cm off the midline with an angle of convergence of 25 degrees encompassing the facet joint.

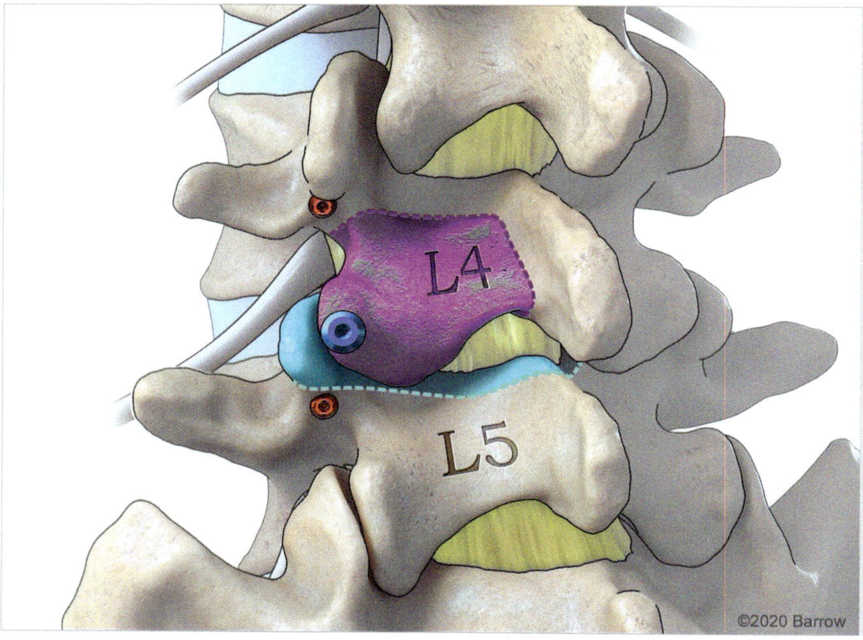

Fig. 4.2 The North Star of the minimally invasive transforaminal lumbar interbody fusion: the facet joint. The blue fiducial indicates the docking point for the first dilator. Pedicle screw entry points (marked with red fiducials) are only millimeters away from the blue fiducial as are the osteotomy cuts (*dotted lines*). The transforaminal access into the disc space is relative to this joint.

that one particular approach was a philosophical one. Throughout this book, I have emphasized that the procedures performed with a minimally invasive approach should be indistinguishable from the same procedure performed with an open approach. Applying that criterion implies that the decompression performed through a minimal access port would need to be indistinguishable from its open equivalent. The same would apply to the actual fusion construct, which includes the interbody and posterolateral arthrodesis. I was also mindful of the various criticisms of the minimally invasive TLIF, specifically that the procedure takes far too long, exposes the surgeons to too much ionizing radiation because of the reliance on fluoroscopy, does not adequately restore segmental lordosis, and does not allow for adequate central decompression. As I evolved my surgical technique, I incorporated these criticisms of the minimally invasive TLIF along with my philosophical standard that whatever procedure I performed in a minimally invasive manner should be indistinguishable from that of the open procedure. The procedure that I believe allowed me to meet all of these criteria while simultaneously addressing the perceived shortcomings of minimally invasive surgery (MIS) was a TLIF performed through direct bilateral exposure of the requisite anatomical structures using expandable minimal access ports.

Direct exposure of the facets and pars interarticularis bilaterally eliminated the need for excessive fluoroscopy, which is associated with percutaneous pedicle screws. Direct visualization of the anatomy for pedicle screw placement reduced radiation exposure to levels lower than what is reported for instrumenting the lumbar spine through open midline exposures. I found that a fixed 22-mm access port did not offer me the exposure to complete a wide decompression and that using larger diameters, such as a fixed 26-mm access port, provided more exposure but not necessarily in the dimensions that I needed. Minor adjustments to the expandable minimal access port and rotation of the patient away from me facilitated complete central decompressions of the neural elements and expedited the procedure. Through this process of thoughtful evaluation of the various options to complete the procedure, ultimately one technique emerged with which I could accomplish all of my goals for the operation, expedite the procedure, and minimize fluoroscopy. Although there are several perfectly acceptable techniques with which to perform the minimally invasive TLIF procedure, this chapter details the rationale and the technique of a minimally invasive TLIF performed in this manner. Given the circuitous journey to the technique I present in this chapter, it is helpful to discuss the rationale behind this approach. The following two sections address the reasoning and justification behind opting for direct instead of percutaneous pedicle screw placement and the selection of an expandable minimal access port over the selection of one with a fixed diameter.

4.3 Rationale: Percutaneous versus Direct Placement of Pedicle Screws

There is nothing more familiar to a spine surgeon than directly looking upon the junction of the pars interarticularis, transverse process and inferior lateral aspect of the lumbar facet to envision the entry point for a pedicle screw in the lumbar spine (▶ Fig. 4.3). The direct exposure of these anatomical landmarks allows for anatomical certainty that a fluoroscopic image or even a computer-generated navigation image cannot supplant. Medial to these landmarks are the lamina and the spinous process, which house the compressed thecal sac and nerve roots. While I am exposing entry points for the pedicle screws, I am simultaneously exposing the requisite anatomy for a decompression and transforaminal access to the disc space. Thus, two elements of the operation occur concurrently, moving the whole operation forward.

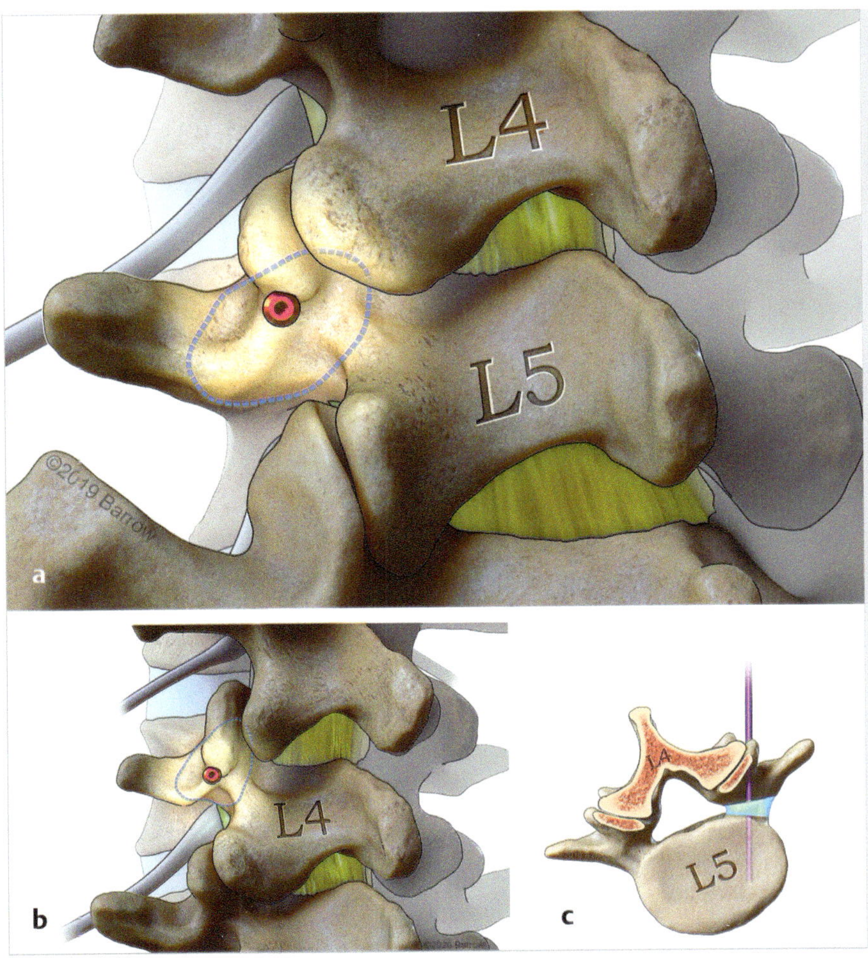

Fig. 4.3 The anatomy of the lumbar pedicle. Illustration demonstrating the pedicle screw entry point for L5 **(a)** and L4 **(b)** at the junction of the pars interarticularis, transverse process and facet denoted by the red fiducial. **(c)** The trajectory for an L5 pedicle screw converging at 25 degrees into the pedicle.

Equally important, the minimal access ports may be secured into their ideal position with two or three fluoroscopic images. It would take me as many fluoroscopic images just to select where to make the stab incision for one percutaneous pedicle screw entry point.

I secure the expandable minimal access ports over the top of the facets on either side and begin the exposure of the pedicle screw entry points. No further fluoroscopy is immediately necessary. In fact, the fluoroscope may be moved away from the operative field until the exposure is complete. I identify the four pedicle screw entry points with direct visualization of the anatomical landmarks within the first 15 minutes of the operation through two well-positioned access ports. With the exposure complete, the fluoroscope is rolled back into the operative field so that I can confirm entry points and trajectories into the pedicles. I drill the entry points, probe through the cancellous bone with a pedicle probe and ensure the integrity of the cortical wall of the pedicle with a ball-tipped probe. I tap the pedicle, determine the width and length of the pedicle and place the screws with only a few lateral fluoroscopic images. On average, there will be no more than four or five fluoroscopic images obtained per instrumented pedicle.

Percutaneous placement of pedicle screws, on the other hand, is either a fluoroscopically driven or image-guided process. The absence of direct visualization of the bony anatomy precludes the ability to use the skill set that we all developed in open surgery. It eliminates our tactile feel of the pedicle that allows us to ensure the integrity of the pedicle and replaces it with anteroposterior (AP) and lateral fluoroscopic images of a Jamshidi needle advancing a K-wire. The absence of direct visualization of the bony anatomy mandates the need for additional fluoroscopic images to guide the placement of the instruments, thereby increasing the radiation exposure to the patient, surgeon and operative team. I readily concede that use of image guidance nullifies this point; however, the absence of tactile feedback remains an issue, at least for me.

The lack of access to the facets and transverse processes is another concern I have with percutaneous techniques. The inability to perform a posterolateral fusion, facetectomy or Smith–Petersen osteotomy is a considerable limitation. With a paramedian incision and direct visualization of the pedicle screw entry points, the transverse processes come fully into view, allowing the drill to thoroughly decorticate and then heap a bounteous amount of morselized autograft, allograft or both onto them to achieve a posterolateral arthrodesis. Paramedian exposures of the transverse process are vastly superior to a midline approach for access to the posterolateral space. I am routinely able to drill the entire transverse process with direct visualization all the way to its lateral tip. An equivalent exposure in an open midline approach would be quite a feat requiring extensive dissection and added length to what is already a sizeable incision.

Finally, the importance of achieving segmental lordosis in transforaminal approaches cannot be overemphasized. One of the weaknesses identified in the literature with transforaminal approaches is the limitation to restore lordosis.[4] In patients with either iatrogenic or degenerative flat back, restoration of segmental lordosis is a vital objective of the operation. A percutaneous approach to the pedicles creates an inherent limitation to achieve segmental lordosis because the contralateral facet remains entirely unexposed and intact. The absence of bilateral facetectomies or the capacity to perform a Smith–Petersen osteotomy on the side contralateral to the transforaminal corridor limits the degree of compression you can achieve and thereby limits the restoration of lumbar lordosis.[5,6,7]

The distinct advantage of an expandable minimal access port is that it permits simultaneous exposure of the entire facet, lamina and pars interarticularis with the port in the same position that was used for the instrumentation. A complete facetectomy on the side of the transforaminal approach and a Smith–Petersen osteotomy on the opposite side, as recommended by Shaffrey and colleagues,[8] optimize the restoration of the lordosis that would be difficult to achieve when one facet remains unexposed.

The advantages of percutaneous technology surpass minimal access direct visualization approaches in multilevel operations, specifically for three or more levels. Although the minimal access approaches described in this chapter become untenable after two levels, the percutaneous techniques offer the possibility for the least disruption of the native spine in the stabilization of multiple levels. In a five-level fusion, direct visualization through a paramedian approach no longer plays to the strength of that technique. Percutaneously placed pedicle screws in that circumstance offer a distinct advantage, and it is always wise to play to the strengths of an individual technique.

4.4 Rationale: Decompression—Fixed Tube versus Expandable Retractor

For guidance regarding the type of minimal access port to use, I look no further than the anatomy. In my estimation, the decompression in any TLIF, whether minimally invasive or open, should include a pedicle-to-beyond-pedicle decompression. The entire thecal sac should be decompressed along with the exiting and traversing roots at the operative segment. As seen in Chapter 2 and shown in ▶ Fig. 4.4, the interpedicular distances range from 36 mm at L3–4 to 28 mm at L5–S1. Therefore, to achieve a pedicle-to-beyond-pedicle decompression, one would need exposure from the inferior aspect of the rostral pedicle to the superior aspect of the caudal pedicle. In most circumstances in the lumbosacral spine, this would require 26 to 32 mm of exposure. The minimal access port that allows for such an exposure all at once is the logical one to use.

Early in my experience, I used a 22-mm fixed access port for decompression and interbody placement. I could readily decompress the traversing root but had difficulty exposing and visualizing the exiting root within the same field of view. Decompression of the entire thecal sac was possible by angling the tube medially, but I found myself making multiple adjustments to fully expose the anatomy that required decompression. When the decompression was completed, I was unable to visualize all the anatomy that I had decompressed within one field of view. Regardless of the trajectory of the port, some element of the anatomy was always outside of that field of view. Although this limited visualization is acceptable for a simple decompression, the inability to visualize all the anatomy, specifically the exiting nerve root, when placing an interbody

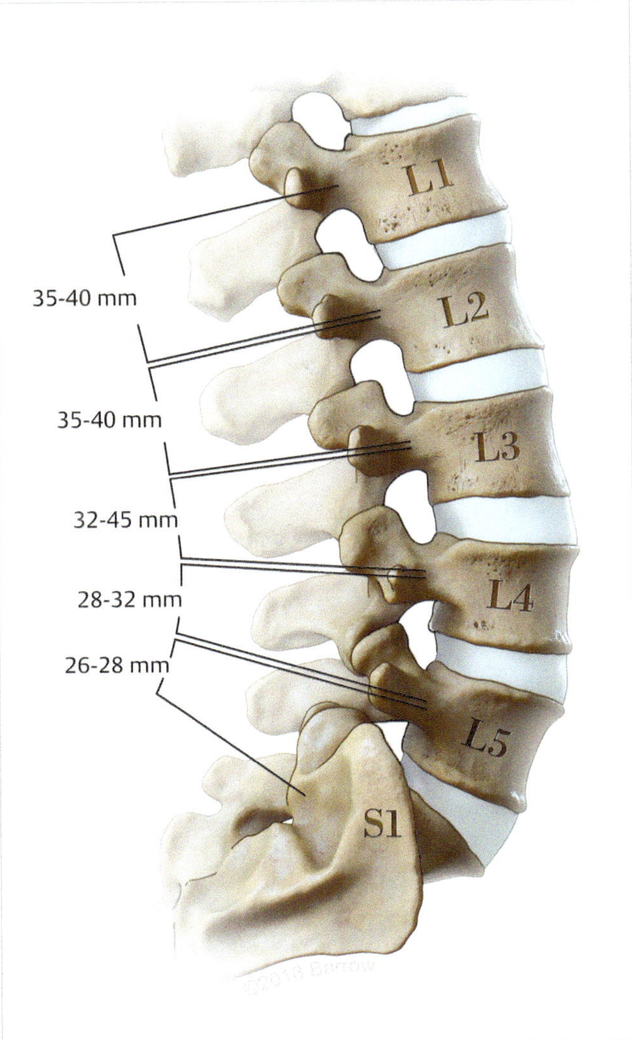

Fig. 4.4 Illustration of the interpedicular distances in the lumbar spine. This illustration from Chapter 2, Minimally Invasive Microdiscetomy, is especially relevant not only for the anatomical basis of the minimally invasive transforaminal lumbar interbody fusion but also for the selection of the minimal access port. The access port that can simultaneously encompass the relevant anatomy of an entire segment is the logical access port to employ for the procedure.

through a transforaminal approach, presented some potential hazards to that exiting root.

Placement of the interbody spacer through a fixed access port became another issue. Such a feat was technically difficult because of the constraints of a fixed diameter. I found that the access port dictated the geometry of the interbody spacer that I would place, specifically the straight spacers designed for posterior lumbar interbody fusions (PLIFs), instead of those with curved geometry, which better occupy the apophyseal ring in the anterior aspect of the disc space. Finally, visualization during placement of the interbody was limited. I was unable to feel comfortable blindly retracting the nerve root while simultaneously securing the interbody into position. For these reasons, I began to explore the role of an expandable minimal access port through which to perform the decompression and secure the interbody spacer.

I found a unique learning curve with the use of an expandable minimal access port, but it did resolve nearly all the issues I was having with a fixed access port. I could simultaneously expose all my pedicle screw entry points along with the bony anatomy that would be needed for an adequate decompression. The capacity to simultaneously expose the anatomy for instrumentation, decompression, and interbody work lent itself to a more efficient work flow. I found myself able to seamlessly transition from one phase of the operation to the next.

I also found that I was better able to visualize the base of the spinous process with a well-placed mediolateral retractor and thereby achieve a midline and contralateral decompression. The exposure that I could achieve with an expandable minimal access port allowed for a pedicle-to-beyond-pedicle decompression of the thecal sac, along with the decompression of both the exiting and traversing nerve roots. The exposure further allowed me to use a curved interbody geometry without compromising my visualization of the neural elements. Finally, I felt much more comfortable retracting the traversing nerve root under direct visualization while securing the interbody into position.

In the final analysis, the rationale for the technique that I describe in this chapter evolved to optimize visualization and decompression of the neural elements and facilitate placement of the interbody while minimizing the need for fluoroscopy for placement of pedicle screws on the ipsilateral side. On the contralateral side, an expandable minimal access port allows for placement of pedicle screws with minimal fluoroscopy and offers access to the transverse processes for a posterolateral fusion and for a facetectomy or Smith–Petersen osteotomy to restore segmental lordosis. Collectively, I feel that employment of a combination of these techniques increases the efficiency of the operation and is more consistent with performing these procedures in ambulatory surgical centers, where computer-assisted navigation may be cost prohibitive. But most importantly, achieving all these objectives optimizes the long-term outcomes.[7]

4.5 Requisite Anatomy

The requisite anatomy for a single-level TLIF that allows for transforaminal access on one side, a posterior column osteotomy and a posterior lateral fusion on the other, is demonstrated in ▶ Fig. 4.5. Whether you are performing the procedure through a traditional midline approach or a minimally invasive one, the requisite anatomy includes access to the pedicle screw entry points, pars interarticularis, facets, lamina and transverse processes of a segment. Notably absent from the list of the requisite anatomy are the spinous processes, whose exposure in a midline approach is the inevitable consequence of the location of the incision. Access to the pedicles employing percutaneous techniques slightly narrows that exposure but comes with the inherent limitations detailed above. For a two-level TLIF, the exposure includes another set of pedicles, laminae, and facets. I believe that a three-level minimally invasive TLIF resides outside of the strengths of MIS with direct visualization as described in this chapter. Multiple levels of interbody and pedicle instrumentation cross into a realm where percutaneous technology now offers greater advantages than disadvantages.

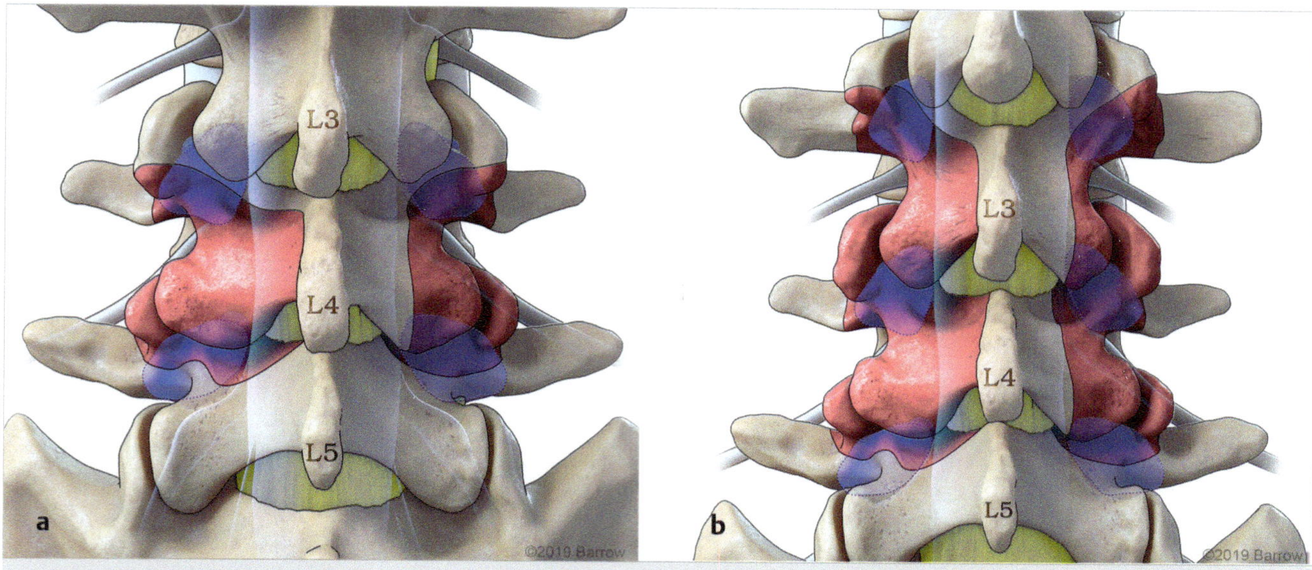

Fig. 4.5 Requisite anatomy for a **(a)** single-level and **(b)** two-level transforaminal lumbar interbody fusion. Whether performed minimally invasively or through a traditional, midline open approach, the pedicles, facets, medial aspect of the lamina and the pars interarticularis are all needed for the operation. In both of these illustrations, the requisite anatomy is demarcated in red, and the pedicles are demarcated in blue.

4.6 Anatomical Basis

The anatomical basis for the minimally invasive TLIF is determined by the angle of convergence into the pedicle. In Section 4.4, Rationale: Decompression: Fixed Tube Versus Expandable Retractor, I touched on the anatomical basis for using an expandable minimal access port for minimally invasive TLIFs, but not the anatomical basis for applying minimally invasive techniques for the TLIF itself. However, one glance at the requisite anatomy highlighted in ▶ Fig. 4.5 begins to build that argument for me. After all, ▶ Fig. 4.5 demonstrates that all the requisite anatomy is lateral, not medial. Beginning in the midline will require a considerably longer incision not only for exposure of the requisite anatomy but also to attain the converging angles into the pedicle. The optimal angle into the pedicle is from lateral to medial as seen in ▶ Fig. 4.6. From that standpoint, the most direct and efficient access to a segment would be from a paramedian starting point that converges onto the epicenter of the requisite anatomy, which is the facet. From there, the surgeon has ready access to the pedicles that are only millimeters away. Finally, the trajectory into the pedicle would be parallel to the trajectory of the access port. It has been my experience with a midline approach that I am waging a battle against the skin and muscle to reach the lateral aspect of the exposure to accomplish the same angle.

Once the surgeon is untethered from the midline and instead working directly over the requisite anatomy, the anatomy determines the extent of the exposure and the length of the incision. ▶ Fig. 4.6 illustrates the interpedicular distance at the various segments from L3 to S1. Limiting the exposure to what the anatomy dictates adheres to the principle set forth by Caspar regarding the ratio of the surgical target to the surgical exposure. A 25-mm incision at L5–S1 on either side of the midline allows for the 26- to 28-mm exposure needed for the operation. A 28-mm incision at L4–5 and a 32- to 35-mm incision at L3–4 accomplish the same. The surgical target defined by the requisite anatomy in ▶ Fig. 4.5 and the exposure determined by ▶ Fig. 4.6 result in a favorable Caspar ratio.

4.7 Preoperative Considerations

In addition to a clinical history and neurologic examination, magnetic resonance imaging (MRI) and AP and lateral radiographs, along with flexion–extension radiographs, are essential. The MRI unveils the level or levels of compression of the neural elements, which should correlate with the patient's neurological examination findings and subjective complaints, both of which guide surgical decision making and the extent of the surgery. MRIs also demonstrate alignment and allow for grading of spondylolisthesis.

I have found that most patients present to the clinic with their MRIs, but a set of static and dynamic radiographs is seldom provided. In the preoperative surgical planning phase, radiographs are equally as important as the MRIs. Flexion and extension studies are helpful in determining the degree of stability of the segment. Extension studies are particularly helpful in determining how much reduction of spondylolisthesis will be obtainable by positioning. The AP and lateral radiographs are predictive of the type of imaging that can be obtained with fluoroscopy in surgery. It is valuable to appreciate a severe coronal imbalance before surgery, so that necessary adjustments can be made to the fluoroscope and incision. ▶ Fig. 4.7 illustrates a case where the preoperative imaging prompted adjustment of the fluoroscope for surgery. In this patient, a severe leftward coronal imbalance on an AP preoperative radiograph prompted a preoperative AP fluoroscopic image. That image defined the angle through the disc space and determined the optimal location for the incisions over the requisite anatomy.

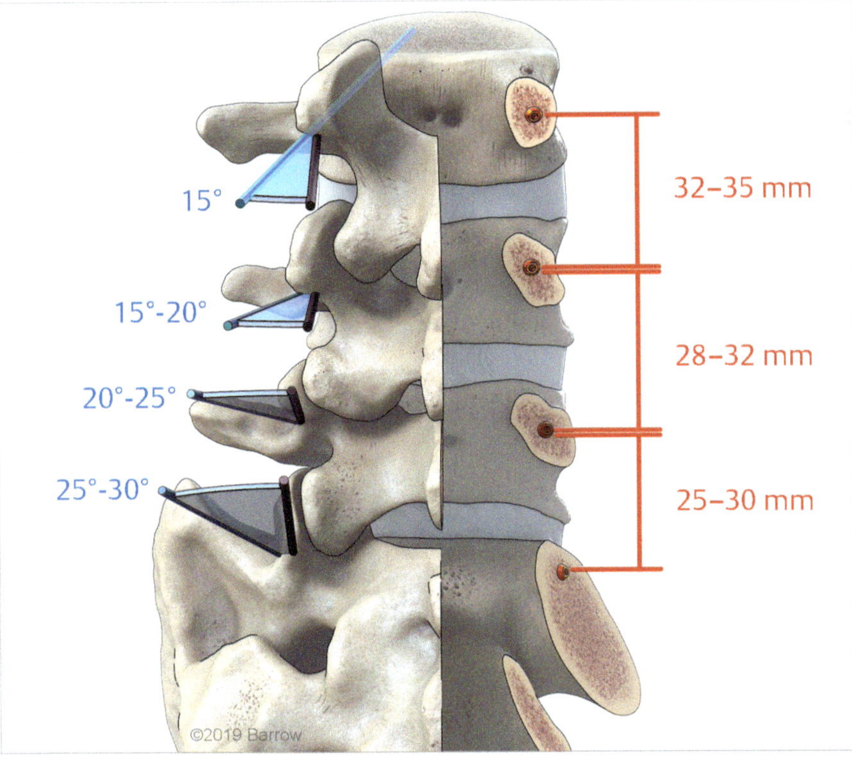

Fig. 4.6 The anatomical basis of a minimally invasive transforaminal lumbar interbody fusion. In this posterior view of the spine, the optimal angle into each pedicle from L3 to S1 is demonstrated on the left side of the spine illustration. A lateral to medial converging angle into the pedicle is most effectively accomplished with a paramedian incision converging onto the facet instead of beginning in the midline and attempting to accomplish that medially converging angle by working in an increasingly lateral direction. The right side of the spine has the posterior elements removed to demonstrate the interpedicular distances in the lumbosacral spine. A midline incision mandates a longer exposure to reach the lateral aspects of the requisite anatomy. In a minimally invasive approach centered over the requisite anatomy, the incision is determined by the interpedicular distance. When the surgeon is untethered from a midline approach, the exposure may be focused and defined by the anatomy itself instead of the constraints of the exposure.

Patients may present with either unilateral symptoms or bilateral symptoms. Unilateral symptoms mandate a transforaminal approach from the symptomatic side. Bilateral symptoms, in the presence of bilateral foraminal stenosis, may mandate bilateral facetectomies. Even in the setting of bilateral facetectomies, although bilateral access to the disc space may be considered, my preference remains to access the interbody space only from one side. Careful analysis of the parasagittal T1-weighted MRIs is critical in assessing the extent of neural foraminal stenosis. In the case of central stenosis with symptoms of neurogenic claudication, severe foraminal stenosis on one side alone may prompt a transforaminal approach from that side.

Any concern for degenerative scoliosis on AP or lateral imaging should prompt standing 36-inch scoliosis radiographs. It is important to recognize that there is an inherent limitation to the amount of lumbar lordosis that may be restored in a single-level minimally invasive TLIF. It has been my experience that 12 degrees of lordosis is at the upper threshold that I can reliably achieve per segment after an ipsilateral complete facetectomy and contralateral Smith–Petersen osteotomy. A significant mismatch in lumbar lordosis and pelvic incidence warrants careful consideration during operative planning. Patients invariably request a minimally invasive solution to their symptoms, but the anatomical circumstance of their degeneration may reside outside the realm of a single minimally invasive approach. The surgeon must recognize these circumstances and define the surgical objectives that need to be achieved to bring the spine back into balance. I always remind the patient who is fixated on a minimally invasive approach that if they think they are too old for the right operation, then they are far too old for the wrong one (▶ Fig. 4.8).

4.8 Operating Room Setup

I prefer to use a Jackson table with the ability to rotate to perform these operations. The Jackson table accomplishes two objectives: it prevents flattening of the back and decreases blood loss. Having the abdomen freely hanging decreases the intra-abdominal pressure and thereby decreases central venous pressure (▶ Fig. 4.9). In my experience, a patient on a Jackson table tends to have less venous bleeding than a patient on a Wilson frame. In fact, I have had greater blood loss from a microdiscectomy on a Wilson frame when tangling with engorged epidural veins near the pedicle than from a TLIF on a Jackson table. Allowing the abdomen to freely hang allows for a greater capacity to restore lumbar lordosis. Placing the hips in slight hyperextension also captures more lumbar lordosis. As mentioned in Chapter 3 on lumbar laminectomy, the capacity to rotate the patients away from the surgeon allows for an ergonomically sound position to decompress the contralateral recess.

The radiology technologist positions the fluoroscope immediately after positioning the patient with the image intensifier opposite the side of the transforaminal access and parks it at the level of the patient's knees. In this manner, the image intensifier is also opposite the side of the microscope. In the absence of any severe coronal imbalance or degenerative scoliosis seen on preoperative plain radiographs, I defer obtaining any preoperative fluoroscopic images. The operating room team places

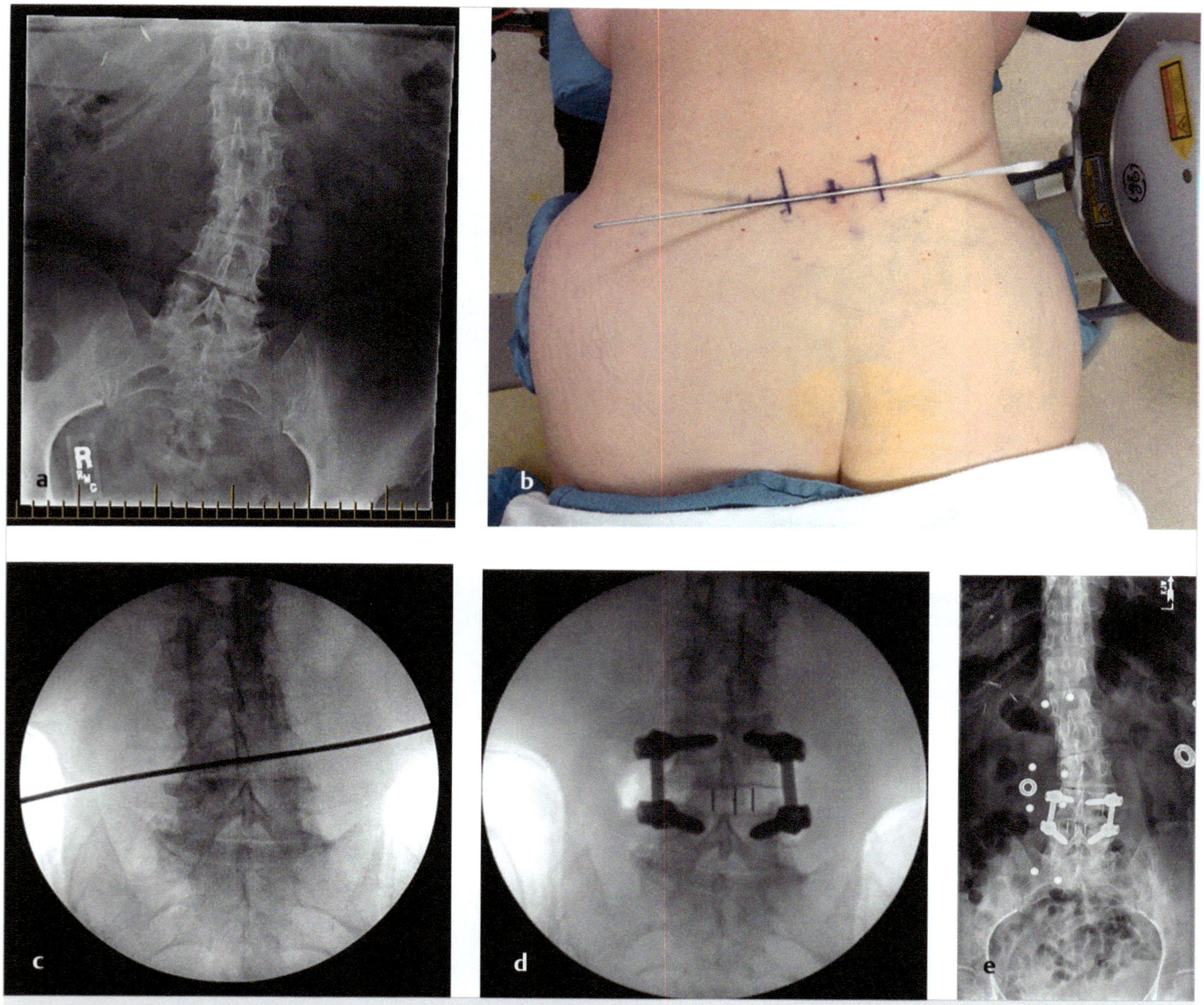

Fig. 4.7 The importance of preoperative radiographs. **(a)** Preoperative radiograph of a patient who presented with a left L4 radiculopathy secondary to a severe coronal imbalance. This preoperative radiograph prompted placement of a Steinman pin over the top of the segment to plan the incision and guide the position and the wag of the fluoroscope as seen in this **(b)** photograph and **(c)** fluoroscopic image. Recognizing the extent of the coronal imbalance, which is not as apparent on magnetic resonance imaging, facilitated planning the incision in a manner that would optimize placement of the pedicle screws as seen in the **(d)** fluoroscopic image and correction of the coronal imbalance as seen in the **(e)** postoperative anteroposterior radiograph.

the microscope on the side of the transforaminal access and the scrub technician drapes it as the patient is anesthetized (▶ Fig. 4.10).

4.9 Operative Technique: The Three Phases of the Operation

I divide the minimally invasive TLIF into three distinct phases. I have found that creating these divisions is helpful to the entire minimally invasive ensemble. It allows the scrub technician to prepare the Mayo stand for each operational phase, that is, pedicle screw phase, decompression phase and interbody phase. The operating room nurse knows to be ready to transition with the microscope after the fourth pedicle screw goes in, and the radiology technologist knows when to be available. Having these distinct phases optimizes the flow of the operation for the entire team and provides targets for increased efficiency.

Phase I entails planning the incision, docking the minimal access ports, exposing the pedicle screw entry points, and securing the pedicle screws into position. I perform this part of the procedure with loupes and a headlight. Phase II entails the laminectomy, facetectomy and decompression of the neural elements, along with the discectomy performed under the operating microscope. If a Smith–Petersen osteotomy is planned for the contralateral side, I perform it during the second phase. Finally phase III, performed under loupes and a headlight,

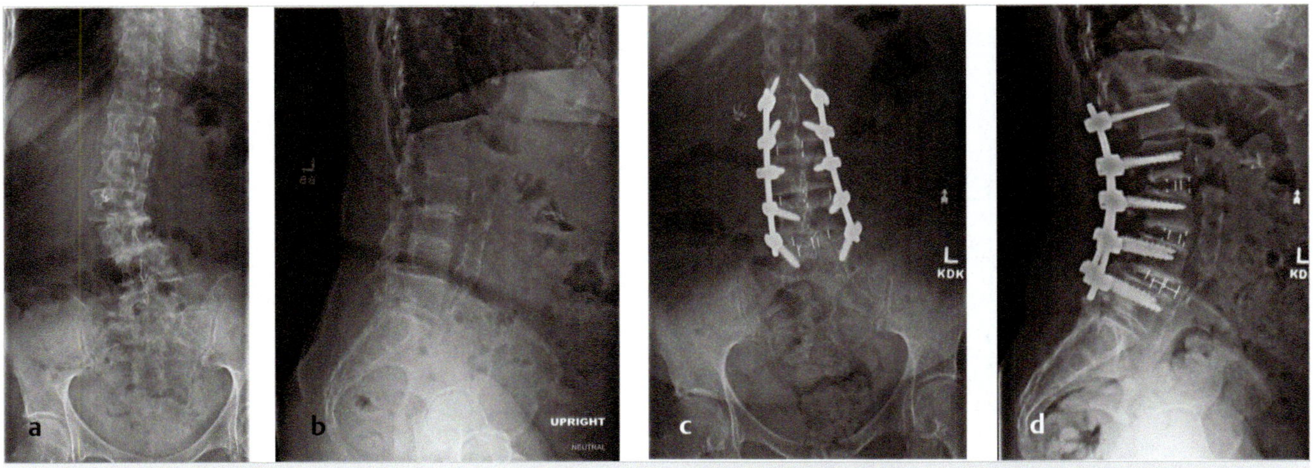

Fig. 4.8 The limitations of a single-level minimally invasive transforaminal lumbar interbody fusion. **(a)** Anteroposterior and lateral radiographs in a patient who presented requesting a minimally invasive operation. The patient had undergone three previous operations over the past decade. **(b)** The pelvic incidence and lumbar lordosis mismatch, degenerative scoliosis, positive sagittal vertical axis (SVA) and multiple levels of spondylolisthesis required the correction of too many parameters and were outside of what could be accomplished with a minimally invasive single-level or two-level operation. **(c)** A more comprehensive surgical plan was offered that would correct these various parameters. Minimally invasive techniques such as transpsoas approaches at L2–3 and L3–4 were used as part of the operative strategy. However, a **(d)** traditional midline approach was needed to allow for multiple levels of Smith–Petersen osteotomies and a transforaminal access to L4–5 to correct the lumbar lordosis and SVA. Clearly defining the objectives that need to be met with the surgery and then deciding whether those objectives can be met with a minimally invasive option is paramount.

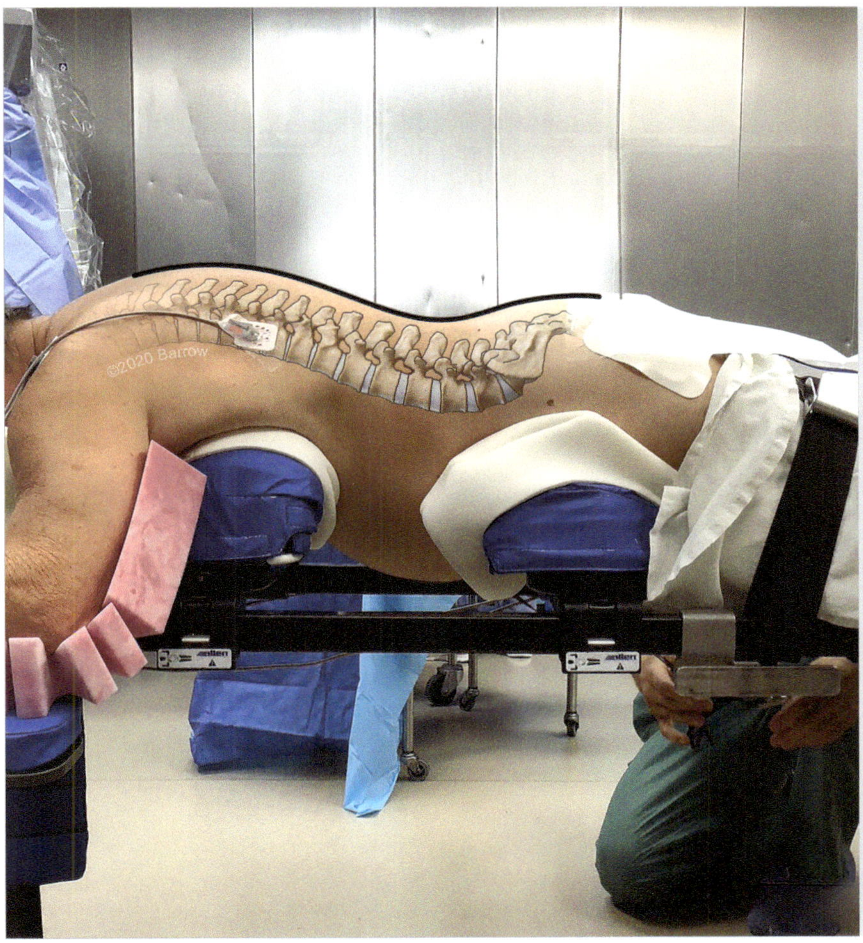

Fig. 4.9 Patient positioning on a Jackson table. The patient in this photograph is undergoing a minimally invasive L4–5 transforaminal lumbar interbody fusion with a right-sided transforaminal approach. The patient is positioned on the Jackson table, where the abdomen can hang freely, thereby decreasing the central venous pressure. With a series of pads, the hips are slightly hyperextended to further optimize lordosis. An artist's rendition of the lumbar spine in lordosis and a contoured black line have been superimposed on the photograph.

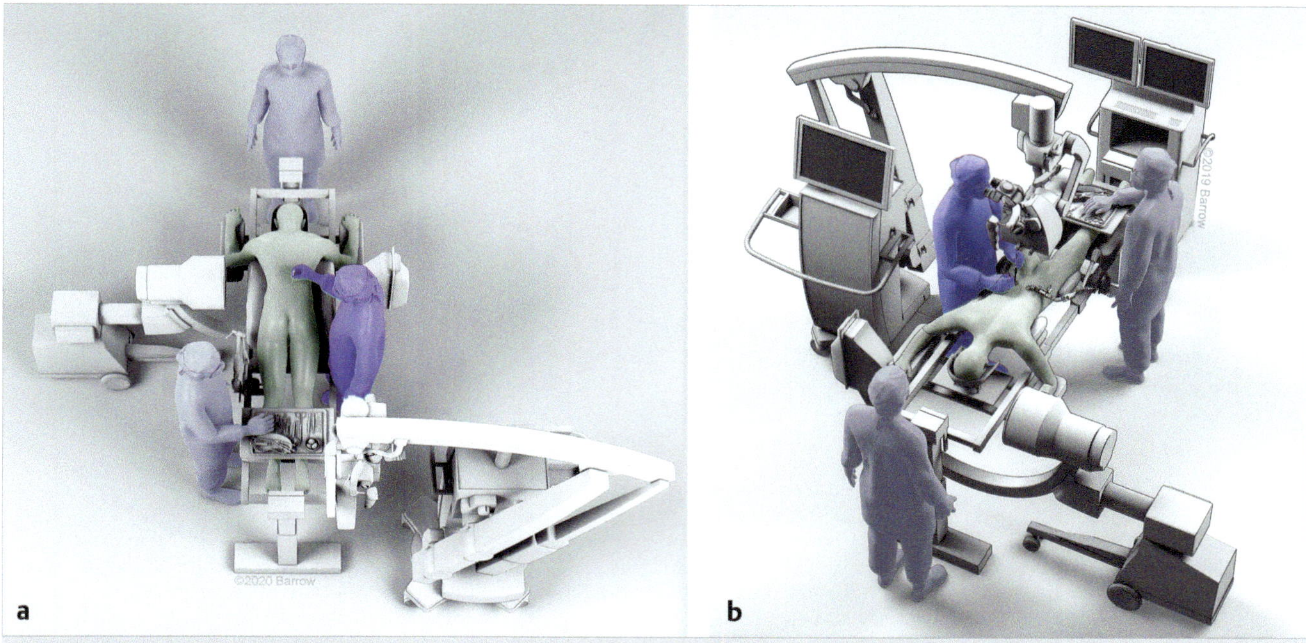

Fig. 4.10 Schematic operating room set up for a minimally invasive transforaminal lumbar interbody fusion. **(a)** Illustration demonstrating the patient positioned on a Jackson table. The microscope is positioned on the symptomatic side of the patient, and the base of the fluoroscope is positioned opposite the microscope. The surgeon performs phase I (pedicle screw placement) and phase III (interbody placement) of the operation with the fluoroscope in position. **(b)** Phase II is performed under the operating microscope with the fluoroscope rolled to the head of the bed, ready to roll back into position for phase III.

entails final preparation of the end plates, identifying the interbody height using a series of trials, rotating the interbody spacer into position, and securing the rods with compression and closure. Each phase will be reviewed in depth in the next sections (Video 4.1).

4.9.1 Phase I: Incision, Docking Minimal Access Ports and Pedicle Screw Placement

After positioning the patient on a Jackson table, I palpate the anterior superior iliac spine to approximate the L4–5 level. I mark the presumptive level, along with the spinous processes above and below, which helps me establish the midline. As described in Chapters 2 and 3, if the level is L2–3, L3–4, L4–5 or L5–S1, I mark what I believe to be the appropriate interspinous process space according to my initial approximation of L4–5. Regarding the length of the incision, I mark 10 mm down from the interspinous process space and 15 to 20 mm up. The rationale is that the interspinous space is indicative of the disc space and the caudal pedicle is closer to the level of the disc space than the rostral pedicle, as seen in ▶ Fig. 4.11. Another glance at ▶ Fig. 4.4 and ▶ Fig. 4.6 reminds us that at L5–S1, the interpedicular distance is seldom more than 28 mm, thereby allowing for a smaller incision of about 25 mm. The pedicles may be reliably accessed with a 28-mm incision at L4–5, where the interpedicular distance increases. At L3–4 and L2–3, the interpedicular distance can be up to 36 mm, mandating a slightly longer incision. I will make these incisions 30 to 35 mm in length at those levels.

The lateral placement of the incision is based on the level operated upon and the body habitus of the patient. At the lower segments of L4–5 and L5–S1, depending on the size and girth of the patient, I plan two incisions on either side of midline approximately 3.5 cm from the spinous process for leaner patients and up to 4.0 cm for larger patients (body mass index [BMI] > 35). That distance off the midline optimizes the trajectory into the pedicle, which must be up to 25 degrees for L5 and up to 30 degrees for S1. For the upper segments of L3–4 and L2–3, I plan the incision 3.0 to 3.5 cm on either side of the midline, again with the rationale that not only is the intrapedicular distance smaller, bringing the facets closer together, but the angle of convergence into the pedicle is also less, about 15 to 20 degrees (▶ Fig. 4.12).

The fluoroscope remains parked at the patient's knees as I plan, measure and mark the incisions (▶ Fig. 4.13). I then prep and drape the patient and include the fluoroscope in the field to have it ready for an immediate image and thereby optimize the workflow of the operation. In a straightforward degenerative case, I am reluctant to obtain a fluoroscopic image before beginning the operation. A preoperative image will not preclude needing to take the same images once the operation has begun. The time invested in evaluating the preoperative AP and lateral radiographs pays immediate dividends at this point. If the AP images demonstrate scoliosis or a significant coronal imbalance, as seen in ▶ Fig. 4.7, then it is worthwhile to obtain an AP image immediately after positioning the patient and prior

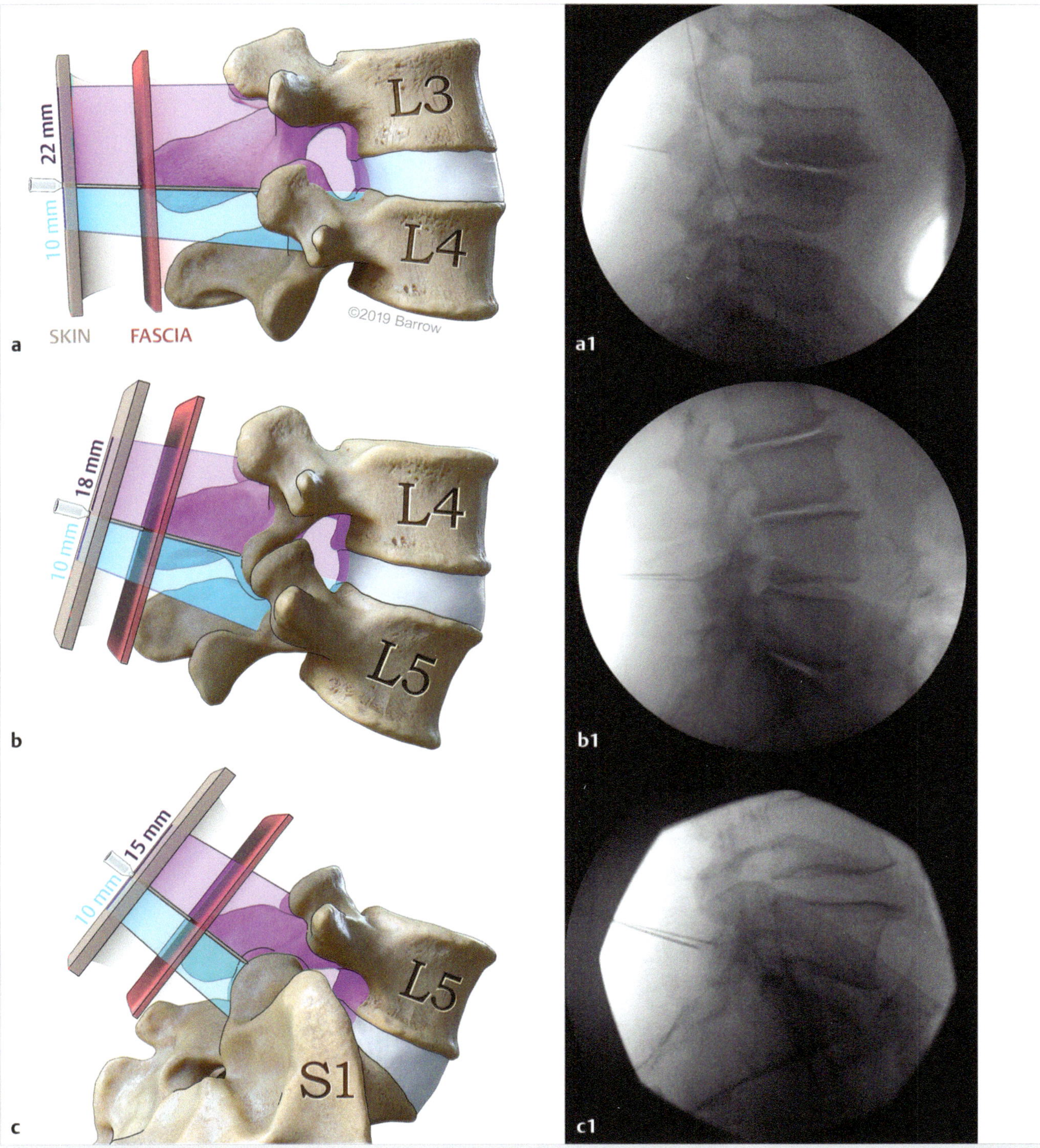

Fig. 4.11 Rationale for the length of the incision depending on the spinal lordosis at various segments of the lumbar spine in a single-level minimally invasive transforaminal lumbar interbody fusion (TLIF). **(a)** Illustration showing the spinal needle at the L3-4 disc space. The distance from the disc space to the L3 pedicle is 22 mm, which requires a longer incision at L3-4 (32 mm) than at L4-5 or L5-S1 because of increasing lordosis. **(a1)** Lateral fluoroscopic image corresponding to **(a)** with a spinal needle in position to plan the incision for an L3-4 TLIF. **(b)** Illustration showing the spinal needle at the L4-5 disc space. The distance from the disc space to the L4 pedicle is 18 mm, requiring a slightly shorter incision at L4-5 (28 mm) than at L3-4. **(b1)** Lateral fluoroscopic image with a spinal needle in position to plan the incision for an L4-5 TLIF. **(c)** Illustration showing the spinal needle at the L5-S1 disc space. The distance from the disc space to the L5 pedicle is 15 mm, requiring an even shorter incision at L5-S1 (25 mm). **(c1)** Lateral fluoroscopic image with a spinal needle in position to plan the incision for an L5-S1 TLIF. In each circumstance, centering the incision on the disc space at each level makes the caudal pedicle readily accessible with an incision that extends downward 10 mm. The rostral component of the incisions is the variable aspect because lumbar lordosis influences the distance to the pedicle.

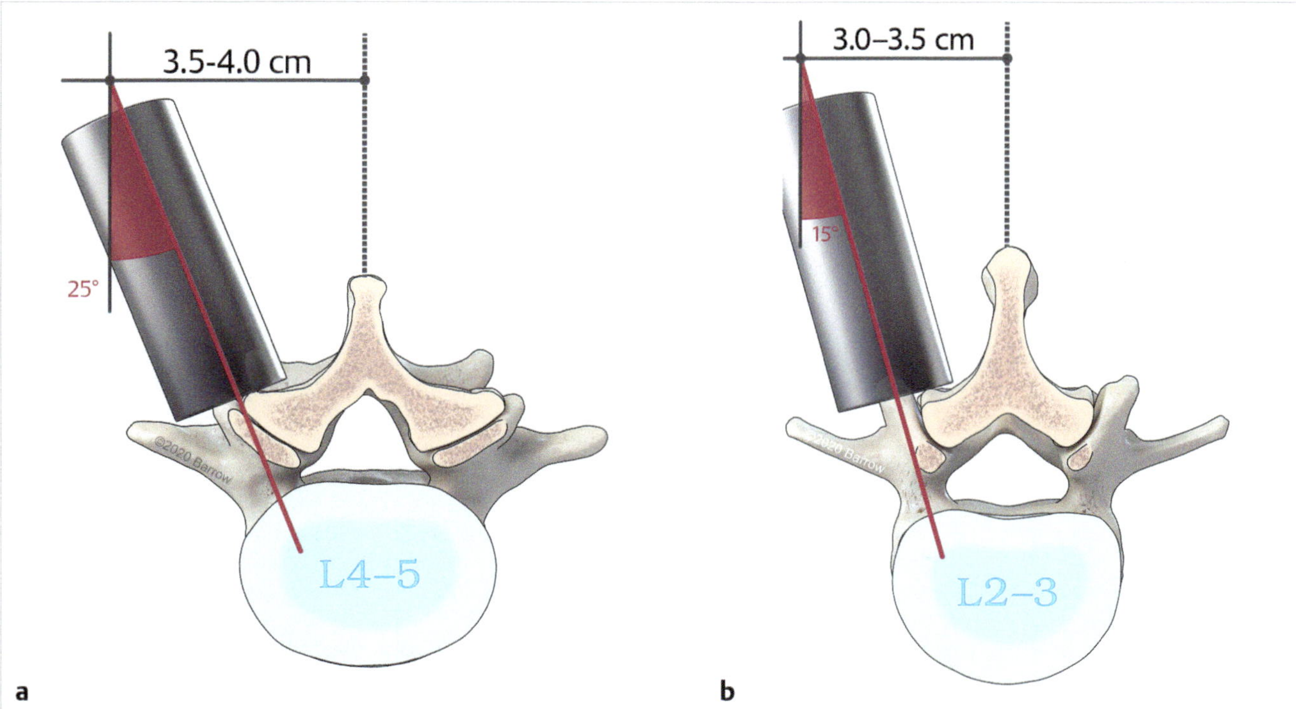

Fig. 4.12 Rationale for the distance from midline of the incision. The distance from the midline is inherently tied to the angle of convergence into the pedicle. **(a)** The larger angles at L5 and S1 mandate a more lateral starting point to ensure the trajectory of the access port is parallel or nearly parallel to the pedicle angle. Therefore, at L4–5 and L5–S1, 4.0 cm is preferred, whereas 3.5 cm is preferred in patients with a lower body mass index. **(b)** The smaller angles and smaller intrapedicular distance make an incision of 3.0 to 3.5 cm the ideal distance from the midline. Capturing the angle that leads into the pedicle vastly facilitates instrumentation of the pedicle.

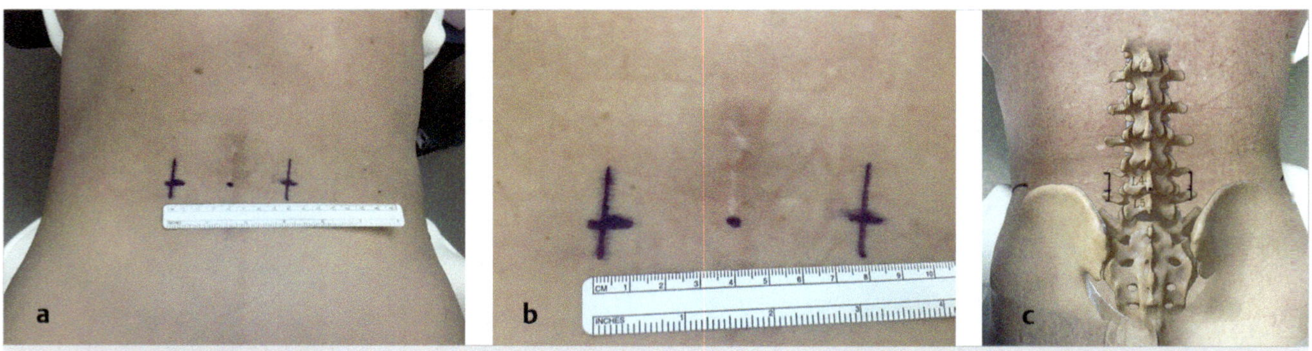

Fig. 4.13 Incision planning for L4–5 minimally invasive transforaminal lumbar interbody fusions. **(a)** Photograph demonstrating the planned incision. The interspinous process space has been marked in the midline (note the incision is no longer than the incision used for a previous midline microdiscectomy). **(b)** At L4–5, two incisions 28 mm in length are marked 4 cm lateral to the midline. **(c)** Artist's depiction of spine superimposed on photograph of proposed skin incision demonstrating the proximity of the requisite anatomy relative to the incisions (different patient).

to prepping and draping. That preoperative image helps guide the position of the C-arm wag for the ideal lateral image, and I incorporate any coronal imbalance into the incision planning. But in the absence of coronal imbalance, the first image awaits the passage of the spinal needle.

Similar to the lumbar microdiscectomy and lumbar laminectomy procedures, I use an infiltration and incision planning set for the MIS TLIF. However, this set is specific for the TLIF. There are two spinal needles, one an 18 gauge and the other a 20 gauge to distinguish between the two on a lateral fluoroscopic image, along with two syringes of local anesthetic and two hypodermic needles (▶ Fig. 4.14). I first pass the 20-gauge spinal needle into the marked incision at the 1-cm mark on one side and dock onto the facet. At 3.5 cm (for low BMI) to 4.0 cm (high BMI) lateral to midline, the risk of a dural puncture is low unless an extreme angle is taken medially toward the interlaminar space. A slight converging angle, typically no more than 15 to 20 degrees, reliably secures the spinal needle onto the facet. The unmistakable tactile sense of the metal of the spinal needle encountering the bone of the facet prompts the first lateral fluoroscopic image, not only to confirm the operative segment but also to provide an ideal trajectory into the disc space

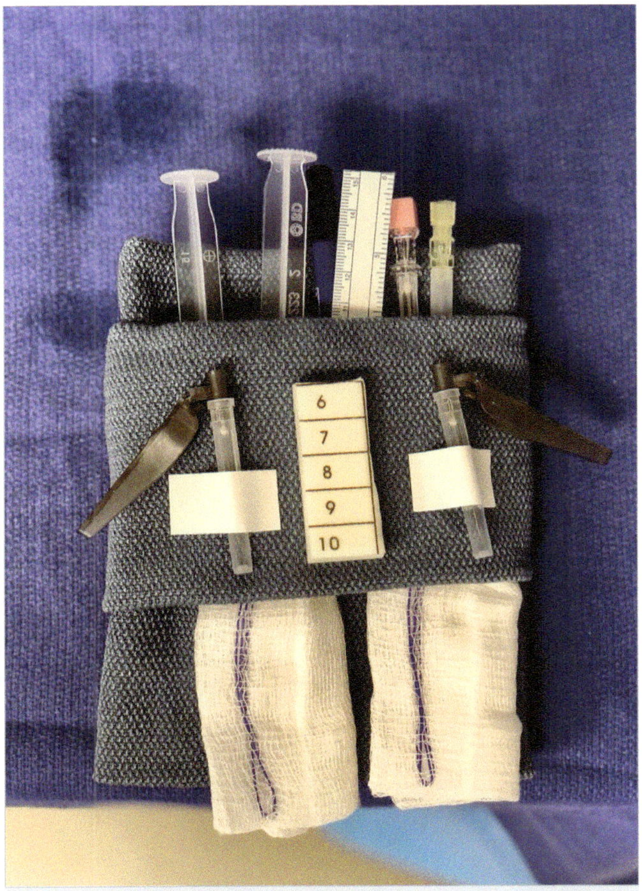

Fig. 4.14 Infiltration and incision-planning set for a minimally invasive transforaminal lumbar interbody fusion. The contents include two syringes filled with local anesthetic, two spinal needles (18 and 20 gauge so that they can be distinguished from each other on a lateral fluoroscopic image), two hypodermic needles to infiltrate the skin and superficial muscles, a marking pen and a ruler in case the incision needs to be adjusted and remarked. Two Ray-Tec sponges (Johnson & Johnson, New Brunswick, NJ) and a foam needle counter for the four needles used in this process. This set may be handed to the surgeon to confirm and optimize the incision as the scrub technician passes the wires for cautery and the tubing for suction. In that manner, the surgeon moves the operation forward, confirming and remarking the incision while the scrub technician passes suction tubing, cautery and bipolar wires to be connected.

(▶ Fig. 4.15). If needed, I reposition the spinal needle to optimize the incision. It is at this point where any adjustments with regard to the wag of the fluoroscope need to be made to optimize visualization of the pedicles.

The radiology technologist should make every effort to eliminate any double shadow through the pedicle. Optimal visualization of the pedicles at each vertebral body and disc space may actually involve two different angles of the fluoroscope, depending on the degenerative pattern of the segment. Such a coronal imbalance needs to be determined and recorded by the radiology technologist at this point. For this reason, a dedicated radiology technologist is imperative for the entire procedure because of the difficulty in achieving the same image with the same angle with a new radiology technologist in the middle of a case. Although the theme of any minimally invasive operation should be to minimize fluoroscopy, optimization of the image at this point with additional fluoroscopy is an investment in the efficiency of the operation.

I confirm the ideal entry point and trajectory over the disc space and onto the facet and remark the incision again 10 mm down from the spinal needle entry point and 15 mm above for L5–S1 (total length: 25 mm), 18 mm for L4–5 (total length: 28 mm), 20 mm for L3–4 and 22 mm for L2–3 (total length: 32 mm) (Fig. 4.11). I place an 18-gauge spinal needle on the opposite side to confirm the incision and the trajectory for that incision. The larger gauge needle is readily distinguishable from the 20-gauge spinal needle, so there is no confusion regarding which needle is confirming which incision (▶ Fig. 4.16).

I remove the stylets from the spinal needles and infuse lidocaine with epinephrine mixed with bupivacaine as I slowly remove the needles. The infusion anesthetizes the future path of the dilators and the access port while the epinephrine mitigates paraspinal muscle bleeding along that same path. Once the spinal needles are removed, I use a hypodermic needle to infiltrate the skin and paraspinal muscles. I make the two incisions with a No. 15 blade and dissect onto the lumbosacral fascia with cautery. I have the radiology technologist roll the fluoroscope to just above the hips of the patient for the exposure of the pedicle screw entry points. It will only be 15 minutes or so before the fluoroscope is needed again, so I ask the radiology technologist to remain in the room.

The fascial opening determines the trajectory that I will have for pedicle screw and interbody placement. Before opening the thoracolumbar fascia, I reorient my mind with regard to the midline. As with lumbar microdiscectomies and laminectomies, palpating the spinous process from within the incision provides you with a sense of where the midline resides. At times, despite adequate surgical planning, what was marked as the midline may not necessarily be the exact midline. In patients with a BMI greater than 35, marking the midline from the level of the skin is especially challenging. Thus, confirming the midline by palpation of the spinous process is essential to ensure an ideal fascial opening immediately over the facet joint and optimal trajectory into the pedicle.

A poorly placed fascial opening will not allow for the ideal trajectory needed for ideal pedicle screw placement and has the potential to make a case long and frustrating. Furthermore, the trajectory needs to afford access to the confluence of the lamina and base of the spinous process for an optimal decompression and placement of the interbody. The ideal trajectory will be from lateral to medial onto the facet. If the skin incision turns out to be too medial and you find yourself less than 2 cm from the spinous process, you will need to make a fascial opening lateral to where the skin incision was made to provide the ideal trajectory for pedicle screw placement. If, when palpating the spinous process, you appreciate that the midline is a good distance away, the fascial opening will need to be medial to your skin incision. The skin is more accommodating than the thoracolumbar fascia for these adjustments. Under ideal circumstances, the fascial opening is slightly medial to the skin incision, creating a lateral to medial converging trajectory onto the facet and into the pedicles.

I make the fascial opening with cautery, just as I would in traditional open surgery. The fascial opening needs to be

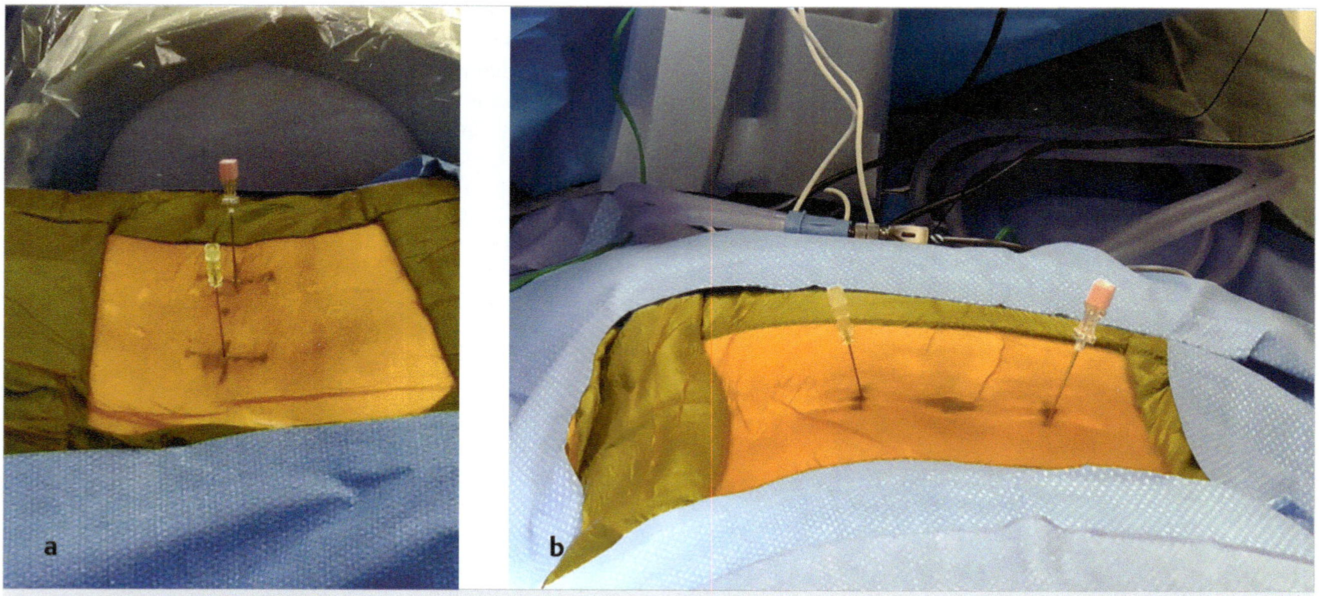

Fig. 4.15 Intraoperative photograph of spinal needle localization. **(a)** A lateral view of two spinal needles in position at the L4–5 segment docked onto the facets. **(b)** View from the head of the bed demonstrating the convergence of 15 to 20 degrees onto the spine.

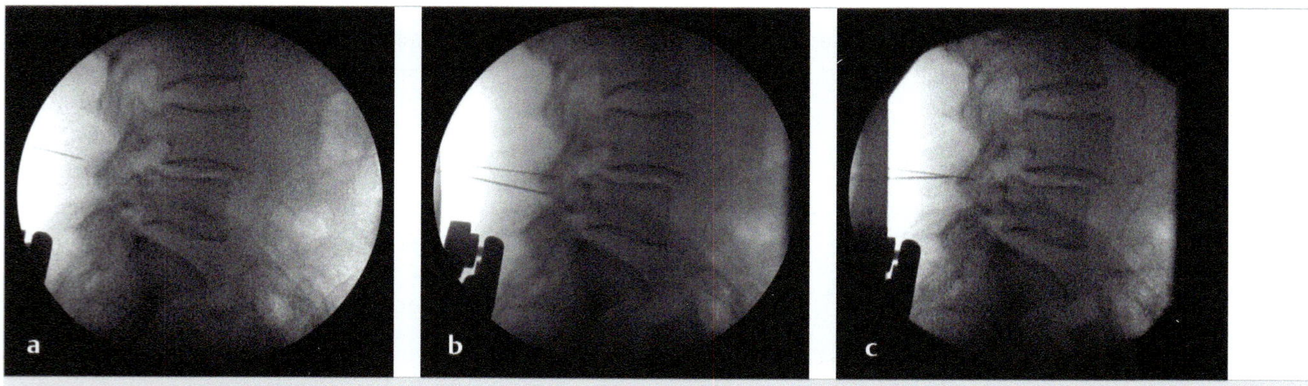

Fig. 4.16 Confirming the planned incision for an L4–5 minimally invasive transforaminal lumbar interbody fusion in the management of a grade I L4–5 spondylolisthesis. Lateral fluoroscopic images demonstrating a 20-gauge spinal needle passed through the 1-cm line of the incision and docked onto the facet. **(a)** The spinal needle has a suboptimal trajectory, indicating the need to adjust the incision lower so that a trajectory completely parallel to the disc space can be achieved with the access port. **(b)** The position of the 20-gauge needle was adjusted before obtaining the second image, and the second spinal needle (an 18-gauge needle) was docked onto the facet on the opposite side and in need of adjustment as well. **(c)** The 18-gauge needle was adjusted before the final fluoroscopic image, which shows both needles at an optimal trajectory to position the access port to instrument and decompress the spine. The incision is re-marked according to these confirmed entry points into the skin.

approximately 10% longer than the skin incision. Keep in mind that the skin incision for an L4–5 minimally invasive TLIF is only 28 mm, but the distance between pedicles may be as much as 32 to 34 mm. Therefore, a slightly larger fascial opening will allow angling of the blades in a rostral-caudal direction. Failure to open the fascia adequately will result in a struggle to identify either the rostral or caudal pedicle screw entry points or both.

4.9.2 Docking the Minimal Access Ports

As the cautery tip opens the fascia, I look for a natural plane of dissection onto the facet, similar to the plane of dissection medial to the sternocleidomastoid muscle that leads directly to the spine in an anterior cervical discectomy with fusion. A well-placed fascial opening allows for blunt dissection lateral to the multifidus and directly onto the facet. Immediate palpation of the facet dome with the tip of my index finger indicates that I have found the right plane. The transverse processes of the levels above and below should be immediately palpable along that same plane. Early in your learning curve, it may be helpful to place a dilator onto the rostral and caudal transverse processes to ensure the adequate release of the fascia for pedicle screw placement. Confirming the range of the exposure may be accomplished within a few minutes after making the incision for placement of the first dilator.

The facet of the segment to be operated upon is the target of the dilatation, since it is the central reference point for the entire procedure. I guide the first dilator onto the facet with my index finger, anchor it firmly in place and obtain a confirmatory fluoroscopic image (▶ Fig. 4.17). I use a converging trajectory onto the spine from a mediolateral perspective at this point. It is crucial to set the appropriate angle when docking the dilators to prevent struggling with the blades of the access port when instrumenting the spine. If I secure an access port into position with a converging angle of only 10 degrees, it will be difficult, if not impossible, to achieve an angle of 25 degrees for the pedicle screw. Angulation of the minimal access port that does not match the angulation of the pedicle will entail wrangling with the blades of the access port and the pedicle screwdriver. To prevent this mismatch, I invest the requisite time to carefully set the trajectory of the minimal access port.

As demonstrated in ▶ Fig. 4.6, each pedicle of the lumbar spine has an ideal angle of convergence. I strive to match that angle with the minimal access port. The ideal angle at L5–S1 is 30 degrees; at L4–5, 25 degrees; at L3–4, 20 degrees; and at L2–3, 15 degrees. Setting the access port along the ideal angle of convergence facilitates pedicle screw placement, decompression and interbody spacer placement.

I determine the sagittal trajectory with a fluoroscopic image to ensure that I capture a trajectory parallel to the disc space. The position of the first dilator should correlate precisely with the 1-cm line marking of the planned skin incision (▶ Fig. 4.17). I set the ideal trajectory, firmly anchor the access port against the facet and dilate the surgical corridor up to 22 mm. Provided that I maintain the same trajectory, there is no need to obtain further fluoroscopic images, fulfilling our prerequisite to minimize radiation exposure. As I dilate to the larger diameters, my hands receive the tactile sense of the dilators swallowing the facet. The concept is that of a cylinder over the top of a sphere (▶ Fig. 4.18).

The precise placement of the larger diameter dilators facilitates stabilization of the final few dilators. The diameter of the dilator now exceeds the diameter of the dome of the facet. The number on the side of the last dilator determines the length of the minimal access blades needed for the access port. The scrub technician assembles the expandable minimal access port with the appropriate blade length. I slip the minimal access port over the dilators and onto the facet. An additional fluoroscopic image at this point ensures that the access port is completely parallel to the disc space. Once I have captured the ideal position and trajectory, I secure the minimal access port onto the table-mounted frame with downward pressure to mitigate muscle creep (▶ Fig. 4.19).

4.9.3 Exposure

Suboptimal trajectories of the access port and inadequate exposure of the anatomy are the root causes of difficulty that may arise during the placement of pedicle screws. Very early in my experience I recognized that the exposure of the pedicle screw entry points was technically easier in a paramedian minimally invasive approach than in an exposure that begins in the midline. After all, the access port is immediately over the relevant anatomy, which places the entry points in my direct line of sight and offers me an optimal trajectory onto the pedicle. In contrast, a midline approach presents a constant struggle to reach the lateral margins of the spine and capture a converging angle. Minimizing the extent of muscle creep is the most important operative nuance to keep in mind to optimize the exposure. Constant downward pressure on the minimal access port against the facet is essential when anchoring the retractor to the table mount. Throughout the exposure, should muscle creep begin to occur, reseating the access port again with downward pressure may improve the exposure. I remove the dilators, and if I have proficiently anchored the expandable minimal access port into position over the facet, I will be looking at the facet and its capsule. On a good day, there should be little, if any, muscle creeping around the perimeter of the port.

Early in my experience, the mistake I made was opening the minimal access port too soon. Opening the blades of the access port immediately after removing the dilators will almost assuredly result in muscle creep that will obstruct your view of the relevant anatomy for the rest of the procedure. I quickly learned that it is essential to keep the access port closed until the entire 22-mm diameter within the blades is devoid of muscle and soft tissue.

Similar to the microdiscectomy exposure, I divide the area of exposure for the TLIF into four quadrants, representing the sequence of the exposure, from the lateral safe zones to the more potentially perilous medial zones. The process of exposing the facet begins in a sequential fashion quadrant by quadrant. ▶ Fig. 4.20 demonstrates the exposure through a minimal access port.

Before proceeding further with the technique, it is worthwhile to comment on the area beneath the learning curve regarding exposure and pedicle screw placement. I distinctly remember my first few cases with a paramedian minimally invasive approach where I worked with the greatest trepidation in the medial zones. Exposures for those early cases were painstakingly slow. My uncertainty with the anatomy slowed me down for fear of an errant pass with the cautery into the canal. As I gained experience, I worked with greater certainty. I incorporated the tactile feedback that dilating and securing the access port gave me. I secured the access port with downward pressure to minimize muscle creep. I began to see the anatomy at depth in my mind before exposing it with cautery. I began the process of transitioning my mind from recognition memory of the spinal anatomy to recall memory of the anatomy at depth. My mind adjusted to the angle of the exposure, and soon I was reconstructing the anatomy at depth, filling the holes of visual input offered by a wide exposure with the tactile feel, fluoroscopic images, and direct visualization of the target anatomy. Soon, operative times declined from painstakingly slow to highly efficient. After 50 cases, I was consistently placing four pedicle screws within 30 minutes of making the incision. Relying more on tactile feedback and direct visualization than on fluoroscopic images, I filled in the void of the midline that I could not see to maintain my orientation. Overcoming the obstacles of limited exposure and orientation are the elements of the learning curve with which you must wrestle in your mind to achieve efficiency.

The exposure begins in the safest quadrant away from the neural elements and proceeds caudal to the pedicle screw entry point, where the transverse process and lateral facet can be unmistakably visualized. With a good sense of the facet, the

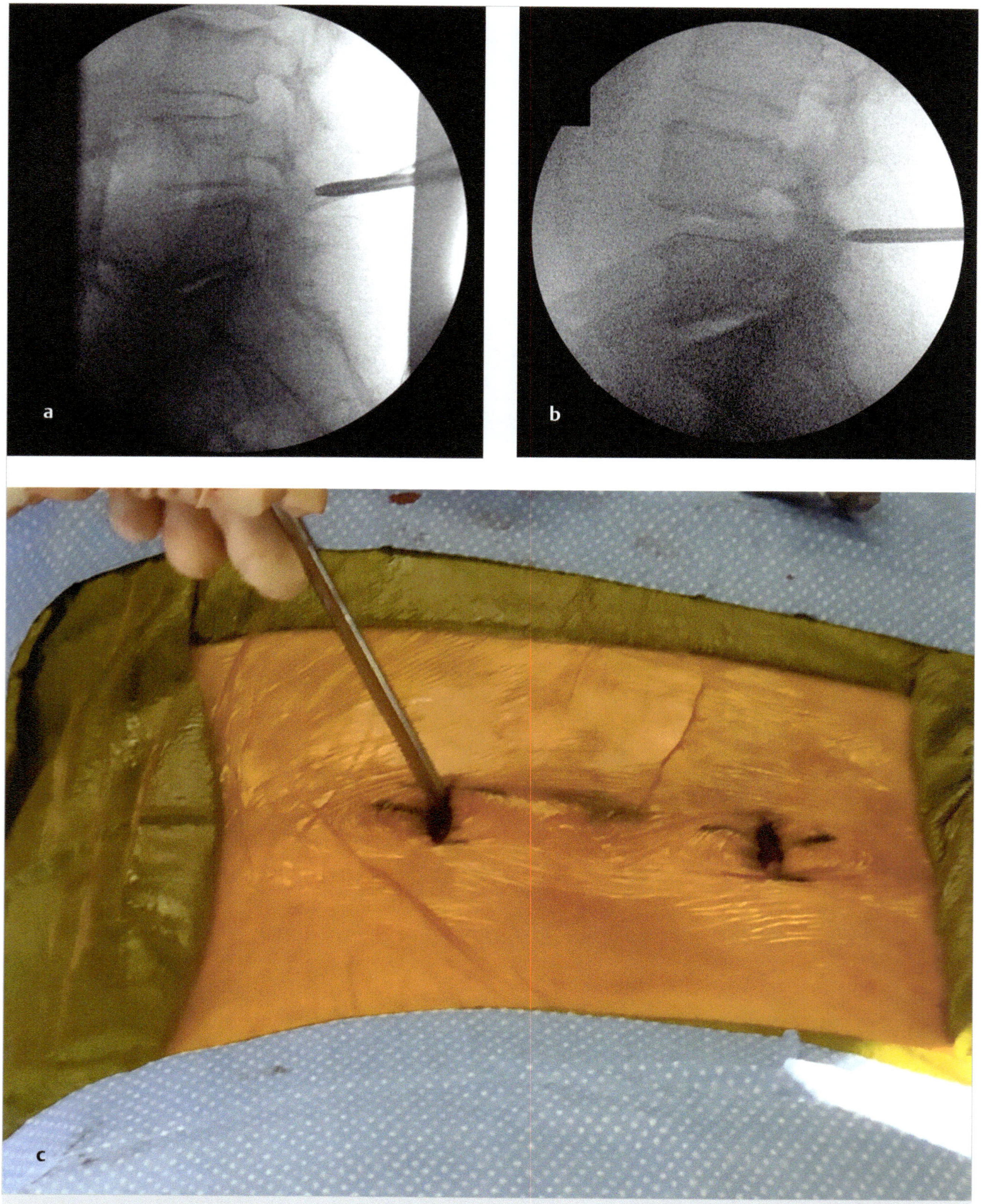

Fig. 4.17 Placement of first dilator. Two examples of initial dilator placement. **(a)** Lateral fluoroscopic image demonstrating the first dilator firmly anchored against the facet and parallel to the disc space. **(b)** Lateral fluoroscopic image of the initial dilator in place for management of a grade I L4–5 spondylolisthesis. The concept is for the dilators to swallow the facet as the dilators increase in size. **(c)** Intraoperative photograph demonstrating utilization of the 1-cm line to guide placement of the initial dilator.

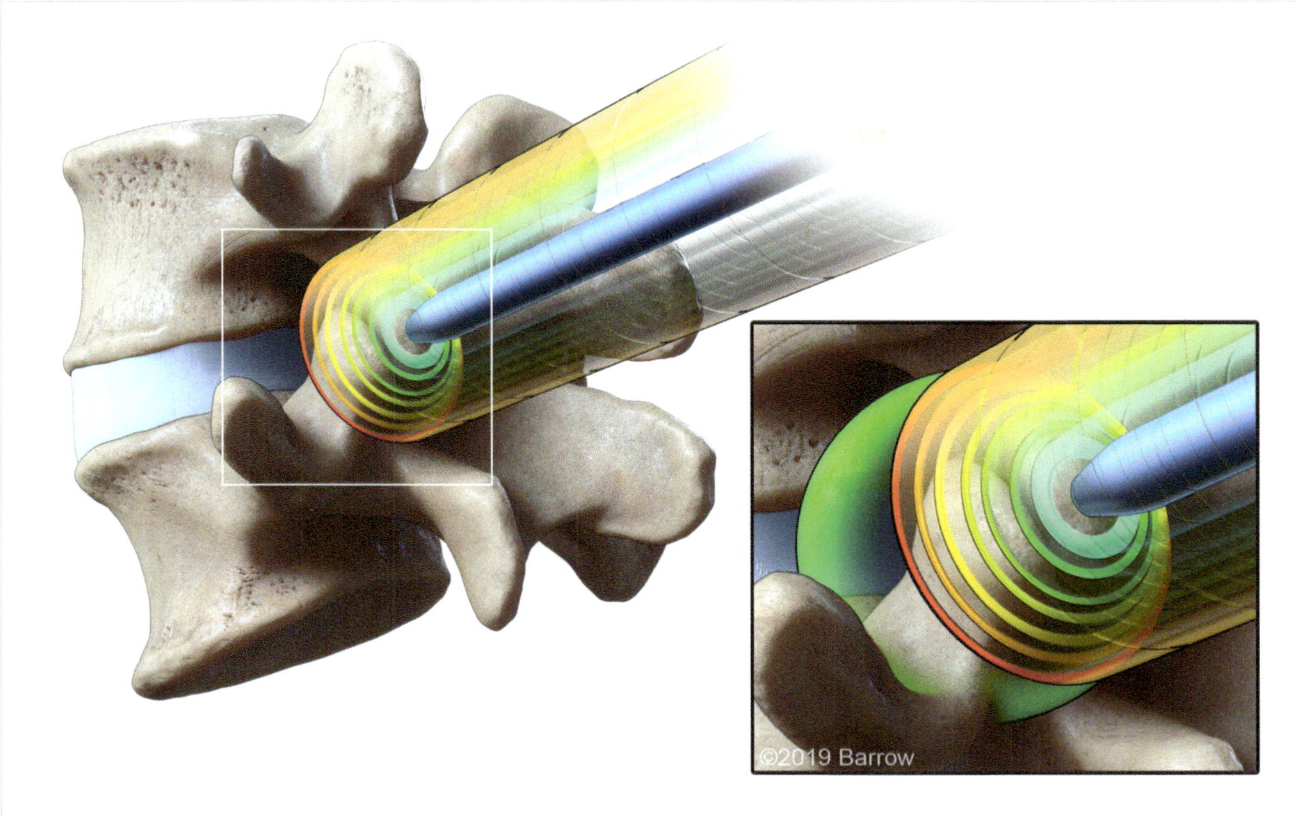

Fig. 4.18 Docking the minimal access port. An illustration of a cylinder over a sphere illustrates the concept of swallowing the facet as the larger dilators are placed. The first dilator anchors the top of the sphere (the facet), and the subsequent dilators begin to swallow the facet and gently displace the muscle and soft tissue.

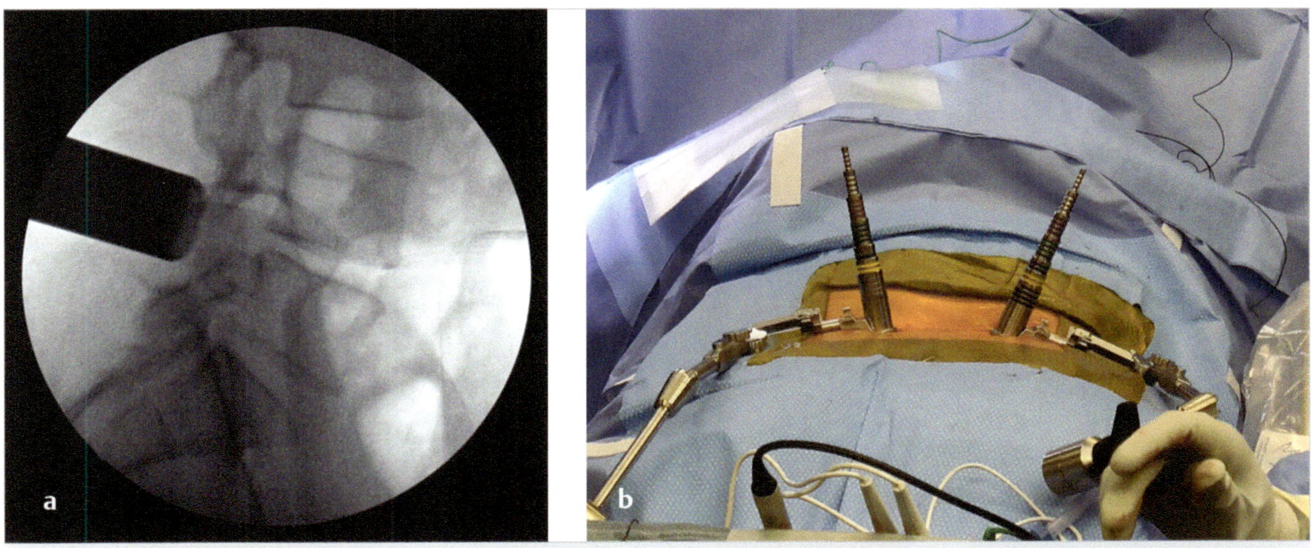

Fig. 4.19 Securing the minimal access ports onto the facets. **(a)** Lateral fluoroscopic image demonstrating a minimal access port in position with the dilators still in place. A trajectory parallel to the disc space is captured in the sagittal plane. Note that the entry point for the caudal pedicle screw is already within the field of view. The entry point for the rostral pedicle screw is only millimeters away. **(b)** Intraoperative photograph demonstrating the converging lateral to medial angle onto the facet.

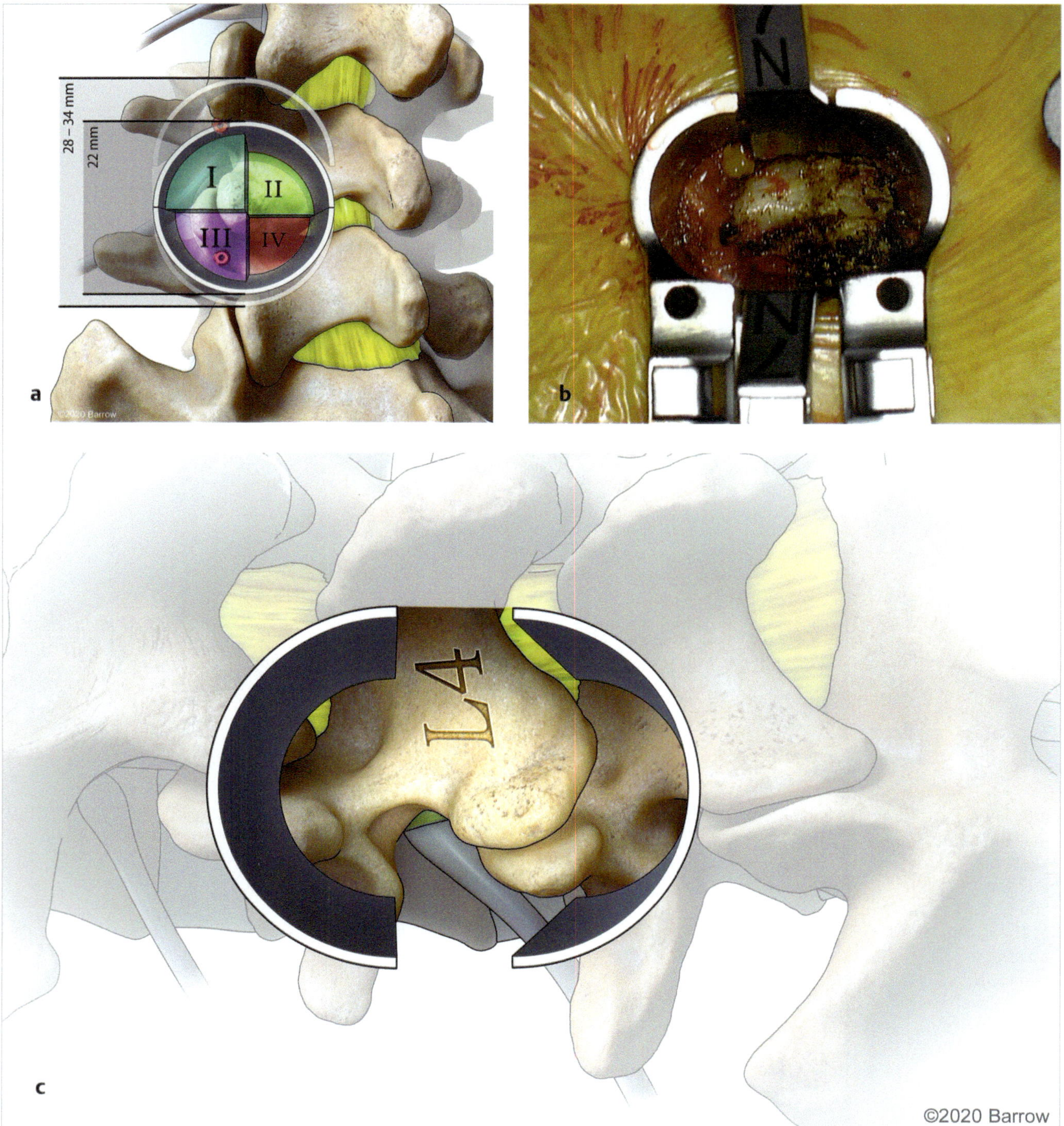

Fig. 4.20 Exposure for a minimally invasive transforaminal lumbar interbody fusion (MIS TLIF). **(a)** Illustration of the sequence for exposing the facet joint. Quadrant I is the safest quadrant in which to begin, proceeding in sequence as illustrated. As the access port is opened, knowledge of the distance from pedicle to pedicle becomes important. As illustrated, the access port may need to encompass up to 34 mm of interpedicular distance. **(b)** Intraoperative photo demonstrating the exposure for an MIS TLIF. The pars interarticularis, entire facet and lamina can be seen through a highly efficient exposure. **(c)** Illustration of the surgical view seen in the intraoperative photograph.

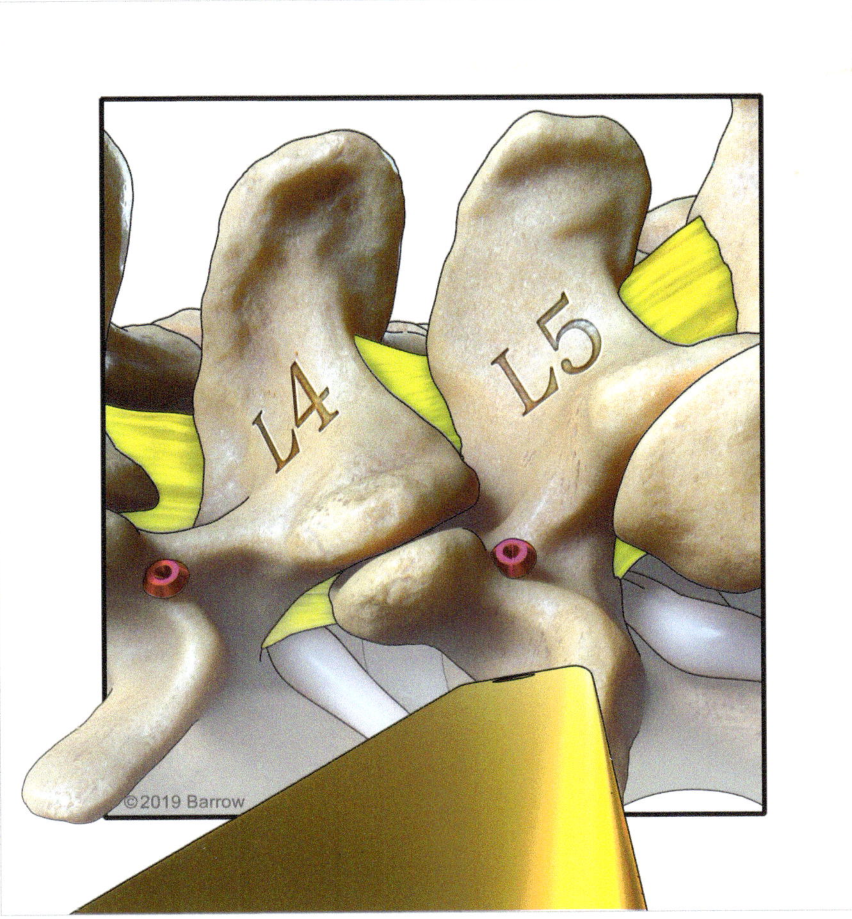

Fig. 4.21 Illustration of the caudal pedicle screw entry point from within the minimal access port in an L4–5 transforaminal lumbar interbody fusion. The suction retractor holds the soft tissue away and reveals the transverse process. When the L4–5 facet is exposed in its entirety, the superior aspect of the L5 pars interarticularis should be readily visible. Unequivocal exposure of the pars interarticularis, transverse process and facet reliably unveils the pedicle screw entry point. With the exposure seen in this illustration, the pedicle screw entry point (demarcated with the magenta fiducial) may be confirmed with nothing more than a single fluoroscopic image.

medial boundaries may be exposed and the interlaminar space may be avoided.

As soon as I have exposed the entire facet of the segment, the access port may be opened in the rostral and caudal direction. You will find that with the muscle swept back to the perimeter of the access port blades, there is less creep as you open the access port. It is essential to remember the distances from pedicle to pedicle at the various segments of the lumbar spine when opening the access port (▶ Fig. 4.4 and ▶ Fig. 4.6). The temptation is to open the access port far wider than the anatomy dictates. The inevitable result is a wall of muscle collapsing down into your exposure. For instance, at L4–5, the distance from the L4 pedicle to L5 pedicle is 28 to 32 mm. The more collapsed the disc space, the closer the pedicles will be to one another. Since the diameter of an unopened minimal access port is 22 mm, the port need not be opened more than 6 to 8 mm to reach the pedicle. Remember, you still have the capacity to angle the blades, which provide several more millimeters of rostral and caudal exposure.

If I expand the access port too widely, muscle invariably creeps into the exposure and obstructs my view of the anatomy. Equally important, an exposure with excessive muscle creep will cause greater postoperative discomfort for the patient. Thus, I emphasize opening the access port only to the amount necessary to expose the pedicle screw entry points. Every effort should be made not to exceed the interpedicular distance. I typically open the expandable access port only enough to fit the blades of a mediolateral retractor. That distance is typically no more than 5 mm.

With the entire facet exposed, my next objective is to expose all the pedicle screw entry points. For the sake of being systematic, the sequence of exposure is caudal to rostral. In a single-level fusion at L4–5, for instance, the L5 transverse process is only millimeters away from the inferior-lateral aspect of the exposed L4–5 facet. Use of a suction retractor is helpful to pull the muscle tissue laterally and complete the exposure of the entire transverse process (of L5 in this example) with cautery (▶ Fig. 4.21). Mediolateral blades added to the access port widen the medial and lateral exposure. I completely expose the caudal transverse process from top to bottom. Based on anatomical landmarks, the pedicle corresponds with the middle of the transverse process. A few bursts of cautery on the superior-most aspect of the pars interarticular of L5 reveal that landmark. The exposed field now includes the L5 transverse process, the superior aspect of the pars interarticularis of L5 and the entire L4–5 facet joint. You are now looking at the first pedicle screw entry point (▶ Fig. 4.21).

I return to the L4–5 facet, the central point of my field of view, and work in the rostral direction. I follow the inferior articular process of L4, as it blends into the pars interarticularis of L4 but stop shy of the L3–4 facet joint. Although the inferolateral aspect of the rostral facet (the L3–4 facet for the L4 pedicle in this case) needs to be exposed for pedicle screw insertion, care should be taken to not disrupt the facet capsule, thereby minimizing the risk of iatrogenic degeneration at that level. The key to preventing inadvertent cautery of the facet capsule is staying lateral. I cannot emphasize this point enough. So instead, I connect the lines of what I can clearly see with my eye (the pars interarticularis of L4) to what I can see only with my mind (the L4 transverse process). I use that mental reconstruction of the anatomy to "leap" onto the transverse process and avoid the L3–4 facet altogether. I accomplish this leap by using a probing suction tip to confirm the location of the L4 transverse process through a thin layer of muscle fibers. The unmistakable sensation of the tip of a metal suction encountering bone confirms the transverse process precisely where my mind has reconstructed it. I use cautery to expose the entire L4 transverse process, and then I nudge medially toward the L3–4 facet without disrupting the facet capsule. Remember, the distinct advantage of the direct visualization of the pedicle screw entry points over percutaneous techniques is the elimination of facet capsule disruption. Leaping from the pars interarticularis to the transverse process ensures that I am playing to the strength of this technique and preserving the rostral facet capsule. I can feel the lateral aspect of the L3–4 facet by nudging the tip of the suction up against the lateral aspect of the facet, which is all that I need to confirm the pedicle screw entry point of L4. Both pedicle screw entry points are now in my field of view (▶ Fig. 4.22).

Completing the exposure for the decompression of the segment is my next objective. I return to the L4–5 facet and continue the exposure medially until I have visualized the pars interarticularis blending into the lamina, which in turn merges into the spinous process. I need to visualize the junction of the lamina and spinous process to accomplish a complete decompression of the segment. I prefer to accomplish all of this exposure at the outset so that after placement of the pedicle screws, I can immediately transition to the decompression phase. However, first I complete the instrumentation component of the operation.

It is a worthwhile mental exercise to go through the difference in sequence between a traditional midline open exposure and a minimally invasive one. A midline open approach provides the spinous process to guide you to the lamina, the facet, the pars interarticularis, and ultimately to the transverse process, all in sequential anatomical fashion. The midline structures are the basis of orientation. A minimally invasive approach has the facet of the operative segment as the center of the field of view. The facet is the first structure that you identify and is the basis of your orientation. All of the relevant structures are only millimeters in each direction: the lamina, the pars interarticularis and the transverse process. Mastery of the anatomical measurements and the topography of the inferior articular process merging into the pars interarticularis allows you to confidently sweep away the soft tissue to complete the exposure for the placement of pedicle screws and decompression. The inability to see the midline structures is no obstacle once you possess the anatomical certainty of the lateral aspect of the lumbar spine. It is this knowledge that is the true organ of sight.

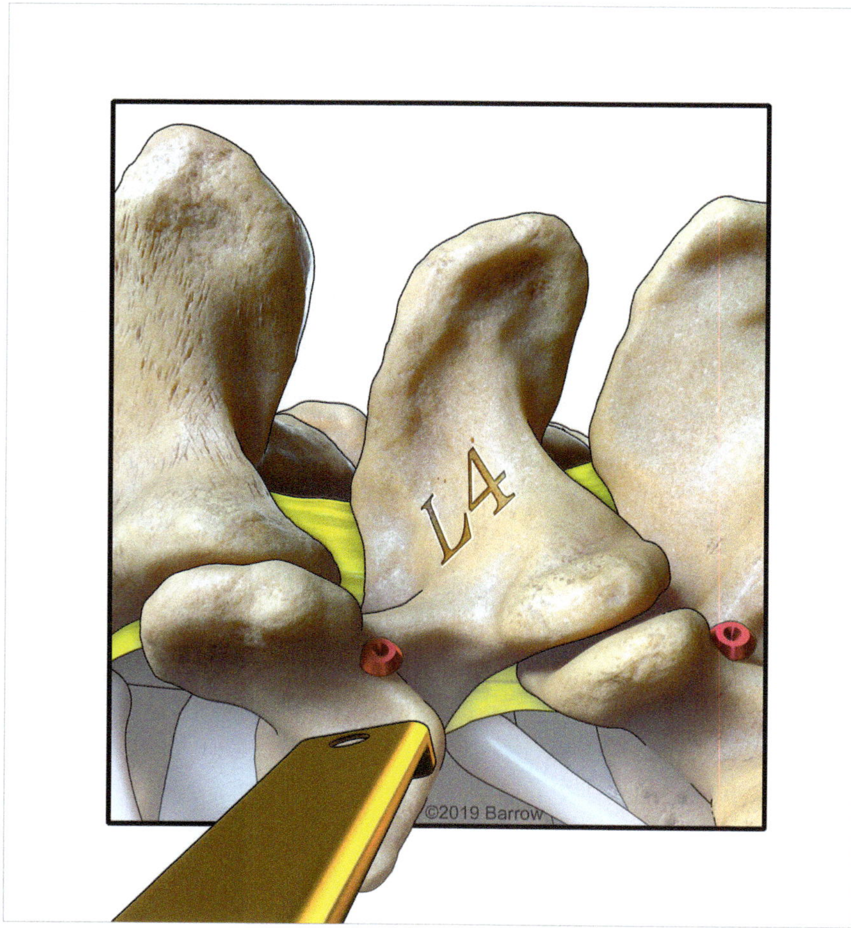

Fig. 4.22 Illustration of the rostral pedicle screw entry point (L4) from within the minimal access port in an L4–5 transforaminal lumbar interbody fusion. After exposure of the caudal pedicle screw entry point, the lamina and pars interarticularis are exposed. Instead of exposing the rostral facet, the focus becomes the rostral transverse process. It is imperative that the capsule of the rostral facet joint be kept intact.

4.9.4 Pedicle Screw Placement

Before the operation, I spend a considerable amount of time reviewing all of the patient's radiographic images while the patient is undergoing anesthesia. I review the AP and lateral radiographs to look for two particular characteristics that make imaging and instrumentation challenging: coronal imbalance and lateral listhesis. A coronal imbalance may make obtaining an ideal lateral fluoroscopic image challenging and prompts me to review this possibility with my radiology technologist before the operation so that they can anticipate wag adjustments with the fluoroscope before even taking the first image. Awareness of a lateral listhesis is valuable when selecting an entry point that seems out of line with the other pedicle screw. Finally, I measure the width of the pedicle and select entry points and angles at the levels I intend to instrument. In my experience, the value of this preoperative planning is without measure, as it begins the reconstruction of the anatomy at depth before ever making an incision.

The technique that I describe below for pedicle screw placement capitalizes on the direct visualization of the anatomy to minimize the amount of fluoroscopy needed to safely instrument the spine. The principles espoused by Lenke and colleagues[9,10] in their free-hand technique are all incorporated into the technique that I describe below. This technique harnesses the advantage of having the minimal access ports to use as a frame of reference to align the trajectory for a pedicle probe, tap or pedicle screw. Using the minimal access ports in this manner helps decrease your exposure to ionizing radiation. I avoid AP imaging and instead carefully assess my angulation throughout the process of probing, tapping and placement of the pedicle screw. Furthermore, I use electrophysiological stimulation at every step of the process to minimize the risk of missing a pedicle breach.

A minimally invasive procedure should not be a license to increase the use of fluoroscopy. Instead, I encourage you to develop a mentality that it is exactly the opposite. You should consider that a direct paramedian exposure of the entry points and minimal access ports offering a trajectory in line with the pedicle decreases the need for fluoroscopy.

It is only after I have exposed all the pedicle screw entry points that I bring the fluoroscope back into the field to its previous mark. Under ideal circumstances with two surgeons operating, the exposures described earlier should be done simultaneously and take no more than 15 minutes to complete. If I am operating by myself, I complete the exposures on both sides before beginning with instrumentation. When I have completed the exposure, the fluoroscope rolls back into position, and I place the drill at the junction of the pars interarticularis, midtransverse process and inferior lateral facet. I confirm the proposed entry point with a single lateral fluoroscopic image. The ideal position for the entry point is in the upper half of the pedicle (▸ Fig. 4.23). Depending on the amount of facet arthropathy, the lateral aspect of the facet may need to be drilled to adequately expose the entry point. I use a drill with a minimally invasive attachment to create a breach through the cortical bone and unveil the blush of cancellous pedicle bone.

With regard to the operative sequence, I prefer to start at the caudal pedicle and then line up the pedicle entry points for ease of rod placement. However, it is not unusual for the fluoroscope position to be ideal for a lateral image of the pedicles of one vertebral body but not for the other. Under those circumstances, I begin with whichever level has an ideal lateral fluoroscopic image with the pedicles lined up, regardless of whether it is the rostral or caudal pedicle (▸ Fig. 4.23). In the case of an L4–5 TLIF, where there is no coronal imbalance, I drill the entry points for both pedicle screws before probing the pedicles. I place the tip of the drill at the junction of the pars interarticularis and the midtransverse process of L5 while nudging into the inferior and lateral aspect of the L4–5 facet. A fluoroscopic image confirms the ideal entry point, and the pilot holes are drilled (▸ Fig. 4.23). I repeat the same process for the L4 pedicle and obtain another fluoroscopic image to confirm the L4 entry point. I then explore the cortical breach with the pedicle probe in search of cancellous bone. Depending on the pedicle being probed, the medial-lateral angulation will vary. For a sacral pedicle trajectory, the angle may be as much as 25 to 30 degrees, whereas for an L3 pedicle trajectory, it may be as little as 5 to 10 degrees.

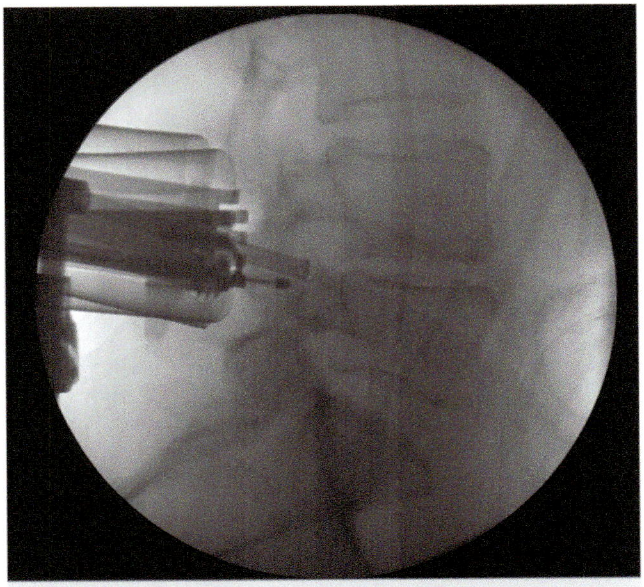

Fig. 4.23 Confirming the pedicle screw entry point. Lateral fluoroscopic image demonstrating confirmation of the entry point. The tip of the drill is positioned at the junction of the pars interarticularis, transverse process and facet. With the entry point clearly visualized, no anteroposterior fluoroscopic image is needed. Although the pedicles of L5 appear to be in perfect alignment, the pedicles of L4 are not. The image shows a double shadow through the pedicle and requires adjusting the wag of the fluoroscope before instrumenting the L4 pedicles.

The term I use to describe the indisputable sensation of a pedicle probe displacing cancellous bone as it advances into the pedicle is "pedicular." When the probe advances with more wiggle than push, delivering a soft haptic sense of crunching cancellous bone to the palm of your hand, you are experiencing the definition of this neologism. Pedicular advancement of the probe provides you with the unmistakable sensation that you are within the cortical walls of the pedicle and advancing in the right direction along the ideal trajectory (▸ Fig. 4.24a). The probe should advance with little resistance. If you encounter stiff resistance, it is likely that the tip of the pedicle probe is abutting the unforgiving cortical bone of the pedicle. Should

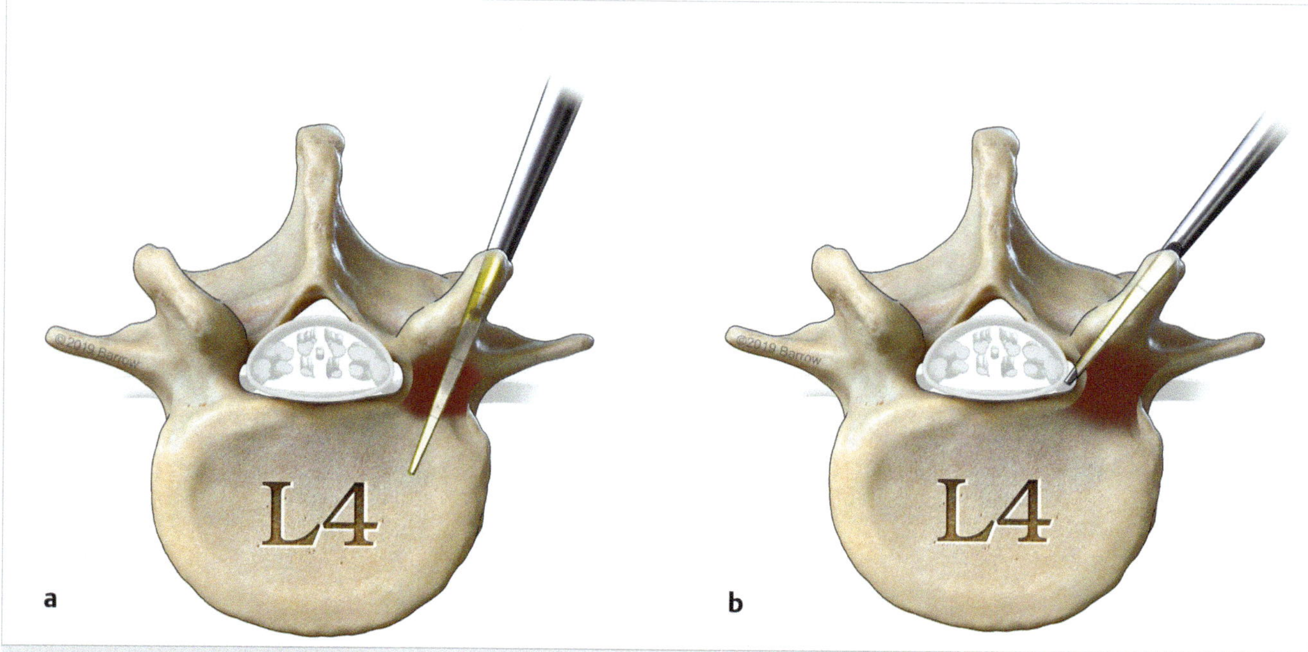

Fig. 4.24 Probing the pedicle. **(a)** Illustration demonstrates probing of the pedicle with an appropriate trajectory. The unmistakable tactile feedback of the tip of the pedicle probe displacing cancellous bone is a distinct tactile feel compared to encountering the stiff resistance of the cortical wall of the pedicle. **(b)** Illustration demonstrates a potential pitfall in probing the pedicle. Encountering stiff resistance when probing the pedicle may be an indication that the tip of the pedicle probe is against the cortical bone of the pedicle. Failing to make an adjustment and instead continuing in that trajectory is a recipe for a breach in the pedicle. Awareness of the pedicular probing sensation and assessment of any resistance allows for adjustment of the trajectory to find the cancellous bone again.

this occur, pause and reassess. Forcing the pedicle probe against resistance is a recipe for a breach. Never ask for a mallet.

The breaches I have caused have come after encountering significant resistance where at first there was none. Convinced I knew the anatomy of the pedicle, I continued to push the probe down the errant path and forced my way through that resistance (▶ Fig. 4.24b). I erroneously reasoned that I had found the cancellous bone of the pedicle again because, after some initial resistance, the probe began to pass easily again. When I stimulated the probe to 20 mA, my jaw dropped as my patient's leg began to fire compound motor action potentials with a sickening rhythmicity. In actuality, I had forced the tip of the pedicle probe through the cortical wall of the pedicle. With the cortical wall breached, I no longer met resistance and the probe advanced once again. For this reason, if you encounter stiff resistance that suddenly gives way, stop. Remove the pedicle probe and check the integrity of the pedicle with a ball-tipped probe. Depending on the entry point, the trajectory, and the shape of the pedicle, the breach may have been medial or lateral. Palpating the pedicle with a ball-tipped probe invariably revealed the breach and confirmed the error in trajectory.

Now that my technique has evolved from the countless miscalculations I have made over the years, any resistance that I encounter gives me pause. I may check an additional lateral fluoroscopic image, reassess my trajectory and entry point, or stimulate the probe (using electrophysiological monitoring) up to 20 mA to see if it generates a compound motor action potential. If I am still unable to probe into the pedicle after reassessing the entry point and my angle, I obtain an AP fluoroscopic image and visualize the pedicle from another view. Regardless, experience has taught me to never force a pedicle probe past significant resistance. Instead, I adjust the angle until the tip of the probe finds the welcoming cancellous bone.

When I have passed the pedicle probe a distance of 30 mm, I obtain an additional fluoroscopic image to ensure an optimal trajectory and to stimulate the probe to 20 mA to ensure that there is no generation of a compound motor action potential. A positive response under 10 mA may be indicative of a breach within the pedicle. Any response under 20 mA automatically prompts an AP image and potentially an "owl's eye" view (an angled view down the pedicle). The positive stimulation is indicative that there is something that I am not appreciating with the anatomy of the pedicle and that I need additional information to proceed.[9,10] If there is no compound motor action potential at 20 mA, I continue instrumenting the pedicle (▶ Fig. 4.25b).

I strive for a trajectory parallel to the end plate. I can still adjust the trajectory as I pass the probe an additional 10 mm to a total distance of 40 mm if the anatomy allows it. I take note of the position of the probe within the minimal access port and use this as a frame of reference for the trajectory of the tap and pedicle screw.

In the absence of any irritation of the traversing nerve root, I use a ball-tipped probe to ensure the integrity of the pedicle. I do not assume an intact pedicle because of the absence of a compound motor action potential. Lenke and colleagues emphasize this principle in perhaps the most comprehensive

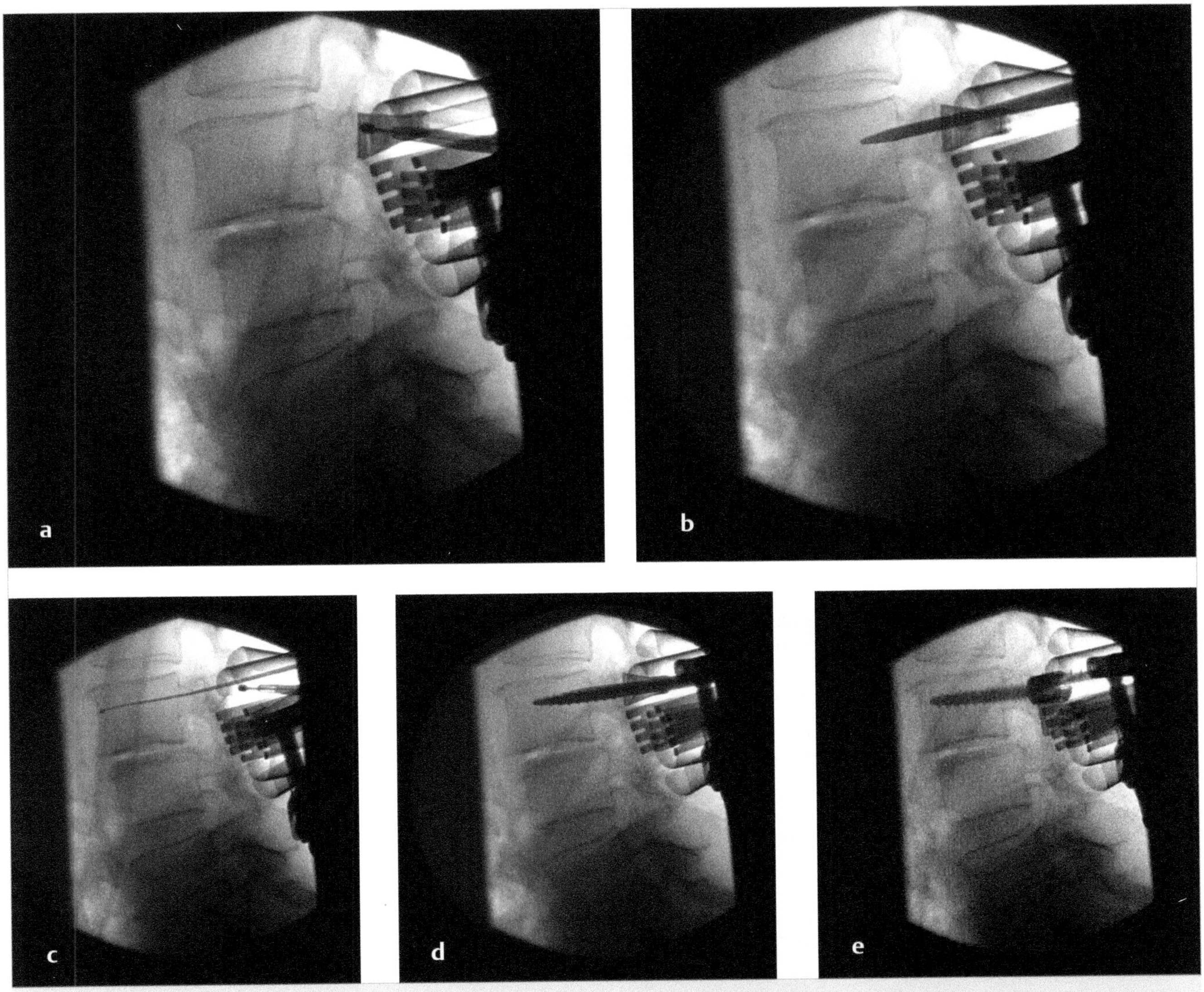

Fig. 4.25 Fluoroscopy sequence of an L3–4 transforaminal lumbar interbody fusion with severe coronal imbalance. (a) Lateral fluoroscopic image demonstrating the drill confirming the pedicle screw entry point. In this circumstance, the wag of the fluoroscope provided an ideal lateral view through the pedicles of L3 but not L4 (note the double shadow of the L4 pedicle). The L3 pedicle was instrumented first, and then the wag of the fluoroscope was adjusted for the L4 pedicles. (b) Lateral fluoroscopic image demonstrating an advancing pedicle probe with a medial angle. Once in position at 30 mm, the pedicle probe is stimulated to rule out a medial breach. The absence of a compound motor action potential does not necessarily rule out a lateral breach. (c) A ball-tipped probe ensures the integrity of all five walls of the pedicle. Note the drill confirming the entry on the contralateral side by the second surgeon working on that side. (d) Knowledge of the length of the tap helps determine the length of the screw when the threads are buried on a lateral fluoroscopic image. In this lateral fluoroscopic image, the tap with the threads buried measures 37.5 mm. Review of the distance to the anterior part of the vertebral body prompted placement of a 45-mm pedicle screw. (Note the pedicle probe advancing in the contralateral pedicle.) (e) Placement of the L3 pedicle screw on the left with the pedicle screw already in position on the right. The pedicle screw is parallel to the end plate and reaches 80% of the depth of the vertebral body.

analysis in the neurosurgical literature of pedicle screws placed with electrophysiological monitoring.[9,10] The ball-tipped probe should be used to confirm all five sides of the pedicle. The “bottom” aspect of the probed pedicle, which represents the anterior aspect of the vertebral body or the floor, is always the first boundary that I check. The absence of a bottom typically suggests a lateral breach, which is the result of inadequate medialization of the trajectory. If the floor of the probed hole is intact, I proceed to confirm the medial, lateral, superior and inferior walls of the pedicle.

I use a pedicle tap with the diameter one size smaller than the proposed width of the pedicle screw as determined in my preoperative planning; that is, if I am planning to place a 7.5-mm screw, I will use 6.5-mm tap. I pass the pedicle tap along the same trajectory as the pedicle probe, with an initial fluoroscopic image obtained to ensure the trajectory within the pedicle and a subsequent fluoroscopic image taken when the threads of the tap are buried. The minimal access port can serve as a frame of reference for the various instruments passing into the pedicle. ▶ Fig. 4.26 demonstrates the relative position of the

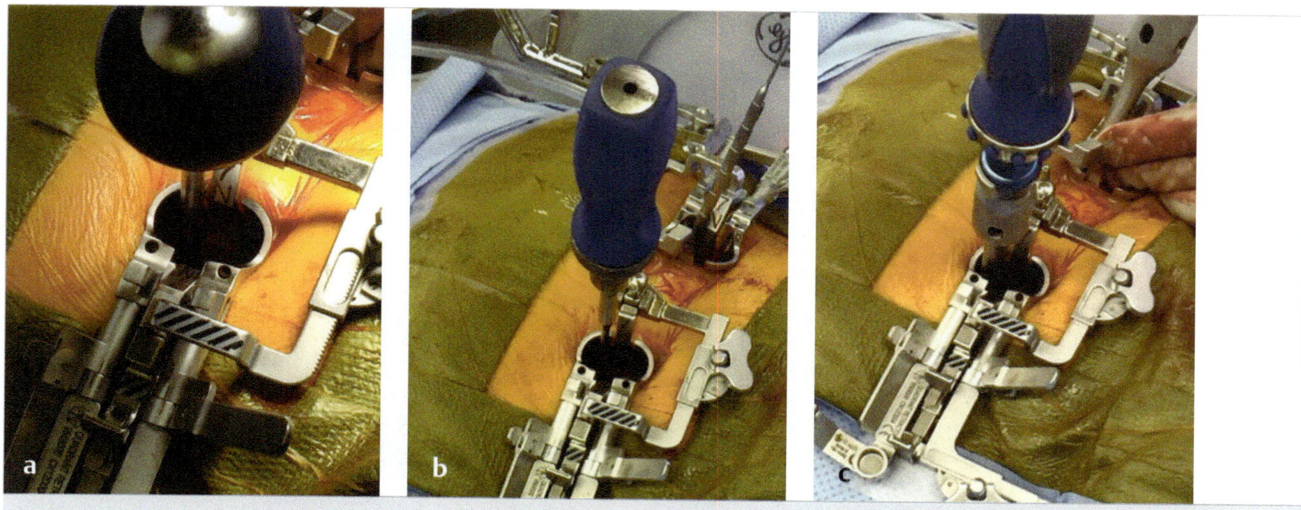

Fig. 4.26 Intraoperative photos demonstrating (a) the pedicle probe, (b) the tap and (c) the pedicle screw driver in the same position relative to the minimal access port. Registering in your mind the position of the instruments within the frame of reference of the retractor helps to decrease the need for fluoroscopy and minimizes radiation exposure to the patient, the surgeon and the operating room staff.

pedicle probe, tap and pedicle screwdriver. In the sequence of those photos, the pedicle probe, tap and pedicle screwdriver are all in the same position relative to the access port. Keeping a mental image of the position of these instruments relative to the access port ensures the same trajectory and has more potential value than any additional fluoroscopic image.

It is essential to know the length of the tap from the tip of the instrument to the end of the threads. That measurement helps you appropriately size the length of the pedicle screw. For instance, knowledge that the threads of a tap end at 37.5 mm from the tip helps determine the length of the screw to be placed. One look at the fluoroscopic image and I can quickly decide between a 40- and a 45-mm screw length.

I stimulate the tap once again, and in the absence of a compound action potential, I probe the tapped hole again with a ball-tipped probe to ensure the integrity of the pedicle. If I am working on the side of the transforaminal approach, I secure the pedicle screw into position again using the frame of reference of the access port and one final fluoroscopic image to set the trajectory. If on the contralateral side, I decorticate the transverse processes and pack graft material onto them before I secure the pedicle screw. I have found that I can decorticate the transverse process and place morselized graft for a posterolateral fusion more proficiently without the pedicle screw in position.

Throughout the placement of the caudal pedicle screw on one side, if a second surgeon is operating, they perform a mirror operation on the contralateral side simultaneously, which has several advantages (► Fig. 4.27). First, it saves fluoroscopic radiation exposure. Second, it allows the pedicle screws to be aligned one with another within the vertebral body and gives the appearance of one pedicle screw on a lateral image, which is an element of craftsmanship. Finally, it allows both surgeons to confirm the degree of convergence by having both taps or both pedicle probes in place at the same time.

When identifying the entry point for the rostral pedicle screw, the surgeon can use the caudal pedicle screw as a frame of reference to set the entry point. In the absence of a lateral listhesis or severe coronal deformity, the entry point will be in line with the caudal pedicle screw. Again, I identify the junction of the pars, transverse process and inferior lateral facet; confirm the proposed entry point with a single lateral fluoroscopic image; and repeat the process of placing the pedicle screw into position.

In a straightforward case, simultaneously docking the access ports and exposing the pedicle screw entry points should take 15 to 20 minutes with two surgeons. Placement of the pedicle screws should take another 15 to 20 minutes. Thus, the total time for phase I should fall within the range of 30 to 40 minutes. Although I strive to complete phase I in 30 minutes, at times, it has taken me well over 1 hour. The causes of these delays were invariably due to poor exposure, poorly placed access ports, suboptimal fascial openings, a pedicle breach that required salvage or a combination of these. Some cases are more challenging than others. Although it is helpful to keep a rhythm to the surgery and a tempo to the steps, trying to keep time should not compromise the safety of the procedure or the basic principles of instrumentation of the spine (Video 4.2).

4.9.5 Minimally Invasive Instrumentation of the Spine and Radiation Exposure

Over the course of a surgeon's experience with minimally invasive TLIFs, there should be a downward trend in the amount of fluoroscopy needed to place four or six pedicle screws. Investing the time directly exposing the pedicle screw entry points and confirming those entry points with certainty have more value than any fluoroscopic image. After all, that is the advantage of direct visualization of the anatomy. It is important to leverage that advantage into decreasing radiation exposure. After gathering some experience, there is seldom a need for more than four to five lateral fluoroscopic images per pedicle in a straightforward case. Thus, phase I may be completed with approximately 25 images. The first 5 images confirm the spinal level and confirm an ideal trajectory for the access ports; the

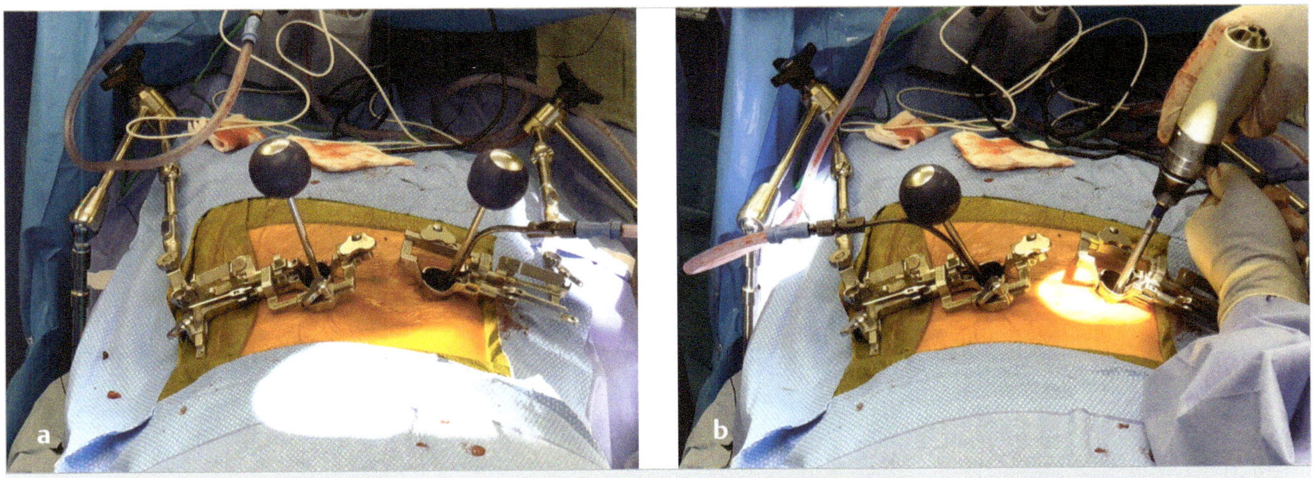

Fig. 4.27 Simultaneous instrumentation of the pedicles. Intraoperative photographs demonstrating simultaneous probing of the pedicles at L5 **(a)** as well as probing the pedicle of L4 on the right while **(b)** tapping the pedicle of L4 on the left.

next 20 images are for pedicle screw preparation and placement (5 images per pedicle). As always, there will be good days and bad days. The times and numbers of images are guiding parameters for the procedure. In the end, you should always take the time and the number of images that you need to perform the procedure safely.

4.10 Provisional Ipsilateral Expandable Rod

The next several paragraphs may seem premature to the reader since the content refers to the interbody phase of the operation, and at this point in the chapter, I have yet to cover the decompression phase. However, placement of an ipsilateral expandable rod needs to occur before the decompression, when the intact lamina, facet, and pars interarticularis still offer protection to the neural elements. Placement of the ipsilateral expandable rod in the intact spine eliminates any risk to the neural elements. In the spirit of describing the actual sequence of the operation, I will present the rationale and technique at this point and elaborate on it further in Section 4.12, Phase III: Trials and Interbody Spacer Placement.

In Harms' description of the TLIF, he advises expansion of the disc space by placement of a provisional rod and distraction off of the pedicle screws.[11] Harms would tighten the set screws on the rod with the pedicle screws distracted and thereby capture and maintain the expanded disc height (▶ Fig. 4.28).[11] Harms felt his technique offered him greater access to the disc space, optimized restoration of the foraminal height and facilitated placement of the interbody spacer. However, Harms described the distraction of the screws on the side of the transforaminal corridor. Such an approach may work with an open exposure, but I have found placement of a rod on the side of the transforaminal approach quite constraining in a minimally invasive approach. The corridor is simply too narrow. The placement of a rod obstructs access to the disc space needed for insertion of the interbody spacer because of the lateral to medial trajectory into the disc space. Nonetheless, I have always recognized the true benefit in distracting the disc space as recommended by Harms for transforaminal approaches. The question is how to bring that component into a limited paramedian minimally invasive corridor. The following section describes a solution to that question. Although I cover some elements of interbody work in this section, the goal is to introduce the concept of a provisional, ipsilateral expandable rod as an option for surgeons working through this corridor. I will present a more detailed description of interbody techniques later in the chapter.

To resolve the conundrum of ipsilateral provisional distraction in a minimally invasive transforaminal approach, I created a list of criteria that the solution would have to meet. First and foremost, whatever the device, it could not obstruct the transforaminal corridor into the disc space along the minimally invasive trajectory. Second, the device would need to engage into the pedicle screw system that was placed. Third, the device would have to be easily placed and removed within a minimally invasive exposure. Finally, there had to be a mechanism to capture the expansion that did not require a distractor like that initially described by Harms. Such a traditional pedicle screw distractor would not fit within a minimally invasive expandable access port.

Turning the tulip heads of the pedicle screws 90 degrees solves the first problem. That displaces the expanding component of the rod out of the transforaminal corridor. Small limbs with the same diameter as the permanent rod slip into the tulip heads of the pedicle screws, which projects the main arm 90 degrees from the limbs so that the transforaminal corridor remains open. A two-component distractor system with a sleeve arm and a distractor latch and spring, along with a rack arm that captures the height as paddle distractors, open the interbody space. The self-capturing sleeve and latch system avoids the need for an additional distractor to expand the device. The first iteration of the device is illustrated in ▶ Fig. 4.29. Although the device was too bulky for placement through an expandable minimal access port, it served as the proof of principle that successfully distracted the disc space and kept the transforaminal corridor open. In the next iteration, I lowered the profile so that it fit through the expandable

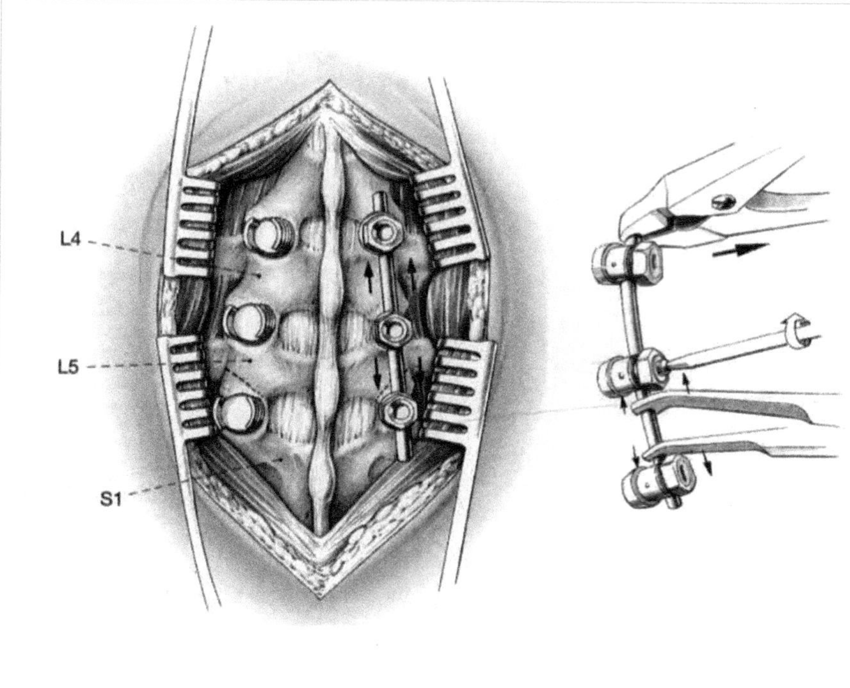

Fig. 4.28 Illustration from Harms' technique description of the transforaminal lumbar interbody fusion.[11] In this illustration, Harms places a distractor on the rod and between the pedicle screws. Tightening of the set screws captures the distraction. Distraction opens the disc space and facilitates interbody work. However, the trajectory into the disc space used in a minimally invasive approach is in the same plane as the rod. As a result, the rod obstructs access to the disc space. (Reproduced with permission from Harms J, Rolinger H. A one-stage procedure in operative treatment of spondylolistheses: dorsal traction-reposition and anterior fusion (author's transl) [in German]. Z Orthop Ihre Grenzgeb. 1982; 120:343–347.)

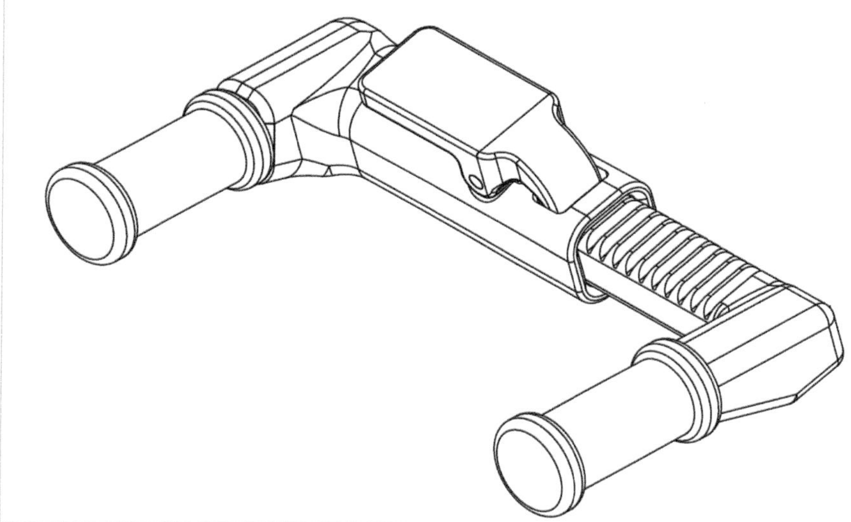

Fig. 4.29 A conceptual drawing of the provisional, expandable, ipsilateral rod that could be used in a minimally invasive approach. Turning the tulip heads of the pedicle screws 90 degrees allows for lateral displacement of the expanding rod away from the transforaminal corridor.

minimal access port as seen in ▶ Fig. 4.30. On the basis of the interpedicular distances discussed earlier in this chapter, I designed the expandable minimally invasive TLIF distractor to collapse to 21 mm from pedicle fixation point to fixation point and to expand to 42 mm.

When applying the expandable retractor at the time of surgery, the tulip heads of the pedicle screws are turned 90 degrees from the vertical position that would be used for permanent rod placement. I secure the provisional ipsilateral provisional rod with a rod holder and a head alignment tool. When inserted into the polyaxial pedicle screw tulip head, I achieve a fixed position with placement of a set screw. ▶ Fig. 4.31 demonstrates that when in position, the expandable rod does not interfere with access to the neural elements or the disc space for completion of the interbody fusion.

Using currently available instrumentation sets, this provisional rod may be easily placed and secured prior to the decompression. I prefer to place the provisional ipsilateral expandable rod before exposing the neural elements. As the interbody height increases with the use of either paddle distractors or trials, the provisional ipsilateral rod captures that height in 1-mm increments. The height captured by the expandable rod directly corresponds to the height of the paddle distractors and trial spacers that I used to expand the disc space. The final height of the trial spacer determines my selection of the height for the final interbody spacer I place into the disc space. Instead of worrying about the collapse of the disc space after removal of the paddle or trial spacer, the expandable rod maintains the height (▶ Fig. 4.32). Upon completion of the interbody placement, the set screws and the ipsilateral expandable rod are removed by hooking one of the limbs of the rod with a reverse angle curet and pulling it up and then removing it with a rod holder.

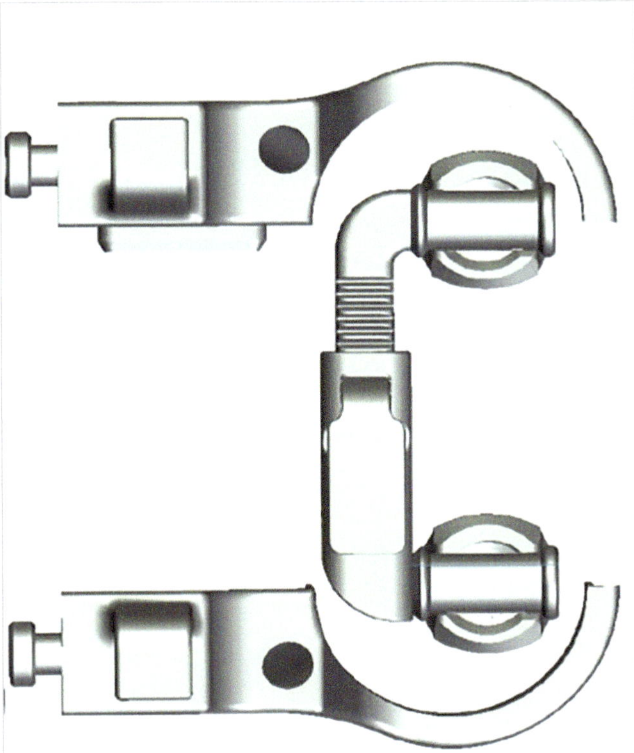

Fig. 4.30 Illustration of a low-profile ipsilateral expandable rod within a minimal access port. The pedicle screws are turned 90 degrees from the vertical position, and the limbs of the expandable rod are slipped into the tulip heads of the pedicle screws. The set screws are then tightened to fixate the rod to the segment. The device is small enough to fit within an expandable minimal access port without obstructing the transforaminal corridor.

As soon as I began to use the provisional expandable ipsilateral rod, I appreciated the wisdom of Harms. The capacity to maintain distraction on the ipsilateral side vastly facilitated preparation of the cortical end plates and insertion of the interbody spacer. Provisional distraction also optimized the interbody height I was able to achieve. Greater interbody height allowed for greater restoration of segmental lordosis when I placed the pedicle screws under compression at the end of the TLIF. The expandable rod used in a transforaminal approach is analogous to the Caspar post distractor used in cervical spine procedures.

Further discussion of interbody techniques awaits the reader in the later sections of this chapter. However, since I secure the ipsilateral expandable provisional rod before beginning the decompression, I feel the need to introduce this concept and present it now to preserve the accuracy of the sequence of events. Therefore, before I proceed to the second phase of the operation, the decompression phase, I place a straight rod on the contralateral side with set screws so that I can capture the increased disc height symmetrically. With the placement of these rods, phase I is complete. The nursing staff removes the loupes and the headlights, while the radiological technologist moves the fluoroscope to the head of the bed. The operating microscope rolls into position, and phase II of the operation begins.

4.11 Phase II. Decompression, Discectomy and End Plate Preparation

To achieve a central decompression, I must expose the lamina until I can see it merge into the base of the spinous process, which is the same exposure I would accomplish in a minimally invasive laminectomy. Since the trajectory for pedicle screw placement is distinct, I routinely readjust the expandable

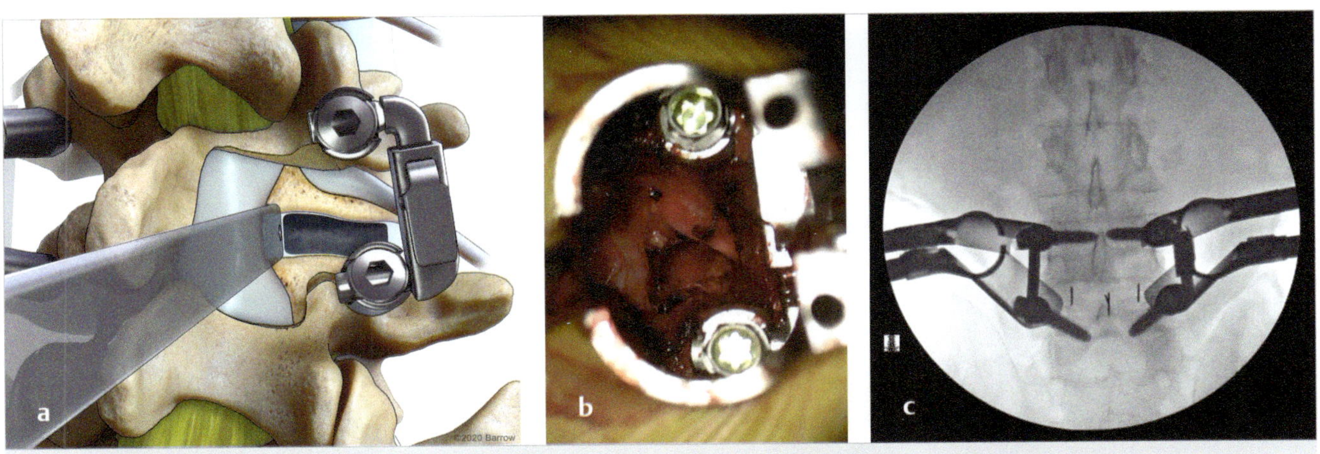

Fig. 4.31 Application of the provisional ipsilateral expandable rod for a minimally invasive transforaminal lumbar interbody fusion. **(a)** Artist's illustration of the provisional ipsilateral expandable rod in position. The transforaminal corridor is readily accessible. **(b)** Intraoperative photograph demonstrating the thecal sac, the exiting nerve root and the expanded disc space held open by the provisional ipsilateral expandable rod. **(c)** Anteroposterior fluoroscopic image demonstrating the provisional ipsilateral expandable rod in position after placement of the interbody spacer. At the end of the procedure, the ipsilateral expandable rod is replaced with a standard permanent rod.

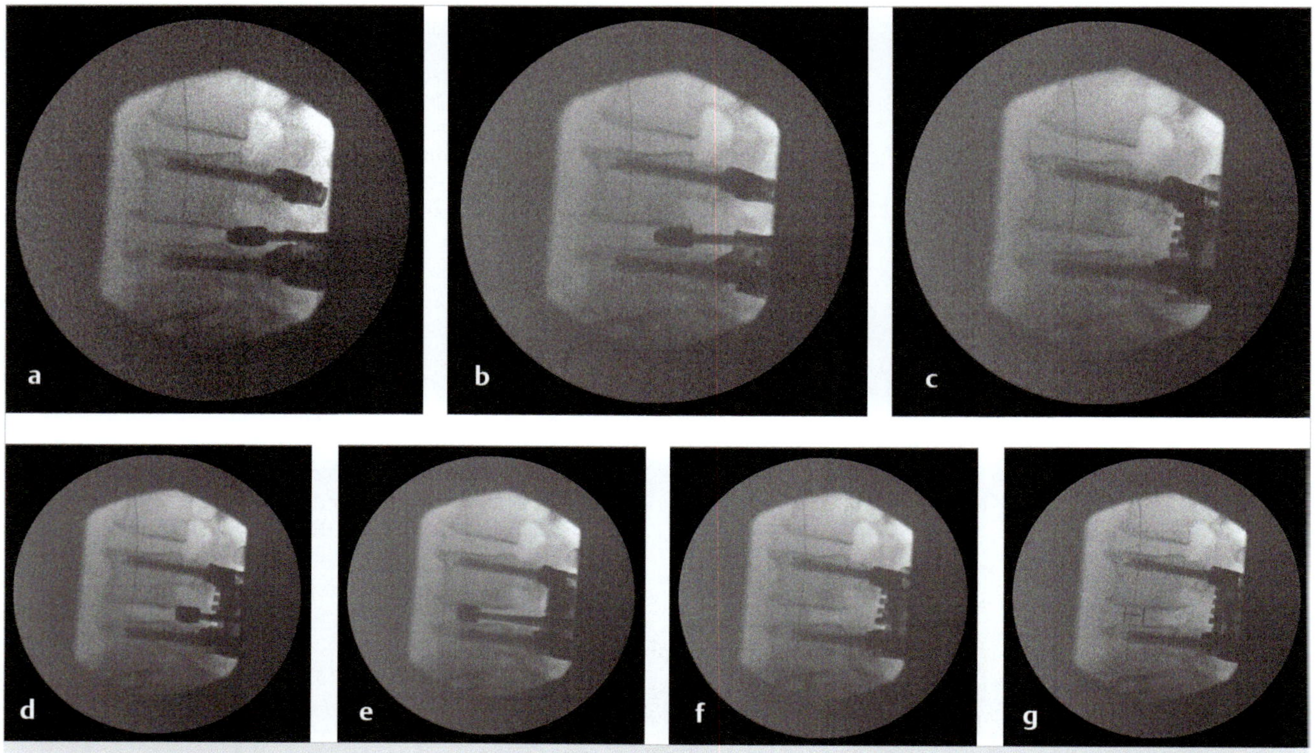

Fig. 4.32 Proof of principle for ipsilateral expandable rod distractor to maintain interbody height in an L3–4 transforaminal lumbar interbody fusion with and without provisional ipsilateral expandable rod. **(a)** Lateral fluoroscopic image demonstrating an 8-mm interbody trial entering the L3–4 disc space without the provisional ipsilateral expandable rod. **(b)** The posterior height of the disc space is restored with the trial in place. **(c)** The height collapses once the trial is removed. Ipsilateral expandable rod now placed to capture trial height. **(d)** When the provisional ipsilateral expandable rod is in position, **(e)** the height restored by the interbody trial is captured and **(f)** maintained. **(g)** Placement of an interbody spacer with 12 mm of foraminal height restoration.

minimal access port more medially at this time. It is equally worthwhile to achieve a more medial angulation of the medial-lateral retractor. Since it is no longer necessary to view the pedicle screws at this point, I loosen the table-mounted arm and then angle the expandable minimally invasive access port with a trajectory onto the junction of the lamina and spinous process and capture this angle by tightening the table-mounted retractor arm (▶ Fig. 4.33).

Once I achieve an optimal medial trajectory onto the lamina that exposes the base of the spinous process, I enlist my anesthesia colleagues to rotate the Jackson table away from me, in a way that is similar to what I describe in Chapter 3. The patient must be securely positioned on the rotating Jackson table to rotate them safely to the ideal angle for decompression. Rotation away from the surgeon creates a more ergonomic operating position and facilitates access to the contralateral side of the canal. ▶ Fig. 4.34 illustrates how access across the midline for complete decompression of the thecal sac is readily achievable when the spine is rotated 30 degrees away from the surgeon.

When viewing the vertebral anatomy under the operating microscope, I must take the time to identify the entire span of the pars interarticularis from its most lateral aspect to the base of the spinous process. All the bone, lamina, facet and pars interarticularis should be visualized from pedicle screw to pedicle screw. When I am satisfied that I have the requisite exposure, I use the drill to make two osteotomy cuts that intersect at the level of pars, the lamina, and the base of the spinous process. As seen in ▶ Fig. 4.35, the first osteotomy cut begins on the lateral aspect of the pars interarticularis and extends toward the base of the spinous process. The second osteotomy cut begins at the junction of the spinous process and lamina and extends toward the interlaminar space. These two osteotomies allow for disarticulation of the entire hemilamina and the inferior articular process (▶ Fig. 4.35). I use a bone mill to morselize the bone removed into a bone graft for placement into the disc space and interbody spacer.

4.11.1 First Osteotomy Cut: Drilling the Pars Interarticularis

A sophisticated understanding of the topography of the pars interarticularis is the most valuable knowledge to have to expedite the first osteotomy. Early in my experience, the initial pars osteotomy cut is where I spent the greatest amount of time. My concern for the exiting nerve root, which traversed just beneath the unfamiliar bone I was drilling, slowed down my progress. Now, with a greater understanding of the subtleties of the anatomy, it is currently where I save the most time. For this reason, it is a worthwhile investment to study the topography of the pars interarticularis in great detail (▶ Fig. 4.36).

At its most lateral aspect, the pars interarticularis is up to 18 mm thick and maintains that thickness for approximately 10 mm before it begins to taper as it blends into the lamina.

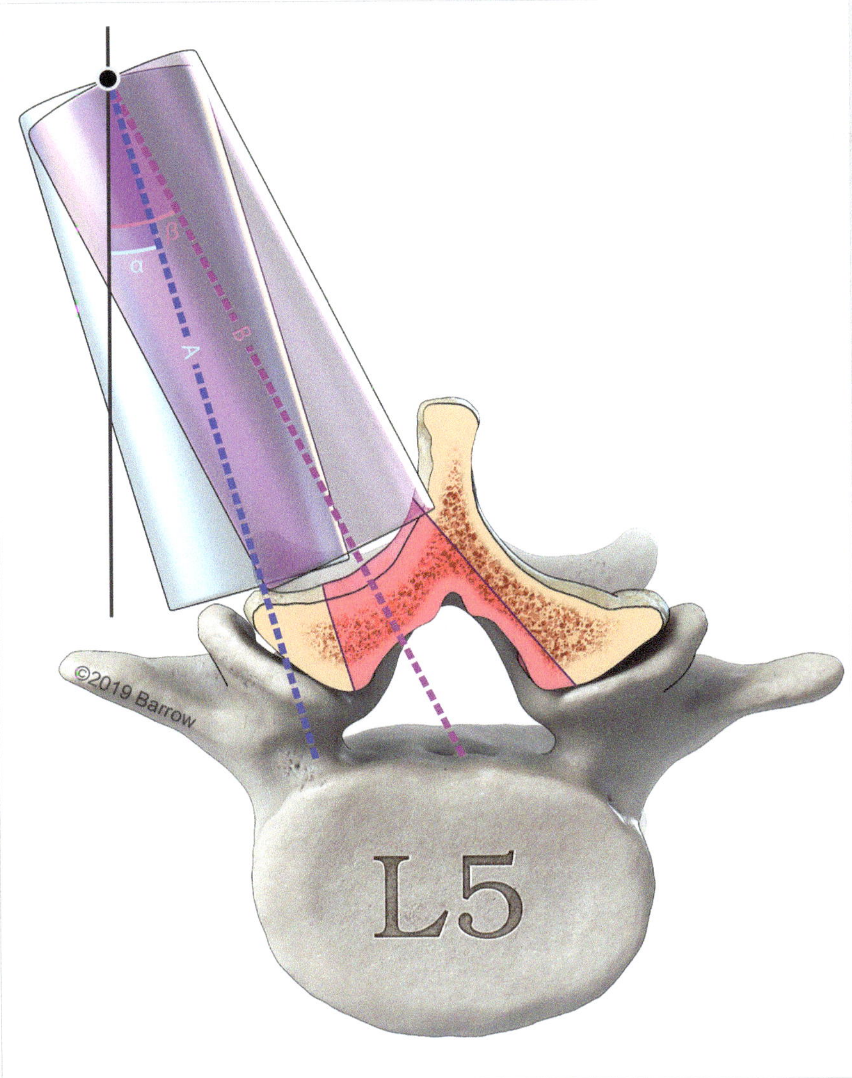

Fig. 4.33 Readjustment of the minimal access port for the decompression phase of the transforaminal lumbar interbody fusion. The illustration demonstrates the difference in the angles for pedicle screw placement (*blue*) and decompression (*purple*). The need to achieve a midline decompression requires repositioning of the minimal access port to converge onto the base of the spinous process.

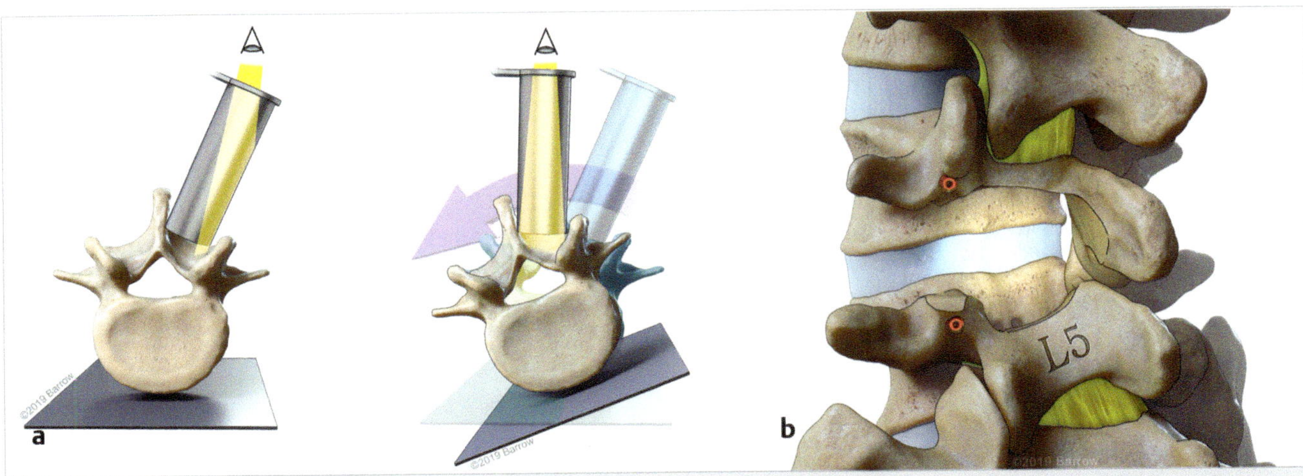

Fig. 4.34 Optimizing the trajectory for decompression. **(a)** Rotation of the bed away from the surgeon allows for a more ergonomic trajectory to the contralateral canal. It is this rotation of the bed that allows for greater facility in achieving a midline decompression. **(b)** The artist's illustration demonstrates the completed bone work for an L4–5 minimally invasive transforaminal lumbar interbody fusion from a 30-degree perspective.

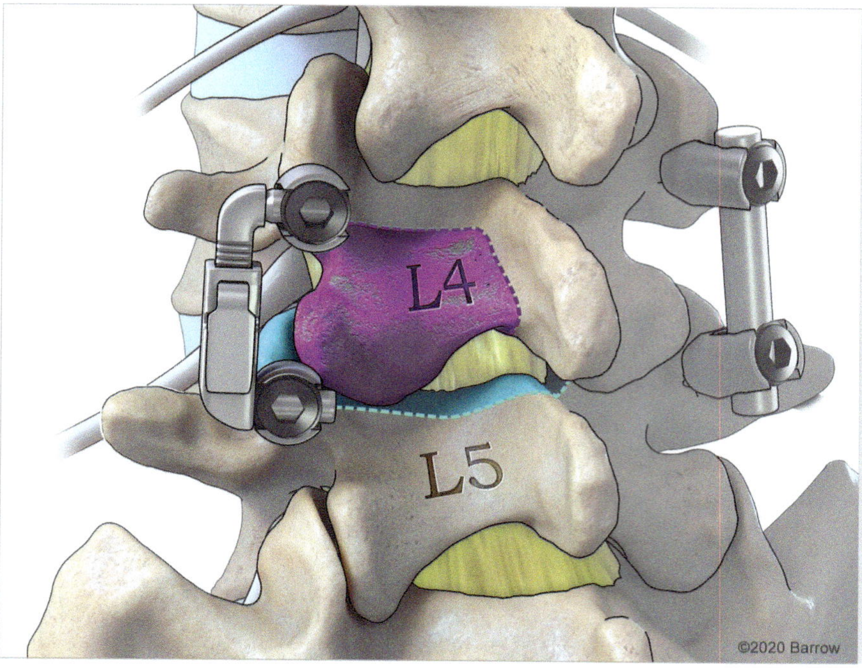

Fig. 4.35 Illustration of the bone work performed for the decompression phase of a minimally invasive transforaminal lumbar interbody fusion. The lamina in *purple* indicates the work performed at the L4 level. The advantage of having the pedicle screws in place is that they demarcate the boundaries of the decompression. The first osteotomy cut is in the pars interarticularis just below the rostral pedicle screw extending to lamina-spinous process junction. The second osteotomy cut is at the junction of the spinous process and the lamina extending to the interlaminar space. With the patient rotated, the cut is oblique, thereby undercutting the spinous process and contralateral lamina. The third osteotomy cut (*aqua*) removes the superior articular process just above the L5 pedicle screw and extends inferiorly to the superior aspect of the caudal lamina.

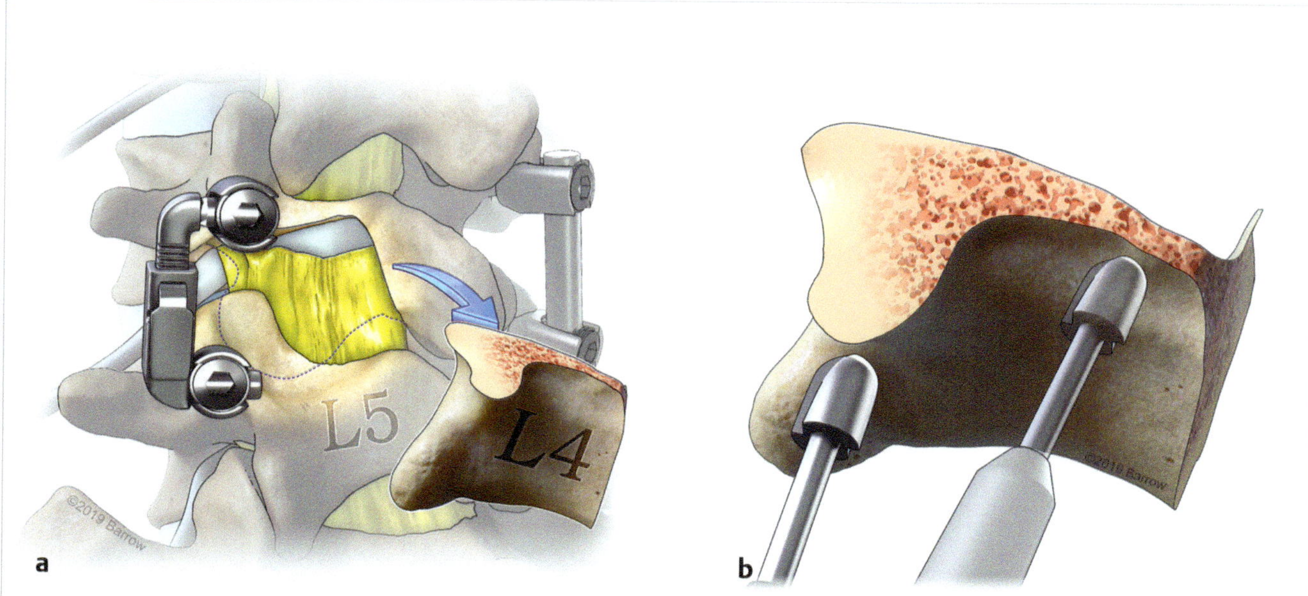

Fig. 4.36 Topography of the pars interarticularis. **(a)** Illustration of the first two osteotomy cuts with removal of the lamina, pars interarticularis and inferior articular facet. **(b)** Illustration showing the variable thickness of the pars interarticularis. When drilling the lateral aspect of the pars, the thickness can be up to 18 mm. When drilling medially toward the spinous process, the thickness tapers considerably to only several millimeters. Understanding the thickness of the pars interarticularis in the lateral aspect of the canal and how that thickness changes toward the central part of the canal minimizes the risk to the neural elements below while expediting the osteotomy cut with the drill.

Keeping the gradient of thickness of the pars in mind, I drill laterally to medially, that is, from the thickest part of the pars to the thinnest, with the intention of creating a breach into which the footplate of a Kerrison can safely fit to complete the work. My preference is to begin the drilling at a point just inferior to the rostral pedicle screw, which is one of the advantages of having the pedicle screws in position prior to the decompression. The screws help delineate the boundaries of the decompression. The ideal decompression for which I strive in every case is from the rostral pedicle to beyond the caudal pedicle.

Drilling a transverse line toward the lamina just below the rostral pedicle reliably places me above the insertion of the ligamentum flavum. Similar to identifying the rostral insertion of the ligamentum flavum that I described in Chapter 3, working above the insertion facilitates the en bloc resection of the ligamentum flavum and decompression of the entire thecal sac. I continue to drill the lateral aspect of the pars until I have thinned it to a shrimp-shell thickness and then continue medially across the entire isthmus of the pars interarticularis and into the lamina until I reach the base of the spinous process. Since there is no ligamentum flavum at this level, I take care to thin the bone enough that I may finish the cut with a Kerrison rongeur. I return to the lateral aspect of the pars interarticularis and drill until I make a small breach in the pars over the top of the nerve root. Although the ligamentum flavum is absent at this level medially within the canal, it lies on top of the nerve root laterally. Thus, the lateral aspect of the pars is an ideal location for the breach and completion of the osteotomy cut with a Kerrison rongeur (▶ Fig. 4.37).

4.11.2 Second Osteotomy Cut: Oblique Cut of the Lamina

I make the second osteotomy cut obliquely through the base of the spinous process down to the interlaminar space (▶ Fig. 4.38). I begin drilling further down on the junction of the spinous process and lamina where the ligamentum flavum is the thickest. I work in a rostral direction until I intersect the transverse cut in the pars interarticularis. As I approach the first osteotomy cut, my objective is to lightly thin the lamina in that area but not to create a breach. With the patient rotated away from me, the osteotomy invariably results in an oblique trajectory beneath the spinous process and into the contralateral lamina.

As I drill the caudal aspect of the lamina, I look for the unmistakable tuft of the ligamentum flavum to unveil itself from within my drill trough. The goal is to make a breach in this area of the lamina and identify the ligamentum flavum that resides immediately below it. After I create the breach, I continue to thin the bone of the lamina in the rostral and caudal directions (▶ Fig. 4.39). I remain cautious when drilling at the most rostral aspect of the bone work where I anticipate the absence of the protective cover of the ligamentum flavum. With the bone thinned, the ligamentum flavum evident, and both osteotomy cuts complete, the footplate of a number 2 Kerrison rongeur fits nicely into the trough above the ligamentum flavum, and I complete the bone work.

As I work the Kerrison rongeur, the entire lamina, pars interarticularis, and inferior articular process disarticulate. A forward-angled curet establishes a plane of dissection between the lamina and the ligamentum flavum. The goal remains to keep the ligamentum flavum in position so that it protects the dura until all the bone work is complete. Invariably, attachments to the most caudal aspect of the inferior articular process require division with a Kerrison rongeur or a forward-angled curet before it is feasible to liberate that entire section of bone. After I have freed all the attachments to the lamina and facet, I remove this entire piece in one fell swoop and then prepare it for the autograft that I will place into the disc space. I ask the scrub technician to remove the synovium and cartilaginous surface from the inferior articular process of the facet and to denude the bone of any soft tissue. The synovium and articular surfaces can be detrimental to optimizing an environment for fusion within the disc space. The scrub technician uses a bone mill to grind this section of bone to create morselized autograft ideal for the interbody space.

When I peer back down through the microscope at the operative field, I see the superior articular process (SAP) and superior aspect of the lamina at L5. Under ideal circumstances, the ligamentum flavum remains intact as seen in ▶ Fig. 4.40.

4.11.3 Third Osteotomy Cut: Superior Articular Process and Conjoined Nerve Roots

I make a point to leave the ligamentum flavum intact as I remove the lamina, pars interarticularis and the inferior articular process of L4 and then turn my attention to the SAP of L5 and the L5 lamina. The caudal pedicle screw is an excellent guide that indicates the location of the osteotomy cut in the SAP (▶ Fig. 4.41). I drill down the base of the SAP just above the pedicle of L5 and thin it to a point that allows an osteotome to disarticulate it with nothing more than a twist. The area above the pedicle is a relatively safe zone, devoid of both the traversing and exiting nerve roots, and so an alternative to drilling is to use a mallet to tap an osteotome through the base of the SAP just above the pedicle screw angled away from the neural elements. However, since it is safest to perform such an osteotomy cut with fluoroscopy, I have settled on using a drill to remove the SAP. I find it to be disruptive to the work flow to bring the fluoroscope into the surgical field while working under the microscope. Drilling the SAP can be just as efficient as cleaving it with an osteotome. The use of the drill further allows work to be done on the caudal lamina, which has an unfavorable topography for an osteotome.

The possibility of a conjoined root is another reason that I prefer the drill to the osteotome. Admittedly, a conjoined root is a rare occurrence. On 4 occasions out of over 600, I have encountered a conjoined root beneath the SAP, which an osteotome would have potentially injured had I used it exclusively to perform the osteotomy. The tip of the drill safely unveiled this anatomical variant just by thinning the bone and creating a breach. The twisting action of an osteotome within the trough disarticulated the SAP, and a Kerrison rongeur completed the bone work. With a conjoined root, there is no safe zone overlying the disc space. In all four of these cases, I looked for the lateral aspect of the thecal sac, but all I saw was one large nerve root with continuous dura on the top of the disc space (▶ Fig. 4.42). The thecal sac, which typically retracts readily with a suction retractor, did not budge. The intraoperative video (Video 4.3) demonstrates the inability to mobilize the thecal sac. The traversing and exiting roots were conjoined. Should you encounter this anatomical variant, no attempt should be made to approach the interbody space from that side. A conjoined root is a contraindication for transforaminal access to the disc space. In each circumstance where I encountered a conjoined root, I successfully accomplished the interbody fusion from the opposite side. I have yet to encounter a bilateral conjoined root at one level.

4.11.4 Final Element of Bone Work: Superior Aspect of the Caudal Lamina

In Chapter 3, I presented the en bloc resection of the ligamentum flavum for the treatment of lumbar stenosis. A key

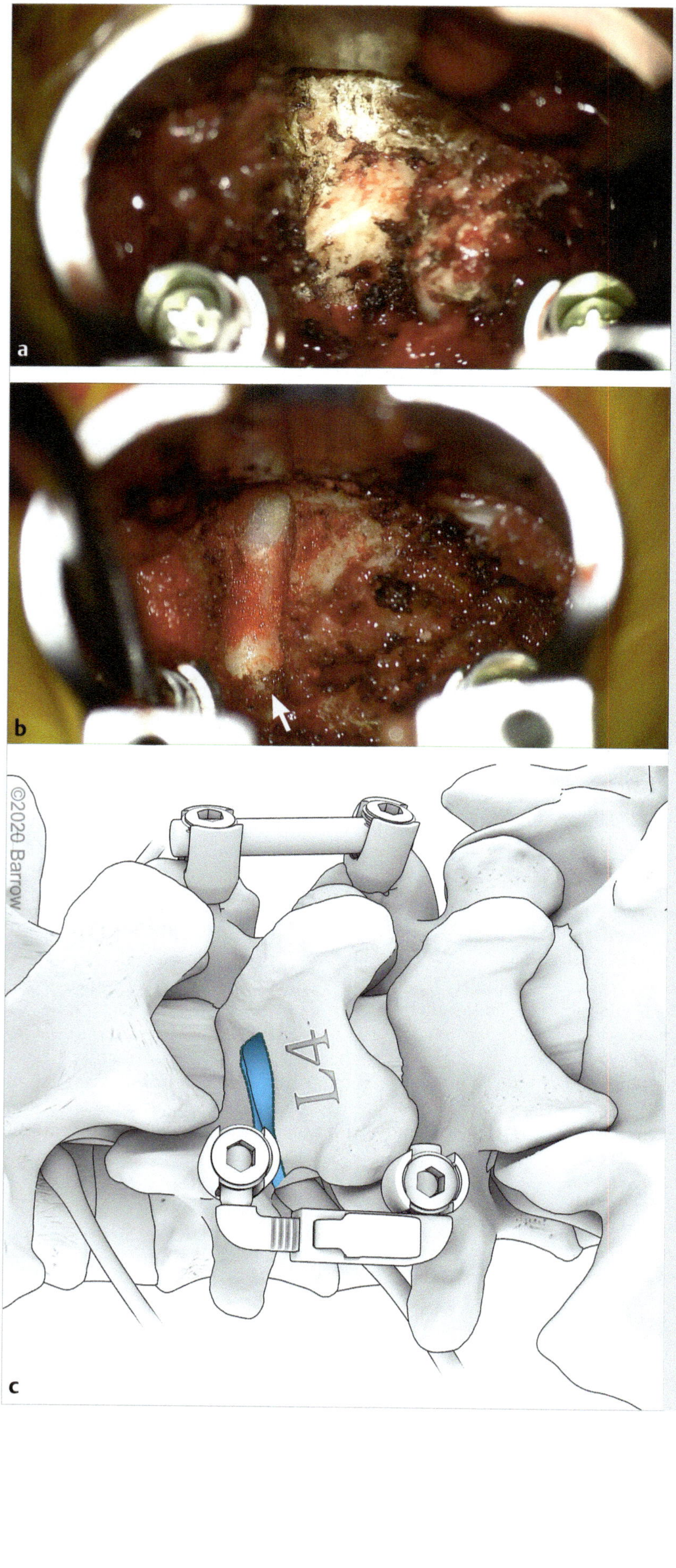

Fig. 4.37 The first osteotomy cut through the pars interarticularis. **(a)** Intraoperative photograph of the exposure of the L4 lamina and pars interarticularis before the osteotomy cut in a left-sided approach to an L4–5 transforaminal lumbar interbody fusion. Note that the medial blade is anchored up against the base of the spinous process. **(b)** Intraoperative photograph showing the thinned lamina with a breach over the lateral-most aspect of the pars interarticularis (*arrow*). **(c)** Illustration of the completed first osteotomy cut showing the orientation of the cut in L4.

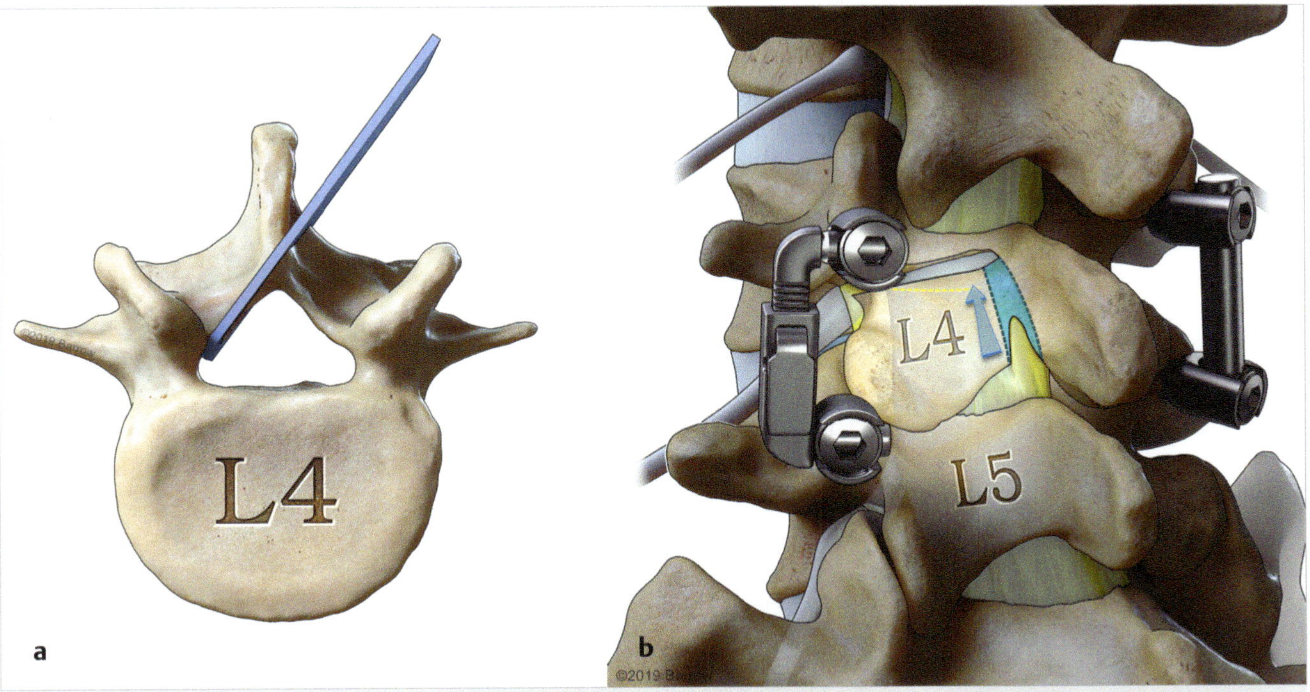

Fig. 4.38 Illustration of the second osteotomy cut through the pars interarticularis. (a) Axial view of the L4 vertebra demonstrating the trajectory of the oblique osteotomy cut that grants access to the contralateral recess. (b) Surgical view demonstrating beginning the osteotomy cut near the interlaminar space and then proceeding in the rostral direction to join the first osteotomy cut.

component of that technique is the exposure of the rostral and caudal insertion points of the ligamentum flavum. I apply a more extensive version of that same technique to the decompression phase of the TLIF. The two osteotomy cuts have freed the ligamentum flavum from its rostral insertion. The complete removal of the SAP has released the lateral insertion point of the ligamentum flavum. The only insertion that remains is the caudal insertion on the underside of the superior aspect of the caudal lamina (▶ Fig. 4.43). Logically, that is the next target for the tip of the drill.

Similar to the lumbar laminectomy, the goal is to reach the caudal insertion of the ligamentum flavum for the segment. Additional exposure of the caudal lamina is necessary to accomplish this task. Bipolar cautery shrinks the soft tissue and reveals the superior aspect of the caudal lamina. At other times, a Kerrison rongeur is needed to remove the facet arthropathy debris that obscures a clear path to the lamina.

The SAP blends into the superior aspect of the lamina and comes into view by following the SAP beyond the pedicle screw in the caudal direction. I use a large straight curet to wipe away the ligamentum flavum overlying the superior aspect of the lamina and to expose the unmistakable ivory of the lamina. With my target in sight, I begin drilling. The objective is to thin the superior aspect of the lamina up to the midline and reveal the insertion of the ligamentum flavum there (in the case of an L4–5 MIS TLIF, it would be L5). As described in Chapter 3, I work beyond the insertion of the ligamentum flavum, which places me in a larger cross-sectional area of the canal, facilitates resection of the ligamentum flavum, and optimizes the central decompression and the foraminotomy for the traversing root. I apply those same principles for the TLIF decompression. Throughout all bone removal, I make it a point to maintain the ligamentum flavum intact. That intact ligamentum flavum serves as the protector of the neural elements from inadvertent injury.

The unmistakable appearance of thin strands of ligamentum and epidural fat becomes evident when I have drilled through the inner cortex of the lamina and have created a breach. If I still encounter thickened ligamentum flavum after creating the breach, I know that I have not drilled beyond the insertion and need to proceed further caudally. I believe that the safest technique for resection of the ligamentum flavum is to prevent the need for the Kerrison bite that encompasses both ligamentum flavum and lamina. Instead, I work through the laminar breach beyond the ligamentum flavum, expand that opening with a Kerrison rongeur, and identify the uncompressed dura below the level of the insertion. Mobilizing the ligamentum flavum upward from there becomes a straightforward exercise. Such an approach entirely prevents the need for a hopeful but blind Kerrison bite of lamina with a mouth already full of thickened ligamentum flavum.

Thinning the lamina, unveiling the epidural fat, or directly visualizing the thecal sac is more inviting to the footplate of a Kerrison rongeur than is the constrained and deep underside of the same lamina. Working from caudal to rostral, I can watch the footplate of the Kerrison pass safely over the top of the thecal sac instead of passing the Kerrison blindly in the rostral to caudal direction. After widening the breach, the bone work continues both medially and laterally. In proceeding laterally, the traversing nerve root comes clearly into view, and I can readily perform a generous foraminotomy over the top of the root well beyond the level of the pedicle, thus fulfilling my objective to achieve a pedicle to beyond pedicle decompression. Proceeding medially, I

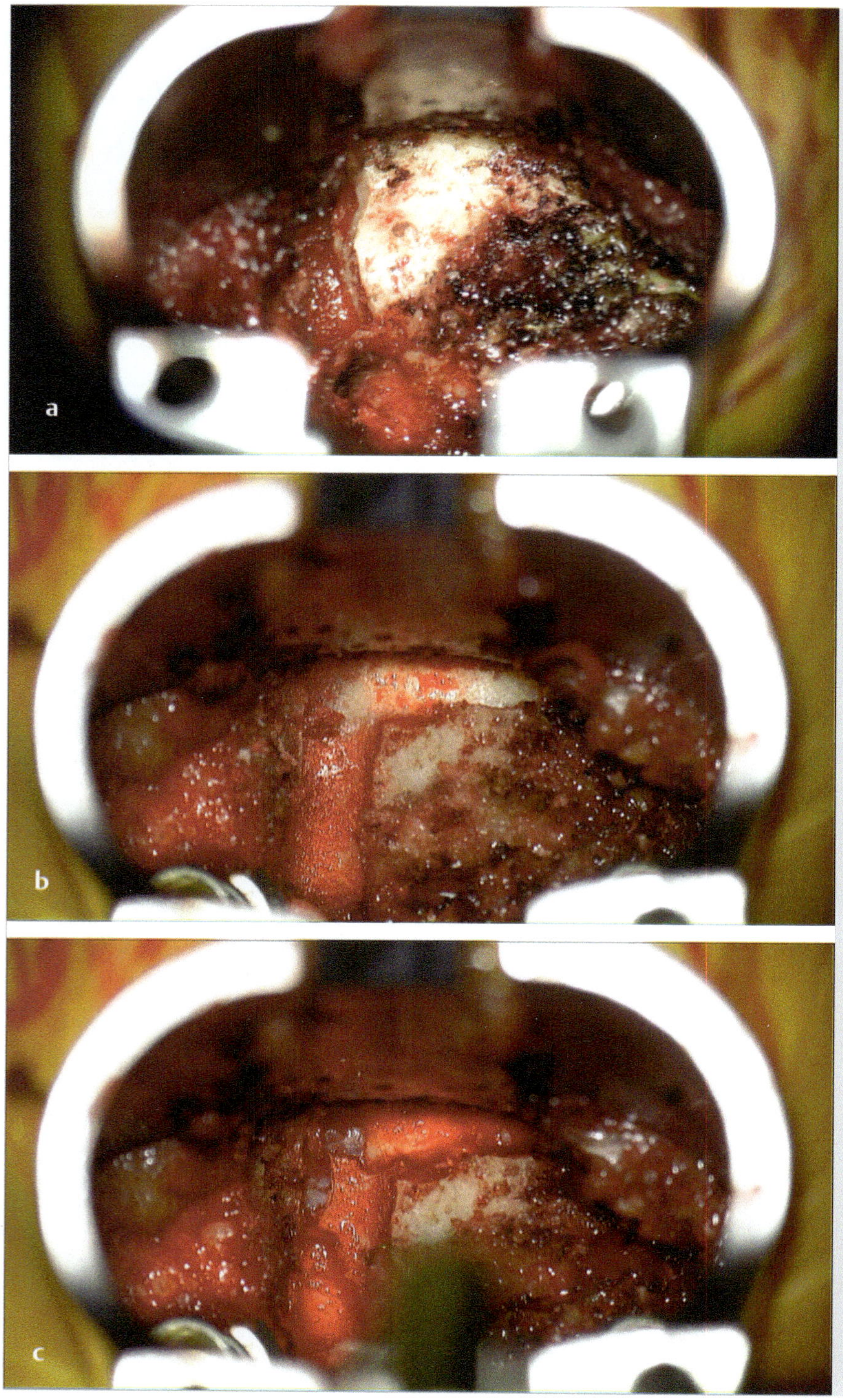

Fig. 4.39 Intraoperative photographs of the second osteotomy cut. **(a)** Exposure of the L4 lamina in a left L4–5 transforaminal lumbar interbody fusion with the first osteotomy cut complete. **(b)** Thinned bone across the entire L4 lamina. **(c)** Connection of the osteotomy cuts at the intersection of the pars interarticularis, lamina and base of the spinous process. Note that the osteotomy cut is beyond the ligamentum flavum as dura may be seen just above the transverse cut.

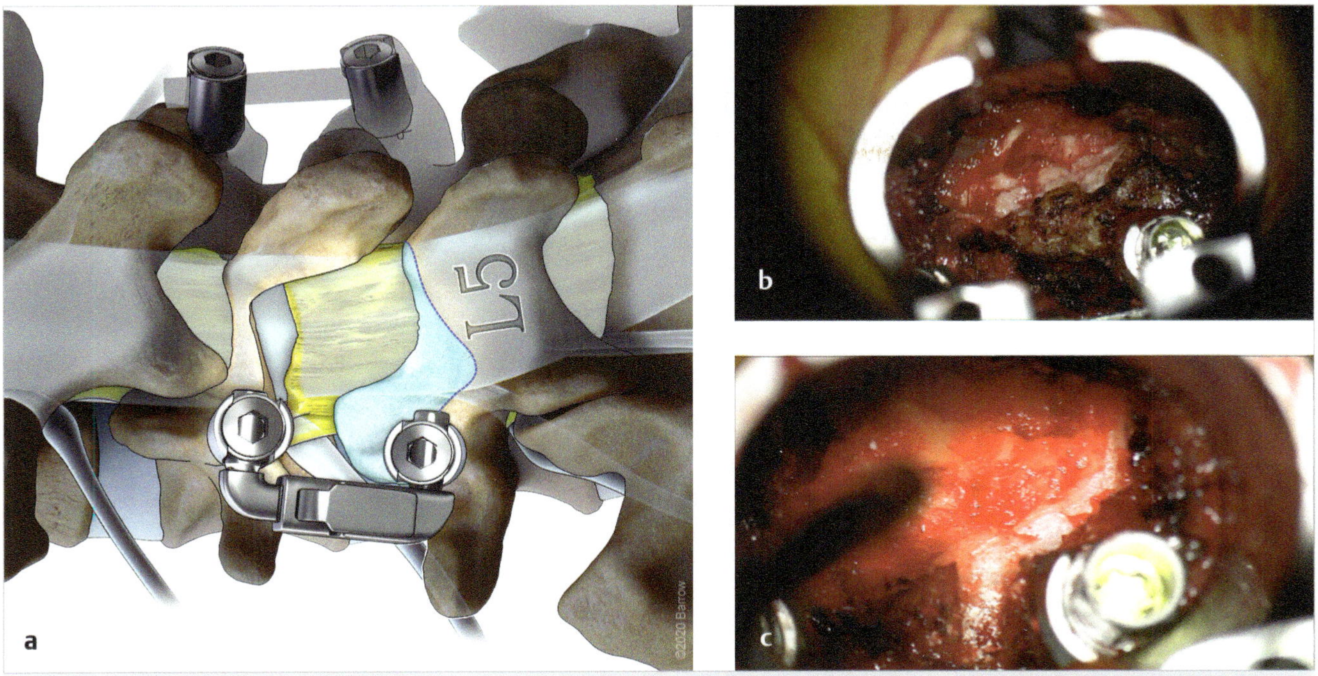

Fig. 4.40 **(a)** Illustration of the anatomy after removal of the pars interarticularis, lamina and inferior articular process. The entire pars interarticularis on the top of the L4 nerve root is removed, thereby decompressing the root. The spinous process is undercut, allowing for a complete decompression of the thecal sac and contralateral recess. The ligamentum flavum remains intact, covering the thecal sac. **(b)** Intraoperative photograph of L4 after the removal of the lamina, pars interarticularis and inferior articular process in a left L4–5 transforaminal lumbar interbody fusion. The superior articular process of L5 and the lamina of L5 are now readily accessible. **(c)** Intraoperative photograph of the ligamentum flavum over the top of the thecal sac and exposure of the superior aspect of the caudal lamina of L5. A preliminary trough has been drilled in preparation to breach the lamina beyond the insertion of the ligamentum flavum, which will facilitate the en bloc resection.

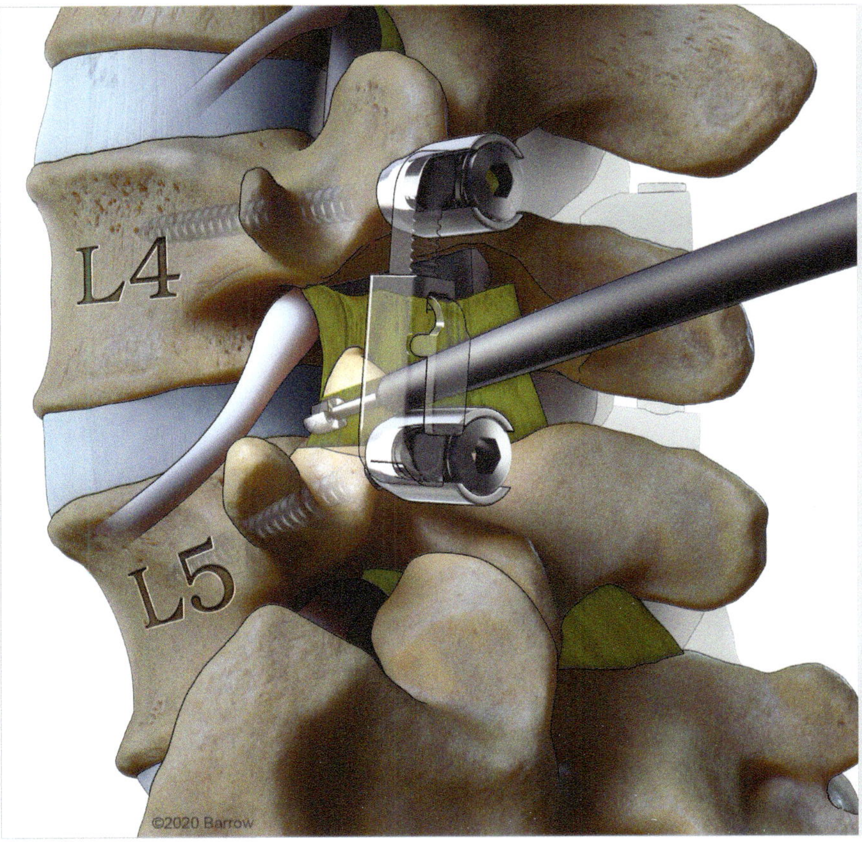

Fig. 4.41 Illustration of the osteotomy cut for the superior articular process (SAP). Lateral image of the L4–5 segment. The caudal pedicle screw serves as a guide to determine the location of the osteotomy cut in the SAP. Removal of the SAP provides access to the disc space. The lateral displacement of the expandable ipsilateral rod (ghosted) as seen in this illustration offers a working corridor to the SAP.

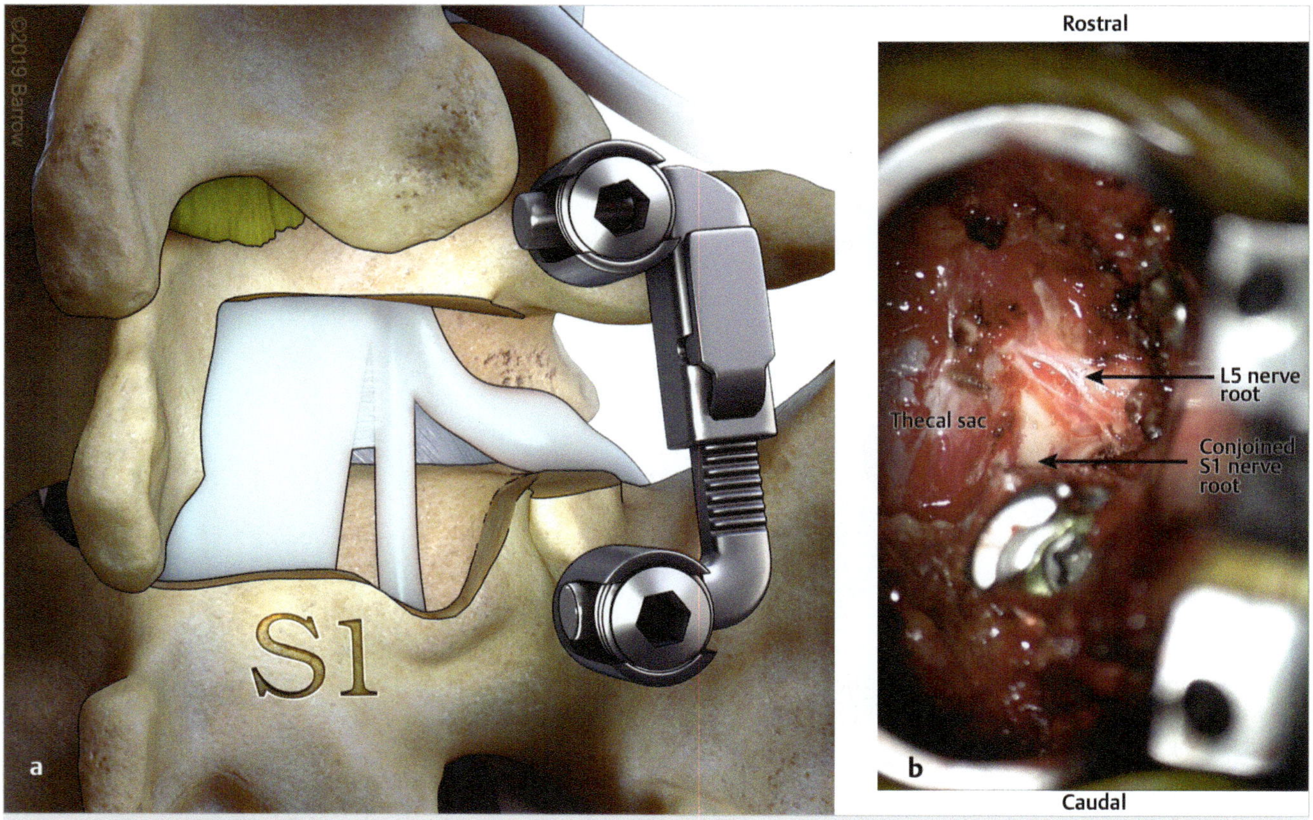

Fig. 4.42 Intraoperative photographs and illustration of a conjoined nerve root at L5–S1 on the right side. **(a)** Conjoined nerve root at L5–S1. The L5 nerve root is tethered to the S1 nerve root preventing access to the transforaminal corridor. **(b)** Intraoperative photograph of a right-sided approach to the L5–S1 segment shows the L5 nerve root directly over the disc space. There is no clear separation of the L5 nerve root from the thecal sac or the traversing nerve root of S1. There was no access to the disc space from the right. Access to the interbody space was successfully accomplished from the left side.

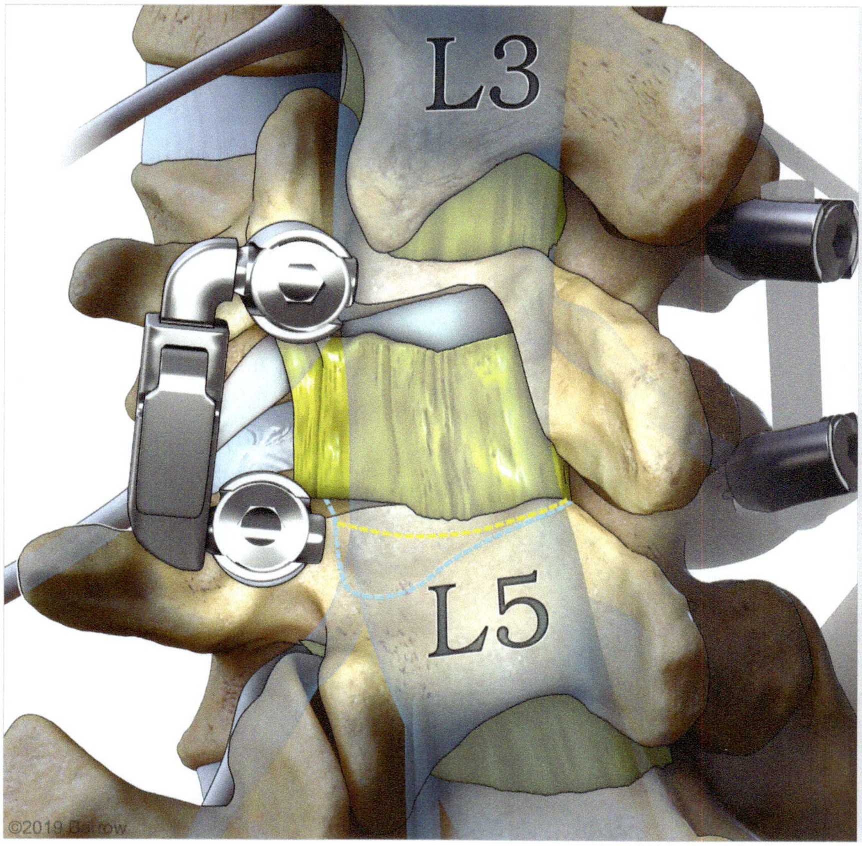

Fig. 4.43 Illustration of the removal of the superior aspect of the caudal lamina. The *aqua* line indicates the section of the lamina to be removed. The *yellow* line indicates the caudal insertion of the ligamentum flavum. In this case, drilling beyond the insertion along the *aqua* line prevents the need to work in the most constrained part of the central canal and releases the caudal insertion of the ligamentum flavum. An en bloc resection of the ligamentum flavum completes the decompression of the entire segment.

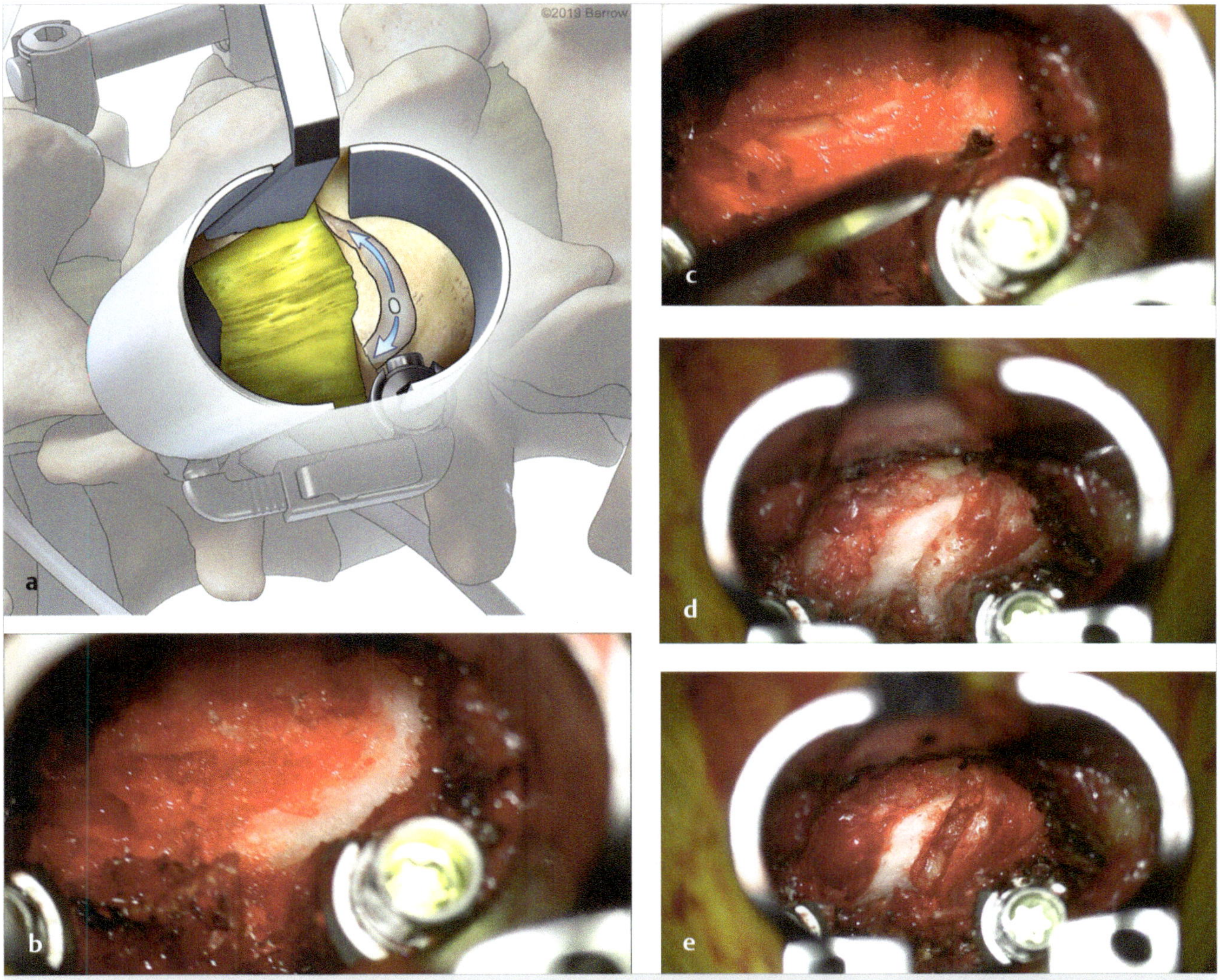

Fig. 4.44 Releasing the inferior insertion of the ligamentum flavum in a left L4–5 transforaminal lumbar interbody fusion. **(a)** Illustration demonstrating the concept of working below the insertion of the ligamentum flavum and beyond the most constrained aspect of the canal. A drill is used to thin the superior aspect of the lamina, and a breach is made exposing the thecal sac. A corridor of lamina is removed medially and laterally, releasing the ligamentum flavum from its inferior insertion. **(b)** Intraoperative photograph demonstrating the trough drilled into the superior aspect of the L5 lamina. **(c)** Intraoperative image demonstrating a forward-angled curet entering the breach to ensure safe passage for a Kerrison rongeur. **(d)** Intraoperative photograph from another operation showing the breach in the superior aspect of the lamina of L5 beyond the ligamentum flavum. **(e)** Intraoperative photograph of the completed osteotomy through the superior articular process of L5; the osteotomy extends into the superior lamina of L5 beyond the insertion of the ligamentum flavum in preparation for the en bloc resection.

use the Kerrison rongeur to access the contralateral recess (▸ Fig. 4.44). With both of these corridors cleared, I remove the SAP that I had previously disarticulated. As with the inferior articular process, there are several attachments that I must divide for the safe and seamless removal of the disarticulated SAP. Because the attachments tethering the SAP tend to be lateral, I use a small forward-angled curet to scrape the tethers free. I then lift out the SAP, clean it, and mill it for additional autograft material.

4.11.5 En Bloc Removal of the Ligamentum Flavum

At this point in the decompression phase, the inferior articular process, lamina, pars interarticularis and the SAP have all been removed. The superior and inferior insertions of the ligamentum flavum have been exposed (▸ Fig. 4.45a, b). To complete the decompression, I lift the entire ligamentum flavum off the dura in an en bloc manner. I use a series of forward angle curets and Kerrison rongeurs to continue to undercut the contralateral lamina, extend the bone work well beneath the spinous process and release the contralateral ligamentum flavum from its lateral insertion. The rotation of the patient 15 to 20 degrees away from me that I had my anesthesia colleagues perform at the outset of the decompression phase has optimized the working trajectory to accomplish this task (▸ Fig. 4.34). I extend the bone work in the rostral direction until the insertion of the ligamentum flavum comes into view. The thickened fibers of the ligament give way to thin strands amidst epidural fat and

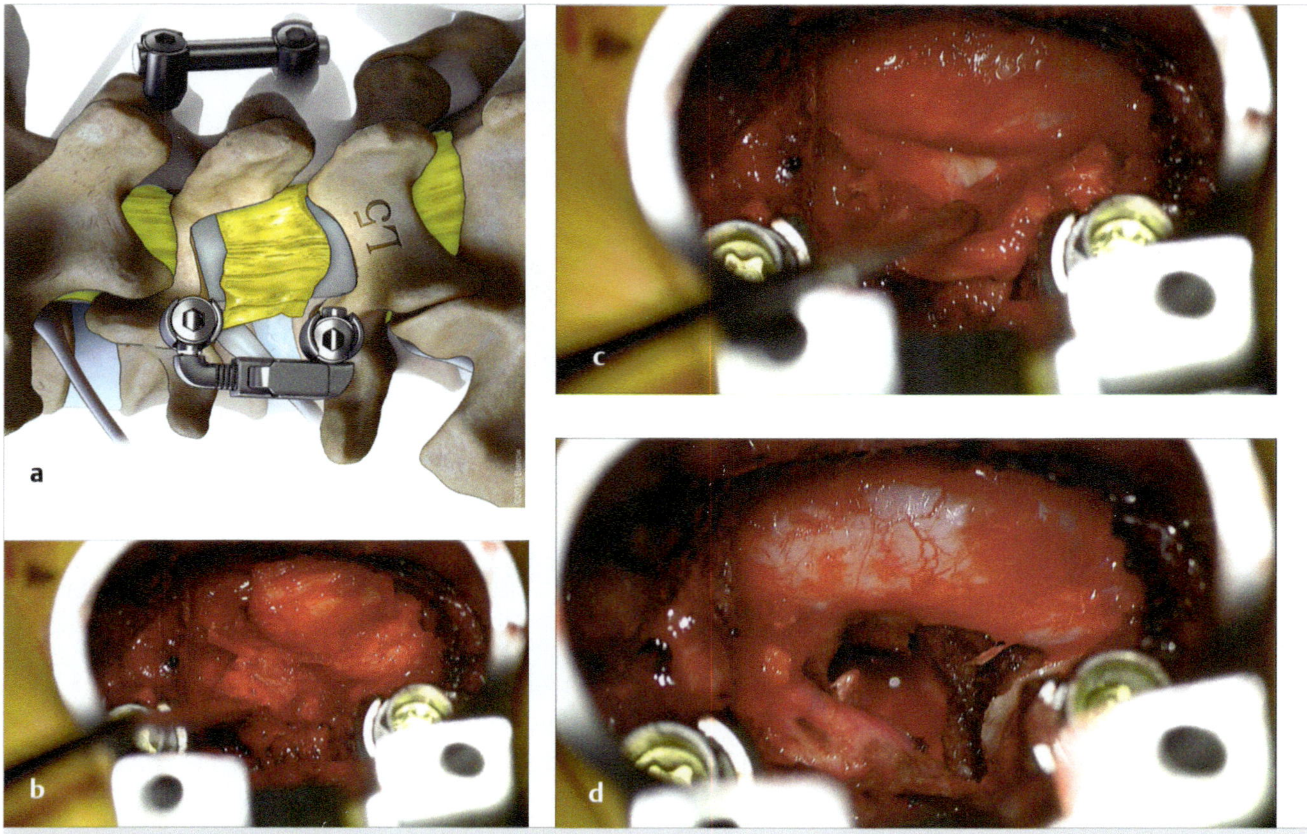

Fig. 4.45 En bloc resection of the ligamentum flavum in an L4–5 transforaminal lumbar interbody fusion. **(a)** Illustration showing the release of the rostral, caudal, lateral and contralateral insertions of the ligamentum flavum. When all these insertions are released, a plane between the dura and the ligamentum flavum is established, and the entire ligamentum flavum is resected from the segment. **(b)** Intraoperative photograph demonstrating the ligamentum flavum released from its rostral, caudal and contralateral insertion. **(c)** Intraoperative photograph showing the ligamentum flavum rolled back, revealing the entire thecal sac. The ipsilateral insertion still needs to be released. **(d)** Intraoperative photograph demonstrating the segmental decompression achieved with en bloc resection of the ligamentum flavum.

epidural veins. Finding those structures is an indication that you have achieved an adequate rostral exposure. Squaring off the exposure that has been achieved completes the rostral bone work. At this point, I have exposed beyond the rostral and caudal insertions of the ligamentum flavum. I have both medial and lateral access to the ligamentum flavum. With these objectives accomplished, I begin the removal of the entire ligamentum flavum of the segment.

I have found the right-angled ball-tipped probe to be the most useful instrument to slip in between the dura and ligamentum flavum and establish a plane. I prefer a forward angle curet to separate the ligamentum flavum from its bony insertion on the contralateral side. The dura comes into view after a few bites with the Kerrison rongeur. After I ensure a safe plane over the top of the dura with a forward-angle curet, I use a right-angle ball-tipped probe or nerve hook to release any adhesions between the ligamentum flavum and the dura. It is now possible to begin resecting the ligamentum flavum with direct visualization of the dura.

Decompression proceeds first from rostral to caudal until I reach the level of the disc space. From there, I proceed caudal to rostral, working from beyond the ligamentum flavum back to the disc space. I then release the contralateral and ipsilateral insertion points. As I begin to work beneath the rostral spinous process and contralateral lamina, the contralateral ligamentum flavum comes into view. I am now looking at the ligament from the inside out. I place a half-inch by half-inch cottonoid over the top of the dura and use a forward-angle curet to divide the fibers of the contralateral ligamentum flavum in the rostral to caudal direction. I sequentially separate the ligamentum from its insertion and intermittently use a Kerrison rongeur to resect the outer boundaries of the ligamentum flavum. I proceed in a circumferential pattern around the insertion points of the ligamentum flavum and eventually encounter the contralateral facet, where I undercut the insertion of the ligamentum flavum to decompress the contralateral lateral recess. There is no need to use the Kerrison rongeur over the superior aspect of the caudal lamina for two reasons. First, working in that corridor is the most constrained part of the canal, and maneuvering a Kerrison from the rostral to caudal direction increases the risk of a dural tear. Second, the bone work done as part of the osteotomy has already been removed to unveil the insertion of the ligamentum flavum; thus, proceeding from caudal to rostral allows for the direct visualization of the ligamentum flavum. I have now decompressed the entire contralateral aspect of the thecal sac and have released the contralateral aspect of the ligamentum flavum from insertion to insertion.

With the contralateral decompression complete, I turn my attention to the ipsilateral foramen. The line of sight needs to be more direct onto the traversing nerve root, so I rotate the bed slightly back toward me and optimize a working trajectory to the ipsilateral recess. A forward-angle curet may be used to identify a plane between the dura and the ligamentum flavum beneath what remains of the SAP, which should be nothing more than a thin shelf of bone. The goal is to remove all the ligamentum flavum and bone from pedicle to beyond pedicle and thereby achieve complete decompression of the entire thecal sac and the exiting and traversing roots. Thus, I skeletonize the caudal ipsilateral pedicle such that a Kerrison may pass both medially and laterally to the pedicle.

At each step in the removal of the ligamentum flavum, I meticulously release only the insertion points without resecting the main body of the ligamentum. Instead, I let it lay over the thecal sac for protection (▶ Fig. 4.45b, c). Resection of the ligamentum over the pedicle and the exiting nerve root completes the release of the ligamentum flavum from the entire segment, and I remove the entire swath of the ligamentum flavum en bloc. The entire thecal sac, with its traversing and exiting nerve roots, is now completely decompressed (▶ Fig. 4.45d). Over the years, I have found that en bloc resection is more efficient than piecemeal resection. The en bloc technique minimizes the number of actions with Kerrison rongeurs over the top of the dura and thereby decreases the risk of an inadvertent dural tear. Especially important is the elimination of the perilous bites of ligamentum flavum beneath the caudal lamina, which are avoided by drilling past the caudal insertion of the ligamentum. Finally, this particular technique creates a systematic approach for decompression from pedicle to beyond pedicle (Video 4.3).

4.11.6 Kambin Triangle versus Expanded Transforaminal Corridor: A Historical Point of Clarification

Before proceeding with the discectomy and interbody fusion phase of the operation, I feel that a discussion regarding the historical nomenclature of the triangular transforaminal working zone into the disc space is relevant. Textbook chapters and technique papers alike have blurred the lines between the transforaminal working corridor defined by Harms[11,12] and what has become known as the Kambin triangle. The overlap in the boundaries between these two distinct corridors has led to an openhanded but inappropriate application of the term "Kambin triangle."[13,14,15] Although the boundaries of the Kambin triangle and the working corridor defined by Harms are the same, these corridors represent two completely distinct anatomical entities with one notable difference in their boundaries: the SAP. The next few paragraphs explain how these lines became blurred and introduce a new perspective on what is undoubtedly the most misunderstood eponym in spine surgery.

History of the Triangular Working Zone in the Intact Spine

The terminology that we currently apply to the corridor into the disc space began with pioneering spine surgeons in the 1970s and 1980s who began exploring alternate corridors into the lumbar disc space that avoided midline traditional open techniques to manage disc herniations. Wielding endoscopes with the intention of aspirating the disc herniations from within the disc space, these early endoscopic spine surgeons defined the anatomical corridor that allowed access for endoscopic procedures. To access the disc space percutaneously, these early endoscopic surgeons defined a right triangle lateral to the SAP. Kambin[16] in particular demarcated the boundaries of this triangle as the exiting root serving as the hypotenuse, the base of the triangle delineated by the superior end plate of the caudal vertebral body, and the height of the triangle defined by the distance from the base to the intersection of the SAP and the exiting root (▶ Fig. 4.46).[16] Kambin felt that this triangle offered a safe corridor into the disc space since it was devoid of neural and vascular structures.

Now eponymously known as the Kambin triangle after Dr. Parviz Kambin, the triangular corridor was initially conceived for percutaneous endoscopic procedures into the disc space. It is important to note that no removal of the SAP was ever described by Kambin. Interventionalists soon embraced the Kambin triangle as a safe corridor for discography, transforaminal epidurals and selective nerve root injections. It is important to note that the Kambin triangle was never defined as a working corridor for lumbar interbody fusions.

Transforaminal Access to the Disc Space: Removal of the SAP

For transforaminal access to the disc space as defined by Harms (▶ Fig. 4.47),[11] the classic definition of the Kambin triangle would not apply. Nevertheless, the exact definition of the medial border of the Kambin triangle has been an area of frequent misinterpretation in the literature. I believe the origin of this misinterpretation is a misunderstanding of Kambin's original description of his original drawing (▶ Fig. 4.46). In his own words, Kambin defined the working zone:

The triangular working zone is bordered anteriorly by the exiting root, inferiorly by the proximal plate of the lower lumbar segment, posteriorly by the proximal articular process of the inferior vertebra, and medially by the traversing nerve root and dural sac[13] *(▶ Fig. 4.48).*

The first issue with this description that undoubtedly contributed to the misunderstanding and thereby the misapplication of the Kambin triangle is the use of the term "triangular working zone." By name alone, the number of assigned borders is limited to three. However, Kambin goes on to mention four borders: (1) the exiting root, (2) the proximal end plate of the lower lumbar segment, (3) the proximal articular process of the inferior vertebra and (4) the traversing root and dural sac. It is entirely possible that if Kambin had been offered the geometric shape of a prism that could encompass all four of those boundaries, he might have adopted it.

The second potential source of the confusion is that Kambin's definition identified the medial border of the triangle as the "traversing root and dural sac," which is the same border as in a transforaminal approach. That description of the medial border has allowed the Kambin triangle to be understandably grafted into the TLIF vernacular, where after removal of the entire facet as described by Harms, the medial border of the right triangle is indeed the traversing root and thecal sac. Nevertheless, it is the trajectory onto the

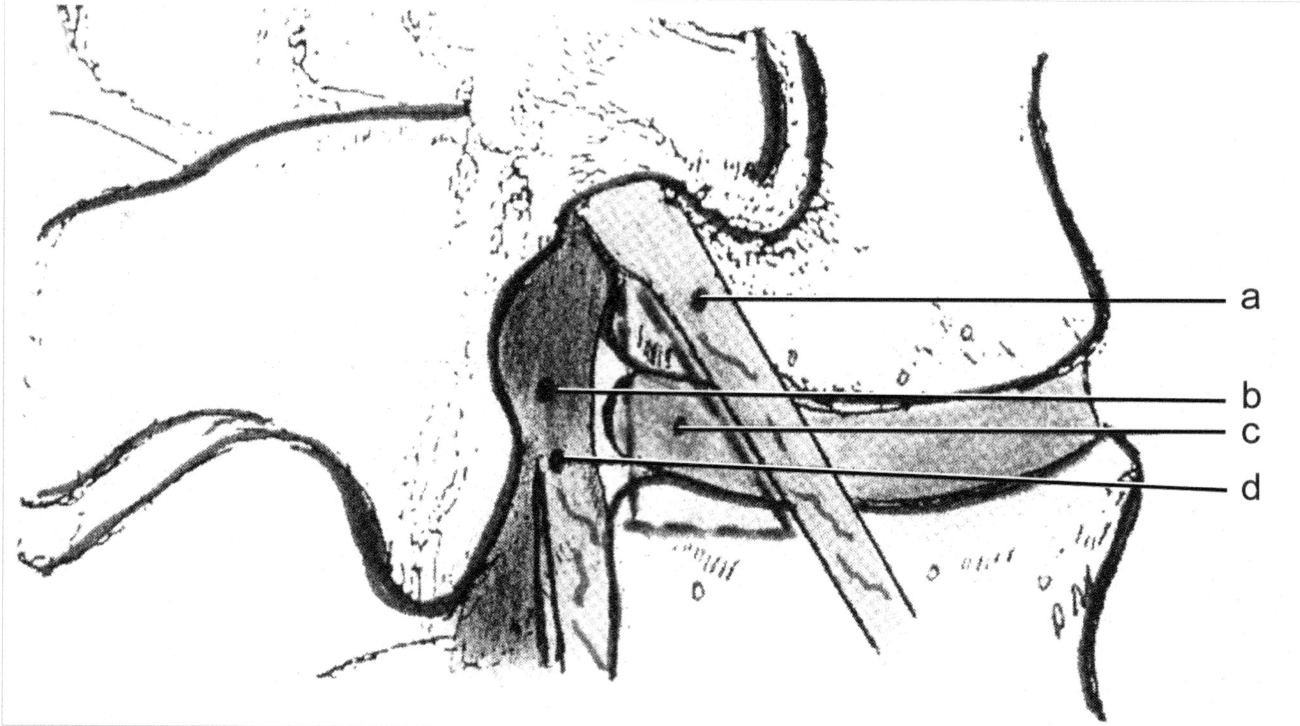

Fig. 4.46 Kambin's drawing of the triangular working zone.[16] The exiting lumbar nerve root, ***a***, represents the anterior aspect of the triangle and its hypotenuse. The thecal sac, ***b***, and the traversing root, ***d***, represent the medial border of the triangle. The superior end plate of the caudal vertebral body represents the base of the triangle. The traversing root, ***d***, is a component of the medial side of the triangle. The center of the triangle is the disc space, ***c***, which represents the target of the endoscope. What is mentioned in the description but not labeled in the diagram is the "fourth" side of the triangle, which is the "proximal articular process of the inferior vertebra" or the superior articular process (SAP); it is the posterior aspect of the triangle. The lateral aspect of the SAP is the fourth side of this three-dimensional triangle, which by definition is a prism. Therein lies the root of the controversy. That "fourth side" is removed in the transforaminal approach described by Harms. In doing so, the boundaries become the same boundaries described by Kambin. (Reproduced with permission from Kambin P. History of surgical management of herniated lumbar discs from cauterization to arthroscopic and endoscopic spinal surgery. In: Kambin P. (ed) Arthroscopic and Endoscopic Spinal Surgery. Humana Press, 2005.)

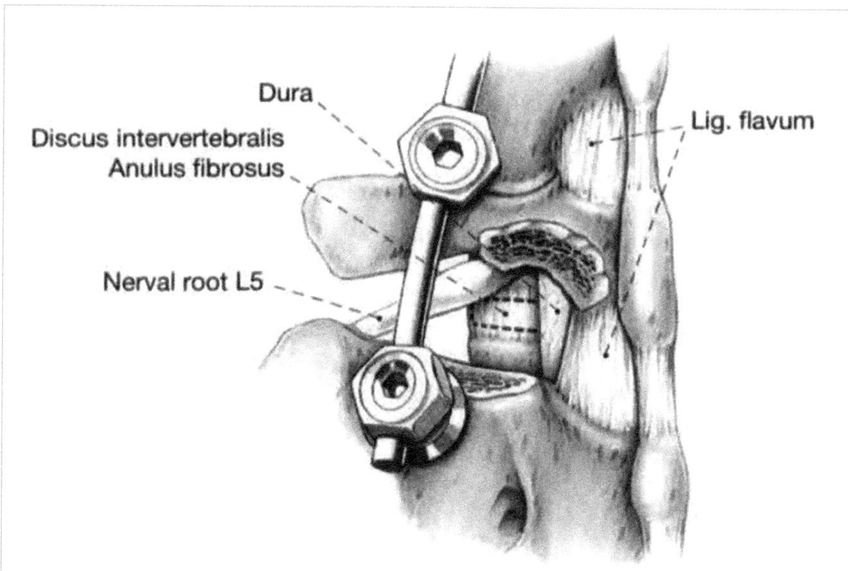

Fig. 4.47 The transforaminal corridor described by Harms. The illustration is from Harms' original description of the transforaminal lumbar interbody fusion in 1998.[11] The borders of the triangle described by Kambin are exactly the same as in Harms' illustration (exiting root: hypotenuse, traversing root and thecal sac: medial border and superior end plate: base of triangle). It is the removal of the facet, as seen in this illustration, that allows these borders to be the same. The illustration is a direct posterior view of the spine. When the facet is intact, a perspective of 35 to 45 degrees is needed to visualize the borders of the Kambin triangle. Abbreviation: Lig., ligamentum. (Reproduced with permission from Harms J, Jeszenszky D. The unilateral, transforaminal approach for posterior lumbar interbody fusion. Orthop Traumatol. 1998; 6:88–99.)

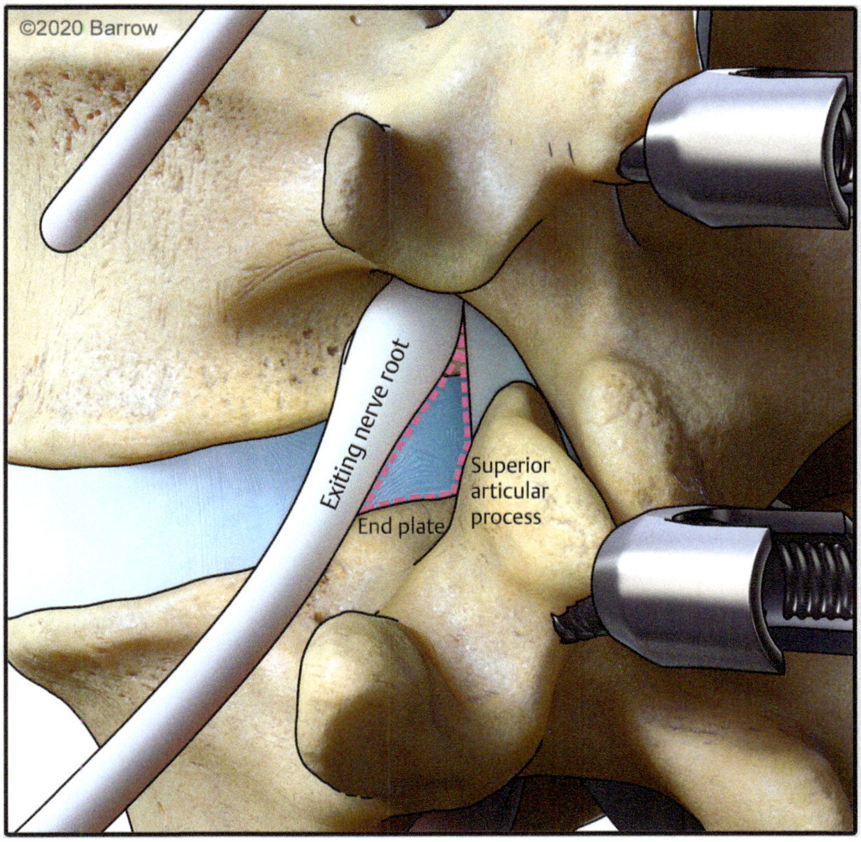

Fig. 4.48 Illustration of the working triangle as described by Kambin. The spine is viewed from a perspective of 35 degrees, allowing us to view the traversing root and thecal sac, exiting root and superior end plate of the inferior vertebral body. The superior articular process, which is a vital structure to navigate to access the disc space, is left unassigned. The Kambin triangle would be a constrained corridor to access the disc space for the interbody fusion described by Harms. In the end, the three sides of a triangle are an inherent limitation to describe a corridor that has four boundaries. A three-dimensional shape is needed.

spine that Kambin employed that accounts for his definition of the medial border and the overlap in these corridors.

In his operative technique, Kambin planned an entry point 10 to 12 cm off the midline with an angle of 35 to 45 degrees onto the spine. It is only from that vantage point that the SAP becomes the posterior border of the triangle, and the thecal sac and traversing root become the medial border in an otherwise intact spine. When we consider a minimally invasive transforaminal approach as I have described in this chapter, the incision is 4 cm off the midline and the angle of convergence is 25 degrees, the superior articular facet now becomes the medial border of the triangle, and the corridor into the disc space is quite different. It is not until the SAP is removed that the thecal sac and traversing root come into view and the borders of the triangle become identical to the triangle that Kambin described.

In reality, it would be an anatomical impossibility to secure an implant 10 mm wide through a corridor with the SAP intact. The anatomical corridor to access the disc space is simply not there without the removal of the facet. Kambin actually worked through cannulas with an outer diameter of 6.4 mm because of the constraints of the anatomy.[15]

Reconciling the Difference between the Kambin Triangle and Harms' Transforaminal Access Corridor

For transforaminal access to the disc space as described by Harms, the medial aspect of the working zone is not bound by the SAP but rather by the medial aspect of the thecal sac. So, to distinguish the two working corridors, we need to assign a boundary to the "fourth" side of the triangle that was described by Kambin. That fourth side is the SAP, an important structure by any account, since the lateral border of the SAP is one of the major limitations to accessing the disc space. The omission of designating a boundary for that structure carries implications for access to the disc space. The only way to assign all of the anatomical structures in the working triangle of the intact spine is to shift from the two-dimensional shape of a triangle with three sides to the three-dimensional shape of a prism that has four sides. Placing that geometric shape of a prism into the working triangle now incorporates all of the important boundaries and provides uniform boundaries that distinguish the Kambin triangle from the transforaminal working corridor. It is the back wall of the prism that is the difference between these two corridors (▶ Fig. 4.49).[11,12,16]

The term "Kambin triangle" or "Kambin prism" should not be applied to TLIFs when the facet, pars interarticularis and lamina have been removed. That was never Kambin's intent, nor did he ever write such a description. The use of the Kambin triangle should be limited to the description of percutaneous access to the disc space for endoscopic, diagnostic and interventional procedures in the intact spine.

When it comes to transforaminal access to the disc space where the SAP has been removed, the term "expanded transforaminal corridor or prism" should be used. Removing the SAP shifts the back wall of the prism medially and considerably expands the corridor for preparation of the disc space and insertion of an interbody spacer (▶ Fig. 4.50).[16] I will use this

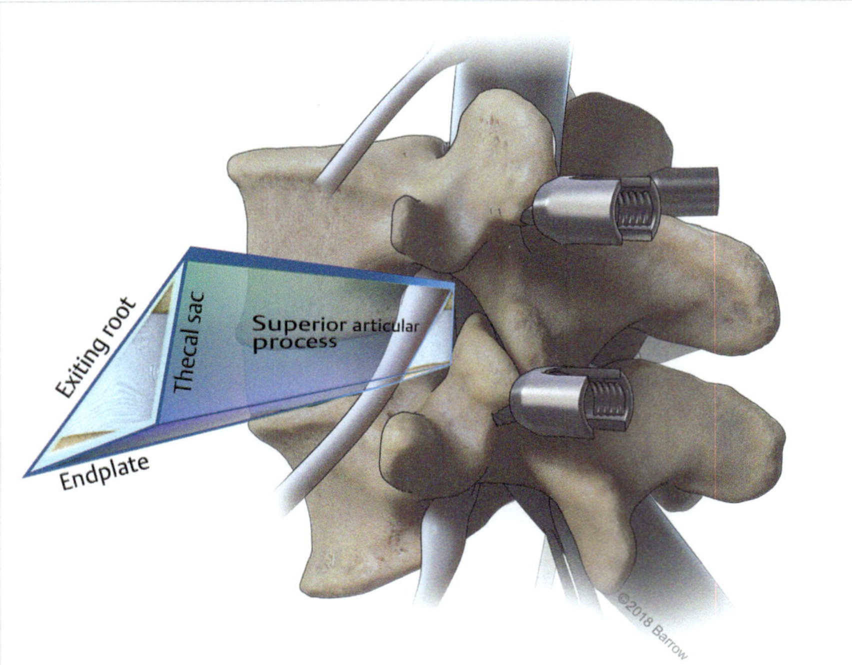

Fig. 4.49 Kambin prism. The three-dimensional shape of the prism incorporates all of the structures initially described by Kambin to include the superior articular process (SAP), which was left unassigned in Kambin's[16] original description. The use of a prism allows us to reconcile the difference between the Kambin triangle and the prism-shaped transforaminal corridor described by Harms.[11,12] When the SAP is removed, the back wall of the prism moves to the traversing nerve root and thecal sac, and the working corridor becomes considerably larger.

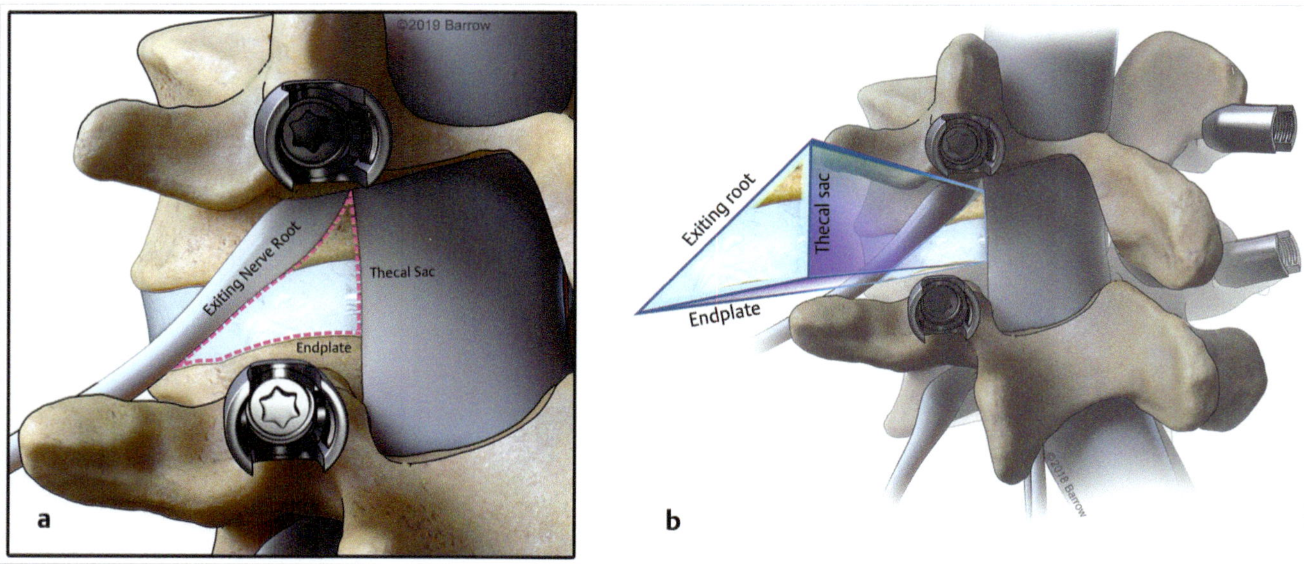

Fig. 4.50 The expanded transforaminal corridor. **(a)** The expanded transforaminal corridor is distinct from the Kambin triangle[16] and should be used when describing access to the disc space when the facet is removed. The creation of that corridor involves the various osteotomy cuts described in this chapter, which was never part of Kambin's initial description. **(b)** Applying the concept of a prism allows for a uniform assignment of the medial border when discussing Kambin's working zone and the expanded transforaminal corridor.

terminology for the remaining description of the MIS TLIF in this chapter.

4.11.7 Discectomy and Preparation of the End Plates

At this point in the operation, with the entire ligamentum flavum of the segment removed, the thecal sac and traversing and exiting roots should be evident, along with the disc space (▶ Fig. 4.51). Invariably, there will be a nest of crimson veins beneath the thecal sac and the traversing nerve awaiting your arrival into the expanded transforaminal corridor. These veins represent the dorsal epidural venous plexus. I have found that the more compression present at the level, the more robust and engorged these veins are. A wide suction retractor is the instrument of choice to retract the neural elements and expose the veins over the disc space and along the pedicle. The suction retractor in one hand and the right-angled bipolar forceps in the other hand are essential to cauterize the veins before their interruption. Once cauterized, I sharply divide them with

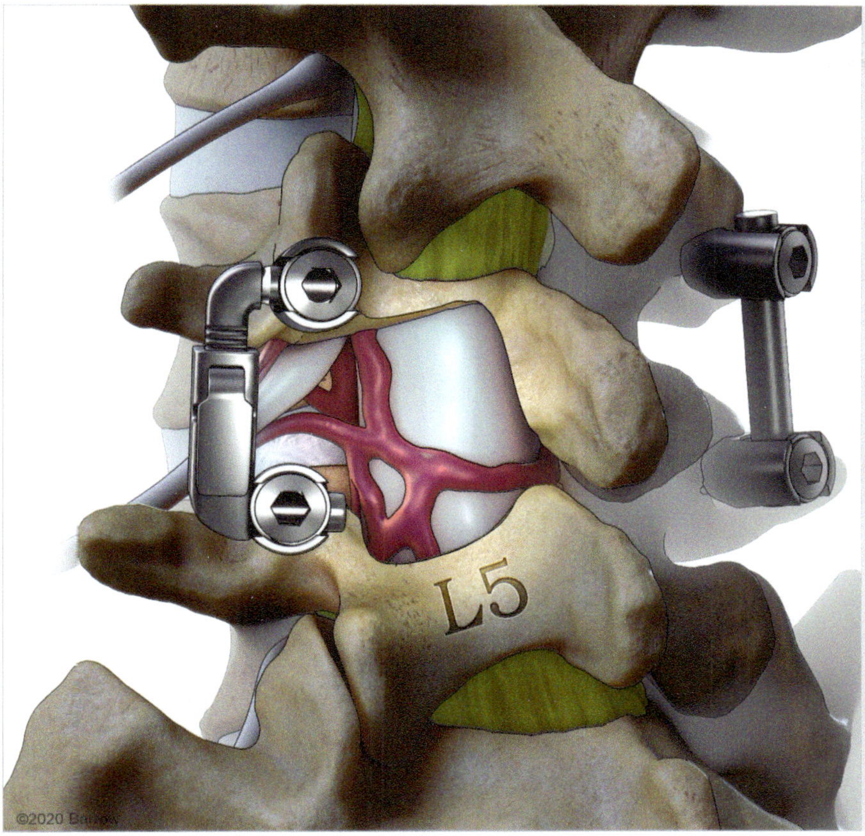

Fig. 4.51 Exposure before discectomy. Illustration demonstrating a widely decompressed thecal sac, traversing nerve root and exiting nerve root. The entire ligamentum flavum has been resected. Before beginning the discectomy, cauterization of the engorged veins of the dorsal epidural venous plexus will mitigate bleeding during insertion of the interbody.

microscissors to prevent these veins from rebleeding during the placement of the interbody. I prefer using the blunt-tipped microscissors or a No. 1 Kerrison rongeur for this task. In my experience, the sharp-tipped microscissors should be kept on the back table at all times.

Meticulous cauterization of any vein along the path of the disc space is a valuable preemptive strike in controlling bleeding before beginning the interbody phase of the operation. Mobilizing the nerve root, along with the thecal sac, allows for the exposure needed to further skeletonize the caudal pedicle and complete the pedicle-to-beyond-pedicle decompression. With the resection of the ligamentum flavum complete, a right-angle ball-tipped probe passes effortlessly over the top of the dura, lateral to the thecal sac, and into and out of the ipsilateral and contralateral neural foramen. Palpating the limits of the decompression with a ball-tipped probe is part of a systems check for the decompression phase of the operation that helps to ensure the same operation every time.

After a systems check, I remove any remaining ligament on top of the exiting ipsilateral nerve root. Sometimes, the ipsilateral exiting root hangs prominently in the transforaminal corridor. Other times, the exiting root remains hidden. An unfurled disc may push the root into the rostral pedicle and keep it out of view. However, at this point, it is not necessary to directly identify the exiting nerve root, which is nestled within a bed of crimson veins. In my experience, the exiting nerve unveils itself after the disc height is restored and the discectomy complete. Removing the unfurled disc, which is actually displacing the nerve root, invariably unveils the exiting root.

4.11.8 Discectomy and End Plate Preparation

I begin the discectomy and end plate preparation with visualization through the operating microscope and complete the work with loupes and a headlight before placement of the interbody spacer. I start with the use of a suction retractor to retract the thecal sac and nerve root, and, at times, with another suction retractor to retract the exiting nerve root. Working within the expanded transforaminal corridor, a No. 11 blade incises the disc space and creates a generous annulotomy as medial as can be safely performed with the thecal sac and nerve root protected by the suction retractor. The annulotomy extends in the lateral direction at least to the mid-pedicular line (▶ Fig. 4.52). For the lateral incision of the disc, the suction retractor shifts into the vicinity of the exiting root to lift it away from the disc space and shield it from potential harm from the No. 11 blade.

I extend the annulotomy with a series of Kerrison rongeurs and remove the annulus up to the end plate of the vertebral body. I begin to remove the disc material with pituitary rongeurs and remove the cartilaginous end plates with a series of curets. With the preliminary discectomy completed, the disc height may now begin to be restored with paddle distractors. The ipsilateral provisional expandable rod, which is already in position, is of tremendous value at this point.

The provisional rod on the contralateral side captures the restored disc height when my assistant intermittently tightens

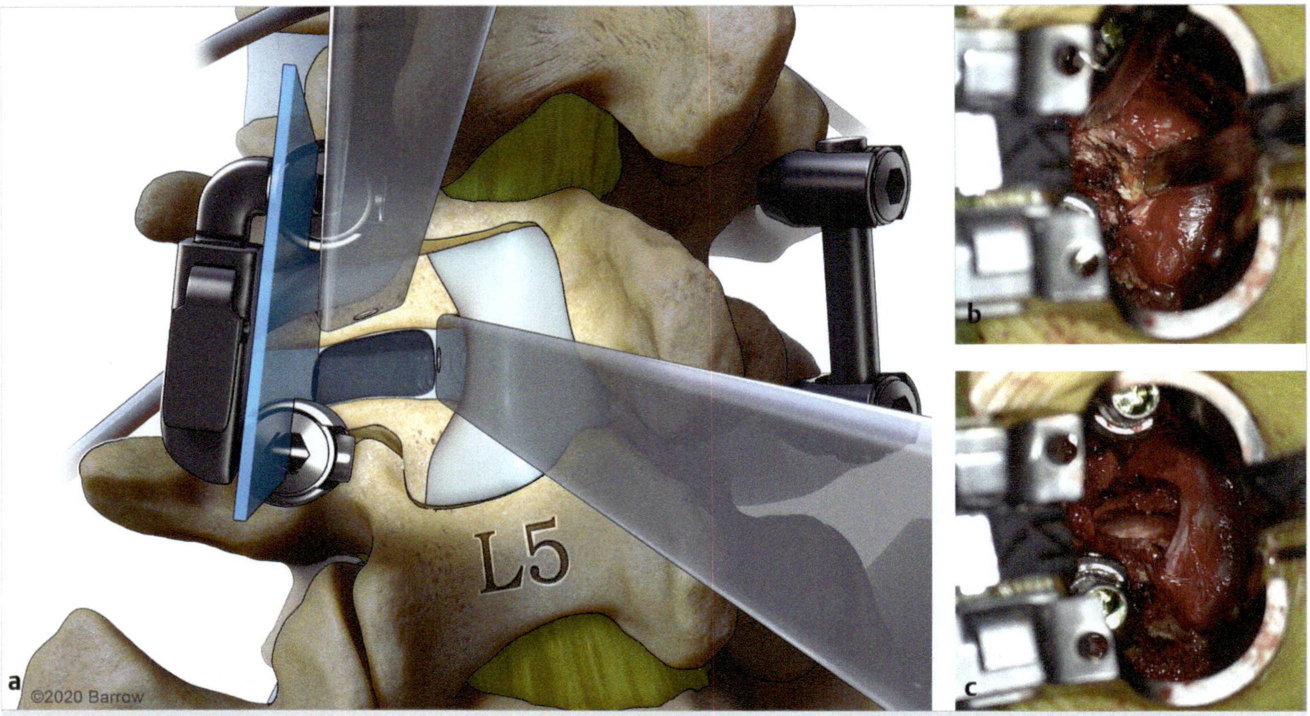

Fig. 4.52 Annulotomy for L4–5 transforaminal lumbar interbody fusion (TLIF). **(a)** Illustration of the expanded transforaminal corridor into the disc space. Note that the annulotomy extends medially beneath the thecal sac and laterally to the midpedicular line as demarcated by the blue plane. **(b)** Intraoperative photograph demonstrating the exposure for the discectomy in an L4–5 TLIF. **(c)** Intraoperative photograph demonstrating the wide annulotomy and discectomy that extends to the midpedicular line. A wide annulotomy facilitates the placement of the interbody spacer through the expanded transforaminal corridor.

the rostral set screw that had remained loose. If the ipsilateral provisional expandable rod is in position, it captures the height without any additional action. With each paddle distractor sequentially restoring the disc height, it becomes increasingly easier to access the disc space. The restoration of the disc space also begins to reduce the slip of the spondylolisthesis. However, care must be taken throughout the restoration of the disc height to use the appropriate trajectory to prevent injury to the cortical end plate. Violation of the cortical end plate of either the rostral or caudal vertebral body has implications for the interbody spacer placement and, even more concerning, can result in subsidence of the implant during the postoperative period.

I avoid the sharp paddle-disc space preparation instruments out of concern for violation of the cortical end plate. The purpose of these sharp paddles is to remove the cartilaginous end plates that overlie the cortical end plate, without disrupting the integrity of the cortical end plate. However, in my experience, these sharp paddles have the capacity to cut into the cortical end plate, especially in collapsed disc spaces. Instead, I use only blunt paddle distractors to restore the height and reserve the interbody curets for the preparation of the cortical end plates and removal of cartilaginous end plates.

The various interbody curets help to ensure that an adequate amount of disc and cartilaginous end plate have been removed and that the cortical end plate has been prepared to optimize the environment for an interbody arthrodesis. These interbody curets have graduated markings that indicate the distance within the disc space. I strive to be able to insert the angled curet 40 mm into the disc space, which ensures that I have the capability to place the largest curved interbody spacer across the disc space.

There is a characteristic sound created when metal scrapes a well-prepared cortical end plate. It is the unmistakable sound of "fusion." My ears must unequivocally hear that sound before I consider the end plate prepared so that I do not hear the sounds of a pseudarthrosis in the months that come. Preparation of the disc space can reach a point of diminishing returns. After 15 minutes of methodically scraping, resecting disc material and preparing the end plate, it is unlikely that anything more meaningful is being accomplished. Before I complete the disc preparation and remove the microscope from the field, I systematically check my blind spots. Specifically, I make sure that there is no disc material in the foramen of the traversing root or behind the thecal sac. Finally, I ensure that no disc material has migrated onto the exiting nerve root, which has finally revealed itself after the combination of decompression, discectomy and retraction.

If the anatomical circumstance calls for a bilateral facetectomy, I adjust the microscope and move to the other side. If the patient does not have a symptomatic radiculopathy or profound facet arthropathy that requires removal on the other side, I limit the bone work to a Smith–Petersen osteotomy. Creation of a gap on the contralateral side allows for restoration of segmental lordosis when the construct is placed under compression. It is essential to remove the rostral aspect of the SAP to prevent compromise of the neural foramen with compression. I decorticate the transverse processes on the side of the Smith–Petersen osteotomy and pack autograft into the posterolateral space for a posterolateral arthrodesis. If I have performed bilateral decompressions with complete facetectomies and exposure of the exiting nerve roots, I refrain from a posterolateral fusion on either side out of concern that the bone graft will come into contact with the exiting root. I continue the discussion regarding the creation of segmental lordosis with compression in the description of phase III below.

Once I complete a systems check on the decompression, the Smith–Petersen osteotomy and posterolateral fusion, phase II is complete. I remove the microscope from the field, and I ask my anesthesia colleague to rotate the bed back to the level position. I don operating loupes and headlight once again as the fluoroscope rolls back into its previous position to image the trials entering the disc space. Phase II of the operation is complete, and the final phase of the operation begins.

4.11.9 Duration of the Second Phase

Under the best circumstances, the second phase of the operation takes 30 to 45 minutes. But in a patient with a previous decompression, it can take upward of 1 hour. Obviously, if a bilateral facetectomy is needed it will take longer unless two surgeons are working simultaneously to advance the bone work. Recently, my average time for this phase of the operation is just less than 45 minutes. In my experience, the decompression is the phase of the operation that takes the longest to perform and requires the greatest technical skill and attention. The anatomy at depth dictates the length of this phase. Some decompressions are more straightforward than others. Patients with previous discectomies or laminectomies with significant scarring may take significantly more time than *de novo* cases. Regardless of the time, this operation is not complete until the neural elements are decompressed from pedicle to beyond pedicle and the interbody space prepared. The times provided here are guidelines. No two surgeries are ever the same.

4.12 Phase III: Trials and Interbody Spacer Placement

Although the second phase of the operation tends to be the longest, the third phase has the potential to be the shortest. Once the fluoroscope is back in its previous position, I am ready to begin placing trials into the disc space. The final paddle distractor may determine the size of the trial spacer to be placed. It is a good idea to use a paddle distractor that is one size larger than the trial you intend to insert into the disc space. While the paddle distractor enters the disc space at a smaller height and then rotates to a larger height to achieve restoration of the disc space, the trial enters the disc space at a uniform height. For instance, an 11-mm paddle distractor enters the disc space at 6 mm, and only after occupying the entire disc space does it rotate to the full height of 11 mm. As a result, it is quite easy to place the paddle distractor. The interbody trial, on the other hand, has to enter at 11 mm from the outset. Therefore, having a slightly greater opening in the disc space facilitates its insertion (▶ Fig. 4.53).

Concave end plates introduce an element of complexity when attempting to secure a well-fitting graft. One glance at the lateral fluoroscopic image (▶ Fig. 4.54) tells you whether this issue should concern you. In patients with a significant concavity to the end plates, the center of the disc space will be considerably taller than the posterior entry into the disc space, through which the interbody needs to traverse. A trial spacer may be inserted with great difficulty past the posterior aspect of the disc space but then end up floating in the middle of the disc space. If an interbody of the same height is selected, then pseudarthrosis is the predictable outcome.

Managing the geometry of the intervertebral body space for interbody grafts and fusion is nothing new. In his original manuscript in 1953, Cloward[17] identified this problem and set forth the criteria that I strive for when preparing the interbody space. Cloward writes:

There is always an overhanging lip on the posterosuperior margin of the vertebral body. Removal of this ledge of bone makes it possible to visualize the entire superior surface of the vertebral body which may otherwise be obscured. This bone removal, which is also carried laterally to include part of the base of the vertebral pedicle increases the width of the intervertebral space.

There are several options available to meet the criteria set forth by Cloward.[17] One approach to overcome this anatomical challenge is with expandable interbody spacers (see discussion below). Inserting an interbody spacer at a height smaller than the height of the concavity and then expanding it to a greater height once it is within the disc space circumvents the need to address the concavity altogether. The second option is using an osteotome or a box cutting osteotome. This particular technique essentially equalizes the height of the concavity on the periphery of the disc space with the height at the center of the interbody space by cutting away the bone. Therefore, the trial and the subsequent interbody will pass through the path created by the box cutter at one uniform height. Although this is an effective manner to handle this anatomical scenario, it also has the capacity to fracture or violate the end plate. Wielding this instrument with the guidance of fluoroscopy minimizes the risk of end plate violation. However, from my perspective, brandishing such an instrument in the vicinity of the neural elements in such a narrow corridor gives me pause. Nonetheless, I have found it to be a valuable adjunct in my interbody access armamentarium, especially for deeply concave disc spaces. For the majority of the cases, I have had success using a large Kerrison to remove the posterosuperior lip of the caudal vertebral body and the posteroinferior lip of the rostral vertebral body. Removal of these lips equalizes the disc space height and optimizes the environment for placement of the interbody graft (▶ Fig. 4.55 and ▶ Fig. 4.56).[17]

Another alternative to meet Cloward's criteria[17]—"to visualize the entire superior surface of the (caudal) vertebral body"—is by distracting the posterior aspect of the disc space. Such a configuration facilitates the placement of the interbody spacer. A combination of a provisional rod on the contralateral side and the expandable rod on the ipsilateral side (discussed earlier) captures the restoration of the disc height as the paddle distractors are rotated and the trials are placed. The capture of the disc height with the provisional ipsilateral expandable rod is analogous to that of the Caspar post distractor used in the cervical spine, where the distraction of the posts not only facilitates placement of the interbody spacer but also optimizes the cortical end plate to interbody interface when the distraction is released.

Using the ipsilateral expandable provisional rod allows the height of the final trial to be captured. Instead of a collapsed

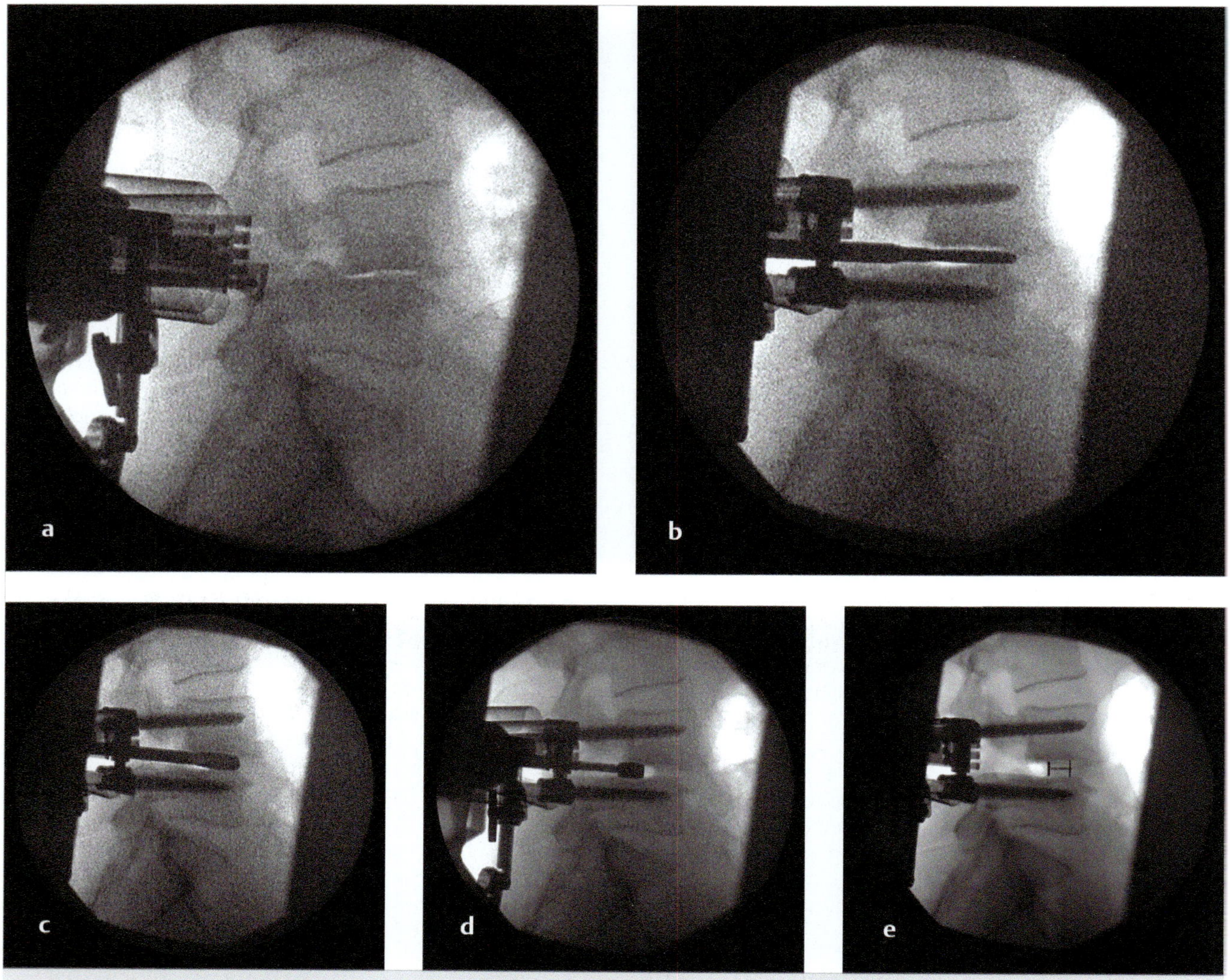

Fig. 4.53 Management of grade II L4–5 spondylolisthesis. (a) Lateral fluoroscopic image demonstrating grade II L4–5 spondylolisthesis with complete collapse of the disc space. (b) A paddle distractor enters at 6 mm but rotates to 11 mm, making it easier to insert than a trial. (c) A trial has a uniform height that needs to enter the annulotomy. In this case, a 10-mm trial was inserted after an 11-mm paddle was used to open the space. (d) The combination of the ipsilateral expandable rod, paddle distraction and trials allowed for restoration of the disc height and reduction of the listhesis. (e) Lateral fluoroscopic image after insertion and rotation of a banana-shaped interbody spacer 10 mm in height.

disc space resisting placement of a large interbody spacer, the distracted disc space welcomes it. Placement of the interbody spacer proceeds without any difficulty. After successful placement of the interbody, the provisional distraction is released, similar to a Caspar post distractor in the cervical spine. In this way, you have optimized the interbody spacer to cortical end plate interface and thereby achieved an ideal environment for arthrodesis (▶ Fig. 4.57).

Regardless of the technique employed to restore and maintain the disc height, the primary objective of this phase is to size and secure an interbody spacer that restores the height of a collapsed disc space, occupies the disc space from apophyseal ring to apophyseal ring, and creates an ideal environment for fusion. An appropriately sized interbody trial firmly wedges in between the vertebral bodies in the middle to anterior aspect of the disc space and is difficult to dislodge without a slap-hammer, as seen in the operative video (Video 4.4). Once I have determined the height of the interbody spacer to be placed, it is time to secure the interbody into position. Before describing that technique, a discussion regarding the optimal type of interbody spacer is germane.

4.12.1 Biomechanics of the Vertebral Body End Plate

The options for objects one can insert into the interbody space are becoming endless. With so many viable options, I turn to an anatomical and historical perspective for guidance. Again, the end goals of interbody work remain the same regardless of the interbody spacer: to restore disc height and thereby foraminal height as well as to create an environment for a robust fusion and restore segmental lordosis. Working in tandem with these goals is the necessity to minimize the risk of short-term and long-term complications. The short-term risks include subsidence

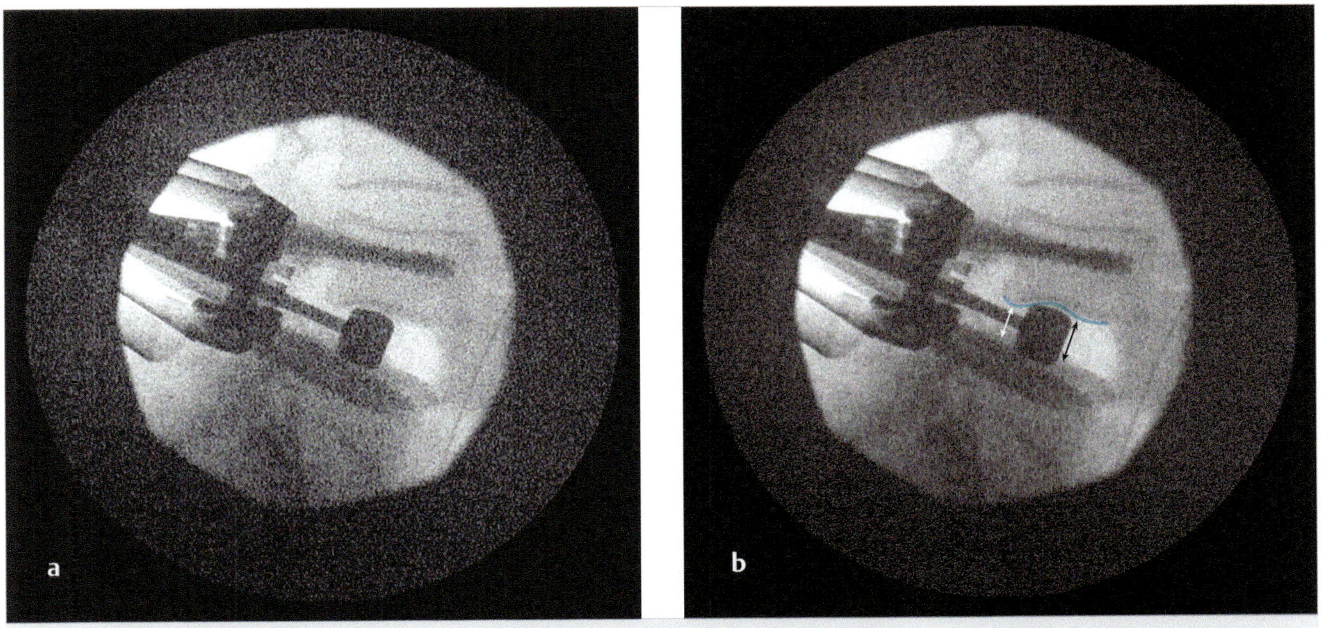

Fig. 4.54 Concave end plates and interbody fusion. **(a)** Lateral fluoroscopic image of a concave end plate at L4–5 (*blue line*). The posterior height of the disc space is several millimeters shorter than the center of the disc space. **(b)** Modified lateral fluoroscopic image highlighting the difference between the center (*black arrow*) of the disc space and the posterior aspect (*white arrow*) of the disc space.

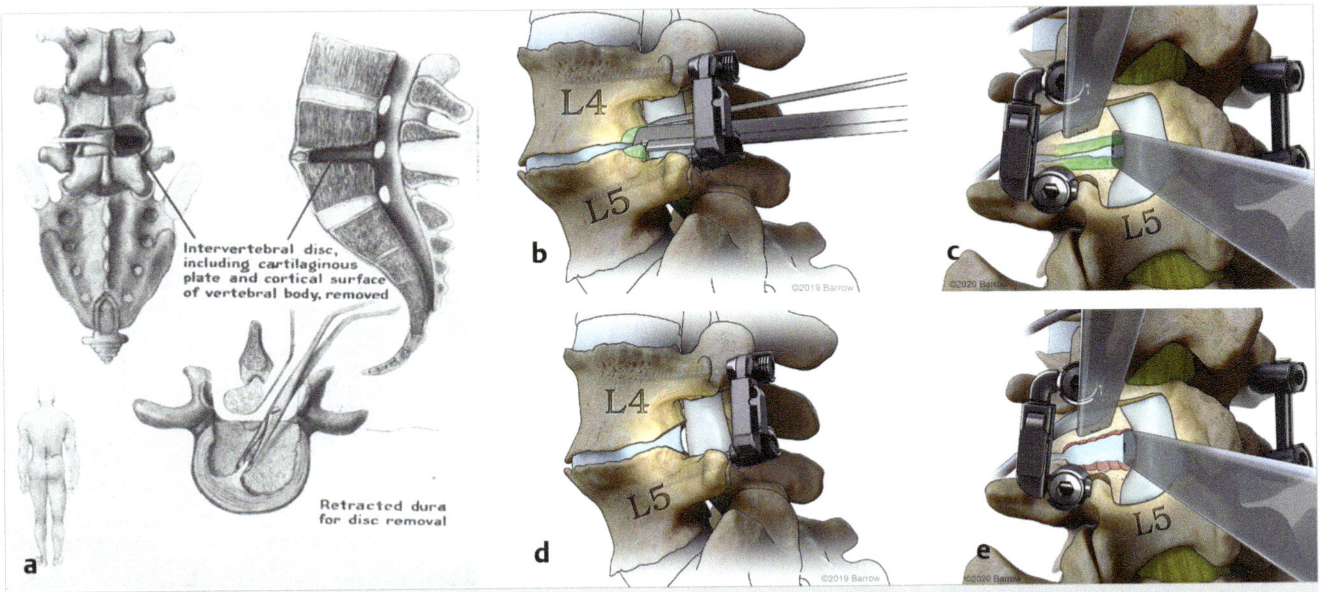

Fig. 4.55 The Cloward criteria for interbody preparation. Before considering the insertion of an interbody spacer, Cloward advised us "to visualize the entire superior surface of the (caudal) vertebral body." **(a)** Illustration demonstrating the criteria set forth by Cloward in 1953.[17] Series of illustrations demonstrating the various techniques to achieve Cloward's criteria of visualization of the end plates. **(b)** Illustration of the spine in the lateral perspective. The use of a large Kerrison rongeur helps to equalize the height differential created by a concave end plate. The posterior aspect of the disc space, denoted in *green*, is the target of the Kerrison. **(c)** Illustration of the spine from a posterior surgical view revealing osteophytes and concave end plates. The *green* demarcates the bone that needs to be removed to facilitate the placement of an ideally sized interbody. **(d)** Illustration of the lateral view of the spine showing the reduction in the concavity of the end plate. **(e)** Illustration showing the posterior surgical view of the interbody space that meets Cloward's criteria. (► Fig. 4.55**a** is reproduced with permission from Cloward RB. The treatment of ruptured lumbar intervertebral discs by vertebral body fusion: I. Indications, operative technique, after care. J Neurosurg. 1953; 10:154–168.)

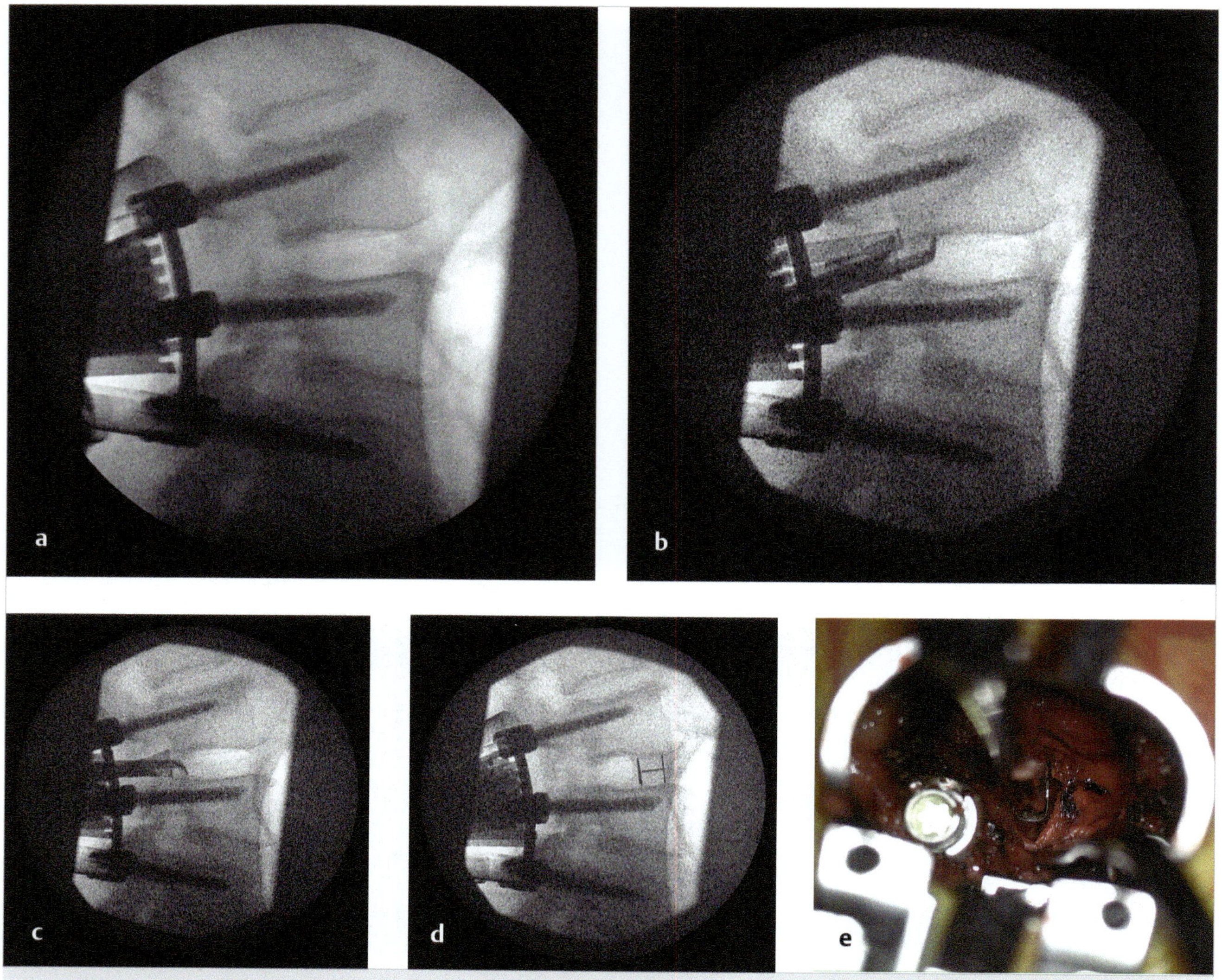

Fig. 4.56 Application of Cloward's criteria.[17] (a) Lateral fluoroscopic image of a two-level transforaminal lumbar interbody fusion at L3–4 and L4–5, where the L3–4 disk space has a deep concavity. (b) A No. 4 Kerrison rongeur removes the posterior superior aspect of the concavity and (c) the posterior inferior aspect of the concavity. (d) Removal of the posterior end plate facilitates placement of the ideal interbody spacer for the disc space. (e) Intraoperative photograph showing the use of a Kerrison to open the posterior aspect of the disc space. With the exiting nerve root retracted, a Kerrison may be safely used to enter the disc space and remove the posterior aspect of the end plate, thereby reducing the concavity.

and migration of the implant. The long-term risks include pseudarthrosis and iatrogenic flat back. For best accomplishing these goals, the ideal interbody spacer is one that occupies the disk space from apophyseal ring to apophyseal ring, with as much surface area of the disc space as anatomically feasible, and rests on the hardest part of the end plate. Cloward[17] espoused these principles 60 years ago and routinely performed this operation, reliably achieving fusions without instrumentation. These principles were reiterated by Harms in his TLIF procedure 40 years later.[11,17] I see no reason to venture far from what these master surgeons recommended.

From a structural standpoint, the cortical end plate of the lumbar vertebral body is quite similar in shape to the bottom of a can of cola. Using this analogy, if one desired to poke a hole in the bottom of the can, one would aim for the center, where the least resistance would be met. Basic biomechanics tells us to apply that same principle to the cortical end plate when considering the ideal location for the placement of an interbody spacer. It would be a fool's errand to attempt to poke a hole into the outer perimeter of the can, where the greatest resistance would be met. When applying this analogy to the cortical end plate of the vertebral body, the weakest point of the cortical end plate is the center of the disc space, whereas the strongest point would be in the outer perimeter of the cortical end plate or the apophyseal ring. Several biomechanical studies have independently confirmed that the geometric center of the end plate is the weakest, whereas the outer and lateral aspects of the end plate are the strongest (▶ Fig. 4.58).[18,19] Therefore, the outer perimeter of the end plate is the ideal target for the interbody spacer to land within the disc space.

When Cloward initially conceived of the posterior interbody fusion, it was the lateral margins of the disc space that he targeted with his cortical grafts. It was subsequently proven through biomechanical studies that these lateral margins have

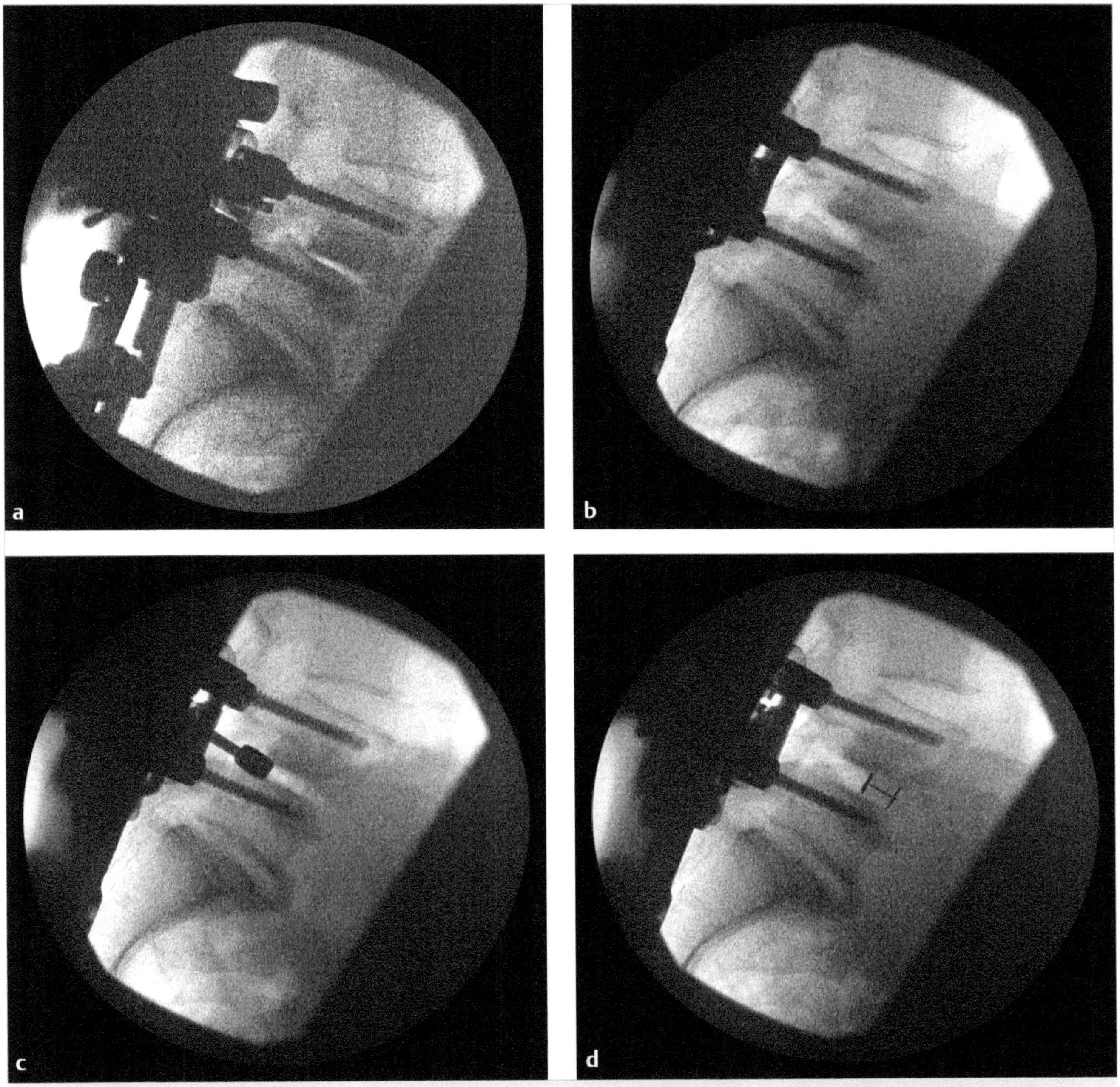

Fig. 4.57 Provisional ipsilateral expandable rod and restoration of the disc height. **(a)** Lateral fluoroscopic image of grade II spondylolisthesis at L4–5 managed with a minimally invasive transforaminal lumbar interbody fusion. Pedicle screws are in position. **(b)** Provisional ipsilateral expandable rod allows for the distraction to be captured and maintained to facilitate the placement of the trials. **(c)** A 10-mm trial may access the disc space with the height maintained at 10 mm. Provisional distraction allowed the disc height to be restored from complete collapse. **(d)** A 10-mm interbody spacer was secured into the interbody space with the help of provisional distraction.

the greatest structural strength and, therefore, the least risk of interbody subsidence (▶ Fig. 4.59).[17] After removing as much of the disc and cartilaginous end plate as possible from a bilateral approach, Cloward espoused the principle of occupying as much of the disc space as possible, "as many bone wedges as possible are driven into the interspace."[17] As a result, Cloward occupied more of the disc space in 1953 than I did with my initial attempts at this operation in 2008. Ever since reviewing his manuscript, I have taken measures to match Cloward's occupancy of the intervertebral space with graft material and spacers. I also strive to place these interbody spacers into the hardest part of the end plate.

With the evolution of the transforaminal approach by Harms,[11] unilateral access to the disc space allowed for interbody fusion with substantially less retraction and, at times, no retraction on the traversing nerve root (▶ Fig. 4.60).[11] However, instead of a trajectory directed to the lateral margins of the disc space on either side, the trajectory was obliquely toward the center. The straight PLIF interbody geometries that surgeons were accustomed to using still fit naturally into their hands as

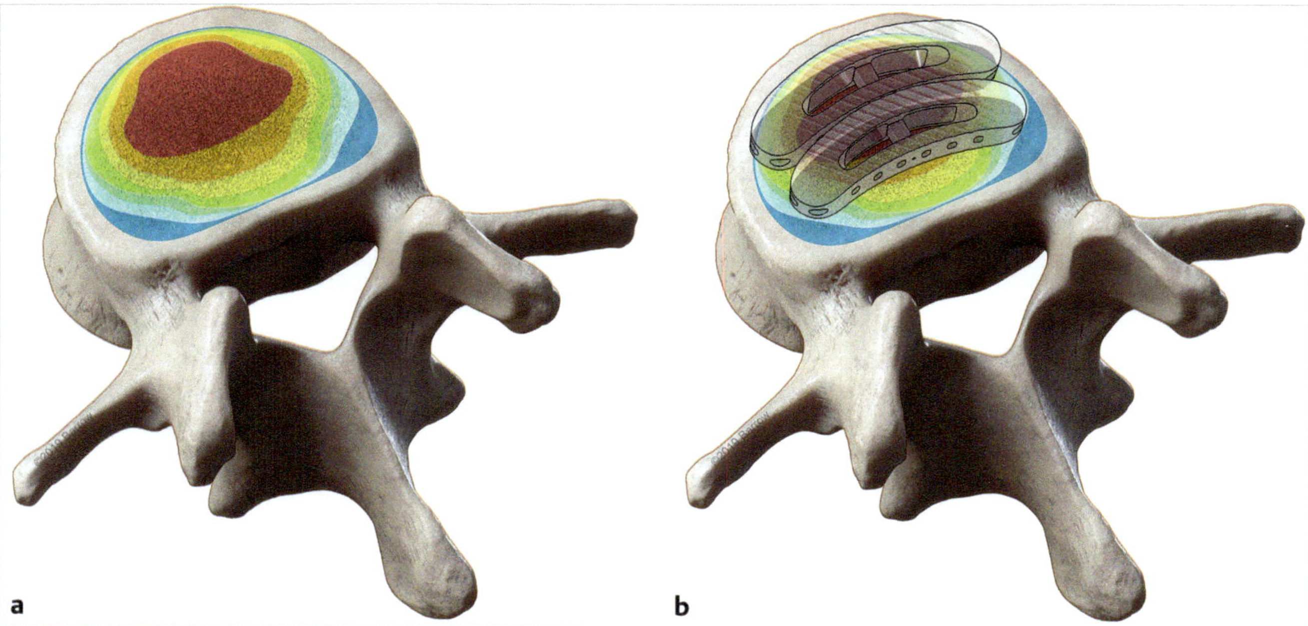

Fig. 4.58 Regional vertebral body end plate strength based on the work by Grant et al and Lowe et al.[18,19] **(a)** Illustration showing the regional differences in end plate strength using a gradient color scheme. The dark blue in the posterior aspect of the vertebral body and in the vicinity of the pedicle represents the strongest part of the end plate, whereas the red color in the center of the disc space represents the weakest and, therefore, the area most susceptible to subsidence. **(b)** Illustration showing an interbody geometry that occupies the disc space spanning the stronger aspects of the end plate.

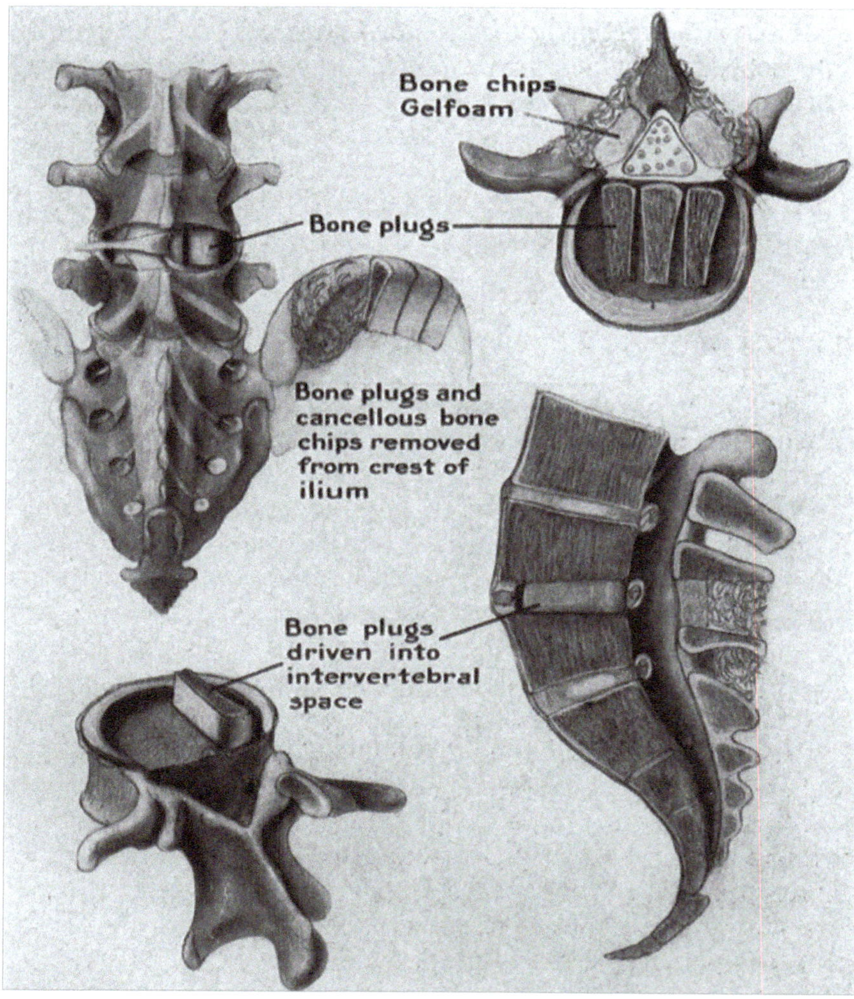

Fig. 4.59 Illustration from Cloward's original publication on the interbody fusion.[17] Note the extent of coverage of the disc space achieved with placement of the autograft "bone plugs." (Reproduced with permission from Cloward RB. The treatment of ruptured lumbar intervertebral discs by vertebral body fusion: I. Indications, operative technique, after care. J Neurosurg. 1953; 10:154–168.)

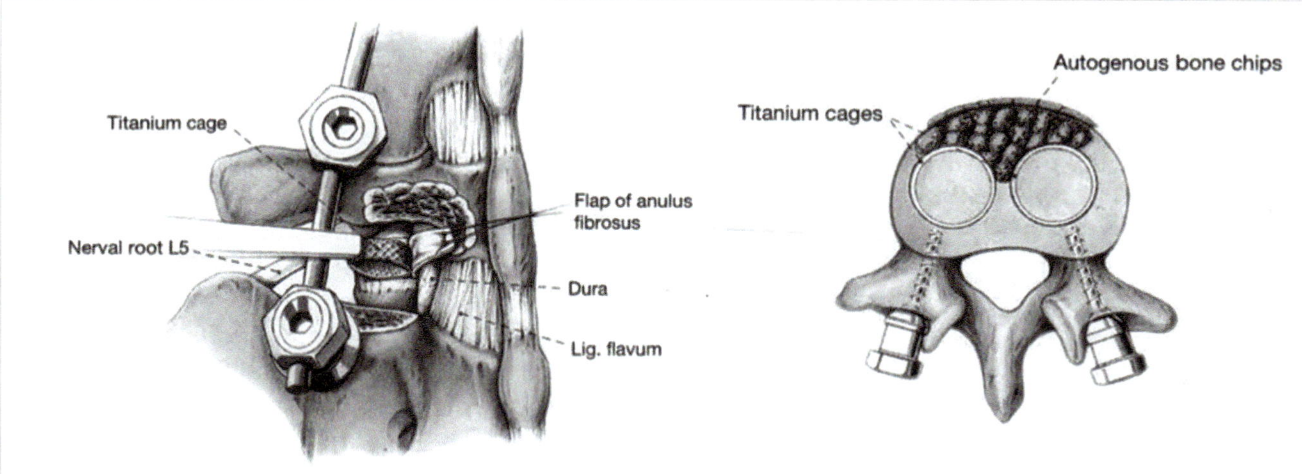

Fig. 4.60 An illustration from Harms' transforaminal lumbar interbody fusion technique.[11] Harms advocated full occupancy of the disc space through a unilateral approach by tamping the cage across the midline. The unilateral approach to the disc space eventually led to the development of semicircular interbody spacers or banana-shaped interbody spacers. Abbreviation: Lig., ligamentum. (Reproduced with permission from Harms J, Jeszenszky D. The unilateral, transforaminal approach for posterior lumbar interbody fusion. Orthop Traumatol. 1998; 6:88–99.)

they migrated from PLIFs to TLIFs. The familiarity and relative simplicity of a straight interbody spacer resulted in their continued use in transforaminal approaches, even though they were never intended to traverse an oblique trajectory. As a result, straight PLIF interbody spacers remain commonplace. Meanwhile, surgeons who recognized the unique aspects offered by the transforaminal approach developed interbody geometries that conformed to the disc space and capitalized on the trajectory of insertion. The unilateral transforaminal approach spawned the semicircular or "banana"-type grafts, which when inserted obliquely rotate into position to conform to the disc space and occupy the lateral margins of the end plate.

Several surgeons continue to use single, straight "PLIF" grafts in transforaminal approaches, and with the appropriate craftsmanship, end plate preparation, and grafting technique, this type of interbody works perfectly well. However, from an anatomical standpoint, I prefer an interbody spacer that rests upon the most structurally sound element of the vertebral body end plate, the apophyseal ring. I want to avoid the center of the end plate. In the analysis of my experience with obliquely placed PLIF interbody spacers, I found that they all rested on the structurally weakest part of the end plate, the center. I came to the conclusion that if the lateral margins of the vertebral body end plate were the ideal position for the interbody spacer, then a spacer with a semicircular geometry that matches the curvature of the disk space as it rotates into position on the outer margins of the end plate would be conceptually the most alluring. The semicircular or banana-shaped geometry fits that standard. Striving for the largest interbody spacer along the apophyseal ring is my rationale for using the semicircular interbody spacer in transforaminal approaches.

4.12.2 The Ideal Interbody: A Concept Based on Surface Area

If we were to set the criteria for the ideal interbody graft, we would desire the tallest and widest interbody spacer that we could safely secure in the disc space. It would rest upon the lateral margins of the apophyseal ring, restore segmental lordosis and minimize the risk of migration and subsidence. The graft we would select would likely resemble an interbody graft used in a transpsoas approach. With these criteria as a framework, it is worthwhile to examine the anatomy of the disc space in greater detail.

▶ Fig. 4.61 shows the L4–5 disc space of a patient who presented with pseudarthrosis after an L4–5 TLIF with a straight interbody spacer placed obliquely. Compared with Cloward's four "bone plugs" seen in ▶ Fig. 4.62,[24] the coverage of the disc space is miniscule. Let us begin with basic geometry. The dimensions of the disc space are approximately 50 × 40 mm. The interbody spacer measures 25 × 10 mm. If we were to approximate the surface area of the disc space, assuming the disc space is encompassed by a circle with a radius of 20 mm, the surface area (πr^2) would be approximately 1,500 mm^2. The surface area covered by the interbody spacer, on the other hand, would be the length times the width of the rectangle covered by the spacer or 250 mm^2, or approximately 16% of the disc space is covered by that implant. Because the goal remains to occupy as much of the disc space as possible, other alternatives to that interbody spacer are worthy of consideration. Bilateral access to the disc space would allow a second interbody spacer to be inserted, thereby doubling the surface area covered to 32%. However, this would require significantly more work and add a significant amount of time to the operation.

Another approach would be to increase the surface area of the interbody spacer placed in a unilateral approach. Returning to the dimensions of the disc space, which measures approximately 50 × 40 mm, we know that a semicircular 36-mm implant that is rotated into position would comfortably fit into the anterior aspect of the disc space. Such a spacer, if well centered and positioned anteriorly, will rest upon the apophyseal ring. Even though the implant could be better positioned from an anatomical standpoint, it would result in only a modest increase in surface area from 16 to 23% of the disc space. However, the geometry of this implant affords the possibility of

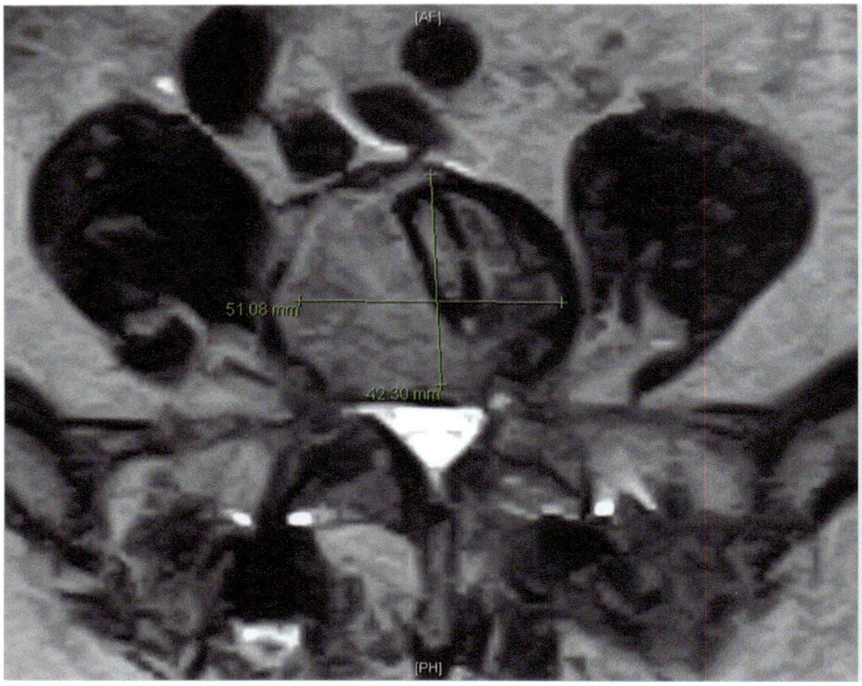

Fig. 4.61 Axial T2-weighted magnetic resonance imaging shows a straight interbody spacer inserted obliquely through a transforaminal approach during a posterior lumbar interbody fusion. The patient developed symptomatic pseudarthrosis and required a revision surgery. The dimensions of the disc space measure 51 × 42 mm.

placement of additional spacers through the same annulotomy, which is not tenable with a straight interbody graft placed obliquely. With 40 mm of anterior-posterior distance, there remains 30 mm of disc space that may still be occupied. The geometry of semicircular interbody spacers capitalizes on the remaining surface area that exists in the disc space. The distance that remains has the possibility of being occupied by an additional semicircular spacer that may be rotated into position. It is the appreciation of the distances within the disc space that prompted me to consider the possibility of additional spacers, which, if nested, would occupy more of the disc space without adding significant technical complexity or increasing the risk of injury to the neural elements. Placing two nested interbody spacers increases the surface area covered from 16 to 43%. If the length of the interbody spacer increases from 36 to 40 mm or even 45 mm, then I have covered over 50% of the end plate with a structural graft. The surface area available within the disc space and the biomechanics of the cortical end plate have led me to insert two semicircular interbody spacers into the disc space whenever possible (▶ Fig. 4.63).

The additional benefit of a second interbody spacer is the ability to place the spacer on compression without causing any significant compromise to the foraminal height. A single interbody placed in the anterior aspect of the disc space may act as a fulcrum upon which compression causes foraminal narrowing, whereas adding a second interbody creates a greater surface area that eliminates the fulcrum effect. The second interbody spacer distributes the forces of the compression while maintaining the foraminal height. Furthermore, a biomechanical analysis of the nested interbody technique demonstrated greater resistance to compression and greater maintenance of foraminal height than that of a single interbody spacer (▶ Fig. 4.64).[20]

4.12.3 Technique for Curved Interbody Spacer Insertion

The placement of a curved interbody spacer is more technically demanding than that of a straight PLIF interbody spacer. There are nuances to consistently securing the spacer in the ideal position. The interbody spacer must be inserted into the disc space and then rotated into position so that it lies in the anterior third of the disc space and in the midline. The prevention of problems with interbody insertion begins with an awareness of their origins. The root causes of the vast majority of problems I have encountered over the years have been associated with violation of the cortical end plate and inadequate disc removal.

The operating microscope is a wonderful tool for decompression but distorts your perspective of the interbody spacer work, especially when the bed has been rotated away from the surgeon. Thus, after the microscope has been removed and the fluoroscope brought back into the field, I critically evaluate the boundaries of the expanded transforaminal corridor that I have created to insert the interbody spacers. More often than not, I use a Kerrison punch to extend the annulotomy both medially and laterally to open the disc space further. My assistant surgeon typically holds the suction retractor up against the thecal sac, traversing nerve root while I retract the exiting root, which is now visible. Retraction of the exiting and traversing nerve roots allows me to safely widen the corridor into the disc space (▶ Fig. 4.65). Once I feel that I have optimized the corridor, I begin the interbody trials.

Assessing the height of the first normal level (i.e., no significant degeneration) above or below is a starting point for determining the ideal interbody height of the segment. In my estimation, there is seldom need to exceed the height of one of the normal levels in the lumbosacral spine. One of the elements I use to identify the appropriate height of the interbody spacer

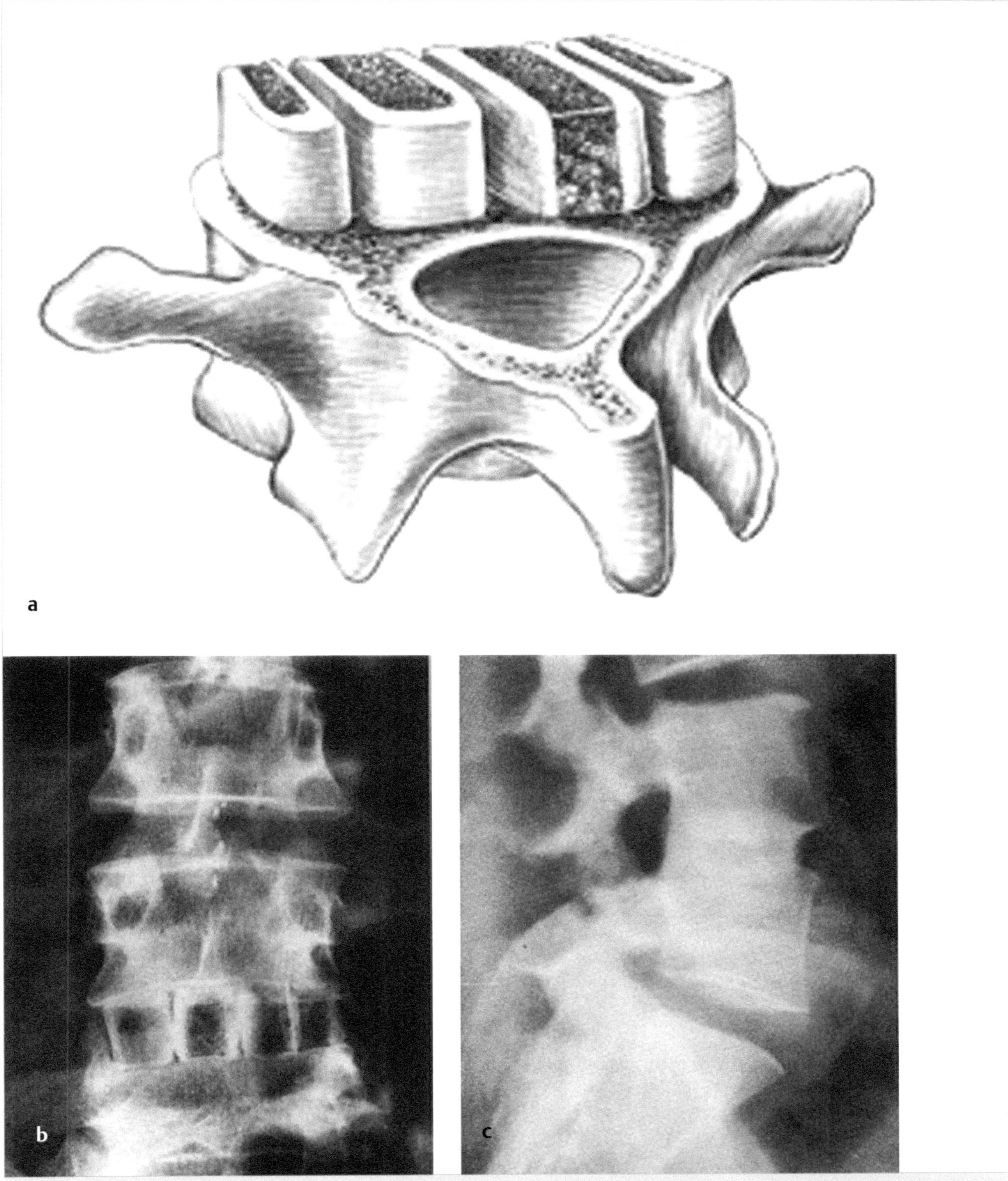

Fig. 4.62 The Cloward posterior lumbar interbody fusion procedure.[24] **(a)** An illustration from Cloward's technique guide where the straight geometry of the graft that Cloward envisioned would occupy the entire disc space with multiple grafts that span the entire cortical end plate. **(b)** Immediate postoperative anteroposterior radiograph showing the extent of coverage with 4 interbody grafts. **(c)** Postoperative lateral radiograph showing complete incorporation of Cloward's "bone plugs." The coverage accomplished by Cloward is the standard for which we strive in interbody fusion operations. The extent of this coverage stands in stark contrast to the minimal coverage of the single interbody spacer placed obliquely and shown in ▶ Fig. 4.61. (▶ Fig. 4.62a is reproduced with permission from Cloward RB. Posterior Lumbar Interbody Fusion (P.L.I.F.) Surgical Techniques. Honolulu, HI: Cloward Instrument Corporation.)

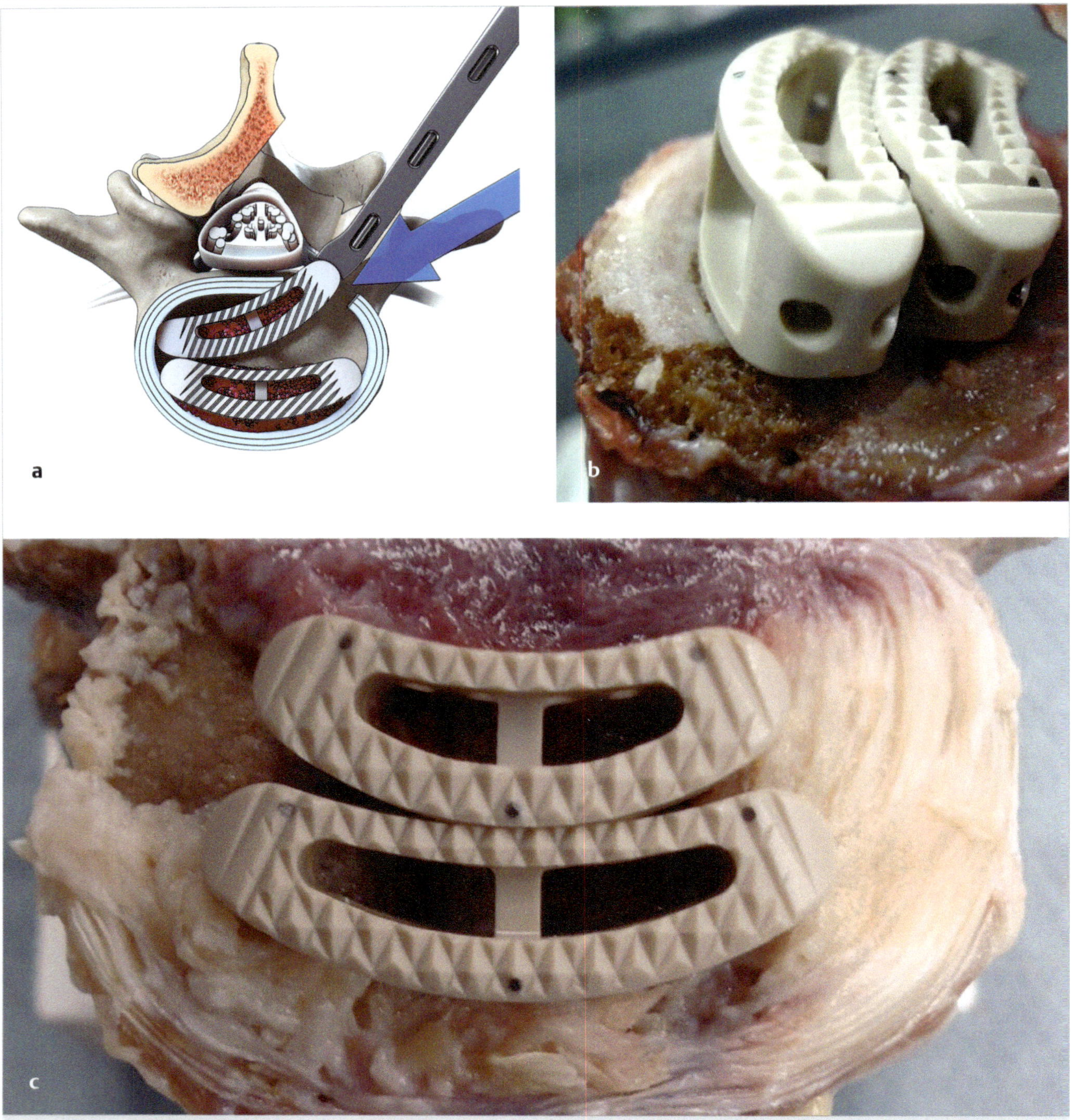

Fig. 4.63 Nested interbody spacers for a transforaminal lumbar interbody fusion. (a) Illustration demonstrating the concept of two nested interbody spacers. Sequential placement of semicircular-type grafts significantly increases the surface area covered within the disc space. (b) Photograph of a lateral oblique view of a disarticulated cadaveric specimen with nested interbody spacers resting on the end plate. (c) Photograph of the cadaveric specimen showing the increased coverage of the disc space with a 36 × 10 mm and a 30 × 10 mm interbody spacer. When using interbody spacers that are 40 mm in length, the coverage of the disc space exceeds 50%.[20] (Reproduced with permission from Soriano-Baron H, Newcomb AG, Malhotra D, et al. Biomechanics of nested transforaminal lumbar interbody cages. Neurosurgery. 2016; 78:297–304.)

is the feel of the trial spacer within the disc space, which should feel firmly secured within the disc space. Insertion of the trial should require the use of a mallet to secure it in position and a slap hammer to remove it. A loose-fitting interbody trial leads to a loose-fitting interbody spacer, and the stage has been set for a pseudarthrosis in the months to come.

It is important to ensure that the interbody trial can completely cross the midline of the disc space to reach the contralateral aspect of the disc space. Tapping the trial in at various trajectories will ensure that the contralateral aspect of the disc space will not limit the ability to rotate a 36-, 40-, or even a 45-mm interbody spacer into the anterior and center part of the disc (▶ Fig. 4.66). The

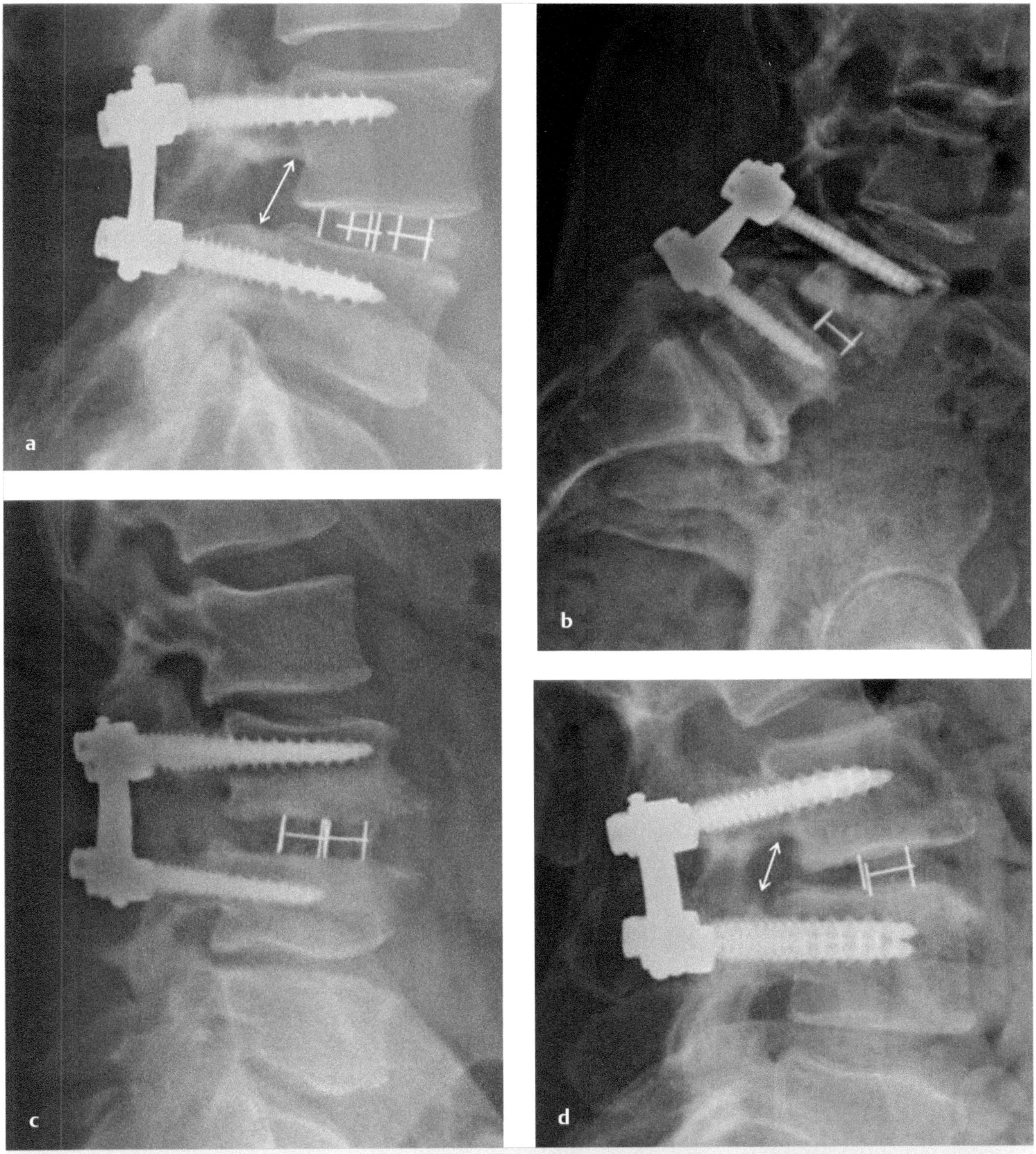

Fig. 4.64 Lateral postoperative standing radiographs showing the difference in foraminal heights with nested interbody spacers compared with a single interbody spacer. All constructs in this figure had interbody spacers 10 mm in height. **(a)** Two nested interbody spacers in an L4–5 transforaminal lumbar interbody fusion (TLIF). The second interbody maintains the foraminal height despite compression of the construct to restore segmental lordosis (*arrow*). **(b)** The single-spacer construct in an L4-5 TLIF provides shorter foraminal height than that of the nested construct. **(c)** An example of a construct at L3–4 in a patient who presented with grade I spondylolisthesis. The second interbody spacer maintained the posterior disc height compared to **(d)** the single interbody spacer, which maintains the anterior disc height but not the posterior disc height. One can imagine that a second 10-mm interbody spacer in **d** would also have maintained greater foraminal height.

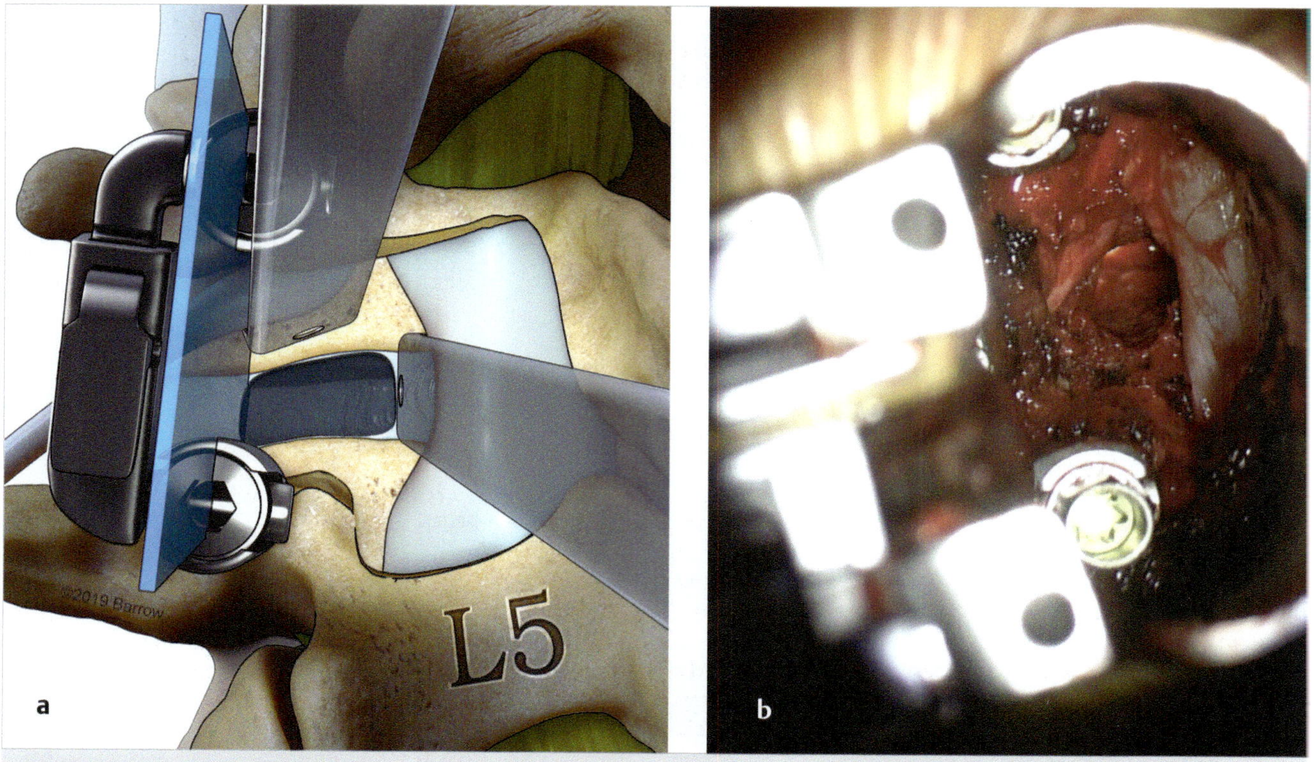

Fig. 4.65 Optimizing the expanded transforaminal corridor. **(a)** Illustration focusing on the expanded transforaminal corridor during interbody preparation. The annulotomy should extend medially at least to the medial aspect of the thecal sac and laterally to the midpedicular line (*blue plane*). **(b)** Intraoperative photograph demonstrating the expanded transforaminal corridor. Note the annulotomy in this case goes beyond the midpedicular line. The exiting root may be clearly seen beneath the L4 pedicle screw.

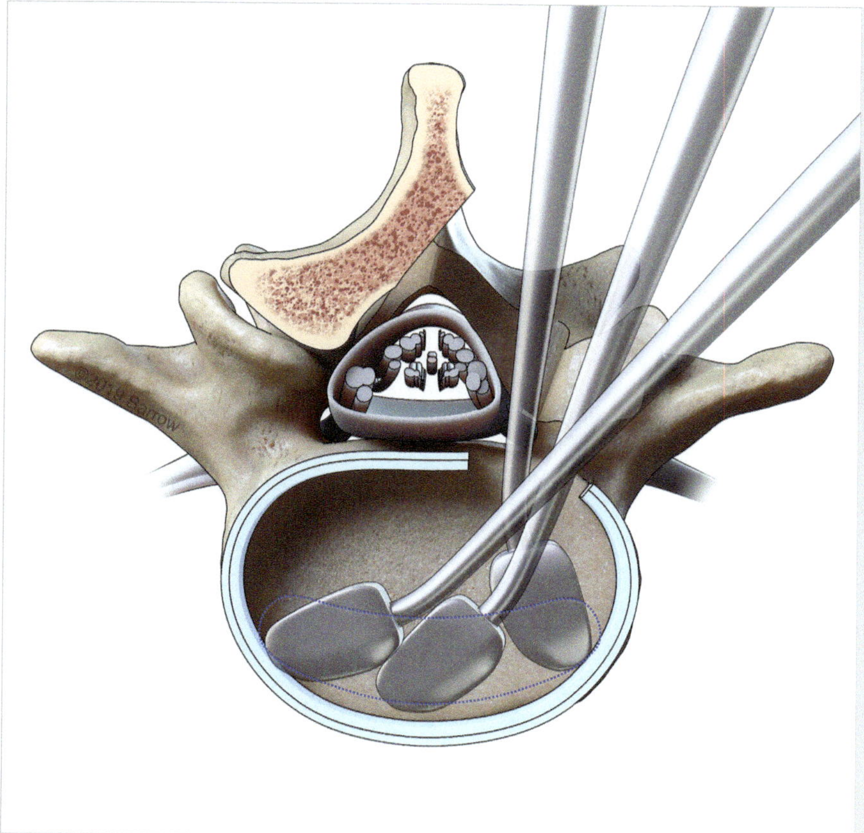

Fig. 4.66 Illustration of the various trajectories of the trial demonstrating the process of securing the trial into the contralateral aspect of the disc space across the midline, the center of the disc space and the ipsilateral aspect of the disc space. Once the height of the interbody has been selected, placement of the trial in these three trajectories ensures the disc space has been adequately prepared for an implant that can cover up to 40 mm of the anterior aspect of the disc space as denoted by the outline (*dark blue dotted line*) of the interbody.

process of using the interbody trials will inevitably free up more disc material and cartilaginous end plate. Irrigating out the disc space will deliver errant pieces of disc and cartilaginous end plate. It is worthwhile to use a pituitary for one final sweep within the disc space before placing the morselized graft and interbody spacer.

4.12.4 Lateral Dimension of an Interbody Spacer

Once I have selected the height of the interbody spacers, I assess the width of the available disc space. The goal is always to insert the widest interbody spacer that the disc space will allow. I do this by passing a calibrated angled interbody curet into the disc space, which allows me to reach across the disc space and ensure that I have enough room. As I pass the angled curet into the disc space, I nudge it up against the thecal sac and ensure that I can see the 40-mm mark on the curet. If the curet easily passes to the 40-mm mark, I know that I can place the widest spacer available into the disc space. At this point, even though I have done this previously while under the microscope, I repeat this as part of my systems check before I secure the interbody spacer into position.

It is rare that I do not use the widest implant available. My confidence in inserting the widest implant stems from my knowledge of the dimensions of the disc space. Anthropometric studies suggest those dimensions are rarely less than 40 mm in width and typically up to 50 mm.[21] My experience with transpsoas interbody spacers also serves as a frame of reference. Transpsoas interbody widths begin at 45 mm and may be as wide as 60 mm. The widest commercially available transforaminal interbody spacers now reach 40 mm, which pales in comparison even though it may occupy the same interspace. In the years to come, as facility with transforaminal approaches increases, I predict wider interbody spacers with widths of 45 and 50 mm will become commercially available. In the well-prepared disc space, the only limitation to securing the widest implant is the comfort of passing the implant around the neural elements and rotating it into position.

4.12.5 Placement of Autograft

With the height and length of the interbody spacer selected, I pack the now empty disc space with morselized autograft and allograft anteriorly as described by Harms.[11] The amount of autograft always varies. Sometimes the morselized autograft harvest is plentiful; other times, it is scant. In cases with an abundant harvest, it is important not to pack too much of that bone into the interbody space. Overpacking the space may impede the ability to place the interbody spacer into the ideal location. Too much bone graft in one location—that is, not equally distributed across the disc space—will also interfere with the ability to completely rotate the interbody spacer. I have encountered this problem and remedied it only with removal of the interbody spacer and removal or redistribution of graft. To deliver the autograft, I use a funnel-shaped trumpet-like device that the scrub technician packs with the morselized graft and pass it into the disc space. I then use the large Epstein interbody curet to distribute the graft equally across the anterior aspect of the disc space. Although there may be a liability for too much bone graft in the disc space, there is equal liability for too little. An inadequate quantity of graft material could allow the interbody spacer to move too far forward and up against the annulus. In my estimation, it is the ideal circumstance for the autograft to occupy the anterior one-fourth to one-fifth of the disc space. Therefore, in situations where there is an inadequate amount of autograft, I add morselized allograft and ensure equal distribution throughout the anterior aspect of the disc space up against the annulus. The annulus serves as an important bolster against which the morselized graft will be compressed by the rotated interbody spacer. The compression of the graft between the annulus and the interbody spacer will fully allow loading of the graft and thereby the application of Wolff's law (▶ Fig. 4.67).

4.12.6 Interbody Insertion

There are a variety of insertion instruments available from several manufacturers that will accomplish the objective of rotating the curved interbody into the anterior third and the center of the disc space. It is important to learn the various nuances of the particular insertion device you choose to use. Achieving that mastery is best done over and over in the setting of a cadaver lab until you have acquired proficiency with the instruments and the techniques. It is imperative to become comfortable with all the instruments for insertion and extraction of the implant. You should become comfortable inserting, rotating and extracting an implant in cadavers before applying these skills in your patients. Regardless of the implant you choose, the technique remains the same: set an oblique trajectory, advance the interbody spacer into the disc space and rotate it into the center and anterior third of the disc space (▶ Fig. 4.68). The following description is a generic technique for the insertion of any commercially available curved interbody.

With the autograft and allograft packed into the disc space, the curved spacer is loaded into the inserter and also packed with bone graft. The nerve root and thecal sac are slightly retracted by the assistant surgeon. Retraction is to protect the root and the thecal sac more than any genuine need to expose more of the disc space, which is readily accessible in transforaminal approaches. There are times when the expanded transforaminal corridor is so capacious that retraction of the traversing root is unnecessary. On other occasions, a constrained corridor may prompt the need to retract the exiting root upward with one hand while securing the interbody spacer into the disc space with the other. I shoehorn the interbody spacer into the disc space and clear the exiting root, which I am retracting with the suction retractor as it enters the disc space. Once the tip of the spacer enters the annulotomy, I release the retraction on the exiting root. I now have a free hand to tap the interbody spacer into the disc space in an oblique trajectory with a mallet. Before tapping the spacer, I obtain a fluoroscopic image to ensure that I have a good trajectory parallel to the disc space. An errant trajectory can damage the cortical end plate and derail any possibility of perfect placement.

When I have set the ideal trajectory, I begin tapping the interbody spacer obliquely across the disc space. I continue advancing the implant obliquely until it has cleared the posterior aspect of the disc space. As it proceeds obliquely, the implant needs to cross the midline as seen in ▶ Fig. 4.68. I confirm the clearance of the posterior aspect of the disc space

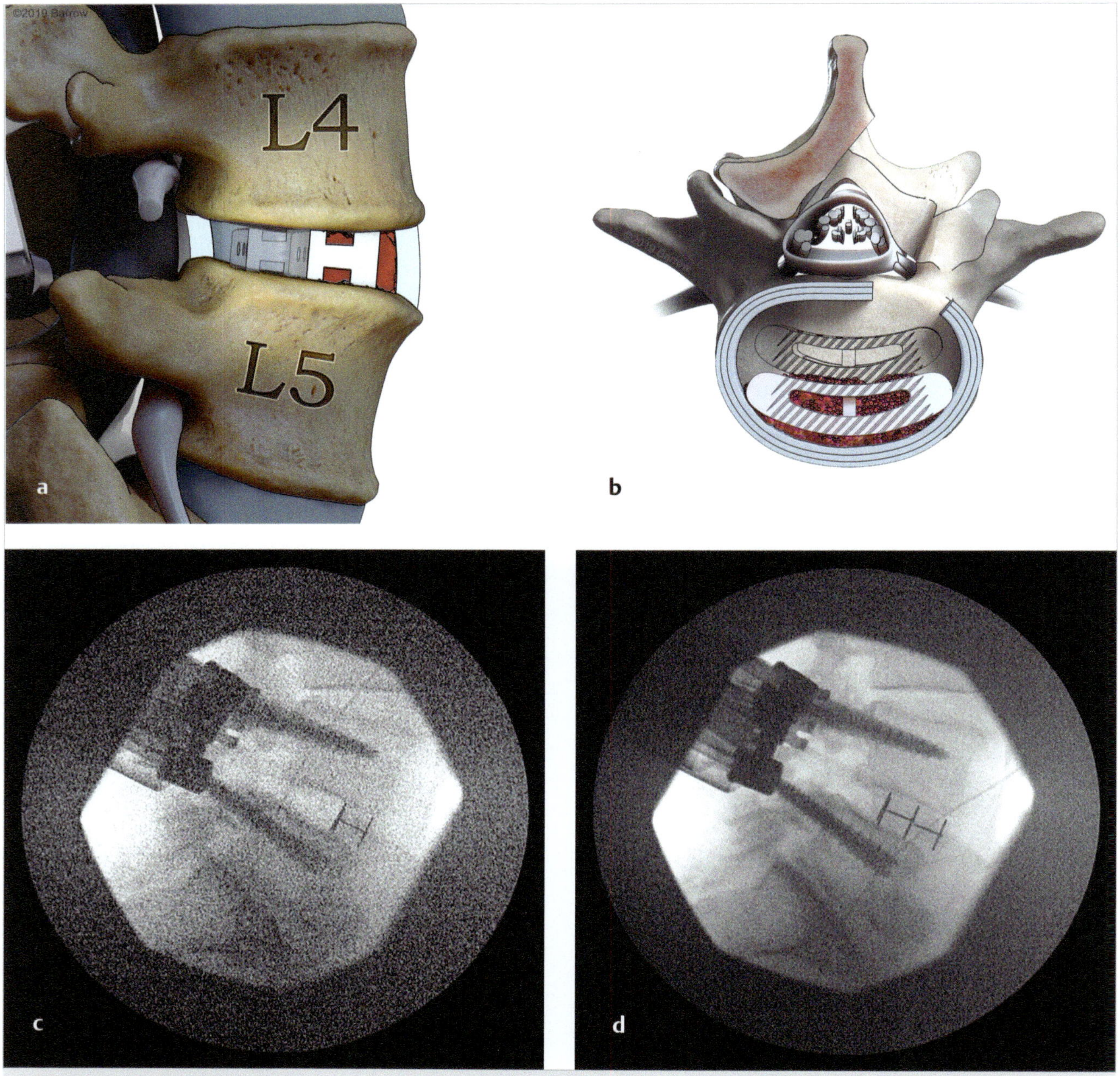

Fig. 4.67 Distribution of graft within the anterior aspect of the disc space. **(a)** Illustration demonstrating the L4–5 disc and interbody fusion of the L4–5 segment. Under ideal circumstances, morselized autograft and allograft are packed into the anterior 20% of the disc space up against the annulus. An interbody spacer occupies another 25% of the disc space, compressing the morselized graft against the annulus as it rests on the apophyseal ring. The geometry of the curved spacer allows for the possibility of an additional interbody spacer to occupy another 25% of the disc space. **(b)** Illustration in the axial place of the placement of an interbody spacer. The bone graft is compressed by the interbody spacer against the annulus. **(c)** Low-dose collimated lateral fluoroscopic image of a 12 × 40 mm interbody spacer in the anterior aspect of the disc space resting on the apophyseal ring. The risk of subsidence with this position is low. Note the increased density within the interbody spacer indicating the degree of compression of the morselized graft between the annulus and the spacer. **(d)** Full-dose fluoroscopic image with second interbody in position. Greater than 50% of the disc space is now occupied with a structural graft.

with direct visualization first and then obtain a fluoroscopic image (▶ Fig. 4.69). All commercially available polyether ether ketone (PEEK) interbody spacers have tantalum markers on the leading and posterior aspects of the implants. Titanium spacers are even more obvious on fluoroscopy. I obtain a fluoroscopic image once my visual inspection confirms that the trailing edge of the interbody is past the posterior aspect of the disc space. That image allows me to reconfirm the trajectory. I have found that as the interbody makes its way into the disc space, the trajectory may alter slightly. Reconfirming the trajectory prevents

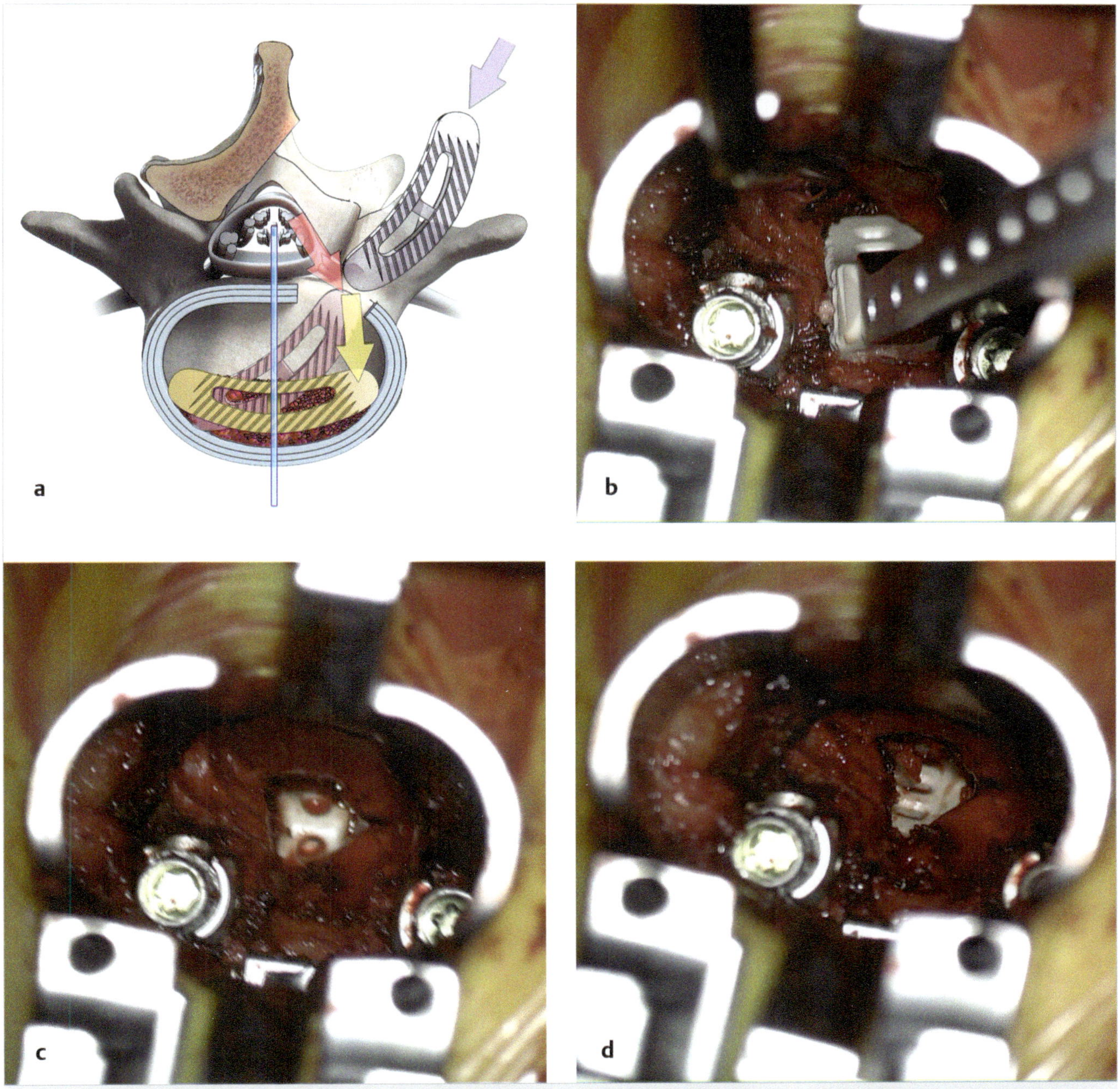

Fig. 4.68 Insertion of the interbody spacer. **(a)** Illustration of interbody spacer insertion. With an oblique trajectory (*lavender arrow*), the implant (*lavender shade*) advances until the posterior margin has cleared the posterior aspect of the disc space (*crimson shade*). The implant (*crimson shade*) needs to cross the midline (*blue plane*) before the trajectory changes from converging toward the disc space to diverging away from the disc space (*crimson arrow*). The final maneuver is to tap the implant down against the annulus into the anterior aspect of the disc space (*gold shade*) with a continued divergent trajectory (*gold arrow*). The interbody spacer in this position compresses the morselized graft against the annulus and thereby loads the graft. The implant is also now resting on the hardest part of the cortical end plate. **(b)** Intraoperative photograph demonstrating the interbody spacer entering the disc space with an oblique trajectory. This image matches the lavender-shaded interbody spacer shown in **a. (c)** The interbody device in this photograph has cleared the posterior margin of the disc space. This image corresponds with the crimson-shaded interbody spacer in **a. (d)** Changing the vector force rotates the interbody and drives it to the front of the vertebral body. This image corresponds with the gold interbody spacer shown in **a**.

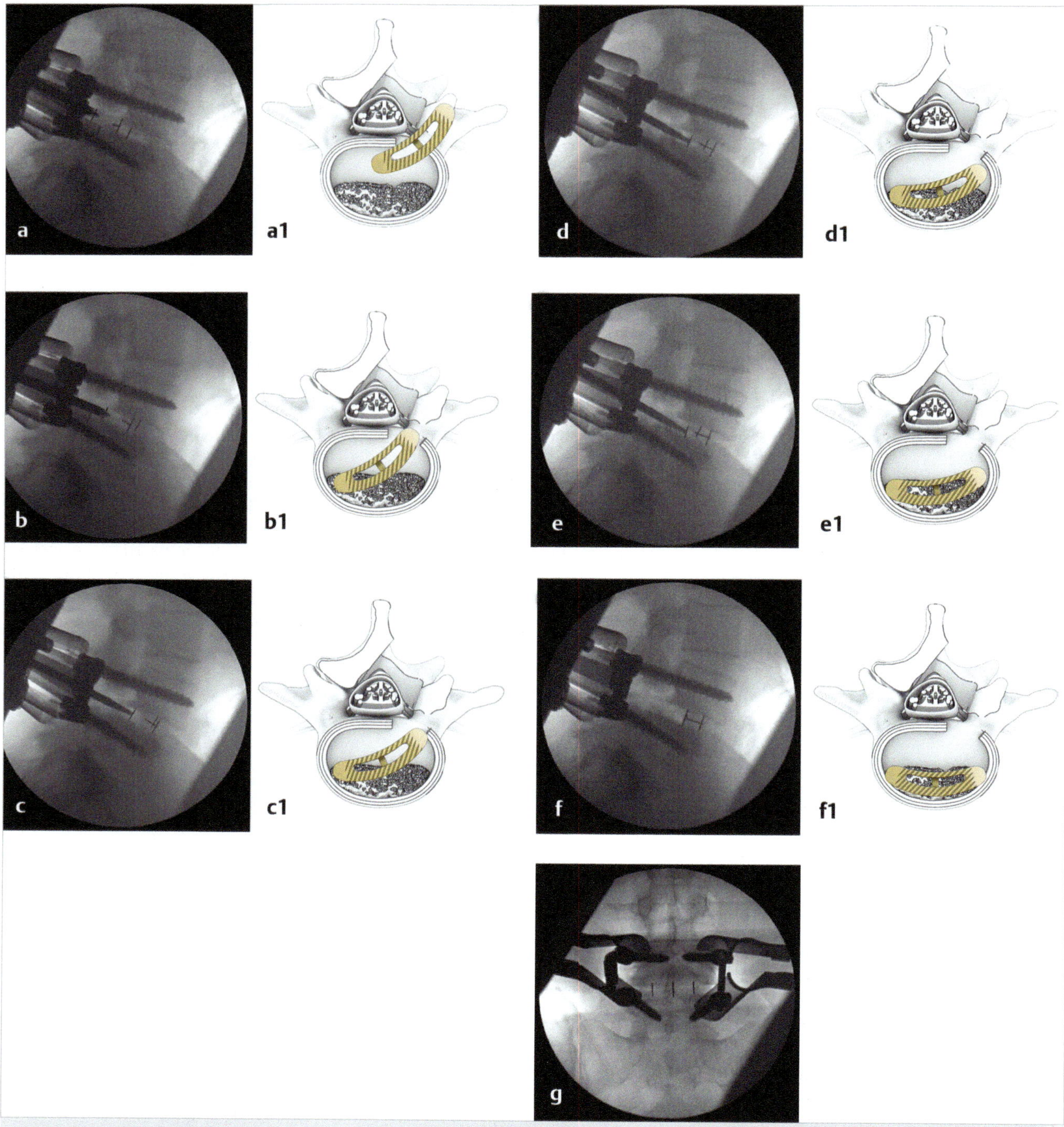

Fig. 4.69 A series of lateral fluoroscopic images showing the insertion of a curved interbody spacer into the disc space. **(a)** Establishing the ideal trajectory into the disc space to prevent end plate violation; **(a1)** corresponding axial illustration demonstrating the oblique trajectory for insertion. **(b)** Advancing the interbody spacer into the disc space obliquely; **(b1)** corresponding axial illustration showing the spacer crossing the midline. **(c)** Before beginning the rotation of the interbody spacer, a fluoroscopic image confirms that the spacer has cleared the posterior aspect of the disc space; **(c1)** corresponding axial illustration depicting that the spacer has cleared the posterior aspect of the disc space. **(d,e)** Changing the vector force is essential to rotating the interbody spacer into position; **(d1,e1)** corresponding axial illustration demonstrating the point that changing the vector force is essential to rotate the interbody into position. **(f)** A fully rotated interbody spacer resting on the apophyseal ring of L5 in a patient with grade II spondylolisthesis reduced to grade I; **(f1)** corresponding axial illustration. **(g)** Anteroposterior image demonstrating placement of the interbody spacer across the midline.

driving the implant into an end plate. It is difficult to recover from a damaged end plate. Implants always find the path of least resistance into the disc space during insertion, and once an end plate is damaged, the implant tends to settle into this defect. Rotating the implant into the ideal position in this circumstance is exceedingly challenging, and the inability to work around the end plate violation almost always results in subsidence in the coming weeks to months but does not preclude fusion from occurring. Implants into the end plate may not be radiographically pleasing to the eye, but may still offer a satisfactory clinical outcome. Still, it is a worthwhile investment to take every measure to optimize the implant position.

When the posterior aspect of the interbody spacer clears the posterior aspect of the disc space, the rotation of the implant begins. I loosen the inserter and begin to rotate the graft. Regardless of the implant used, the vector force needs to be adjusted to allow for continued rotation of the device. Rotation may be accomplished with any number of instruments designed for such a purpose. Some systems attempt to automate the rotation of the implant with the insertion device. Becoming familiar with the appearance of the tantalum markers on lateral fluoroscopic images for the particular implant that is used is essential to master the insertion process. I check an occasional fluoroscopic image as I rotate the implant to ensure that it remains parallel to the disc space. My goal is to achieve a perfect lateral configuration of the implant within the disc space.

As the implant begins to turn, I begin to look past the inserter, through the annulotomy and into the disc space to assess the center of the interbody relative to the thecal sac. Most curved interbody spacers have a midline marker that can be seen even after insertion. I draw an imaginary line from what I perceive to be the center of the thecal sac down to the implant (▶ Fig. 4.68). If I feel I have not centered the implant well, I begin to make minor adjustments, a task that is significantly easier to do before completing the rotation. There are a number of instruments that can engage the posterior aspect of the interbody that allow a vector force to push the implant across the midline. Although it is difficult to overshoot the midline of the disc space with a 36- or 40-mm spacer, it is not impossible, and pulling it back is hard to do because the optimal vector force for that direction is difficult to achieve.

Making minor adjustments toward the midline tends to de-rotate the implant, and so after repositioning the implant, instruments might be needed to rotate the implant back into the ideal configuration (▶ Fig. 4.69).

Over-rotation of the interbody spacer is a relatively easy problem to solve by inserting a de-rotation instrument beneath the thecal sac, across the midline and onto the far side of the spacer. Once in position, the instrument can de-rotate the spacer with just a few taps. In the event that I am unable to completely rotate the implant, it is likely that the graft or ipsilateral disc is preventing me from doing so. At this point, I need to determine whether the implant is sufficiently rotated and whether the implant is in the midline. One of the criteria that I use is the posterior tantalum marker, which should be at least 1 cm away from the posterior aspect of the disc space as seen on the lateral fluoroscopic image. Visual inspection may also confirm a safe distance from the neural elements. If this distance is less than 1 cm and the implant will not rotate any further, it needs to be removed and the disc space reassessed. It is either disc material on the ipsilateral side or graft material that is precluding its rotation. If the posterior tantalum marker is greater than 1 cm from the posterior aspect of the disc space but not completely rotated, I obtain an AP fluoroscopic image to determine if a midline position has been achieved. The final decision on what is acceptable ultimately rests with the operating surgeon.

4.12.7 Nested Interbody Spacers

A well-positioned and well-centered interbody implant that rests in the anterior one-fourth of the disc space merits consideration of the placement of a second interbody spacer. As I noted in Section 4.12.2, The Ideal Interbody: A Concept Based on Surface Area (particularly ▶ Fig. 4.63), a second implant increases the surface area that can be loaded under compression between the vertebral bodies to embrace Wolff's law and more reliably achieve fusion. The second implant also maintains the foraminal height under compression, which may otherwise become compromised with a single implant in the anterior disc space.[20]

The second interbody spacer that I select is typically the same height and length as the initial spacer. After all, the disc space has only become wider at its midpoint compared to the anterior aspect. The first step in the placement of the second interbody is tapping a trial into position, which is how I determine if there is adequate room available in the disc space (▶ Fig. 4.70). With the first interbody in position, the trial and subsequent interbody spacer are easier to place because the disc space height is maintained by the first interbody spacer. Once the trial is tapped into position up against the first interbody, I check a lateral fluoroscopic image (▶ Fig. 4.70a). The distance from the posterior aspect of the trial to the posterior aspect of the disc space should be at least 1 cm. If the distance is less than 1 cm, I forgo the second interbody. If this distance is more than 1 cm, a second interbody may be placed.

The key to placement of the second interbody spacer is early rotation. Thus, once I pack the interbody with autograft and load it onto the inserter, I place a suction retractor on the thecal sac and traversing root more for protection than retraction. With a direct line of sight into the disc space, I place the implant into the annulotomy and begin to tap the second interbody spacer into the disc space. Once half of the interbody spacer has cleared the posterior aspect of the disc space, I obtain a fluoroscopic image to determine the distance from the leading edge of the implant to the back of the implant already in position. That image gives me an idea how much room there is for rotation. A potential pitfall is driving the leading edge of the second interbody spacer into the first before rotation. Any contact of the second spacer with the first limits the capacity to rotate and thereby nest the interbody spacers. If this happens, it will be necessary to extract the interbody and begin again. Attempting to continue to rotate the interbody at this point will alter the position of the first interbody (▶ Fig. 4.71).

Rotation of the second interbody spacer should begin once half of it has cleared the disc space. Beginning the rotation early allows the implant to fully rotate and settle into the posterior curvature of the first interbody. Tapping the inserter with a divergent trajectory away from the disk space will nest the interbody spacers. The path of least resistance and geometry

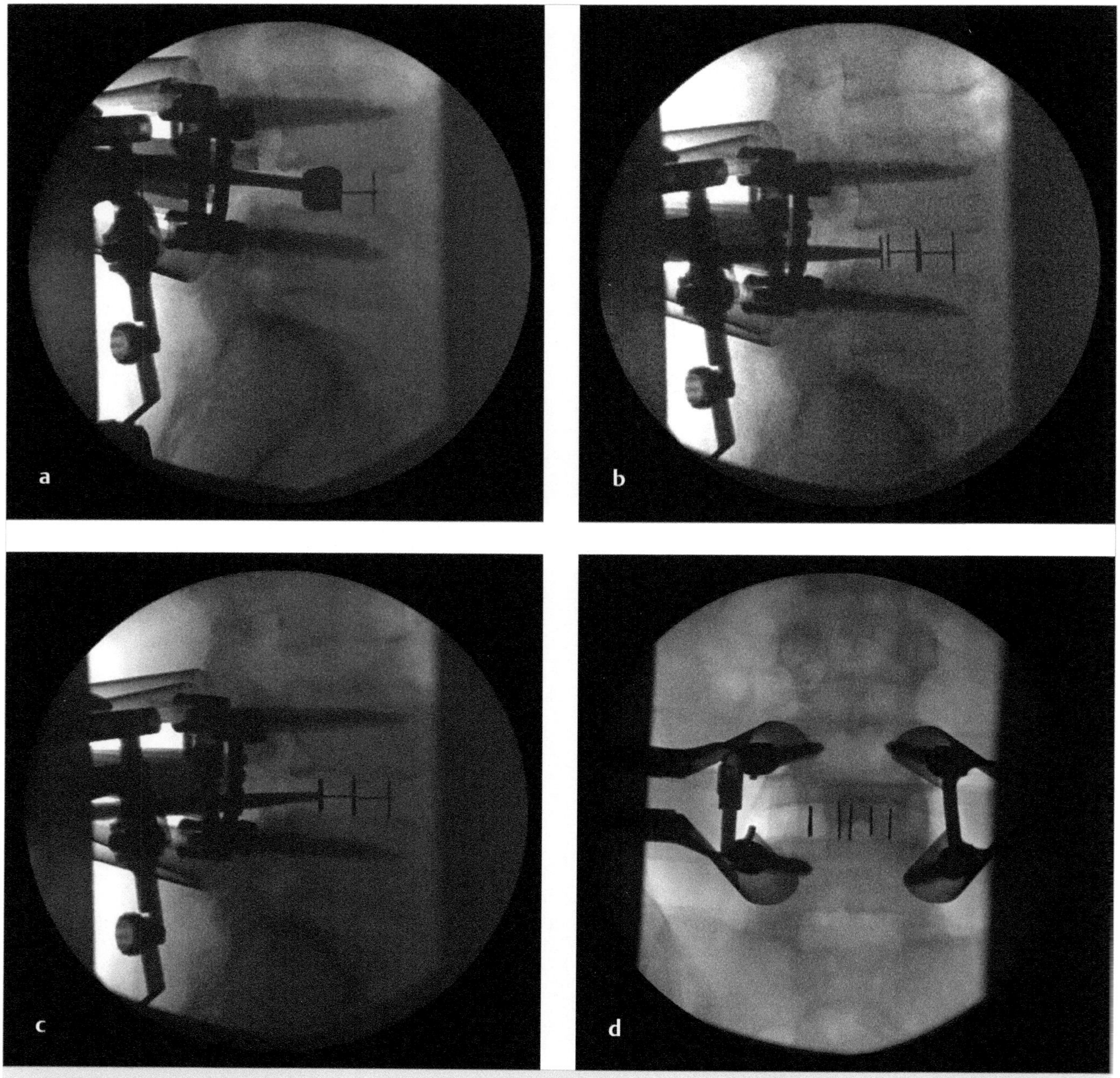

Fig. 4.70 Nested interbody spacers. A series of fluoroscopic images demonstrating placement of a second interbody spacer. **(a)** A trial is inserted to determine if there is adequate room within the disc space for a second interbody. The clearance of 1 cm indicates adequate room for the placement of a second spacer. **(b)** Insertion of the second spacer tends to be straightforward because the second spacer nests into the first one. **(c)** Final rotation of the interbody spacer into the full lateral configuration across the disc space. **(d)** Anteroposterior fluoroscopic image demonstrating the interbody spacers spanning the disc space.

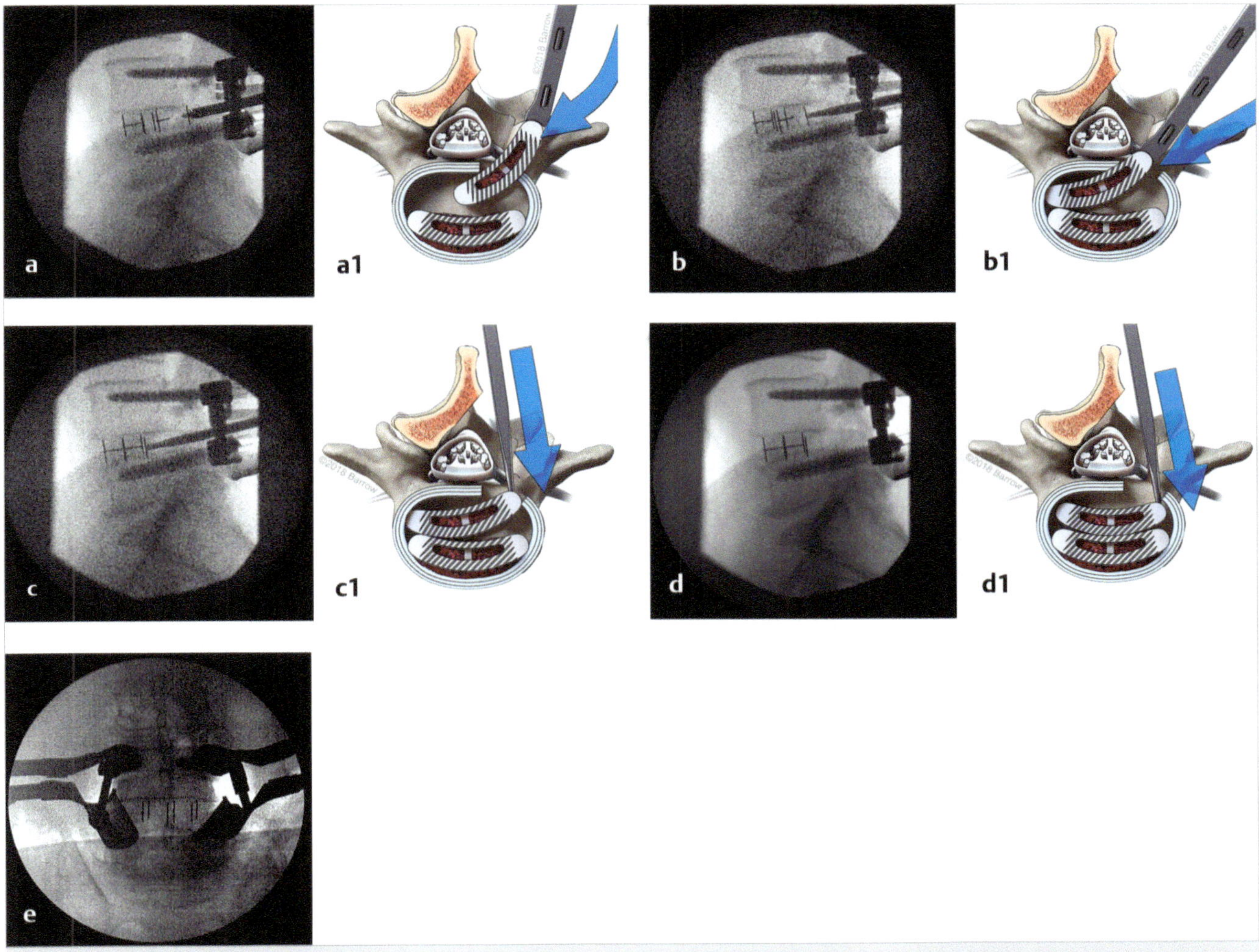

Fig. 4.71 Technique for insertion of an interbody spacer. Fluoroscopic images juxtaposed with axial illustrations that show the advancement of the interbody spacer, with an emphasis on the vector force for the advancement and rotation of the spacer. The first two fluoroscopic images **(a,b)** and corresponding axial illustrations **(a1,b1)** demonstrate an oblique vector force across the disc space. Once advanced obliquely into the disc space, the vector force is in the opposite direction to complete the rotation, as shown in fluoroscopic images **(c,d)** and the corresponding axial illustrations **(c1, d1)**. Once in contact with the first interbody spacer, the downward force will result in the interbody spacers nesting with corresponding axial illustrations. The final anteroposterior fluoroscopic image **(e)** demonstrates two 15 × 40-mm interbody spacers nested in the L4–5 disc space.

guide the front part of the second spacer into the posterior aspect of the spacer already in position (▸ Fig. 4.71). Final lateral and AP fluoroscopic images confirm a well-positioned and well-centered construct.

4.12.8 Placement of Permanent Rods and Compression

If the provisional ipsilateral expandable retractor was used for distraction, I release it by pressing down on the release lever with a curet, remove the set screws and remove the provisional expandable rod by hooking it with a reverse angled curet. The tulip heads of the pedicle screw are rotated 90 degrees so that I can place the permanent rod in position. After I have centered the permanent rod onto the tulip heads of the pedicles, I secure the rods with the set screws.

By convention, I set the permanent rod so that it protrudes slightly more from the caudal pedicle screw than the rostral screw. Hardly any of the rods should protrude from the rostral pedicle screw to minimize any encroachment of the rod onto the rostral facet complex. I provisionally tighten the rostral set screw without breaking it off so that it does not rotate away from me when I break off the caudal set screw. Next, I final-tighten and break off the torque-limiting set screw on the caudal pedicle screw before using the compressor to place the interbody spacers under compression and break off the rostral set screw. I place the final tightener on the rostral screw while simultaneously wrapping the minimally invasive compressor around the caudal screw. In a minimally invasive exposure, the compressor works by bringing the caudal pedicle screw toward the rostral screw with the use of a lever arm. A manual squeeze on the lever arm brings the pedicle screws together, thereby compressing the interbody spacers with the end plates of the vertebral bodies. To capture the compression, I tighten and break off the rostral set screw. I confirm compression by comparing the protrusion of the rod above the rostral pedicle screw before and after compression. There should be an obvious change in the amount of rod protruding above the tulip head of the rostral pedicle screw, which will reflect how much compression I have accomplished. I compress and break off the torque-limiting set screws on the left and right sides, and the operation is now complete. I may now begin to close the incisions.

The rationale for compressing the construct is threefold. The first reason is figuratively to shut the door of entry behind the interbody spacers. With compression, the migration of an interbody spacer becomes almost a mechanical impossibility. In Fessler's series of 513 MIS TLIFs, he identified five cases of interbody spacer migration, two of which required additional surgery.[22] In my current series of 600 MIS TLIFs, I have had three cases of interbody spacer migration after the use of my current compression technique; two cases occurred in patients actively using tobacco. Of these two cases, one case involved nested interbody spacers; in the third case, the patient had osteoporosis. Two of the three cases required additional surgery.

The second reason to put the construct under compression is to apply the principles of Wolff's law. Compression loads the graft material within the spacer, prevents stress shielding from the pedicle screws and optimizes the environment for arthrodesis to take place.

The final reason to compress the construct is to restore segmental lordosis. With the transforaminal bone work on one side and a Smith–Petersen osteotomy on the other, I can reliably achieve up to 12 degrees of lordosis. Placing the construct under compression without completing the Smith–Petersen osteotomy has the potential to compromise the foramen and cause radiculopathy (▶ Fig. 4.72).

4.12.9 Closure

Before I begin the multilayered closure, I infiltrate the muscle, fascia and subcutaneous tissue with the maximum dose of 0.5% bupivacaine as determined by the anesthesiologist. I distribute this volume equally between the two incisions and throughout the various layers to be closed.

The closure of a deep 28-mm incision with conventional suture needles is impractical. For the fascial closure, I use size 0 polyglactin-910 (Vicryl, Ethicon Inc., Somerville, NJ) on a UR-6 needle, which is designed for closure of laparoscopic incisions. A hyper-curved needle that forms five-eighths of a circle allows for easy rotation at the surgical depth within the confined space for approximation of the fascial edges. I approximate the tendinous sheath over the paraspinal muscles with running 0 polyglactin sutures. I use interrupted sutures for reapproximation of the thoracolumbar fascia and place all the stitches before tying them. I then close the subcutaneous layer with interrupted 2.0 polyglactin on an X-1 needle, which forms a half circle for easy rotation. Finally, I bring the skin edges together with 3.0 polyglactin suture on a 17-mm RB-1 needle. I apply Mastisol (Eloquest Healthcare, Inc., Ferndale, MI) and Nexcare Steri-Strips (3 M, Maplewood, MN) to the wound surfaces, a piece of Telfa to cover the Steri-Strips (3M) and 5% lidocaine dressings to both wounds to help with pain control.

4.13 Postoperative Management

Immediately after surgery, patients are given a muscle relaxant and an immediate release narcotic. Patients are weaned from all narcotics between 10 and 14 days after surgery. It is rare for me to use a Foley catheter, but if one is used, it is removed immediately after surgery, unless there is an underlying prostate issue, in which case it is removed on the first postoperative day. When the mean operative time is consistently less than 2 hours, a Foley catheter is no longer necessary. I have refrained from using a Foley catheter in my last 400 single-level minimally invasive TLIFs without an untoward event. The mean hospitalization time is 1.4 days (range, same-day discharge to 4 days). Patients who present with a predominance of radicular leg pain and who are not on preoperative narcotics stand a reasonable chance of same-day discharge if the operative time was less than 2 hours. Standing postoperative AP and lateral radiographs are obtained on the afternoon of the surgery or on the first postoperative day. The lidocaine dressing is removed on the first postoperative day. Patients are evaluated at 1 month postoperatively with AP and lateral radiographs. Flexion-extension radiographs are taken at the 3-month follow-up. Mature fusions can typically be seen between 6 and 12 months on plain radiographs (▶ Fig. 4.73).

4.14 Case Illustrations

Although this Primer focuses on techniques and not on indications, I would be remiss if I do not include a discussion on the indications for this procedure. In a review of my last 600 cases, the leading indication for surgery was spondylolisthesis (61%) followed by advanced degenerative disc disease years after a microdiscectomy or laminectomy with recurrent stenosis and radiculopathy from foraminal compromise (21%). A third-time re-herniation was the indication in 10% of the cases, and recurrent facet cyst formation was the least common indication, representing only 8% of the cases.

The case illustrations below provide a brief clinical history, operative management, postoperative images, and the clinical outcomes for the two leading diagnoses.`

4.14.1 Spondylolisthesis

A 48-year-old man with a long-standing history of axial back pain and a more recent history of radicular leg pain presented after 4 years of successful nonoperative measures. The patient had been successfully managed with an annual epidural injection. More recently, the epidural injections had not provided him any meaningful or sustained relief. The patient was missing days of work because of radicular leg pain. The preoperative Oswestry Disability Index (ODI) was 43, the 36-item short form health survey (SF-36) score was 19, the visual analog scale (VAS) for leg pain was 80 mm and the VAS for back pain was 45 mm. On examination, the patient had a blunted right patellar reflex, along with decreased strength in the right tibialis anterior, extensor hallucis longus and quadriceps, all of which were 4/5 compared to 5/5 on the left side. The sensory examination findings were normal. MRI demonstrated grade I spondylolisthesis with severe foraminal narrowing on the right, and

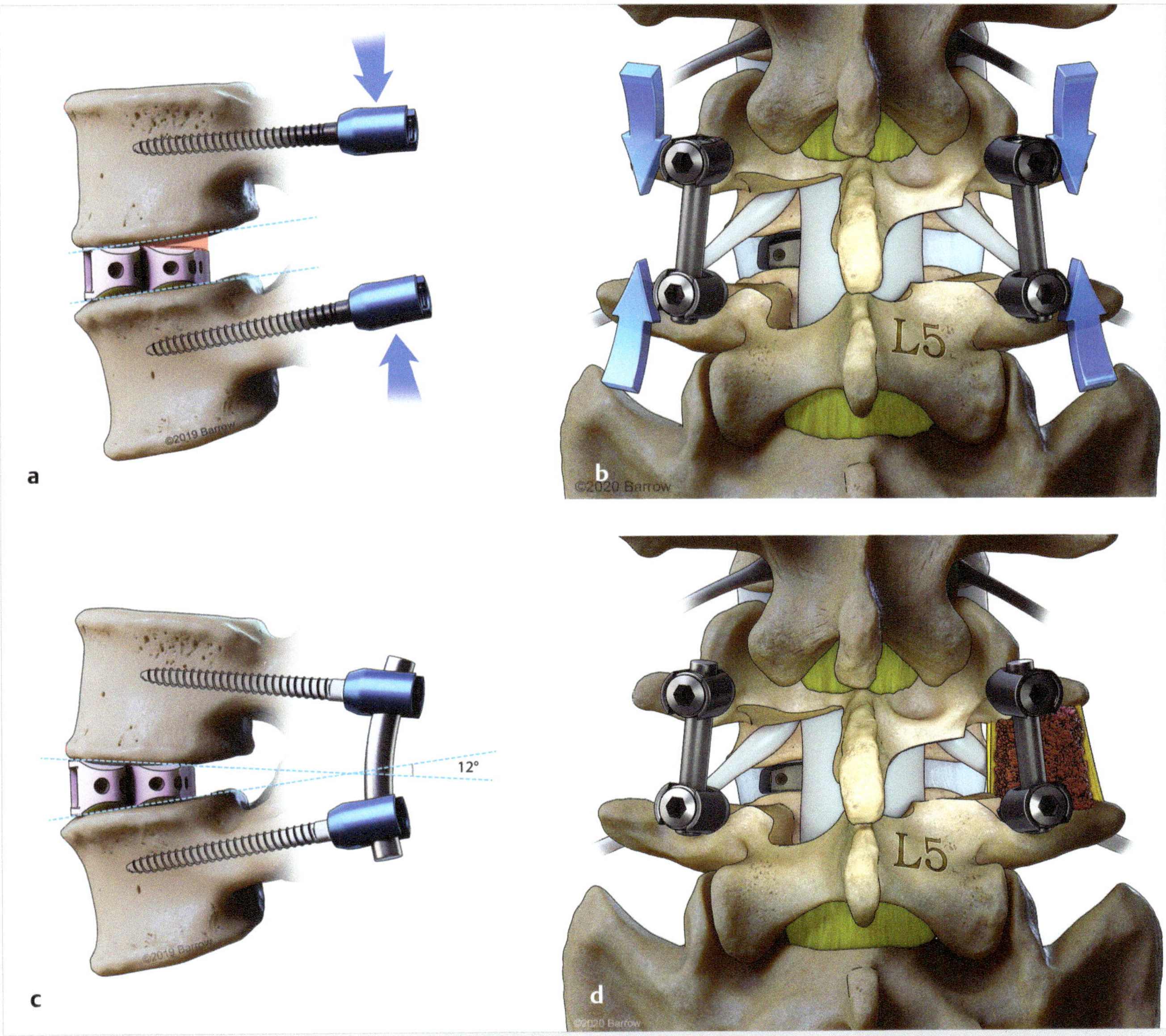

Fig. 4.72 Restoring segmental lordosis with compression. **(a)** Illustration of a lateral projection demonstrating nested interbody spacers. The *blue arrows* indicate the compression that will be accomplished. **(b)** Illustration of surgical view demonstrating the transforaminal bone work on the left and the Smith–Petersen osteotomy on the right before compression. **(c)** Illustration of a lateral projection demonstrating the construct in **b** under compression. Up to 12 degrees of lumbar lordosis may be achieved with the combination of disc height restoration, osteotomies and compression. **(d)** Illustration of the surgical view showing the construct after compression and breaking off the set screws. Note that the gap created by the Smith–Petersen osteotomy has narrowed. The transverse processes on the side of the Smith–Petersen osteotomies have been decorticated, and allograft and autograft have been placed in the posterolateral space. Note the illustration shows the preservation of the intertransverse process ligament where the bone graft is placed. When I perform bilateral decompressions, I do not perform a posterolateral fusion because I do not want the nerve root to become enveloped in the bone graft.

flexion-extension radiography confirmed the instability of the segment (▶ Fig. 4.74).

4.14.2 Operative Intervention

The predominance of symptoms on the right prompted a right transforaminal approach to the disc space. Two 28-mm incisions were made over the L4–5 segment 4 cm lateral to midline. Two expandable minimal access ports were secured over the top of the L4–5 facets. The pedicle screw entry points were exposed, and four pedicle screws were secured using the techniques described earlier. A Smith–Petersen osteotomy was performed on the left side to allow for greater reduction of the slip.[5] A complete right facetectomy at L4–5 and an L4 hemilaminectomy and removal of the superior aspect of the L5 lamina were performed. The right L4 nerve root was directly visualized and decompressed by removing the L4–5 disc that had unfurled into the L4 nerve root. The entire thecal sac was decompressed

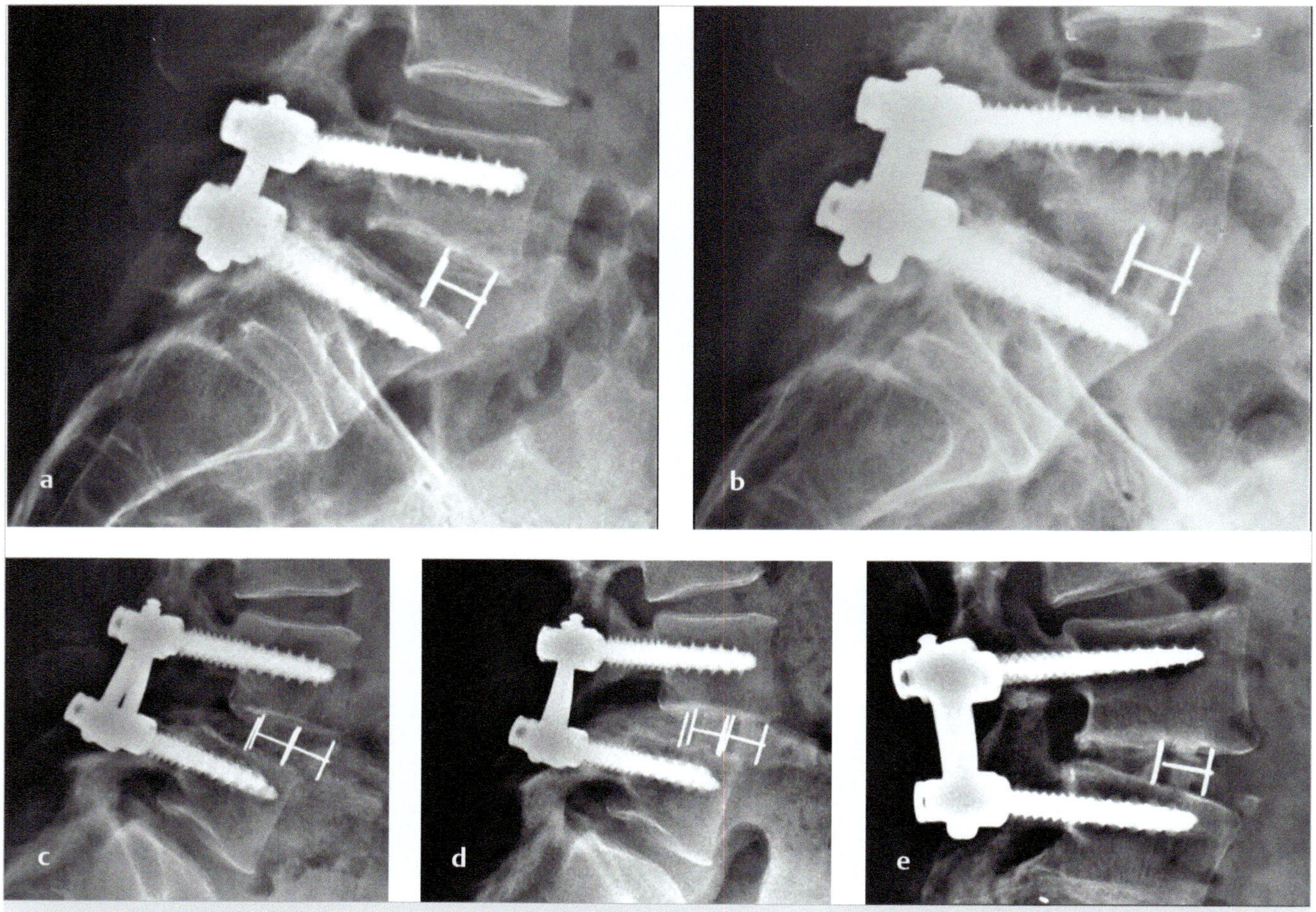

Fig. 4.73 Radiographic unions in minimally invasive transforaminal lumbar interbody fusions (TLIFs). **(a)** Lateral radiograph of an L5–S1 minimally invasive TLIF 30 days after surgery and at **(b)** 11 months after surgery. Note the outline of the spacer is determined by the bone growth. **(c)** Lateral radiograph of an L4–5 minimally invasive TLIF at 30 days and at **(d)** 7 months after surgery. Again, robust bone formation seen through the spacer and posterior to the spacer 1 year after surgery. **(e)** Lateral radiograph showing bone formation revealing a cast of the interbody spacer in an L3–4 TLIF at 6 months. Bridging bone from end plate to end plate is clearly seen within the interbody spacer.

with resection of the ligamentum flavum. The disc space was prepared, and the height was restored with paddle distractors and trials. Upon completion of preparing the cortical end plates, morselized autograft was packed into the anterior aspect of the disc space, and a 36 × 12-mm interbody spacer was rotated into position behind the autograft (▶ Fig. 4.75).

4.14.3 Postoperative Course

Immediately after surgery, the patient noted complete resolution of his right radicular leg pain. He was discharged on the first postoperative day and weaned off of all narcotic pain medications after 1 week. He returned to work in his office 2 weeks after surgery. At 1 year, the patient had an ODI of 9, SF-36 of 65, VAS for leg pain of 0 mm and VAS for back pain of 20 mm. The 1-year postoperative radiographs demonstrate robust interbody fusion (▶ Fig. 4.76).

4.14.4 Previous Microdiscectomy with Facet Arthropathy and Foraminal Stenosis

A 51-year-old former collegiate swimmer presented 11 years after undergoing an L4–5 microdiscectomy for management of left L5 radiculopathy. At the time of presentation, the patient described left knee pain and left medial calf pain. He also reported more recent symptoms of neurogenic claudication, but the predominance of symptoms embodied left radicular leg pain. The patient had intact strength and normal sensory examination findings. He had a positive left straight leg raise test result and a negative right straight leg raise test result. His patellar and Achilles reflexes were 1 + bilaterally. A left L4 selective nerve root block alleviated a significant portion of his left-sided symptoms. A left L5 selective nerve root block also offered

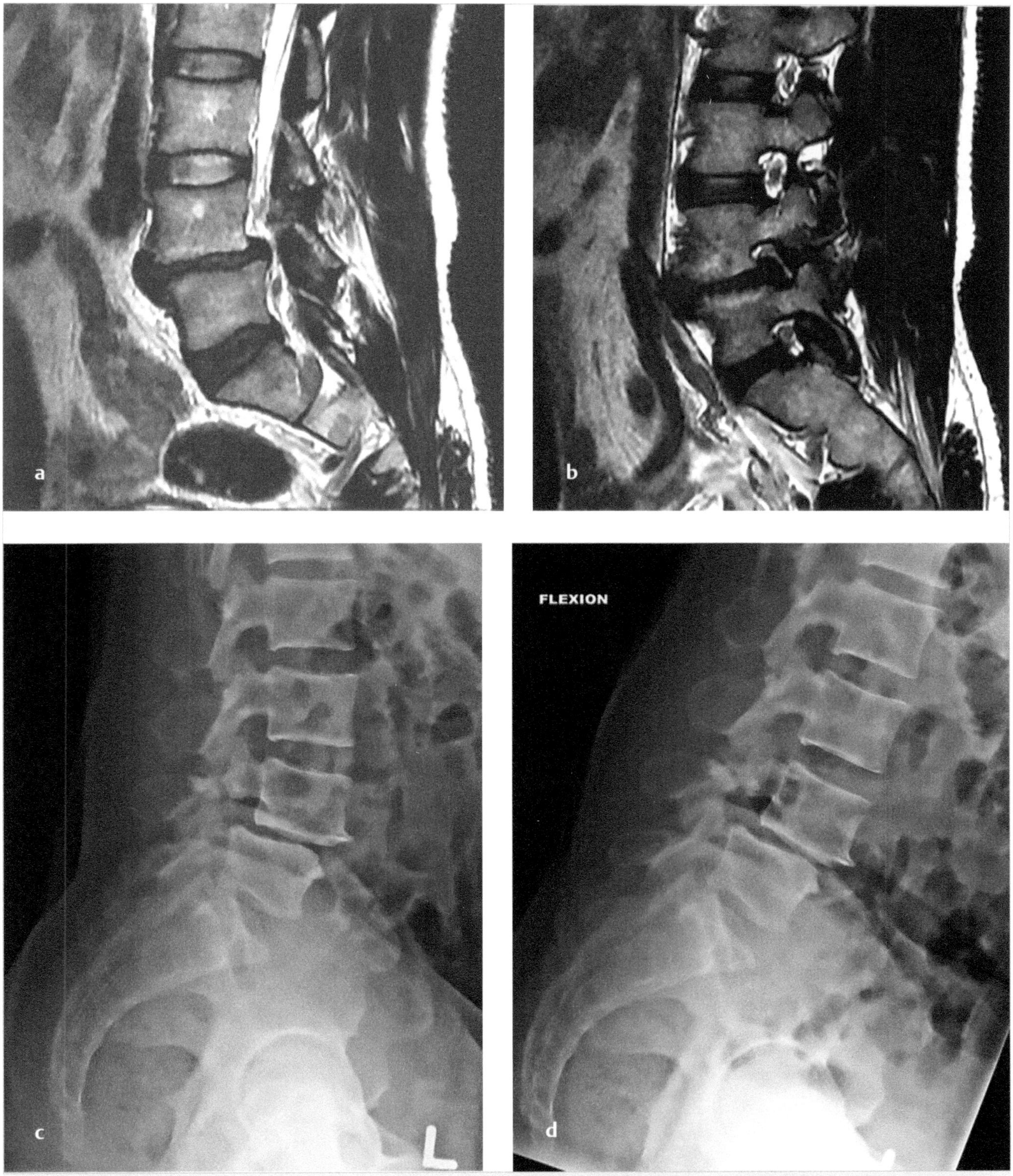

Fig. 4.74 Grade I mobile spondylolisthesis at L4-5. **(a)** Sagittal T2-weighted magnetic resonance imaging (MRI) demonstrating a grade I L4–5 spondylolisthesis resulting in moderate central stenosis. **(b)** Parasagittal T2-weighted MRI demonstrating severe foraminal compromise affecting the exiting nerve root of L4. **(c)** Extension and **(d)** flexion radiographs demonstrating subtle translation of the L4 vertebral body on L5, distraction of the posterior aspect of the disc space and collapse at the anterior aspect of the disc space.

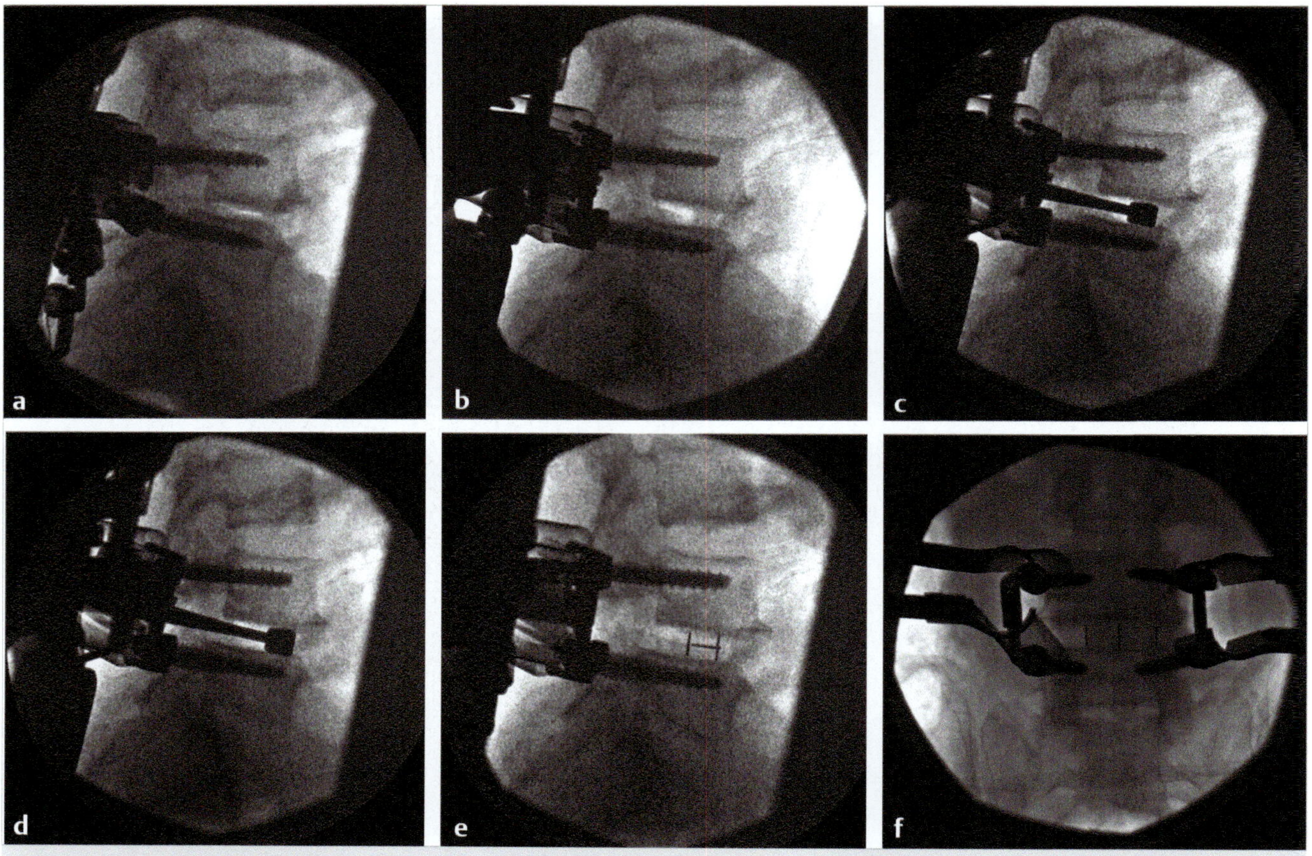

Fig. 4.75 Minimally invasive transforaminal lumbar interbody fusion for mobile grade I spondylolisthesis. **(a)** Lateral fluoroscopic image obtained after placement of pedicle screws into L4 and L5. **(b)** Lateral fluoroscopic image obtained after completing the discectomy and using a series of paddle distractors to restore disc space height. The ipsilateral provisional expandable rod is in position, capturing the restoration in disc height. **(c)** An 11-mm interbody trial is inserted to restore height. The trial is tapped across the disc space to the contralateral side, and the height is captured by tightening the set screw of L4; the L5 set screw had been tightened at the time of placement. **(d)** A larger 12-mm trial is tried to capture height and simultaneously restore alignment. The tactile feel of the 12-mm trial, along with comparing the height to the L3-4 segment, confirm that a 12-mm spacer is the ideal height to restore this interbody space. **(e)** Lateral fluoroscopic image demonstrating a 12-mm interbody spacer in position with morselized autograft anterior to the spacer. **(f)** Anteroposterior fluoroscopic image demonstrating a 36 × 12-mm spacer centered within the disc space. The ipsilateral expandable provisional rod is in position, maintaining the disc height captured by the trials.

relief. The preoperative ODI was 34, the VAS for leg pain was 80 mm and the VAS for back pain was 40 mm. Radiographic studies demonstrated stenosis at the L4–5 segment from facet arthropathy and foraminal compromise that affected the exiting nerve root of L4 on the left (▶ Fig. 4.77). Dynamic imaging confirmed instability (▶ Fig. 4.78).

4.14.5 Operative Intervention

The majority of the patient's symptoms were on the left side. The selective nerve root blocks at L4 and L5 demonstrated that his symptoms emanated from both nerve roots. Left transforaminal access would allow for decompression of the exiting L4 nerve root and the traversing L5 nerve root. The axial images demonstrate a facet cyst on the right, which can be readily accessed by undercutting the lamina and contralateral facet. A right-side Smith–Petersen osteotomy was performed at the L4–5 facet to allow for further reduction. A left transforaminal approach was undertaken with the technique described earlier. The disc space was restored to a 12-mm height. The size of the disc space and the position of the first interbody spacer allowed for nested interbody spacers to be placed (▶ Fig. 4.79).

4.14.6 Postoperative Course

The patient reported near-complete relief of his left radicular leg pain immediately after surgery. He was discharged later that same evening after ambulating and urinating without difficulty. He returned to working at his office 2 weeks after surgery. At 1 year, his ODI was 11, the VAS for back pain was 25 mm, and the VAS for leg pain was 10 mm, with radiographic evidence of union (▶ Fig. 4.80).

4.15 Complication Avoidance

Complications can arise at three distinct times in a minimally invasive TLIF: during surgery, in the early postoperative stage, and in the late postoperative stage. Understanding what these complications are and at what point they can potentially occur is the surest path to their avoidance.

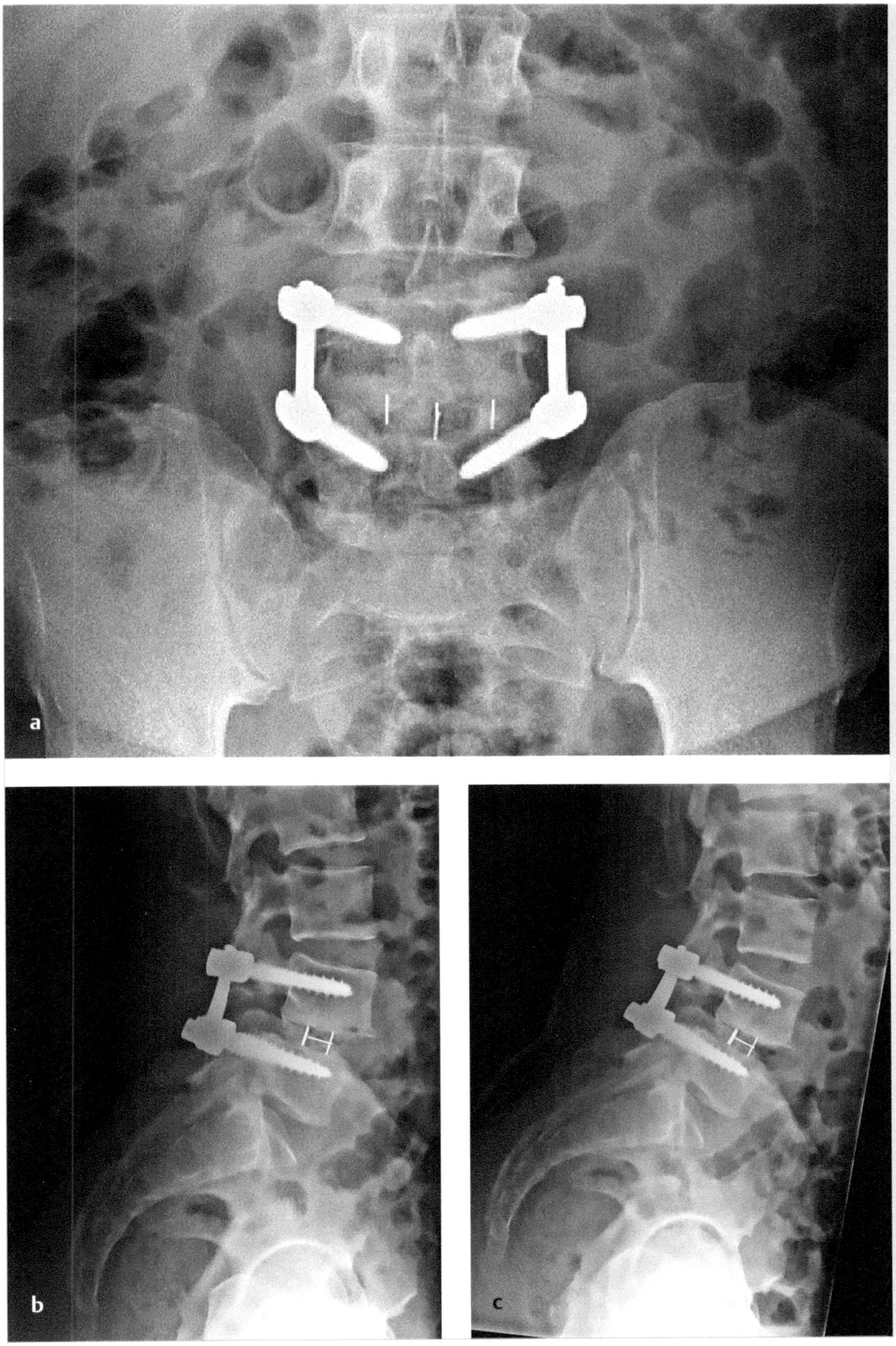

Fig. 4.76 Radiographic follow-up at 1 year for an L4–5 minimally invasive transforaminal lumbar interbody fusion. **(a)** Anteroposterior radiograph showing fusion within the interbody space. **(b)** Extension and **(c)** flexion radiographs showing the formation of a fusion mass within the interbody space and near anatomical alignment of the vertebral bodies.

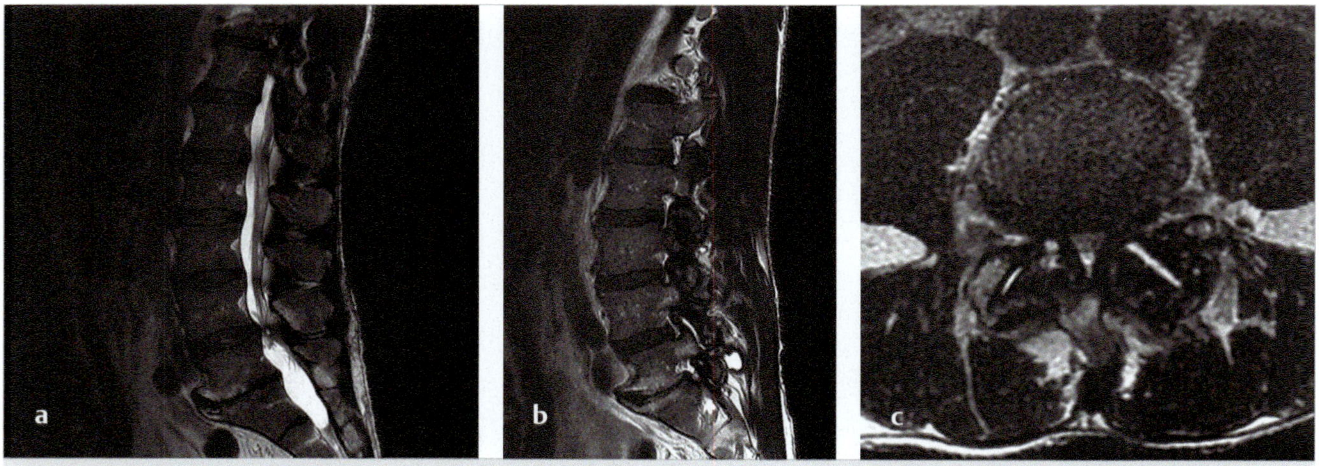

Fig. 4.77 Advanced facet arthropathy at L4–5 11 years after microdiscectomy. (a) Sagittal T2-weighted magnetic resonance imaging (MRI) demonstrating compression of the neural elements predominantly from the facet arthropathy and a facet cyst at L4–5. L5–S1 also shows advanced degeneration, but there was no correlation with clinical symptoms related to this level. (b) Parasagittal T2-weighted MRI revealing the extent of foraminal compression of the exiting nerve root of L4 on the left. The compression was due in large part to the overgrowth of the superior articular process. (c) Axial T2-weighted MRI at the L4–5 level showing central stenosis from ligamentum flavum hypertrophy and a right-sided facet cyst.

4.15.1 Avoidance of Immediate Complications

Immediate complications are those that occur at the time of surgery. These include errant placement of instrumentation, a dural tear and suboptimal decompression. A misplaced pedicle screw tends to be a consequence of exposure. The direct visualization of the junction of the pars interarticularis, inferolateral facet and mid-transverse process is essential. Proceeding with instrumentation without unequivocal visualization of that junction places you on a trajectory for a misplaced pedicle screw. Although I emphasize minimizing the use of fluoroscopy, in the beginning of your learning curve, you should always take the necessary images to safely instrument the spine. However, no amount of fluoroscopy will replace the information that direct visualization of the bony anatomy will provide, nor will it replace your capacity to reconstruct the anatomy at depth. Remember that the pedicle screw entry point will always be lateral to the pars interarticularis. When you clearly expose the pars interarticularis, the likelihood of a medial breach plummets.

There are several strategies I employ to mitigate the risk of a cerebrospinal fluid (CSF) leak. The first strategy is to perform all of the instrumentation prior to decompression. I drill, probe, tap and place all of the pedicle screws with the neural elements fully protected by the intact lamina, facets and pars interarticularis. Wielding sharp instruments with the neural elements exposed never made any sense to me. One inadvertent slip with the neural elements exposed changes the entire mood of the operation.

The second strategy is keeping the ligamentum flavum intact for all of the bone work. I hope by now I have been able to convince you of the benefit of the en bloc resection of the ligamentum flavum. As described in Section 4.11.3, Third Osteotomy Cut: Superior Articular Process and Conjoined Nerve Roots, I make every effort to keep the ligamentum flavum intact until I have completed all of the bone work. Working in the periphery of the canal with the drill and then completing an en bloc resection minimizes the number of passes with a Kerrison and therefore decreases the risk of an inadvertent durotomy. Drilling the superior aspect of the caudal lamina beyond the caudal insertion of the ligamentum flavum as described in Section 4.11.3, Third Osteotomy Cut: Superior Articular Process and Conjoined Nerve Roots, eliminates the risk of a Kerrison bite in the most constrained part of the canal. In my first 500 minimally invasive TLIFs, I have caused eight CSF leaks, five of which were caused when completing the decompression on the caudal aspect of the segment. Modifying my technique to expose and drill the superior aspect of the caudal lamina has further decreased the rate of CSF leaks.

Equally interesting is that six of the eight CSF leaks occurred between case 100 and 200. The caution I had during my first 100 cases was replaced by perhaps some overconfidence. Although my operative times went down, my complication rate went up. The increased rate of CSF leaks quickly put that confidence into check. I reassessed my technique and approach. I began to drill the lamina beyond the ligamentum flavum. I also found a better balance between my caution and confidence for my next few hundred cases, and my CSF leak rate declined once again. We all must remember that our next potential CSF leak is only one case away, and every effort should be made to mitigate that risk.

A suboptimal decompression is obvious immediately after surgery. The patient has persistent symptoms. Such a circumstance is painful for both the patient and the surgeon. A complete resection of the ligamentum flavum from insertion point to insertion point and pedicle to pedicle avoids a suboptimal decompression. Completing the systems check before proceeding to interbody spacer placement, specifically, palpating the pedicle and completing the foraminotomies over the nerve roots, mitigates the chances of overlooking persistent compression of the nerve root or thecal sac. Although rare, it is

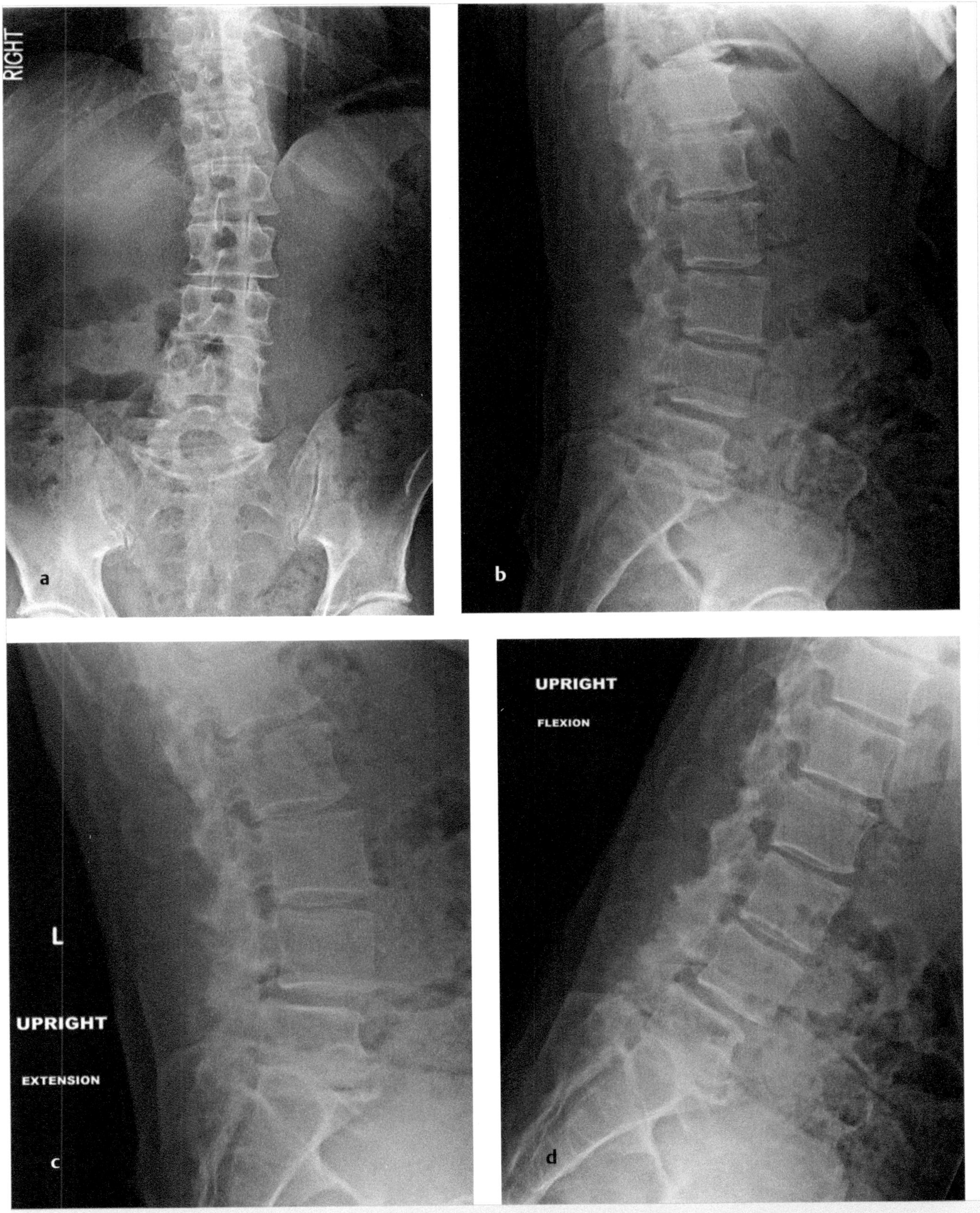

Fig. 4.78 Preoperative radiographs. **(a)** Anteroposterior radiograph demonstrating advanced degenerative disc disease at L4–5 with coronal imbalance to the left. **(b)** Lateral radiograph showing anterolisthesis of L4 on L5 and advanced degeneration at L5–S1. **(c)** Extension and **(d)** flexion radiographs demonstrating anterior translation of L4 on L5.

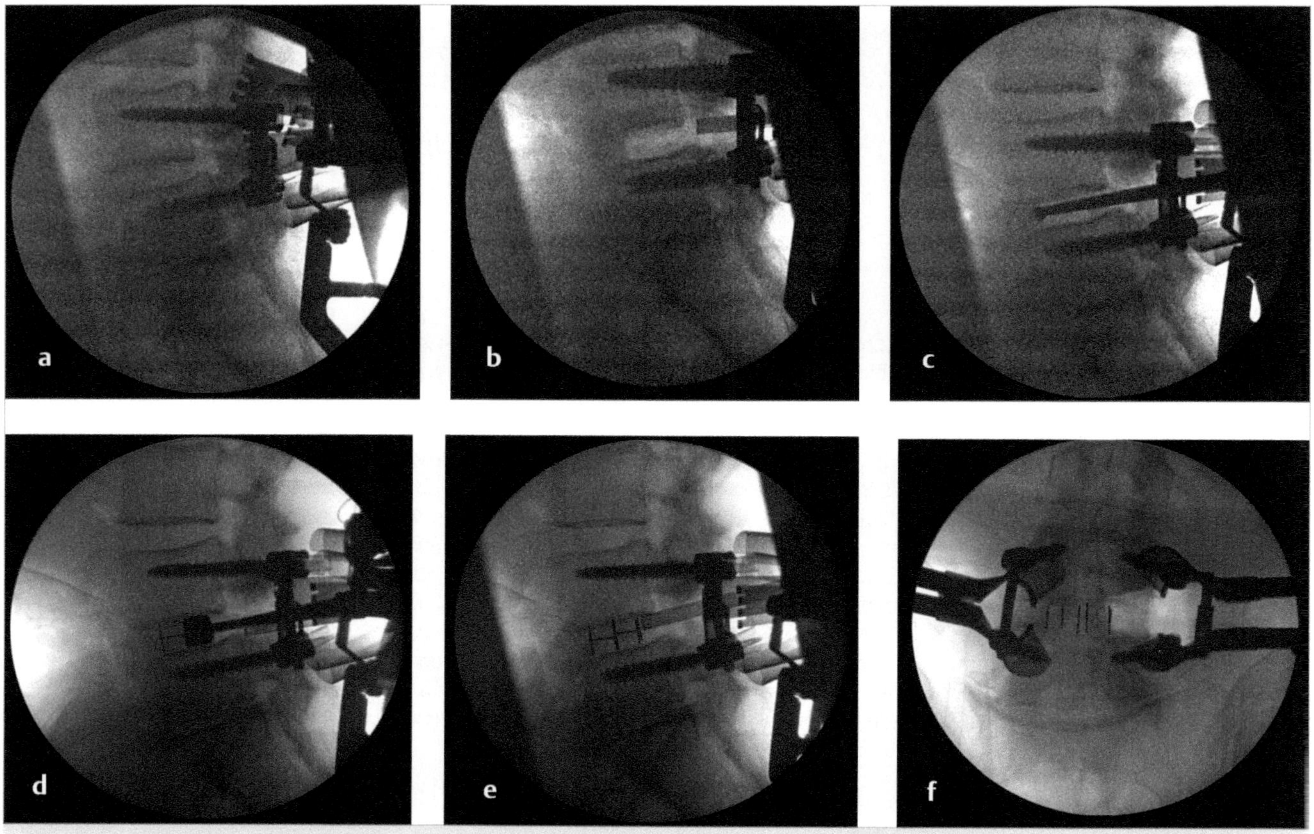

Fig. 4.79 Operative sequence for interbody placement. **(a)** Lateral fluoroscopic image demonstrating the L4–5 segment after placement of the pedicle screws. **(b)** Lateral fluoroscopic image showing the distraction of the disc space after discectomy. Note the segment has been distracted into kyphosis by the ipsilateral provisional expandable rod to meet the criteria set forth by Cloward regarding visualization of the end plates. A more complete preparation may be performed under direct visualization, and a larger interbody may be more easily placed. **(c)** Autograft harvested from the lamina and the facet may be secured in the anterior half of the disc space. **(d)** Given the position of the interbody spacer in the anterior aspect of the disc space, a second spacer may be inserted to occupy more disc space. **(e)** Lateral fluoroscopic image demonstrating two 12-mm nested interbody spacers in position. **(f)** Anteroposterior fluoroscopic image showing the centered interbody spacers.

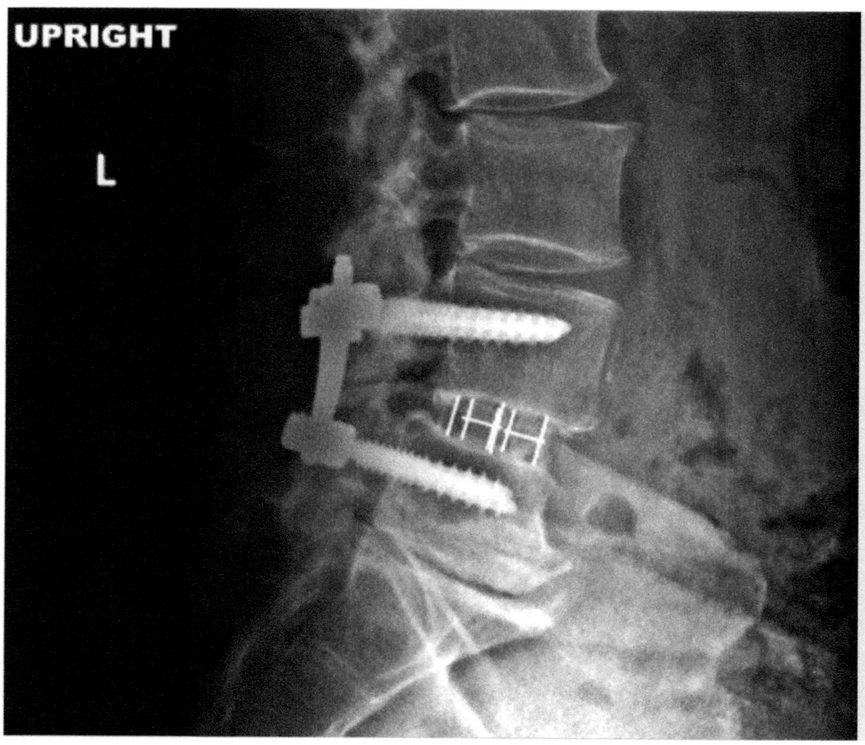

Fig. 4.80 Lateral radiograph 1 year postoperatively shows mature interbody fusion.

sometimes necessary to perform bilateral decompressions that include bilateral facetectomies to adequately address the extent of compression of the neural elements. Such a complication may be avoided by careful history taking, thorough neurological examination and careful review of the parasagittal T1-weighted MRIs showing the foramen.

4.15.2 Early Postoperative Phase

Migration of the interbody graft is a potential complication in the early postoperative phase. Migration occurs for two reasons. The first is an undersized graft and the second is a violation of the cortical end plate. It is vital to sense a firm placement of the interbody trial. It is worth repeating that it should require a slap hammer to dislodge the trial from its position to deem the height to be appropriate. You should not be able to pull it out by hand. In my experience, it is much less likely that a curved interbody spacer rotated into position will migrate than a straight spacer, especially when placed under compression. The action of compression further engages the graft–end-plate interface. Bullet-shaped grafts may extrude along the same path they were inserted. A curved graft rotated into position is much less likely to do so because it is inserted along various vector paths that would be difficult to re-create in reverse. Finally, distracting the pedicle screws, as recommended by Harms, opens the disc space and allows for a larger interbody spacer. Similar to distraction of the Caspar posts in the cervical spine that allow for a tight-fitting graft when the distraction is released, provisional distraction of the disc space facilitates placement of a larger interbody spacer and a tighter fit when the distraction is released. The combination of a larger implant rotated into position under distraction followed by release of the distraction and compression of the implant creates an environment very resistant to migration.

4.15.3 Late Postoperative Phase

Pseudarthrosis and adjacent level degeneration are late-stage complications of the TLIF regardless of the technique chosen. Pseudarthrosis and migration of the graft often walk hand in hand. The measures mentioned in the previous section, 4.15.2, Early Postoperative Phase, to mitigate the risk of graft migration and extrusion are the same measures needed to prevent pseudarthrosis. It is important to recognize that a pseudarthrosis may occur with a well-positioned interbody graft that has not migrated. Under that circumstance, it is likely that the cartilaginous end plate was not completely removed from either the inferior or superior end plate or both. In such a case, the interbody is wedged between two sheets of cartilaginous end plate, which reliably blocks the growth of bone. The preparation of the end plate requires a tactile feel and also has a visual component. Although it is difficult to directly visualize the end plate, in the process of removing the disc material and preparing the end plate, you may experience entire sheets of the cartilaginous end plates coming out of the disc space. When you can feel the unmistakable tactile feeling of rasping against cortical bone compared to cartilaginous end plate, you know end plate preparation is complete. The end plate preparation phase should never be rushed. The time invested in end plate preparation pays immediate dividends by mitigating the risk of a pseudarthrosis.

Adjacent segment degeneration may be difficult to avoid altogether since it is an element of the natural history of lumbar disc degeneration. Still, certain measures may be taken to mitigate that risk. Minimizing the extent of exposure is the first measure. The advantage of a minimally invasive approach is the capacity to perform a procedure without the wide exposures that can weaken muscle and cause inadvertent injury to the surrounding structures. The second measure is respecting the integrity of the facet capsule of the rostral level. Although it is essential to expose the inferior and lateral aspects of the rostral facet to expose the pedicle screw entry point, that exposure does not require violating the facet capsule. Beginning on the transverse process and working in the lateral to medial direction is the surest way to prevent inadvertent disruption of the facet capsule.

Lastly, you must incorporate the spinopelvic parameters into your operative plan. Every effort must be taken to optimize segmental lordosis. A pelvic incidence and lumbar lordosis mismatch should be a central component of your operative plan. Biomechanical and clinical studies have both demonstrated the importance of segmental lordosis.[7,23] The combination of a large interbody spacer, complete facetectomy on one side and a Smith–Petersen osteotomy on the other is the surest technique to optimize lordosis, and it bolsters the argument for bilateral minimal access ports to complete bilateral posterior column osteotomies.

4.16 Conclusions

In my experience, the frustrations faced by surgeons when performing a minimally invasive TLIF come as a consequence of not having a purposeful familiarity with the anatomy from a paramedian approach. The eye cannot see what the unprepared mind is not yet capable of comprehending. Staring downward into a narrow corridor at an unfamiliar angle and looking at a limited field of view consisting of equal parts of muscle and bony prominence is harrowing. Nothing replaces the familiarity that can only be achieved by working through small-diameter minimal access ports at various angles, first by decompressing a single nerve root and then decompressing the entire thecal sac. This familiarity becomes the foothold from which the surgeon may step in and feel comfortable within a more lateral exposure and begin to instrument the spine. Performing a minimally invasive lumbar interbody fusion is the realization of a skill set developed through those microdiscectomies and then laminectomies discussed in the previous two chapters. It is this experience that ultimately produces the confidence and reliability with the procedure so that it can be safely and efficiently performed as effectively as its open counterpart. The minimally invasive TLIF also becomes the firmest of footholds for the next chapter, Minimally Invasive Far Lateral Microdiscectomy. Your eyes will now see what your mind has been well prepared to comprehend.

References

[1] Isaacs RE, Podichetty VK, Santiago P, et al. Minimally invasive microendoscopy-assisted transforaminal lumbar interbody fusion with instrumentation. J Neurosurg Spine. 2005; 3(2):98–105

[2] Holly LT, Schwender JD, Rouben DP, Foley KT. Minimally invasive transforaminal lumbar interbody fusion: indications, technique, and complications. Neurosurg Focus. 2006; 20(3):E6

[3] Mummaneni PV, Rodts GE, Jr. The mini-open transforaminal lumbar interbody fusion. Neurosurgery. 2005; 57(4) Suppl:256–261, discussion 256–261
[4] Hsieh PC, Koski TR, O'Shaughnessy BA, et al. Anterior lumbar interbody fusion in comparison with transforaminal lumbar interbody fusion: implications for the restoration of foraminal height, local disc angle, lumbar lordosis, and sagittal balance. J Neurosurg Spine. 2007; 7(4):379–386
[5] La Marca F, Brumblay H. Smith-Petersen osteotomy in thoracolumbar deformity surgery. Neurosurgery. 2008; 63(3) Suppl:163–170
[6] Smith-Petersen MN, Larson CB, Aufranc OE. Osteotomy of the spine for correction of flexion deformity in rheumatoid arthritis. Clin Orthop Relat Res. 1969; 66(66):6–9
[7] Tempel ZJ, Gandhoke GS, Bolinger BD, et al. The influence of pelvic incidence and lumbar lordosis mismatch on development of symptomatic adjacent level disease following single-level transforaminal lumbar interbody fusion. Neurosurgery. 2017; 80(6):880–886
[8] Jagannathan J, Sansur CA, Oskouian RJ, Jr, Fu KM, Shaffrey CI. Radiographic restoration of lumbar alignment after transforaminal lumbar interbody fusion. Neurosurgery. 2009; 64(5):955–963, discussion 963–964
[9] Lenke LG, Padberg AM, Russo MH, Bridwell KH, Gelb DE. Triggered electromyographic threshold for accuracy of pedicle screw placement. An animal model and clinical correlation. Spine. 1995; 20(14):1585–1591
[10] Raynor BL, Lenke LG, Bridwell KH, Taylor BA, Padberg AM. Correlation between low triggered electromyographic thresholds and lumbar pedicle screw malposition: analysis of 4857 screws. Spine. 2007; 32(24):2673–2678
[11] Harms J, Jeszenszky D. The unilateral, transforaminal approach for posterior lumbar interbody fusion. Orthop Traumatol. 1998; 6(2):88–99
[12] Harms J, Rolinger H. A one-stager procedure in operative treatment of spondylolistheses: dorsal traction-reposition and anterior fusion (author's transl) [in German]. Z Orthop Ihre Grenzgeb. 1982; 120(3):343–347
[13] Kambin P, Casey K, O'Brien E, Zhou L. Transforaminal arthroscopic decompression of lateral recess stenosis. J Neurosurg. 1996; 84(3):462–467
[14] Tumialán LM, Madhavan K, Godzik J, Wang MY. The history of and controversy over Kambin's triangle: a historical analysis of the lumbar transforaminal corridor for endoscopic and surgical approaches. World Neurosurg. 2019; 123:402–408
[15] Kambin P, Gennarelli T, Hermantin F. Minimally invasive techniques in spinal surgery: current practice. Neurosurg Focus. 1998; 4(2):e8
[16] Kambin P. History of surgical management of herniated lumbar discs from cauterization to arthroscopic and endoscopic spinal surgery. In: Kambin P. (ed) Arthroscopic and Endoscopic Spinal Surgery. Humana Press, 2005.
[17] Cloward RB. The treatment of ruptured lumbar intervertebral discs by vertebral body fusion. I. Indications, operative technique, after care. J Neurosurg. 1953; 10(2):154–168
[18] Grant JP, Oxland TR, Dvorak MF. Mapping the structural properties of the lumbosacral vertebral endplates. Spine. 2001; 26(8):889–896
[19] Lowe TG, Hashim S, Wilson LA, et al. A biomechanical study of regional endplate strength and cage morphology as it relates to structural interbody support. Spine. 2004; 29(21):2389–2394
[20] Soriano-Baron H, Newcomb AG, Malhotra D, et al. Biomechanics of nested transforaminal lumbar interbody cages. Neurosurgery. 2016; 78(2):297–304
[21] Panjabi MM, Goel V, Oxland T, et al. Human lumbar vertebrae. Quantitative three-dimensional anatomy. Spine. 1992; 17(3):299–306
[22] Wong AP, Smith ZA, Nixon AT, et al. Intraoperative and perioperative complications in minimally invasive transforaminal lumbar interbody fusion: a review of 513 patients. J Neurosurg Spine. 2015; 22(5):487–495
[23] Zhao X, Du L, Xie Y, Zhao J. Effect of lumbar lordosis on the adjacent segment in transforaminal lumbar interbody fusion: a finite element analysis. World Neurosurg. 2018; 114(Feb):e114–e120
[24] Cloward RB. Posterior Lumbar Interbody Fusion (P.L.I.F.) Surgical Techniques. 1988; Honolulu, HI: Cloward Instrument Corporation

5 Minimally Invasive Far Lateral Microdiscectomy

Abstract
The minimally invasive far lateral microdiscectomy takes the surgeon far from the midline of the spine. The inevitable result is the greatest potential for disorientation of all of the minimally invasive procedures I have described thus far in this Primer. However, expertise with the minimally invasive transforaminal lumbar interbody fusion lays the foundation for a level of immediate comfort and familiarity working within a focal but limited exposure of the lateral lumbar spine that is immediately on top of the neural foramen. This chapter details the evolution, anatomical basis and operative techniques of the minimally invasive far lateral microdiscectomy. Case illustrations are presented to reinforce the concepts introduced in the chapter.

Keywords: far lateral disc herniation, foramen, lumbar, pars interarticularis, radiculopathy, transforaminal lumbar interbody fusion

Man cannot discover new oceans unless he has the courage to lose sight of the shore.

Andre Gide

5.1 Introduction

It is no accident that this chapter falls immediately after the chapter on transforaminal lumbar interbody fusion (TLIF) instead of after the chapter on microdiscectomy. After all, it was the transforaminal approach that made me comfortable working lateral to the pars, in the vicinity of the transverse process and immediately over the top of the exiting nerve root. Admittedly, the first few times I endeavored upon this approach, I was lost, completely lost. The principle I introduced earlier in this Primer regarding the distance from the midline and the capacity to maintain your orientation rings especially true for this procedure. Of all the minimally invasive procedures, it is the far lateral microdiscectomy that takes you farthest from the midline, with limited exposure of the target. It is that combination that has the potential to disorient the uninitiated mind. The root cause of this disorientation is the complete absence of the orienting midline structures. For example, with transforaminal exposures, the confluence of the lamina into the spinous process and visualization of the entire facet help you keep your bearings. For a far lateral microdiscectomy, a limited glimpse of the lateral pars interarticularis and the inferior aspect of the transverse process are all you have to orient your mind to the anatomy that lies before you. The far lateral microdiscectomy is the one case in which you undeniably lose sight of the shore. You must navigate by something other than the structures of the midline. Even the familiar paramedian structure of the facet, which guides the entire basis of the exposure for the minimally invasive TLIF, is not in the field of view, nor should it be.

Over the years, I have found that it is the facility that I developed with transforaminal approaches that taught me the far lateral microdiscectomy technique. The transforaminal approaches helped familiarize my mind with the unique topography of the lateral lumbar spine. As I became more comfortable exposing the pars interarticularis and decompressing the exiting nerve root in TLIFs, decompression of the exiting nerve root without removal of the pars became a more feasible concept for my mind to grasp. Working under the microscope case after case, I gained an appreciation for the way that the pars interarticularis blended into the transverse process and the superior articular process (▶ Fig. 5.1). Alongside the comfort I had with the exposure, I applied the principles of the medial microdiscectomy to the far lateral microdiscectomy. In particular, I sought to preserve as much of the native spine as possible while safely exposing and mobilizing the neural elements to decompress them.

One of the challenges I encountered was that far lateral disc herniations were much less common than medial disc herniations in my practice. I found the ratio of medial microdiscectomies to far lateral microdiscectomies over 10 years of practice was 30:1. I thought the scarcity of these cases would limit my ability to rapidly gain a facility with this technique. I soon realized that the paucity of far lateral disc extrusions would not affect my ability to acquire proficiency with this operation. The skill set for this operation originates from the transforaminal approach more so than the medial microdiscectomy. Developing that transforaminal skill set provided me with the foundation to achieve a greater understanding of the subtleties of the anatomy of the far lateral recess and readily translate that knowledge to the far lateral microdiscectomy. This procedure is effectively a miniature and lateral form of the transforaminal approach. The goal of the procedure is to identify the exiting root and remove the far lateral disc herniation while preserving as much of the lateral bony anatomy as possible. This chapter describes how to do just that. I begin by discussing the remarkable history of radiculopathy caused by a far lateral disc herniation, before describing in detail the anatomy of the foramen and the lateral lumbar spine. Finally, I present the operative technique with representative case presentations. Although this procedure builds on the familiarity of the transforaminal approach, it has its unique subtleties and nuances, which I describe in detail in the upcoming pages to help you navigate those unfamiliar waters so far off the shore.

5.2 Far Lateral Microdiscectomy: A Perspective

When it comes to the far lateral microdiscectomy with a lateral extraforaminal approach, I can no longer fathom an open operation that begins in the midline. I recall the two traditional open Wiltse approaches I performed during my residency, one for a schwannoma and the other for a far lateral disc extrusion. Both of these exposures were extensive, bloody, and disorienting. I recall the degree of discomfort that each of these patients had in the aftermath of the operation, and I cannot help but think of the wise words written by Caspar four decades ago regarding the ratio of a surgical target to a surgical exposure. Even my colleagues who question whether there is a benefit to a minimally invasive microdiscectomy for a paracentral disc

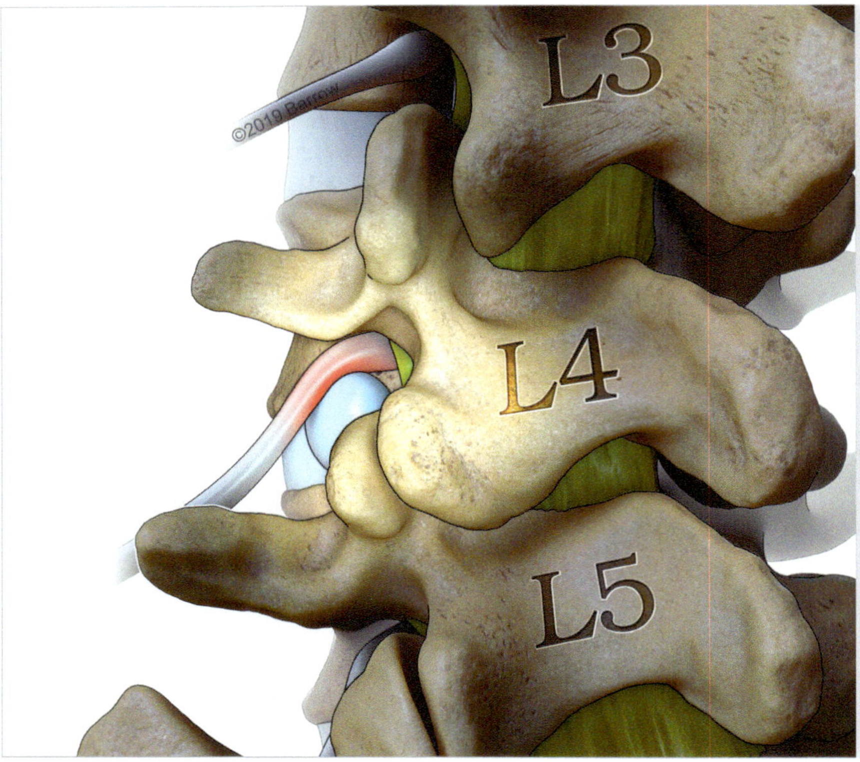

Fig. 5.1 Anatomy of the far lateral recess of the lumbar spine. Illustration demonstrating the compression of the nerve root in the far lateral recess at L4–5 on the left. The key to the entire operation is the pedicle, but the pedicle cannot be immediately appreciated from the surface anatomy. The junction of the pars interarticularis, transverse process and the inferior lateral facet are the surface anatomical landmarks that guide you to the pedicle. The lateral aspect of the pars interarticularis safely guides you into the foramen. In this manner, identification and mobilization of the nerve root allow for a safe corridor onto the far lateral disc herniation.

herniation readily concede that the best manner to address pathology in the far lateral recess of the lumbar spine is with a minimally invasive approach. Docking a minimal access port on the far lateral aspect of the spine immediately over the affected exiting root is perhaps the most efficient and effective manner to decompress a nerve root flattened by a far lateral disc herniation. The exposure of the surgical target may be reliably achieved through a 16-mm access port and results in a favorable Caspar ratio of nearly 1:1. In comparison, a traditional Wiltse approach, where the exposure would be several times the size of the surgical target, becomes difficult to conceive. Nevertheless, every operation has its own story of evolution, which reflects the challenges that faced surgeons attempting to treat patients suffering from radiculopathies. Buried within that history are kernels of insight that provide perspective for your study of the far lateral microdiscectomy. With that statement in mind, I feel that the next few pages are an invaluable element of understanding the far lateral microdiscectomy.

5.3 Historical Perspective

What a diagnostic conundrum far lateral disc herniations must have been at the dawn of our specialty. In the early 20th century, the rudimentary diagnostic imaging with intrathecal Lipiodol (Guerbet, Villepinte, France) or air as contrast media provided surgeons a limited view of the thecal sac, nerve roots, and potential sights of compression relative to the bony anatomy. Such imaging offered a line of sight limited to neural elements in the midline and just off the midline. In light of these limitations and the potential morbidity of the diagnostic imaging itself, the emphasis was on the localization of the nerve root compression by clinical examination. A patient who had classic L4 radiculopathy would undergo an L3–4 midline microdiscectomy by a well-intended surgeon whose clinical examination unequivocally demonstrated an L4 nerve root compression syndrome. That empty feeling created by retracting the nerve root without extrusion of a disc fragment revealing itself is a feeling only a spine surgeon knows. I can sympathetically envision that early spine surgeon taking time to reassess whatever primitive imaging they had, perhaps asking the operating room nurse to read aloud the clinical note to ensure the correct laterality. All the while, that surgeon was correct in his clinical assessment. The L4 nerve root was indeed compressed, but not as it traversed the L3–4 disc space. The compression was in the far lateral recess as the nerve root exited beneath the pedicle. A far lateral disc herniation had unfurled from the L4–5 segment and compressed the exiting L4 nerve root. The surgeon's assessment of the nerve root compression syndrome was correct. The surgeon was just looking in the wrong place. However, in the early 20th century, there was no imaging capability to unveil that blind spot.

Walter Dandy's[1] mention of "concealed discs" in his 1942 publication regarding the advancements in the management of disc herniations may have been the first acknowledgment of the existence of far lateral disc herniations, although certainly not recognized as such at the time. Dandy, along with his early pioneering colleagues, identified a group of patients who presented with classic nerve root compression syndromes, yet had negative findings at the time of surgery. Consistent with our current knowledge of far lateral disc herniations, the incidence was in the vicinity of 10%.[1,2,3] With our current technology, it is almost impossible to imagine venturing into the operating room with nothing more than a clinical examination and 5 mL of intrathecal ethiodized oil (Lipiodol) injected before an X-ray of the lumbar spine. At the time, surgeons looked where they could see, and they could see compression only in the vicinity of the central canal. Contrast media in the thecal sac could reveal compression of the midline and structures in the lateral recess. No imaging at that time shed light on the far lateral recess; therefore, surgeons did not venture into that vicinity, at least at first.

The simple law of percentages suggests that a number of those segments exposed based on the clinical examination and limited radiographic imaging may have indeed harbored a disc herniation that resided in the far lateral recess. In 1949, Echols and Rehfeldt[2] suggested the possibility of foraminal compression by a far lateral disc herniation. In their thoughtful analysis of 32 patients who had negative findings at the time of surgery, these surgeons concluded that in the event of a negative exploration, the nerve root should be explored outside of the foramen. Of course, that particular approach would require a facetectomy and the potential need for fusion.

It was not until 1971, when Macnab[3] wrote an article entitled "Negative disc exploration," that the first formal description of extraforaminal disc extrusions entered the literature. Macnab described a patient with a clear L5 nerve root compression syndrome who had complete relief with a selective nerve root block at L5. An L4–5 microdiscectomy failed to reveal the expected disc herniation, but confident in his diagnosis, he ventured into the foramen after removing the entire facet and found "the root engulfed and almost buried in a diffuse lateral bulge of the disc." Macnab[3] appropriately labeled the location of the far lateral disc herniation the "hidden zone." The sacrifice of the facet required a posterolateral fusion, but the operation relieved the patient's radiculopathy. ▶ Fig. 5.2[3] from Macnab's study captures the essence of the anatomical circumstance beautifully.

Despite the recognition of this clinical entity, diagnostic challenges remained in the era before magnetic resonance imaging (MRI) and computed tomography (CT). In 1974, Abdullah and colleagues[4] published a compelling argument for using discography for the diagnosis of far lateral disc herniations. Despite the absence of a surgical technique section in their study, they appear to be the first who recommended a simple discectomy instead of a complete facetectomy.

The introduction of CT vastly facilitated the recognition and diagnosis of far lateral disc herniation, and as a result, several technique papers began to populate the literature. A 1988 publication, again by Abdullah and colleagues,[5] details the operative technique, which they applied to 138 cases. Not surprisingly, the recommended approach was medial to lateral, an approach that builds on the familiarity of the midline structures and extends laterally (▶ Fig. 5.3).[5] In subsequent years, authors began to explore lateral to medial approaches. Surgical series describing the various surgical approaches began to populate the literature. The medial facetectomy, trans-pars interarticularis and extraforaminal and intertransverse process approaches were all reported for the management of far lateral disc herniation.[6,7,8]

Wiltse and Spencer,[9] Maroon et al[10] and Jane et al[11] were among the first to recommend a lateral to medial approach for the management of far lateral disc herniations via an extraforaminal inter-transverse process approach. One look at the illustrations from their technique brings immediately to mind the statement made by Caspar[12] regarding the ratio of exposure to the surgical target (▶ Fig. 5.4).[10,12] With the surgical target defined as the area from the pedicle to the disc space, the surgical exposure required with conventional retractors far exceeds the 10 × 6 mm of the surgical target as determined by Reulen and colleagues[13] in their anatomical study of the lateral approach, which had a very unfavorable Caspar ratio.

By 1997, Foley and Smith[14] had already introduced the use of minimal access ports for the management of paramedian disc herniations. Applying that same technique and those access ports to the lateral spine would be the natural solution to reconcile the unfavorable Caspar ratio for the exposure needed to treat a far lateral disc herniation. Foley and colleagues[15] turned

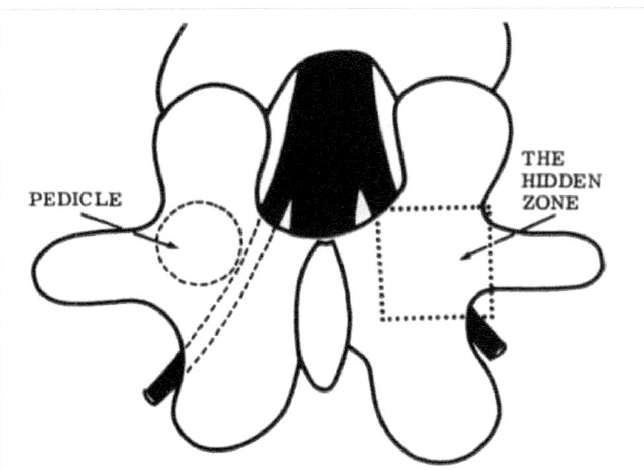

Fig. 5.2 The hidden zone. Illustration from Macnab[3] (1971), where he identifies the hidden zone as the location where a far lateral disc herniation would be found. (Reproduced with permission from Macnab I. Negative disc exploration. An analysis of the causes of nerve-root involvement in sixty-eight patients. J Bone Joint Surg Am. 1971; 53:891–903.)

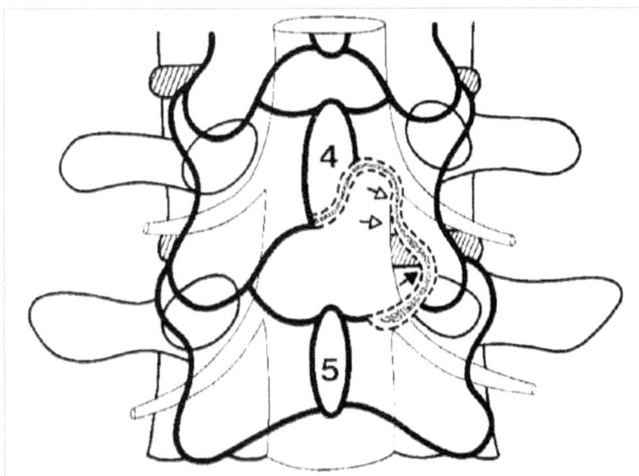

Fig. 5.3 Surgical management of a far lateral disc herniation. Illustration of the medial-to-lateral surgical technique employed by Abdullah and colleagues[5] in 1988. (Reproduced with permission from Abdullah AF, Wolber PG, Warfield JR, et al. Surgical management of extreme lateral lumbar disc herniations: review of 138 cases. Neurosurgery. 1988; 22:648–653.)

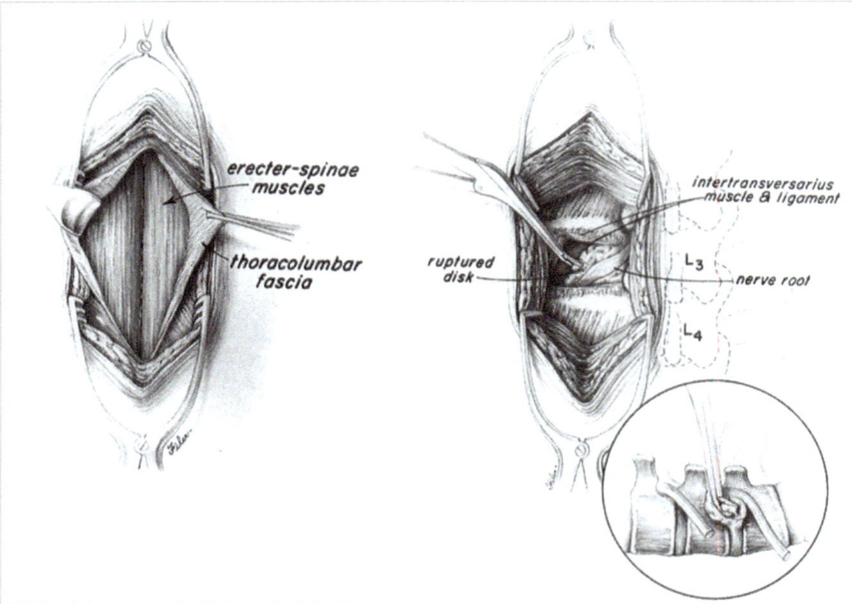

Fig. 5.4 Illustration of the far lateral technique through a paramedian incision as described by Maroon et al.[10] Adhering to the principle of the Caspar ratio[12] (i.e., minimizing the ratio of surgical target to the surgical exposure), one must consider a more focal exposure of the lateral spine. (Reproduced with permission from Maroon JC, Kopitnik TA, Schulhof LA, et al. Diagnosis and microsurgical approach to far-lateral disc herniation in the lumbar spine. J Neurosurg. 1990; 72:378–382.)

their access ports to the far lateral recess and 2 short years after their initial manuscript, they published their series on the minimally invasive management of far lateral disc herniations. They demonstrated the efficacy and, especially, the efficiency of a minimally invasive far lateral approach. Since that publication, surgeons have populated the literature with several series applying minimally invasive techniques to the treatment of far lateral disc herniation. The use of the minimal access port to approach the lateral spine for removal of a far lateral disc herniation through an extraforaminal approach is the focus of this chapter.

5.4 Anatomical Basis of the Minimally Invasive Approach

The key to the far lateral microdiscectomy is the pedicle that corresponds to the compressed nerve root. Identification of that pedicle brings into focus the orientation, confirms the boundaries of the foramen, helps identify the nerve root safely and unveils the disc extrusion. For this operation, the pedicle is the North Star in the absence of the shoreline. In symptomatic far lateral disc herniations, the disc herniation typically displaces the nerve root upward against the pedicle (▶ Fig. 5.1). In the lumbar spine, the nerve root exits below its like-numbered pedicle (i.e., the L4 nerve root exits below the L4 pedicle). Therefore, one must find the pedicle first and sift through a sea of epidural fat and engorged crimson veins after resecting the lateral aspect of the ligamentum flavum to identify the symptomatic nerve root. The final element of the exposure is to identify the disc extrusion and the actual disc space. A thoughtful examination of the anatomical basis of the minimally invasive approach provides the framework for understanding, learning and applying this technique.

The ideal diameter for the access port in the far lateral microdiscectomy is 16 mm. That diameter provides a metric to compare to the anatomy at depth relative to the diameter of the exposure. Knowledge of the various anatomical distances will help reconstruct the anatomy of the spine at depth in your mind's eye. An aptitude for mental reconstruction of the spinal anatomy is helpful in all cases, but this mental ability is especially advantageous in the far lateral microdiscectomy. In the absence of the midline structures, the potential for disorientation through such a limited field of view remains high. The anatomical studies by Reulen et al[13] and Schlesinger et al[16] fill the void of our limited experience in the lateral spine and are essential reading for this procedure.

If one were to deconstruct the anatomy of the lumbar spine in the lateral and AP projections, one could examine the far lateral microdiscectomy from the inside out (▶ Fig. 5.5). In particular, we could begin with the anatomic measurements of the neural foramen of the affected root.

5.5 Anatomy of the Lumbar Neural Foramen

The distance between the pedicles above and below a nerve root determines the rostrocaudal dimension of the neural foramen (▶ Fig. 5.6). Logically, the distance between the pedicles becomes the first measurement we need to examine to establish the anatomical basis for the far lateral microdiscectomy. That interpedicular distance, as measured from the bottom of the rostral pedicle to the top of the caudal pedicle, is seldom greater than 18 mm (range, 14–20 mm from caudal to rostral). Although this distance is inherently linked to the disc space height, because of lordosis, the level has a bigger impact than one might think (i.e., it is less at L5–S1 and more at L3–4). Intuitively, we know that the interpedicular distance is greater in the upper segments of the spine and decreases as we proceed to the sacrum. For instance, we know that we will likely need a 40- or 45-mm rod to connect the L3 pedicle to the L4 pedicle, whereas at L5–S1, a 30-mm rod will be more than adequate. Various anatomical studies have confirmed that intuition.

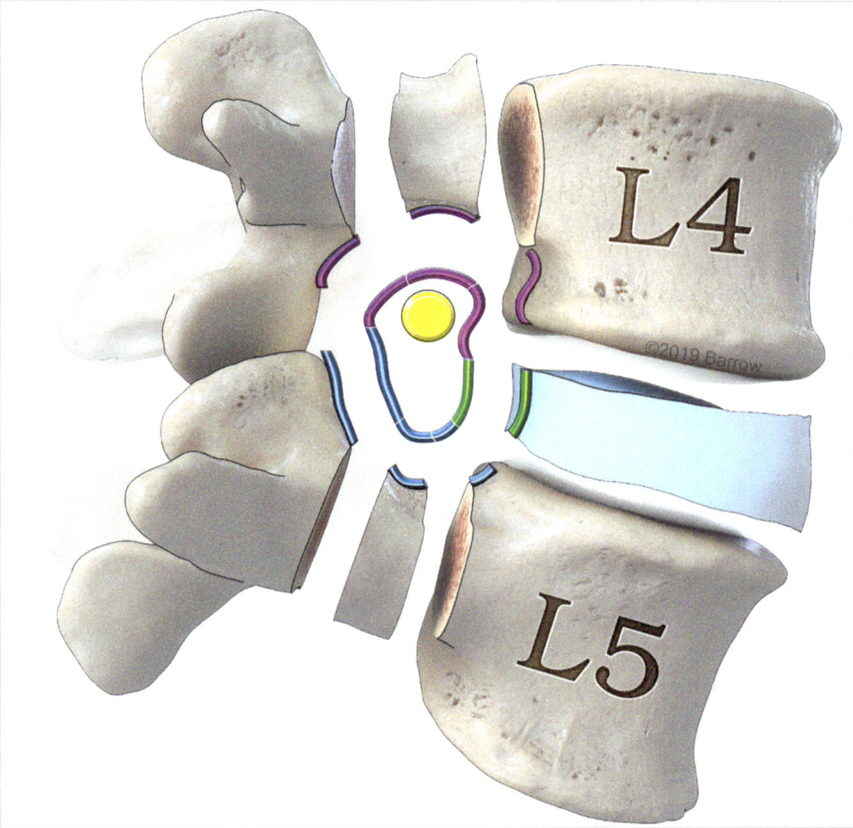

Fig. 5.5 Illustration of the deconstructed neural foramen of L4 represented by a multicolored ring. Each color represents the relative contributions of the rostral and caudal vertebral bodies, as well as the disc space, to the foramen. The posterior wall of the rostral vertebral body and disc space make up most of the anterior neuroforamen. There is little contribution to the neuroforamen by the posterior wall of the caudal vertebral body. The superior and inferior pedicles correspond with the superior and inferior boundaries of the neuroforamen. The superior articular and inferior articular processes make up the posterior aspect of the neuroforamen. The *turquoise* color of the ring represents the contribution from the L5 vertebral body, pedicle and superior articular process. The *magenta* color of the ring represents the contribution from the L4 pedicle, vertebral body and inferior articular facet. The *emerald* color of the ring represents the contribution from the disc space.

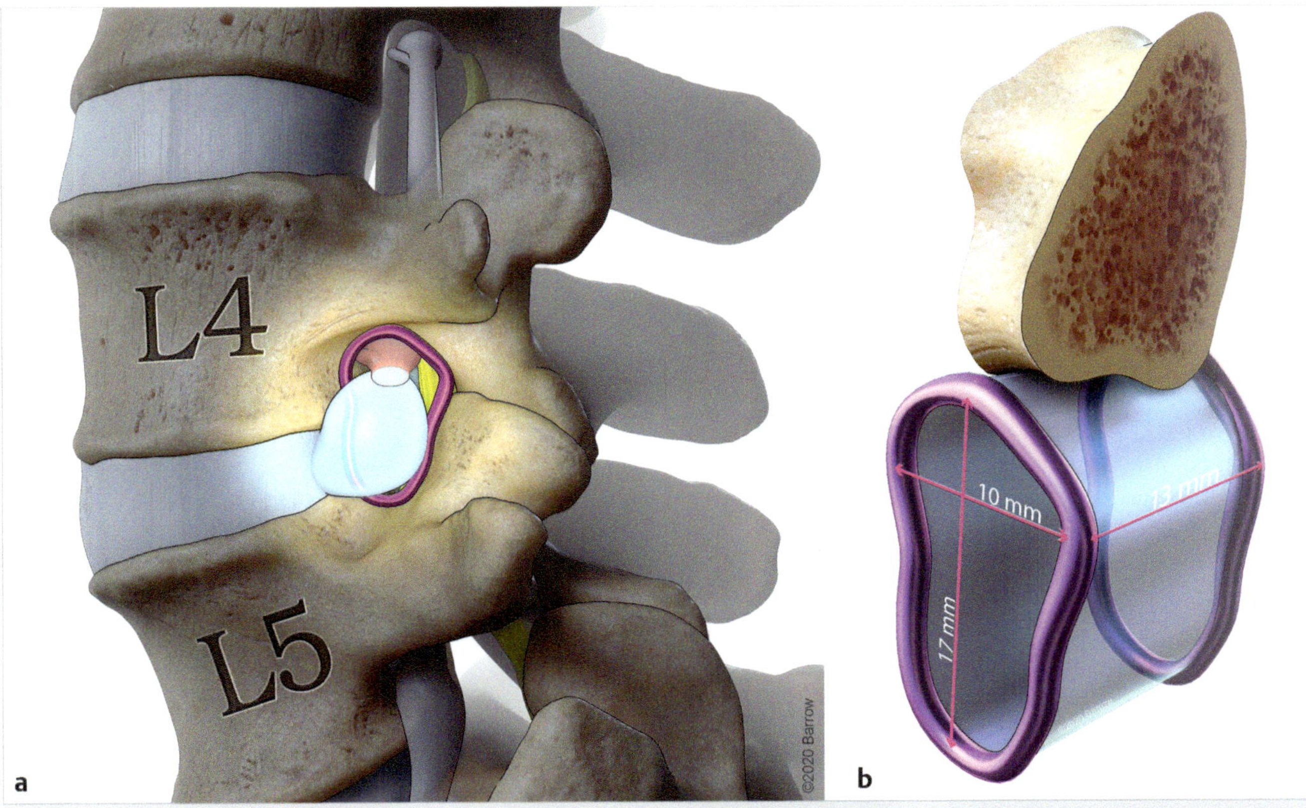

Fig. 5.6 (a) Anatomy of the neural foramen. Illustration of the L4–5 segment where a lateral disc extrusion has occurred. The exiting nerve root of L4 has been displaced against the L4 pedicle. The rostrocaudal dimension of the foramen, depending on the disc height, tends to be less than 18 mm, which establishes the anatomical basis for the use of the 16-mm diameter minimal access port. **(b)** The *magenta* ring demarcates the foramen; the foraminal height is determined by the inferior aspect of the L4 pedicle and the superior aspect of the L5 pedicle. The anteroposterior dimension is the distance from the superior articular process to the posterior vertebral body line, which is seldom more than 10 mm. The depth of the neural foramen corresponds to the width of the pedicle.

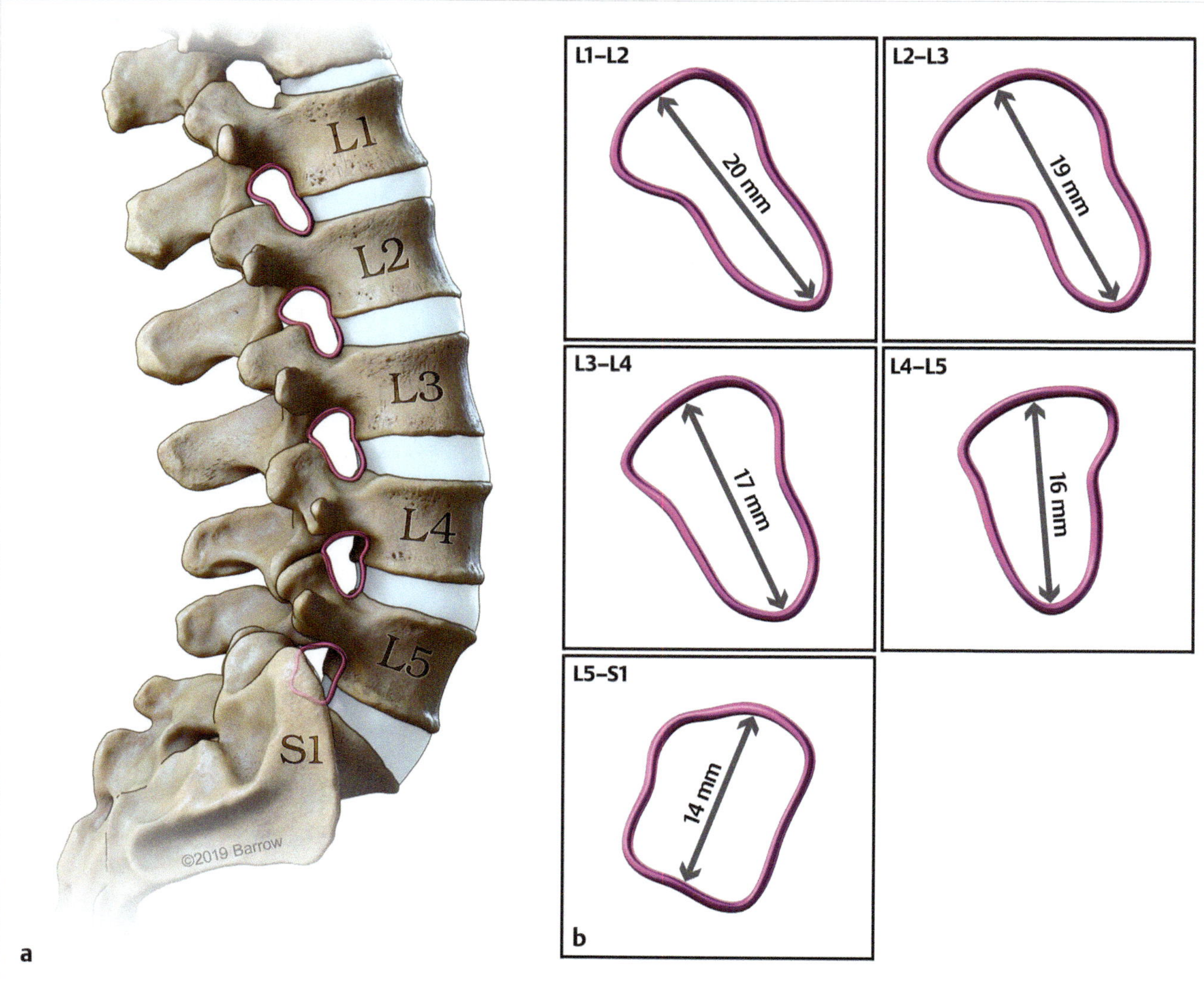

Fig. 5.7 Foraminal height of the neural foramen from L1–S1. **(a)** Illustration of the lumbosacral spine; the *magenta* rings indicate the neural foramen at each segment. **(b)** The foraminal height from L1–S1 decreases from rostral to caudal and the foraminal height of the L5–S1 segment is the smallest.

▶ Fig. 5.7 illustrates the foraminal height for the different segments of the lumbar spine. It is important to note that ▶ Fig. 5.6 is an idealized illustration without degeneration of the disc space incorporated into the measurement. Any collapse of the disc directly affects the foraminal height to some extent.

Reulen and colleagues were among the first to precisely define the operative window as the lateral aspect of the pars interarticularis (the isthmus), the inferior aspect of the pedicle, the transverse process, and the superior aspect of the facet joint. At segment L1–2, L2–3 and L3–4, they found this distance to be approximately 10 mm (range, 5–16 mm). At L4–5, this distance decreased to 7.9 mm (range, 3–14 mm), and at L5–S1, the operative window was a paltry 5.1 mm (range, 0–11 mm; ▶ Fig. 5.8).[13] The L5–S1 far lateral disc herniation is therefore almost a separate entity that requires careful consideration before endeavoring to treat it with a minimally invasive procedure.

The disc space of the segment where the far lateral disc herniations originate is between the pedicles and closest to the caudal pedicle by only a few millimeters. The anatomical studies of Reulen and colleagues show that distance from the rostral pedicle, the North Star of this operation, to the disc space is seldom more than 10 mm. This distance is essential to keep in mind so that once you have identified the pedicle, you have a sense of how far it is to the disc space below.

The anterior aspect of the foramen is primarily made up of the posterior aspects of the rostral vertebral body and disc space. There is only a modest contribution from the caudal vertebral body, as shown in ▶ Fig. 5.5. Consequently, the exiting nerve root is in the direct path of a lateral disc herniation. Far lateral disc herniations can therefore result in severe compromise of the foramen and compression of the nerve root. The posterior aspect of the foramen is made up of the pars interarticularis and the superior articular process (▶ Fig. 5.5). The anteroposterior (AP) dimension of the neural foramen is a meager 8 to 10 mm, which is not much room for a disc extrusion and exiting nerve root to coexist in that space.

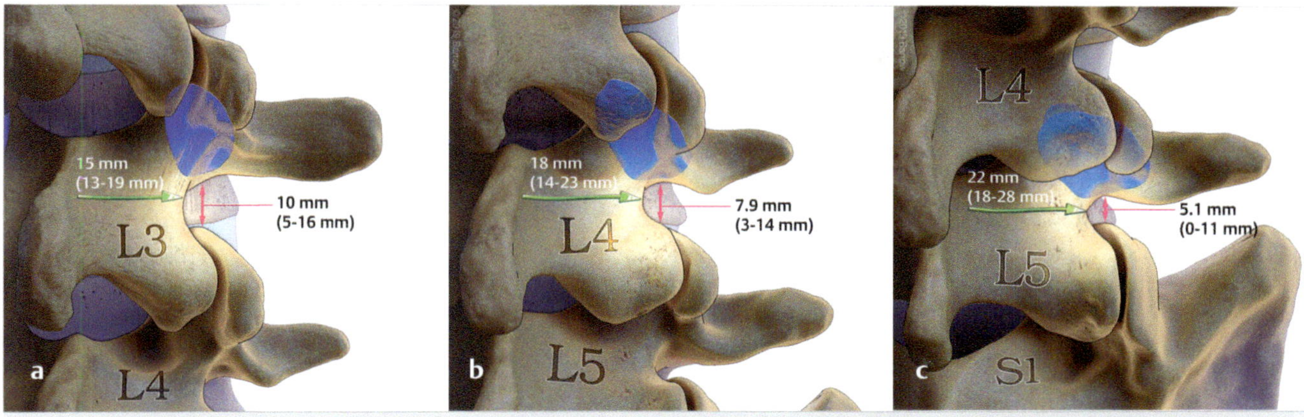

Fig. 5.8 Defining the operative window. Illustrations showing the values reported by Reulen et al,[13] who defined the operative window for a far lateral microdiscectomy as the lateral aspect of the pars interarticularis (the isthmus), the inferior aspect of the pedicle, the transverse process and the superior aspect of the facet joint. The measurements shown are essential when exposing and performing a far lateral microdiscectomy at **(a)** L3–4, **(b)** L4–5 and **(c)** L5–S1. Although the anatomy is not immediately visible, in-depth knowledge of the neural foramen provides you with the confidence to expose, identify and decompress a nerve root within the neural foramen with minimal disruption of the native spine. Thus, knowledge is the true organ of sight.

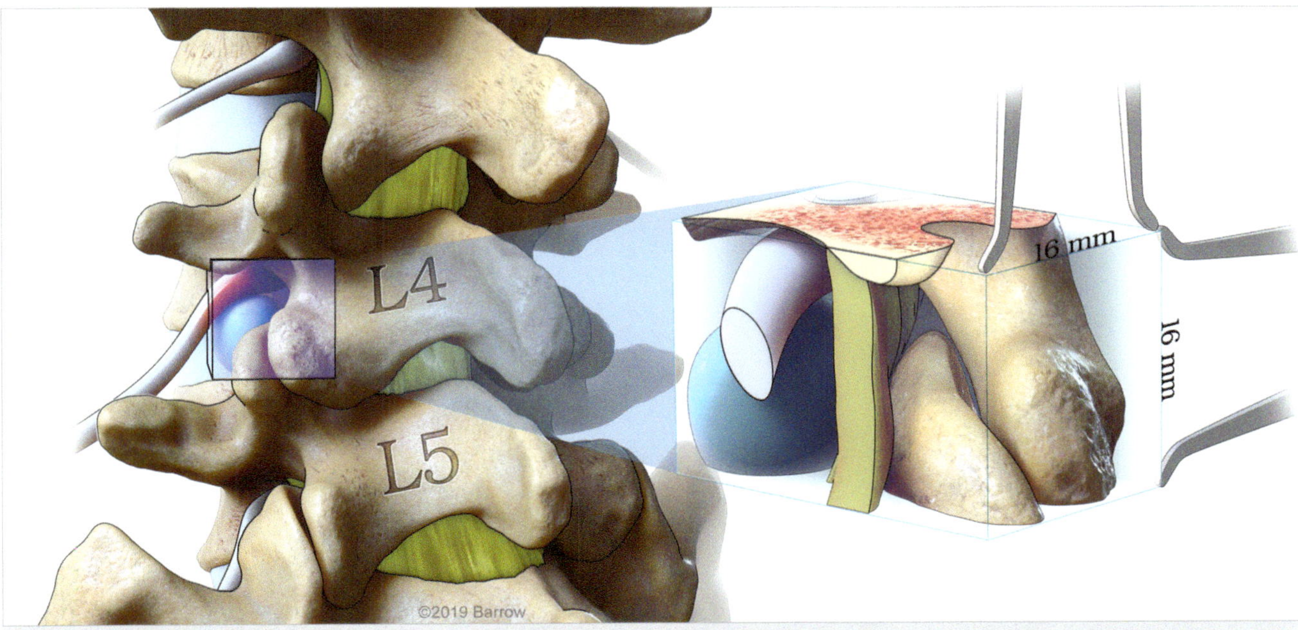

Fig. 5.9 A volumetric representation of the requisite anatomy for a far lateral microdiscectomy. The requisite anatomy is extracted from the lumbar spine into the cube (*inset*) to demonstrate the capacity of a 16-mm diameter to encompass the pars interarticularis, superior and inferior articular processes, the inferior aspect of the transverse process and the rostral pedicle.

It is equally important to recognize the path of the exiting root relative to the surface anatomy of the spine. Although we know that the nerve root exits beneath its like-numbered pedicle, we cannot see the pedicle from the surface anatomy. The pars interarticularis, on the other hand, can be readily visualized on the surface anatomy of the lateral spine. The nerve root traverses immediately beneath the rostral aspect of the pars interarticularis as it blends into the transverse process and pedicle. ▶ Fig. 5.9 demonstrates how the exiting root leaves the neuroforamen at the level of the rostral pars interarticularis just beneath its like-numbered pedicle. Thus, the pars interarticularis becomes a valuable anatomical landmark on the surface of the spine to target for the exposure. Both Reulen et al[13] and Schlesinger et al[16] have elegantly described this anatomy in their studies of the lateral spine for extraforaminal approaches. Again, I emphasize the importance of reading these classic articles alongside this chapter to achieve an understanding of the anatomy required for the procedure. The distance from the midline to the limited field of view requires mastery of the anatomy and a sophisticated capacity to readily reconstruct the lateral anatomy of the spine at depth in your mind's eye, with only limited glimpses of the bony structures.

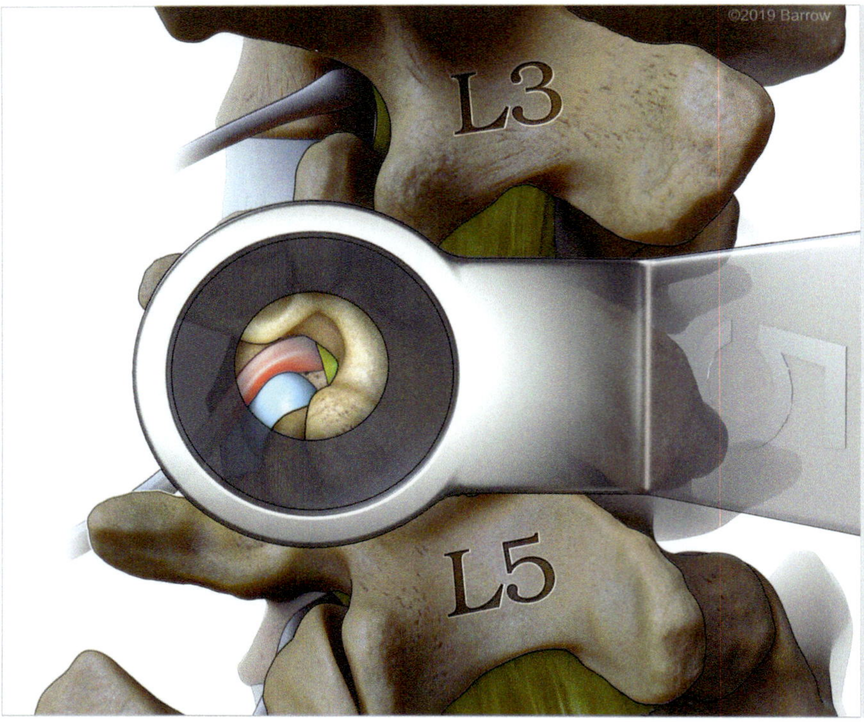

Fig. 5.10 Exposure of the requisite anatomy. Illustration of the surgical view through a 16-mm access port. The port is docked onto the pars interarticularis of L4 for removal of a far lateral disc extrusion at L4–5. All of the requisite anatomy to perform the operation falls within the field of view offered by the 16-mm access port.

From these anatomical measurements, it becomes evident that a 16-mm diameter encompasses the rostrocaudal exposure needed to reveal the affected nerve root and the disc space (▶ Fig. 5.9).

5.6 Anatomical Basis of the Distance from Midline for the Incision

The distance from the midline to the lateral aspect of the pars is seldom more than 20 mm in the upper segments of L1–2 and L2–3, scarcely more than 25 mm at the L3–4 and L4–5 segments and up to 30 mm at the L5–S1 segment (▶ Fig. 5.8).[13] Therefore, an incision of 25 to 30 mm lateral to the midline for the upper segments and 35 to 40 mm lateral to the midline for the lower segments allows for a converging trajectory onto the lateral pars interarticularis and the neural foramen. With the center of the diameter at the junction of the lateral pars and superior facet, it becomes readily apparent how all the requisite anatomy for a far lateral microdiscectomy comes into view with a well-positioned 16-mm diameter access port (▶ Fig. 5.10). Such a diameter encompasses the entire operative window defined by Reulen and colleagues.[13]

The measurements of the foramen and the position of the pars interarticularis relative to midline establish the anatomical basis for the minimal access port and offer guidance for selection of the diameter of the minimal access port. The 16-mm diameter access port assures a favorable Caspar ratio of almost 1:1, which is in step with the guiding principles of minimally invasive spine surgery. A firm grasp of the knowledge of these dimensions and measurements will increase your confidence as you peer through the microscope at the anatomy at the bottom of the access port. Early in my experience, I routinely used 18-mm diameter ports, thinking that a wider exposure was of greater value. As my experience with this approach grew, I found the value of 16-mm diameter ports. A smaller diameter was easier to secure into the extraforaminal corridor and less disruptive of the lateral musculature and facet. The larger diameters were more of a liability than an asset. Based on all the measurements of the neural foramen, the precise placement of a 16-mm access port over the lateral aspect of the pars interarticularis provides all the necessary exposure needed for the procedure.

The pars interarticularis is the first beacon to identify so that you remain oriented to the anatomy. From there, you will locate the pedicle that will guide you safely into the lumbar neural foramen so that you may safely and efficiently identify and then decompress the exiting nerve root by removing the far lateral disc extrusion.

5.7 Operating Room Setup

There is no difference between the operating room set up for a paramedian microdiscectomy and a far lateral microdiscectomy (▶ Fig. 5.11). The Jackson table and Wilson frame are equally as valuable for a far lateral discectomy as they are for a paramedian discectomy. The microscope stands sterilely draped and ready on the symptomatic side of the prone patient while the fluoroscope remains initially parked at the knees of the patient so that the scrub technician can drape it into the field. The operating room nurse secures the clamp for the table-mounted arm at the base of the Wilson frame to prevent any delay in securing the minimal access port after the operation begins.

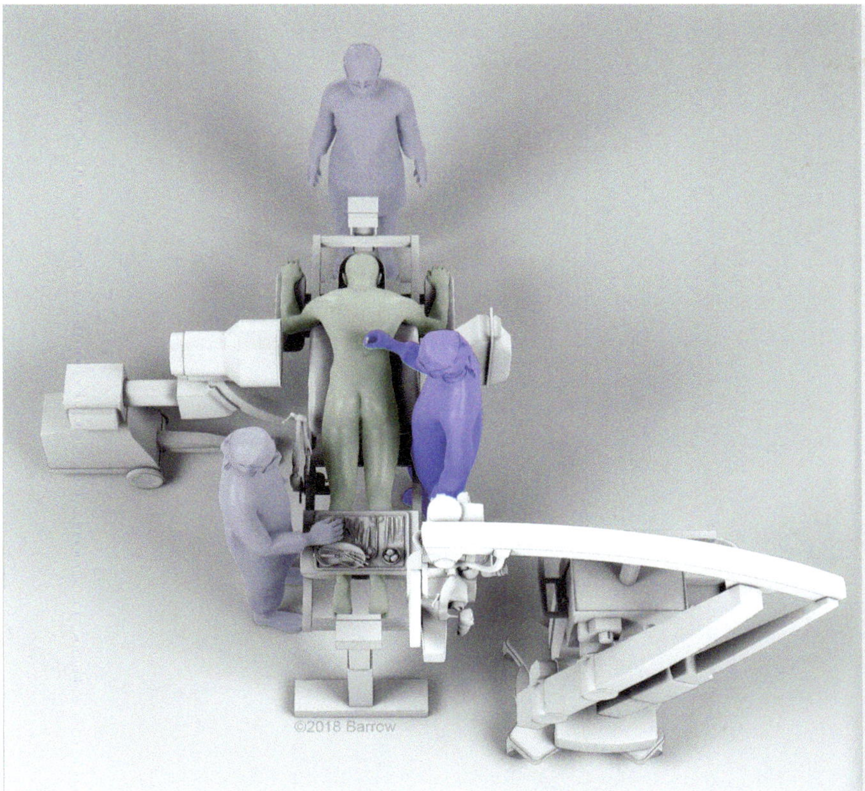

Fig. 5.11 Operating room set up for far lateral microdiscectomy. Illustration demonstrating the exact same set up for the operating room as used in a paramedian microdiscectomy.

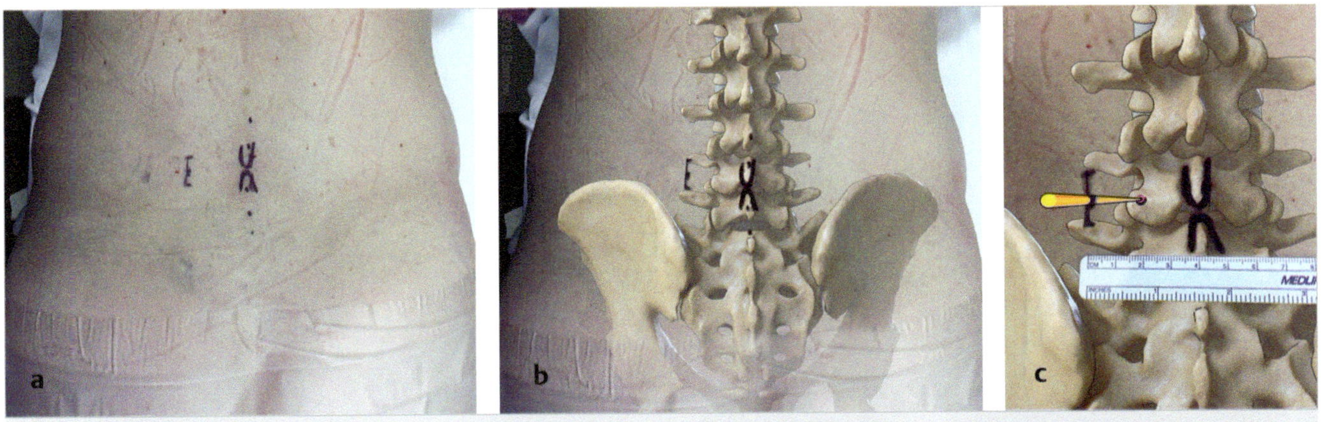

Fig. 5.12 Planning the incision for an L4–5 far lateral microdiscectomy. (a) Interoperative photograph demonstrating the measurement 40 mm from the midline for a left-sided L4–5 far lateral microdiscectomy. (b) The anterior superior iliac spine approximates the L4–5 interspace as shown. The ghosted anatomy superimposed on the image reveals the lamina, pars interarticularis, and spinous process and demonstrates the importance of the 35–40 mm offset from the midline at the L4–5 level. (c) Enlarged photograph with anatomy overlay showing the planned incision. In this image, a spinal needle (*goldenrod*) converges onto the initial target of the rostral aspect of the inferior articular facet. The *magenta* fiducial indicates the initial target on the inferior articular process, which is a safe initial target. As the dilatation process continues, the eventual target will be the lateral pars interarticularis. A converging trajectory onto the spine allows for an ideal working corridor into the neural foramen.

5.8 Planning the Incision

With the patient positioned prone on a Jackson table atop a Wilson frame, I palpate the bony landmarks to mark the symptomatic side. Approximating the L4–5 level by palpating the interspinous process space that corresponds with the anterior superior iliac spine, I mark what I feel to be the appropriate level. I then make a midline mark based on the palpation of the spinous processes so that I can measure off the midline and mark my incision (▶ Fig. 5.12). I bring the fluoroscope into position before prepping the incision so that I can drape the fluoroscope at the same time as the patient. Similar to the standard minimally invasive microdiscectomy, I refrain from using preoperative fluoroscopy to minimize the use of ionizing radiation. I mark an 18-mm-long incision 25 to 40 mm lateral to the midline at the symptomatic level. I make an incision 25 mm lateral to the midline at L1–2 and L2–3. When I am operating at L3–4, I expand that distance to 30 mm, and when I operate at L4–5, I

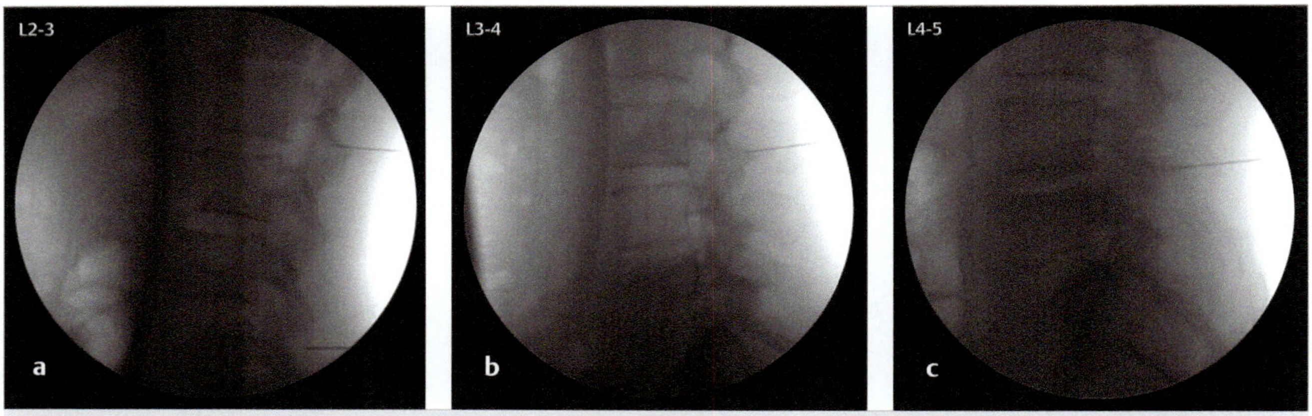

Fig. 5.13 Localization for a far lateral microdiscectomy at L2–3, L3–4, and L4–5. **(a)** Lateral fluoroscopic image demonstrating a spinal needle localizing the L2–3 segment. Note the spinal needle is docked at the upper lateral aspect of the facet. Since the sacrum cannot be visualized, an image was captured confirming the spinal needle pointing to the L5 pedicle. This spinal needle becomes the reference point for confirming the L2–3 segment. **(b)** Lateral fluoroscopic image with a spinal needle localizing the L3–4 segment. **(c)** Lateral fluoroscopic image demonstrating a spinal needle localizing the L4–5 segment.

make an incision 35 to 40 mm from the midline. I make the incision a full 40 mm from the midline when I operate at L5–S1. The L5–S1 segment is a distinctive anatomical circumstance that merits a separate section in this chapter.

I prep and drape the incision area before passing a spinal needle onto the lateral and superior aspect of the facet. I do not attempt to target the pars interarticularis for localization because of its depth. There is some risk inherent in targeting the pars interarticularis with the use of landmarks only. I believe the superior aspect of the facet is a safer, larger and more superficial target with a more familiar trajectory than that of the pars interarticularis.

Unlike with the standard minimally invasive microdiscectomy and laminectomy, I allow the spinal needle to converge onto the spine, as it looks to encounter the lateral aspect of the inferior articular process. With a starting point 30 to 40 mm lateral to the spinous process, the risk of a dural puncture by the localizing needle is very low, if not absent. Slight convergence of the spinal needle, as seen in ► Fig. 5.12c, reliably enables the tip to encounter the lateral aspect of the lamina or inferior articular facet. Without convergence, the needle runs the risk of passing laterally to the spine altogether. As I pass the needle, I keep in mind Reulen's measurements of the distance from the spinous process to the lateral aspect of the pars interarticularis at each level (► Fig. 5.8).

Once in contact with the spine, I obtain my first lateral fluoroscopic image (► Fig. 5.13). Ideally, I want the spinal needle to be pointing to the upper aspect of the disc space. I make the necessary adjustments to ensure that the spinal needle is in the axial plane of the neural foramen to provide an adequate working trajectory to decompress the nerve root. When I have the spinal needle in the ideal position, I pull the needle back from the facet, remove the stylet, and infiltrate the proposed trajectory with a lidocaine–bupivacaine–epinephrine mixture.

5.9 Docking the Minimal Access Port

Since the incision for the access port is 30 to 40 mm lateral to the midline, it is vital to commit early to a medial trajectory to have a working corridor that converges onto the spine. You can ensure an ideal trajectory by making the fascial opening just medial to the skin incision. Use cautery to divide the fascia and then blunt dissection with your index finger, as described by Wiltse and Spencer,[9] to effortlessly cleave a plane between the multifidus and longissimus muscles. With minimal dissection, the tip of your index finger immediately encounters the superior aspect of the facet complex. Then, with your index finger still in position, shoehorn the first dilator onto the superior aspect of the facet complex and allow it to slide onto the pars interarticularis. I have found it imperative to guide the tip of the dilator with my index finger, lest it fall lateral to the spine. Once I confirm its placement onto the spine, I hold it firmly in place for the fluoroscopic image and the subsequent dilatation (► Fig. 5.14).

I always keep in mind that the topography of the lateral spine is not as welcoming to the dilators as that of the medial spine. Although I can firmly anchor a dilator onto the medial lamina in a laminectomy or microdiscectomy without concern for the tip of the dilator migrating off the target, the lateral pars interarticularis and lateral lamina are more inhospitable to the tip of the dilator. The topography of the lateral aspect of the pars interarticularis does not offer the same surface interface to anchor a dilator with the same confidence and firmness that the medial lamina provides. As a result, the tip of the dilator tends to slip off the lateral aspect of the pars interarticularis. If at any time I feel like the dilators have slipped off the pars, I do not attempt to reposition them. Instead, I begin anew, starting with the first dilator. As shown in ► Fig. 5.14, the tip of the dilator slides up the inferior articular process and probes the lateral aspect of the pars interarticularis. Thus begins the reconstruction of the anatomy at depth in the surgeon's mind without ever catching a glimpse of the bony structures. Since far lateral disc extrusion at L2–3, L3–4 and L4–5 represents the vast majority of cases, the fluoroscopic images in ► Fig. 5.15 demonstrate the sequence of positioning the access port at each level.

It is not feasible to place subsequent dilators that remain in contact with the pars interarticularis. In fact, after the second dilator, it is untenable that the dilators would stay in contact with the pars interarticularis because the diameter of the

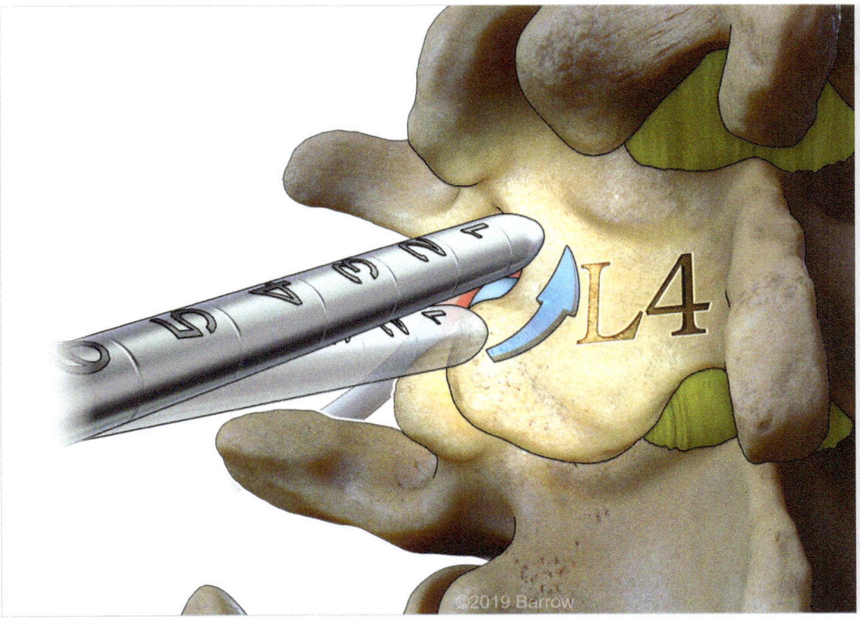

Fig. 5.14 Securing the first dilator onto the pars interarticularis. The initial target for the first dilator is the inferior articular process. Once in position, the first dilator slides onto the pars interarticularis, which places it immediately over the top of the neural foramen. The subsequent dilators prepare the way for the 16-mm access port to be secured into position.

dilatation encounters the inferior articular process of the facet, which is at a shallower depth (▶ Fig. 5.16).

After the preliminary exploration probing with the tip of the first dilator, I reconstruct the location of the pars interarticularis in my mind. With that mental image, I firmly anchor the first dilator against the superior aspect of the facet and sequentially dilate the working corridor. Unlike a medial microdiscectomy or laminectomy, where the smooth surface of the lamina is conducive to wanding, there is no such bony anatomy in the far lateral spine. The topography is less favorable for wanding because the pars interarticularis and facet are in different planes. Therefore, the dilators are best kept firmly anchored to the superior facet. A well-positioned 16-mm diameter access port reliably encompasses the requisite anatomy for the procedure.

Once I have the minimal access port in what I feel to be the ideal position, I obtain another lateral fluoroscopic image before anchoring it into its final position. This image allows me to make the necessary minor adjustments that optimize the trajectory onto the far lateral disc and the neural foramen. After optimizing the trajectory, I capture a 15- to 20-degree angle of convergence onto the spine with the table-mounted arm (▶ Fig. 5.17).

I obtain a final lateral fluoroscopic image followed by an AP image. Although the AP image in a medial microdiscectomy or laminectomy is of limited value, the AP image at this stage in a far lateral microdiscectomy is of tremendous value. Working with a constrained channel and limited visibility of bony landmarks, I find this AP image indispensable for showing where the diameter of the access port is relative to the rostral pedicle, which is the guiding star of the operation (▶ Fig. 5.18).

The far lateral microdiscectomy is one of the circumstances in which I have found tremendous value in a fluoroscopic image that is obtained looking down into the access port. This image provides me with a view in line with the pedicle, or what has become known as an owl's eye view (▶ Fig. 5.19).

With imaging complete and the minimal access port secured, I remove the fluoroscopy unit from the field and bring in the operating microscope. As I peer down into the minimal access port, I immediately begin to establish my bearings with the AP and lateral fluoroscopic images fresh in my mind. On a good day, I see a hint of the superior facet amid the fibers of the paraspinal muscle as I begin to probe the anatomy with the suction catheter. The smooth and relatively flat pars interarticularis resides on a lower plane than the prominent inferior articular process. As a result, there is a tuft of muscle and soft tissue over the top of the pars interarticularis. I use a bayoneted extended cautery tip to brush away this tuft of muscle and reveal the superior, lateral and rostral aspects of the inferior articular processes of the facet (▶ Fig. 5.20).

Proceeding with the dissection slightly medially on the inferior articular process allows a safe passage onto the lateral aspect of the pars interarticularis. Once I have the entire lateral aspect of the pars interarticularis exposed (▶ Fig. 5.20b), I probe superiorly and laterally with the suction tip to identify the inferior aspect of the transverse process of the like-numbered nerve root that I intend to decompress. After I am convinced that I have unequivocally palpated the transverse process, I expose the inferior medial aspect of that bony prominence. For instance, if I am performing an L4–5 far lateral microdiscectomy to decompress the L4 nerve root, upon completion of the exposure, I would be looking at the inferior aspect of the L4 transverse process, the pars interarticularis of L4 and the superior and lateral aspects of the inferior articular process of L4. Only after these elements of the anatomy have been exposed should one begin drilling the pars interarticularis. As always, if I am not certain of the anatomy, I reassess, reimage and reposition the access port. No good comes of drilling bone when you are uncertain of what lies beneath it. Proceeding in such a manner only adds to your disorientation by distorting the anatomy further.

5.10 Bone Work: Drilling the Lateral Pars Interarticularis

The location of the disc herniation relative to the pedicle determines the extent of bone work that is needed. For a far lateral disc herniation that resides lateral to the pedicle, there is no

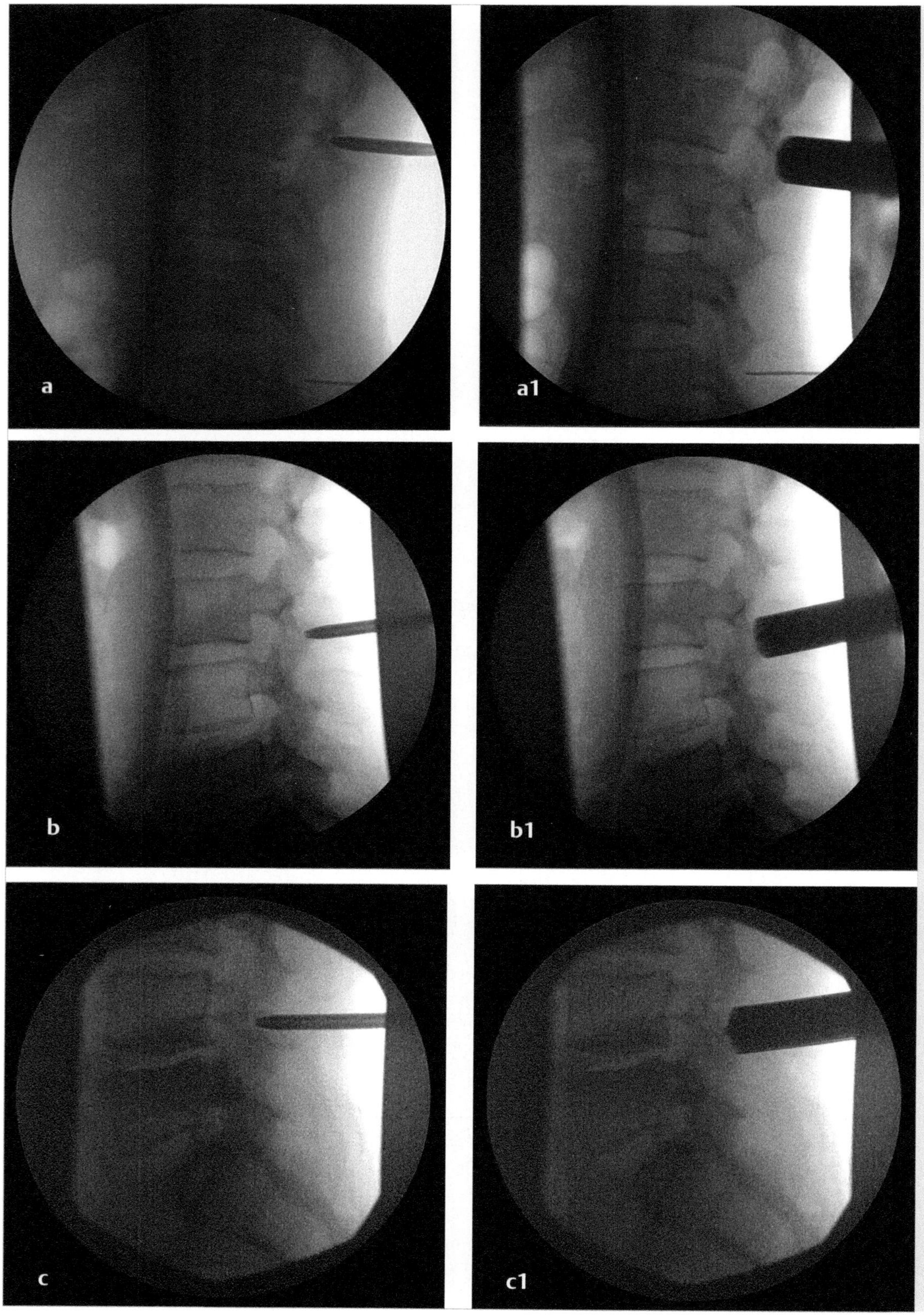

Fig. 5.15 Dilators on the lateral spine at L2–3, L3–4, and L4–5. **(a)** Lateral fluoroscopic image demonstrating the first dilator up against the L2 pars interarticularis. Sounding the pars interarticularis with the first dilator is feasible. **(a1)** The prominence of the inferior articular process of the facet precludes the ability to remain anchored against the pars interarticularis as the diameter of the dilators increases. **(b)** Lateral fluoroscopic image of the first dilator sounding the anatomy at L3–4. **(b1)** The minimal access port over the top of the superior aspect of the facet complex. **(c)** Lateral fluoroscopic image demonstrating the first dilator at the pars interarticularis of L4. **(c1)** The minimal access port over the top of the facet complex at L4–5.

need for bone work, whereas a disc herniation in line with the pedicle or even slightly medial to the pedicle requires removal of the lateral pars interarticularis. Early in your experience, I advise you always to drill the lateral pars interarticularis to enter the foramen and to identify the pedicle, which is the most reliable manner to identify your landmarks and minimize the risk of nerve root injury. As you build experience, you develop the facility to achieve and maintain your orientation. With that experience, you will find less of a need to remove bone from the pars interarticularis to enter the foramen and decompress

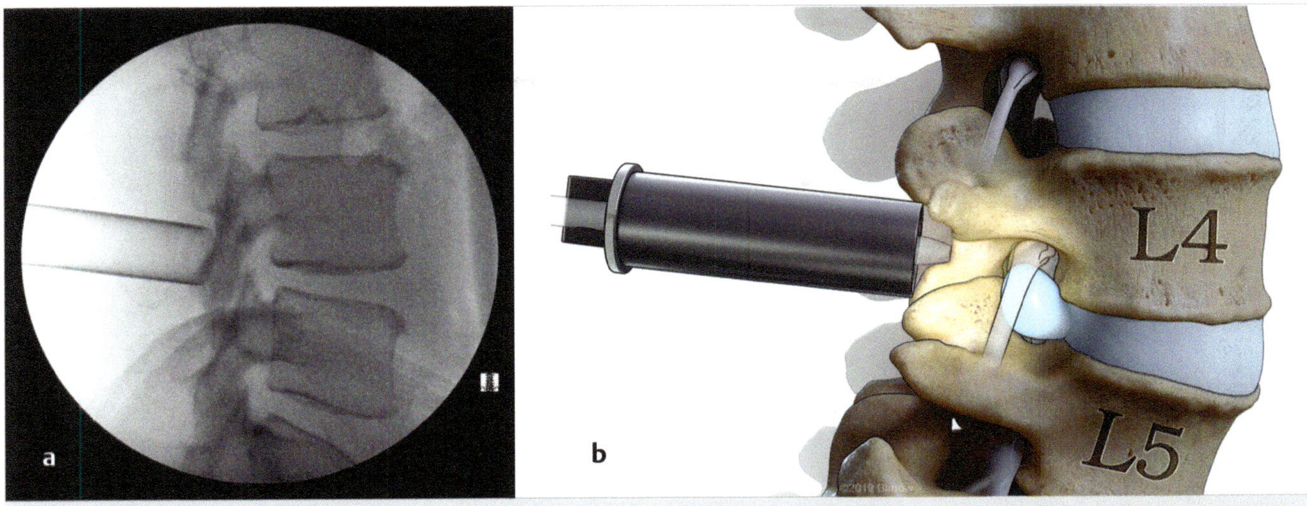

Fig. 5.16 (a) Lateral fluoroscopic image of an access port secured onto the lateral aspect of the L4–5 segment. The prominence of the inferior articular process precludes the capacity for the access port to remain flush against the pars interarticularis. (b) Illustration of the fluoroscopic image in (a) demonstrating the inability to maintain the minimal access port up against the pars interarticularis. The flat pars interarticularis is at a deeper depth than the prominent inferior articular process of the facet, which makes anchoring the access port up against the pars interarticularis an anatomical impossibility. The result is a tuft of soft tissue covering the pars interarticularis that needs to be removed.

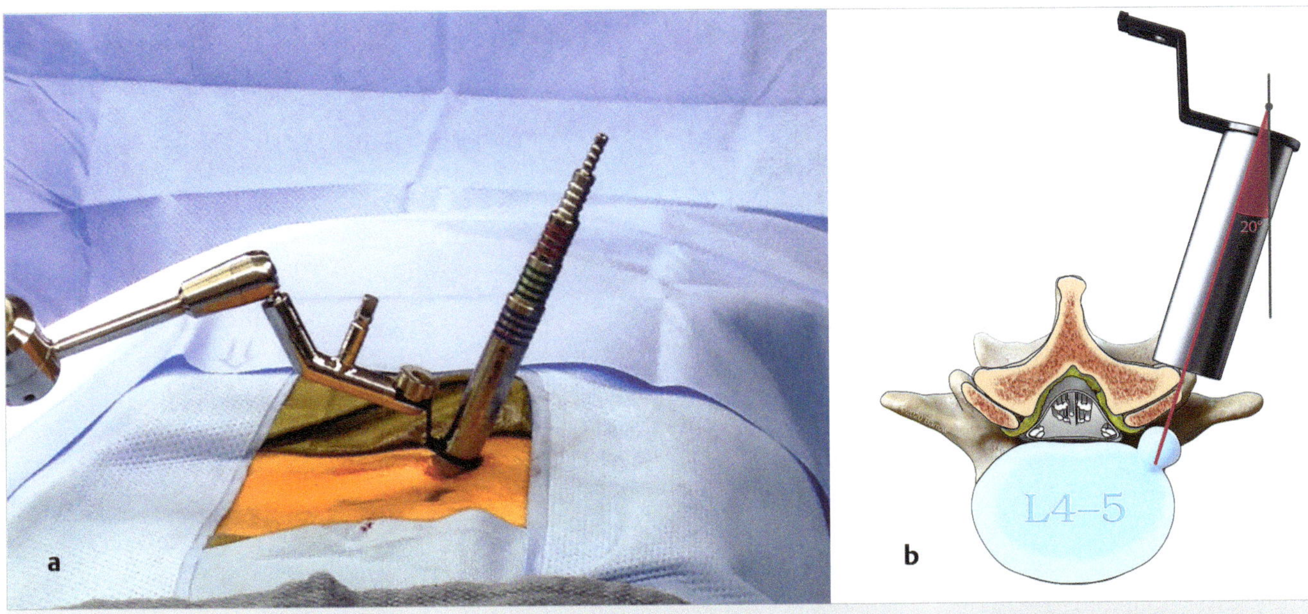

Fig. 5.17 (a) Photograph of the minimal access port in position for a far lateral microdiscectomy. Note the convergence, which places the field of view over the pars interarticularis providing an optimal trajectory into the neural foramen. (b) Illustration of an axial view demonstrating the convergence onto the neural foramen.

the nerve root in extraforaminal disc herniations. The amount of bone removed from lateral pars interarticularis will only be a function of the location of the disc extrusion.

I begin the bone work by drilling the superior lateral aspect of the pars interarticularis just beneath the transverse process. I have seldom found a need to remove more than 1 to 2 mm of the lateral aspect of the pars interarticularis. The thickness of the 2-mm matchstick head of the drill bit is a reliable guide to ensure that I drill the least amount of bone that still safely provides access to the neural foramen. Removal of 2 mm of the lateral aspect of the pars interarticularis provides reliable access to the requisite anatomy. I drill the entire length of the pars interarticularis from the transverse process to just shy of the lateral and superior aspects of the inferior articular facet, a distance no greater than 10 mm. I continue to drill until I reach the depth of the intertransverse process ligament, which represents the lateral extension of the ligamentum flavum (► Fig. 5.21).

I maintain the intertransverse process ligament intact at this time and extend my bone work toward the inferior aspect of the transverse process, which provides access to the insertion

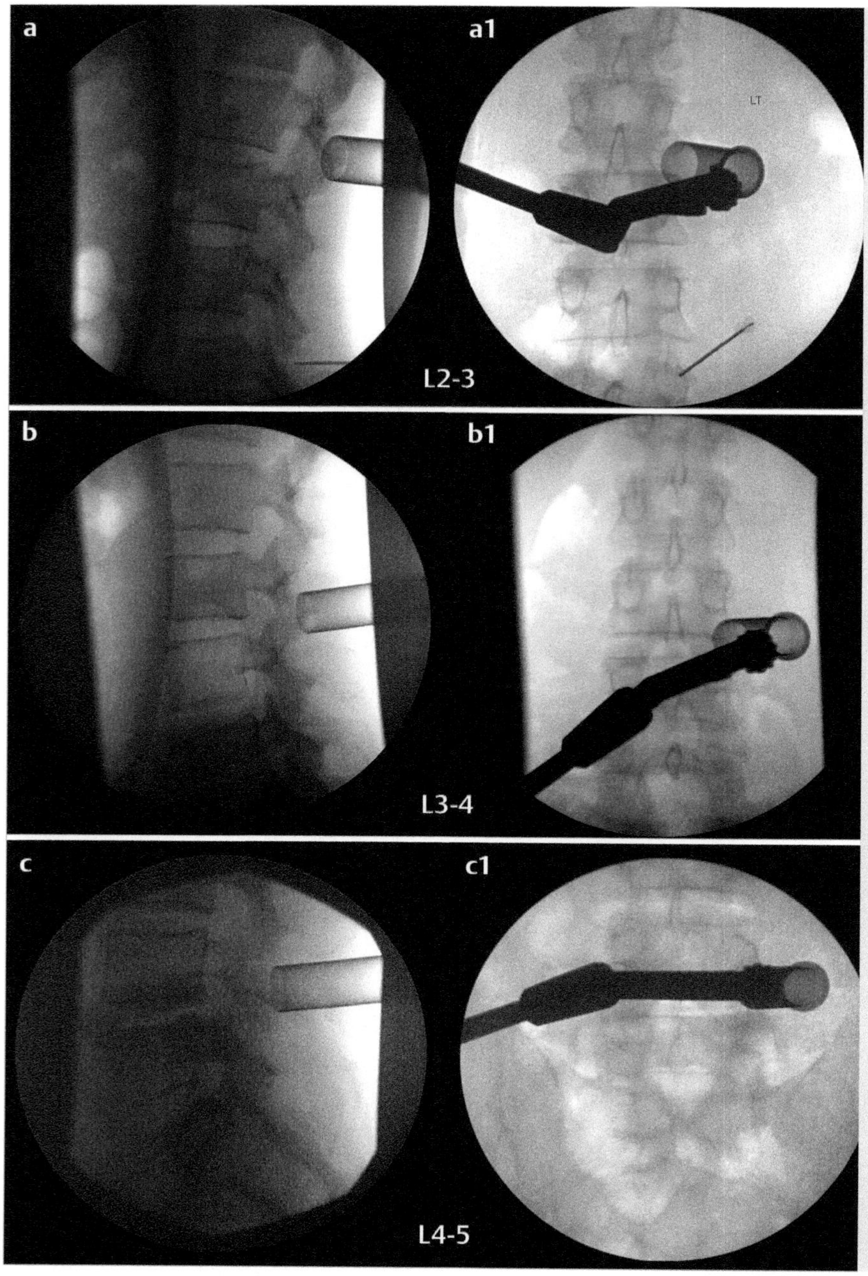

Fig. 5.18 Final positioning of the minimal access port for L2–3, L3–4 and L4–5 far lateral microdiscectomies. **(a)** Lateral fluoroscopic image demonstrating the access port over the top of the superior and lateral aspect of the L2–3 facet. **(a1)** Anteroposterior (AP) fluoroscopic image demonstrating the minimal access port in position over the top of the lateral aspect of the facet encompassing the pars interarticularis at L2. The isthmus of the pars interarticularis in this circumstance is narrow, requiring greater convergence of the access port. Note the spinal needle remains in position at L5 for reference until the localization is complete. **(b)** Final lateral and **(b1)** AP fluoroscopic images at L3–4. **(c)** Final lateral and **(c1)** AP fluoroscopic image at L4–5.

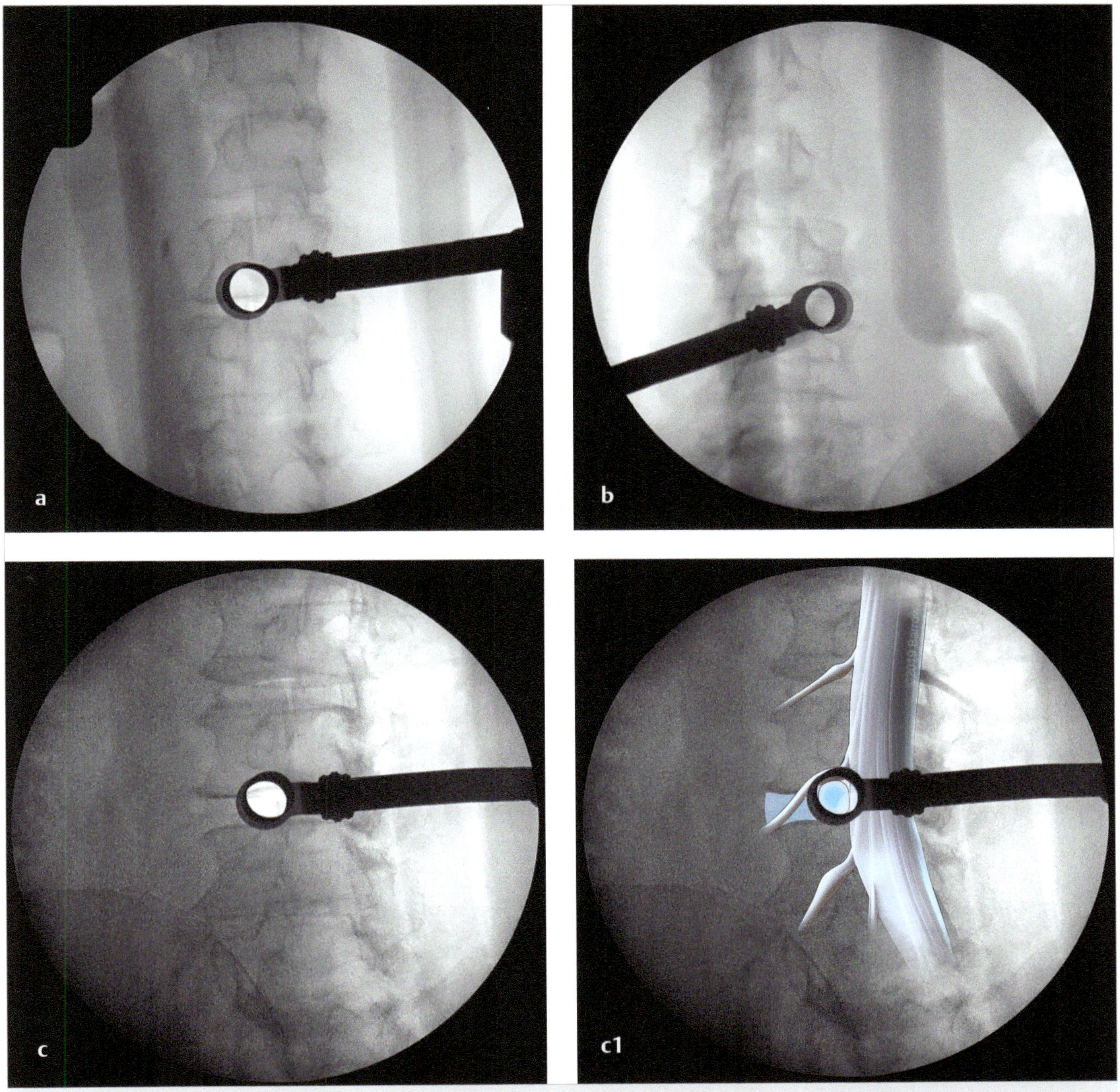

Fig. 5.19 Fluoroscopic images of the owl's eye view showing the minimal access port in position over the top of the neural foramen in L2–3, L3–4 and L4–5 far lateral microdiscectomies. **(a)** Owl's eye fluoroscopic image demonstrating the diameter of the access port just below the pedicle of L2 in a left L2–3 far lateral microdiscectomy. **(b)** Owl's eye fluoroscopic image demonstrating the diameter of the access port just below the pedicle of L3 in a right L3–4 far lateral microdiscectomy. **(c)** Owl's eye fluoroscopic image demonstrating the diameter of the access port just below the pedicle of L4 in a left L4–5 far lateral microdiscectomy. **(c1)** The neural structures superimposed onto the fluoroscopic image in **c**. The overlay shows the L4 nerve root displaced into the L4 pedicle by a far lateral disc herniation.

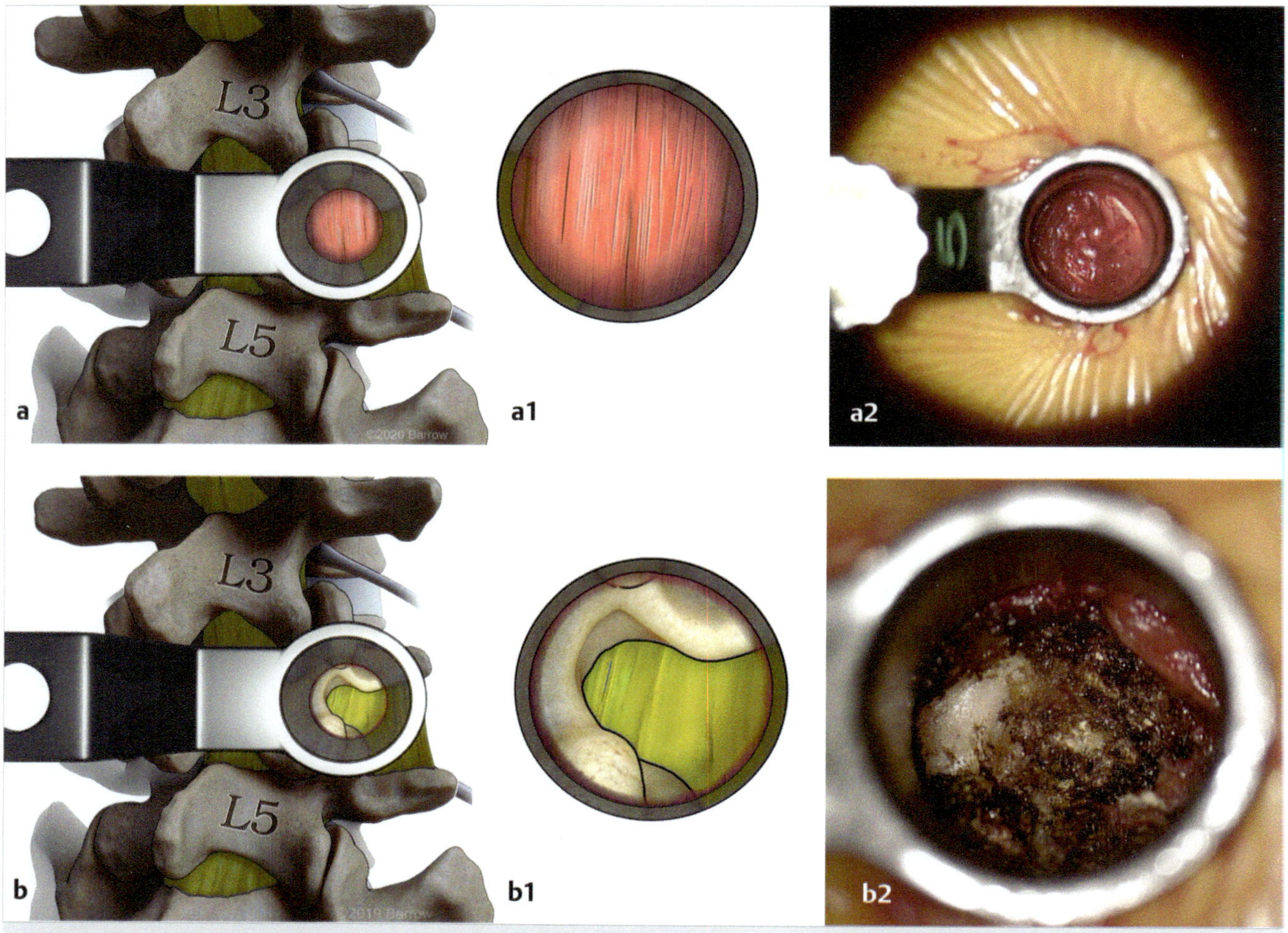

Fig. 5.20 Exposure of the lateral lumbar spine. **(a)** Illustration of the surgical view through a 16-mm access port over the top of the pars interarticularis. The uneven topography of the lateral lumbar spine prevents a tight interface between the minimal access port and the pars interarticularis. The inevitable result is a tuft of muscle at the bottom of the access port. **(a1)** Magnified view of **a**. **(a2)** Intraoperative photograph of a view through the access port before exposure. **(b)** Illustration of the exposure before drilling the lateral aspect of the pars interarticularis after sweeping away the muscle. **(b1)** Magnified view of **b**. **(b2)** Intraoperative photograph of a view through the access port after exposure.

of the intertransverse process ligament and a safe corridor into the foramen. Finally, I turn my attention to the lateral aspect of the superior articular facet. The inferior bone work on the facet provides access to the disc space. I drill only the lateral-most aspect of the superior articular process and make every effort to stay out of the facet joint.

5.11 Identification of the Pedicle

I divide the fibers of the intertransverse process ligament at its insertion on the underside of the transverse process. With the division of these fibers, the perineural fat becomes readily evident. I resect several millimeters of the ligament medially to facilitate access into and out of the foramen with instruments. Next, I confirm the location of the pedicle with absolute certainty. I use a right-angled ball-tipped probe and confirm that I feel the rostral pedicle of the segment. Since the junction of the pars interarticularis and the transverse process of the rostral level is in plain sight, the pedicle that corresponds to these two elements will be readily palpable if not visible. If it is not palpable, I keep drilling the pars in a rostral direction until I can unequivocally palpate or see the inferior lateral wall of the pedicle. The pedicle is the North Star of this operation, and its palpation leads directly to the exiting nerve root, which is the target of our decompression. The pedicle always leads you to the nerve root (▶ Fig. 5.22).

As soon as I palpate the pedicle, I know with certainty where the nerve root resides. I can confidently continue to divide and resect the fibers of the intertransverse process ligament and unveil the exiting nerve root. By detaching the fibers of the ligamentum flavum from the inferior and lateral aspect of the pars interarticularis, I establish a safe plane over the top of the nerve root and continue to resect more of the intertransverse process ligament to gain a better view of the contents of the foramen. Typically, there is an abundance of perineural fat engulfing the nerve root. Within this perineural fat, an abundance of epidural veins become evident. I employ a preemptive strike policy and immediately deal with any veins encountered in this region with bipolar cautery. Experience has taught me that it is easier to identify, cauterize and divide these vessels when meeting

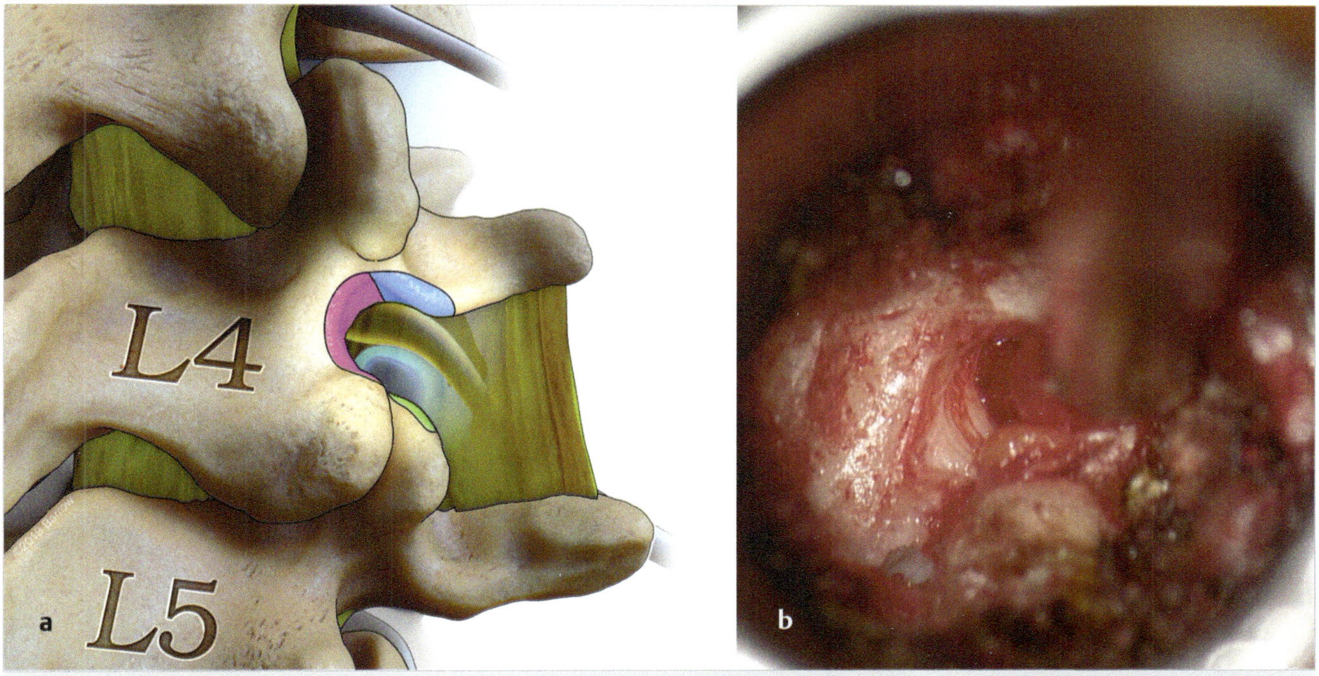

Fig. 5.21 Bone removal for a far lateral microdiscectomy. **(a)** Illustration demonstrating the sequence of drilling the pars interarticularis, the transverse process and the superolateral aspect of the inferior articular process. Removal of the bone reveals the lateral extension of the ligamentum flavum and the intertransverse process ligament. Dividing the ligamentum flavum allows for entry into the foramen. The sequence of drilling begins with the pars interarticularis first (*magenta*), followed by the inferior aspect of the transverse process (*blue*). If necessary, the superolateral aspect of the superior articular (*green*) process is drilled to access the disc space. **(b)** Intraoperative photograph of a view through the access port after the completion of the bone work.

them for the first time than to await the troublesome bleeding that arises from sweeping a right-angled ball-tipped probe over the pedicle. Because the nerve root is in the immediate vicinity, I use right-angled bipolar cautery and turn down the energy. I hook the epidural veins and apply very slight upward traction away from the nerve root and cauterize them. I always remain keenly aware of any leg movement during these preemptive vein cauterizations. To divide the cauterized veins, I use a right-angled nerve hook and hold upward traction away from the nerve root to allow the safe use of blunt-tipped microscissors. As an alternative to the microscissors, I sometimes use a Kerrison No. 1 rongeur to accomplish the same task. The critical point is the sharp division of the veins instead of blunt traction to prevent a deluge of epidural bleeding in such a confined space.

The artery of the pars interarticularis is also in this immediate vicinity. Throughout the process of exposing the nerve root, a Kerrison rongeur may encounter and inadvertently interrupt this vessel. A hemostatic agent and pressure will not stop the bleeding from the artery of the pars, which is a branch of a segmental vessel. Direct visualization of the lumen and cauterization is straightforward and imperative.

5.12 Identification of the Nerve Root

With the veins cauterized and divided, I use a blunt medium Penfield dissector and sweep down from the pedicle. That particular maneuver reliably unveils the affected nerve root. Teasing through the perineural fat with the Penfield and the suction tip may also reveal the root. If the anatomy is not clearly visible, I use a light stream of irrigation, which has the uncanny ability to reveal the unseen anatomy below. Lightly pulsing the irrigation separates the perineural fat and uncovers the white tubular structure of the nerve root.

Upon unequivocally identifying the root, I clear away any soft tissue and intertransverse process ligament caudal to the nerve root. Sweeping a right-angled ball-tipped probe over the top of the root accomplishes this task. Once the ball-tipped probe passes freely, I use a Kerrison punch to extend the exposure in the caudal direction. The goal is to identify the disc space. I remove soft tissue, ligament and bone until the inferior aspect of the root comes clearly into view. I can now use a suction retractor in one hand to sweep the nerve root rostrally and keep it out of harm's way while a Kerrison rongeur in the other hand continues caudally to resect any remaining ligament obscuring the disc space. The annulus comes into view with dissection in this direction, and along with it, the far lateral disc herniation (▶ Fig. 5.23).

5.13 Far Lateral Microdiscectomy

More often than not, a far lateral disc herniation is a free, extruded disc fragment. These free disc fragments are brought into view by doing little more than displacing the nerve root with a suction retractor. After some minimal dissection with either the right-angled ball-tipped probe or small forward-angled curet, the disc fragments are easily removed, and the

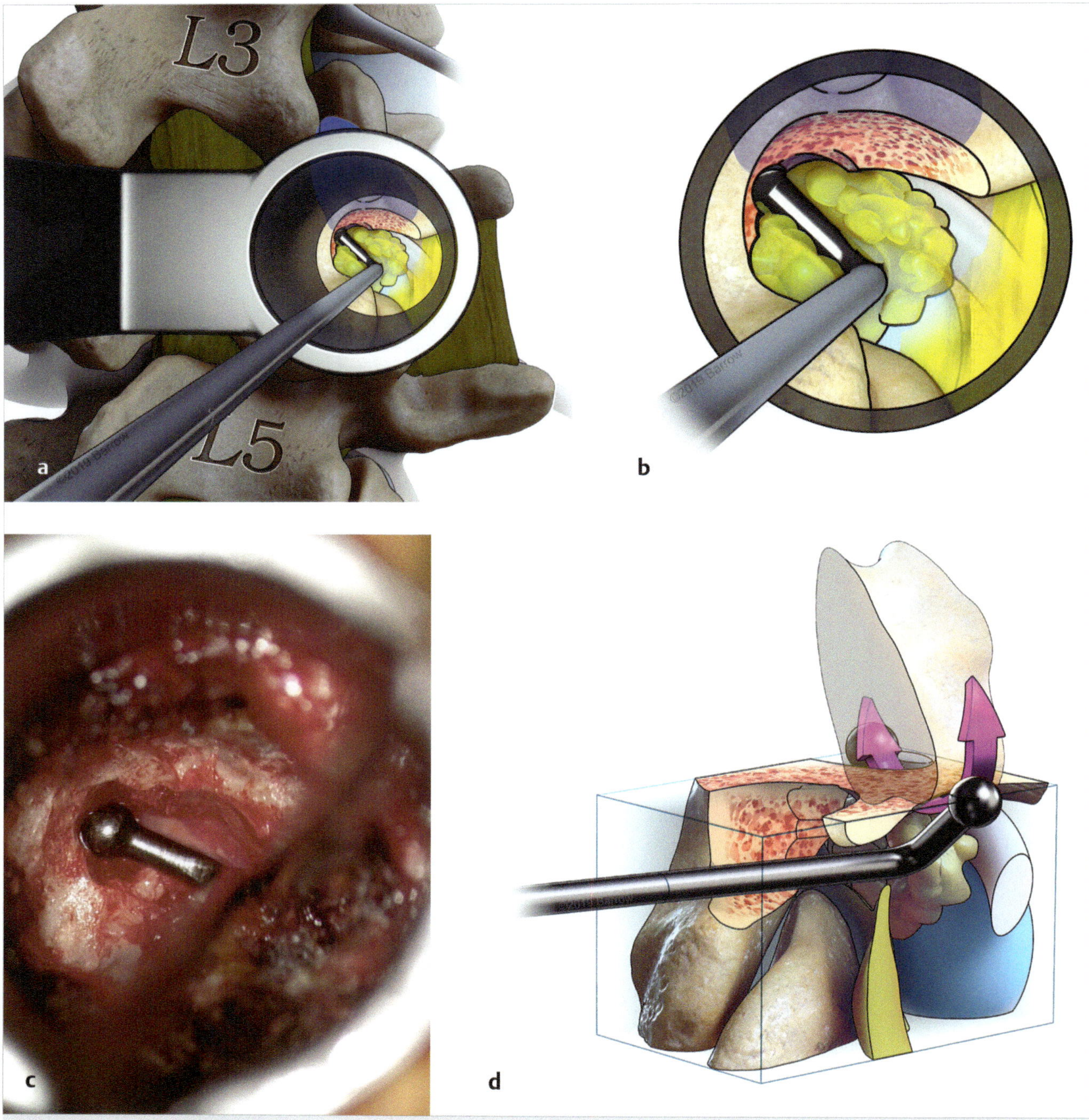

Fig. 5.22 Identification of the pedicle within the foramen. **(a)** Illustration demonstrating the operative field after the division of the intertransverse process ligament. The field of view is notable for the perineural fat and epidural veins overlying the nerve root. **(b)** Once in the foramen, identification of the pedicle establishes the location of the nerve root. The illustration shows a right-angled ball-tipped probe palpating the inferior medial aspect of the pedicle (*lavender*). **(c)** Intraoperative photograph demonstrating the palpation of the pedicle. **(d)** Illustration limited to the volumetrically extracted requisite anatomy. The pars interarticularis has been drilled along with the inferior aspect of the transverse process. The illustration demonstrates the process of confirming the pedicle by sweeping the probe medially and laterally to it within the foramen (*magenta arrows*).

operation is nearly done. On rare occasions, I must create an annulotomy with a No. 11 blade and retrieve the disc material through the defect I have created. Regardless, similar to medial disc herniations, a systematic approach to the decompression ensures adequate decompression and consistent outcomes.

The first step in the far lateral microdiscectomy is the adequate mobilization of the exiting nerve root. I ensure that nothing is tethering the root to preclude its safe retraction. A right-angled ball-tipped probe is the ideal instrument to accomplish this objective. I pass the probe over the top of the nerve root and then laterally and sweep it beneath the nerve root from above and below the root. These maneuvers unveil the compression caused by the disc herniation, if they do not deliver the herniation altogether.

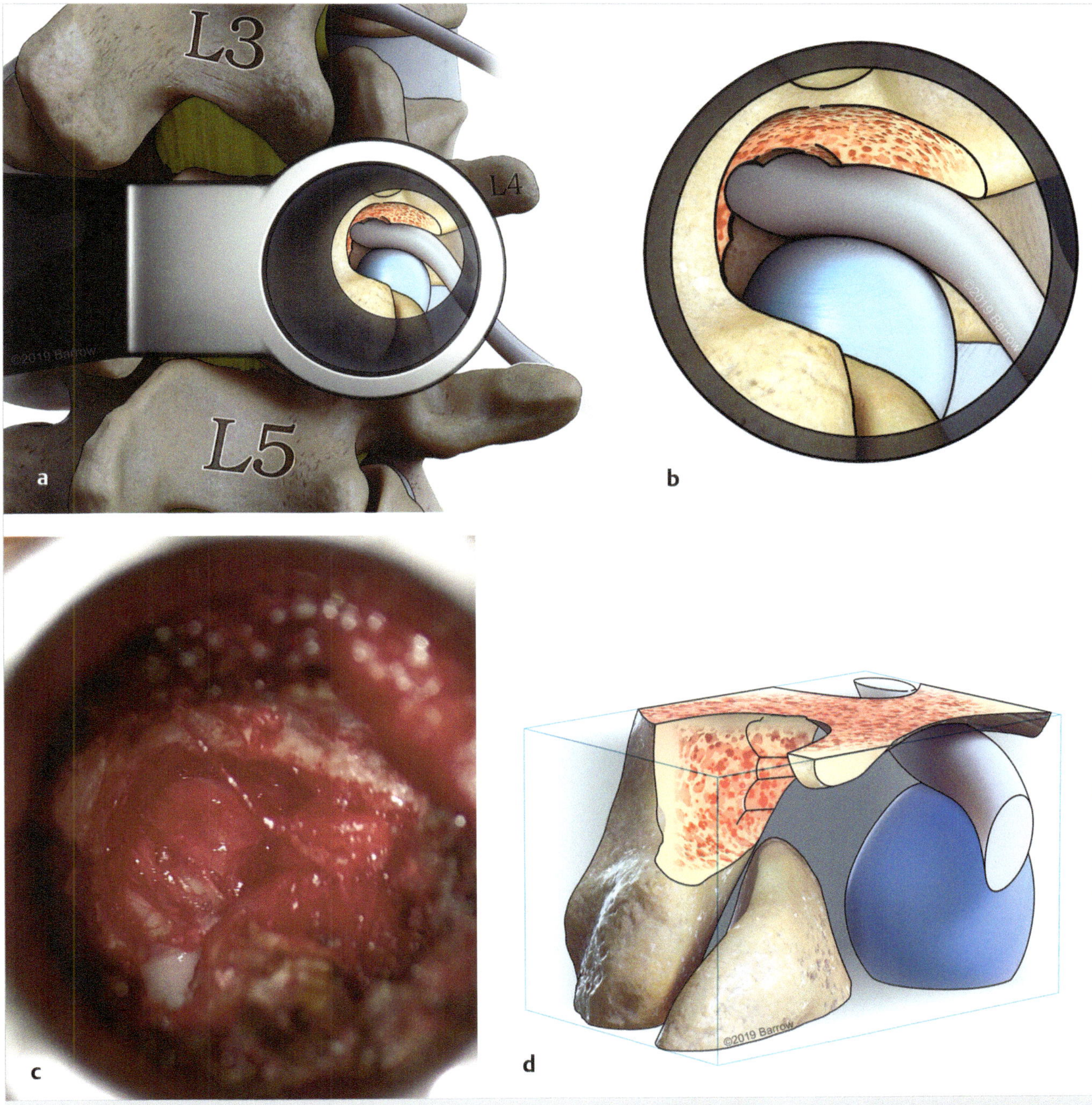

Fig. 5.23 Exposure of the nerve root and the far lateral disc extrusion. **(a)** Illustration demonstrating the surgical view through a 16-mm access port where 2 mm of the lateral pars interarticularis has been removed along with the inferior aspect of the transverse process to allow the intertransverse process ligament to be resected and the pedicle identified. The combination of these steps allows for the safe exposure of the nerve root and the far lateral disc extrusion. **(b)** Illustration of the surgical view through the operating microscope. **(c)** Intraoperative photograph after exposure of the nerve root. **(d)** Illustration limited to the volumetrically extracted requisite anatomy—oblique view demonstrating the pedicle and pars interarticularis relative to the nerve root and disc extrusion.

In the various cases I have managed, I have found the majority of far lateral disc herniations have displaced the root superiorly into the pedicle. At times, it may be difficult to find the nerve root. One reason for this difficulty is that the disc herniation has the perplexing ability to resemble the nerve root itself in this region, particularly when it occupies the entire foramen. I reemphasize that identifying and palpating the pedicle resolves this dilemma. Sweeping down from the pedicle allows me to identify the nerve root reliably and mitigate the risk of nerve root injury. I always identify and establish a distinct plane between the nerve root and the disc herniation, which is impossible without a clear delineation of the nerve root. I emphatically stress that it is imperative to identify the nerve root before ever wielding a No. 11 blade in this region for an annulotomy. In some circumstances, a Penfield dissector effortlessly establishes the plane beneath the nerve root as a suction retractor lightly retracts the root (▶ Fig. 5.24). At other times, I find myself meticulously dissecting to separate the root from the disc.

With a plane established between the nerve root and the disc, doing nothing more than mobilizing the extruded disc material with a right-angled ball-tipped probe delivers the fragment into view. Once in view, I use a pituitary forceps to reach into the annulotomy and grab ahold of and remove the wayward disc fragment that is compressing the nerve root.

On occasion, opening the annulus is necessary to retrieve the contained disc fragment. Before using the No. 11 blade near the annulus, I always confirm the nerve root relative to the disc space. A small annulotomy is all that is needed to access the disc herniation. A right-angled ball-tipped probe rotated within the annulotomy reliably delivers the disc fragment (Video 5.1).

The moment I feel that I have removed an adequate amount of disc and have completely decompressed the nerve root, I go through my final systems check. I use a right-angle ball-tipped probe to sweep beneath the nerve from above and below, which ensures that there is no disc material left behind that may be out of my field of view because of the nerve root. Next, I use the right-angled ball-tipped probe and sweep it medially beneath the pars interarticularis, which is an area out of my field of view and a potential hiding place for disc material. Time and time again, a sweep in this vicinity has offered me generous amounts of disc material that would have undoubtedly kept the patient symptomatic had I not retrieved it. Finally, I take the right-angled ball-tipped probe and sweep downward from above the nerve root. Going through this systems check invariably stirs up some epidural bleeding. I use a suction retractor to lightly displace the nerve root rostral into the pedicle so that I can safely use a right-angled bipolar cautery tip to cauterize the bleeding epidural veins up against the disc space. A combination of particulate thrombin, a half-inch by half-inch cottonoid and some pressure brings an end to the venous bleeding.

5.14 Closure

With the decompression complete, my assistant slowly removes the minimal access port as I hold the cautery in one hand and suction in another. It is essential to ensure that the artery of the pars interarticularis was not interrupted or was adequately cauterized. Occasionally, I have encountered brisk arterial bleeding after pulling the tubular retractor slightly back. In this situation, the minimal access port acts as a tamponade for the vessel, and its removal releases the pressure and allows the artery to bleed. Slowly removing the access port provides the opportunity to identify and cauterize any vessel that is bleeding. Removing the port too quickly closes the door on an opportunity for a quick remedy and leaves the surgeon searching for bleeding that cannot be seen through an impossibly small opening.

With the access port out, I infiltrate the skin and muscle with a lidocaine and bupivacaine mixture and then reapproximate the fascia with size 0 polyglactin 910 (Vicryl, Ethicon, Bridgewater, NJ) sutures on a UR-6 needle. Next, I suture the subcutaneous tissue with 2.0 polyglactin on an X-1 needle and the skin edges with 3.0 polyglactin sutures on an RB-1 needle. I place Steri-Strips (3 M, Maplewood, MN) and a 5% lidocaine dressing on the top of the incision.

5.15 Postoperative Care

For an unknown reason, I have found that reherniation is rare in far lateral disc herniations. I have managed approximately one dozen per year for the past 10 years, and I have seen only four reherniations or recurrent symptoms, which I subsequently managed with a minimally invasive TLIF. One reason for the modest reherniation rate may be that the number of cases is small, and it could take a larger number of cases before this entity surfaces as a clinically relevant issue. Regardless, I admonish my patients about the risks of reherniation. Most patients are discharged from the hospital on the day of surgery with a weight limit restriction of 5 pounds for the first month. They are encouraged to walk daily but to avoid impact training. Similar to the physical therapy for minimally invasive microdiscectomy of paramedian discs, physical therapy begins 1 month after surgery, and I release the patient without limitations or restrictions after 3 months.

5.16 Far Lateral Disc Herniations at L5–S1: A Unique Anatomic Circumstance

"A special, and sometimes extremely difficult situation to manage may be encountered at level L5-S1." That statement is the first sentence Reulen and colleagues[13] write in the section discussing the lumbosacral junction in their paper on extraforaminal lumbar disc herniations, and I believe it captures the essence of this region perfectly. I only wish I had read that sentence much earlier in my experience with minimally invasive techniques. As I ventured into the far lateral regions in the lumbosacral spine early in my career, I did so blissfully ignorant and thinking it was just another segment in the lumbar spine. Not so.

Nor had I read the technical note by Cervellini et al[17] on minimal access approaches to far lateral disc herniations. The Methods and Materials section of their paper has the admonishing statement, "at L5-S1, this approach is not possible," and the Discussion section ends with the unflinching statement, "we never performed an approach at the level L5-S1 because of the iliac crest."[17] These authors clearly had concerns about the lumbosacral junction and far lateral discs, and their concerns were well warranted.

It is my opinion that a minimally invasive approach to a far lateral disc herniation is, in fact, possible at the lumbosacral junction, but it would be naive to treat it as if it were just another segment of the lumbar spine. The statements made by Reulen et al and Cervellini et al are worth keeping in mind as you consider approaching this level. Notably, the focus should be on understanding the anatomical basis of their statements rather than thoughtlessly obeying their statements. In particular, there are three elements to acknowledge at the lumbosacral junction. The first is the upward slope of the sacral ala, which can compromise access to the foramen (▶ Fig. 5.25). The second is the interpedicular distance, which is the shortest distance

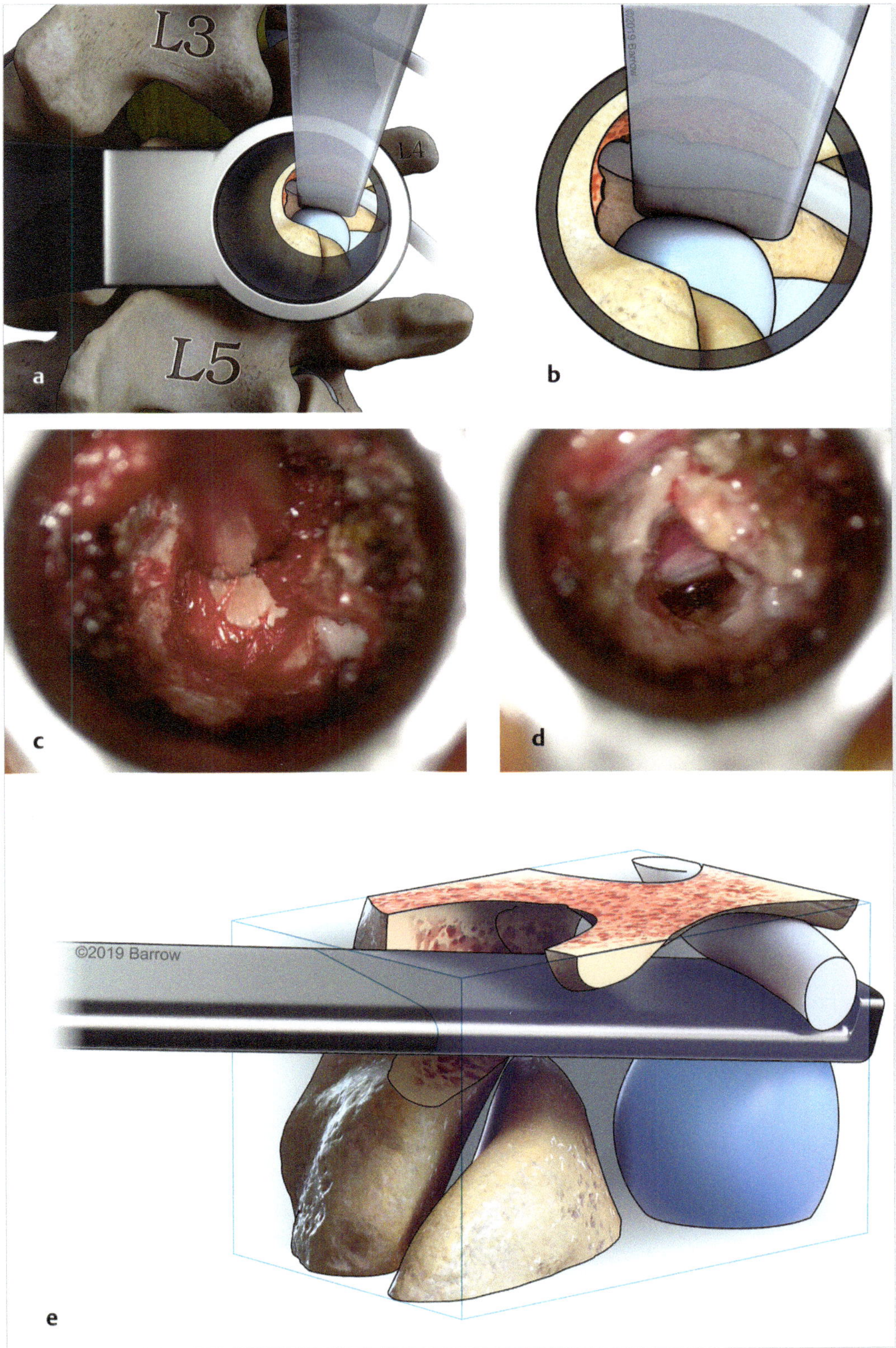

Fig. 5.24 Retracting the nerve root. **(a)** Illustration of the surgical view through a 16-mm minimal access port after resection of the intertransverse ligament and exposure of the nerve root. After mobilizing the nerve root, the disc extrusion may be further exposed with a suction retractor, which also protects the nerve root. **(b)** Magnified surgical view through the operating microscope showing retraction of the nerve root and exposure of the disc extrusion. **(c)** Intraoperative photograph showing retraction of the exiting nerve root with the suction retractor. **(d)** Intraoperative photograph after completion of the microdiscectomy. **(e)** Illustration of the volumetrically extracted requisite anatomy. Oblique view demonstrating the suction retractor relative to the pedicle and the facet.

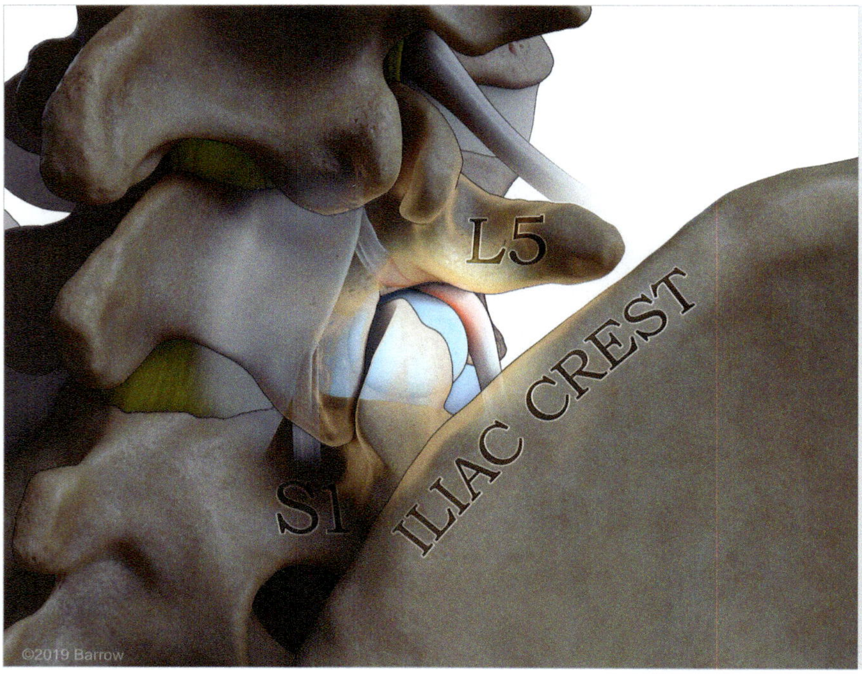

Fig. 5.25 The lumbosacral junction. Illustration of the unique clinical circumstance of the lumbosacral junction. The alar wing, the shortened isthmus of the pars interarticularis and the encroachment of the transverse process into the foramen collectively combine to create a constrained operative window.

between pedicles in the entire lumbar and sacral spine. Such a shortened interpedicular distance places the transverse process squarely in the path of the operative window. The third is the width of the isthmus of L5. Reulen et al demonstrated that the lateral edge of the pars interarticularis could exceed the entire width of the L5 vertebral body (▶ Fig. 5.26).[13] The consequence of this combination is the smallest rostrocaudal dimension of any neural foramen in the lumbar and sacral spine.

The surgical strategy for this segment would have to involve enlargement of the constrained operative corridor. A potential solution is drilling the medial-most aspect of the sacral ala. Although I have not found this to be necessary in every case, it is something that I am prepared to do to access the neural foramen. Bleeding from the cancellous bone can be a potential issue and can be adequately addressed with nothing more than bone wax. The second modification at this segment is the requirement to drill more of the L5 transverse process. Reulen et al appropriately identified that the accessory process of the transverse process might be more prominent at L5, further crowding the constrained working area. At this level more than any other, I find I must drill the inferior medial aspect of the transverse process. Having drilled the sacral ala and inferior transverse process, I find a more generous corridor onto the isthmus of the pars interarticularis.

I have already emphasized the importance of identifying the pedicle in the technique section above. The pedicle is as valuable at this segment as it is elsewhere. The pedicle reliably serves as the North Star that guides you to the nerve root. Given the width of the L5 isthmus, it requires more drilling to reach the intersection of the transverse process, pars interarticularis and the pedicle. O'Toole and colleagues demonstrated the capacity to perform a far lateral microdiscectomy in their cadaveric feasibility study and clinical paper, which I highly recommend reading before embarking on an L5–S1 far lateral microdiscectomy.[18] Understandably, the L5–S1 segment should not be your first foray into minimally invasive far lateral disc extrusions. The two surgical strategies for managing far lateral disc herniation at this level are shown in the operative video that accompanies this chapter (Video 5.2).

5.17 Case Illustrations

In the following case illustration section, I review the clinical presentation and operative techniques at three different spinal levels: L2–3, L4–5, and L5–S1.

5.17.1 Case Illustration 1: L2–3 Far Lateral Disc Herniation

Clinical Presentation and Radiographic Findings

A 68-year-old woman with a previous history of an L4–5 minimally invasive TLIF 4 years prior presented acutely with incapacitating left anterior thigh pain that radiated to the knee. MRI demonstrated a far lateral L2–3 disc herniation affecting the exiting nerve root of L2 (▶ Fig. 5.27). Despite selective nerve root blocks and epidural injections, the patient remained symptomatic and elected to undergo an L2–3 left-sided far lateral microdiscectomy.

Surgical Intervention

The patient was positioned on a Jackson table atop a Wilson frame. An incision was planned 35 mm lateral to the midline over the top of the L2–3 segment (▶ Fig. 5.28).

After the area was prepped and draped, a spinal needle was inserted with a convergent trajectory onto the spine, and a lateral fluoroscopic image confirmed the level and trajectory for

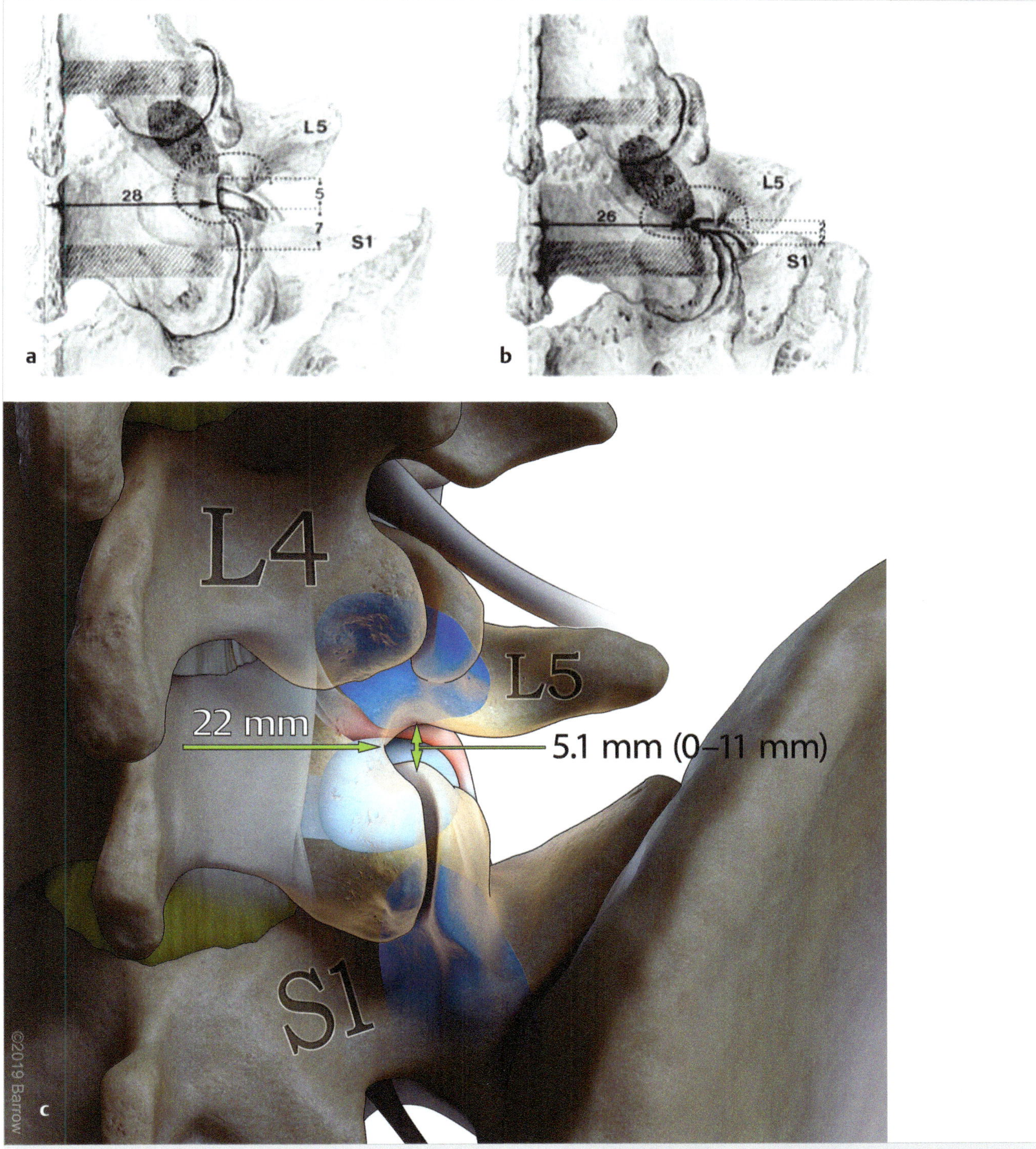

Fig. 5.26 The lumbosacral junction. **(a** and **b)** Illustrations from the anatomical study by Reulen et al of the operative windows at L5–S1.[13] These drawings illustrate two unfavorable anatomical circumstances. **(a)** The first is a flattened sacral alar wing. The isthmus, in this circumstance, measures 28 mm in width. The distance from the inferior aspect of the transverse process to the superior articular facet is 5 mm, which contributes to a constrained operative corridor. The L5 pedicle is shaded and marked with the letter P. **(b)** The second anatomical circumstance is even more constrained by the rising slope of the sacral ala. The operative corridor has narrowed to 2 mm. **(c)** Illustration modernizing the anatomical corridor from Reulen's artwork in **a.** The pedicle of L5 and S1 are shaded in *royal blue*. The far lateral disc extrusion (*sky blue*) displaces the nerve root of L5 into the pedicle of L5. At the L5–S1 segment, the distance from the inferior aspect of the L5 transverse process to the superior articular process of S1 can be as much as 11 mm or may be completely collapsed to 0 mm. The average distance is 5.1 mm, as seen in the illustration. When approaching far lateral L5–S1 disc extrusions, knowledge of the constraints of this corridor is essential to decompress the L5 nerve root.

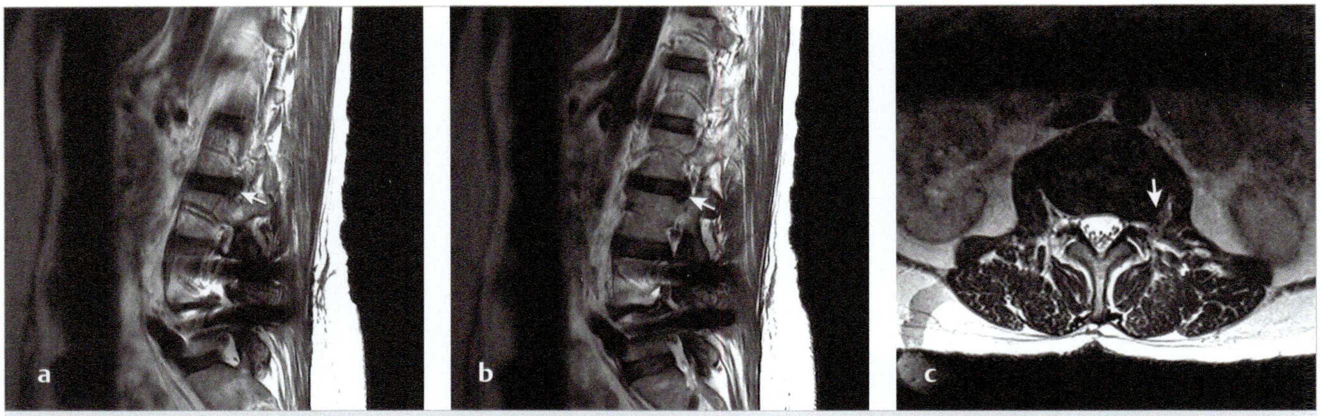

Fig. 5.27 Magnetic resonance imaging (MRI) demonstrating a left far lateral L2–3 disc herniation. **(a)** Parasagittal T2-weighted MRI demonstrating compression of the exiting nerve root (*white arrow*) of the left L2 within the foramen. **(b)** Parasagittal T2-weighted MRI obtained even further lateral in the foramen (*white arrow*) of L2. **(c)** Axial T2-weighted MRI demonstrating compression of the nerve root in the left lateral recess (*white arrow*).

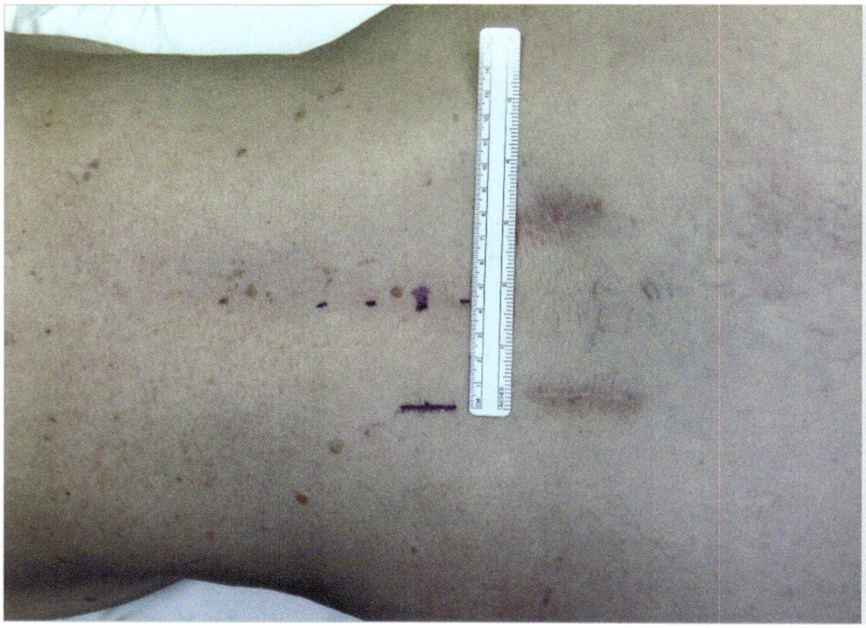

Fig. 5.28 Photograph of incision planning for an L2–3 far lateral microdiscectomy. The midline is palpated and marked. The L2–3 segment is approximated by palpation of the anterior superior iliac spine, and an 18-mm incision is planned 35 mm lateral to the midline. Note the scars from an L4–5 minimally invasive transforaminal lumbar interbody fusion performed previously.

the minimal access port. The incision was infiltrated with a local anesthetic mixture (lidocaine and bupivacaine), and the incision was made with a No. 15 blade. The first dilator was inserted to probe the transverse process and the lateral pars interarticularis. That first dilator was anchored onto the lateral pars pointing directly at the neural foramen. Sequential dilation up to 16 mm displaced the minimal access port from resting directly on the pars interarticularis because of the unique topography of the lateral lumbar spine (▶ Fig. 5.29). After the minimal access port was anchored into position with the table-mounted arm, a lateral and AP fluoroscopic image confirmed an ideal position over the top of the foramen. The operating microscope was then rolled into the field.

After the exposure of the pars interarticularis, 2 mm were drilled off its lateral aspect and the inferior aspect of the transverse process. The intertransverse process ligament was exposed and divided. The L2 pedicle was identified, which led directly to the nerve root. The disc extrusion displaced the nerve rostrally into the pedicle, and a plane of dissection between the nerve root and the disc extrusion was developed to allow for retraction of the nerve root and removal of the disc extrusion.

5.17.2 Case Illustration 2: Far Lateral Facet Cyst Resection

Although the contents of this chapter are focused on the management of lumbar radiculopathy due to a far lateral disc extrusion, the following case illustration demonstrates a unique application of the far lateral technique for the management of lumbar radiculopathy caused by a facet cyst within the foramen.

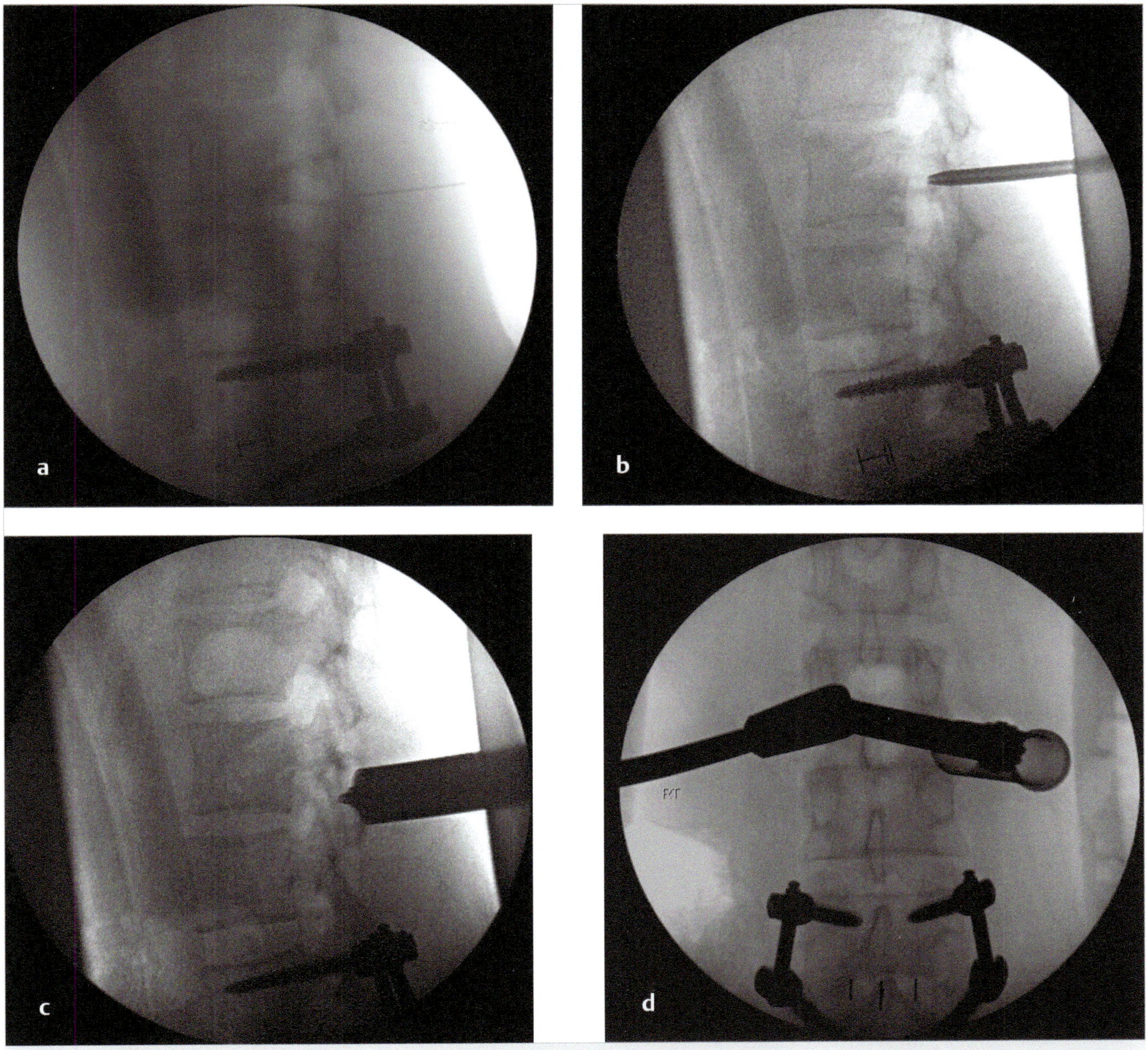

Fig. 5.29 The fluoroscopic sequence for securing the access port for a far lateral microdiscectomy. **(a)** Lateral fluoroscopic image of localization for an L2–3 far lateral microdiscectomy. Note the previous instrumentation at L4–5 facilitating localization of the segment. **(b)** Lateral fluoroscopic image of the first dilator docked onto the pars interarticularis. **(c)** Sequential dilatation to 16 mm. Note the final dilator is unable to dock immediately onto the pars interarticularis because of the uneven topography of the facet. **(d)** AP fluoroscopic image demonstrating the position of the access port over the top of the foramen and immediately beneath the pedicle of L2. In this case, the compression of the nerve root was in the lateral aspect of the foramen, and so the minimal access port was positioned slightly lateral to the pedicle.

Clinical Presentation and Radiographic Findings

A 61-year-old man presented with progressively worsening left radicular leg pain of 6 weeks' duration. He was ambulatory only with a cane since the onset of symptoms. On examination, the patient presented with a weak left quadriceps muscle (4-/5) to the extent that he was able to ascend stairs leading only with his right leg. He was utterly unable to lead with the left leg to climb the stairs. The left patellar reflex was absent. However, it was the pain (VAS leg pain = 91 mm) that was the most debilitating component of his presentation. An attempt to aspirate the cyst was unsuccessful. MRI demonstrated mild facet arthropathy at L4–5, no central canal compromise and the presence of a focal cyst within the foramen on the left at L4 (▶ Fig. 5.30).

Surgical Intervention

With the patient positioned on a Wilson frame atop a Jackson table, an incision 18 mm in length and 40 mm from midline was planned (▶ Fig. 5.31). A spinal needle was docked on to the lateral aspect of the inferior articular process, and the segment

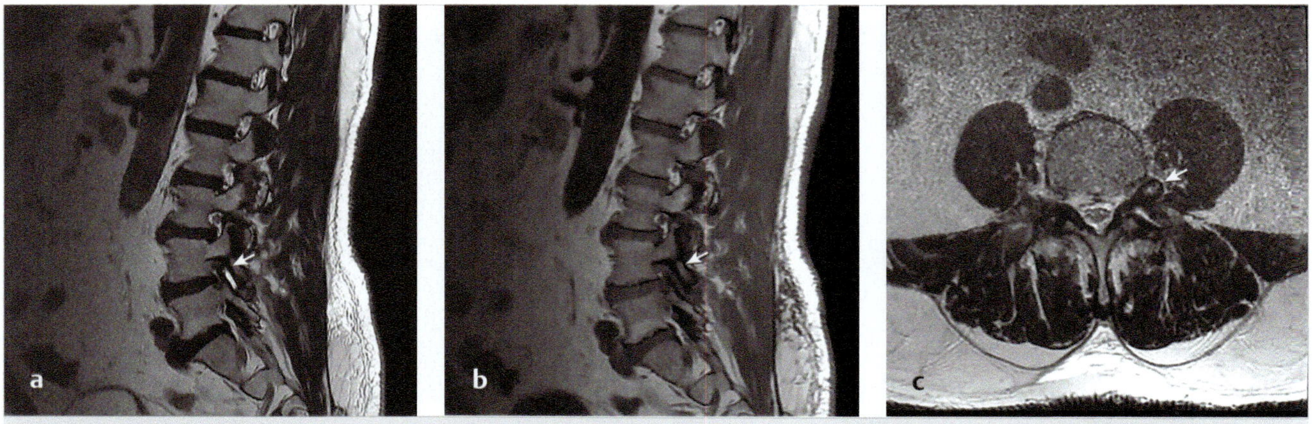

Fig. 5.30 Magnetic resonance imaging (MRI) of the lumbar spine demonstrating a facet cyst in the far lateral recess. **(a)** Parasagittal T2-weighted MRI demonstrates a facet cyst compressing the exiting nerve root of L4 (*white arrow*). **(b)** Parasagittal T2-weighted MRI demonstrates the obliteration of the perineural fat within the lateral recess (*white arrow*). Note the patent neural foramen in the segments above. **(c)** Axial T2-weighted MRI demonstrates a facet cyst (*white arrow*) compressing the exiting nerve root of L4 in the far lateral recess.

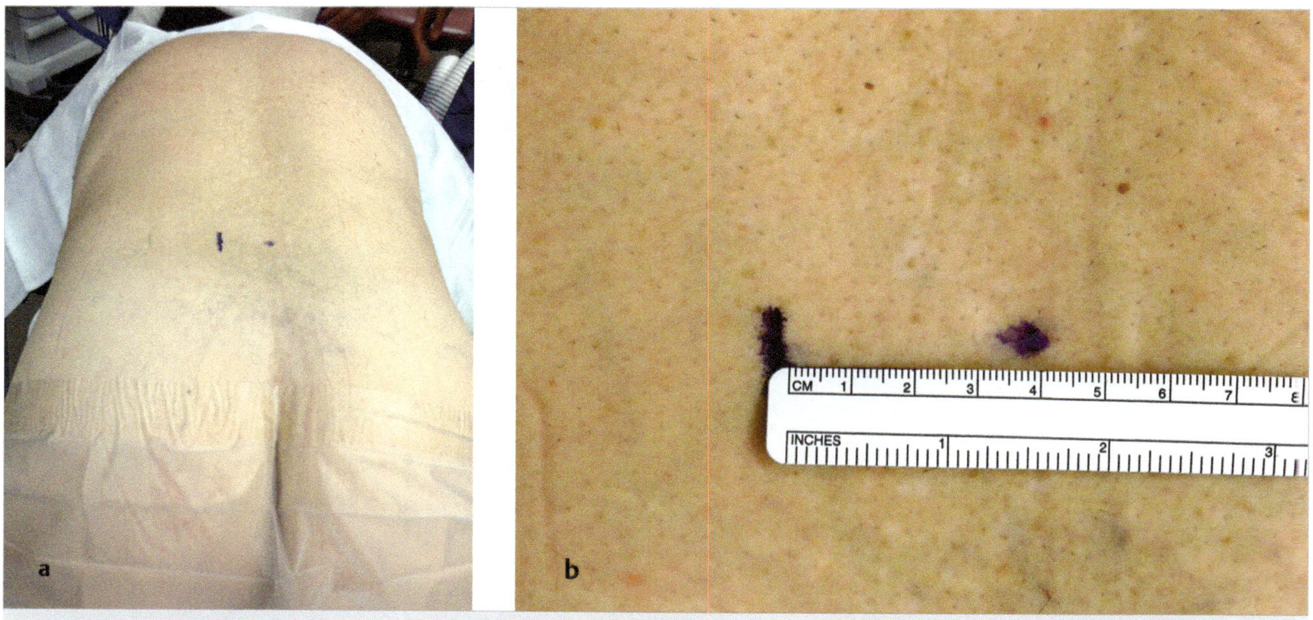

Fig. 5.31 Planning the incision for an L4–5 far lateral facet cyst resection. **(a)** Photograph of the patient positioned for surgery on a Wilson frame atop a Jackson table with the incision marked. **(b)** Enlarged photograph of the incision planned 40 mm lateral to the midline to allow for convergence onto the foramen.

confirmed with a lateral fluoroscopic image. The incision was made with a No. 15 blade, and the fascia was divided with cautery. The first dilator cleaved a plane onto the pars interarticularis, and sequential dilatation proceeded to 16 mm. Lateral and AP fluoroscopic images demonstrate the positioning of the minimal access port over the top of the pedicle (▶ Fig. 5.32).

Under the operating microscope, the lateral aspect of the pars interarticularis was exposed, and then 2 mm were removed with a drill; the intertransverse process ligament was identified and divided. I then used a right-angled ball-tipped probe to palpate the L4 pedicle, which led directly to the exposure of the L4 nerve root. From there, the facet cyst emanating from the facet joint was identified and resected. The patient had a complete and immediate resolution of his radicular leg pain. His quadriceps strength gradually returned over the ensuing months. By the third postoperative month, he was walking independently and fully capable of ascending the stairs.

5.17.3 Case Illustration 3: L5–S1 Far Lateral Microdiscectomy

The final case illustration reviews a far lateral microdiscectomy at L5–S1. The video that accompanies this chapter reviews the various surgical corridors to access the L5 nerve root in the far lateral recess. This particular case illustration focuses on the technique described in this chapter. The surgical video

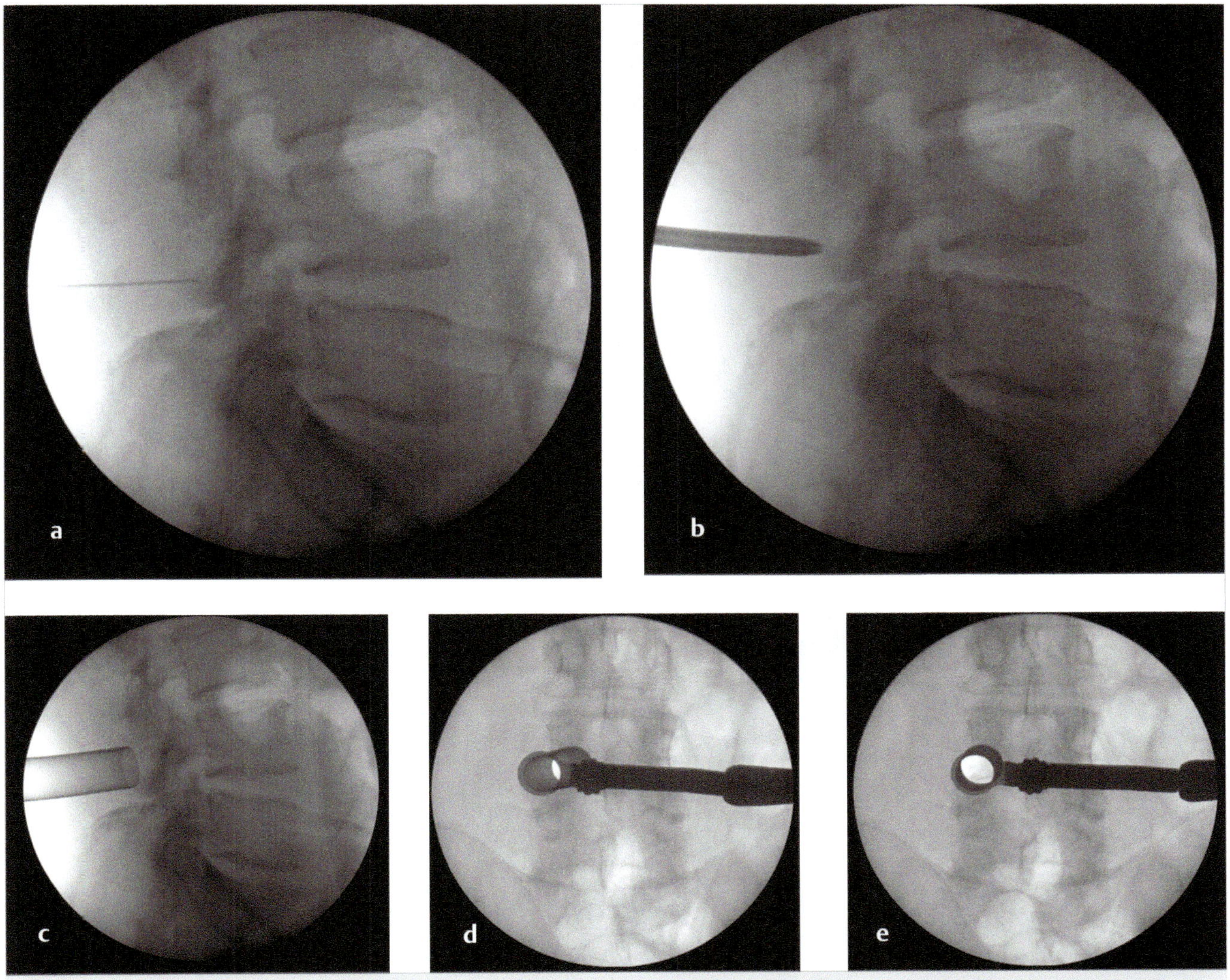

Fig. 5.32 Fluoroscopic sequence of docking the minimal access port. **(a)** Localizing needle confirming the L4–5 segment. **(b)** Palpating the lateral bony anatomy with the first dilator. **(c)** Minimal access port in position aimed directly at the pars interarticularis. **(d)** Anteroposterior (AP) image demonstrating suboptimal placement of the minimal access port. The base of the port is slightly medial to the pedicle. **(e)** AP image demonstrating optimal placement of the minimal access port immediately beneath the pedicle. The last two images (**d** and **e**) demonstrate the value of the AP image in far lateral microdiscectomies.

demonstrates an alternate corridor to decompress the L5 nerve root (Video 5.2).

Clinical Presentation and Radiographic Findings

A 38-year-old man presented to the emergency room with left foot drop, the onset of which occurred while moving a refrigerator 36 hours earlier. The patient had 0/5 tibialis anterior and extensor hallucis longus function along with decreased sensation on the dorsum of the left foot. He was nonambulatory because of the left radicular leg pain. MRI demonstrated bilateral pars interarticularis defects, mild degeneration of the L5–S1 segment, and a far lateral disc extrusion displacing the left L5 nerve root (▶ Fig. 5.33).

Surgical Intervention

Given the 36 hours of complete foot drop, the patient was taken emergently for surgery for a far lateral decompression. The inherent constraints of the corridor to the L5 nerve root were discussed with the patient, including the possibility of a complete facetectomy and fusion, for which the patient consented, if necessary. With the patient on a Wilson frame atop a Jackson table, an 18-mm incision was planned 40 mm lateral to the midline at the L5–S1 segment (▶ Fig. 5.34).

After making the incision and dividing the fascia with cautery, the first dilator was placed onto the inferior articular process. The pars interarticularis had defects that precluded it as the target for the first dilator. Once it became apparent that the iliac crest and sacral ala would not interfere with an ideal trajectory

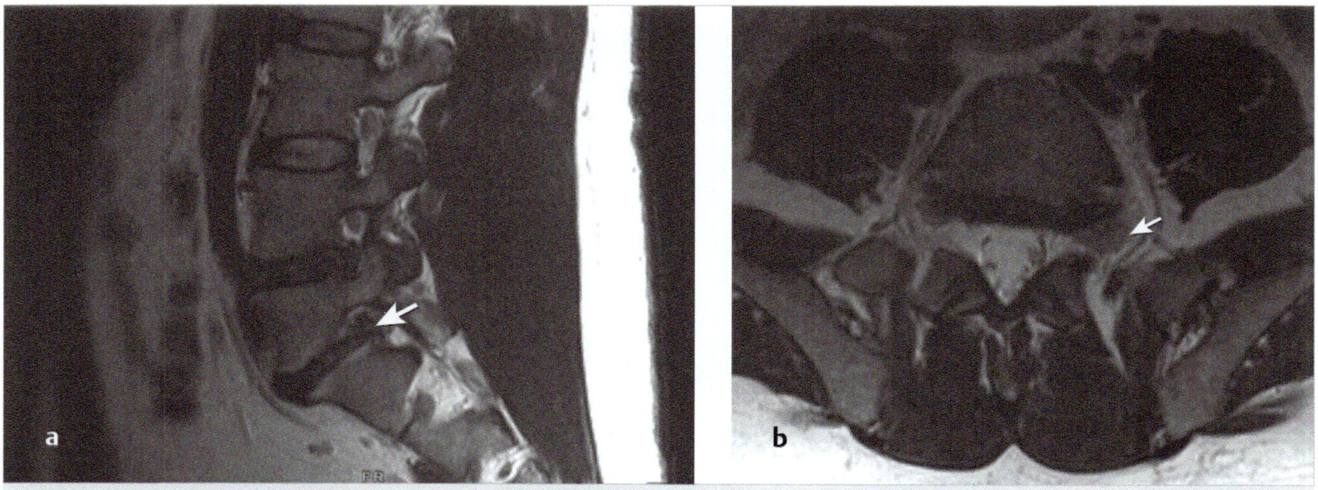

Fig. 5.33 Left L5–S1 far lateral disc herniation, which caused foot drop. **(a)** Parasagittal T2-weighted magnetic resonance image (MRI) demonstrating the far lateral disc extrusion (*arrow*) within the foramen of L5. There is a collapse of the disc space with Modic changes seen on the underside of L5 and the superior aspect of S1. The patient also had bilateral pars defects. **(b)** Axial T2-weighted MRI demonstrating a far lateral disc extrusion in the L5 foramen (*arrow*).

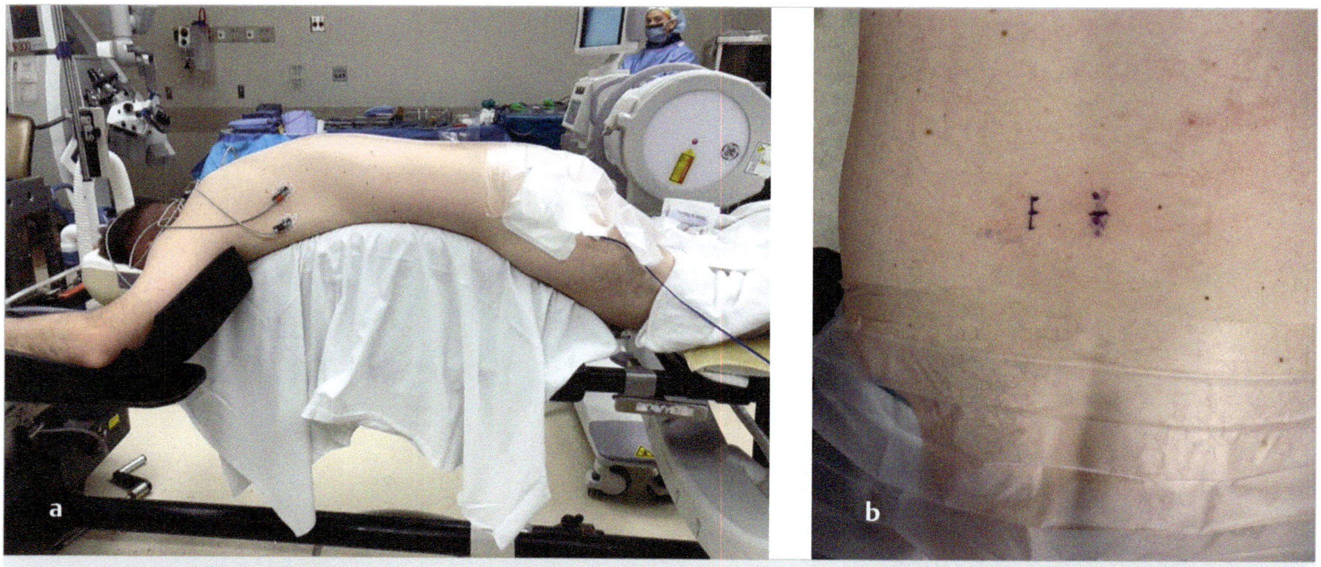

Fig. 5.34 Left L5–S1 far lateral microdiscectomy. **(a)** The patient is positioned on a Jackson table atop a maximally expanded Wilson frame. Note the fluoroscope already in position. Not visualized in this photograph is the microscope draped and at the ready. **(b)** An 18-mm incision 40 mm from the midline is planned based on the anatomical landmarks of the anterior superior iliac spine and the spinous processes.

onto the spine, sequential dilatation proceeded to the 16-mm diameter needed to secure the access port into position (▶ Fig. 5.35).

After the preliminary dissection leading to the pars interarticularis, the pars defect was identified. No bone was drilled to access the foramen in this circumstance. The intertransverse process ligament was identified and divided. The L5 pedicle was confirmed, which led immediately to the L5 nerve root. Mobilization of the nerve root revealed the disc herniation, which was removed (Video 5.2).

Postoperative Course

The patient had strength measurements of 3/5 in the tibialis anterior and extensor hallucis longus muscles immediately after surgery and complete resolution of his radicular symptoms. He was fitted with an ankle-foot-orthosis. By the third postoperative month, he had successfully weaned himself out of the ankle-foot-orthosis and had only mild weakness (4/5) in the tibialis anterior and extensor hallucis longus muscles. The patient demonstrated 2 mm of anterior transla-

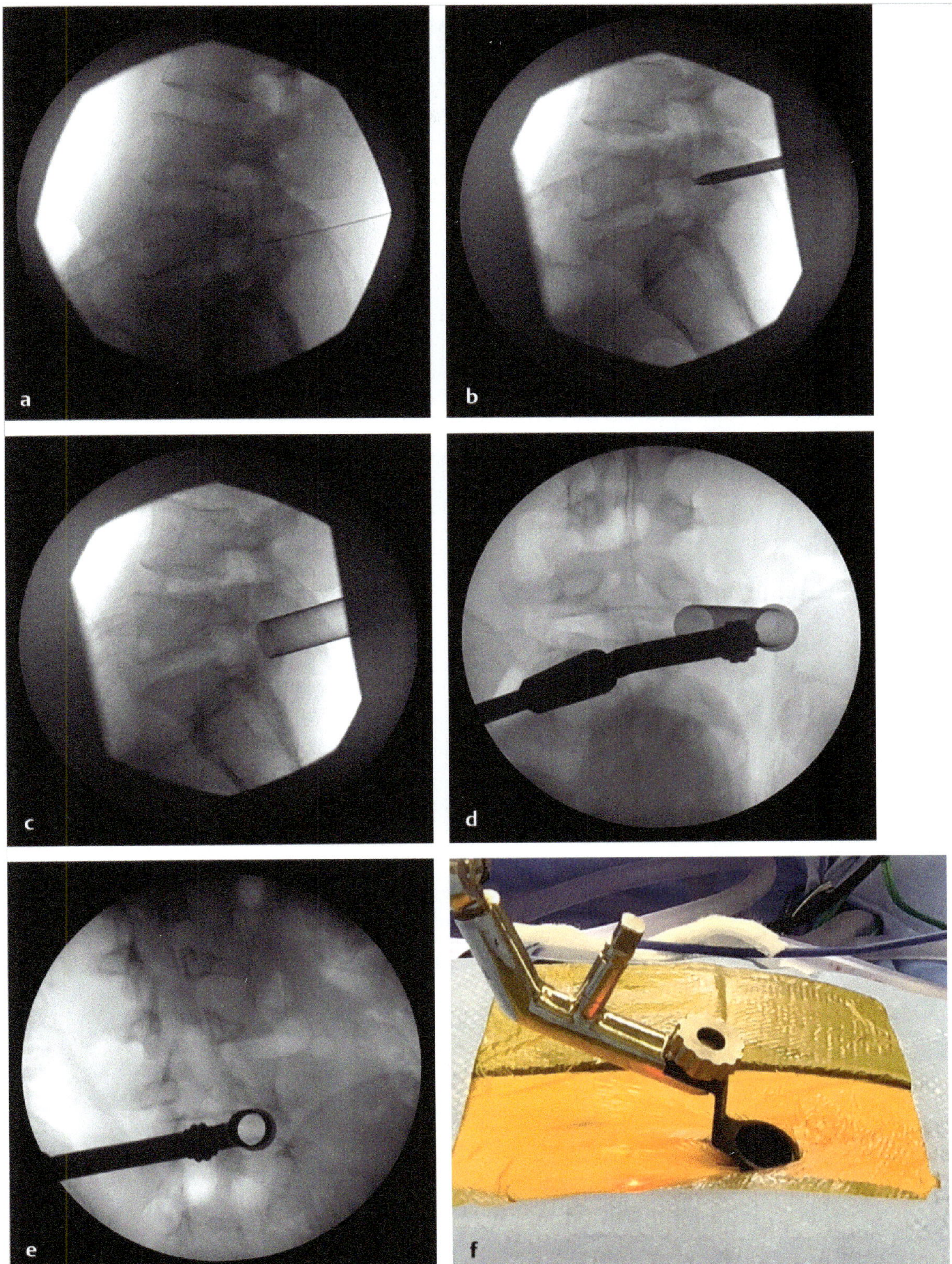

Fig. 5.35 Fluoroscopic sequence securing the access port for the L5–S1 far lateral microdiscectomy. **(a)** Lateral fluoroscopic image demonstrating spinal needle confirmation of the segment. **(b)** Lateral fluoroscopic image with the first dilator in position. **(c)** Lateral fluoroscopic image demonstrating a 16-mm access port in position parallel to the disc space. **(d)** Anteroposterior fluoroscopic image with the distal aspect of the access port immediately beneath the pedicle. **(e)** Owl's eye view of the L5 pedicle confirming the access port has been positioned immediately beneath the pedicle. Note the distance from the access port to the iliac crest. **(f)** Intraoperative photograph taken from the head of the bed demonstrating the converging access port in position.

tion of L5 onto S1 on dynamic radiographs but reported no axial back pain. No intervention was required for the management of his spondylosis 1 year after the surgery. He continues to be under observation.

5.18 Conclusions

Few procedures lend themselves more to a minimally invasive approach than the far lateral microdiscectomy. It is a significant departure from the exposures of the microdiscectomy, laminectomy and transforaminal approaches. At the same time, it is the skill set developed from those procedures, especially minimally invasive transforaminal approaches, that allows your mind to become familiar with the anatomy in the far lateral recess. It is losing sight of the shore (i.e., the midline), in the words of Andre Gide that began this chapter, and establishing your bearings by the tactile feel of the pars interarticularis, the fluoroscopic images and your absolute certainty of the anatomy that allows you to master this procedure. Once mastered, the minimally invasive far lateral microdiscectomy could actually take less time than a standard minimally invasive microdiscectomy.

Throughout the first four chapters of this Primer, the focus has been to develop skills to deftly maneuver instruments in and out of minimal access ports and become familiar with the bony structures from a slightly different vantage point while safely and effectively decompressing the neural elements and instrumenting the spine. The upcoming sections of this Primer now take those skills and apply them to the cervical and thoracic spine. Along the way, the reader takes two detours, one through the psoas muscle and the other through the anterior cervical spine. The first detour is the topic of the next chapter. The transpsoas approach to the lumbar spine is a complete departure from the skill set developed thus far in this Primer. Except for the use of dilators, the operation stands alone in its concept, approach and technique. The transpsoas approach has been a transformative procedure that has ushered in a new era in the management of degenerative disc disease and deformity.

References

[1] Dandy WE. Recent advances in the diagnosis and treatment of ruptured intervertebral disks. Ann Surg. 1942; 115(4):514–520

[2] Echols DH, Rehfeldt FC. Failure to disclose ruptured intervertebral disks in 32 operations for sciatica. J Neurosurg. 1949; 6(5):376–382

[3] Macnab I. Negative disc exploration. An analysis of the causes of nerve-root involvement in sixty-eight patients. J Bone Joint Surg Am. 1971; 53(5):891–903

[4] Abdullah AF, Ditto EW, III, Byrd EB, Williams R. Extreme-lateral lumbar disc herniations. Clinical syndrome and special problems of diagnosis. J Neurosurg. 1974; 41(2):229–234

[5] Abdullah AF, Wolber PG, Warfield JR, Gunadi IK. Surgical management of extreme lateral lumbar disc herniations: review of 138 cases. Neurosurgery 1988; 22(4):648–653

[6] Epstein NE. Different surgical approaches to far lateral lumbar disc herniations. J Spinal Disord. 1995; 8(5):383–394

[7] Darden BV, II, Wade JF, Alexander R, Wood KE, Rhyne AL, III, Hicks JR. Far lateral disc herniations treated by microscopic fragment excision. Techniques and results. Spine. 1995; 20(13):1500–1505

[8] Donaldson WF, III, Star MJ, Thorne RP. Surgical treatment for the far lateral herniated lumbar disc. Spine. 1993; 18(10):1263–1267

[9] Wiltse LL, Spencer CW. New uses and refinements of the paraspinal approach to the lumbar spine. Spine. 1988; 13(6):696–706

[10] Maroon JC, Kopitnik TA, Schulhof LA, Abla A, Wilberger JE. Diagnosis and microsurgical approach to far-lateral disc herniation in the lumbar spine. J Neurosurg. 1990; 72(3):378–382

[11] Jane JA, Haworth CS, Broaddus WC, Lee JH, Malik J. A neurosurgical approach to far-lateral disc herniation. Technical note. J Neurosurg. 1990; 72(1):143–144

[12] Caspar W. A new surgical procedure for lumbar disc herniation causing less tissue damage through a microsurgical approach. Advances in Neurosurgery. Berlin: Springer-Verlag; 1977

[13] Reulen HJ, Müller A, Ebeling U. Microsurgical anatomy of the lateral approach to extraforaminal lumbar disc herniations. Neurosurgery. 1996; 39(2):345–350, discussion 350–351

[14] Foley K, Smith M. Microendoscopic discectomy. Tech Neurosurg. 1997; 3(4): 307–307

[15] Foley KT, Smith MM, Rampersaud YR. Microendoscopic approach to far-lateral lumbar disc herniation. Neurosurg Focus. 1999; 7(5):e5

[16] Schlesinger SM, Fankhauser H, de Tribolet N. Microsurgical anatomy and operative technique for extreme lateral lumbar disc herniations. Acta Neurochir (Wien). 1992; 118(3–4):117–129

[17] Cervellini P, De Luca GP, Mazzetto M, Colombo F. Micro-endoscopic-discectomy (MED) for far lateral disc herniation in the lumbar spine. Technical note. Acta Neurochir Suppl (Wien). 2005; 92:99–101

[18] O'Toole JE, Eichholz KM, Fessler RG. Minimally invasive far lateral microendoscopic discectomy for extraforaminal disc herniation at the lumbosacral junction: cadaveric dissection and technical case report. Spine J. 2007; 7(4):414–421

6 Minimally Invasive Lateral Transpsoas Interbody Lumbar Fusion

Abstract:
Minimally invasive lateral transpsoas interbody lumbar fusion is a direct, 90-degree lateral retroperitoneal transpsoas approach to the lumbar disc space. The procedure itself has made a seismic impact on the management of degenerative scoliosis, adjacent segment degeneration and degeneration in the segments of the upper lumbar spine. Similar to the evolution of the various minimally invasive techniques already presented in this Primer, the transpsoas technique evolved from the familiarity of working through thoracolumbar exposures for the management of burst fractures. Recognizing the safety of the retroperitoneal space, surgeons narrowed their focus to the disc spaces and began exploring the use of a retroperitoneal corridor to directly access the lateral aspect of the lumbar spine. This chapter presents the evolution and application of the lumbar transpsoas interbody fusion, with an emphasis on the anatomy and understanding of the lumbar plexus. From there, the anatomical basis, operating room setup, and patient positioning are presented along with case illustrations that cover three broad categories of the transpsoas application.

Keywords: adjacent segment, femoral nerve, genitofemoral nerve, iliohypogastric nerve, ilioinguinal nerve, interbody fusion, lumbar plexus, scoliosis, transpsoas

The more original a discovery, the more obvious it seems afterwards.
Arthur Koestler

6.1 Introduction

No statement better describes the transpsoas interbody approach to the lumbar spine than Arthur Koestler's astute observation on discovery. For decades of modern spine surgery, surgeons have traversed the paraspinal muscles for posterior approaches, mobilized the peritoneum and the iliac vessels for anterior surgery, and taken down the diaphragm and mobilized the psoas muscle in lateral thoracolumbar approaches. All these procedures were done in the name of accessing the thoracic, lumbar and sacral spine. Initially, none of these exposures were minimal; however, all were safe, comprehensive and reliable. In the end, these approaches were the necessary first steps in the evolution of spine surgery that would ultimately yield an elegant solution for accessing the lumbar interbody space.

The sophisticated understanding of the anatomy and the increasing experience gained from these approaches became the stepping-stone for the development of minimally invasive approaches to the spine. An entire array of minimally invasive techniques began to evolve to accomplish the same goals that were being otherwise accomplished with traditional midline incisions. Lumbar and cervical decompressions could now be reliably achieved through minimal access ports. Soon after, the access ports allowed for instrumentation of the lumbar spine. Building upon these maturing minimally invasive platforms, innovative surgeons pioneered a solution to a problem that had been staring all of us in the face for decades. Spine surgery then took a colossal step forward with the straightforward and well-conceived transpsoas approach to the lumbar interbody space.

At the end of the last century, the trend toward minimizing the extent of exposure required to accomplish the same goals of traditional midline surgeries quickly gathered momentum. Adhering to the principle introduced by Caspar regarding the ratio of the surgical target to the surgical exposure, a series of dilators passed through a paramedian incision expanded a corridor for a minimal access port and became a viable alternative to traditional larger midline exposures with self-retaining retractors. These techniques began by addressing more straightforward pathologies such as herniated discs and lumbar stenosis. The skill sets developed to deal with these pathologies were, in turn, translated to instrumentation of the lumbar spine and lumbar interbody approaches. By the mid-2000s, a firm foothold and comfort level had been established using dilators, table-mounted arms, and fixed diameter and expandable minimal access ports in the posterior lumbar and posterior cervical spine. These new techniques would lay the foundation for a more direct lateral approach to the lumbar interbody space.

Interest in a more direct approach to the spine from a lateral approach may be traced back to as early as 1985 when McAfee and colleagues[1] described decompression and stabilization of thoracolumbar burst fractures. Comfort with the thoracolumbar exposures eventually enabled these authors to explore a more focused exposure within the retroperitoneal space, which led directly to one of the first descriptions of lateral lumbar interbody fusions by Mayer[2] and McAfee et al[3] in the late 1990s. Running in parallel with spine surgeons' increasing interest and comfort in the retroperitoneal space were continued improvements in minimally invasive techniques. Building upon the existing platforms of both endoscopic and minimal access port-based approaches, surgeons now began to narrow their focus on one target: the disc space. As early as 2004, Bergey and colleagues[4] described an endoscopic transpsoas interbody approach to the lumbar spine. In due time, a transpsoas approach built upon the muscle dilating tubular retractor platforms would follow. In 2006, Ozgur and colleagues[5] reported the current technique of the lateral transpsoas approach and thus commenced the decade of lateral transpsoas interbody lumbar fusions.

I still remember learning about the transpsoas interbody approaches to the lumbar spine as a fifth-year resident. My first reaction was, "Why did it take so long to think of that?" It seemed like such an obvious solution to the upper lumbar spine, especially in cases of adjacent segment degeneration at L2–3 or L3–4. I recalled case after case where I painstakingly exposed and then extended previous fusions, an operation that caused equal discomfort to the patient and the surgeon alike. All those cases now fell into the precinct of a transpsoas approach, which avoided the previous posterior surgery altogether, restored the disc height, corrected the coronal imbalance and indirectly decompressed the neural elements. I marveled as I considered the implications of this clear answer to a difficult circumstance that, as spine surgeons, we had been facing all this time. Again, the more original the solution, the more obvious it seems afterward. My second reaction was concern. I had completed my spine rotation, and I feared that the opportunity to learn this technique in residency might have passed. I dreaded the possibility that I might stumble through a career in spine surgery without this procedure in my arsenal.

Fortunately, the orthopedic surgeons at the institution where I was trained brought the transpsoas technique immediately into the fold and gave me ample opportunity to observe. While I never scrubbed a case in residency, the transpsoas approach is a procedure similar to the odontoid screw, where positioning the patient and setting up the operating room represents 90% of the case. It was in these early cases that I began to appreciate the nuances of positioning the patient in a perfectly orthogonal lateral position as well as the importance of the ideal fluoroscopic image. After I left residency, I found myself at the Naval Medical Center in San Diego just a stone's throw away from the University of California at San Diego, where Dr. William Taylor had been pioneering the lateral transpsoas approach for years. Dr. Taylor welcomed my interest in the lateral approach and mentored me through case after case. This chapter in large part represents the technique taught to me by Dr. Taylor.

6.2 Advantages of the Transpsoas Approach

A lateral exposure avoids all the consequences of a posterior exposure, specifically iatrogenic instability from resection of the bony elements and disruption and denervation of the paraspinal muscles. The distinct advantage of the transpsoas approach to the interbody space is that it is a minimally invasive approach in the purest sense. An access corridor in the safety of the retroperitoneal space allows for direct exposure of the disc space through the psoas muscle without the need for any significant dissection or disruption of the musculature. The very nature of a retroperitoneal corridor onto the lateral spine makes the risk of vessel injury substantially less than in anterior approaches, where the aorta and vena cava need to be directly exposed and mobilized. The decreased risk of vessel injury is especially true in the upper lumbar segments where anterior exposures require extensive mobilization of the great vessels (▶ Fig. 6.1).

In an anterior approach, the iliac vessels, the veins in particular, have the potential to constrain access to the disc space. In a posterior transforaminal approach, access to the disc space is constrained by the exiting and traversing nerve roots (▶ Fig. 6.2). The single greatest advantage of the transpsoas approach is the unconstrained wide corridor into the disc space. A direct trajectory into this wide corridor provides the ability to span the entire breadth of the disc space and cover a substantial amount of the apophyseal ring. The correction of a coronal imbalance within a segment is unparalleled with this approach.[6]

6.3 Disadvantages

The main limitation of the transpsoas approach is the unseen formation of the lumbar plexus and its branches within the psoas muscle. Navigating around these unseen branches of the plexus while traversing the psoas muscle to reach the disc space is the most technically demanding aspect of the operation. The lower the segment on the lumbar spine, the more anterior the lumbar plexus becomes and the greater the risk of neurologic injury. One lumbar plexus branch in particular that remains at risk with this approach is the genitofemoral nerve, which has the uncanny ability to unveil itself immediately over the disc space that requires the operation. A common course for the genitofemoral nerve is to travel within the psoas major muscle over the top of the L2–3 disc space. Identification and

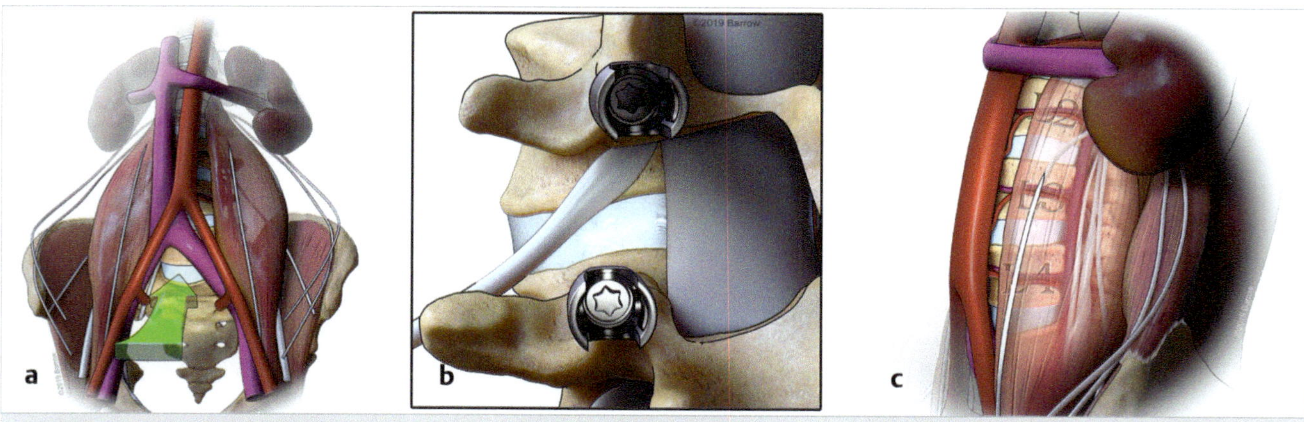

Fig. 6.1 Illustration demonstrating the various corridors to the lumbar disc space. (a) Anterior view of the vascular anatomy of the lumbar spine. At L5–S1 a generous corridor becomes available with minimal mobilization of the iliac arteries and veins. However, the anterior corridor to the disc space becomes constrained in the upper segments of the lumbar spine because of the aorta and vena cava. Mobilization of these vessels is necessary to access the upper levels of the lumbar spine but with a subsequently increased risk of vascular injury. (b) Illustration showing the transforaminal corridor at L4–5. Access to the disc space is constrained by the exiting and traversing nerve roots. (c) Lateral view of the lumbar spine demonstrating the vascular anatomy. The aorta and vena cava remain anterior, and the trajectory of approach does not require visualization or mobilization of these vessels. The segmental vessels course over the lateral vertebral body and remain vascular structures at risk with a lateral approach, but these vessels do not course over the disc space. The main disadvantage is the need to traverse the psoas muscle and navigate the lumbar plexus. The combination of a thinner psoas muscle and more posteriorly located lumbar plexus makes the upper segments of the lumbar spine ideal for the transpsoas approach.

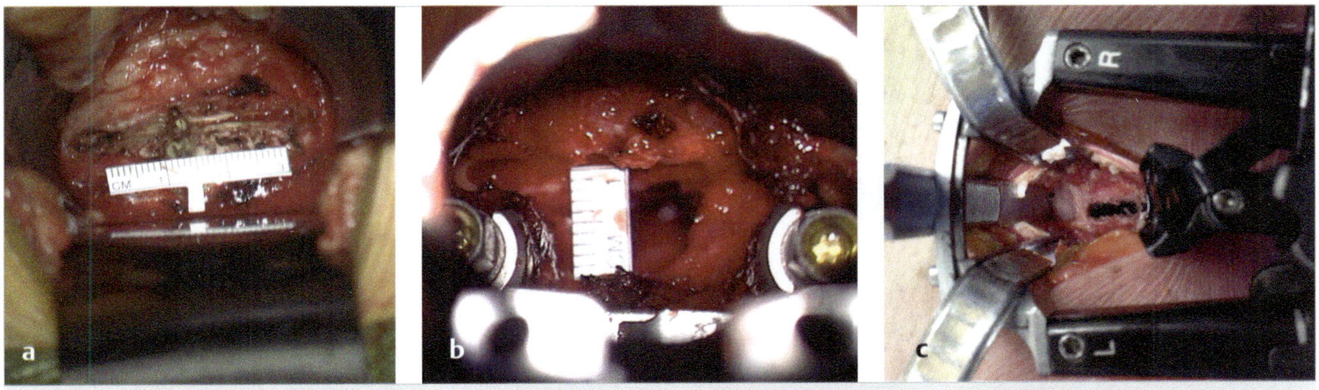

Fig. 6.2 Access corridors to the lumbar disc space. **(a)** Intraoperative photograph of an anterior lumbar interbody fusion at L5–S1. The vascular anatomy at L5–S1 level offers a generous corridor into the disc space of up to 40 mm. The corridor becomes more constrained at the levels above L5, resulting in a greater vascular risk, especially because of the proximity of the vena cava. **(b)** Intraoperative photograph of a transforaminal corridor on the right at L4–5. The access to the disc space is constrained by the traversing nerve root and exiting nerve root. The resulting corridor is 10–12 mm. **(c)** Intraoperative photograph of a transpsoas approach at L2–3. The corridor into the disc space is not constrained by vascular or neural anatomy. After a safe corridor has been established through the psoas with electrophysiologic monitoring, and the genitofemoral nerve has been safely mobilized, there are over 20 mm of access to the disc space. (Photograph (c) is provided courtesy of Juan S. Uribe, MD.)

mobilization of the nerve are essential to mitigate the risk of neuropraxia or disruption. But it is not only the lumbar plexus that is a concern in this approach. The lower one descends in the lumbar spine, the thicker the psoas becomes, adding to the distance that one has to traverse to reach the spine. Traversing the psoas comes at the consequence of hip flexion weakness and soreness in the coming weeks after the operation. Discussions with patients regarding these risks are an important part of the patient education and informed consent for this operation.

Patients with previous abdominal surgery, specifically colon surgery, may have significant scarring in the retroperitoneal space. Although I have not encountered any significant difficulty in patients with previous laparoscopic cholecystectomies or appendectomies, it has been my practice to defer the transpsoas approach in those individuals with colon resections, where the retroperitoneal space has been obliterated by the previous surgery and at times by radiation.

6.4 Patient Selection and Lumbar Segment Selection

Ideal patients present in three broad categories: an isolated degeneration at one of these levels (L1–2 or L2–3), multiple levels of degeneration that include these segments resulting in deformity or an adjacent segment degeneration above a previous fusion construct. The upper lumbar segments, L1–2 and L2–3 in particular, are ideal for a transpsoas interbody approach. At both of these levels, the psoas is thin, and the lumbar plexus has yet to become fully formed, and what has formed is in the posterior aspect of the disc space. This arrangement leaves the anterior two-thirds of disc space as a corridor for entry, once one has appropriately identified and mobilized the genitofemoral nerve.

While single-level degeneration of the upper lumbar spine is not common, when these patients do present, a minimally invasive same-day, standalone surgical option is a valuable intervention to offer (▶ Fig. 6.3).[7] The most common scenario is the involvement of L1–2 and L2–3 within a multilevel degenerative deformity. The transpsoas technique in that circumstance is part of a more comprehensive strategy to address the deformity. A single incision can offer access to up to three levels as the first phase of the operation. Posterior instrumentation, posterior column osteotomies, and additional lower lumbar segments are addressed during the second phase of the operation (▶ Fig. 6.4).[8,9]

The third category of patients that is ideal for the transpsoas technique is patients with extensive constructs in the lower lumbar spine with a symptomatic adjacent segment. In these patients, the transpsoas approach is an appealing alternative to exploration, explantation and extension of the fusion construct (▶ Fig. 6.5). In the absence of a severe coronal imbalance or instability, a standalone construct for the management of the adjacent segment is an option.[10,11,12] Relying primarily on the principle of indirect decompression by restoring the disc height, the adjacent segment may be adequately treated. Patients are then observed for the coming weeks and months. It becomes evident when and if a posterior operation will be necessary for additional decompression and stabilization. In this scenario, the transpsoas approach transforms a 3- to 4-hour operation with a 3- to 4-day hospital stay into a procedure performed in less than 1 hour with a 23-hour admission period.

6.5 Transpsoas at L4–5

A transpsoas approach to the L4–5 segment presents unique challenges that are not present in the upper segments of the spine (L1–2, L2–3 and L3–4). The iliac crest, the thickness of the psoas and the femoral nerve are all factors that need to be considered. Anteroposterior (AP) and lateral radiographs provide the information needed regarding the iliac crest. The lateral radiograph, in particular, shows whether the iliac crest prevents access or limits an ideal trajectory to the disc space. If the

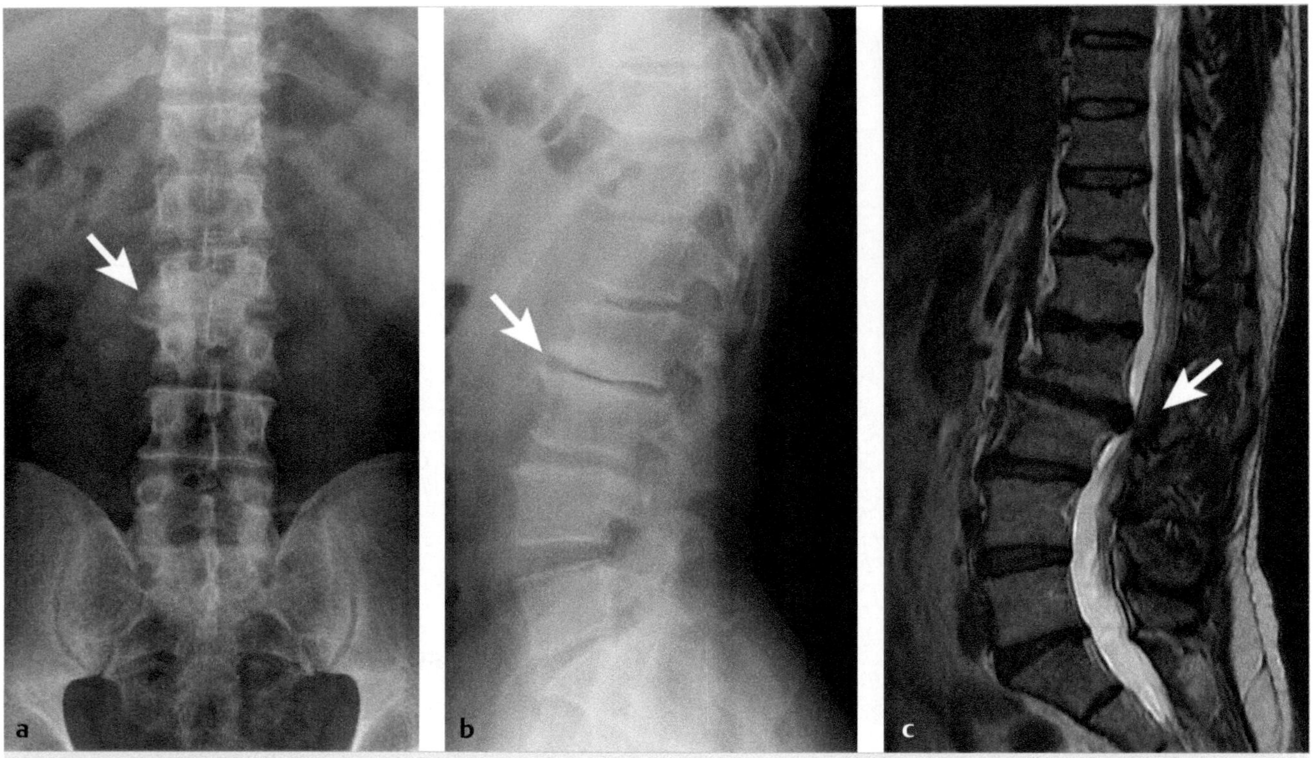

Fig. 6.3 Isolated degeneration at the L2–3 segment. The ideal candidate for a transpsoas approach is an individual with a degenerative segment in the upper lumbar segments. In this case illustration, the patient presents with single-level disc degeneration at L2–3. The location of the lumbosacral plexus and the thin psoas muscle at this level makes a transpsoas approach ideal. **(a)** Anteroposterior radiograph of the lumbar spine showing no coronal deformity. Note the lateral osteophyte on the right at L2–3 (*arrow*). **(b)** Lateral radiograph of the lumbar spine showing single level degeneration at L2–3. The collapse of the disc space has resulted in a loss of the segmental lordosis. The presence of the vacuum disc phenomenon that is evident within the disc space (*arrow*) assures the ability to reliably restore disc height and segmental lordosis with an interbody spacer. **(c)** Sagittal T2-weighted magnetic resonance imaging of the lumbar spine showing the focal stenosis at the segment of L2–3 (*arrow*). This patient presented with elements of neurogenic claudication and L2 radiculopathy.

patient has a favorable iliac crest for a transpsoas approach, then the focus of the operation becomes navigating the lumbar plexus through the psoas muscle, with particular attention to the femoral nerve. The experience in the literature has demonstrated the safety and efficacy of the transpsoas approach at the L4–5 segment.[13] As I consider the anatomy of the lumbar plexus at L4–5 and its branches, and the femoral nerve in particular, I admire the thickness of the psoas muscle and assess the corridor provided to me by the iliac crest, and I take pause. The L4–5 transpsoas approaches that I have performed have resulted in substantially more discomfort in the hip flexors for a longer duration than at the segments above it. I readily concede that there are techniques that mitigate the risk to the lumbar plexus and the disruption of the psoas muscle, such as shallow docking of the access port. With experience comes efficiency, and there is little doubt as to the impact of retraction time on the psoas muscle. I have several colleagues who have mastered a transpsoas interbody technique at the L4–5 segment.

However, it is difficult for me to approach the L4–5 segment with a transpsoas approach when, in my hands, the transforaminal approach is a perfectly viable option. Furthermore, the degenerative pathology that is addressed at L4–5 is typically posterior, specifically spondylolisthesis, facet arthropathy or lumbar stenosis. While distraction of the disc space allows for indirect decompression of the neural elements, I find great comfort in direct visualization and direct decompression of the symptomatic nerve roots and the thecal sac. In cases of a mobile spondylolisthesis at L4–5, it is difficult to have a standalone construct. In these cases, the transpsoas approach is typically augmented with the placement of pedicle screws and at times, additional decompression. Although a transpsoas approach is a perfectly viable surgical solution, from a philosophical standpoint, if there is one comprehensive solution to a problem with a single approach that accomplishes all of the goals of surgery in a 1.5-hour procedure from one position, that would be the approach I would intuitively favor. Finally, I have not had transient or permanent motor or sensory deficits in my L4–5 transforaminal approaches at the rate reported for the transpsoas approach.[13]

The L3–4 segment falls somewhere in between. For single-level L3–4 degeneration, even in the context of a coronal imbalance, I tend to favor a transforaminal approach. Where the transpsoas interbody approach has become transformational is in cases of adjacent segment degeneration, specifically in those patients who have had L4–S1 instrumented fusions (▶ Fig. 6.6).

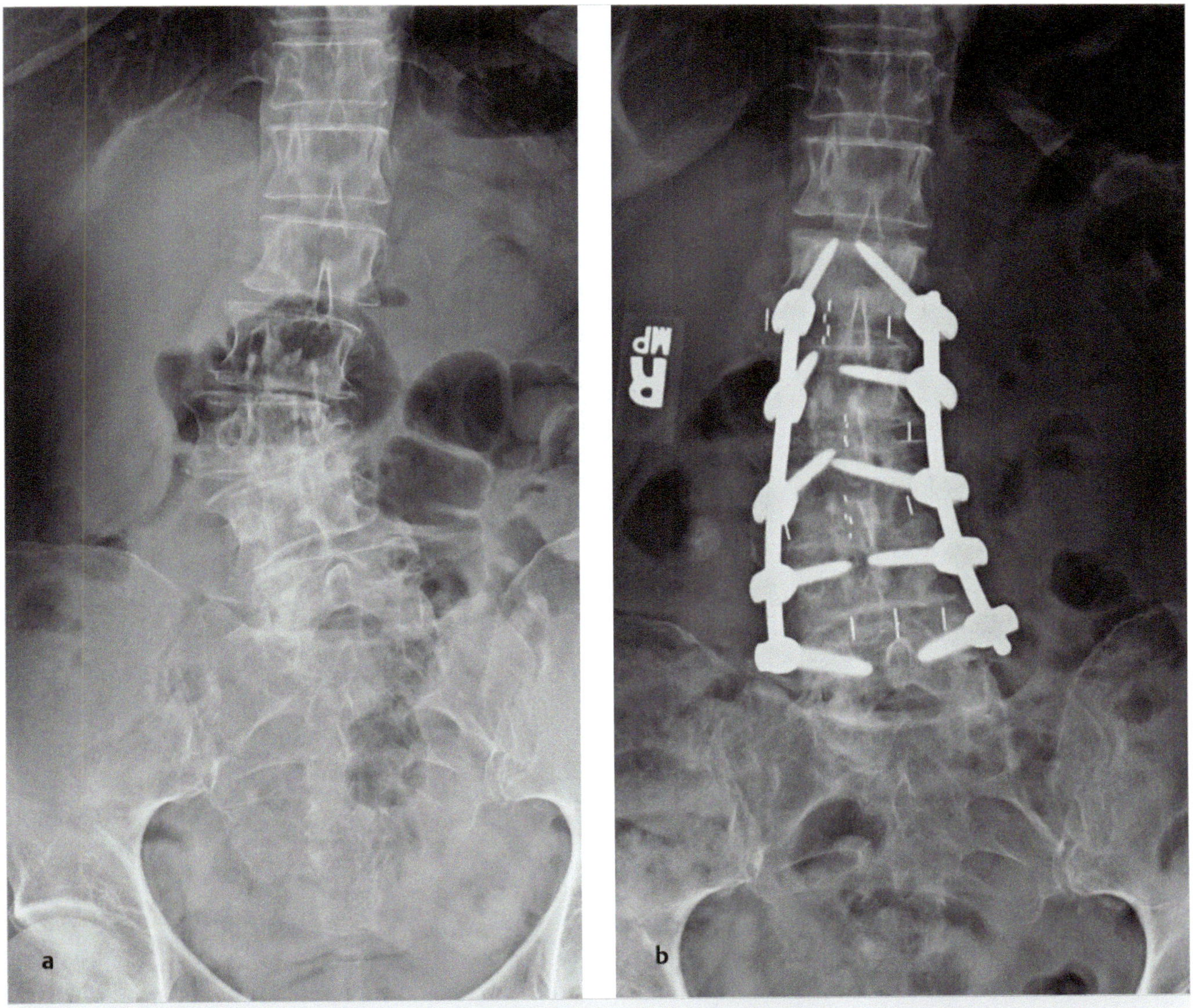

Fig. 6.4 Transpsoas approach as part of deformity correction. **(a)** Preoperative anteroposterior (AP) radiograph demonstrating severe coronal imbalance, lateral listhesis and focal deformity in the lumbar spine. The patient has a Cobb angle of 32 degrees. **(b)** Postoperative AP radiograph demonstrating the application of the transpsoas approach as part of a more comprehensive strategy to correct the coronal imbalance at multiple levels (L1–2, L2–3 and L3–4). The patient underwent pedicle screw fixation from L1 to L5, transforaminal lumbar interbody fusion at L4–5 and posterior column osteotomies at L1–2, L2–3, L3–4 and L4–5.

6.6 The Literature and the Lumbar Plexus

I began my forays through the psoas muscle and into the disc space with a less than adequate understanding of the lumbar plexus anatomy. At that particular time, I was more capable drawing out the brachial plexus and its branches, an area I had not operated upon in years, than the lumbar plexus, where I found myself going with increasing frequency. The reality is that my understanding of this anatomy as I began to perform these procedures mirrored the literature on this topic at the time: it was limited. In 2006, when the transpsoas approach was introduced, the literature expounding upon the implications of navigating the lumbar plexus and its branches through the psoas major muscle was narrow at best. One thing I can readily admit is that the surgeries that I performed early in my career relied more on neurophysiological monitoring than my rudimentary understanding of the lumbar plexus anatomy.

As experience among surgeons grew, and complications became increasingly recognized, the literature began to reflect a more sophisticated understanding of the anatomy of the lumbar plexus. As I read these manuscripts over the years, I breathed a sigh of relief that, except for one genitofemoral injury and an abdominal hernia, my undeveloped understanding of the lumbar plexus did not lead to an irreversible catastrophic injury to the plexus or one of its branches.

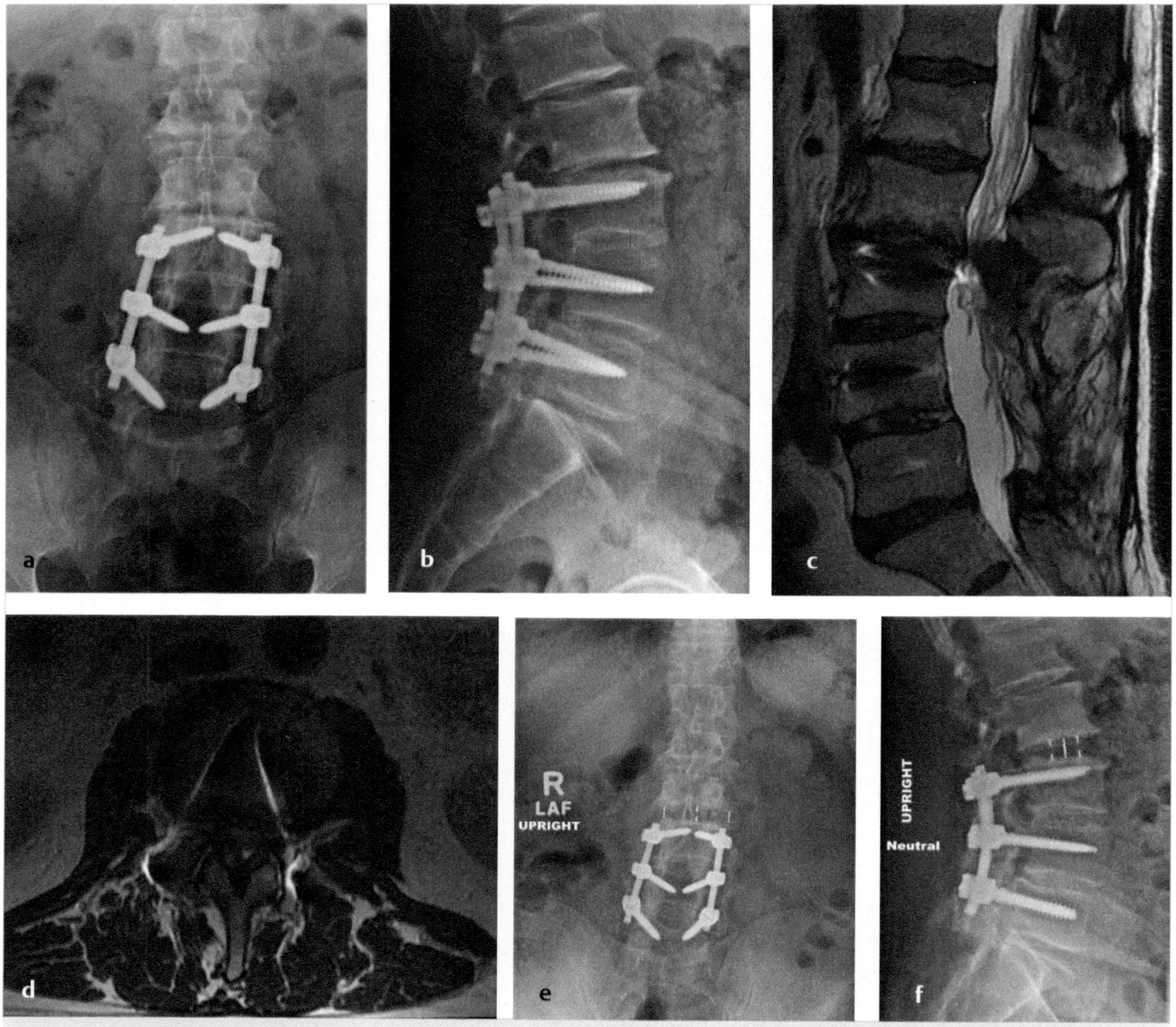

Fig. 6.5 Transpsoas approach for the management of adjacent segment degeneration. Adjacent segment degeneration is seen at L2–3 above the level of an instrumented decompression and fusion at L3–4 and L4–5 on **(a)** an anteroposterior (AP) standing radiograph and **(b)** a lateral standing neutral radiograph. **(c)** Sagittal T2-weighted magnetic resonance imaging (MRI) demonstrating severe stenosis at the L2–3 segment. The redundancy of nerve roots is clearly evident. **(d)** Axial T2-weighted MRI revealing the ligamentum flavum and facet arthropathy contributing to the central stenosis. **(e)** Postoperative AP radiograph after placement of interbody placed through a transpsoas approach. **(f)** Lateral radiograph demonstrating correction of segmental lordosis and restoration of disc height. No additional surgery was needed for this patient.

In the current transpsoas literature, surgeons have reported their extensive breadth of experience and their complications, along with comprehensive anatomical studies of the lumbar plexus.[8,14,15,16,17,18,19] Reviewing these experiences and studying this anatomy enable you to possess a sophisticated understanding of the lumbar plexus in the context of a transpsoas approach that was not available when this procedure was first introduced. Take full advantage of that body of literature, which represents the growing pains of a novel technique. That knowledge is a key component of complication avoidance. A high-level understanding of the lumbar plexus positively impacts your decision-making to proceed with this technique for surgery, during surgery, and even after surgery as you guide patients through the postoperative course. Whether it is mobilizing the genitofemoral nerve or recognizing that a safe corridor into the L4–5 disc space is not feasible because of the location of the femoral nerve, it is anatomical certainty that empowers you to make a decision.

In the paragraphs below, I highlight some of the most valuable aspects of this anatomy. Still, I encourage you to read the anatomical studies in the bibliography of this chapter. Those manuscripts filled the void of my knowledge and served as a foundation for my understanding of the lumbar plexus and its branches. That knowledge has given me the

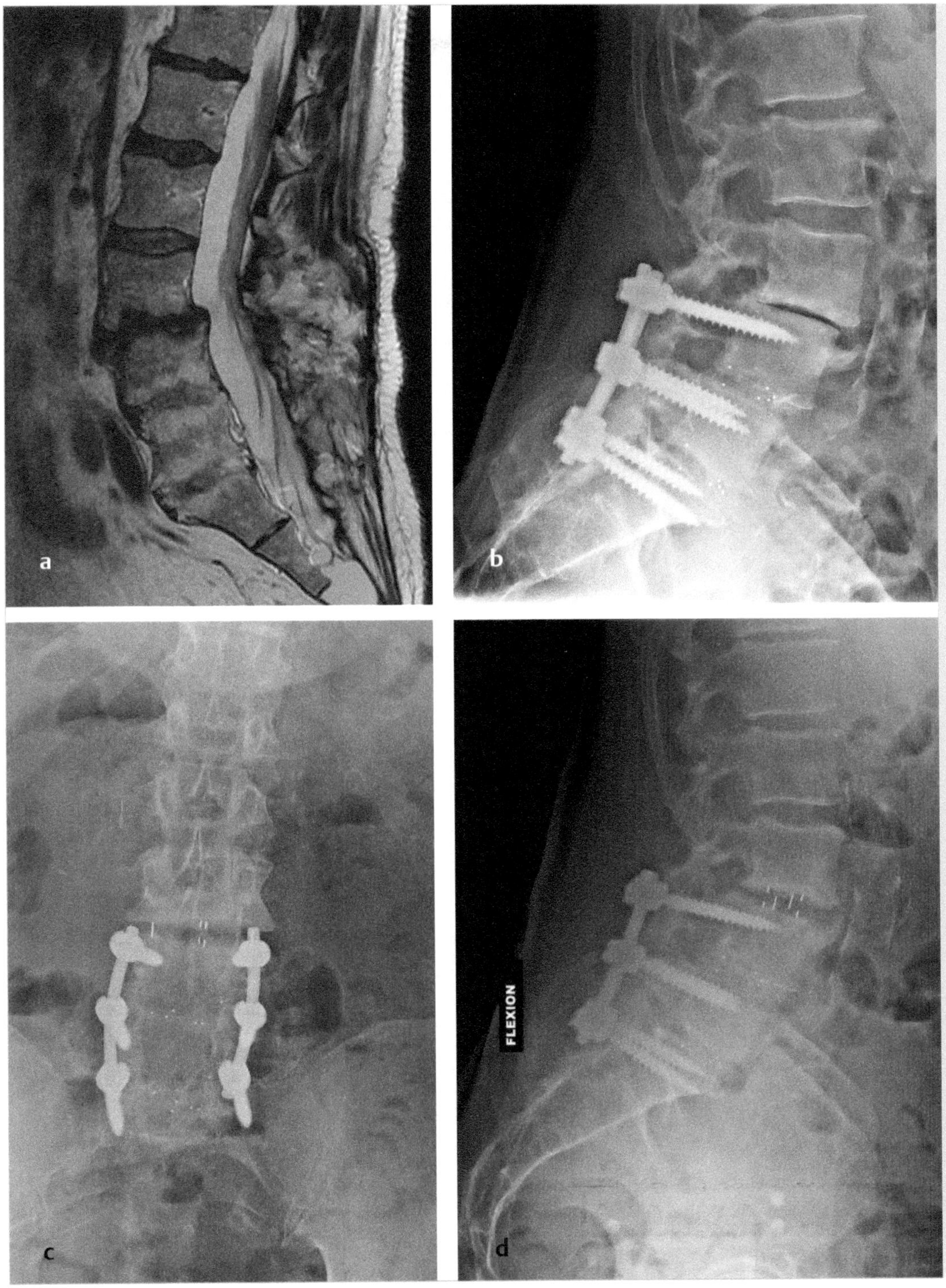

Fig. 6.6 Transpsoas approach at L3–4. A patient who presents 12 years after an L4–5, L5–S1 instrumented interbody fusion with adjacent segment degeneration at L3–4. The patient had been fused without lordosis at L4–5 or L5–S1, likely contributing to the adjacent segment issue. **(a)** Sagittal T2-weighted magnetic resonance imaging (MRI) showing anterolisthesis of L3 on L4. The MRI primarily shows foraminal stenosis, and the patient presented with L3 and L4 symptoms exacerbated by any degree of ambulation. **(b)** Lateral radiograph again demonstrating the collapse and anterolisthesis of L3 on L4. Note the vacuum disc phenomenon, which is indicative of the ability to restore disc height and alignment. An exploration of the previous fusion, explantation of hardware and extension to L3–4 is an extensive operation for this particular patient with multiple comorbidities. By comparison, a transpsoas approach is an efficient minimally invasive option. **(c)** Anteroposterior radiograph demonstrating the restoration in disc height with a transpsoas approach. **(d)** Lateral radiograph demonstrating disc height restoration, reduction of the listhesis and the return of some segmental lordosis. In this case, the patient was discharged 23 hours after management of the adjacent segment with a transpsoas approach.

confidence to manage the complications that have arisen from this technique and, at other times, to altogether avoid complications for patients who have trusted me with their care. You have the distinct advantage of reading about the learning curve of a novel surgical technique that occurred in real time. That literature accurately describes the evolving understanding of the innervation of the psoas muscle,[20] the implications of the sensory branches,[13,21] which cannot be monitored and the potential motor deficits that arise based on the surgical level.[13] Harness all that literature to your advantage for the benefit of your patients. One thing is certain: your mind should be able to visualize the lumbar plexus and its branches far better than the brachial plexus and its branches.

6.7 Anatomy of the Lumbar Plexus

The occasion invariably arises where you peer down into the minimal access port at the substance of the psoas major muscle and find the unmistakable white sheen of a nerve shining back at you. The goal of this section is to describe the various branches of the lumbar plexus in a manner that is valuable so that when you encounter that white sheen of a nerve in your path to the disc space, you know what it is and how to navigate safely around it.

The lumbar nerve is numbered the same as its vertebra and courses beneath the vertebral pedicle. It then exits its foramen to merge with other lumbar nerve roots at several points. The confluence of these nerves that occurs at several points both outside and within the substance of the psoas muscle forms the lumbar plexus. The following section describes the plexus and its branches, first in the abdominal wall and then in the psoas muscle (Video 6.1).

6.8 Branches of the Lumbar Plexus in the Abdominal Wall

Early in my transpsoas experience, I placed all my emphasis on the branches of the lumbar plexus within the psoas muscle itself and not enough emphasis on the nerves coursing outside of the psoas muscle. The reality is that the nerves that course outside of the plexus and instead through the abdominal wall may be at greater risk. Unlike the plexus in the psoas major muscle, no electrophysiologic monitoring identifies these nerves. The nerves of the abdominal wall include the subcostal, iliohypogastric, ilioinguinal and lateral femoral cutaneous nerves, and they are the first nerves that you have the potential to encounter as you make your way through the various muscle layers of the abdominal wall and into the retroperitoneal space.

6.9 Subcostal Nerve

The first nerve to consider is not even a part of the lumbar plexus. Instead, it is a branch of the ventral ramus of the T12 nerve root, which forms the subcostal nerve. The nerve courses anteriorly to the upper part of the quadratus lumborum and then travels in between the transversus abdominis muscle and internal oblique. It is important to recognize that the subcostal nerve has a motor and sensory component, supplying the muscles to the anterior abdominal wall, especially the external oblique. Injury to this nerve may result in weakness to the musculature of the anterior abdominal wall, anterior abdominal numbness and even painful paresthesias.

6.10 Iliohypogastric and Ilioinguinal Nerves

The iliohypogastric and ilioinguinal nerves represent the first branches of the lumbar plexus. Both of these branches originate from the ventral rami of the T12 and L1 nerve root (▶ Fig. 6.7). The iliohypogastric nerve emerges from the lateral border of the psoas major muscle, continues anteriorly to the quadratus lumborum and then travels anteriorly between the muscle layers of the transversus abdominis and internal oblique muscles, eventually completing its course in between the internal and external oblique muscles (▶ Fig. 6.8). The ilioinguinal nerve travels along a similar path caudal to the iliohypogastric nerve with the main difference between these two nerves being the site of termination. The ilioinguinal nerve travels to the inguinal canal and emerges superficially to the inguinal ring.

Similar to the subcostal nerve, both of these nerves have motor and sensory components. The iliohypogastric nerve gives rise to an anterior cutaneous branch that innervates the suprapubic skin. The ilioinguinal nerve provides sensation to the medial skin of the thigh. In women, it provides sensation to the mons pubis and labia majora, while in men it provides sensation to the base of the penis and upper part of the

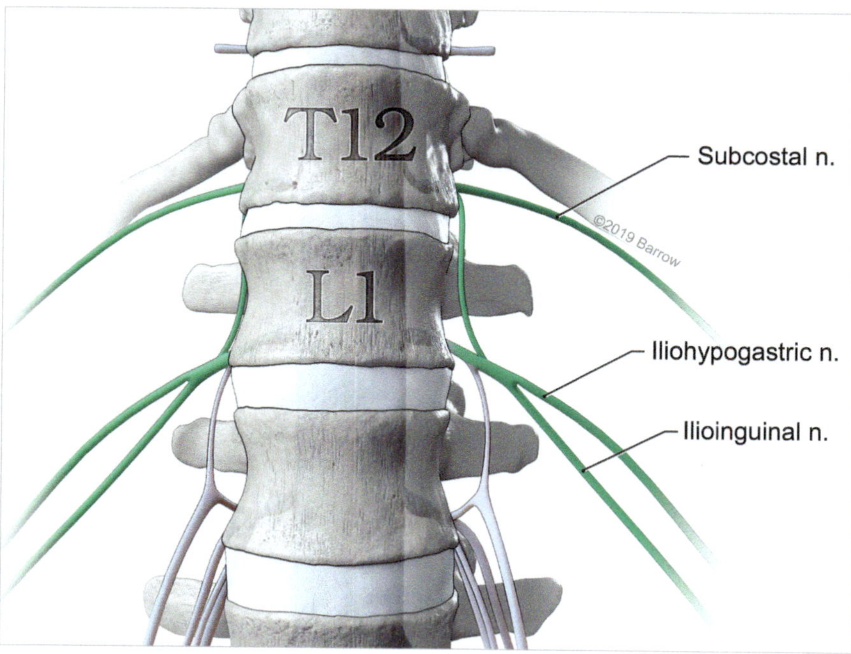

Fig. 6.7 The formation of the subcostal, iliohypogastric and ilioinguinal nerves (*emerald green*). The T12 ventral ramus branches to give rise to the subcostal nerve and a second branch that merges with the ventral ramus of the L1 nerve root and gives off the iliohypogastric and ilioinguinal nerves.

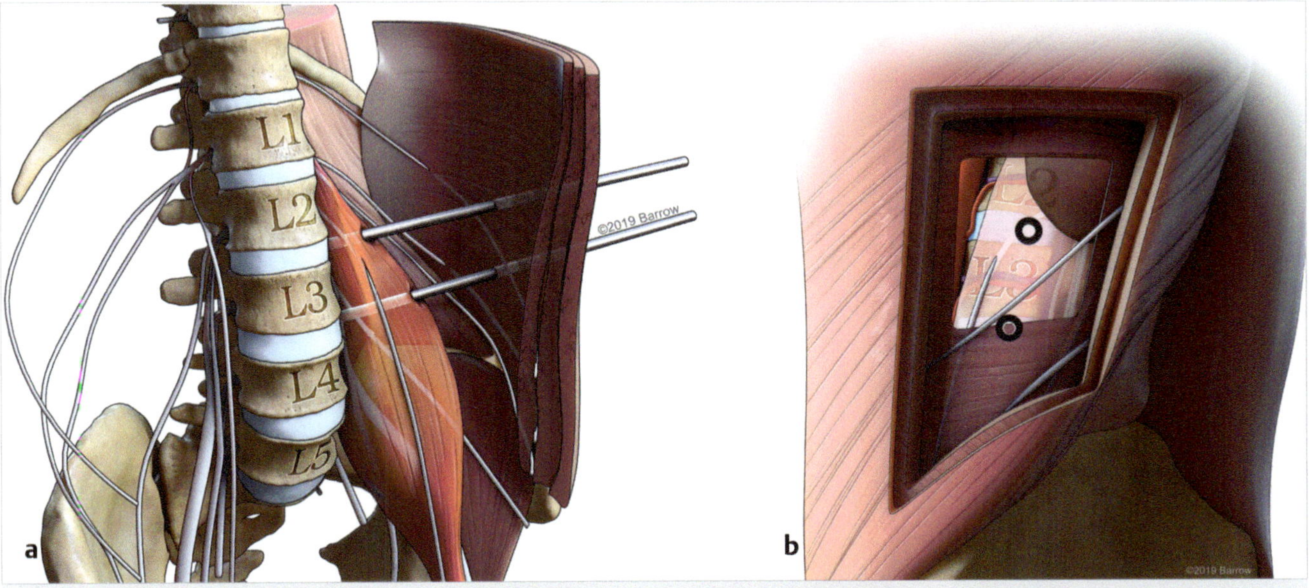

Fig. 6.8 Illustration demonstrating the course of the subcostal, iliohypogastric and ilioinguinal nerves as they leave the spine and traverse through the muscle layers of the abdominal wall. **(a)** An oblique illustration of the lumbar spine and the abdominal wall muscles with the subcostal, iliohypogastric, and ilioinguinal nerves leaving the spine and entering the abdominal wall. The dilators are seen traversing the abdominal wall en route to the lumbar disc spaces of L2–3 and L3–4. Blunt dissection and avoiding cautery minimizes the risk of injury to these nerves. **(b)** A lateral illustration of the image in **a** showing the abdominal wall and lumbar spine where the three muscle layers have been cut away. The *black rings* represent the position of the dilator over the disc spaces of L2–3 and L3–4. The iliohypogastric nerve courses just above the L3–4 dilator. The ilioinguinal courses well below the iliohypogastric. Note the genitofemoral nerve courses within the psoas just anterior to the dilator over the L2–3 disc space and then pierces through the psoas muscle and continues on the surface of the muscle.

scrotum. Both of these nerves supply the muscles of the anterior abdominal wall, and injury may result in paresis of the abdominal wall that may lead to herniation.

6.11 Lateral Femoral Cutaneous Nerve

The lateral femoral cutaneous nerve originates from the dorsal branches of the ventral rami of the L2 and L3 nerve roots. Similar to the nerves described earlier, it emerges from the lateral border of the psoas major muscle at approximately the L4 level and courses much lower than the subcostal, iliohypogastric and ilioinguinal nerves. The nerve continues obliquely across the iliacus muscle toward the anterior superior iliac spine before branching into anterior and posterior branches. The lateral femoral cutaneous nerve is a purely sensory nerve and innervates the anterior and lateral aspects of the thigh. Fortunately, its lower course places this nerve at a lower risk of injury than the others discussed, especially in the management of the L2–3 and L3–4 segments. Injury to this nerve root results in meralgia paresthetica.

6.12 Lumbar Plexus within the Psoas Major Muscle

6.12.1 Genitofemoral Nerve

Branches of the ventral rami of L1 and L2 combine within the substance of the psoas major muscle to form the genitofemoral nerve (▶ Fig. 6.9) as it descends through the psoas and tends to emerge on the medial border opposite L3 or L4. It proceeds beneath the peritoneum on the psoas major muscle and divides into its genital and femoral components above the inguinal ligament. However, it is not uncommon to see both branches coursing on top of the psoas major muscle. As the name implies, it provides sensation to the femoral and genital areas. The femoral component provides sensation to the upper medial thigh and skin over the femoral vessels. The genital branch enters the inguinal canal and supplies the cremaster and the skin of the scrotum in men, whereas in women, it follows the round ligament to supply sensation to the mons pubis and labia majora. Injury to this nerve results in decreased sensation or painful paresthesia, or both in these distributions.

When performing the dilatation through the psoas, it is important to recognize that the genitofemoral nerve courses on the medial aspect of the psoas and more often than not, you will be approaching the nerve blindly. Second, electrophysiologic monitoring does not identify the location of this cutaneous nerve. In my experience, I have found this particular nerve to be the most variable nerve of the lumbar plexus, and as such, I always take a moment or two to bluntly dissect through the psoas muscle in search of this nerve before proceeding to the disc space. If I have exposed an adequate amount of disc space for the discectomy and have not found it, I proceed with the interbody work. If during my dissection, I do identify it, I take the time to mobilize it out of the way of the working corridor to the disc space.

6.12.2 Femoral Nerve

The dorsal branches of the ventral rami of the L2, L3 and L4 combine within the substance of the psoas major muscle to

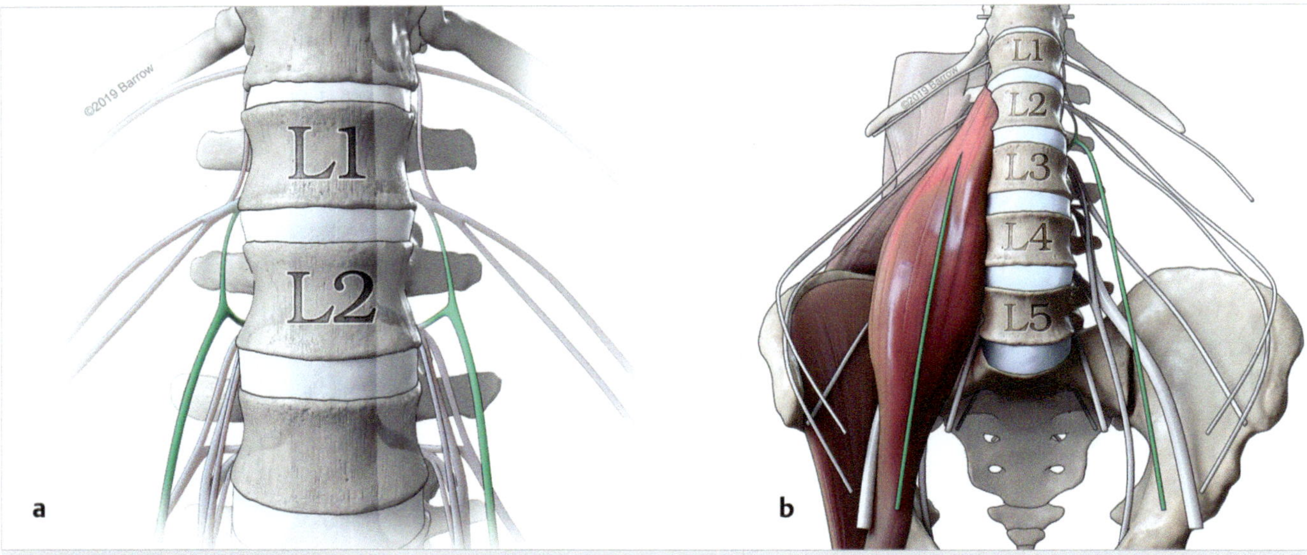

Fig. 6.9 The genitofemoral nerve. **(a)** Schematic illustration demonstrating the branches of L1 and L2 combining to form the genitofemoral nerve. **(b)** Anatomical illustration demonstrating the course of the genitofemoral nerve (*emerald green*) with the psoas illustrated on the right of the spine and without the psoas illustrated on the left of the spine. The course of the genitofemoral nerve is on the medial border of the psoas major, which means that in a transpsoas approach, the genitofemoral nerve is approached blindly. Electrophysiologic monitoring does not reveal the location of this nerve. It is worthwhile to dissect through the psoas to identify this nerve to avoid injury to it. The left side of the spine shows the course of the genitofemoral nerve (*emerald green*) relative to the other nerves of the lumbar plexus.

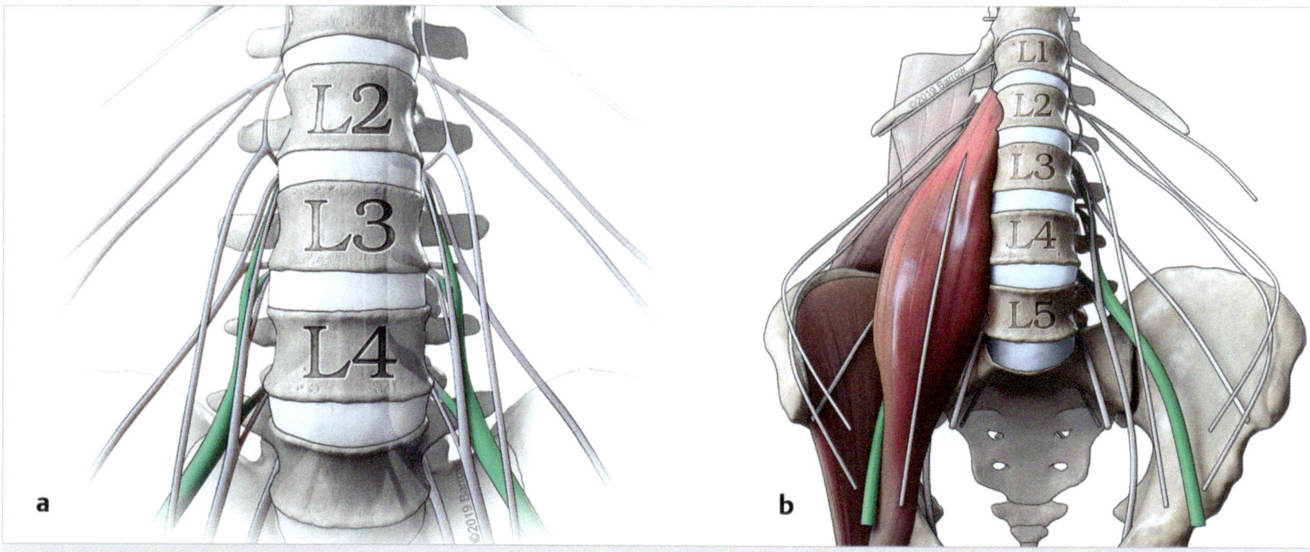

Fig. 6.10 The femoral nerve. **(a)** Schematic illustration demonstrating the branches of L2, L3 and L4 (*emerald green*) combining to form the femoral nerve. **(b)** Anatomical illustration demonstrating the course of the femoral nerve (*emerald green*) within the substance of the psoas on the right of the illustration emerging only after outside the surgical window of the transpsoas approach. The nerve emerges on the inferolateral aspect of the psoas muscle just above the inguinal ligament. The branches contributing to the femoral nerve and the femoral nerve itself must be identified with electrophysiologic monitoring to avoid injury. The left side of the illustration shows the course of the femoral nerve relative to the other nerves of the lumbar plexus.

form the femoral nerve, which is the largest branch of the lumbar plexus (▶ Fig. 6.10). Even after it is fully formed, the femoral nerve continues within the psoas major muscle and does not emerge within the corridor provided by transpsoas access. The nerve continues beneath the inguinal ligament and then divides into its anterior and posterior branches to innervate the quadriceps and provide sensation to the leg. Since it remains unseen, identification of the nerve relative to the access corridor into the disc space is essential and is discussed in greater detail later.

6.12.3 Practical Application of the Lumbar Plexus Anatomy to Traverse the Psoas

With the anatomy of the lumbar plexus having been covered, the next section transitions to the application of the anatomy in the context of the transpsoas approach. As you perform this procedure, it should not be surprising to catch a glimpse of some of these nerves in the upper lumbar segments as they make their way within the psoas muscle, and at times, find them emerging in the posterior aspect of the lumbar disc spaces. These findings should not concern you but instead help you identify a safe corridor into the disc space.

Moro and colleagues[22] published one of the first anatomical studies in the literature, specifically assessing the lumbar plexus relative to the psoas. Interestingly, the study was written in 2003 with endoscopic approaches to the lumbar disc space in mind and predated the landmark 2006 publication by Ozgur and colleagues[5] describing the current transpsoas interbody technique. Regardless, it represents the first study to analyze the lumbar plexus and its branches relative to the psoas muscle and the disc space. Therefore, it was immediately applicable to the transpsoas approach, which had no other anatomical study that provided the necessary information. Moro and colleagues divided the vertebral bodies and the disc space into four quadrants (▶ Fig. 6.11).[22] The most anterior quadrant has been designated zone I and the most posterior quadrant has been designated zone IV.[15] The authors sectioned their specimens and reported the frequency of finding one of the branches of the lumbar plexus within a particular zone. There is no question as to the value of this grid system for anatomical probabilities of the location of the various branches, especially when considering that the study was not even written with the transpsoas interbody technique in mind. However, there is a limitation to its practical application in surgery.

Application of the four-quadrant system locates the branches that make up the ilioinguinal and iliohypogastric nerves in zone IV at the L2–3 disc space. When moving from rostral to caudal, the next branch is the lateral femoral cutaneous nerve. The lateral femoral cutaneous nerve arises from the posterolateral border of the psoas at L3–4 in zone IV. As mentioned earlier, these nerves may be more at risk from the preliminary exposure through the abdominal wall at the distal end of their course than traversing the psoas muscle into the disc space and encountering them at the beginning of their course.

Branches from the L1 and L2 nerve root form the genitofemoral nerve. The L1 branch tends to cross the L1–2 disc space on a course in the anterior half of the vertebral body. The L2 contribution joins the L1 branch on its anterior course. Several anatomical studies corroborate my experience with reliably identifying this nerve over the top of the middle or anterior aspect of the L2–3 disc space (zone II). When this nerve is identified, it is essential to mobilize and protect it from the corridor that is being used to access the interbody.

Finally, the branches of L2, L3 and L4 coalesce to form the femoral nerve, which is the largest caliber branch of the lumbar plexus that resides deep within the psoas muscle. It courses along a trajectory gradually proceeding from its posterior to anterior position and can reach the midvertebral body (zone III) at the L4–5 disc space.

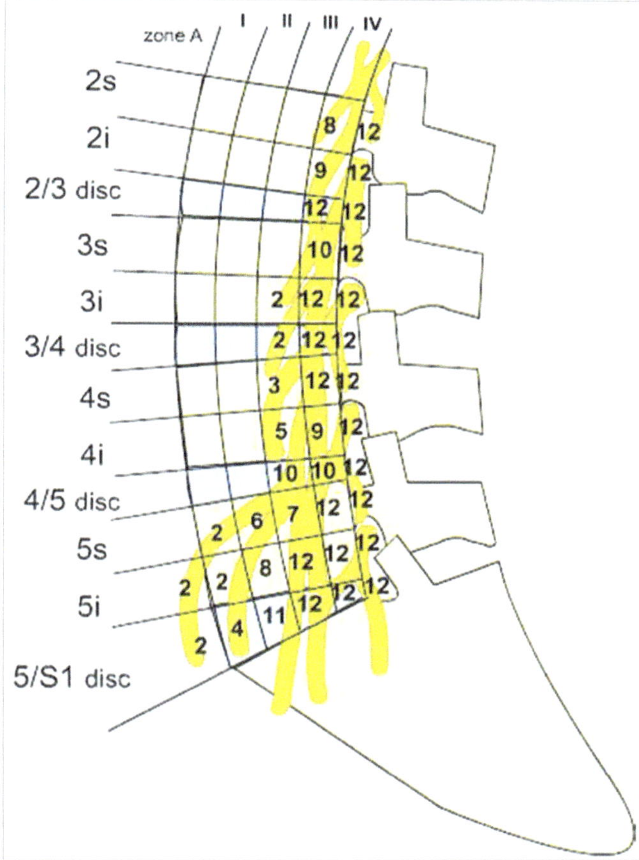

Fig. 6.11 Illustration from Moro and colleagues[22] determining the frequency of occurrence of the branches of the lumbar plexus in the four zones. The number correlates with the vertebral body. The "s" is indicative of the superior aspect of the vertebral body, and the "i" is indicative of the inferior aspect of the vertebral body. The disc spaces are labelled. It is important to note that the authors did not incorporate the genitofemoral nerve into this illustration. (Reproduced with permission from Moro T, Kikuchi S, Konno S, Yaginuma H. An anatomic study of the lumbar plexus with respect to retroperitoneal endoscopic surgery. Spine. 2003; 28(5):423–428, discussion 427–428.)

6.12.4 Major Sensory and Motor Nerves Relative to the Disc Space

Since the objective of the transpsoas interbody approach revolves entirely around accessing the disc space, the concept that you must master is the anatomical location of the lumbar plexus and its branches in the retroperitoneal space relative to the disc spaces that you intend to access. Uribe and colleagues[15] evolved the four-quadrant system into a more practical anatomical study of the lumbar plexus along with its branches relative to the disc spaces from L1–2 to L4–5 (▶ Fig. 6.12). Identifying the safe zone is tremendously helpful as a starting point when performing the dilation phase through the psoas muscle. To this day, as I traverse the psoas to access the disc space, I keep in mind the observations made by these authors, which I have summarized below.[15]

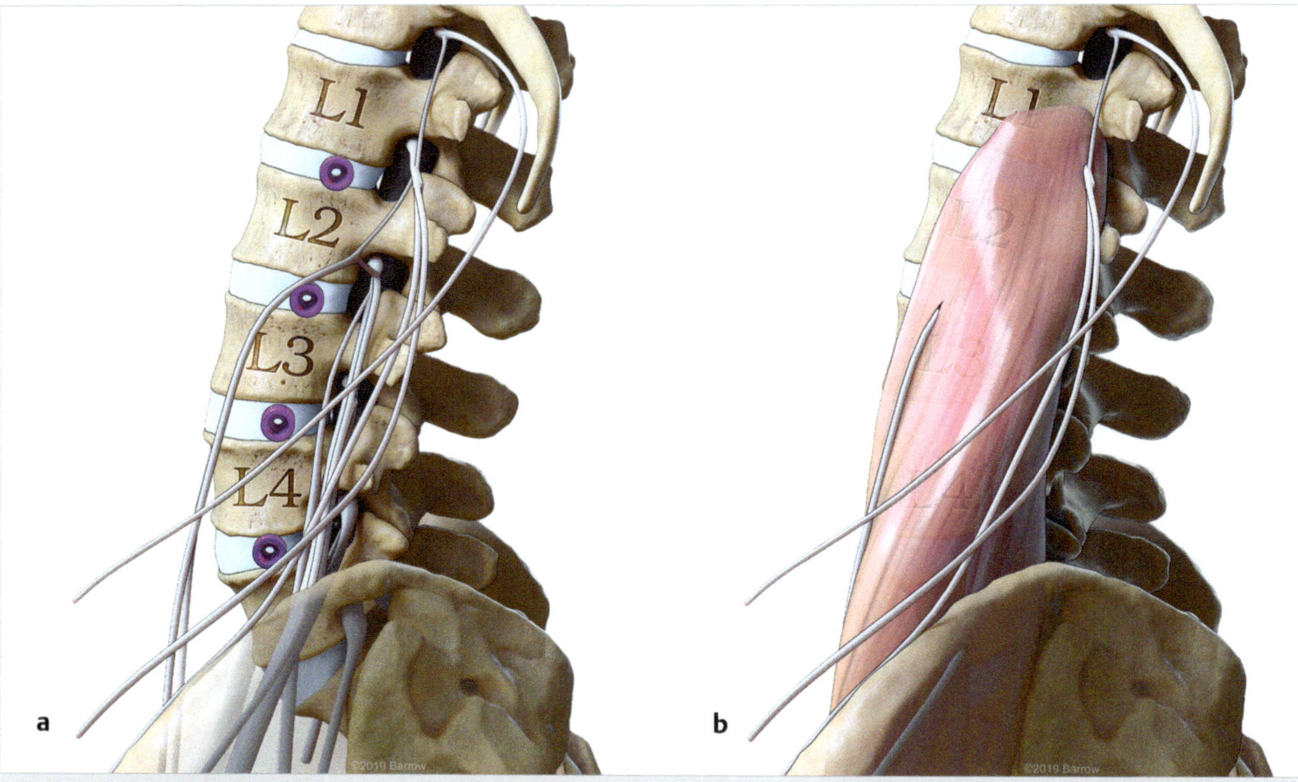

Fig. 6.12 The transpsoas safe working zones to access the disc space. Illustration incorporating the safe working zones as reported by Uribe and colleagues.[15] The safe working zones at the various disc spaces have been marked with a magenta fiducial with the branches of the lumbar plexus in full view (**a**) without the psoas (**b**) and with the psoas. It is important to be able to visualize the image in **a** in your mind's eye during surgery when, in reality, all you see is the image in **b**.

L1–2: All nerve roots are in the posterior quadrant of the disc space (zone IV). The risk is low for injury to a nerve root, lumbar plexus or its branches (ilioinguinal and iliohypogastric).

L2–3: The genitofemoral nerve can take a course in the midportion of the disc space (zone II). The remaining nerve roots and divisions all course in the posterior aspect of the disc space (zone IV).

L3–4: The variable genitofemoral nerve may traverse in the mid to anterior portion of the disc space (zone II) or even the anterior aspect of the disc space. The remaining nerves traverse the disc space posterior to the mid vertebral body line (zone IV). Dissection through the psoas muscle to identify and mobilize the genitofemoral nerve should be considered.

L4–5: The femoral nerve and the obturator nerves may course right up to the mid vertebral body line (zone III). Once again, the genitofemoral nerve may be found in the anterior aspect of the disc space (zone I).

Having in your possession the knowledge of all the anatomical studies in the literature does not change the reality of surgical anatomy that lay before you or the information provided by intraoperative monitoring. Nothing replaces what you can see directly with your own eyes. The anatomical studies and electrophysiologic monitoring serve as guides through the psoas and into the disc space, but it is the anatomy at depth that dictates your surgical decision-making, especially in the case of the genitofemoral nerve, which does not reveal its position with electrophysiologic monitoring.

6.13 Vascular Anatomy

Understanding the vascular anatomy of the lumbar segment is as important as understanding the lumbar plexus, especially on the rare occasion that you encounter vigorous bleeding. I did not have that perspective when I first began performing these procedures, but bleeding from a lumbar segmental artery quickly cured my myopic focus on the lumbar plexus and expanded my vision to include the vascular structures. Review of ▶ Fig. 6.13 reveals the lumbar segmental arteries branching off the aorta and coursing with a slightly upward slope before settling into the midvertebral body. The lumbar vein runs in parallel to the segmental artery draining into the vena cava. It is important to recognize the ascending lumbar vein, which courses in the posterior aspect of the vertebral body within the substance of the psoas muscle. Examination of the vascularity leads to the intuitive conclusion that the safest corridor devoid of vascular structures is the center of the disc space. In the event of bleeding, identifying its nature (i.e., arterial or venous) leads to its control and resolution. A bleeding segmental artery cannot be controlled with a hemostatic agent and tamponade, whereas venous bleeding can. Direct visualization and cauterization are needed for the control of arterial bleeding. Hemostatic agents, pressure and patience are needed for venous bleeding. At times, visualization through the operating microscope and dissection through the psoas onto the vertebral body vastly facilitate identification and cauterization of the bleeding vessel.

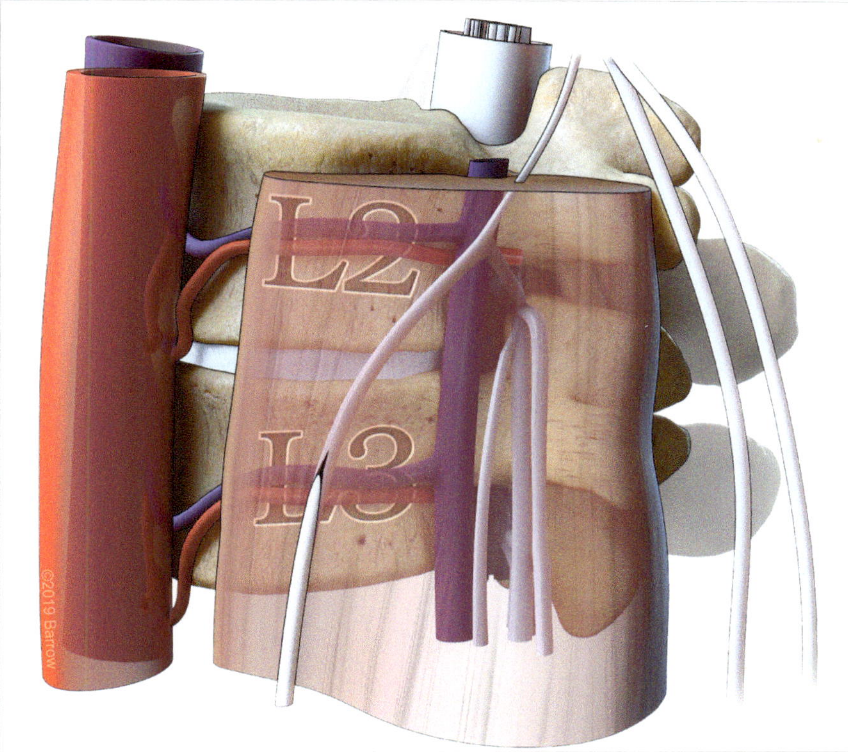

Fig. 6.13 Vascular anatomy of the lumbar segment. Illustration of the arterial and venous structures at the L2–3 lumbar segment. The psoas muscle is diaphanous in this image to reveal the vascular anatomy. The lumbar segmental artery comes directly off the aorta, tends to have an upward slope and course in the midvertebral body. The segmental artery is accompanied by the vein that drains into the vena cava. The ascending lumbar vein courses in the rostrocaudal direction along the posterior aspect of the disc space within the substance of the psoas. The nerves of the lumbar plexus are also illustrated in this image. Note the genitofemoral nerve piercing the psoas muscle and then coursing on its surface.

6.14 Anatomical Basis and the Requisite Anatomical Unit

Assembling the dimensional values of the lumbar vertebrae reported by Panjabi and colleagues,[23] incorporating the safe working zones reported by Uribe and colleagues,[15] and finally superimposing the lumbar plexus and vascular anatomy establish the anatomical basis for the transpsoas procedure (▶ Fig. 6.14). Even more specific is establishing what anatomy must be exposed for a seamless, efficient and low-risk procedure. What I refer to as the requisite anatomical unit for the procedure centers within 20 to 22 mm on the anterior two-thirds of the disc space, which I have evaluated to be devoid of the structures of the lumbar plexus with electrophysiologic monitoring (▶ Fig. 6.14). The exposure encompasses at most 10 mm of the rostral and caudal vertebral body, keeping the working corridor a safe distance from the vascular anatomy. The next section describes the technique for placement of the access port within the ideal requisite anatomical unit.

6.15 Room Setup

A standard operating table that can slide and break at the middle is ideal for this procedure. The image intensifier component of the fluoroscope is opposite the side of the approach (▶ Fig. 6.15). A special C-arm drape that maintains sterility while allowing the fluoroscope to alternate from AP to lateral is invaluable for this procedure (C-Armor; CFI Medical, Fenton, MI). The C-Armor drape eliminates the need for multiple sterile C-arm covers and adds efficiency to the operation.

6.16 Patient Positioning

After induction of anesthesia, I position the patient in the lateral position. In the context of scoliosis or severe coronal imbalance, it is the convexity of the deformity curve that is accessed and therefore is positioned up to facilitate the approach. All other aspects being equal, I prefer a left-sided approach because of the vascular anatomy, specifically keeping the vena cava as far away from the working corridor as possible. The anterior superior iliac spine of the patient should rest just below where the table breaks. Early in my career, I always broke the table to an acute angle to facilitate access to the disc space. The observation made by surgeons that excessive breaking of the table could stretch the femoral nerve and make it more vulnerable to injury resonated with me as I listened to patients reporting their subjective complaints in the days and weeks after surgery.

One valuable article on positioning written by Molinares and colleagues[24] examined the effect of positioning on 50 healthy individuals. The subjects were placed into one of two positions: straight lateral or lateral jackknife for 60 minutes. None of the patients in the straight lateral position experienced a neurologic deficit, but all the patients in the lateral jackknife position did. These results provide compelling evidence that it may be the position more so than the dilatation through the psoas that leads to neurologic deficits.[24] For a time after reviewing this article, I refrained from breaking the table altogether to prevent tension on the psoas muscle, lumbar plexus and, in particular, the femoral nerve. However, I soon discovered that a patient in a purely lateral position does not provide for an adequate access corridor. I found that without a break in the table, the ribs are a more prominent factor limiting the access to the disc space. I

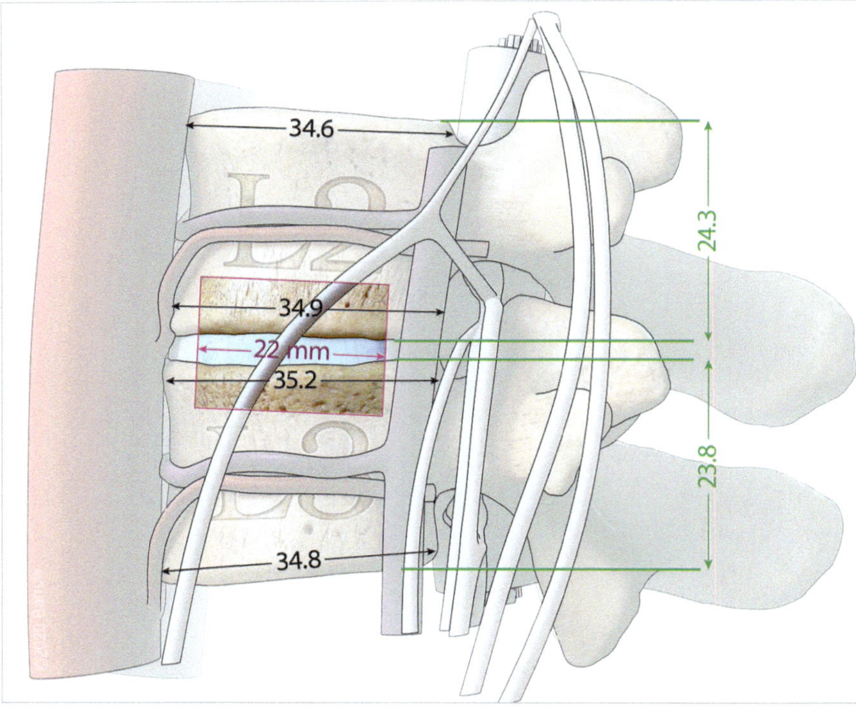

Fig. 6.14 The requisite anatomical unit for a transpsoas approach at L2–3. Illustration of a lateral view of the L2–3 level with the vascular and neural anatomy in place. The dimensions (mm) reported by Panjabi and colleagues[23] demonstrate the anatomical basis for 22 mm of exposure of the lateral aspect of the disc space, which when centered over the disc space is a safe distance from the segmental artery and vein as well as from the various branches of the lumbar plexus. A posteriorly placed access port increases the risk of an injury not only to the branches of the lumbar plexus but also to the ascending lumbar vein. Note the genitofemoral nerve coursing within the requisite anatomical unit at L2–3. Identification and mobilization may be necessary.

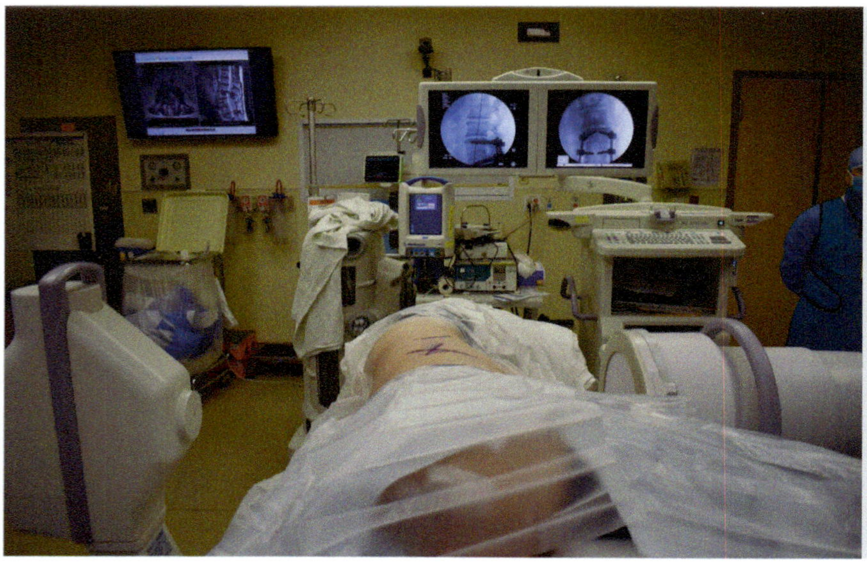

Fig. 6.15 Operating room setup. Photograph of the operation room setup. The patient is positioned laterally on a standard operating table that can break with the left side up for management of an adjacent segment issue at L3–4, which can be seen on the screens of the fluoroscope. The surgeon stands on the posterior side of the patient, and the image intensifier is opposite the surgeon.

have since returned to breaking the table to facilitate access, but I limit the extent to which I do it. Equally important is that I limit the time that the patient is in that position (▶ Fig. 6.16).[24]

In certain cases, however, the anatomical circumstance requires breaking the table at a significant angle to allow for adequate access to the disc space. Whether there is a need to break the table or not, flexions of hip and leg reduce the tension on the psoas and thereby the lumbar plexus (▶ Fig. 6.17).

A gel roll is placed in the axilla to minimize compression on the brachial plexus for the arm that is down. A well-padded arm board or Mayo stand may be used to support the arm that is elevated (▶ Fig. 6.18). The knees are bent, and the hips are ever so slightly flexed to decrease the tension on the psoas muscle. The patient needs to be positioned perfectly lateral to be able to obtain the ideal fluoroscopic images.

Once the ideal position is captured, I secure the patient firmly to the bed with tape above and below the operative site. The goal is to minimize movement of the spine once the patient is positioned. I have long stopped using a bean bag, which complicates the fluoroscopic imaging. I have replaced the bean bag with Dr. William Taylor's creation of the "sticky roll," which is nothing more than rolled-up blankets secured with the adhesive component of the tape facing outward (▶ Fig. 6.19). These rolls are placed on either side of the patient and provide

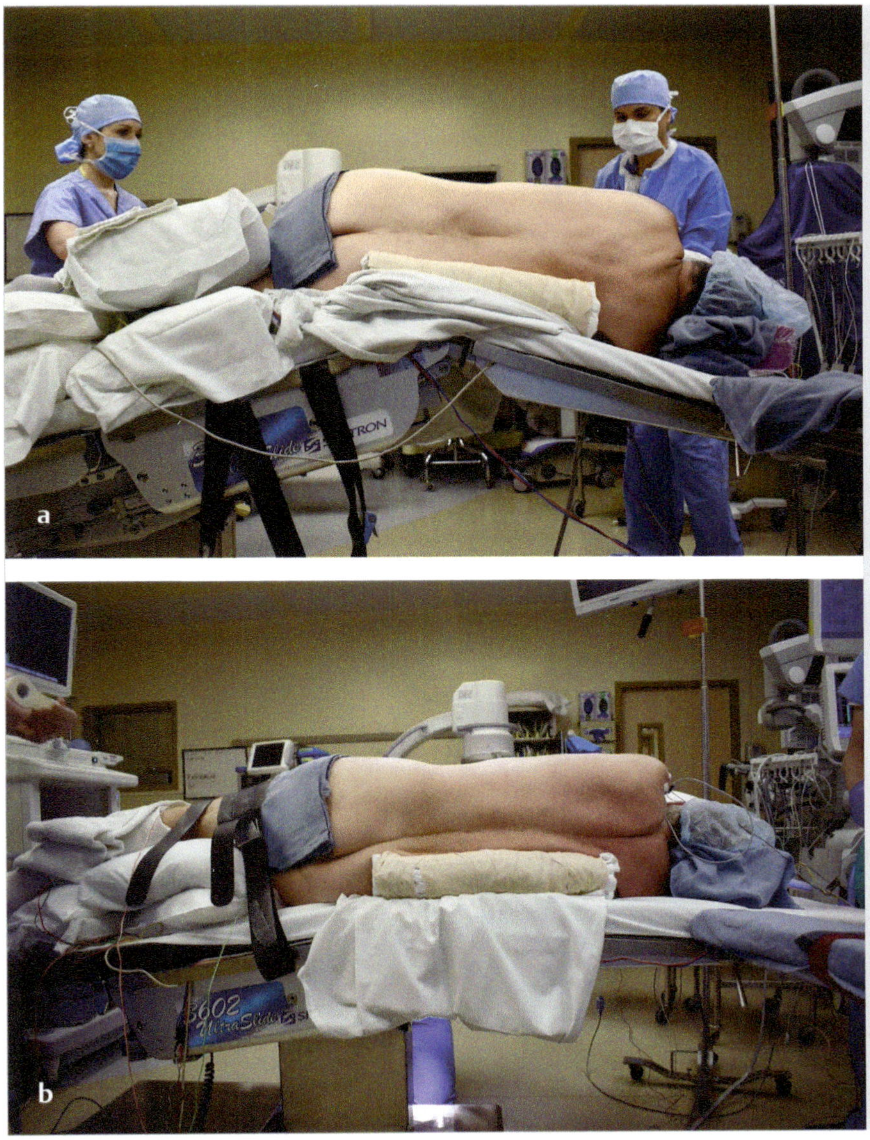

Fig. 6.16 Patient positioning: breaking the table. Photograph of two different patients positioned for an L2–3 transpsoas interbody approach. **(a)** The first patient is positioned in a lateral jackknife position at 25 degrees. Molinares and colleagues[24] identified that patients in this position are at risk for a neurologic deficit after 60 minutes. The positioning was modified to eliminate such an extreme angle in the table. **(b)** The second patient is positioned lateral, with only a modest break in the table to displace the ribs rostral enough to optimize a corridor to the lateral spine but decrease, if not eliminate, the tension on the lumbar plexus.

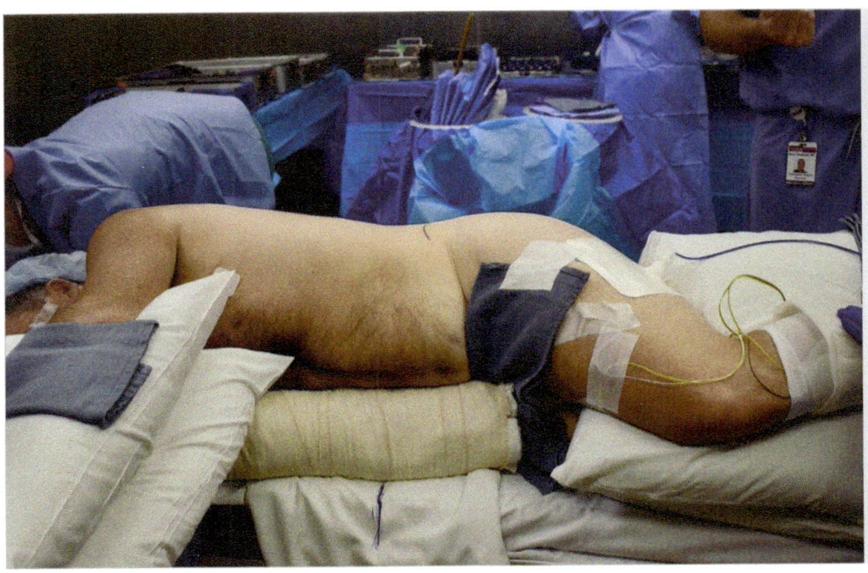

Fig. 6.17 Patient positioning: hip flexion. Photograph demonstrating flexion of the hip and knee to reduce tension on the psoas and the lumbar plexus.

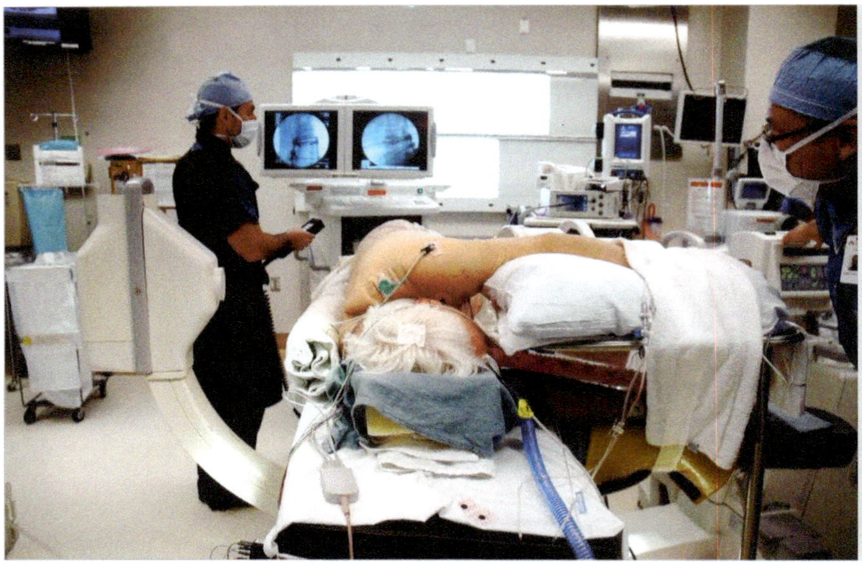

Fig. 6.18 Patient positioning: positioning the arms. Photograph showing a superior view of the patient positioned for an L3–4 transpsoas approach for management of adjacent segment degeneration above an L4–S1 construct. In this circumstance, a well-padded Mayo stand is used to support the arm that is up. An axillary roll is placed in the axilla to protect the brachial plexus of the arm that is down.

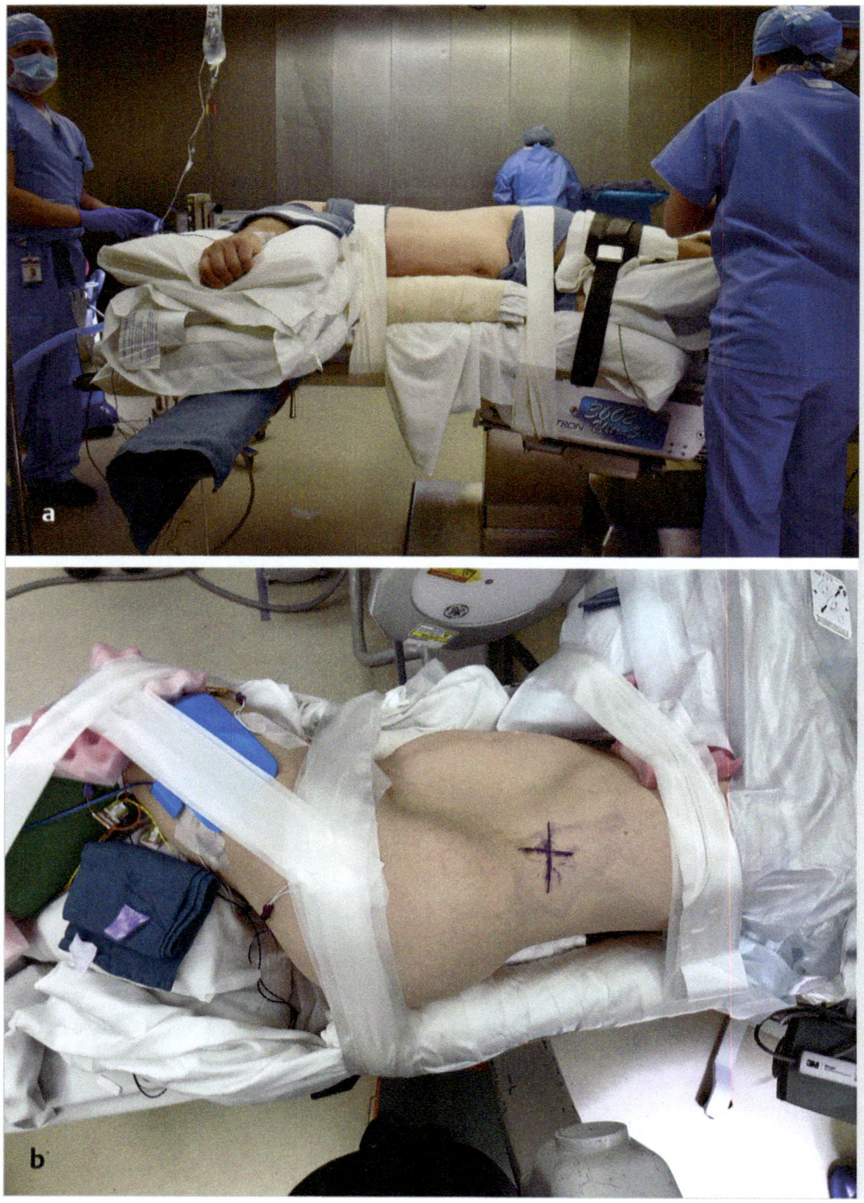

Fig. 6.19 Securing the patient's position. **(a)** Photograph of a patient positioned for an L3–4 transpsoas interbody fusion. The "sticky rolls" are placed on the abdomen and the lumbar spine and then included in the taping to firmly secure the patient to the bed in the ideal lateral position. **(b)** Photograph with a bird's eye view of a patient positioned for an L2–3 transpsoas interbody approach. The fluoroscope is in position to confirm a perfectly orthogonal position of the spine that, when captured, is secured with the tape.

valuable additional support without interfering with fluoroscopic imaging. The bed is then minimally flexed to no more than 15 degrees in the middle, allowing the torso and the legs to flex and open the disc space. A break in the table of 15 degrees makes the ribs less of a factor in the approach to the disc space. I continue to adjust the bed further (with Trendelenburg maneuvers) to keep the long axis of the spine parallel to the floor; in particular, the operative segment needs to be perfectly orthogonal to the floor. After I have optimized the patient's position and secured that position with tape, I roll in the fluoroscope.

6.17 Fluoroscopy and Localization

When the patient is in the lateral position, the vertical position of the fluoroscope generates a lateral image of the spine, where we are accustomed to seeing an AP image instead. Similarly, an AP image of the spine is acquired with the fluoroscope in the horizontal position, which would typically have produced a lateral image. Thus, the nomenclature of AP and lateral has the potential to be confusing when communicating among the operating team, surgeon and fluoroscopic technician. To mentally remedy the reversal of AP and lateral images in the lateral position with the vertical and horizontal position of the fluoroscope, I now use the terms "vertical" and "horizontal" in reference to the position of the fluoroscope. The vertically positioned fluoroscope generates the lateral images, whereas the horizontally positioned fluoroscope generates the AP images. Applying that terminology makes the request for imaging more straightforward for the operative team (▶ Fig. 6.20).

The cardinal rule of fluoroscopy in the transpsoas approach is that the X-ray tube and image intensifier are to remain perfectly orthogonal to the spine throughout the entire case. The first step in accomplishing that task is positioning the patient's spine, specifically the target disc space, in a perfectly lateral position relative to the operating room floor. Any manipulation to obtain an AP or lateral image should be done by repositioning the patient or rotating the operating table rather than the fluoroscope. Keeping the fluoroscope orthogonal to the spine at all times allows the surgeon to maintain all instruments in the orthogonal plane throughout the surgery. If the angle were changed in the fluoroscope, it would be impossible for the surgeon to adjust the trajectory of the instruments that are entering the disc space to match that angle. As the spine shifts throughout the procedure, it is imperative to make any changes with the operative bed to minimize the risk of vascular or neurologic injury and optimize the placement of the interbody spacer.

6.18 Planning the Incision

With the fluoroscope in position, preliminary images of the spinal segment are obtained, and the patient's position is fine-tuned until the ideal AP and lateral images are obtained. Fine-tuning involves altering the bed or readjusting the patient or both. Again, there should be no movement of the cant, the oblique or the wag of the fluoroscope, which must remain perfectly orthogonal to the floor of the operating room. It is the spinal segments that need to be positioned so that they are orthogonal to the floor of the operating room. The base of the fluoroscope should be such that a horizontal configuration of the fluoroscope generates a perfectly orthogonal AP image of the spine without adjusting the wag, and a vertical configuration of the fluoroscope generates a perfectly orthogonal lateral image. The ideal AP image has the spinous process in the geometric center of its like-numbered two pedicles and crisp end plates at the segment targeted for the operation. The distance from the pedicle to the spinous process is equidistant at each level (▶ Fig. 6.21).

The ideal lateral image also has crisp end plates at the segment to be operated upon and a single pedicle (i.e., no double

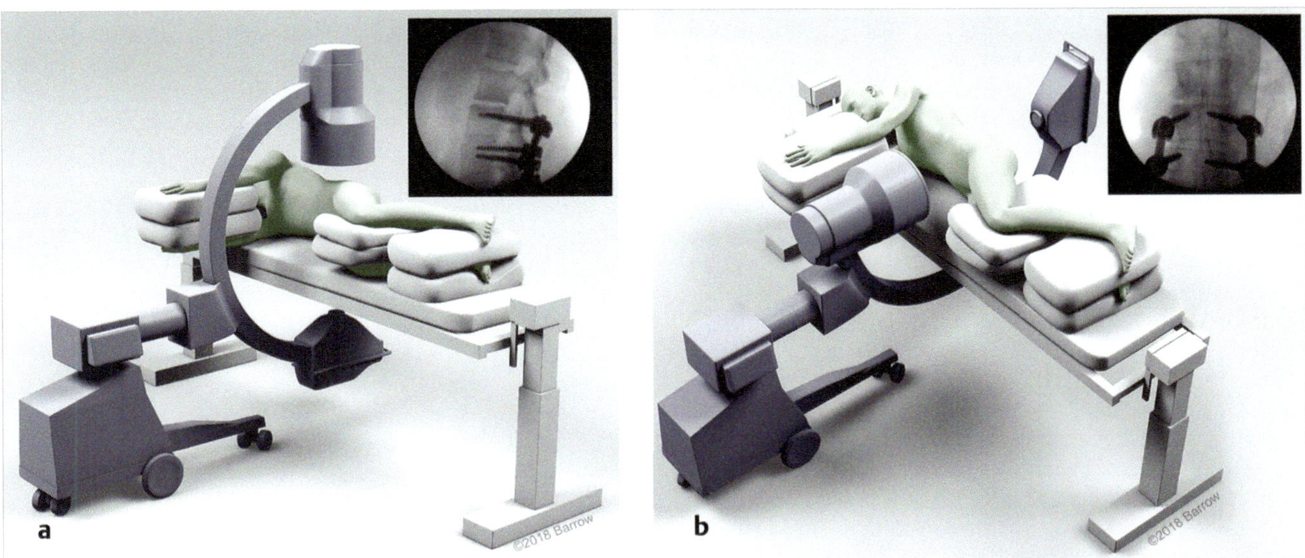

Fig. 6.20 Fluoroscopic nomenclature for a transpsoas interbody fusion. **(a)** Illustration of a patient in the lateral position with the fluoroscope in a vertical configuration, which generates a lateral image (fluoroscopic inset). **(b)** Illustration of a patient in the lateral position with the fluoroscope in a horizontal configuration, which generates an anteroposterior (AP) image. By convention, an AP image is requested by using the term "horizontal" and a lateral image is requested by using the term "vertical" to prevent confusion in communication.

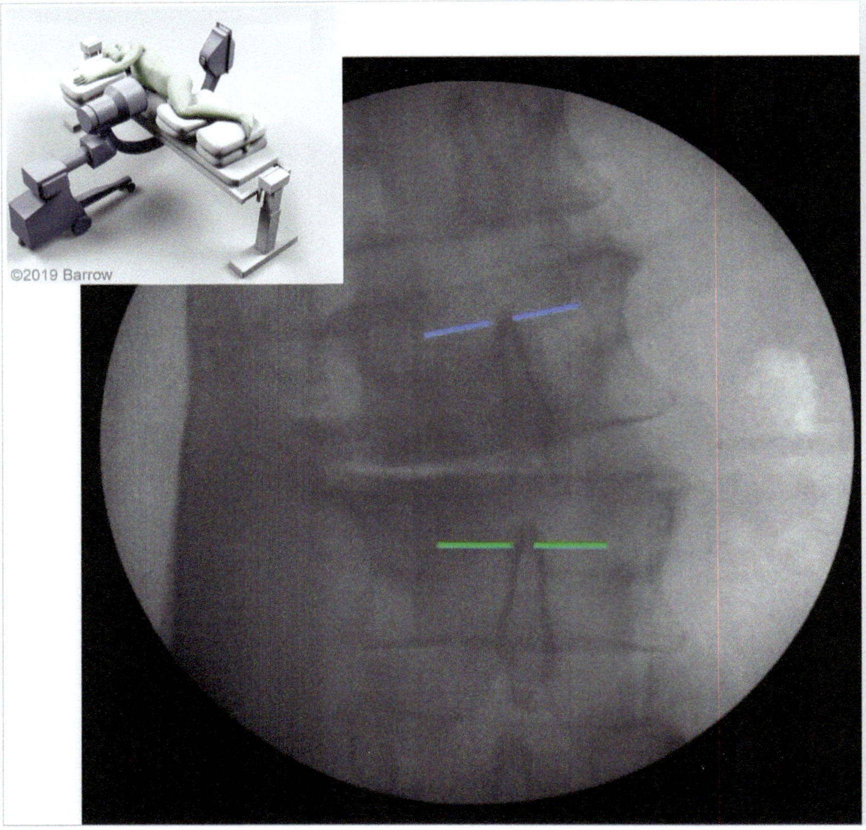

Fig. 6.21 Ideal horizontal (anteroposterior) image. Fine-tuning of the horizontal image for an L2–3 transpsoas interbody fusion. The blue lines in this image are equidistant from the pedicles of L2 to the spinous process of the L2, and the green lines are equidistant from the pedicles of L3 to the spinous process of L3. Once this image is captured, the patient is further reinforced with additional tape to secure the spine in this position.

shadow of the pedicles). For the pedicles to be in line for the fluoroscopic image, only the bed is altered to change the degree of Trendelenburg, which brings the level into the orthogonal position (▶ Fig. 6.22). It is an investment in time to obtain the perfect lateral images before marking the incision and then reinforcing the patient's position with additional tape to capture the position. It is also a worthwhile investment to position the fluoroscopic unit in a position relative to the operating table where it can transition from the horizontal position (AP) to the vertical position (lateral) without having to do anything other than release one lever and rotate it 90 degrees. Having the radiology technologist ensure there is a seamless transition from the horizontal to the vertical position before draping the patient identifies areas where a problem can occur. Practicing these transitions once or twice before draping identifies potential snags that occur with the 90-degree transition and adds tremendously to the efficiency of the procedure.

Once I have the ideal horizontal (AP) and vertical (lateral) images, I further secure the patient to the bed to minimize movement of the spine. With the fluoroscope in the vertical position, I mark the incision. There are a variety of ways to mark the proposed incision. One way is to use two Kirschner wires, one along the long axis of the spine and the other along the disc space (▶ Fig. 6.23). The intersection of these two wires indicates the central point for the incision. Marking a long line to indicate the long axis of the spine and a second line to indicate the disc space is of continued value throughout the procedure as reference points to align the instruments along the center of the disc space and the long axis of the spine.

I strive to achieve precise placement of the two Kirschner wires to intersect where I want my final implant to reside. As shown in ▶ Fig. 6.23, these wires may be cut or uncut. The advantage of the cut wires is that I can tape them to the skin and apply the principle of the inverse square law that governs radiation: create distance between myself and the X-ray source. I base the preliminary target on the transpsoas safe zones described by Uribe and colleagues and mentioned earlier in this chapter and illustrated in ▶ Fig. 6.12.[15] At L1–2 and L2–3, I mark the center of the disc space. At L3–4, I shift that mark slightly away from and anterior to from the lumbar plexus. All these markings are based on the anatomy of the lumbar plexus and its branches, which occupy more and more of the psoas as one descends. At L4–5, the target would be slightly anterior still; however, as mentioned earlier, I prefer a transforaminal approach at this level.

I mark a 30-mm incision in line with the disc space centered on the long axis of the spine (▶ Fig. 6.24). I prep and drape the patient widely, including the fluoroscope in the horizontal position. The patient should be connected to electrophysiologic monitoring before draping to ensure an optimal flow to the operation.

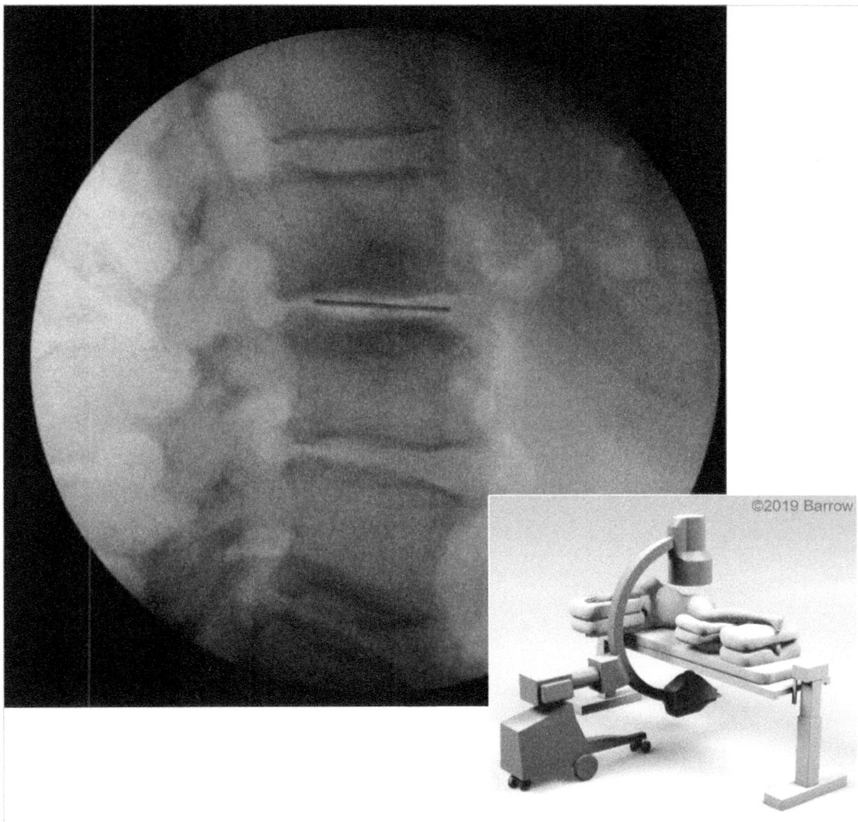

Fig. 6.22 Ideal vertical (lateral) image. Vertical image (inset) for a patient undergoing an L2–3 transpsoas interbody fusion. After ensuring an ideal horizontal image, the degree of Trendelenburg was adjusted to bring the pedicles of L2 and L3 into alignment. Clear visualization of the L2 and L3 end plates is the result. Note, while there is a double shadow at the pedicle of L4, there are no double shadows at the pedicles of L2 and L3. In this fluoroscopic image, a trimmed Kirschner wire was placed over the top of the L2–3 disc space to help plan the incision.

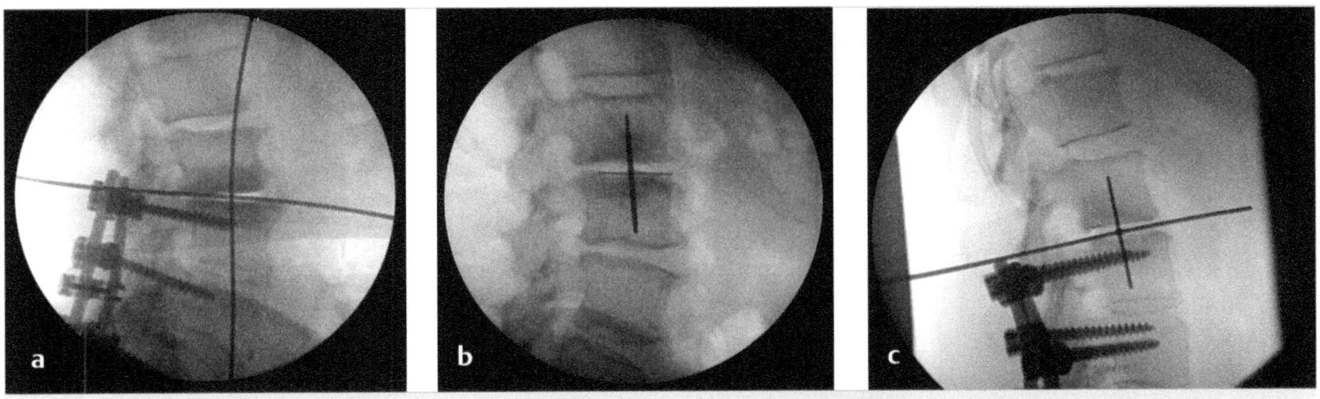

Fig. 6.23 Planning the incision. **(a)** Localizing fluoroscopic image with the Kirschner wires in a patient with adjacent segment degeneration at L3–4. The incision is planned over the top of the desired position of the interbody spacer. Note the ideal lateral image with crisp end plates is accomplished with rotation of the bed, not the fluoroscope. The "safe-zone" at L3–4 is in the anterior half of the disc space. **(b)** Planning an incision with trimmed Kirschner's wires that are taped over the top of the L2–3 disc space. The advantage of this approach is that it allows the surgeon to avoid proximity to the radiation source. **(c)** Vertical fluoroscopic image demonstrating the use of a localizing tool, provided by the vendor, to plan the incision.

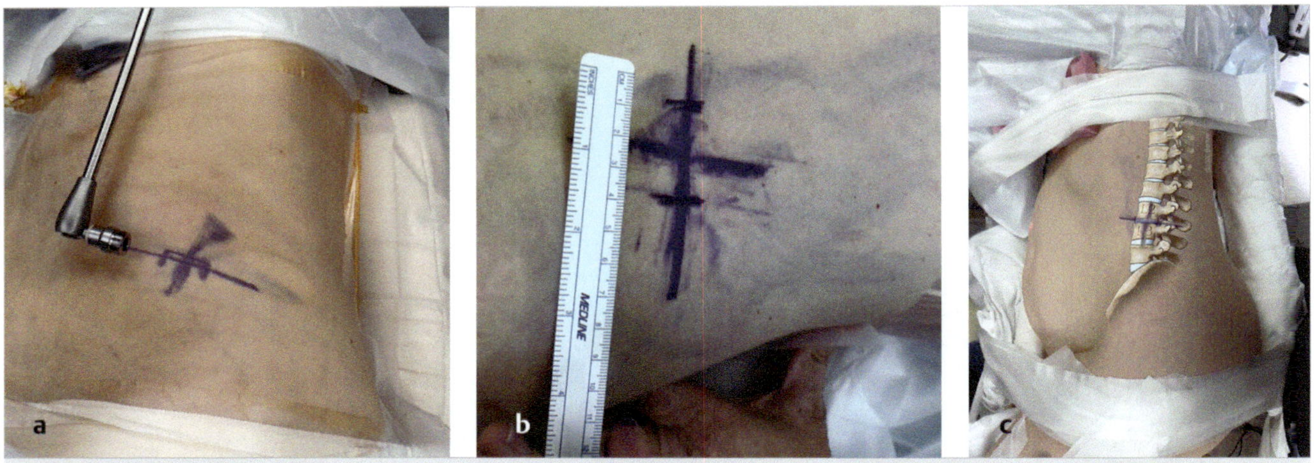

Fig. 6.24 Planning the incision. (a) Photograph taken from the foot of the bed of an incision for an L2–3 transpsoas interbody fusion. The intersection of the Kirschner wires is used to mark the disc space and the long axis of the spine. Those marks are valuable references during the operation to ensure that the instruments are centered on the disc space. (b) Photograph taken from the back of the patient immediately over the top of the incision. A 30-mm incision centered on the long axis of the spine and along the level of the disc space is marked. (c) Illustration of the spine superimposed onto the skin incision for an L2–3 transpsoas approach.

6.19 Electrophysiologic Monitoring

Electrophysiologic monitoring is the sine qua non of the transpsoas approach. The patient should be appropriately connected for free-running electromyography (EMG) and triggered evoked motor potentials. Whether using a neuromonitoring console or an electrophysiologist, the necessary preparations regarding anesthesia and connectivity should be ensured. To that end, the anesthesiologist should avoid long-acting paralytics, and a train of four twitches must be present before making the incision. It is also important to note that regardless of normal electrophysiologic signals throughout the case, nerve injury may occur. Real-time, discrete threshold responses provide feedback only for branches of the lumbar plexus that contribute to motor nerves, not sensory nerves. Thus, the genitofemoral nerve remains vulnerable. It is a combination of taking into account the threshold responses from the triggered EMG, the vertical (lateral) fluoroscopic image and the direct visualization of the anatomy that allows you to traverse the psoas safely. Nothing replaces the anatomical certainty provided by the knowledge of the lumbar plexus, which your mind's eye superimposes onto the direct visualization of the anatomy. Knowledge is the true organ of sight.

6.20 Surgical Technique

6.20.1 Incision and Traversing the Layers of the Abdominal Wall

With the incision marked, the area is prepped and draped. I always mark and include the spinous process into the field so that I have another palpable reference point. I find it helpful at times to palpate the spinous process with my nondominant hand as I begin my preliminary dissection. Palpation of the spinous process helps my mind triangulate onto the spine.

There are two techniques reported for the transpsoas approach. The first is the two-incision technique.[5] In that technique, an incision is made in the posterior abdominal wall to guide the dissection plane onto the psoas muscle. I have never found the added value in this "orienting" incision to warrant the increased risk of infection and discomfort to the patient. In this chapter, I describe the single-incision technique only.

For a single-level operation, I plan a single horizontal incision immediately over the disc space as determined by my preoperative fluoroscopic images. That incision tends to be just lateral to the erector spinae and latissimus dorsi muscles and immediately below the ribs. For a single-level operation, the length of the incision need not be longer than 30 mm, which is the approximate dimension of the vertebral body (▶ Fig. 6.14). For a two-level operation, I plan a vertical incision along the long axis of the spine and make distinct openings in the lateral abdominal wall onto the spine through that one incision.

Before the incision, I infiltrate generously with a lidocaine and bupivacaine mixture and then make the incision with a No. 15 blade. I use cautery to dissect through Camper fascia and Scarpa fascia, both of which lie superficial to the lateral abdominal muscle layer (▶ Fig. 6.25). Once I reach the layer superficial to the external oblique muscle, I stop using cautery altogether to mitigate risk to the nerves of the abdominal wall. I remind myself of branches of the lumbar plexus which course outside of the psoas and instead run their course within the layers of the abdominal musculature. The subcostal, iliohypogastric and ilioinguinal nerve are all at risk when dissecting through the muscle layers of the abdominal wall into the retroperitoneal space.

The first muscle layer that I encounter is the external oblique. I work to establish a plane of dissection in line with the disc space using two tonsil hemostats that spread the crossing fibers

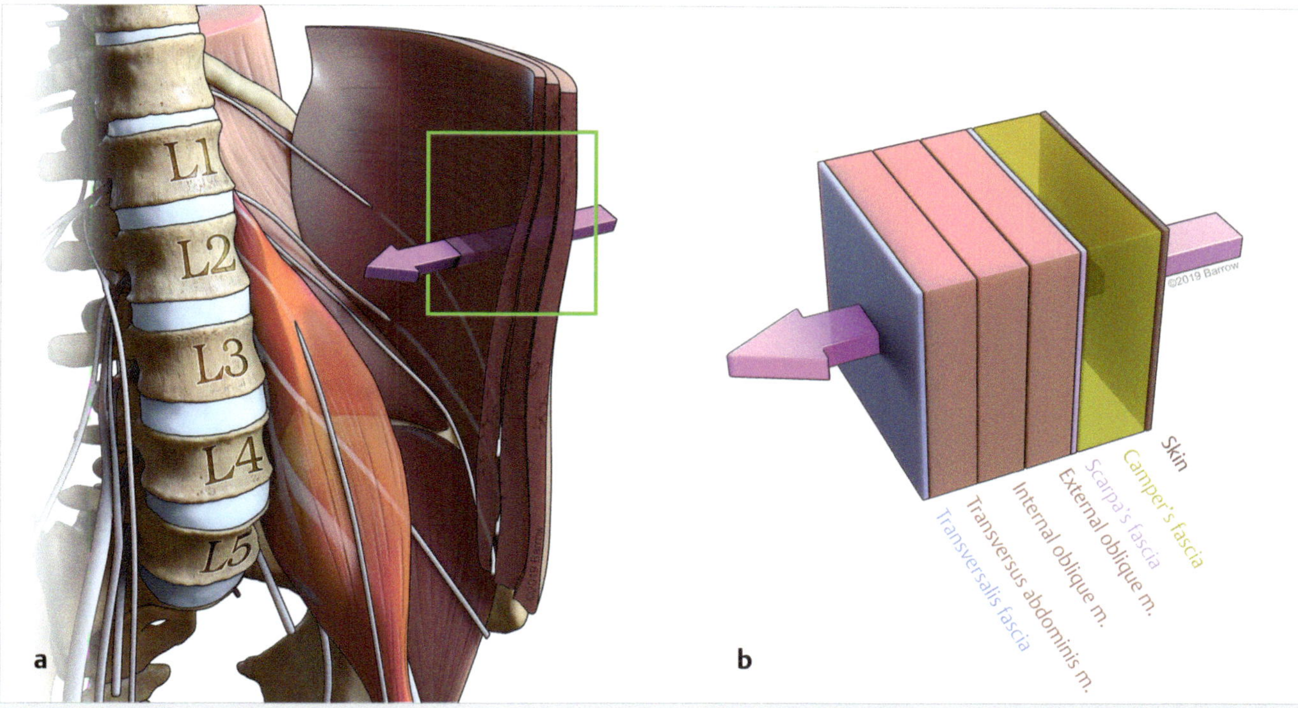

Fig. 6.25 The layers of the abdominal wall. **(a)** Location of the section of the abdominal wall shown in **b**. **(b)** The layers are shown from the outermost skin layer to the interior transversalis fascia layer. After the incision is made, the Camper fascia and then Scarpa fascia need to be traversed to reach the musculature of the abdominal wall. From there, the muscular layers of the external oblique, internal oblique and transversus abdominis muscle need to be traversed before reaching the transversalis fascia.

of the muscle. Again, in the interest of preserving the subcostal, iliohypogastric and ilioinguinal nerves, I limit my dissection to spreading of the 30-mm incision and remaining parallel to the disc space. The next layer is the internal oblique, which is identified by the crossing fibers that are opposite to the external oblique. During this dissection, I am especially mindful of the iliohypogastric and ilioinguinal, which course in between these two muscle layers. As discussed in the lumbar plexus section, injury to these nerves is not inconsequential to the patient, and care should be taken to preserve them. The final muscle layer is the transversus abdominis. By continuing the systematic approach of spreading the tips of the tonsillar hemostats, I encounter the transversalis fascia. Slightly more downward pressure needs to be applied for the tips of the hemostat to create an opening in the transversalis fascia. Peering down as I spread the hemostat, I see the unmistakable appearance of retroperitoneal fat. I now know for certain that I am in the retroperitoneal space. The transversalis fascia can be quite limiting, and so I ensure that I create an opening in line with the disc space that spans the entire length of the incision.

6.20.2 Orientation in the Retroperitoneal Space

Upon entry into the retroperitoneal space, I proceed to orient my mind and begin the reconstruction of the anatomy at depth with blunt finger dissection. I palpate the quadratus lumborum and proceed from there to the transverse process. I find it helpful to identify the transverse process with my dominant hand and palpate the interspinous process space with my nondominant hand at the level of the skin. The combination of these two tactile inputs helps me orient my mind and triangulate onto the disc space. The most prominent transverse process is consistently L3, and more often than not, this location is where I would find myself if I were to take a fluoroscopic image at this point. If I am operating on the L2–3 level, then I slide my finger upward from that long transverse process and confirm the L2–3 interspace with an endoscopic Kittner. If I am operating at L3–4, I slide my finger downward and confirm the L3–4 interspace. For L1–2, the 12th rib is a factor, and the pleura is undoubtedly seen. On occasion, I have found the need to remove at least a part of the rib. Although the rib might not necessarily block my access to the disc space, it does alter the trajectory of the access port, which affects the trajectory of the instruments into the disc space.

Once on the transverse process, I carefully slide my finger over the psoas muscle and palpate the anterior aspect of the disc space and vertebral body. It is important to ensure a free plane over the psoas muscle to prevent any injury to the peritoneum. I now palpate the surgical target: the disc space. The vertebral body and disc space are evident by palpation. The combination of the skin markings, the preoperative fluoroscopy and the palpation of the anatomy reconstruct the anatomy at depth and help me keep my bearings through the remainder of the procedure (▶ Fig. 6.26).

There should always be a concern for the peritoneum and its contents. However, there should also be confidence that the patient's position has shifted the abdominal contents in a manner that creates a safe corridor onto the lateral spine. The morphometric study on the effect that the lateral position has on

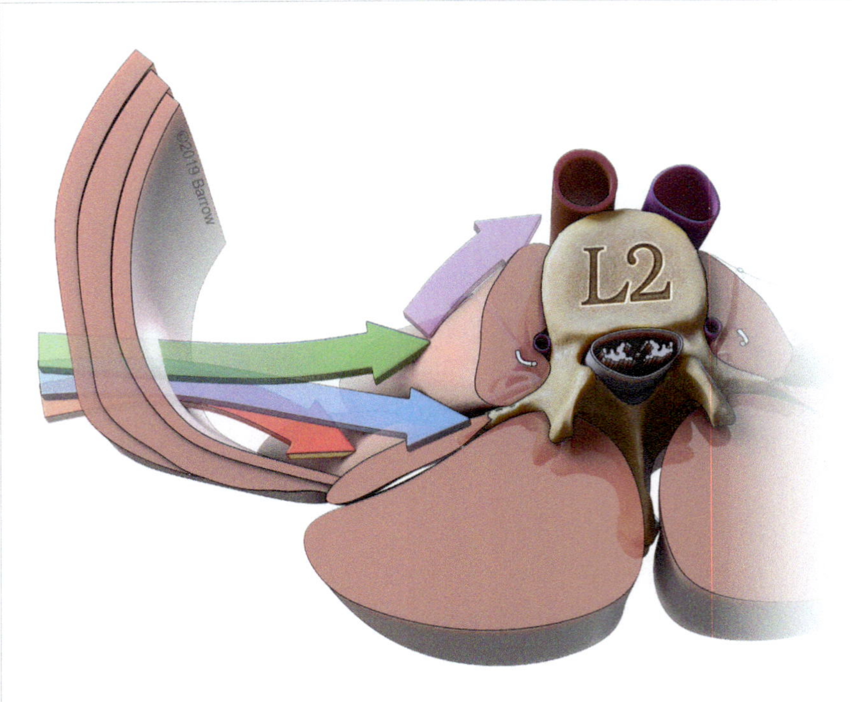

Fig. 6.26 Reconstructing the anatomy at depth in a transpsoas approach. Illustration of an axial view of a retroperitoneal transpsoas approach. After traversing the muscular layers of the abdominal wall and the transversalis fascia, the retroperitoneal space is entered. The quadratus lumborum is palpated first (*crimson arrow*) then the transverse process (*blue arrow*). From there the psoas is gently palpated (*emerald arrow*), and a plane is created over the top of the psoas (*purple arrow*) to ensure free access to the muscle. When palpating the psoas, it is important to keep in mind that the genitofemoral nerve courses over the top and should not be mistaken for an adhesion.

the abdominal contents by Deukmedjian et al[25] is a must-read article for the transpsoas approach that instills confidence in your ability to navigate the retroperitoneal space. The axial magnetic resonance imaging (MRI) figures in that article demonstrate the position of the great vessels and the peritoneum in the supine position and the degree of shift that occurs in the left and right lateral decubitus positions. These are powerful images to become familiar with and have registered in your mind for this procedure.

6.20.3 Traversing the Psoas

Palpation of the disc space in line with my preoperative skin marks reliably places me on my surgical target. I find it helpful to use endoscopic Kittner blunt dissectors for this part of the operation. These instruments are long, slender and straight with a gauze tip that will not dislodge and are of tremendous help holding the peritoneum anterior to the transpsoas corridor. With one finger on the anterior aspect of the disc space, I guide the endoscopic Kittner onto the disc space and hold it there. As I do, I am fully cognizant of the vascular anatomy anterior to my position. With the peritoneum safely swept and maintained forward with the endoscopic Kittner, I can now begin the process of traversing the psoas (▶ Fig. 6.27).

The common denominator in all the commercially available systems is some form of triggered-EMG stimulation delivered to the distal end of the initial introducer or dilator. I pass the introducer or the dilator onto the surface of the psoas muscle with continuous, triggered EMG stimulation running. The lower the thresholds, the closer the dilator is to the femoral nerve. Some systems offer a directional stimulation that helps localize the femoral nerve. In those systems, when the thresholds change from low to high, the direction of the single quadrant stimulation is anterior to the femoral nerve and a safe corridor has been identified. Regardless of the system used, the objective is to traverse the psoas without any nerve depolarization at a low threshold. Before traversing the psoas with the introducer, I get a sense of the disc space by palpating the topography with my index finger (▶ Fig. 6.27). I remind myself of the location of the transverse process and then palpate the anterior aspect of the disc space until I can begin to feel the fall off of the anterior vertebral body begin to occur. In this manner, I orient myself to the anteroposterior boundaries of the disc space. I then slide my index finger back several millimeters and place the tip of the introducer onto the psoas muscle with continuous stimulation. The position of the introducer should be completely orthogonal to the spine and along the line on the skin that marks the long axis of the spine. A horizontal (AP) image confirms my level and my trajectory (▶ Fig. 6.27b). Before passing through the psoas muscle, I obtain a vertical (lateral) image to confirm the level and location of my introducer relative to the posterior aspect of the disc space.

With the level confirmed and neuromonitoring silent, I rest the introducer or initial dilator onto the surface of the psoas muscle and obtain a vertical image to confirm my location within the disc space (▶ Fig. 6.28). Any irritation of the lumbar plexus before or during this process reliably indicates that I am too posterior within the psoas. If this situation were to happen, I do not obtain an image at this point; instead, I shift the introducer or initial dilator and begin again more anterior. I do not advance the introducer or dilator until I obtain an AP (horizontal) and lateral (vertical) image. The ideal position is for the tip to be within the safe zones reported by Uribe et al[15] and illustrated in ▶ Fig. 6.12. At this point, on the basis of what I see on fluoroscopy, I may make minor adjustments, whether anterior or posterior, to achieve ideal placement. Satisfied with the

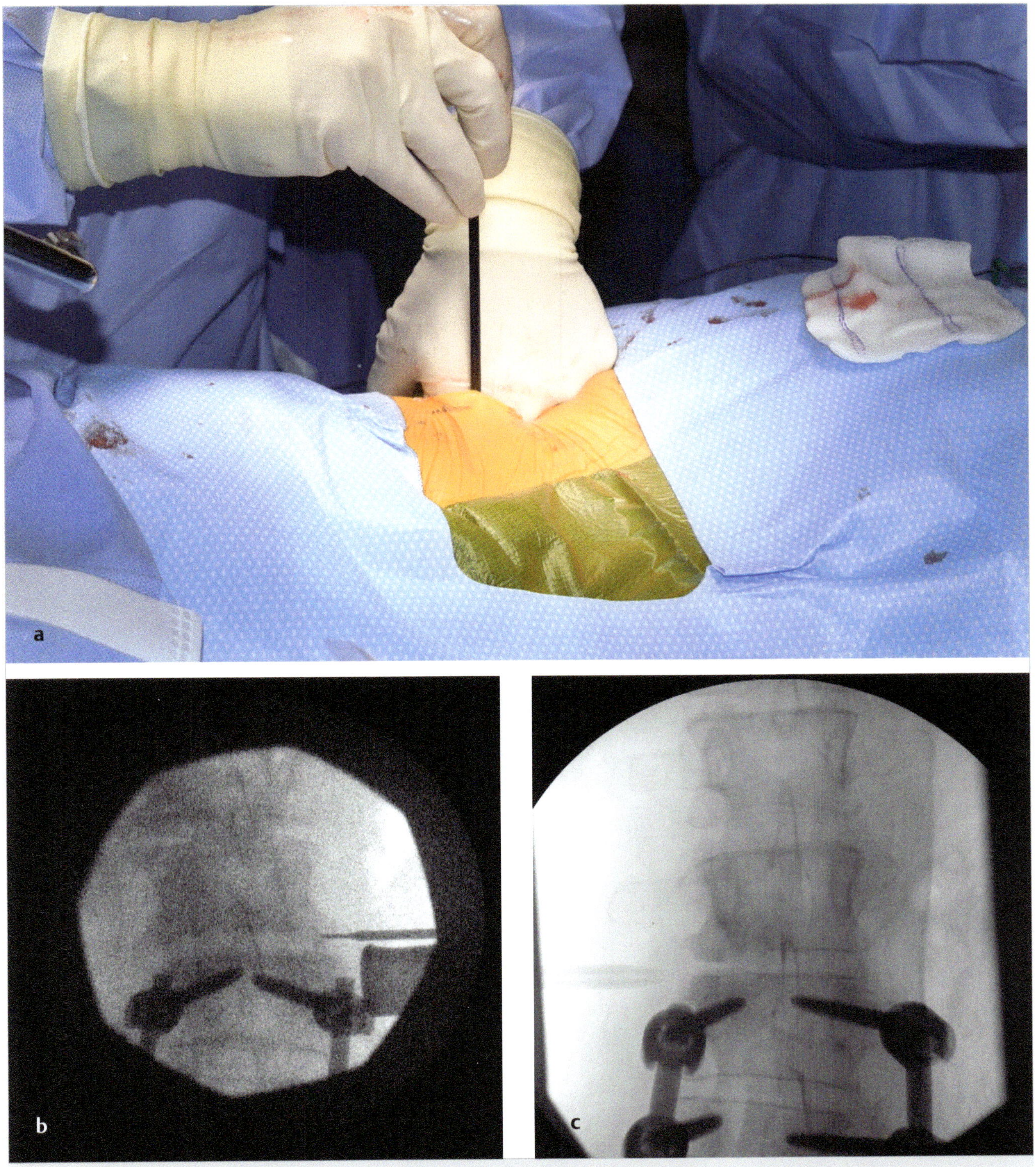

Fig. 6.27 Endoscopic Kittner for blunt dissection and palpation of the disc space. (a) Intraoperative photograph demonstrating the use of an endoscopic Kittner and palpation of the disc space with the index finger. Note that the endoscopic Kittner is maintained orthogonal to the spine and in line with the incision. Such a position reliably assures that Kittner is on the intended surgical target. (b) Horizontal (anteroposterior [AP]) image confirming the location of the initial introducer. Note that when the introducer is passed along the lines that demarcate the long axis of the spine and is maintained in an orthogonal position, the target level that was marked from the outset is reliably localized in one image. (c) Horizontal (AP) image demonstrating the use of a dilator resting on the psoas. Before traversing the psoas, a vertical image is obtained to confirm a safe zone of entry to traverse the psoas and enter the disc space.

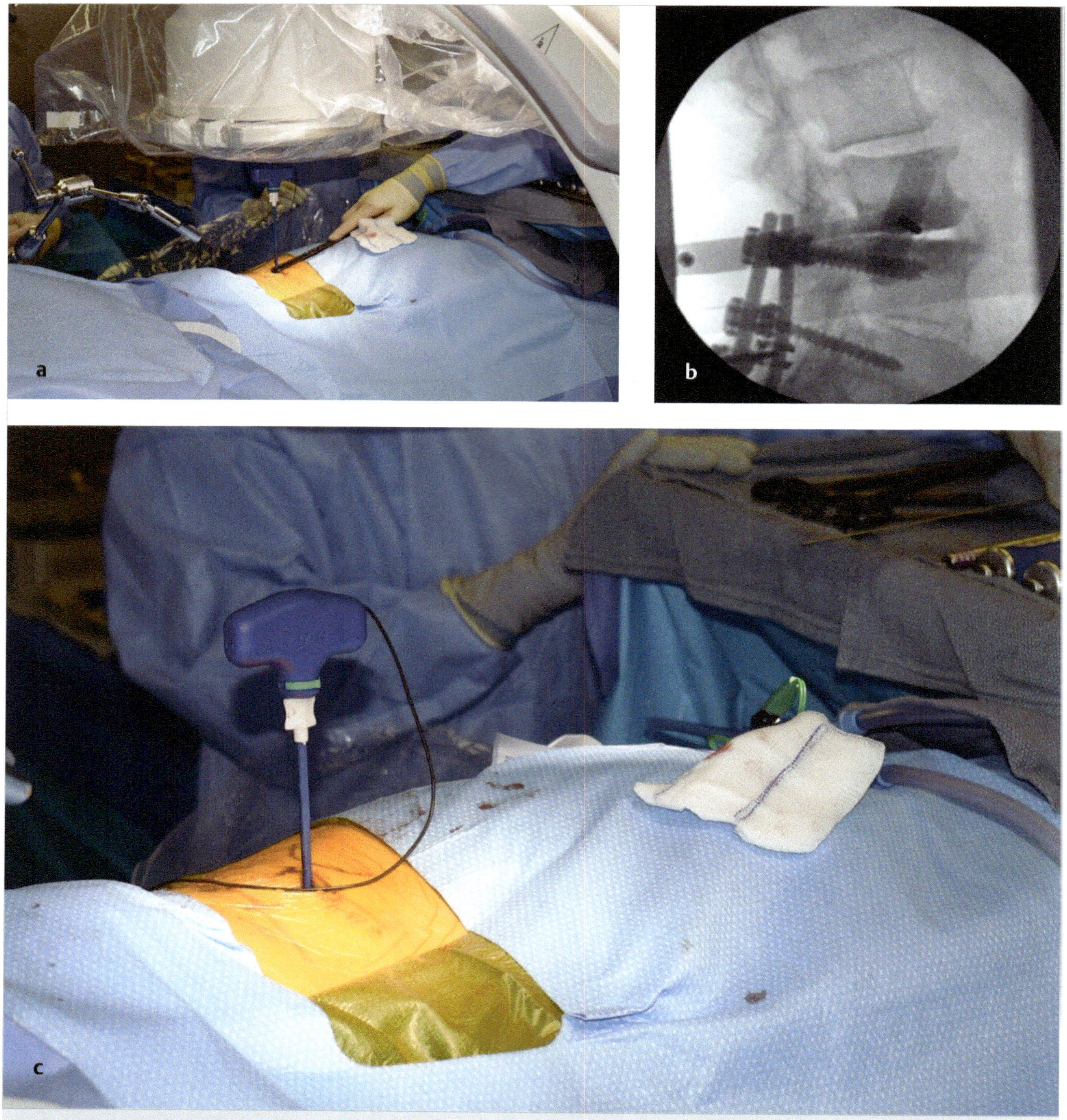

Fig. 6.28 Traversing the psoas with an introducer. Continuously triggered electromyography stimulation ensures a safe corridor through the psoas muscle. **(a)** A vertical (lateral) image confirms the location within the disc space before puncturing the annulus. **(b)** Collimated low dose vertical fluoroscopic image demonstrating the location of the introducer relative to the posterior aspect of the disc space. **(c)** The introducer is advanced when the ideal position in the disc space is confirmed. Note the orthogonal position of the instrument.

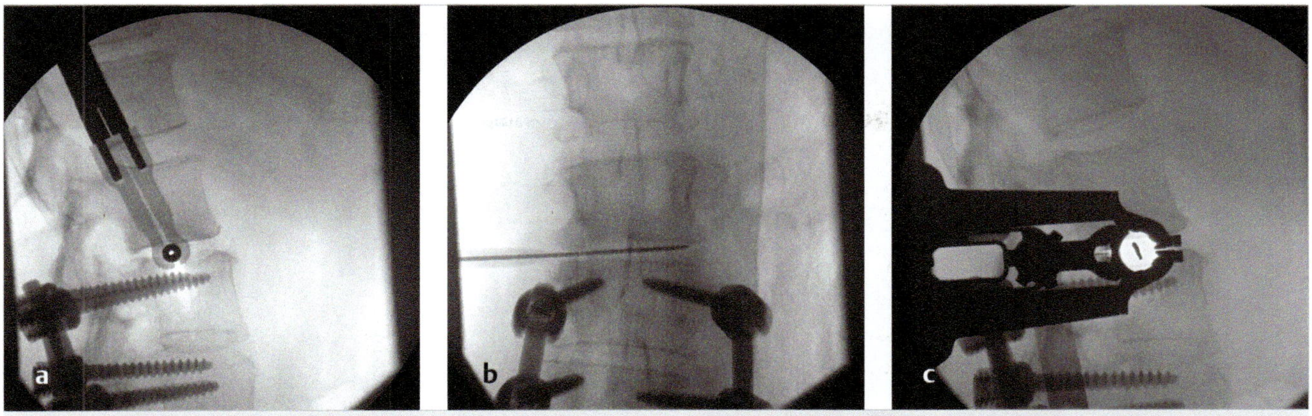

Fig. 6.29 Passage of the Kirschner wire into the L2–3 disc space for management of a patient with adjacent segment degeneration above an L3 to L5 construct. **(a)** Horizontal (anteroposterior, AP) fluoroscopic image of initial dilator resting on top of the psoas to confirm the location of a safe zone of entry to begin to dilate the psoas with continuous free-running electromyography. With a safe zone confirmed, I pass the Kirschner wire into the disc space. **(b)** Horizontal (AP) image demonstrating passage of the Kirschner wire into the disc space. **(c)** One final additional vertical (lateral) fluoroscopic image confirming the position of the access port relative to the safe zone established by the Kirschner wire position.

position of the initial dilator or introducer, I safely navigate through the psoas without irritation of the lumbar plexus, puncture the annulus and enter the disc space. Any repositioning after this step will require repetition of the aforementioned steps to minimize the risk to the lumbar plexus.

With the ideal position achieved and in the absence of any depolarization of the lumbar plexus, depending on the system I am using, I either remove the tip of the introducer and pass the Kirschner wire into the disc space or pass the wire through the first dilator. I pass the wire well into the disc space but short of the contralateral annulus (▶ Fig. 6.29). I pass the dilators one over the other to dilate the psoas muscle. Meticulous dilatation against the disc space is required to expose the requisite anatomical unit. Distinct from the various other procedures described in this Primer, there is no wanding with a transpsoas approach. Instead, circumferential rotation of each dilator with sustained downward pressure and continuous EMG monitoring are imperative to optimize the access port–spine interface. Once the final diameter dilator passes through the psoas, the perimeter of the diameter may be stimulated to ensure no depolarization of the femoral nerve at a low threshold. The depth is measured by the markings on the final dilator, and the expandable minimal access port is secured in position. The table-mounted arm is typically secured on the opposite side of the table above the operative site to minimize the profile. The dilators are removed while the Kirschner wire is kept in position until AP and lateral fluoroscopy confirm ideal placement (▶ Fig. 6.30).

6.20.4 Exposing the Requisite Anatomical Unit

I connect the light source to the access port and peer into the retractor to ensure no concerning structures are within the working corridor, specifically the genitofemoral nerve. I look for this nerve regardless of the level, but I am keenly aware of its presence when I am working at L2–3. A dissection with a long Penfield gently along the fibers of the psoas muscle is all that is needed to rule in or rule out the presence of the genitofemoral nerve in your corridor to the disc space. I distinctly remember encountering the genitofemoral nerve during one of my early cases. I attempted to stimulate it and questioned my electrophysiologist when he did not find any irritation of a nerve root with stimulation. In actuality, I did not have an appreciation of what I was looking at, which in hindsight seems obvious (but the anatomical articles on the lumbar plexus had not been written in 2008). The genitofemoral nerve is a sensory nerve and does not show stimulation on electrophysiologic monitoring. I have found that traction on the root, however, can increase both heart rate and blood pressure when the patient is lightly anesthetized, which may represent an indirect form of neurologic monitoring.

If the genitofemoral nerve is identified, the question then becomes in which direction to mobilize it. It is in attempting to answer this question that my knowledge of anatomy first became a liability. I reasoned that at L2–3 since the genitofemoral nerve courses from zone II to zone I at L3–4, the nerve should be mobilized anteriorly. Early in my experience, I went great lengths to sweep the nerve forward. Such a dogmatic approach is wrongminded. The answer is that the nerve should be mobilized in the direction where it can be kept out of harm's way with the least amount of traction. When I encounter this nerve now, I mobilize it either anterior or posterior, whichever direction seems most conducive to securing it behind the access port blade without traction or holding it back with a Penfield dissector. I also evaluate the position of the access port relative to the disc space on both horizontal (AP) and vertical (lateral) images. If the access port needs to be moved a millimeter or so anterior, posterior, rostral or caudal, I can then make minor adjustments and capture them by loosening and tightening the table-mounted arm.

Some systems have a vertebral body screw that fixates the access port firmly to the spine; other systems have a shim that enters the disc space and secures the access port in that manner. Familiarity with the techniques and the ability to problem

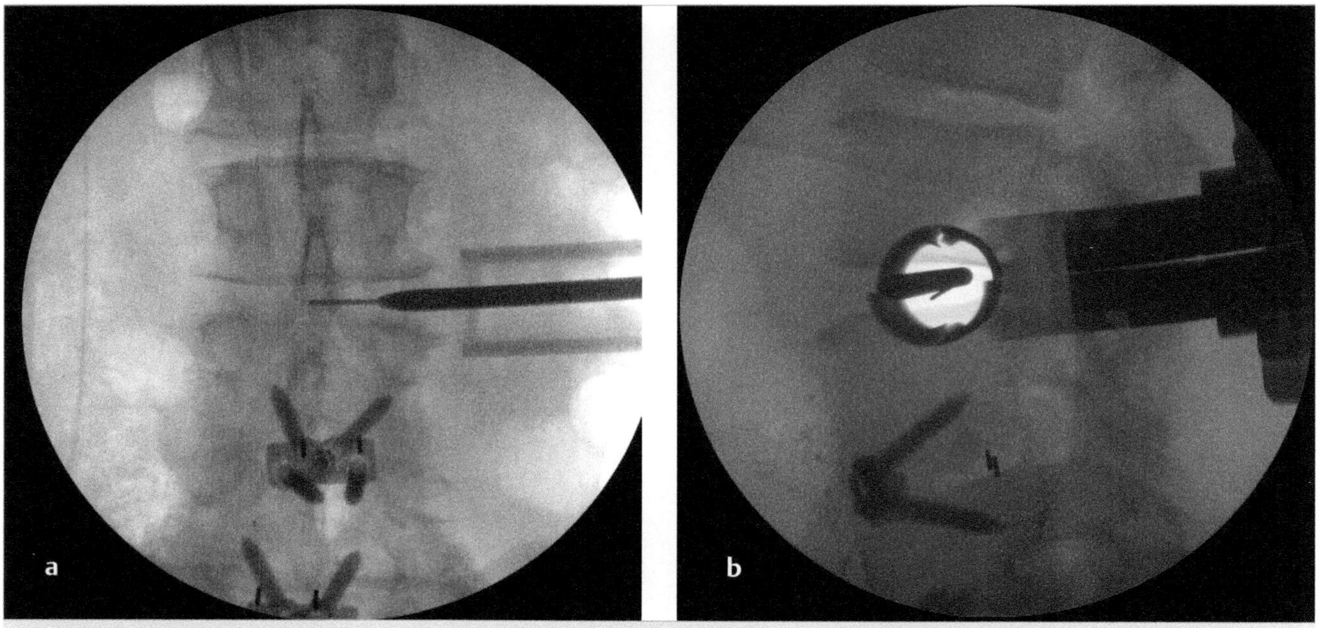

Fig. 6.30 Confirmation of the position of the access port for L3–4 transpsoas interbody. **(a)** Horizontal (anteroposterior) fluoroscopic image demonstrating the orthogonal placement of the access port. **(b)** Vertical (lateral) image demonstrating a slightly posterior position of the access port; however, there was no depolarization of the lumbar plexus with triggered electromyography stimulation. The first dilator and the Kirschner wire remain in position for both of these images.

solve is more important than the type of access port itself (▶ Fig. 6.31).

Traversing the psoas and securing the access port is the most technically demanding part of this procedure. That early phase of the operation is analogous to placing a Kirschner wire across an odontoid fracture for an odontoid screw procedure. Once that wire is across the odontoid fracture, the technically demanding and high-risk component of the procedure is complete. Similarly, once the access port is secured into the optimal position, the technically demanding component of the procedure is behind you. The discectomy and interbody work have the potential to be the most straightforward parts of the procedure.

A Penfield dissector cleaves a plane within the psoas muscle, and the unmistakable appearance of the annulus comes immediately into view. As mentioned earlier, upon peering through the access port, I again ensure that I do not see any branches of the lumbar plexus. On a good day, I am looking at a few thin strands of the psoas muscle covering the annular fibers of the disc. The amount of psoas muscle encountered at this point will be directly proportional to the lumbar level. At L1–2, there will be a strand or two of muscle. At L2–3, the psoas will begin to take shape but remains relatively thin. At L3–4, there is now a potential for a significant amount of muscle mass. Again, my philosophy regarding the L4–5 segment has been made clear earlier.

At this point, a gentle sweeping motion with an endoscopic Kittner or Penfield dissector is all that is needed to expose the disc space further. A more challenging circumstance arises when the entire disc space is covered with the psoas muscle. Under these conditions, a large Penfield is used to cleave a plane through the psoas and establish a plane of dissection into the disc space. Continuously stimulating and restimulating is essential throughout such a dissection because that is the time where neural elements may be encountered. As mentioned earlier, it is typically the genitofemoral nerve that will need to be safely mobilized outside of the working corridor that leads into the disc space. At times, because of the size of the psoas (especially at L3–4), a large Penfield or endoscopic Kittner will be needed to retract the psoas. Under these circumstances, I achieve a preliminary exposure of the disc space and repeat the dilatation process. I place the initial dilator onto the disc space with direct visualization and dilate to the diameter of the access port once again. Iterative dilatation under direct visualization is an investment in time. Optimizing the access port–disc space interface will offer increased efficiency to the operation, optimal visualization of the disc space and decreased postoperative discomfort.

Before incising the disc space, the stimulating probe is used to assess the perimeter and, of course, the vicinity of the annulotomy. I will march the probe around the entire perimeter of the exposure, ensuring that there is no stimulation of the lumbar plexus. I create a generous annulotomy with a bayoneted No. 11 blade that spans the entire exposure provided by the retractor (▶ Fig. 6.32). As mentioned throughout this book, it is vital for a minimally invasive surgeon to know the exact dimensions of the various access ports in use. In this case, the access ports that I use have a diameter that ranges from 16 to 22 mm. With a well-positioned access port, it is seldom necessary to open the retractor at all in the rostrocaudal dimension. However, for access ports with a third blade, several clicks of the third blade sweep the psoas anteriorly and provide further

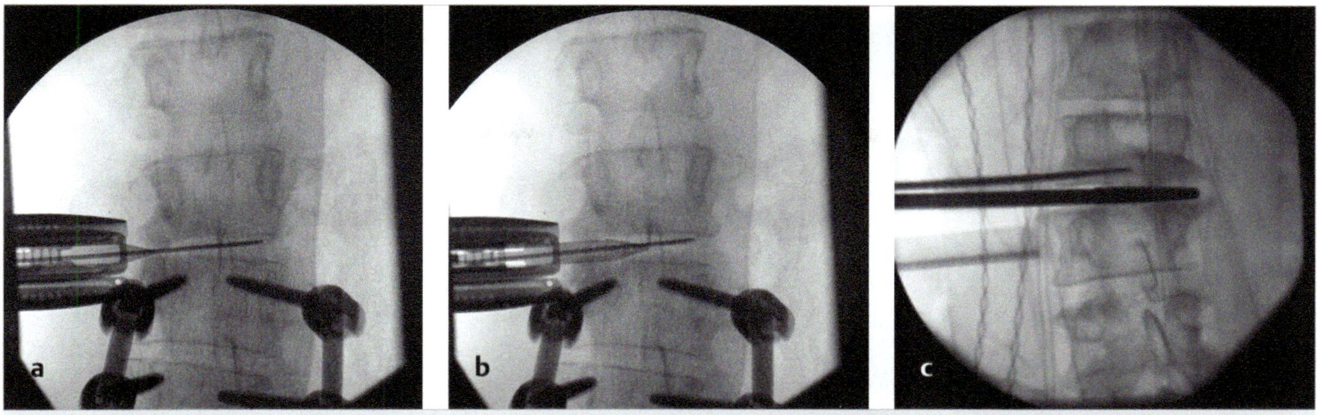

Fig. 6.31 Further securing the access port with a shim or vertebral body screw. **(a)** Horizontal (anteroposterior) fluoroscopic image demonstrating the use of a shim. The proposed path of the shim needs to be explored with monitoring and direct visualization before placement of the shim. **(b)** Once a safe corridor is established, the shim is advanced. **(c)** An alternative to a shim is a vertebral body screw that is used in other systems. Both of these options prevent migration of the access port off the requisite anatomical unit.

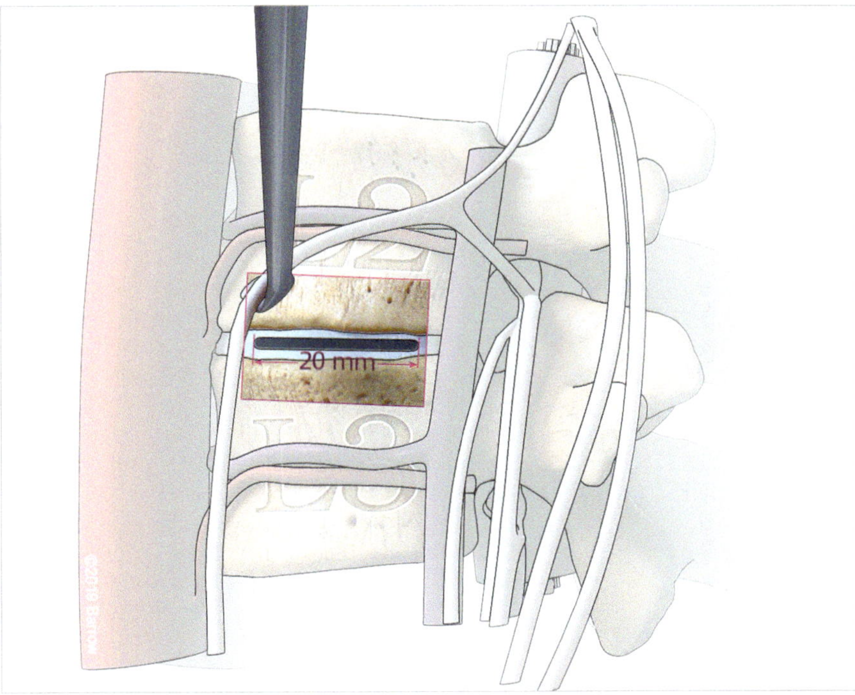

Fig. 6.32 Annulotomy for transpsoas interbody fusion. A generous annulotomy of 20 mm has been performed, which is almost two-thirds of the disc space. Completing the discectomy, preparing the end plates for arthrodesis and placing the interbody remain.

access to the anterior aspect of the disc space. During the discectomy, muscle creep from the psoas may not allow exposure of the disc space all at once. The use of endoscopic Kittner dissectors or a long-bayoneted Penfield dissector allows for sweeping the psoas further posteriorly, which enables the safe extension of the annulotomy.

6.20.5 End Plate Protection

As I begin to prepare the disc space, at the forefront in my mind is the integrity of the rostral and caudal cortical end plates. Violation of either one of the cortical end plates is an irreversible event. In my experience, end plate violation sends the patient down a very different postoperative trajectory with increased discomfort, risk of subsidence of the interbody graft and a suboptimal outcome. Therefore, I take definitive measures to mitigate the risk of cortical end plate violation. To begin with, I avoid the use of the interbody shavers capable of cutting bone, just as I do when I am performing a minimally invasive transforaminal lumbar interbody fusion. These shavers are sharp, and in a disc space with a severe coronal imbalance, they can gouge out the cortical end plate of the most collapsed aspect of the disc space. Instead, I use blunt disc space distractors to open the space. These instruments can still violate the cortical end plate, but to a lesser degree than when used parallel to the end plate. Second, despite my disdain for ionizing radiation, I use

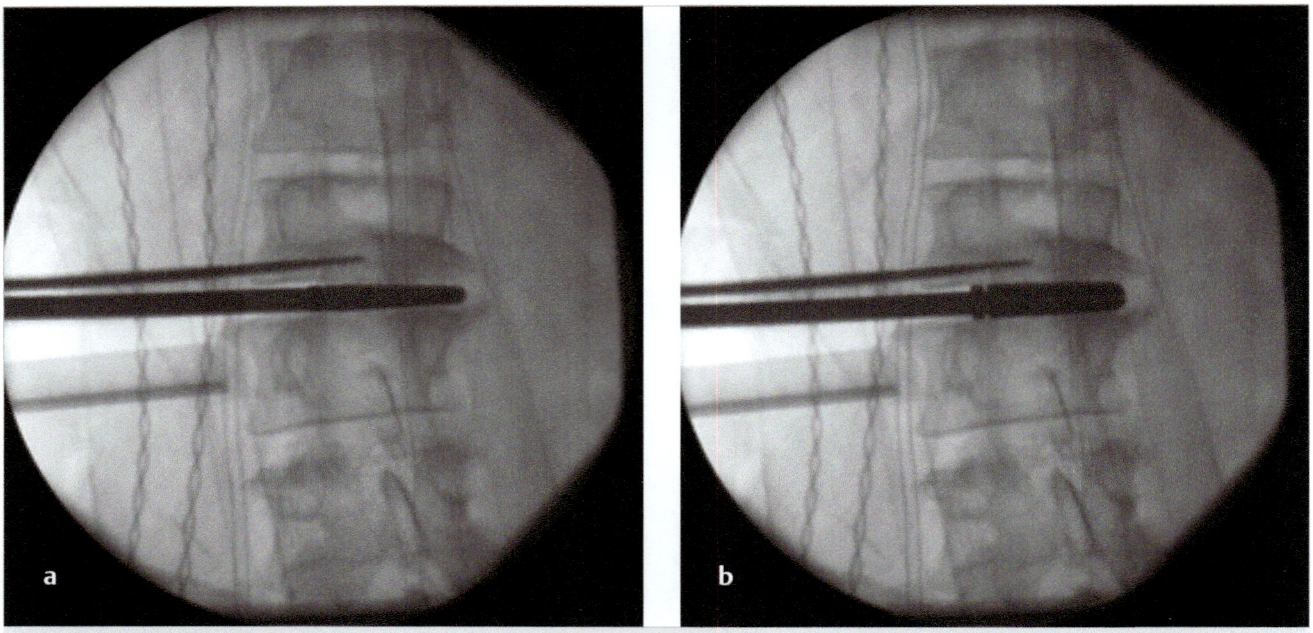

Fig. 6.33 Intraoperative anteroposterior fluoroscopic images demonstrating **(a)** the wedge distractor position under fluoroscopy to prevent violation of the end plate. Once in position, **(b)** the distractor is rotated to expand the interbody space. Note that despite starting with an ideal image, this image is not ideal. Careful analysis of the spinous process of L3 relative to the pedicles indicates that the patient has rotated away from the surgeon. This rotation routinely happens during the operation. The operating table was rotated back toward the surgeon to idealize the image as the interbody work continued.

additional fluoroscopy when wielding an osteotome or wedge distractor to ensure that I am completely parallel to the disc space. Those additional doses of radiation prevent an errant trajectory into the end plate.

Once an annulotomy has been made, pituitary and Kerrison rongeurs are used to remove the disc material. At times, in severely collapsed disc spaces, even the smaller Kerrison and pituitary rongeurs will not fit into the disc space. Under these circumstances, the osteotome or wedge distractor is needed to begin the preliminary distraction of the disc space (▶ Fig. 6.33). Again, caution needs to be taken when using these instruments not to violate the end plate. As mentioned earlier, I align the trajectory of these instruments completely parallel to the disc space with fluoroscopy to minimize the risk of such an event.

The sequential increase in disc height with wedge distractors and blunt rotating distractors is deferred until the release of the contralateral annulus. The objective at this point in the disc preparation phase is to create a working corridor to pass the instruments.

6.20.6 Release of the Contralateral Annulus

It is imperative to release the contralateral annulus to optimize the restoration of the coronal balance and the interbody height. In doing so, it is never lost on me that on the other side of the contralateral annulus reside the contralateral psoas muscle and the contralateral lumbar plexus. I always make the electrophysiology technician aware when I am releasing the contralateral annulus so they can remain vigilant and notify me of any activity on the contralateral lumbar plexus. We spent a great deal of time only moments before doing everything in our power to protect the ipsilateral lumbar plexus and minimize disruption of the ipsilateral psoas. I am now wielding a large Cobb elevator and a mallet with the intention of dividing the fibers of the contralateral annulus with the contralateral psoas and lumbar plexus immediately on the other side. Such an event has the potential to cause injury to the contralateral lumbar plexus and the psoas. And so again, despite my disdain for ionizing radiation, this circumstance is one of the times I use more fluoroscopy than in other phases of the operation.

Releasing the contralateral annulus involves becoming familiar with the haptic feel of the contralateral release and confirming the release with a horizontal (AP) fluoroscopic image. I place a greater emphasis on the haptic feel of the release, thus limiting the fluoroscopic imaging to confirmation of that release when the sensation in my hands informs me that it is done. I begin using an interbody long-handled Cobb, which I insert into the disc space and nudge up against the contralateral annulus with a tap or two of the mallet. There is a slight angle on the Cobb that allows me to focus on the superior aspect of the annulus first. A horizontal (AP) fluoroscopic image confirms that I am clear of the end plate and within the lateral aspect of the disc space. I then begin to tap with the mallet until I feel the unmistakable haptic feedback of heightened resistance. The tip of the Cobb is now firmly against the superior insertion of the contralateral annulus of the disc space and on the verge of dividing it. One or two more increasingly harder taps with the mallet on the handle of the Cobb provide yet another distinct haptic feedback as the Cobb divides the contralateral annulus,

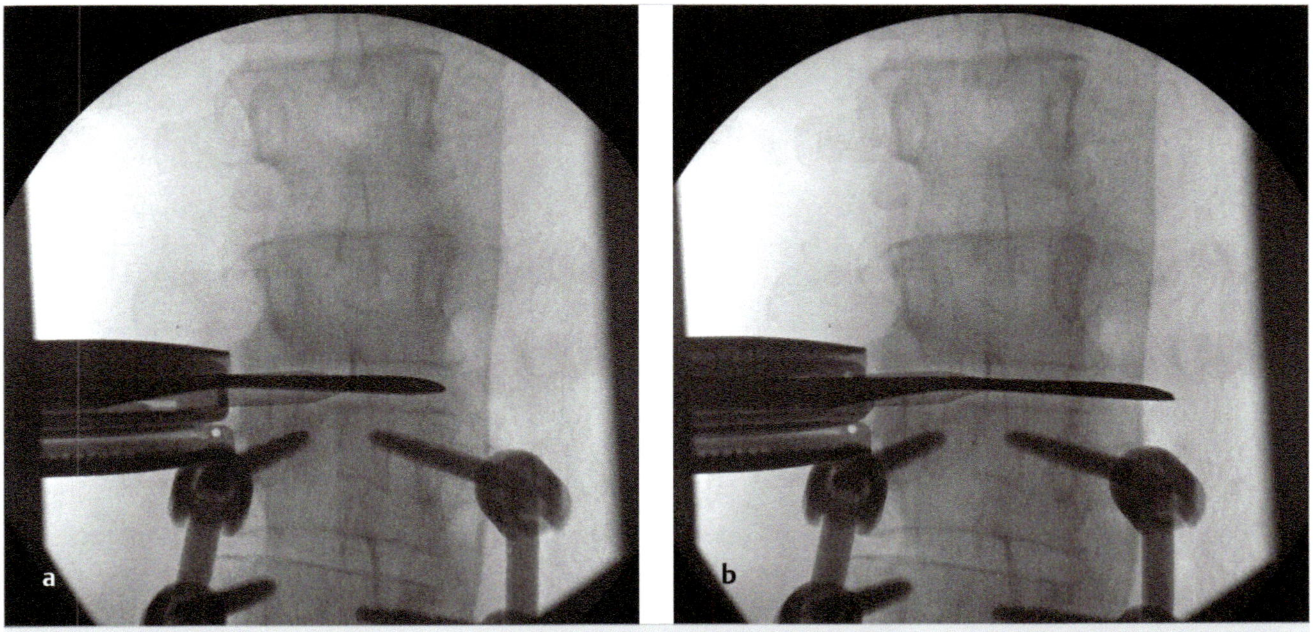

Fig. 6.34 Contralateral release of the annulus in an L2–3 transpsoas for management of adjacent segment degeneration. Horizontal (anteroposterior) fluoroscopic images demonstrating the division of the contralateral annulus with a Cobb elevator, which is accomplished primarily by feel more than by fluoroscopic guidance. **(a)** Cobb up against the contralateral annulus. Despite multiple taps, there is little advancement of the tip of the Cobb. **(b)** The contralateral annulus is released by a few taps on the Cobb with a mallet. The sensation of the release is a sudden advancement of the Cobb within your hands.

and the heightened resistance all of a sudden gives way, like a trap door collapsing beneath my feet.

Similarly, a sequence of fluoroscopic images throughout this process would demonstrate very little change in the position of the Cobb, perhaps an advancement of a few millimeters. Once the trap door has collapsed, and the annulus has been traversed, the appearance on fluoroscopy will be far from subtle. From one image to the next, the advancement of the Cobb will be over a centimeter (▶ Fig. 6.34).

With the superior insertion on the contralateral annulus now divided, I direct my attention to the division of the inferior insertion. To do so, I place the angle of the Cobb elevator toward the inferior insertion of the annulus into the disc space and repeat the process. Admittedly, the haptic feel is different when the superior insertion of the annulus has already been released than in the initial opening because the contralateral annulus has been weakened by its initial division. Again, fluoroscopy is a tremendously valuable guide to minimize risk to the end plate and the contralateral lumbosacral plexus.

The release of the contralateral annulus allows for the restoration of the disc space height and, as a result, greater access to the disc space for curets to remove the cartilaginous end plate and for pituitary rongeurs to remove disc material. If the disc collapse persists after the release of the contralateral annulus, and the passage of instruments in and out of the disc space remains difficult if not impossible, I will insert a paddle distractor into the collapsed section of the disc space and rotate it. I remove the handle and work within the disc space, either in front or behind the paddle, which facilitates passage of the instruments and optimizes the preparation of the disc space.

6.20.7 Interbody Spacer

The unparalleled advantage of the transpsoas approach is the capacity to span the entire disc space from apophyseal ring to apophyseal ring. A well-positioned interbody spacer can rest on the hardest part of the vertebral body, thereby minimizing the risk of subsidence. The interbody spacer has the load of the body weight resting upon it and thereby reliably achieves fusion in a well-prepared disc space. Once the cartilaginous end plates have been removed, the cortical end plate prepared, and the contralateral annulus released, it is time to trial for the interbody size.

6.20.8 Interbody Spacer Dimensions

The lateral dimension of the interbody spacer is seldom less than 45 mm and at times may be as long as 55 mm. The disc space anatomy determines the height, which can be as little as 8 mm and as much as 14 mm. However, years of clinical practice have steered me away from being overzealous in the restoration of the disc space height. The patients in whom I have restored a considerable amount of height have been more susceptible to subsidence in the months after surgery. The requisite anatomical unit offers a safe exposure of two-thirds of the disc space. In a larger patient with vertebral bodies that measure 40 mm in the lateral dimension, approximately 26 mm of the disc space may be exposed. With such a corridor, a wide interbody up to 22 mm in dimension may be safely secured. In a smaller patient with a lateral dimension of the vertebral body that measures 30 mm, the corridor is narrower. In these patients, an 18-mm spacer may be safer. I am less dogmatic about adhering to one width. Instead, I carefully analyze the anatomical corridor to determine my selection. At times, the genitofemoral nerve takes a circuitous path, and a smaller implant allows for safe retraction of the genitofemoral nerve during placement of the interbody, which would not be possible with a larger one. Our first and foremost priority is the preservation of neurologic function.

6.20.9 Interbody Trials

Time and time again, I have found that the final resting place of the interbody spacer is precisely where the trial rested. From this observation, I have developed a rule of thumb: how the trial goes into the disc space is how the interbody spacer goes into the disc space. Experience has validated that rule in case after case. Anytime the interbody graft has appeared in a suboptimal position, hindsight has revealed that the position was reliably predicted by how the trial went in. And so, when I begin placement of the trials, I take special care to ensure the trial is going in perfectly orthogonal to the disc space. In the end, the position of the interbody is a direct reflection of my craftsmanship. It will be something that the patient, my colleagues and I will be looking at for a long time. The placement of the interbody spacer is the core element of the operation, so strive for perfection.

Before I begin placing the interbody trials, I go through a systems check. I want to ensure that I still have a perfect horizontal (AP) and vertical (lateral) image. At times, the manipulation of the spine during the discectomy, contralateral annulotomy and especially the placement or removal of the trials shifts the vertebral segments. Using the mallet to release the contralateral annulus or simply the progress of the procedure may have slightly altered the position of the patient on the table. I make all adjustments by shifting the patient with the bed control. No changes are made to optimize the image by altering the fluoroscope. Only after I have reconfirmed the ideal fluoroscopic imaging do I insert the trial, with intermittent horizontal (AP) fluoroscopic imaging. It is worthwhile to obtain another vertical (lateral) image at this point to confirm the position of the access port. The combination of these two images at this point in the operation helps confirm in your mind's eye the ideal target for the interbody to reside. After the confirmation of ideal imaging, the passage of the trials begins.

The interbody trials have a hole or a slit in the center, which give them a characteristic appearance on AP fluoroscopy. The appearance of the trial is of tremendous value when tapping it into position. Assuming an ideal horizontal (AP) fluoroscopic image, any obscuration or asymmetry of the hole or the slit indicates a suboptimal trajectory. The goal is to maintain a symmetrical appearance of the trial at all times when tapping into position. The hole and the slit are also helpful to align with the spinous process and achieve a perfectly centered position (▶ Fig. 6.35).

The decision regarding the height of the interbody is made purely by feel. You do not want to overdistract the disc space, place undue stress on the segments above and below and potentially create an environment for subsidence. At the same time, you do not want to place a spacer that will not be under sufficient annular tension and thereby risk pseudoarthrosis and migration. I typically begin with one size down from the last blunt intradiscal retractor that was used. For example, if the last blunt intradiscal distractor I used measured 12 mm, then I begin with a 10-mm trial (assuming the trials are provided in 2-mm increments). I tap the trial into position with intermittent fluoroscopy to ensure an optimal trajectory and avoid injury to the end plates. Keep in mind that even though the trial is undersized relative to the blunt distractor that achieved a certain interbody height, tapping the trial of the same height into position may require some forceful tapping with the mallet. However, if you find yourself using a significant amount of force without advancement of the trial, you should stop and reassess to prevent injury to the end plate or vertebral bodies. Under these circumstances, I will go down another trial size and keep sequentially decreasing until the trial advances into the disc space with greater ease.

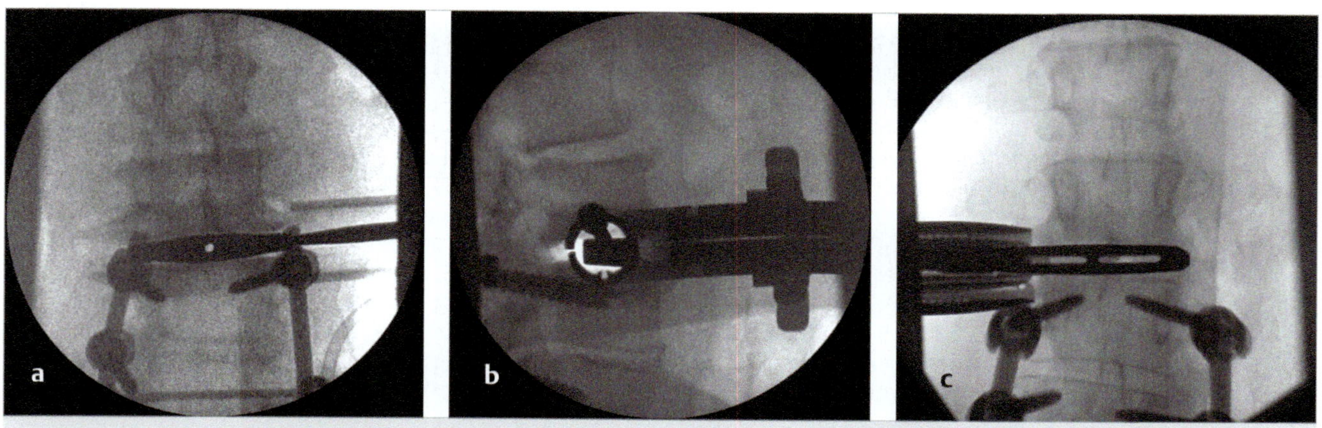

Fig. 6.35 Trial insertion into the interbody space. **(a)** Horizontal (anteroposterior, AP) fluoroscopic image demonstrating the trial in the geometric center of the disc space. **(b)** Vertical (lateral) fluoroscopic image demonstrating ideal placement of trial in the anterior half of the disc space. **(c)** Horizontal (AP) image demonstrating the advancement of a trial into the disc space.

Once I find a trial that traverses the disc space, I return to the trial that I initially attempted, and that trial will now reliably advance into the disc space. I repeat this process until I have identified the ideal interbody height. The final step in sizing the interbody is a horizontal (AP) and vertical (lateral) fluoroscopic image. The position of the interbody trial on this image should be exactly where you want the interbody spacer to reside (▶ Fig. 6.35).

The "appropriate" size for an interbody is a difficult term to define. In essence, the "appropriate" size is a combination of feel, appearance on the horizontal (AP) and vertical (lateral) fluoroscopic imaging and, equally important, a comparison to the disc heights of the normal segments in the lumbosacral spine. Simply having the capacity to insert an interbody twice the size of a normal disc height does not make such an insertion efficacious for the patient.

6.20.10 Insertion of the Interbody Device

With the interbody size selected, it is loaded onto the inserter and packed with graft material. I place the tip of the spacer up against the annulotomy with the inserter perfectly orthogonal to the floor and begin to tap the interbody spacer into position. I typically begin this phase by keeping the interbody trial in position until the implant is ready for insertion, which will continue to relax the annular fibers in the anterior and posterior aspects of the disc space and facilitate the insertion of the interbody. For the insertion of the interbody, I will use every piece of information that confirms my trajectory and position relative to the spine. Fluoroscopic imaging, the initial markings I made on the skin marking the axis of the spine and the orthogonality to the table are all valuable components that will help me with the insertion.

The scrub technician loads the interbody onto the inserter as I remove the trial from the interbody space with a slap hammer. I confirm a trajectory parallel to the disc space with fluoroscopy and the position of the inserter relative to the marks previously made on the skin, and I begin tapping the interbody device into position (▶ Fig. 6.36). The main pitfall at this point is not following the trajectory made by the trial.

6.20.11 Closure

With the interbody in a satisfactory position, I examine the area to ensure no graft material migrated outside of the disc space. At times when I do nothing more than tap the interbody into the disc space, graft material migrates out and needs to be placed back into the interbody spacer. There should be no graft material left on the psoas muscle. Once the interbody has been inspected and the graft material appropriately policed, I close the blades of the access port as the scrub technician loosens the table-mounted arm. Before pulling out the access port, the operative site is meticulously inspected for any bleeding. In my experience, any bleeding should be minimal and easily managed with nothing more than short bursts of bipolar cautery.

I had one occasion where the collapse of the blades unveiled profuse arterial bleeding. It was a segmental vessel that had been interrupted. Control of the bleeding in this circumstance required draping the microscope, using two suctions, and having an inordinate amount of patience to identify and cauterize the vessel. The possibility of such an event is something to keep in mind before pulling out the blades too quickly. Fortunately, to encounter such bleeding is exceptionally rare. The familiarity of the vascular anatomy on the lateral aspect of the spine allows for the confidence to manage such an event should it happen. Recognition that arterial bleeding is likely from the segmental artery and venous bleeding is likely from the ascending lumbar

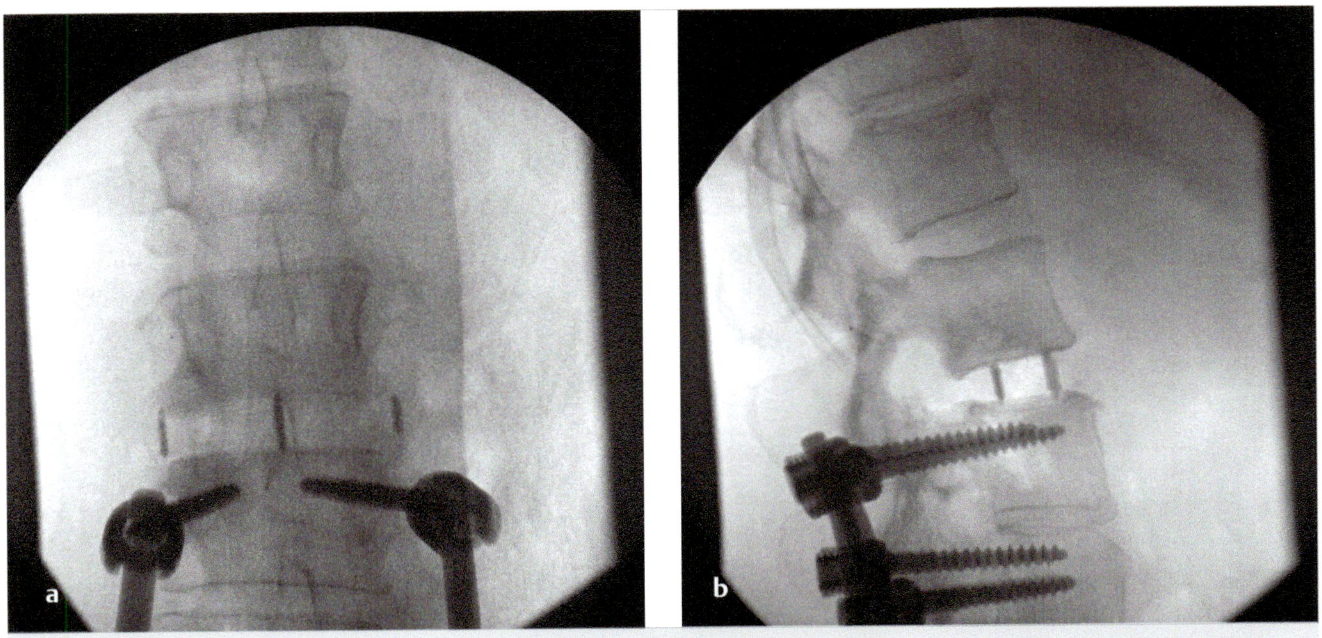

Fig. 6.36 Management of adjacent segment degeneration at L2–3 above an L3–5 construct. **(a)** Horizontal (anteroposterior) and **(b)** vertical (lateral) fluoroscopic images demonstrating ideal placement of the interbody at L2–3.

vein provides the certainty needed to control the bleeding, regardless of the source.

Once hemostasis has been achieved and the access port removed, I identify each side of the transversalis fascia and approximate it in an interrupted fashion using a 0 polyglactin 910 suture on a UR-6 needle. Closure of this fascial layer is essential to prevent an abdominal wall hernia. The various muscle layers are identified and closed. I would be misrepresenting the case if I told the reader that I identify each distinct muscle layer of the abdominal wall and close it. Instead, I approximate the muscle layers that unveil themselves with a size 0 polyglactin 910 suture on a UR-6 needle to the best of my ability. Scarpa fascia is then reapproximated with a size 2–0 polyglactin 910 suture on an X-1 needle, and finally, the subcuticular layer is closed with a size 3–0 polyglactin 910 suture. Benzoin and a single 1-inch Steri-Strip is placed over the incision, and a lidocaine patch is placed over that.

If the transpsoas interbody is part of a larger strategy to address a deformity, I reposition the patient prone at this point for the second phase of the operation. If the procedure was for management of an adjacent segment issue or single-level degeneration, then the patient is awakened and taken to the postanesthesia care unit.

6.21 Postoperative Care

Despite the absence of any abnormalities on electrophysiologic monitoring, a neurologic deficit may occur. The most catastrophic deficit is a femoral nerve deficit. I always examine patients in the recovery room immediately after awakening from anesthesia, specifically examining hip and leg flexion and extension. Patients are prepared to expect some discomfort in the leg on the side of the approach, which may especially limit the examination. Patients are also prepared to expect anterior thigh numbness that may extend into the groin. My main objective with the recovery room examination is to rule out a femoral nerve deficit, which is quite distinct from the earlier-mentioned deficits with profound quadriceps weakness.

Patients are admitted into an observation unit. If the procedure is performed as the first or second case, they may be discharged at the end of the day. Cases done later in the afternoon are typically kept overnight. Multilevel cases are always admitted at least for 23 hours. Patients are asked to wear a lumbar corset for the first month anytime when they are out of bed. Postoperative standing 36-inch radiographs are obtained on the day of surgery or the first postoperative day, and they become the reference radiographs that are compared to the 1-month postoperative radiograph. In particular, I am looking for any evidence of migration of the graft or subsidence. Sagittal balance is again assessed and, if positive, prompts scheduling of posterior instrumentation. Patients who had a positive sagittal balance on a preoperative study, even when corrected with the transpsoas approach, also have posterior instrumentation scheduled, if not performed, under the same anesthesia. The concept that the degenerative spine tends to return to its previous state applies to these circumstances. I query the patient as to whether or not the radicular symptoms or neurogenic claudication symptoms have resolved entirely after a focused neurologic examination. Any persistent radicular symptoms lead me to plan decompression in addition to the posterior instrumentation.

6.22 Posterior or Lateral Instrumentation

Biomechanical studies have exhaustively examined the stability of interbody devices within the disc space. Side plates have been examined and compared to pedicle screw instrumentation, which in turn have been compared to standalone devices with vertebral body screws.[26,27] In my estimation, all these options are viable alternatives for fixation. The goal is to provide enough fixation for an interbody fusion to occur. The question becomes the timing. Over the years, I have evolved from percutaneous posterior pedicle screws (which require an inordinate amount of fluoroscopy in addition to the fluoroscopy used for the transpsoas placement of the interbody) to side plates to dabbling with standalone devices before simply just deferring instrumentation of the spine for a later time. Especially in the management of adjacent segment degeneration, where there resides a sizeable construct below the affected level, the intervention has the potential to be quite extensive. The current body of literature is building a case for a standalone option, but the answer to that question is far from settled.[10,11,12] The question for the need of additional instrumentation is one that may find a definitive answer in the years to come. However, in those patients with a positive sagittal balance, immediate posterior support may be essential to prevent further kyphosis.

6.23 Case Illustrations

In my current practice, I find the transpsoas interbody fusion technique ideal for the management of patients in one of three categories: isolated disc degeneration in the upper lumbar spine; adjacent segment degeneration at L1–2, L2–3 or L3–4 with a two- or three-level construct below; or degenerative deformity where the transpsoas interbody approach is part of a larger strategy. I have included a case illustration on each below.

6.23.1 Case Illustration 1: Single-Level L2–3 Degenerative Disc Disease

Clinical History

A 44-year-old police officer with a work-related trauma to the lumbar spine 7 years prior presented with progressively worsening of axial back pain, right hip pain and gluteal pain refractory to nonoperative measures. He reported a visual analog scale (VAS; back) of 77 mm, VAS (leg) of 57 mm and an Oswestry Disability Index (ODI) of 44. Symptoms reached a level where he was unable to remain on full-duty, limiting his capacity to advance in his profession. At the time of presentation to my clinic, the patient had already been scheduled for an L5–S1 anterior lumbar interbody fusion by another provider.

Neurologic Examination

Motor examination by confrontation demonstrated 4/5 in the right quadriceps; 5/5 in the left quadriceps; and 5/5 in the tibialis anterior, gastrocnemius and extensor hallucis longus muscle bilaterally. The patient demonstrated intact patellar and Achilles reflexes bilaterally. No sensory abnormalities were identified on pinprick or light touch.

Radiographic Data

Standing AP and lateral radiographs demonstrated advanced degeneration at L5–S1 with a vacuum disc phenomenon evident on the standing lateral radiograph. The patient also had a coronal imbalance at L2–3 off to the right and focal degeneration at the L2–3 segment (▶ Fig. 6.37). MRI confirmed the degeneration at L5–S1 with Modic changes on the inferior aspect of L5 and the superior aspect of S1 as well as the degeneration at L2–3 with foraminal compromise of the exiting nerve root of L2 (▶ Fig. 6.38). Given the degenerative pattern at both L2–3 and L5–S1, a computed tomography (CT) spectroscopy was obtained to add further clarity regarding the impact that the degeneration of each segment was contributing to the patient's symptoms (▶ Fig. 6.38).

Rationale for Transpsoas Approach at L2–3

In this case, the radiographic data raise concern for both L5–S1 and L2–3 levels as the cause of symptoms. It would be difficult to categorically dismiss some contribution of discomfort from each one of these segments. The CT spectroscopy distinguishes the L2–3 level from the L5–S1 level with regard to osteoblastic activity. A selective nerve root block at L2 offered the patient symptomatic but only temporary relief. That shifted the focus of my attention to the L2–3 level. The coronal imbalance, foraminal compromise without significant central stenosis and instability in a level of the upper lumbar spine led to the logical conclusion that a transpsoas approach would be the best surgical option that would offer a minimally invasive solution for the anatomical circumstance of two nonadjacent lumbosacral levels with advanced degeneration.

Operative Management

After the patient underwent a confirmatory L2 selective nerve root block with a temporary improvement of his radicular symptoms, a left-sided L2–3 transpsoas standalone approach was performed (▶ Fig. 6.39), with the possibility of posterior stabilization in the weeks or months to come discussed with

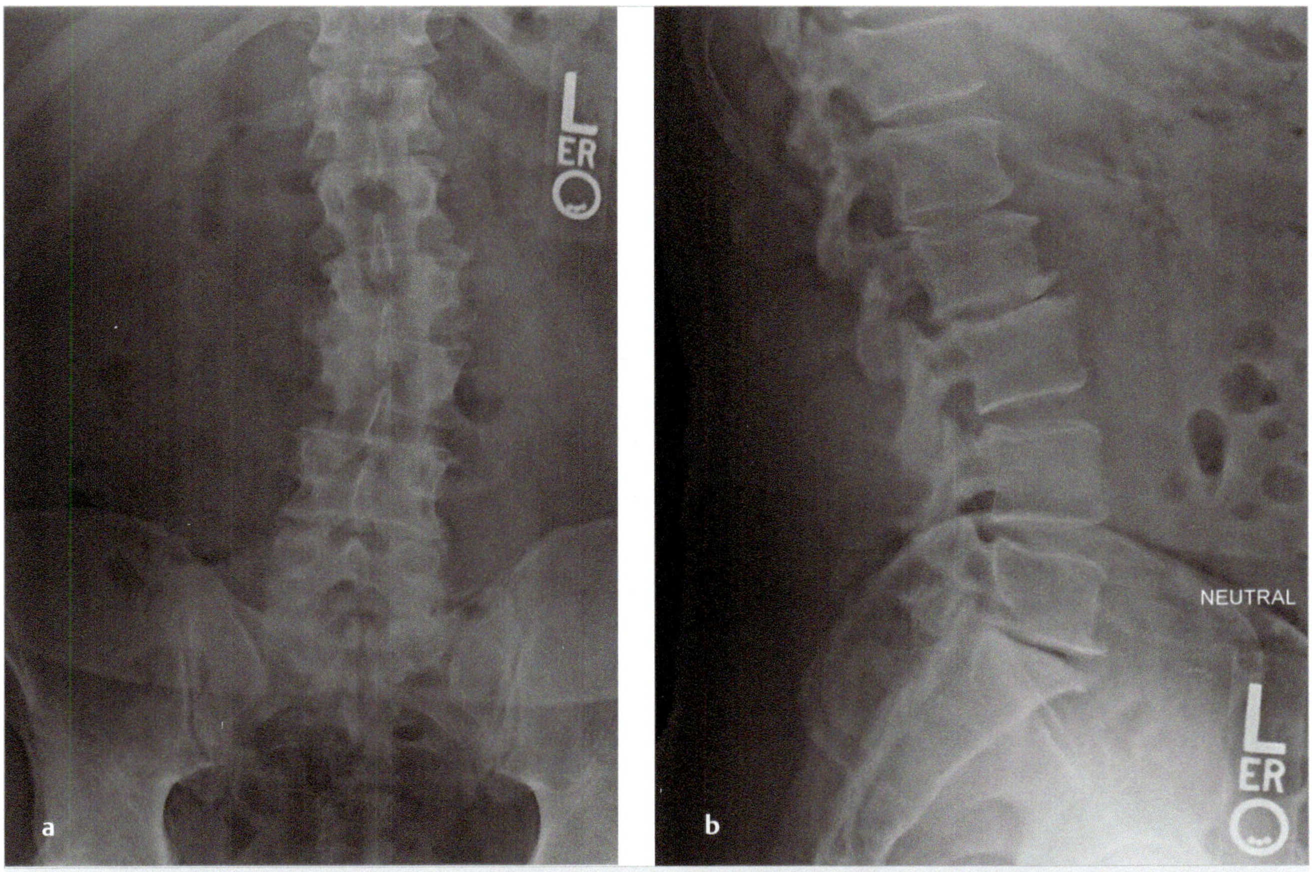

Fig. 6.37 Standing (a) anteroposterior and (b) lateral radiographs demonstrating a focal coronal imbalance at L2–3 and degeneration at L5–S1. The patient had lost lordosis at L5–S1 secondary to advanced degeneration.

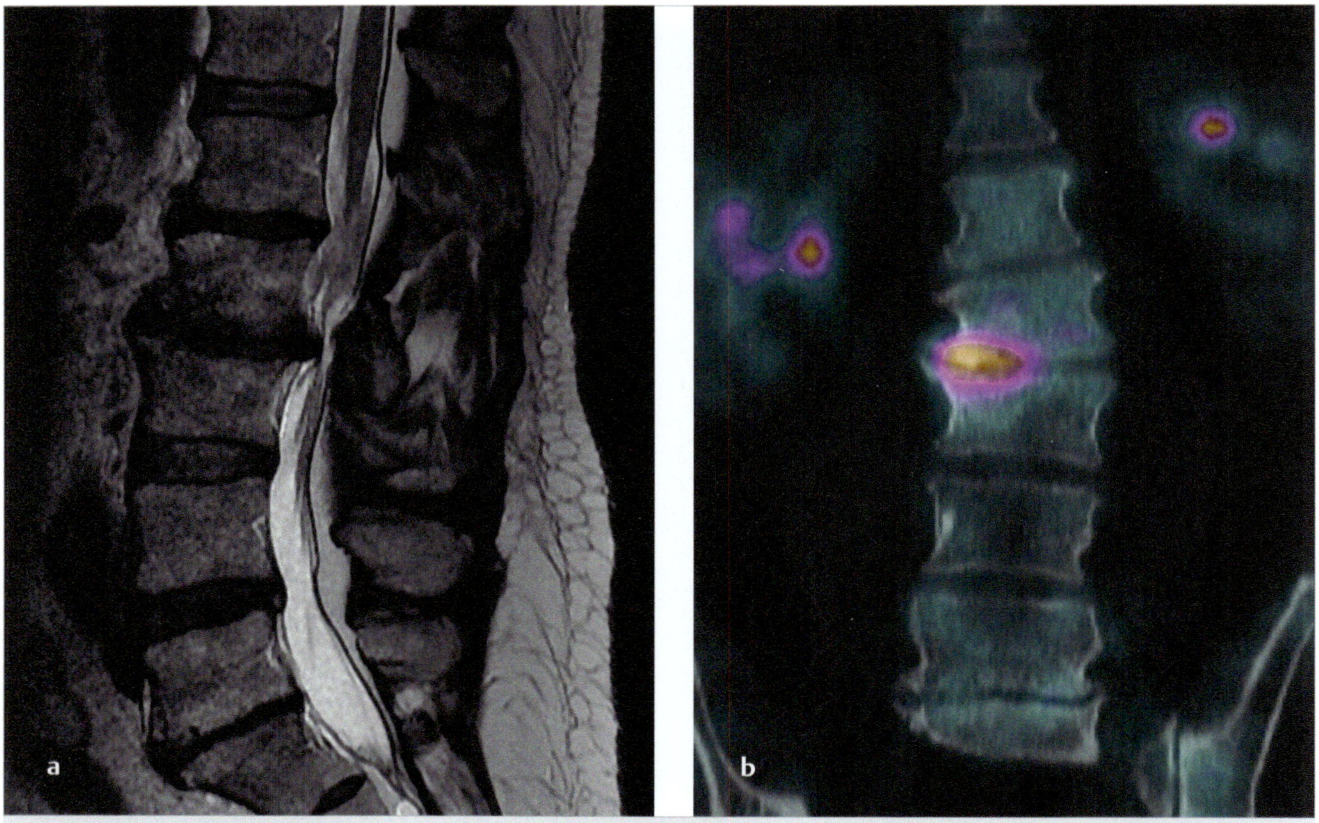

Fig. 6.38 Magnetic resonance imaging (MRI) and computed tomography (CT) spectroscopy in two nonadjacent segments of degeneration. **(a)** Sagittal T2-weighted MRI of the lumbar spine demonstrated coronal imbalance and foraminal compromise at L2–3. No significant stenosis at L5–S1. **(b)** CT spectroscopy demonstrates increased tracer activity in the lateral aspect of the L2–3 disc space without any activity at the L5–S1 segment.

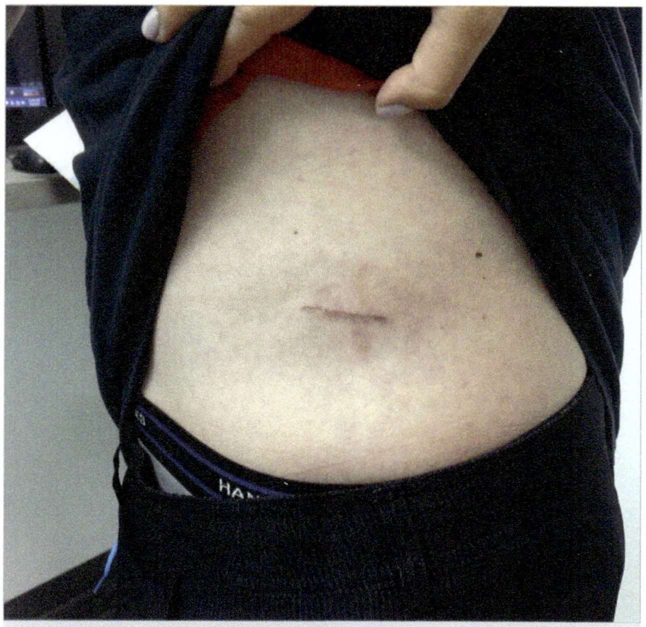

Fig. 6.39 Postoperative incision. Photograph of the incision of the patient in case illustration 1. A 30-mm incision provides more than adequate access to the requisite anatomical unit. The abdomen is examined for any signs of abdominal wall weakness using a Valsalva maneuver.

the patient depending on the radiographic progression toward fusion. The patient was discharged after an uneventful 23-hour stay with immediate improvement of his right radicular symptoms but some left anterior thigh discomfort. Thirty days after the surgery, the patient reported complete resolution of his radicular leg pain, resolution of his left thigh numbness and a significant difference in his axial back pain. His incision was well healed without evidence of abdominal wall weakness (▶ Fig. 6.40).

The patient returned to light-duty work 1 month after surgery. By the sixth postoperative month, the patient demonstrated radiographic fusion on lateral radiographs without evidence of subsidence and returned to unrestricted full duty as a police officer without the need for additional stabilization (▶ Fig. 6.40). At 6 months, his postoperative VAS (back) was 12 mm, the VAS (leg) was 8 mm and the ODI was 14.

6.23.2 Case Illustration 2: Adjacent Segment Degeneration

Clinical History

A 64-year-old attorney presented 16 years after undergoing an instrumented decompression and fusion at L4–5. The patient reported progressively worsening axial back pain and left radicular leg pain. As a litigator, he needed to be able to stand 20 to 30 minutes at a time, but the left radicular leg pain limited his ability to stand for more than 10 minutes, at which point he

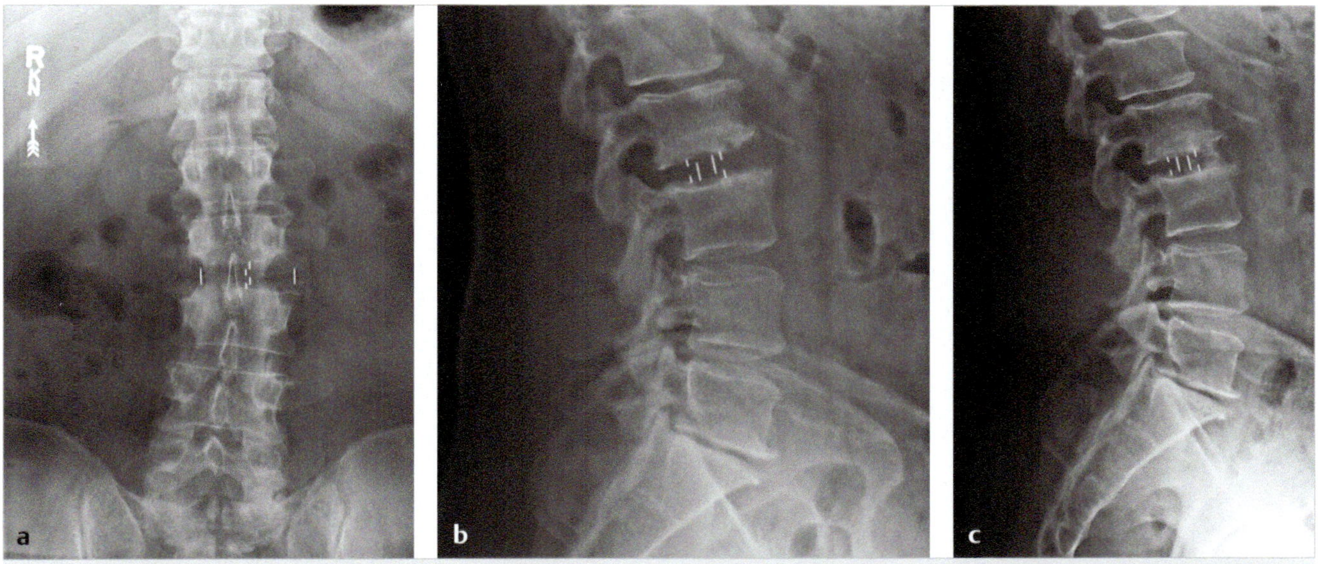

Fig. 6.40 Postoperative standing radiographs. (a) Anteroposterior image demonstrating the interbody in position and partial correction of the coronal imbalance. (b) Lateral radiograph at 30 days without any evidence of bone formation and at (c) 6 months demonstrating the development of a radiographic union without evidence of subsidence. Note: bridging bone can be seen mostly in front of the interbody spacer.

would need to sit and lean forward to alleviate his symptoms. He reported a VAS (back) of 64 mm, VAS (leg) of 78 mm and ODI of 48.

Neurologic Examination

Motor examination by confrontation demonstrated 4/5 in the left quadriceps; 5/5 in the right quadriceps; and 5/5 in the tibialis anterior, gastrocnemius and extensor hallucis longus muscle bilaterally. There was an absent patellar on the left, 2 + patellar reflex on the right and 2 + Achilles reflexes bilaterally. The patient demonstrated nondermatomal sensory loss in the lower extremities bilaterally.

Radiographic Studies

Standing AP and lateral radiographs demonstrate an L4–5 interbody fusion (▶ Fig. 6.41). Evident on both the AP and the lateral radiographs is the degree of disc collapse and foraminal narrowing secondary to the formation of a disc osteophyte complex. MRI confirmed the degree of the degeneration of the L3–4 level, and the parasagittal images confirmed the foraminal compromise of L3 on the left side (▶ Fig. 6.42). CT spectroscopy demonstrated increased tracer activity on the left side of the disc space at L3–4 (▶ Fig. 6.43).

Rationale for Transpsoas Approach at L3–4

I typically reserve a transpsoas interbody approach in adjacent segment degeneration for those circumstances where a multilevel construct resides below the affected segment. For single-level constructs, I typically explant the existing construct through a paramedian minimally invasive approach and address the adjacent segment. However, in this circumstance, the archaic construct did not lend itself well to the trajectories provided by a minimally invasive approach for explantation. My options were for a midline exposure for explantation of the construct and management of the adjacent or indirect decompression with a transpsoas approach, with the possibility of supplemental posterior fixation.

Operative Management

The patient underwent a left-sided transpsoas approach to the L3–4 level. A standalone interbody was placed, and the patient was discharged after an uneventful 23-hour stay (▶ Fig. 6.44). Immediately after surgery, the patient reported the ability to stand for long periods without left radicular symptoms. At 1 month, the patient had returned to his work as a litigator with only minimal symptoms and, at 6 months, was not limited in his ability to stand. The patient reported a 6-month postoperative VAS (back) of 22 mm, VAS (leg) of 11 mm and ODI of 21. Consistent with the reports in the literature, no further stabilization was needed.[10,11,12]

6.23.3 Case Illustration 3: Multiple Levels of Degeneration in the Context of Deformity

Clinical History

A 76-year-old woman presented with incapacitating axial back pain and right greater than left radicular leg pain covering multiple dermatomes in distribution. The patient had past surgical history significant for multiple minimally invasive decompressions (L2–3, L3–4 and L4–5) that were performed at an outside facility over the span of the last 10 years. Over the past year, the patient experienced a progressive decline in her functional mobility. She was dependent on a walker for short distances

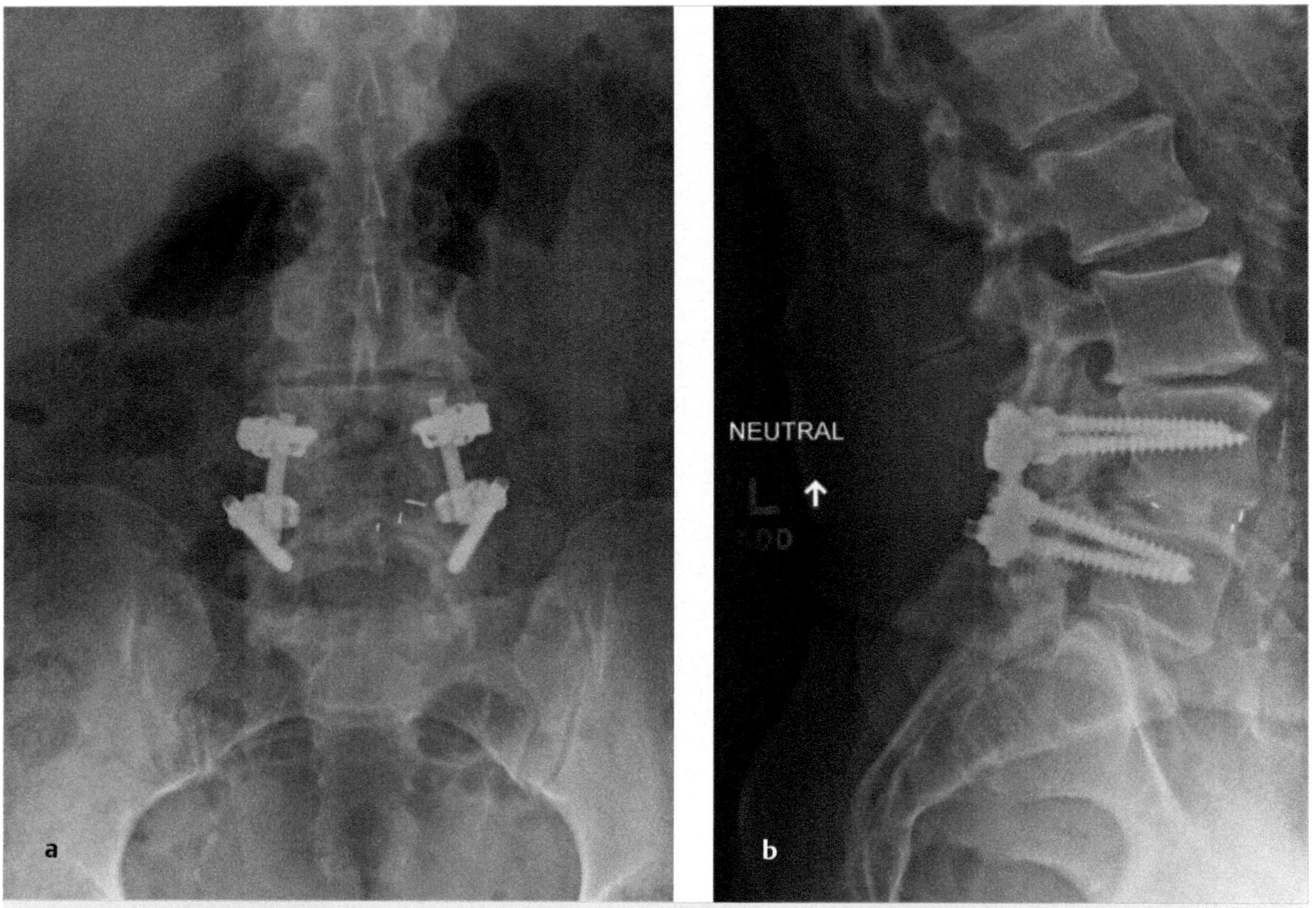

Fig. 6.41 Adjacent segment degeneration at L3–4, 16 years after lumbar fusion. (a) Standing radiograph demonstrating an instrumented lumbar fusion with interbody fusion at L4–5 and advanced degeneration of the L3–4 level. (b) Standing neutral lateral radiograph demonstrating the degree of collapse resulting in foraminal narrowing.

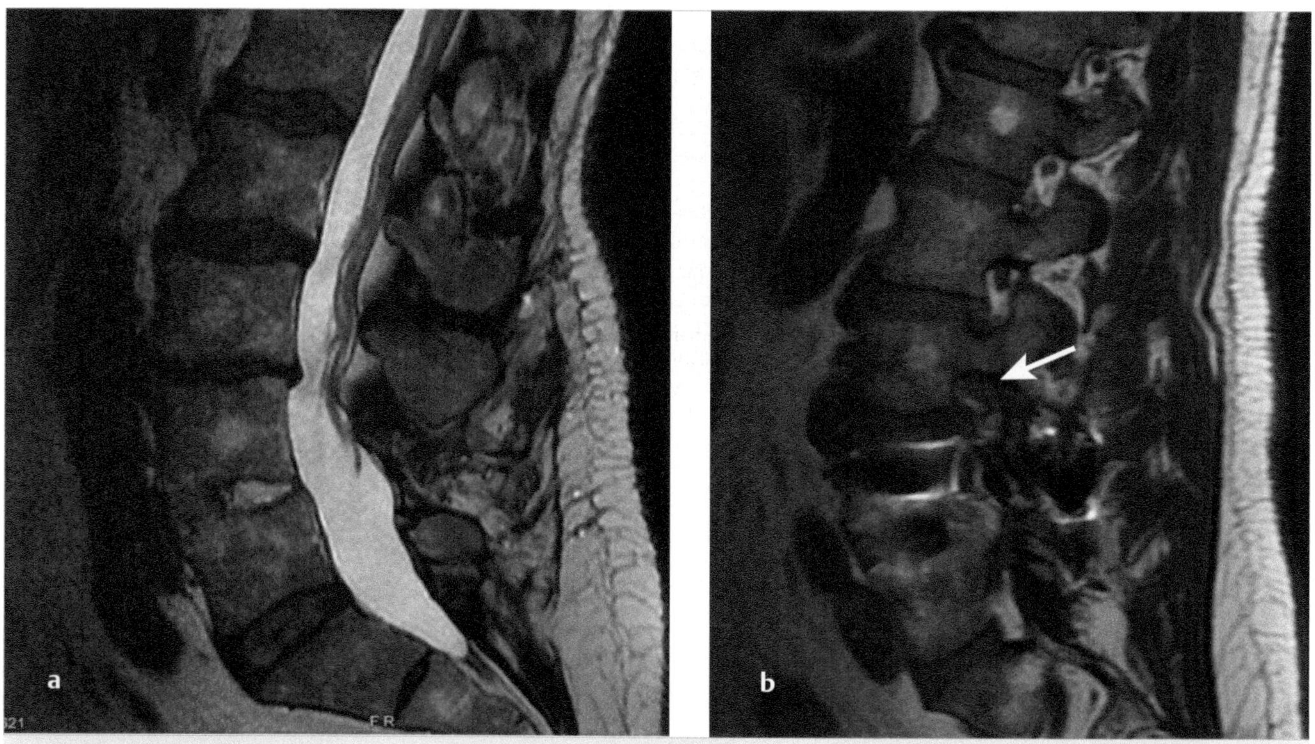

Fig. 6.42 Adjacent segment degeneration at L3–4, 16 years after lumbar fusion. (a) Sagittal T2-weighted magnetic resonance imaging (MRI) demonstrating adjacent segment degeneration at L3–4 without significant foraminal compromise. (b) Parasagittal T1-weighted MRI demonstrating foraminal compromise at L3 on the left (*arrow*).

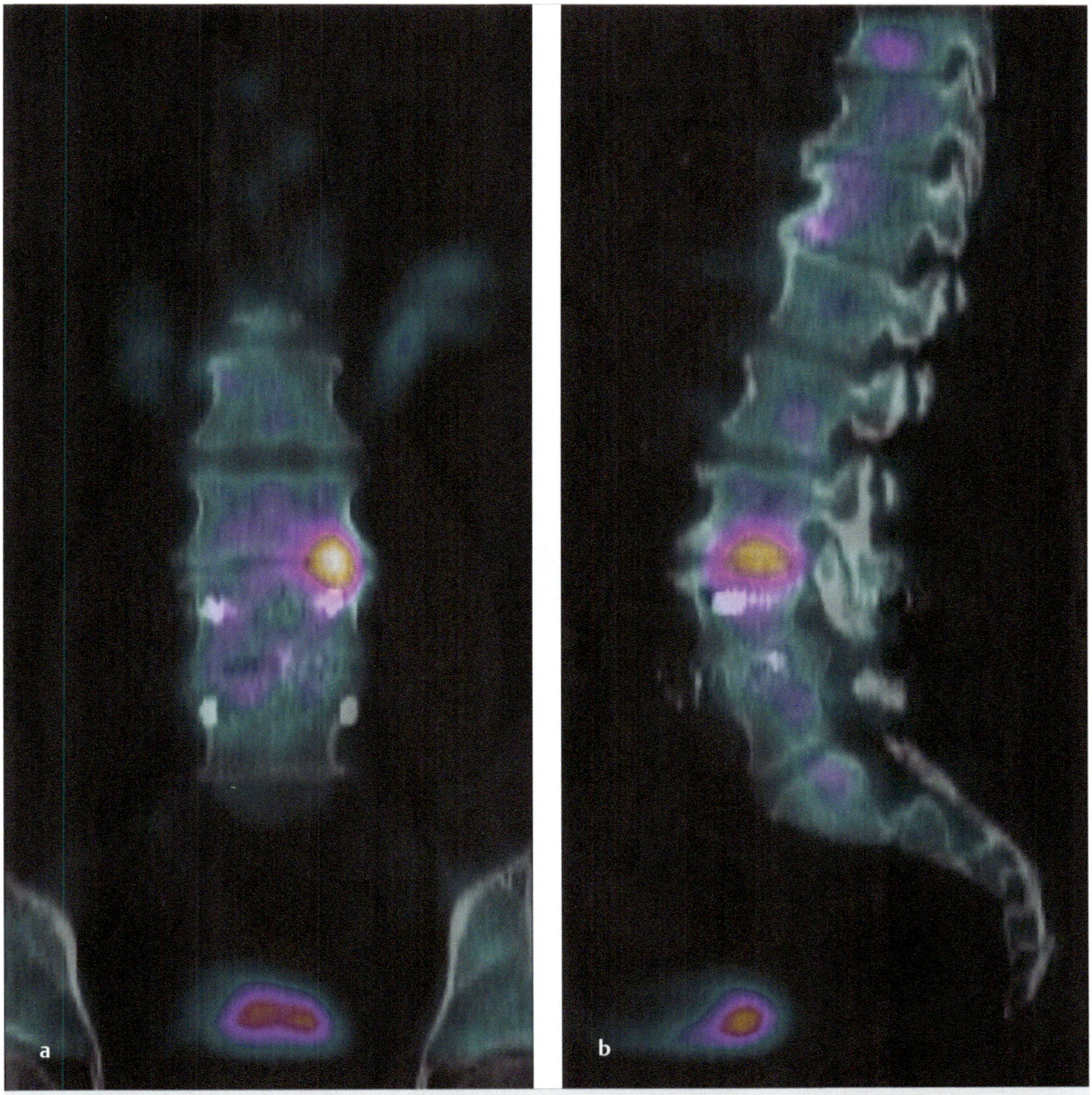

Fig. 6.43 Computed tomography (CT) spectroscopy in adjacent segment degeneration. **(a)** Coronal and **(b)** sagittal reconstruction of the CT spectroscopy that demonstrates increased tracer activity in the left lateral aspect of the L3–4 disc space.

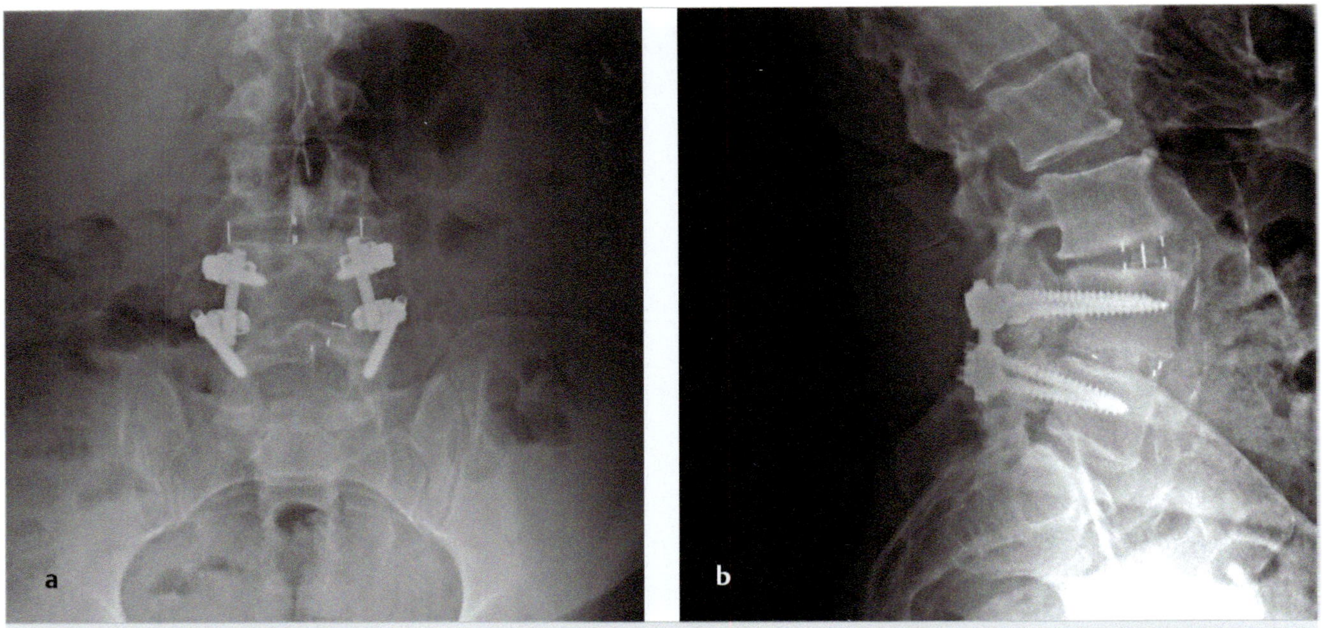

Fig. 6.44 Transpsoas management of adjacent segment degeneration. (a) Anteroposterior standing radiograph demonstrating a standalone interbody spacer in position. (b) Lateral standing neutral radiograph demonstrating the restoration of disc height, segmental lordosis and maturing interbody fusion within the interbody spacer.

and a wheelchair for distances greater than 100 feet. The patient had a preoperative ODI of 72, VAS for back pain of 80 mm and VAS for leg pain of 80 mm.

Neurologic Examination

The patient was areflexic in the patellar and Achilles tendons bilaterally. She was profoundly deconditioned, demonstrating only 4-/5 strength in the muscle groups of the lower extremities. She had a decrease in pinprick and light touch that covered multiple dermatomes of the lower extremities.

Radiographic Studies

AP standing radiographs demonstrated a Cobb angle of 24 degrees, multiple levels of coronal imbalance and a progressive lateral listhesis. Lateral standing neutral radiographs demonstrated a grade I spondylolisthesis at L2–3 and an iatrogenic flat back deformity from L3 to L5. Spinopelvic parameters were as follows: pelvic incidence, 53 degrees; pelvic tilt, 25 degrees; lumbar lordosis, -31 degrees; and pelvic incidence of lumbar lordosis, 22 degrees (▶ Fig. 6.45).

Rationale for the Transpsoas Approach as Part of the Operative Strategy

The patient and her husband were specifically requesting yet another minimally invasive operation for the management of her symptoms out of the concern that she was too advanced in years and too deconditioned for a larger operation. However, in this case, there was no single level or even two levels that if targeted with a minimally invasive technique would accomplish all the objectives of meaningful surgical intervention. I reminded the patient that if she felt she was too old for the right operation, then she was far too old for the wrong one. The patient needed correction of the spondylolisthesis at L2–3, the lateral listhesis at L3–4, the flat back deformity from L3 to L5 and the Cobb angle of 24 degrees. Transpsoas interbody approaches would play a role, but only as part of a larger strategy to accomplish all the surgical objectives in the correction of the deformity.

Operative Management

In the lateral position, the patient underwent placement of interbody spacers using the transpsoas approach at L2–3 and L3–4. The patient was then positioned prone for pedicle screw instrumentation from L1 to L5, Smith–Petersen osteotomies at L2–3, L3–4 and L4–5 with a transforaminal approach using the nested interbody technique at L4–5 (▶ Fig. 6.46). The patient was discharged to a rehab facility after 3 days, ambulating with a walker. At 1 month, the patient was ambulating with the assistance of a cane and ambulating independently at 6 months. Postoperatively, the VAS for leg pain was 24 mm, the VAS for back pain was 34 mm and the ODI was 22 at 6 months.

6.24 Complication Avoidance

The complication profile for the transpsoas interbody approach to the lumbar spine is distinct from any other procedure thus far presented in this Primer. As such, there has been an emphasis throughout the technique sections in this chapter already on how to avoid complications at the various phases of the operation. I cannot emphasize enough that in this operation, complication avoidance begins at the time of patient positioning, and

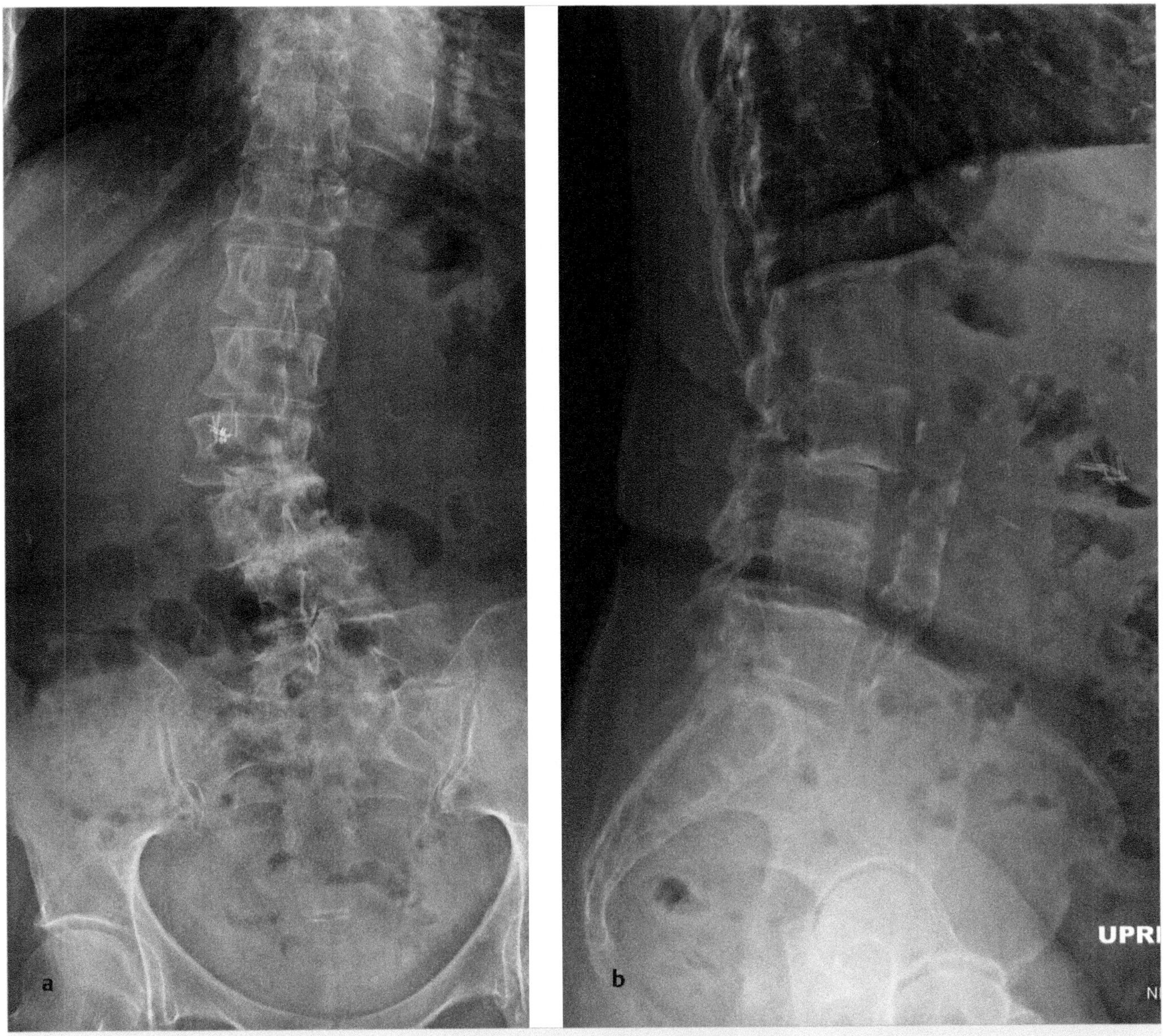

Fig. 6.45 Degenerative scoliosis, iatrogenic flat back deformity and spondylolisthesis. **(a)** Anteroposterior standing radiograph demonstrating a Cobb angle of 24 degrees. A lateral listhesis of L3 on L4 and multiple levels of coronal imbalance. **(b)** Lateral standing radiograph demonstrating an L2–3 spondylolisthesis, multiple levels of the degenerative disc disease, loss of lumbar lordosis and a positive sagittal vertical axis. Spinopelvic parameters were pelvic incidence: 53 degrees, pelvic tilt: 25 degrees, lumbar lordosis: −31 degrees, and pelvic incidence–lumbar lordosis: 22 degrees.

the recognition of complications continues well into the postoperative period. Traversing the abdominal wall alone has the potential to cause complications that may not surface for weeks, if not months.[28,29] Navigating through the psoas muscle and into the disc space may lead to neuropraxia of sensory roots, which goes undetected by free-running EMG. Although the knowledge of the lumbar plexus and its branches is the essential foundation for complication avoidance, that anatomical understanding needs to be placed within the framework of the procedure itself at the various time points before, during and after the procedure to avoid complications. The most important aspect of complication management for postoperative patients who have undergone the transpsoas approach is recognizing the complication itself, explaining its origins to the patient and deciding whether further intervention or evaluation is necessary. Fortunately, the vast majority of complications are self-limiting and improve with nothing more than the tincture of time. Nevertheless, educating the patient regarding the symptoms that they are experiencing and the likelihood that those symptoms will resolve has a psychological value without

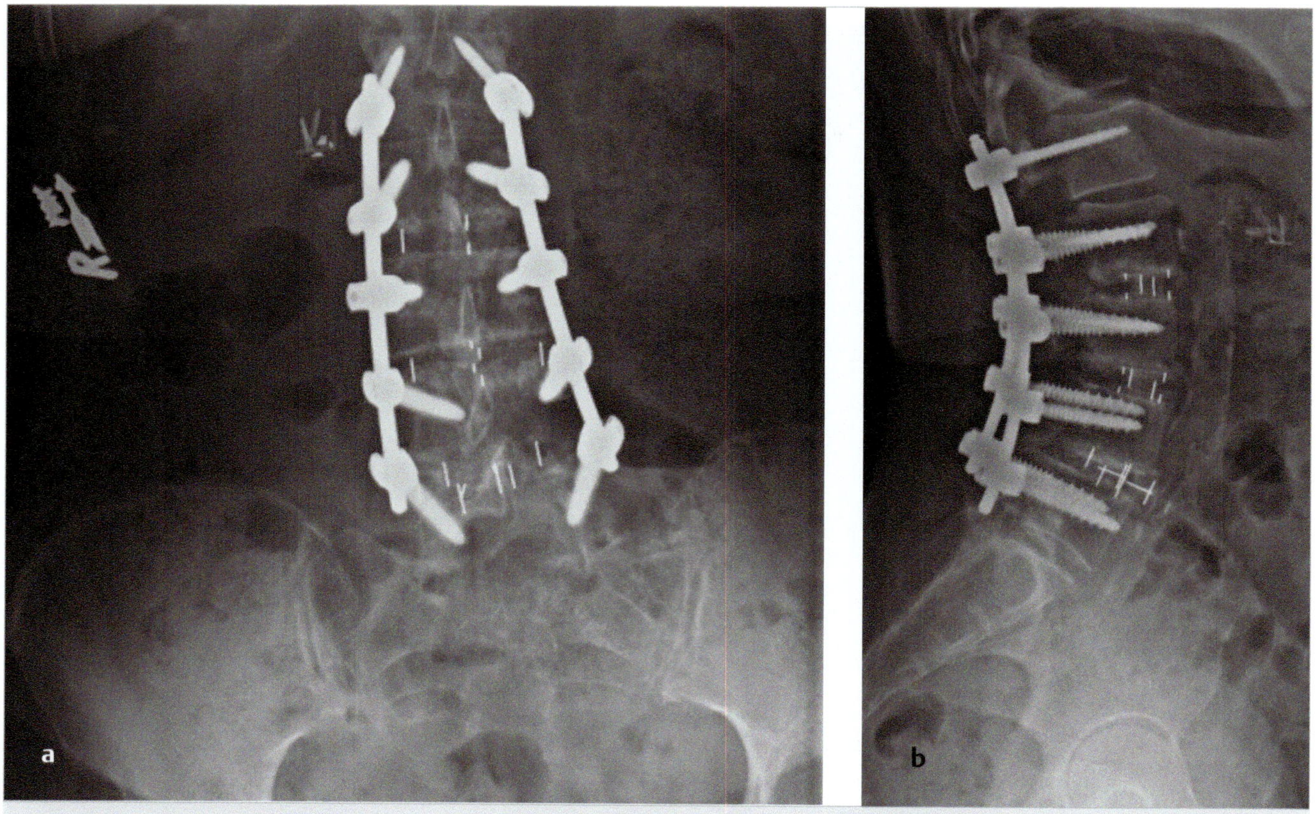

Fig. 6.46 Postoperative radiographs at 6 months after L2–3, L3–4 transpsoas interbody placement with correction of lateral listhesis at L3–4 as seen on **(a)** the anteroposterior radiograph and correction of the spondylolisthesis at L2–3 with the restoration of the lumbar lordosis and sagittal vertical axis as seen on **(b)** the standing neutral lateral radiograph. Bridging bone may be seen within the interbody spacers.

measure for the patient. ▶ Table 6.1 provides the most comprehensive list of complications and their incidence that is available in the literature at this writing.[30]

6.24.1 Complication Case Illustration

The area of greatest controversy is defining the immediate need for posterior stabilization. There is a growing body of literature defining that timing and the need for that intervention. Several of the cases that I have presented in this chapter demonstrate a standalone technique. In the setting of adjacent segment degeneration where there is a sizable construct below the affected segment, the transpsoas interbody fusion offers the most elegant, minimally invasive solution with a standalone interbody spacer. However, instability, a positive sagittal vertical axis or a spondylolisthesis make such a patient a suboptimal candidate for such an approach. The following case illustration demonstrates such an example.

A 46-year-old woman had undergone an L3–4 and L4–5 transforaminal lumbar interbody fusion for the management of advanced degenerative disc disease with a severe coronal imbalance. Five years later, the patient presented with worsening axial back pain and radiculopathy. Radiographic workup demonstrated adjacent segment degeneration at L2–3 (▶ Fig. 6.47). The patient had a grade I spondylolisthesis and instability confirmed by flexion-extension radiographs. She underwent an uncomplicated L2–3 transpsoas approach and had a near-complete resolution of her symptoms (▶ Fig. 6.48).

The patient had been staged for posterior stabilization in the coming weeks, but given her clinical response to the operation, she canceled the posterior instrumentation. At the 3-month mark, the patient's clinical condition deteriorated. She reported increasing back pain and the return of bilateral radicular symptoms. Radiographs demonstrated further slip of the L2 vertebral body relative to L3. The patient then underwent posterior fixation with reduction of the listhesis at the 4-month mark and

Table 6.1 Complication rates from a systematic review and meta-analysis reported by Walker et al[30] on the transpsoas interbody approach

Complication	Transpsoas studies ($n = 39$)			
	No. of events	Total no. of patients	Incidence, % (95% CI)	*P* value
Transient thigh or groin numbness/pain	680	2,352	21.7 (17.2–27.0)	**0.002**
Transient hip flexor weakness	262	1,295	19.7 (14.6–26.0)	**0.001**
Permanent motor neurologic deficit (permanent neurologic weakness)	43	2,842	2.8 (1.9–4.0)	**0.005**
Sympathetic plexus injury	0	641	0.0 (0.0–3.2)	**0.03**
Major vascular injury	5	2,709	0.4 (0.2–1.0)	**0.01**
Peritoneal (bowel) injury	3	1,655	1.3 (0.5–3.8)	0.64
Urologic injury (kidney, ureter)	0	1,655	0.0 (0.0–0.9)	0.05
Postop ileus	15	1,199	2.8 (1.3–5.9)	0.79
Infection	13	1,807	3.1 (1.9–5.1)	**0.01**
Hematoma (psoas, subcutaneous)	5	1,196	1.7 (0.7–3.9)	0.13
Subsidence	201	761 (1,537[a])	13.8 (9.4–19.7)	0.78
Pseudarthrosis	103	796 (1,275[a])	7.5 (4.9–11.4)	0.57

Note: Boldface indicates statistical significance.
[a]Number of levels evaluated.

eventually returned to the clinical status she achieved after the initial transpsoas approach (▶ Fig. 6.49).

I have included this case illustration to demonstrate the potential vulnerability of a standalone construct. The reality is that the final radiographic outcome with posterior stabilization is inferior to the immediate radiographic outcome of the transpsoas approach. In the final analysis, this circumstance would have been ideally suited for immediate posterior stabilization. In a meta-analysis of the existing literature on standalone transpsoas interbody arthrodesis, Alvi et al[31] found that immediate posterior instrumentation was associated with decreased reoperations, subsidence and cage migration. The results of that meta-analysis need to be balanced with a growing body of literature identifying successful management of adjacent segment degeneration with standalone constructs.[10,11,12] In the future, artificial intelligence and machine learning will identify the best course of action in these patients using larger radiographic datasets. For the time being, close radiographic and clinical follow-up is needed in those patients selected for a standalone construct.

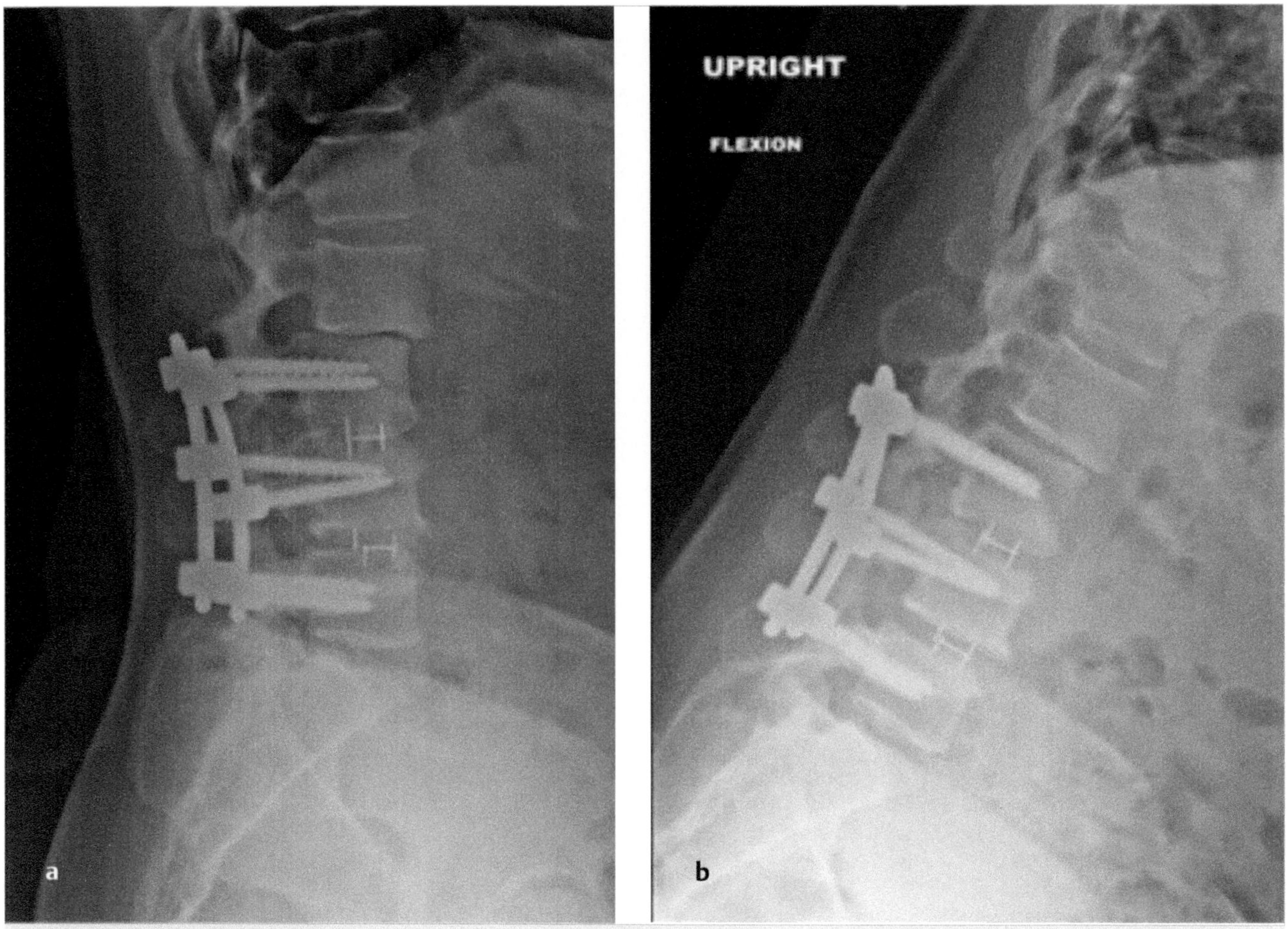

Fig. 6.47 Adjacent segment degeneration at L2–3 with instability 5 years after L3–4 and L4–5 instrumented lumbar interbody fusions. **(a)** Neutral standing lateral radiograph demonstrating a spondylolisthesis at L2–3 with a complete collapse of the disc space. **(b)** Flexion standing lateral radiograph demonstrating instability at the segment.

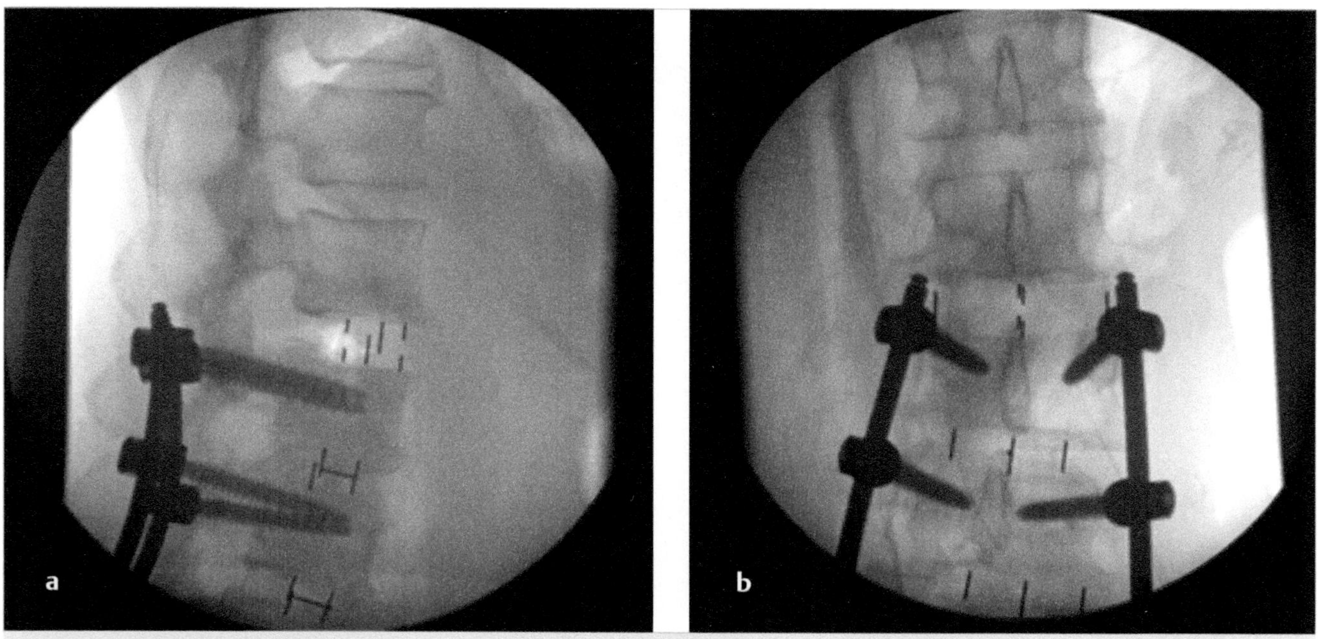

Fig. 6.48 Intraoperative fluoroscopic images of L2–3 transpsoas interbody fusion. **(a)** Vertical (lateral) fluoroscopic image demonstrating reduction of the spondylolisthesis at L2–3 and complete restoration of the disc height. **(b)** Horizontal (anteroposterior) fluoroscopic image again demonstrating restoration of disc height and interbody spacer spanning the entire disc space.

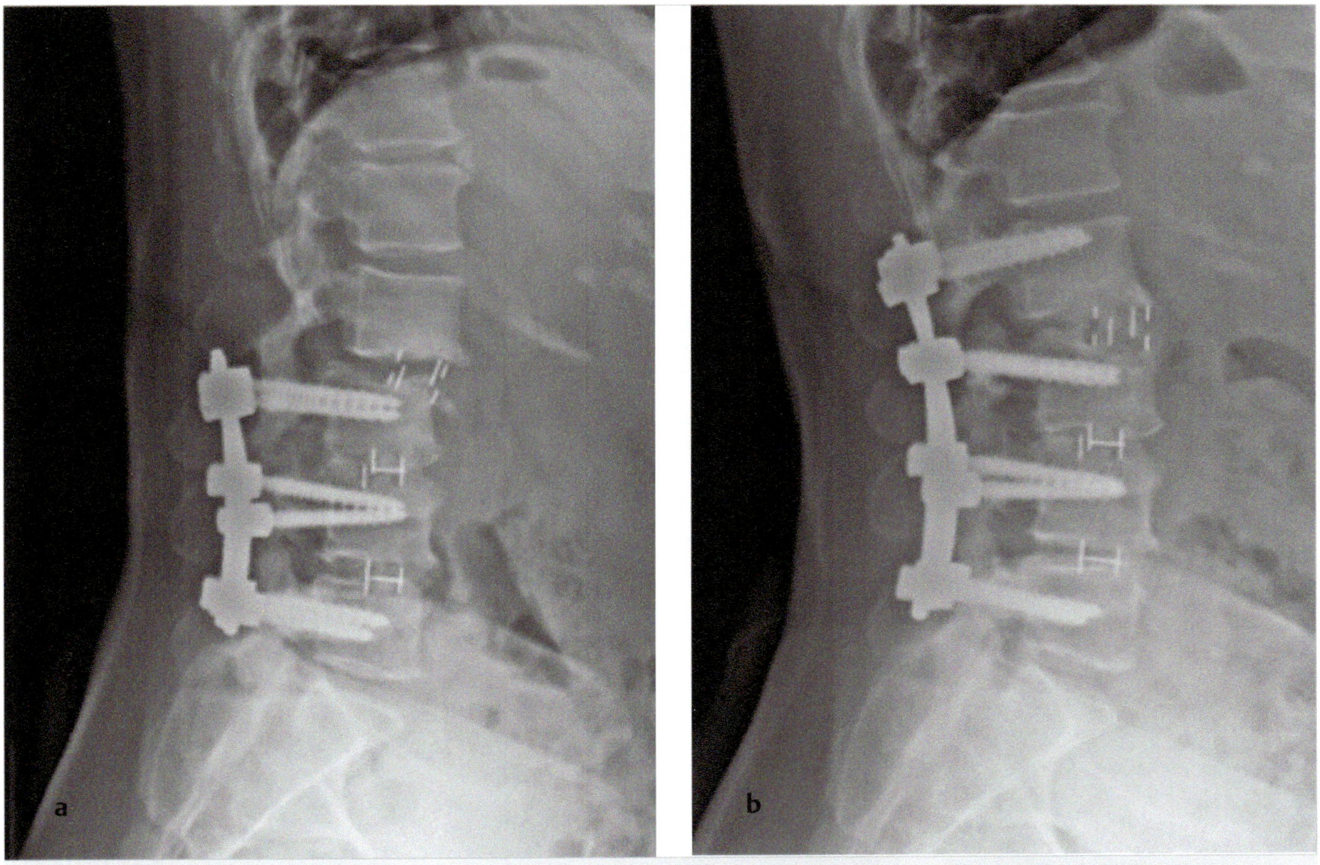

Fig. 6.49 Subsidence of the interbody and loss of reduction of the spondylolisthesis. **(a)** Lateral neutral radiograph demonstrating loss of the correction and progressive slip of L2 on L3. **(b)** Standing neutral radiograph at 4 months after the extension of the posterior instrumentation to L2 to reduce the recurring L2–3 listhesis. Bridging bone is seen within the interbody. Given the radiographic progression of subsidence, this patient would have been ideally managed with immediate posterior instrumentation after transpsoas placement of the interbody spacer.

6.25 Conclusion

The transpsoas interbody approach to the lumbar spine is one of those seismic shifts that occur in a field after the culmination of experience in current techniques leaves clinicians wanting and innovators searching. The preliminary experience with open thoracolumbar approaches offered surgeons a foothold for the development of this transpsoas approach. Within the last decade, a transformation in spine surgery has occurred with the transpsoas approach becoming commonplace in operating rooms across the country. The mechanical and physiological advantages of this approach are many. The very nature of this approach allows for access across the entire disc space from apophyseal ring to apophyseal ring. Comprehensive preparation of the disc space with the removal of the cartilaginous end plate is more readily achievable from a lateral approach than from a posterior one. The coverage of the interbody space by the interbody implant is unparalleled, along with the capacity to restore disc height, foraminal height and coronal balance. All these advantages need to be carefully weighed against the risk of injury to lumbar plexus and its branches. Injury to the genitofemoral nerve can cause significant discomfort to the patient, while injury to the femoral nerve may be catastrophic to functional mobility. The risk of these injuries correlates with the level approached and the experience of the surgeon. At the time of this writing, a pre-psoas technique has entered the surgical arena and has rapidly become the preferred technique at L4–5. Such an approach virtually eliminates the risk to the lumbar plexus and its branches by entering the disc space through a corridor anterior to the psoas. But shifting the working corridor introduces the possibility of a whole new array of complications. And so, the advantages of a pre-psoas technique have to be balanced with increased risk to the vascular tree, sympathetic plexus injury and even urologic complications, in particular, injury to the ureter.[30]

The pre-psoas approach may be a technique described in a future edition of this book. Currently, the limited experience reported in the literature and particularly by the author precludes a chapter on this topic at this writing.

The first six chapters of this Primer have focused exclusively on minimally invasive techniques in the lumbar spine. The next section shifts focus to the cervical spine and explores the application of minimally invasive techniques for the management of cervical radiculopathy, stenosis and spondylosis. The concept of the ratio of the surgical target to the surgical exposure (the Caspar ratio) is a recurring theme in this Primer, along with an emphasis on the anthropometric measurements of the cervical spine that allows for the reconstruction of the anatomy at depth in your mind's eye. You will find that the minimally invasive perspective will allow you to see more through a 14-mm access port placed on the paramedian cervical spine than most surgeons see through a generous midline exposure. All you have to do is turn the page.

References

[1] McAfee PC, Bohlman HH, Yuan HA. Anterior decompression of traumatic thoracolumbar fractures with incomplete neurological deficit using a retroperitoneal approach. J Bone Joint Surg Am. 1985; 67(1):89–104

[2] Mayer HM. A new microsurgical technique for minimally invasive anterior lumbar interbody fusion. Spine. 1997; 22(6):691–699, discussion 700

[3] McAfee PC, Regan JJ, Geis WP, Fedder IL. Minimally invasive anterior retroperitoneal approach to the lumbar spine. Emphasis on the lateral BAK. Spine. 1998; 23(13):1476–1484

[4] Bergey DL, Villavicencio AT, Goldstein T, Regan JJ. Endoscopic lateral transpsoas approach to the lumbar spine. Spine. 2004; 29(15):1681–1688

[5] Ozgur BM, Aryan HE, Pimenta L, Taylor WR. Extreme lateral interbody fusion (XLIF): a novel surgical technique for anterior lumbar interbody fusion. Spine J. 2006; 6(4):435–443

[6] Lowe TG, Hashim S, Wilson LA, et al. A biomechanical study of regional endplate strength and cage morphology as it relates to structural interbody support. Spine. 2004; 29(21):2389–2394

[7] Hartman C, Hemphill C, Godzik J, et al. Analysis of cost and 30-day outcomes in single-level transforaminal lumbar interbody fusion and less invasive, stand-alone lateral transpsoas interbody fusion. World Neurosurg. 2019; 122:e1037–e1040

[8] Dakwar E, Cardona RF, Smith DA, Uribe JS. Early outcomes and safety of the minimally invasive, lateral retroperitoneal transpsoas approach for adult degenerative scoliosis. Neurosurg Focus. 2010; 28(3):E8

[9] Dahdaleh NS, Smith ZA, Snyder LA, Graham RB, Fessler RG, Koski TR. Lateral transpsoas lumbar interbody fusion: outcomes and deformity correction. Neurosurg Clin N Am. 2014; 25(2):353–360

[10] Wang MY, Vasudevan R, Mindea SA. Minimally invasive lateral interbody fusion for the treatment of rostral adjacent-segment lumbar degenerative stenosis without supplemental pedicle screw fixation. J Neurosurg Spine. 2014; 21(6):861–866

[11] Louie PK, Varthi AG, Narain AS, et al. Stand-alone lateral lumbar interbody fusion for the treatment of symptomatic adjacent segment degeneration following previous lumbar fusion. Spine J. 2018; 18(11):2025–2032

[12] Palejwala SK, Sheen WA, Walter CM, Dunn JH, Baaj AA. Minimally invasive lateral transpsoas interbody fusion using a stand-alone construct for the treatment of adjacent segment disease of the lumbar spine: review of the literature and report of three cases. Clin Neurol Neurosurg. 2014; 124:90–96

[13] Januszewski J, Vivas AC, Bach K, Gandhi SV, Paluzzi J. Minimally invasive lateral transpsoas interbody fusion at the L4/5 level: a review of 61 consecutive cases. Oper Neurosurg (Hagerstown). 2018; 15(4):447–453

[14] Benglis DM, Vanni S, Levi AD. An anatomical study of the lumbosacral plexus as related to the minimally invasive transpsoas approach to the lumbar spine. J Neurosurg Spine. 2009; 10(2):139–144

[15] Uribe JS, Arredondo N, Dakwar E, Vale FL. Defining the safe working zones using the minimally invasive lateral retroperitoneal transpsoas approach: an anatomical study. J Neurosurg Spine. 2010; 13(2):260–266

[16] Banagan K, Gelb D, Poelstra K, Ludwig S. Anatomic mapping of lumbar nerve roots during a direct lateral transpsoas approach to the spine: a cadaveric study. Spine. 2011; 36(11):E687–E691

[17] Kepler CK, Bogner EA, Herzog RJ, Huang RC. Anatomy of the psoas muscle and lumbar plexus with respect to the surgical approach for lateral transpsoas interbody fusion. Eur Spine J. 2011; 20(4):550–556

[18] Davis TT, Bae HW, Mok JM, Rasouli A, Delamarter RB. Lumbar plexus anatomy within the psoas muscle: implications for the transpsoas lateral approach to the L4-L5 disc. J Bone Joint Surg Am. 2011; 93(16):1482–1487

[19] Dakwar E, Vale FL, Uribe JS. Trajectory of the main sensory and motor branches of the lumbar plexus outside the psoas muscle related to the lateral retroperitoneal transpsoas approach. J Neurosurg Spine. 2011; 14(2):290–295

[20] Mahan MA, Sanders LE, Guan J, Dailey AT, Taylor W, Morton DA. Anatomy of psoas muscle innervation: cadaveric study. Clin Anat. 2017; 30(4):479–486

[21] Le TV, Burkett CJ, Deukmedjian AR, Uribe JS. Postoperative lumbar plexus injury after lumbar retroperitoneal transpsoas minimally invasive lateral interbody fusion. Spine. 2013; 38(1):E13–E20

[22] Moro T, Kikuchi S, Konno S, Yaginuma H. An anatomic study of the lumbar plexus with respect to retroperitoneal endoscopic surgery. Spine. 2003; 28 (5):423–428, discussion 427–428

[23] Panjabi MM, Goel V, Oxland T, et al. Human lumbar vertebrae. Quantitative three-dimensional anatomy. Spine. 1992; 17(3):299-306

[24] Molinares DM, Davis TT, Fung DA, et al. Is the lateral jack-knife position responsible for cases of transient neurapraxia? J Neurosurg Spine. 2016; 24(1): 189–196

[25] Deukmedjian AR, Le TV, Dakwar E, Martinez CR, Uribe JS. Movement of abdominal structures on magnetic resonance imaging during positioning changes related to lateral lumbar spine surgery: a morphometric study: Clinical article. J Neurosurg Spine. 2012; 16(6):615–623

[26] Fogel GR, Parikh RD, Ryu SI, Turner AW. Biomechanics of lateral lumbar interbody fusion constructs with lateral and posterior plate fixation: laboratory investigation. J Neurosurg Spine. 2014; 20(3):291–297

[27] Nayak AN, Gutierrez S, Billys JB, Santoni BG, Castellvi AE. Biomechanics of lateral plate and pedicle screw constructs in lumbar spines instrumented at two levels with laterally placed interbody cages. Spine J. 2013; 13(10):1331–1338

[28] Vivas AC, Januszewski J, Hajirawala L, Paluzzi JM, Gandhi SV, Uribe JS. Incisional hernia after minimally invasive lateral retroperitoneal surgery: case series and review of the literature. Oper Neurosurg (Hagerstown). 2019; 16 (3):368–373

[29] Dakwar E, Le TV, Baaj AA, et al. Abdominal wall paresis as a complication of minimally invasive lateral transpsoas interbody fusion. Neurosurg Focus. 2011; 31(4):E18

[30] Walker CT, Farber SH, Cole TS, et al. Complications for minimally invasive lateral interbody arthrodesis: a systematic review and meta-analysis comparing prepsoas and transpsoas approaches. J Neurosurg Spine. 2019; 25:1–15

[31] Alvi MA, Alkhataybeh R, Wahood W, et al. The impact of adding posterior instrumentation to transpsoas lateral fusion: a systematic review and meta-analysis. J Neurosurg Spine. 2018; 30(2):211–221

7 Minimally Invasive Posterior Cervical Foraminotomy

Abstract
The posterior cervical foraminotomy builds on the minimally invasive skill set developed for the management of lumbar radiculopathies. Although several of the principles remain the same, it is important to note the differences. Given the complexity of the posterior cervical musculature, the process of dilatation onto the posterior cervical spine has its nuances. Furthermore, unlike the lumbar spine where retraction of the thecal sac may be safely performed to retrieve an extruded disc herniation that resides in the center of the canal, the work of decompression in the cervical spine is limited to the neural foramen and the lateral aspect of the canal. There can be no retraction of the cervical spinal cord to retrieve a midline disc herniation. This inability to retract the spinal cord limits the application of the posterior cervical foraminotomy to compressive pathologies of the cervical foramen. The current chapter reviews the anatomical basis for a minimally invasive posterior cervical foraminotomy before reviewing positioning, the operative technique and case illustrations describing the treatment of a variety of unilateral cervical radiculopathies. Equally important are the final case illustrations detailing the rationale *not* to apply the technique.

Keywords: cervical spine, decompression, discectomy, foraminotomy, herniation, radiculopathy, spinal cord, thecal sac

He who sees through an open window sees less than he who looks through a closed window.

Charles Baudelaire

7.1 Introduction

Throughout the span of my entire residency, I participated in a total of five posterior cervical foraminotomies. The anterior cervical discectomies and fusions that I assisted with or performed, on the other hand, were too many to count. All that would change within my first several weeks at the Naval Medical Center in San Diego where I landed immediately after I completed my residency. I was struck by how many patients were better candidates for a posterior cervical foraminotomy than an anterior cervical approach. Service member after service member presented to my clinic with a unilateral radiculopathy from a cervical disc herniation that was purely within the cervical foramen and nowhere near the spinal cord. Their only symptoms were due to compression of a single cervical nerve root. Although all these patients were candidates for anterior approaches, they all appeared to be even better candidates for a unilateral posterior cervical foraminotomy with discectomy.

A confounding factor that I had to consider in the decision for the surgical approach was the unique patient population with very specific needs. In contradistinction to the older patient population with multiple levels of degeneration seen during residency in Atlanta, the vast majority of my patients in the Navy were young and healthy, with a single symptomatic segment and high motivation to return to unrestricted duty in the military. Surgical approaches in the Navy had consequences regarding timely return to unrestricted duty. If a cervical fusion was recommended, in most cases the service member could not return to unrestricted duty until arthrodesis could be confirmed. Waiting for a radiographic fusion to occur in order to be able to return these service members to full duty did not seem like the best course of action. Furthermore, to take an entire healthy disc and fuse a segment for such a focal problem in a 20- or 30-year-old who presented with a unilateral radiculopathy from a lateral disc herniation without compression of the spinal cord and no significant spondylosis did not play to the strengths of the various surgical options available. Although arthroplasty was a wonderful alternative, I reserved that operation for more central disc herniations, which were out of the reach of the posterior cervical foraminotomy approach.

It became clear working with my colleagues that from a clinical, practical and military standpoint, a posterior cervical foraminotomy was the most logical path forward.[1] However, I had to balance this perspective with my ability to adequately perform the operation given my limited experience. In reality, at that time in my career, I felt more comfortable clipping a posterior communicating artery aneurysm than performing a posterior cervical foraminotomy, much less a minimally invasive one. I have discovered this to be a common theme in the residents and fellows with whom I now work. The posterior cervical foraminotomy is becoming a lost art. The anterior versus the posterior trend is certainly nothing new in the treatment of cervical disc disorders. As long ago as 1990, a concerned Francois Aldrich wrote, "This trend toward anterior discectomy for all types of cervical discs has tended to obscure the progressive development of the posterolateral approach to these lesions."[2]

Of course, there was a reason behind my dearth of experience with the posterior cervical foraminotomy and the decreasing frequency of that operation in clinical practice. The simple answer lay in the fact that the anterior approach is so well tolerated by patients in comparison to an open midline posterior cervical approach. The various things I remember about those five foraminotomies during my residency was the blood loss, the muscle dissection, the inability to see anything clearly and the degree of pain that patients experienced during the postoperative course. It was no wonder my mentors avoided that operation. As I look back at it now, it is a marvel that I saw as many as five of these procedures.

The rise of minimally invasive techniques in the lumbar spine introduced a potential equalizer in this cervical equation of posterior versus anterior. If these same techniques that limited the surgical exposure and thereby postoperative discomfort in the lumbar spine could be applied to the cervical spine, there was the potential for even greater benefit. The question of whether to address a nerve root compression syndrome from a posterior approach or anterior approach would become more balanced. The minimally invasive technique could single-handedly buck the trend of the decreasing application of posterior cervical foraminotomies identified by Aldrich.[2] All of a sudden, all that blood loss, poor visualization and postoperative pain could be replaced by a small incision, a focal area of exposure in a same-day outpatient operation with minimal discomfort for the patient.

A few short years after surgeons began wanding exposures in the lumbar spine with minimal access dilators for microdiscectomies and laminectomies, they ventured with them into the cervical spine. In 2000, Fessler and his colleagues[3] published a cadaveric feasibility study of a transmuscular approach using minimal access ports, effectively translating the techniques from the lumbar spine to the cervical spine. In reading Fessler's statements regarding hemostasis in the discussion of that manuscript, I found his concern to be quite prescient. In 2001, Adamson[4] published the first clinical series in the neurosurgical literature using a minimally invasive approach to access the posterior cervical foramen in 100 consecutive individuals. Perhaps the most important aspect of Adamson's publication[4] was the same-day discharge of 90 of the 100 patients. That data alone demonstrated that the putative benefits of the minimally invasive approach were, in fact, realized. Since Adamson's 2001 publication, the experience reported in the literature regarding the minimal access approach to the posterior cervical foramen has eclipsed that of its open counterpart.

Although some experts may argue that there is little difference between an open and a minimally invasive lumbar microdiscectomy, few would maintain that argument in the cervical spine, where the complex network of insertions in the posterior cervical musculature have to be detached for the exposure in an open approach. The differences between open and minimally invasive exposures for a foraminotomy in the cervical spine are oceans apart.

It was adopting minimally invasive techniques immediately after residency that allowed me to perform more posterior cervical foraminotomies within my first several months in practice as an attending neurosurgeon at the Naval Hospital in San Diego than I did in my entire residency. It is now an operation that I routinely perform several times a month on an outpatient basis. As always, it was the learning curve with the minimally invasive approach that I needed to tackle in order to fully embrace the technique. I emphasize that the minimally invasive posterior cervical foraminotomy is not the operation to begin your conversion to minimally invasive spine surgery. You will need expertise with the skill set that is built by performing the minimally invasive microdiscectomy and laminectomy in the lumbar spine. Comfort with the minimally invasive attachments to the drill and the bayoneted instruments through a minimal access port is imperative since the diameter of the minimal access port with this procedure is even smaller.

Once you have developed a facility with minimally invasive surgery on the lumbar spine, you will be able to readily translate those skills to the posterior cervical foraminotomy, the gateway procedure to managing posterior cervical pathology minimally invasively. Handling the instruments through minimal access ports is only one element of the skill set. Minimally invasive approaches to the posterior cervical spine have their specific learning curve. The posterior cervical fascia is very different to traverse than the lumbar fascia. The posterior cervical muscular planes are more complex and not as distinct as with the lumbar musculature. Docking onto the lamina in the cervical spine is a different experience for the surgeon than docking onto the lumbar lamina. There is something about the cervical spinal cord residing on the other side of the lamina that changes that experience. Although these skill sets are similar, there are nuances specific to the posterior cervical approach.

This chapter began with a quote from Charles Baudelaire who made the comment that individuals peering through an open window see less than individuals who peer through a closed window. Baudelaire's statement, which can be applied to the context of the minimally invasive posterior cervical foraminotomy, resonates with me. The minimal access port that I peer through on the cervical spine forces my mind to reconstruct the anatomy at depth. I have to see the pedicle, the superior articular process (SAP) and the cervical nerve root in my mind's eye before I ever make an incision. The very nature of the limited exposure mandates that I see more through a 14-mm diameter "closed window" than I would otherwise see through a midline "open window." Baudelaire may not have had minimally invasive spine surgery in mind when he wrote these words, but no statement better describes the workings of the minimally invasive mindset.

The goal of this chapter is to describe the anatomical basis, techniques and operative nuances of the minimally invasive posterior cervical foraminotomy. My hope is that you find a greater understanding of the cervical foramen through a limited diameter than you ever would have achieved through a traditional midline exposure. Mastery of this procedure will serve as a platform for the management of other posterior cervical pathologies covered in the next chapter. As always, understanding the anatomical basis for the approach and having at your fingertips the precise measurements serves as the foundation to increase the slope of your learning curve. Once you grasp the nuances of dilatation and exposure, it will be surprising to you how quickly the minimally invasive posterior cervical foraminotomy will become a valuable asset in your armamentarium. But first, given the remarkable and fascinating history of this procedure, it would be difficult not to highlight certain elements of its evolution.

7.2 Evolution of the Posterior Cervical Foraminotomy

Once Mixter and Barr[5] enlightened the world that a lumbar disc herniation can cause radicular leg pain and that surgical removal of that herniation had the potential to alleviate the symptoms, it did not take long before surgeons turned their eyes to the cervical disc as the menacing cause of brachial neuritis. The logical surgical solution to cervical radiculopathy would be to transpose the lumbar operation to the cervical spine. Such a transposition was not a unique idea, and several surgeons went about exploring this possibility. Soon after the publications on the surgical management of lumbar disc herniations made their way into the literature, Love and Camp,[6] Semmes and Murphey,[7] and Spurling and Scoville[8] began reporting their preliminary experience with the clinical diagnosis and surgical treatment of cervical radiculopathy.

In 1943, Semmes and Murphey described their experience in the management of four patients with unilateral radiculopathy treated with posterolateral decompression. Remarkably, these authors report the procedure to have been done under local anesthesia, something I would never entertain even in this day and age.[7] Soon thereafter, two medical officers, a US Army Lieutenant Colonel and a US Army Captain serving on active duty during World War II, published a manuscript in 1944 titled

"Lateral rupture of the cervical intervertebral disc: A common cause of shoulder and arm pain."[8] In that manuscript, Spurling and Scoville described the diagnosis and treatment of cervical radiculopathy. The technique they described required a small dental chisel to remove the lamina and facet to enlarge the cervical foramen before retracting the nerve root and removing the disc herniation (▶ Fig. 7.1).[8] As I read the "Technique" section of this manuscript, I could not help but admire with awe the proficiency these surgeons must have possessed with a chisel and the courage to employ such a technique over the top of the nerve root and spinal cord. The skills that Spurling and Scoville possessed in 1944 far exceed the skill and courage currently in my possession in 2020.

Writing from Stockholm, Sweden, in 1947, Frykholm[9] expressed the same concern I had regarding the use of a chisel over the top of the cervical nerve root and spinal cord. Frykholm's honest assessment of his suboptimal surgical outcomes led him to believe that his surgical technique may have either damaged the nerve by decompression or had resulted in an incomplete decompression. He sought to address the shortcomings of the chisel technique at the time and introduced a dental drill with a cutting drill bit.[9] ▶ Fig. 7.2[9] demonstrates Frykholm's technique with a "spherical vulcanite cutter" drill bit. The change from chiseling to drilling of the bone over the top of the nerve root made the decompression safer and allowed for a more comprehensive decompression. Needless to say, the drill is now the method of choice for this procedure. With advancements in fluoroscopy for localization and general anesthesia, the modern posterior cervical foraminotomy

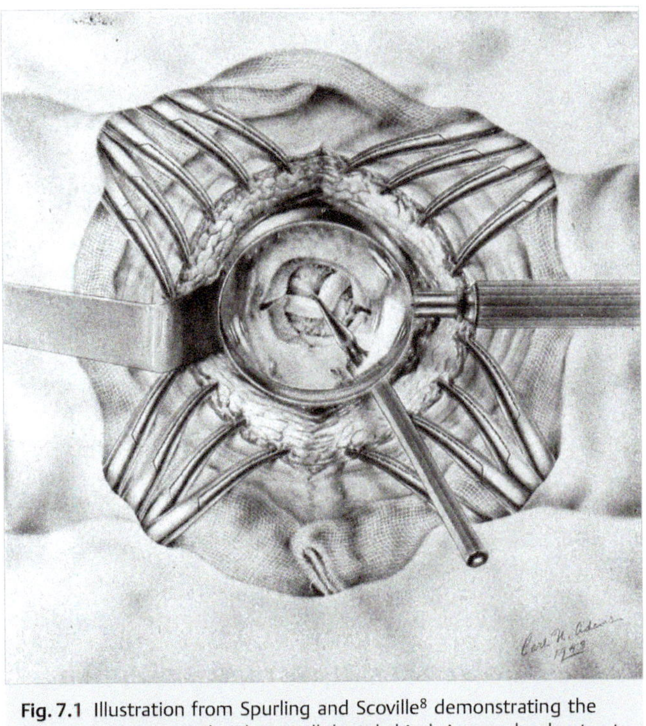

Fig. 7.1 Illustration from Spurling and Scoville[8] demonstrating the foraminotomy created with a small dental chisel. A nerve hook retracts the C6 nerve root downward to reveal a disc herniation. (Reproduced with permission from Spurling RG, Scoville WB. Lateral rupture of the cervical intervertebral disc: a common cause of shoulder and arm pain. Surg Gynecol Obstet. 1944; 78:350–358.)

awaited the development of minimal access ports for its next step in evolution. By the early 2000s, surgeons accustomed to wielding minimal access ports in the lumbar spine began applying them to the cervical spine, just like their predecessors in the 1930s transposed Mixter and Barr's discectomy from the lumbar to the cervical spine. Minimal access ports decreased the surgical exposure relative to the surgical target. The transposition of minimal access ports from the lumbar spine to the cervical spine optimized the Caspar ratio to almost 1:1. Achieving such a Caspar ratio is the essence of a minimally invasive approach.

7.3 Minimally Invasive Posterior Cervical Foraminotomy versus Anterior Cervical Discectomy and Fusion

In this Primer, I have made every effort to make the contents more about technique than about indications for surgery. However, in the case of posterior cervical foraminotomy, it would be difficult not to discuss the topic. An operation like the posterior cervical foraminotomy merits comment regarding the selection of this procedure over an anterior approach. Although an anterior approach tends to be an option for treatment of almost all degenerative pathologies of the cervical spine, the posterior cervical foraminotomy has a much narrower focus.

In my practice, I consider the posterior cervical foraminotomy in patients with unilateral radiculopathy whether from a herniated disc or a disc–osteophyte complex. The ideal patient for this operation is an individual with no significant neck pain, a unilateral radiculopathy with normal lordosis and no significant spondylosis. Magnetic resonance imaging (MRI) should demonstrate compression of the cervical nerve root, whether by foraminal compromise from an osteophyte or a disc herniation. However, patients seldom present in such a clearly delineated category. As such, I apply some additional criteria to further guide my selection. As I review the MRI, I assess whether there is any contact of the disc or disc–osteophyte complex with the spinal cord. The presence of any contact on the ventral aspect of the spinal cord prompts me to consider an anterior approach. Contact by a disc herniation on the lateral aspect of the dura of the spinal cord, provided there is no significant displacement of the spinal cord, is still amenable to a posterior decompression.

As I review the cervical radiographs, focal loss of the cervical lordosis or significant cervical spondylosis, especially at the level where I am considering a foraminotomy, may give me pause. A posterior cervical foraminotomy may not be the best approach in these patients, especially when they present with significant neck pain.

There are three clinical scenarios in which I find the posterior cervical foraminotomy especially valuable. The first is in the patient with multilevel disc degeneration, who is symptomatic at only one level. In this clinical scenario, an anterior approach may mandate a two- or three-level operation, whereas a posterior cervical foraminotomy addresses the symptomatic root. The second clinical scenario involves the patient who has undergone a previous single-level or multilevel cervical fusion and now presents with a unilateral radiculopathy at an adjacent

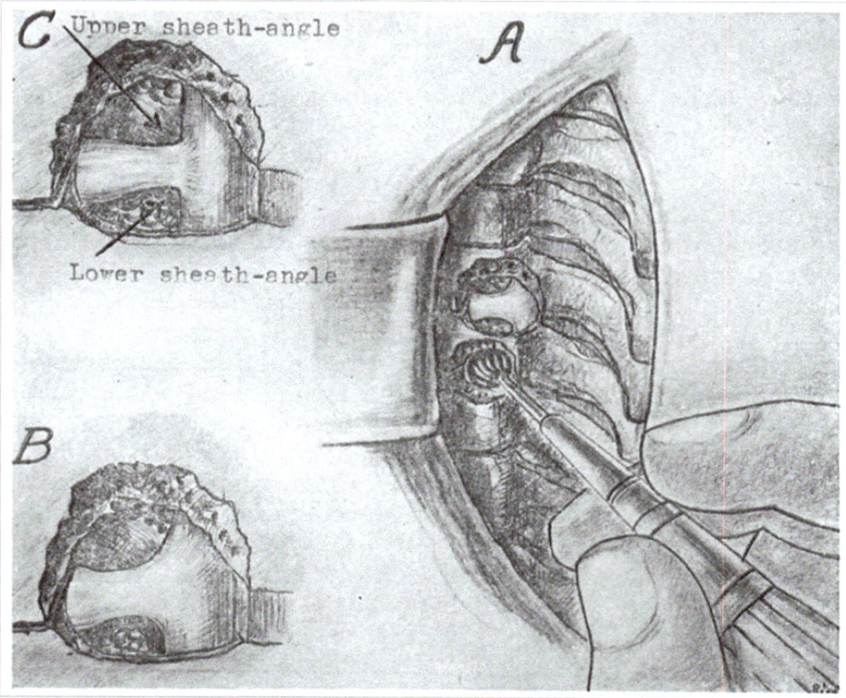

Fig. 7.2 Illustrations of Frykholm's technique[9] for the posterior cervical foraminotomy. Frykholm sought a safer way to remove the lamina and facet and turned to a dental drill to replace the chisels he had used previously. (Reproduced with permission from Frykholm R. Deformities of dural pouches and strictures of dural sheaths in the cervical region producing nerve-root compression; a contribution to the etiology and operative treatment of brachial neuralgia. J Neurosurg. 1947; 4:403–413.)

segment. A posterior cervical foraminotomy vastly facilitates the management of such a patient who would otherwise require an anterior approach with exploration of the previous fusion, possible explantation of the cervical plate and, finally, extension of the fusion to decompress the symptomatic root. With that management strategy, the patient has lost another motion segment. Instead, a posterior minimally invasive approach addresses the symptomatic root and avoids the potential complications of anterior revision surgery while preserving motion. Although a posterior foraminotomy is not a comprehensive solution, it may adequately address the radicular symptoms and potentially delay for years, if not avoid altogether, the need for an anterior approach.

The final clinical scenario is in the patient with persistent symptoms after an anterior cervical discectomy and fusion (ACDF) or cervical arthroplasty. Two or three patients find their way to my clinic every year with incomplete resolution or persistent unilateral radicular symptoms after an anterior approach. Treatment of persistent radiculopathy from an anterior approach has its potential challenges, especially when the patient has already had a fusion. In these patients, a posterior cervical foraminotomy may be the operation of choice.

7.4 Patient Education

When considering one of two procedures for the same condition, setting expectations for the patient is perhaps the most invaluable element of patient education. For a soft disc extrusion causing a unilateral radiculopathy in a patient without spondylosis, preoperative counseling is relatively straightforward. I review the objectives of the procedure and explain the rationale and technique. In the context of spondylosis, I go into greater depth to discuss the natural history of cervical spondylosis in the context of a cervical radiculopathy. I always explain to patients that the most comprehensive way to address a degenerative cervical disc process is to remove the entire disc, restore the disc height and stabilize the segment through an anterior approach. It is the anterior approach that allows for restoration of the disc height and segmental lordosis with decompression of the neural elements while preventing any further degeneration with immobilization. I emphasize to the patient that a minimally invasive posterior cervical foraminotomy is a motion-preserving procedure intended to relieve the compression of the nerve root. It forgoes the need for an implant, whether an arthroplasty device, interbody graft or cervical plate. As a consequence, however, it does not restore foraminal height and does not prevent further degeneration from occurring. I emphasize to the patient that the objective is to decompress a nerve that goes to the arm and, therefore, does not reliably alleviate neck pain. Finally, I specifically mention the potential need for definitive management with an anterior approach in the years or decades to come. I have found that these statements help patients begin to formulate what to expect in the postoperative period and even consolidate their thinking behind their selection of the type of procedure they wish to undergo.

The end of this chapter includes a series of cases regarding the nuances of patient selection, along with a review of the preoperative and postoperative images, to emphasize that careful patient selection is vital to a good outcome. Ultimately, minimally invasive posterior cervical foraminotomy holds a unique place in the armamentarium of a minimally invasive spine surgeon for well-selected patients.

7.5 Anatomical Basis for the Minimally Invasive Approach

The primary objective of a minimally invasive posterior cervical foraminotomy is to decompress the exiting root of a particular cervical segment by opening and expanding the foramen from a posterior approach. In the case of a disc herniation, opening the foramen provides access to the nerve root and canal to remove the disc herniation. As always, it is the anatomy that dictates the procedure, and so it is vital to understand the course of the cervical nerve root relative to the bony anatomy.

In the cervical spine the nerve root exits above its like-numbered pedicle; that is, the C6 nerve roots exit above the C6 pedicle. Thus, the C6 pedicle forms the floor of the foramen for the C6 nerve root, and the C5 pedicle forms the roof. The anterior boundary of the foramen is formed by the disc space (C5–6 disc in this case) and the lateral uncinate process (▶ Fig. 7.3). It is from this aspect of the foramen that the compressive pathology often arises. Discs may herniate and compress the nerve root. The uncovertebral joint may develop osteophyte complexes that result in symptomatic compression of the nerve root.

The posterior wall of the foramen is formed by the SAP of the like-numbered segment; that is, the posterior wall of the C6 nerve root is made up of the SAP of C6. The SAP may also be a source of compression of the nerve root in circumstances of advanced facet arthropathy (▶ Fig. 7.4).

There are three measurements that are of tremendous value when performing a minimally invasive posterior cervical foraminotomy. The first is the interpedicular distance. Depending on the disc height, the interpedicular distance ranges from 9 to 12 mm. It will seldom be more than 12 mm. The second measurement is the anteroposterior (AP) dimension, which is measured from the posterior aspect of the disc space to the anterior aspect of the SAP. This AP dimension ranges from 4 to 6 mm.[10] The final measurement is the lateral dimension of the foramen. This dimension is measured from the lateral aspect of the disc space to the medial aspect of the mid-SAP as it projects forward; this measurement consistently ranges from 8 to 10 mm (▶ Fig. 7.5).

With these measurements in mind, the necessary exposure to perform the operation becomes evident. The rostrocaudal exposure should be from pedicle to pedicle, a distance of at least 12 mm. The mediolateral exposure should be from the medial aspect of the pedicle to the middle of the facet–lateral mass complex, a distance of at least 10 mm. The inherent nature of a posterior approach makes the AP dimension irrelevant for the exposure. Using both of these measurements defines the surgical target as 12 × 10 mm. Applying the principle of the ideal Caspar ratio (surgical target to surgical exposure as 1:1) using a 14-mm-diameter access port fulfills that criterion. It is through a sophisticated understanding of these measurements that it becomes evident how a well-positioned 14-mm-diameter minimal access port can adequately provide the surface area needed for a comprehensive decompression of the cervical nerve root, without exposing unnecessary anatomy (▶ Fig. 7.6).

With this review of the anatomy of the cervical foramen and its anatomical measurements, we have established the anatomical basis of the minimally invasive approach to the cervical spine. Before describing the techniques of the procedure, I want to underscore the words "well positioned" in the previous paragraph. A minimal access port positioned over the lateral aspect

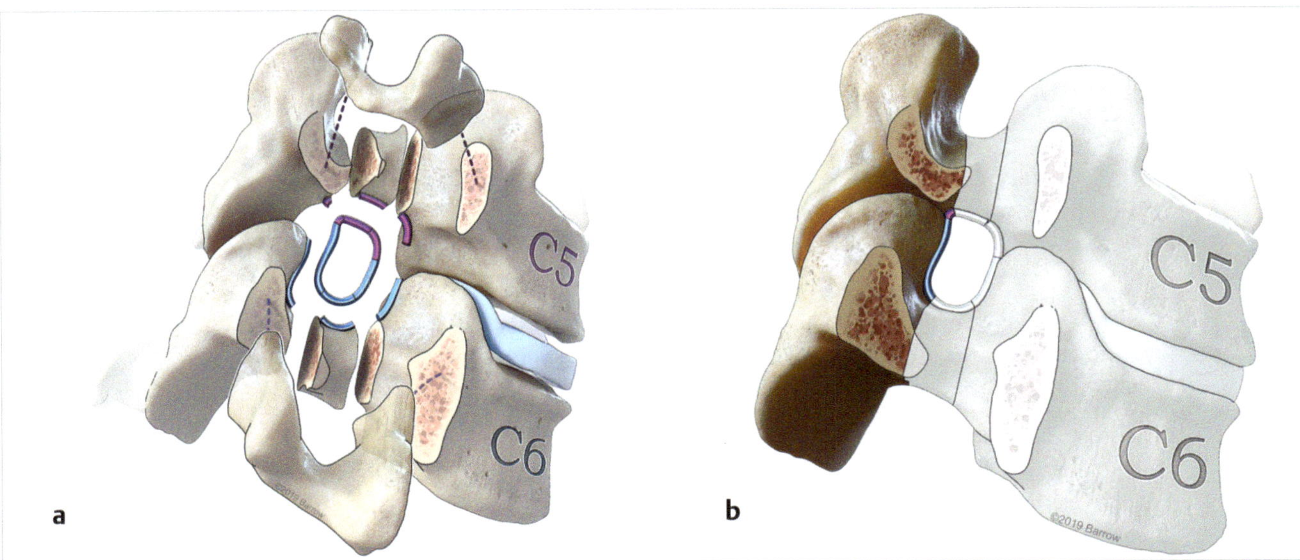

Fig. 7.3 Illustrations of the C6 cervical neural foramen showing the contributions from C5 and C6. **(a)** An exploded version of the cervical foramen demonstrates the contributing boundaries. The components of the *magenta* ring represent the contribution to the foramen by the C5 vertebra. The superior aspect of the foramen is made up of the inferior aspect of the C5 pedicle. The posterior aspect of the C5 vertebral body contributes to the anterosuperior aspect of the foramen. The components of the *turquoise* ring represent the contribution by the C6 vertebra. As can be seen from the illustration, the majority of the C6 neural foramen is made up by elements of the C6 vertebra. The posterior aspect of the vertebra makes up the anteroinferior wall. The superior aspect of the pedicle of C6 makes up the inferior border of the foramen. The superior articular process (SAP) of C6 makes up the majority of the posterior boundary of the neural foramen. **(b)** This illustration demonstrates the main target of the bone work. The emphasis in the posterior cervical foraminotomy is the posterior wall of the foramen (*turquoise*). Therefore, the SAP of C6, in this case, is the main target of the bone work. In this illustration, the foramen transversarium has been removed to demonstrate the contribution of the SAP to the neural foramen.

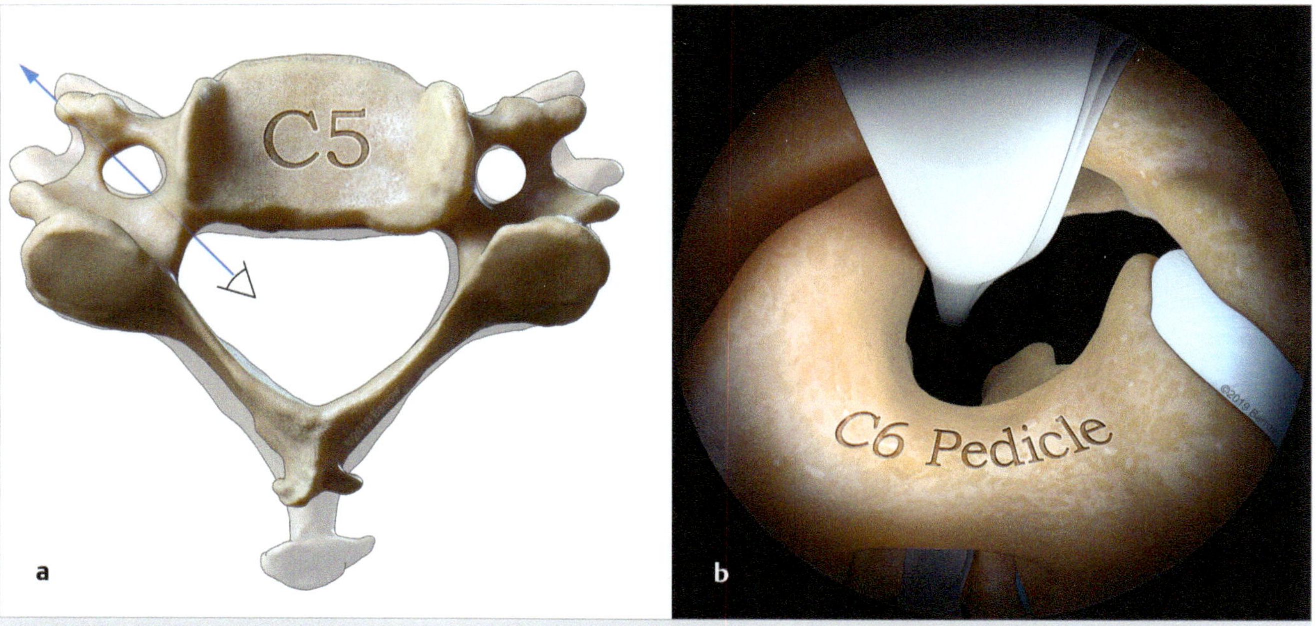

Fig. 7.4 Illustrations of the view of the neural foramen from within the spinal canal. **(a)** Orientation of the view from inside the spinal canal looking out through the C6 neural foramen. The schematic eye within the canal demonstrates the line of sight through the foramen used for the illustration in **b.** **(b)** Looking through the neural foramen of C6, the C6 nerve root is located in the 12 o'clock position. The uncovertebral joint is located at the 3 o'clock position. With this anatomy in mind, it becomes obvious how uncovertebral spurs can result in nerve root compression. At the 6 o'clock position, the pedicle of C6 makes up the floor of the neural foramen. At the 9 o'clock position, the superior articular process makes up the posterior wall, which is the target of the bone work for the posterior cervical foraminotomy.

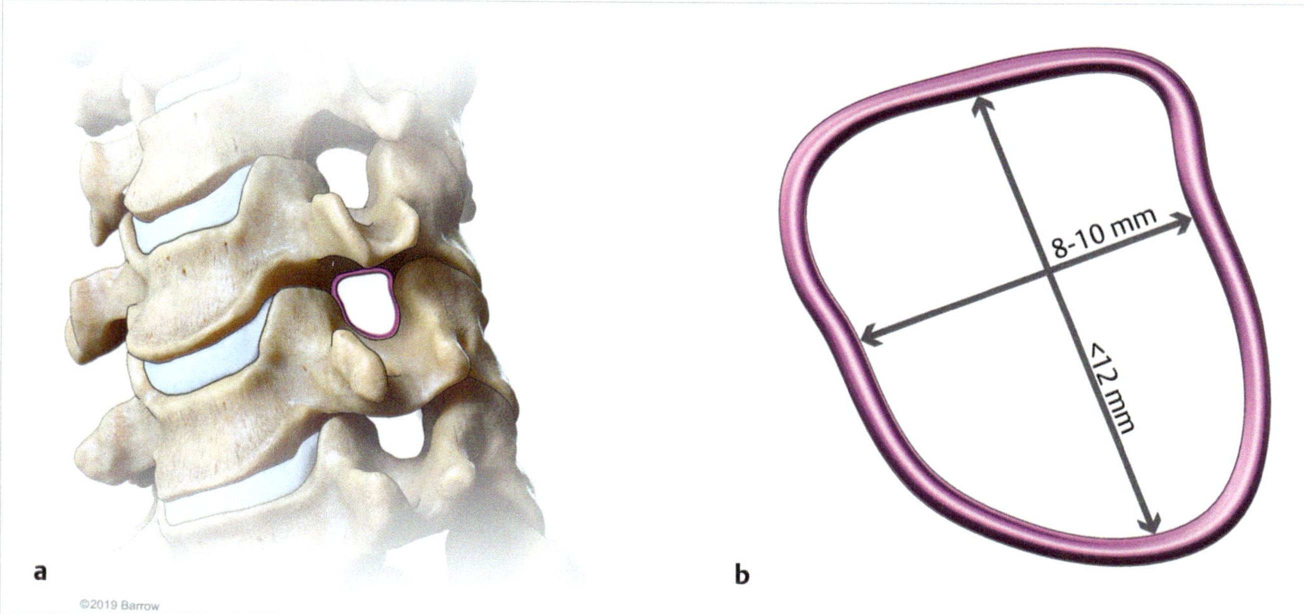

Fig. 7.5 Illustrations showing the dimensions of an average cervical foramen. **(a)** Isolating the boundaries of the cervical foramen (*magenta*). The interpedicular distance is dependent on the disc height. **(b)** The *magenta* ring shows the average dimensions of a cervical foramen. The rostrocaudal dimension is typically less than 12 mm. The medial-lateral dimension ranges from 8 to 10 mm. Osteophytes from the uncinate processes may encroach on the medial aspect of this dimension.

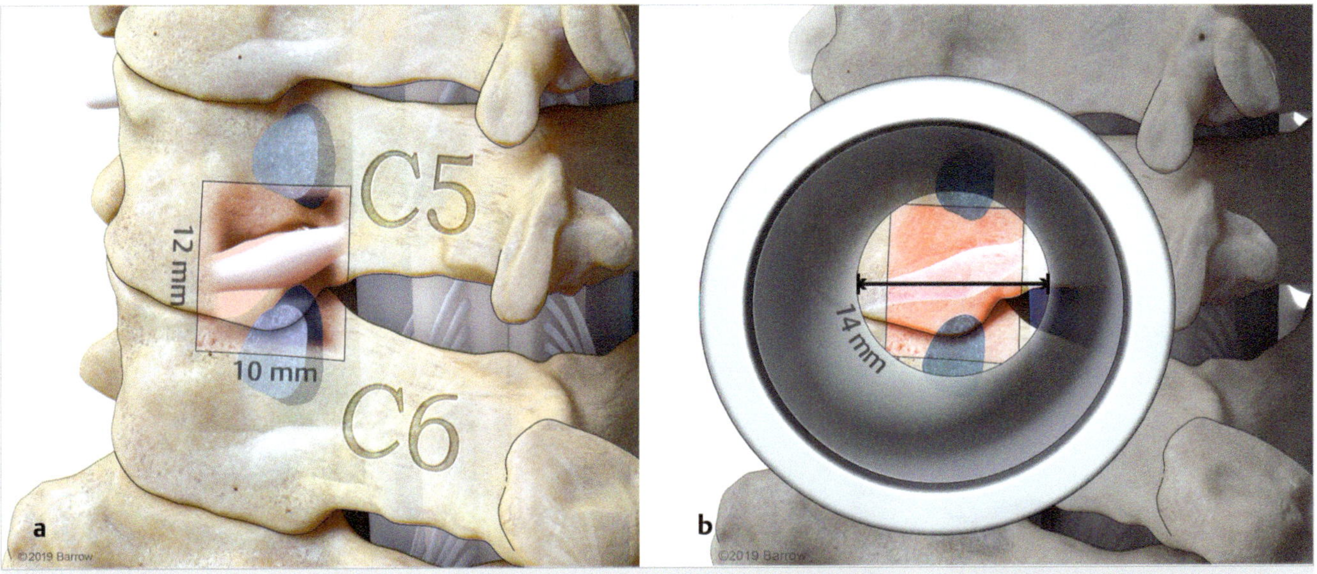

Fig. 7.6 Illustrations of the requisite anatomy and anatomical basis of a minimally invasive posterior cervical foraminotomy. **(a)** The requisite anatomy that is needed for complete decompression of a cervical nerve root. The maximum dimensions of this anatomy are 12 × 10 mm. These dimensions establish the anatomical basis for the use of a 14-mm-diameter access port. **(b)** The Caspar ratio. A 14-mm access port superimposed over the requisite anatomy demonstrates a Caspar ratio of nearly 1:1 and establishes the anatomical basis for the procedure.

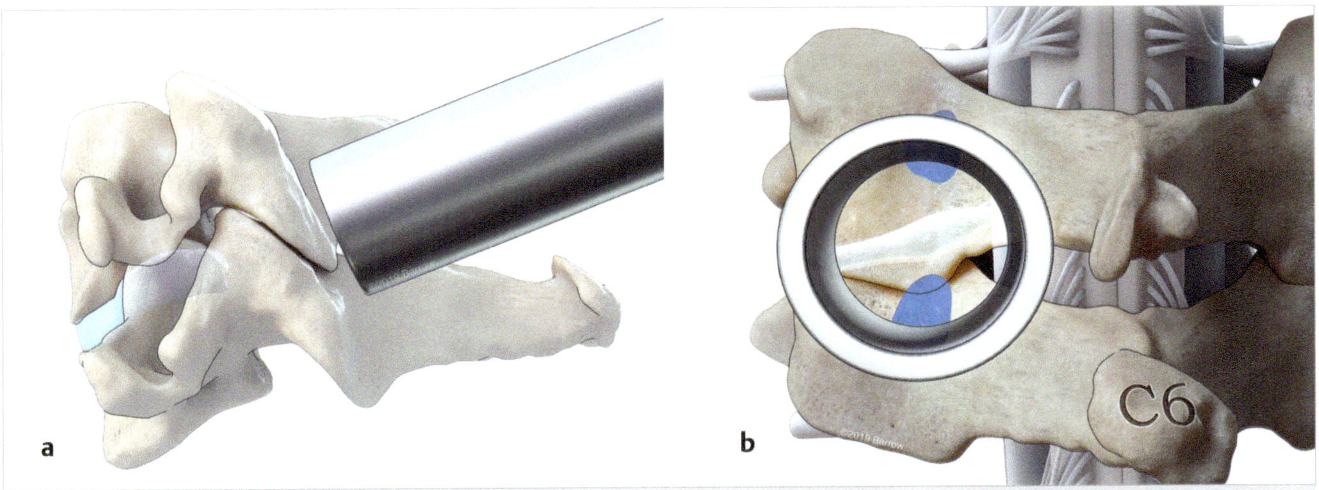

Fig. 7.7 Illustrations of the ideal placement of the minimal access port for a minimally invasive posterior cervical foraminotomy. **(a)** Lateral view of the cervical spine with a 14-mm access port in position, which demonstrates the placement of the minimal access port parallel to the disc space. The inferior and superior articular processes fall within the field of view. **(b)** The posterior view through the access port showing the minimal access port positioned over the midpedicular line to access the medial and lateral aspects of the foramen. The pedicles are demarcated in *blue*.

of the lateral mass will *not* allow you to perform an adequate decompression of the cervical root, and it carries a risk of destabilizing the segment. A minimal access port positioned over the lamina does not destabilize the segment, but it exposes the cervical spinal cord to unnecessary risk as you make your way laterally to the nerve root. The ideal placement of the minimal access port is precisely over the cervical nerve root, and this placement is the central element of this procedure (▶ Fig. 7.7).

7.6 Patient Positioning

There are several elements to positioning a patient for a posterior cervical foraminotomy to optimize visualization of the segment with fluoroscopy, the ergonomics for the surgeon and the comfort of the patient. From the placement of the skull clamp to the position of the chest rolls, this section covers the various nuances of patient positioning.

7.6.1 Application of the Skull Clamp

The ideal position of the skull clamp offers rigid stabilization of the head and cervical spine without causing any significant postoperative discomfort. The key to both is avoiding the temporalis muscle (▶ Fig. 7.8). Pins secured into the temporalis muscle have the potential to cause bleeding once the skull clamp is removed and postoperative discomfort for the patient long after their radiculopathy has resolved. Nonetheless, good purchase into the cranium is an absolute necessity for stability since the dilators exert downward pressure onto the cervical spine. There should never be a circumstance where a patient slips out of the pins because of suboptimal placement. Therefore, the ideal position is to have all the pins at the superior temporal line, which by definition places them above the temporalis muscle.

The clamp should be positioned on the skull so that the pin on one side is in line with the tragus, and the two pins on the opposite side are positioned on either side of the tragus (▶ Fig. 7.8). I apply 60 pounds of pressure onto the skull clamp after confirming the optimal positioning of the pins. As I hold the head of the pinned patient, my operating team rolls the patient onto their chest, and we position the patient in the center of the operating table on chest rolls so that the components of the skull clamp system that connect to the table do not obstruct the eventual AP image I must take to confirm the position of the access port relative to the cervical pedicle. As I hold the patient's head in a neutral position, my assistant secures the articulating arm and locks the skull clamp into position (▶ Fig. 7.9).

7.6.2 Positioning the Patient

Fessler[3] made a very sound argument for performing this operation with the patient in the seated position. The supposition is that the surgeon is more likely to encounter vigorous venous bleeding with the patient in the prone position because of the increased epidural venous pressure that accompanies that position. The greatest advantage of the sitting position is the decrease in epidural venous pressure and, therefore, a decrease in venous bleeding. Even as I type this, certain cases jump immediately to my mind where I was dealing with a venous deluge in patients positioned prone. During those early cases I whispered to myself, "Perhaps I should be doing these operations with the patient in the seated position." At the same time, this argument may be countered by a risk of an air embolism, which, at least in theory, is elevated when the patient is in the seated position. The proponents of the seated position deny this risk is relevant, as they have not seen this entity in the hundreds of cases they have performed.

Acknowledging both the advantages and disadvantages of both the seated and prone position, I perform this operation with the patient in the prone position, but I make a point to place the patient in the reverse Trendelenburg position. In that manner, the head is higher than the heart, which decreases the epidural venous pressure, even if only slightly.

My decision to position patients prone is a practical one. The seated position is not a very popular one among our anesthesia colleagues, and I have found the added struggle to place the patient routinely in the seated position is not worth the putative benefits, which, in large part, may be accomplished in the reverse Trendelenburg position. Although epidural venous bleeding may be less in the seated position, the reality is that bleeding will occur regardless of the patient's position. I have experienced considerable blood loss with the patient in both the seated and prone positions. However, the tipping point for me is the visceral response that is brought about just by alluding to the seated position to our anesthesia colleagues. Even the

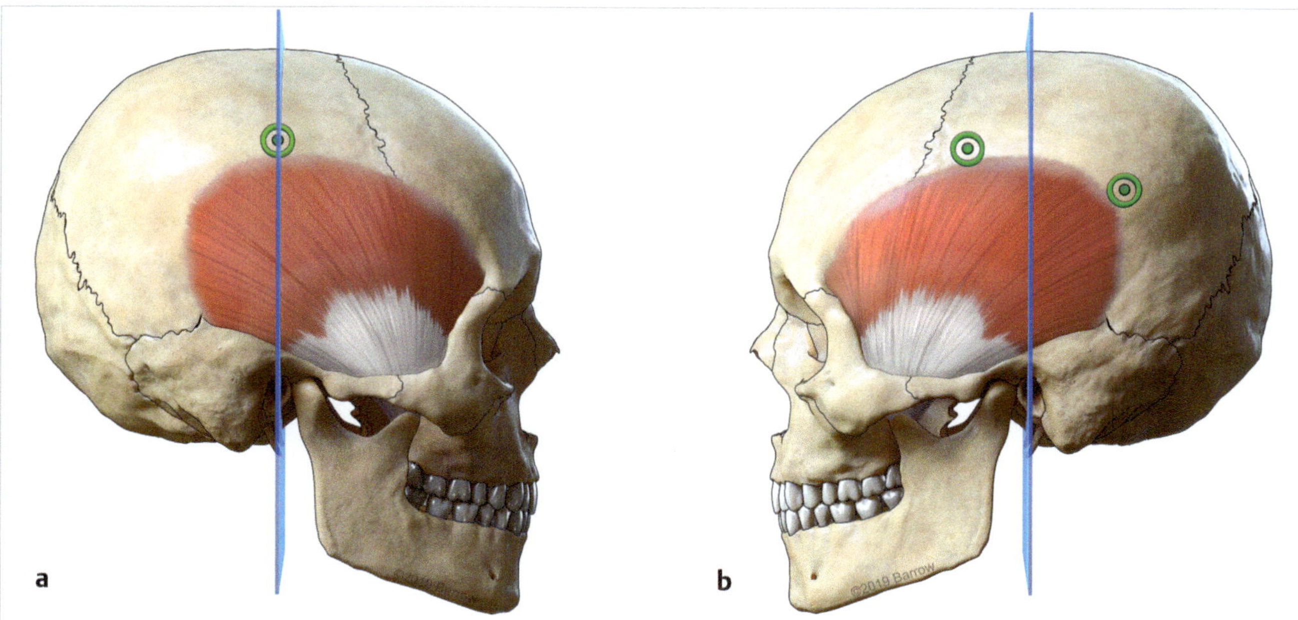

Fig. 7.8 Illustrations of the ideal placement of skull clamp pins in the cranium showing the temporalis muscle, which should be avoided. The pins should be placed above the superior temporal line, which is defined by the rostral insertion point of the temporalis muscle. **(a)** View of the right side of the head with the single pin in line with the external auditory canal and above the temporalis muscle. **(b)** View of the left side of the head with the pin sites denoted as fiducials on either side of the tragus.

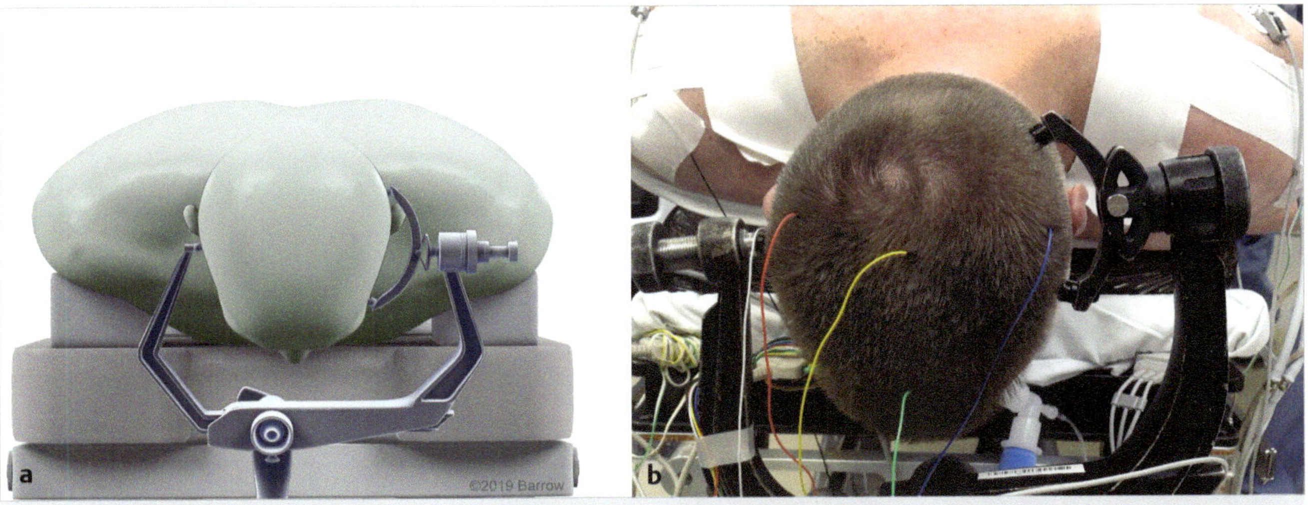

Fig. 7.9 (a) Illustration and (b) photograph of patient positioning. Once the skull clamp has been placed, the patient is rolled onto chest rolls and into the center of the operating table. The skull clamp is then secured to the bed with the articulating arm with the cervical spine positioned in a neutral configuration.

mention of it appears to decrease the efficiency of the anesthesia and thereby, the entire operation. Thus, I have exchanged the potential benefit of decreased cervical epidural venous pressure for the efficiency of positioning and a welcoming and enthusiastic anesthesiologist. I have found that this concession has decreased the time under anesthesia and optimized my time in the operating theater. I seldom have blood losses that exceed 50 mL, but admittedly, on occasion, I do encounter vigorous epidural venous bleeding that once again makes me reconsider the seated position. Fortunately, that type of bleeding does not occur with enough frequency to change my practice.

7.7 Operating Room Setup and Workflow

I set the operating room up to optimize the flow of the operation. I position the operating table well away from the anesthesiologist, almost in the middle of the room, so that I may perform the dilatation and docking of the minimal access port at the head of the bed. The microscope is set on the symptomatic side of the patient. I position the image intensifier of the fluoroscope on the opposite side of the patient's symptoms (▶ Fig. 7.10). Over the years, I have come to realize that the ideal ergonomic position for positioning the access port is at the head of the bed (▶ Fig. 7.11) and not at the side of the patient. Working at the head of the bed optimizes the efficiency of the operation. For this reason, I position the fluoroscope tower with its video screens at the foot of the bed, which provides me with a direct line of sight to the screens as I dilate the muscle and dock the access port.

I place the clamp for the table-mounted arm opposite the side of the symptoms just above the level of the patient's elbow, which is the ideal position for the table-mounted arm to hold the minimal access port for the procedure. By working at the head of the bed, I am not climbing over the fluoroscopy unit to make an incision or position the access port. Instead, I am in the ideal ergonomic position to complete the first phase of the operation.

7.8 Fluoroscopy

The objective of patient positioning is to place the patient in the geometric center of the bed where there is minimal metallic interference with AP fluoroscopic imaging. I make every effort to keep the neck neutral as my assistant tightens the articulating arm of the skull clamp. The first potential positioning pitfall occurs at this moment. The chest rolls need to be high enough on the chest to maintain the neutral position of the neck. If the rolls are positioned too low, the chest settles and the cervical spine goes into extension, with the downward pressure of dilators pushing down against the spine. It is also invaluable to ensure there is no tilt to the head when the skull clamp has been secured into its final position. Any tilt in the position of the head complicates lining up the facets on the lateral fluoroscopic image, which is essential for ideal positioning of the minimal access port. When I keep the anatomy in line without any tilt, the anatomy at depth is predictable for the dissection. When all one has is a 14-mm-diameter exposure, minimizing the variability of the anatomy at depth is crucial to maintain orientation.

Once the patient is positioned, I flex the patient's knees to prevent the patient from sliding down the bed, and then I place the patient in the reverse Trendelenburg position (▶ Fig. 7.12). The shoulders are taped down to facilitate visualization of the level. The fluoroscope rolls into the field for planning and confirming the incision (▶ Fig. 7.13).

A special circumstance arises for visualization for the decompression of the eighth cervical nerve root, given the inherent difficulties of a lateral image at this level. The anatomists of old named the spinous process of C7 *vertebra prominens* because of its long characteristic spinous process that was reliably palpable through the skin. So, I begin by palpating the *vertebra prominens* (C7) and palpate up or down, depending on the level, and approximate the location of the incision by placing a Kelly clamp or a blunted Steinman pin with a protective cover, so as not to puncture the skin (▶ Fig. 7.14). I strive for an ideal lateral fluoroscopic image, with the facets perfectly aligned in the

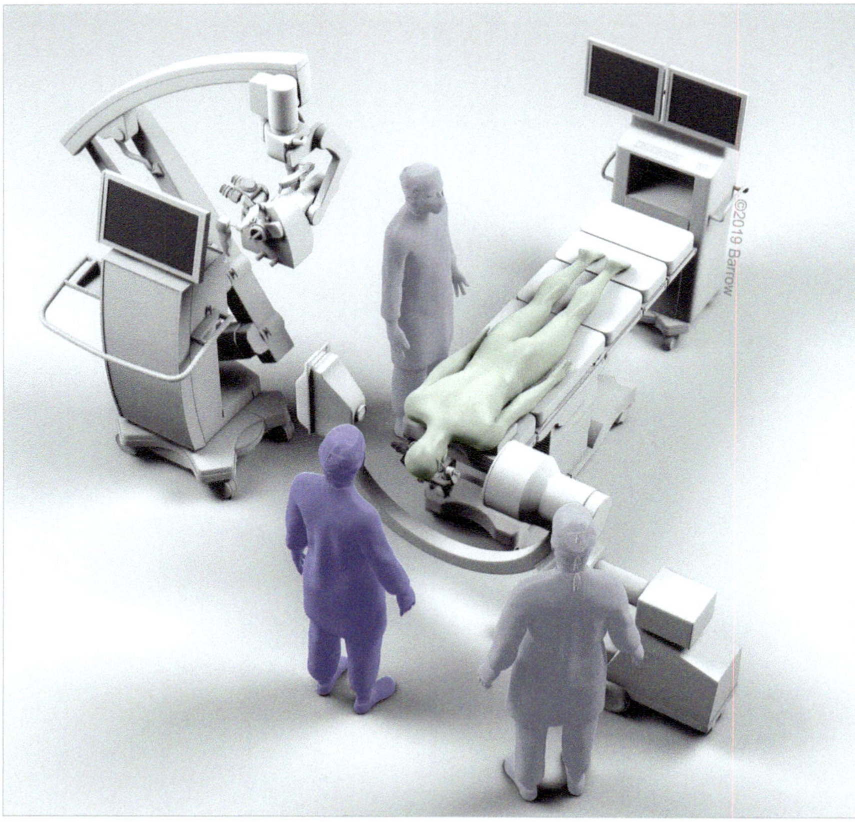

Fig. 7.10 Three-dimensional illustration of the operating room setup. The operating microscope and fluoroscope are all positioned around the patient in a manner that optimizes the flow of the operation. The patient is positioned on a standard operating table on chest rolls. The head and cervical spine are stabilized with a skull clamp fixated to the operating table. The operating microscope is positioned on the side of the patient's symptoms, and the fluoroscope is positioned with the image intensifier opposite the microscope. The fluoroscope tower is at the foot of the bed in the direct line of the surgeon's sight when the surgeon (*dark blue*) is standing at the head of the bed. The scrub technician (*light blue*) stands at the patient's side and the anesthesiologist (*light blue*) stands off to the side at the head of the bed by the airway.

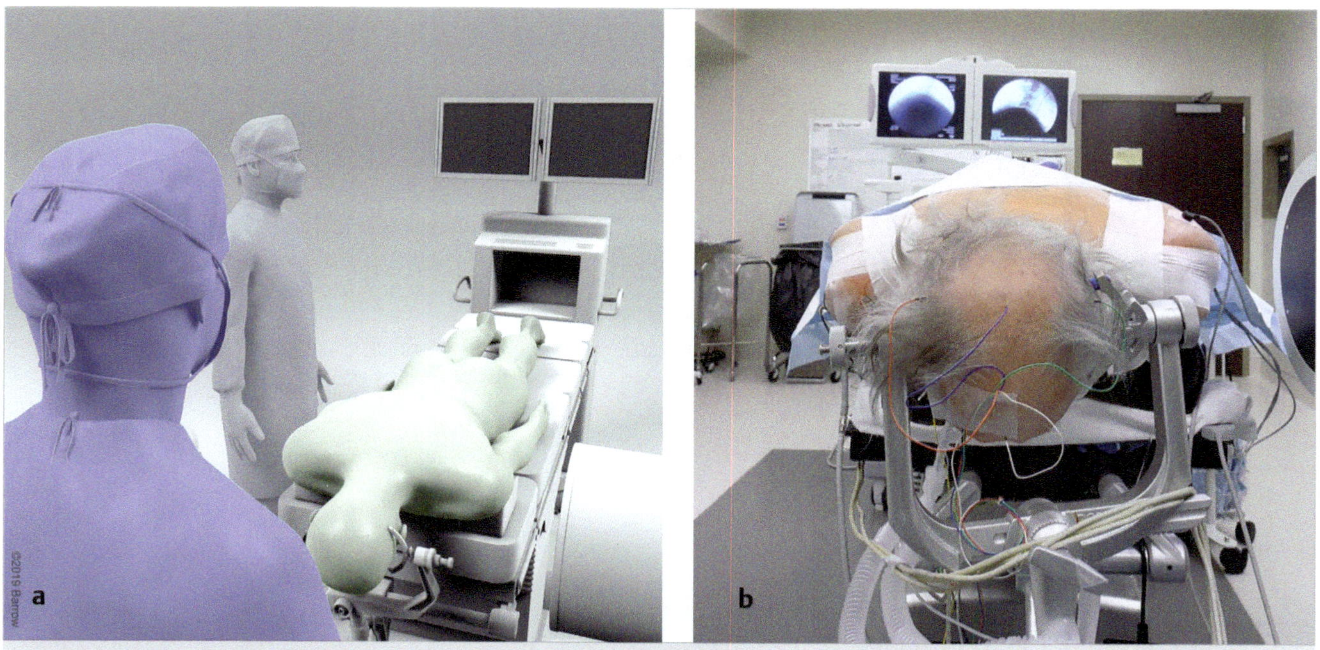

Fig. 7.11 Illustration and intraoperative photograph of patient positioning and operating room set up. **(a)** An illustration of the view over the shoulder of the surgeon. The surgeon stands at the head of the bed with a direct line of sight for the incision, dilatation and docking of the minimal access port. **(b)** Intraoperative photograph with a view from the head of the bed of the operating room setup and patient in a skull clamp positioned on chest rolls. Fluoroscope is in position with the image intensifier opposite the side of the symptoms. The monitors of the fluoroscope are at the foot of the bed. The microscope (not seen) is on the patient's symptomatic side (in this case, the right side), draped and ready to be rolled into place. This photograph is taken from the vantage point of the surgeon working to dock the minimal access port. Working at the head of the bed prevents any obstruction by the fluoroscope when making the incision and securing the minimal access port into position, while optimizing an ergonomic position for the surgeon to work.

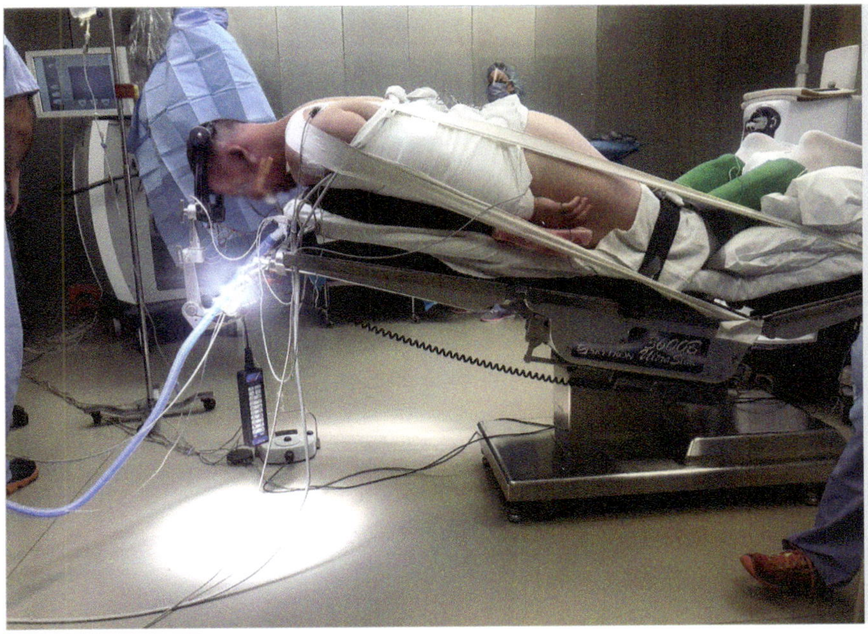

Fig. 7.12 Photograph of a patient positioned prone on chest rolls on a standard operating table with his head in a Mayfield head holder. The bed is reversed in order to facilitate passage of the fluoroscope. The knees are bent first, and then the patient is placed into the reverse Trendelenburg position before taping of the patient's shoulders. The reverse Trendelenburg position decreases the central venous pressure, with the putative benefit of limited venous epidural bleeding from the cervical epidural veins. Once the patient positioning has been finalized, the first fluoroscopic image is obtained.

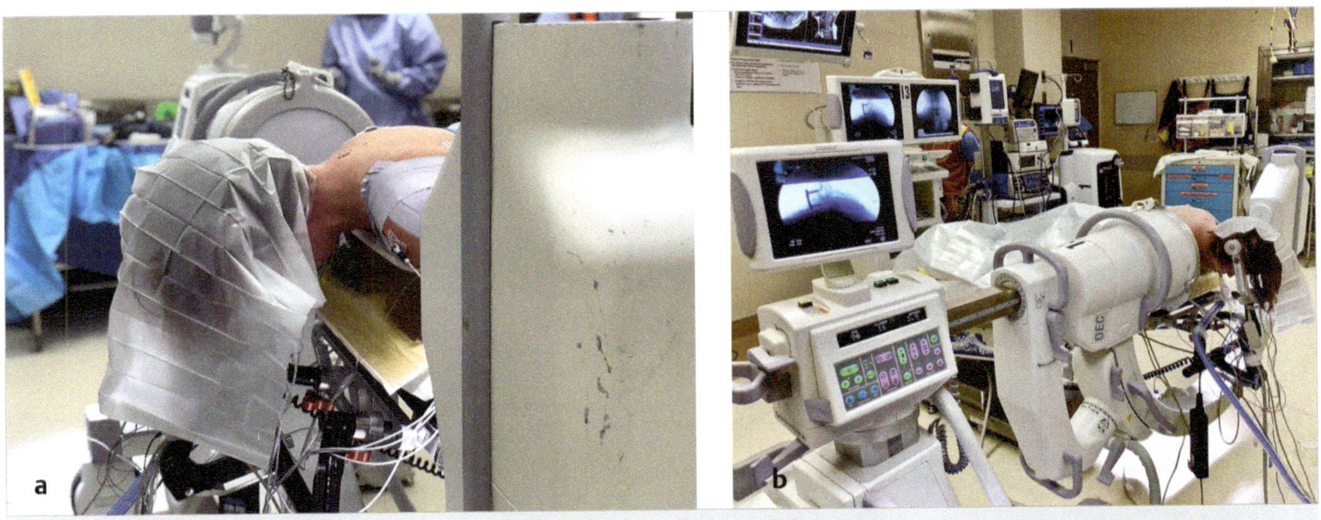

Fig. 7.13 Intraoperative photographs of patient positioning and operating room setup. **(a)** The fluoroscope rolls into the operative field for planning the incision before prepping and draping the patient. **(b)** Intraoperative photograph of the operating room setup for a C7–T1 posterior cervical foraminotomy below the level of a C6–7 anterior cervical discectomy and fusion. Once the ideal image is captured, the fluoroscope will stay in position until the access port is docked to prevent the need to recapture the ideal lateral image.

image. The fluoroscope may need to be wagged and the bed slightly rotated to achieve the ideal image. Unlike the previous procedures described thus far in this Primer, where I defer any imaging until after draping the patient, the time to obtain the perfect image is before prepping and draping the patient. Perfect orthogonal positioning of the patient greatly facilitates radiographic imaging.

Once I have captured the perfect lateral image, I keep the fluoroscope in position until I have secured the minimal access port into position. I may move the table up and down for prepping and draping the patient, but I do not move the base of the fluoroscope. The goal is to save the time of trying to obtain the same image again but only moments later.

I adjust the blunted Steinman pin according to the fluoroscopic image and mark the level (▶ Fig. 7.15). I plan the incision 1.5 cm off the midline. I add 2 mm to the diameter of the port that I will use; that is, for a 14-mm port, I plan a 16-mm incision. I then prep and drape the posterior cervical spine widely. I incorporate the midline markings into the draped field in order to help keep my bearings.

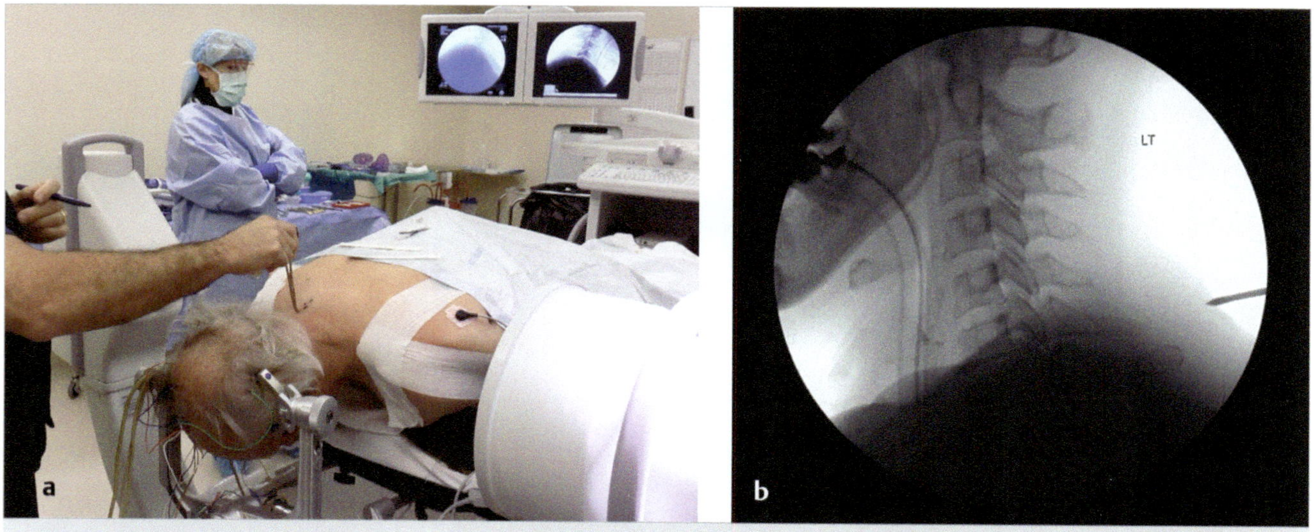

Fig. 7.14 (a) Planning the incision. A Kelly clamp or a protected Steinman pin is used to plan the incision. (b) Lateral fluoroscopic image showing a Steinman pin (with the tip covered by tape to prevent puncture of the skin) at the C6–7 level for planning the incision. The lateral image needs to be adjusted until the facets are perfectly aligned. Note that in this image, the facets of the segment to be operated upon (C6–7) are aligned.

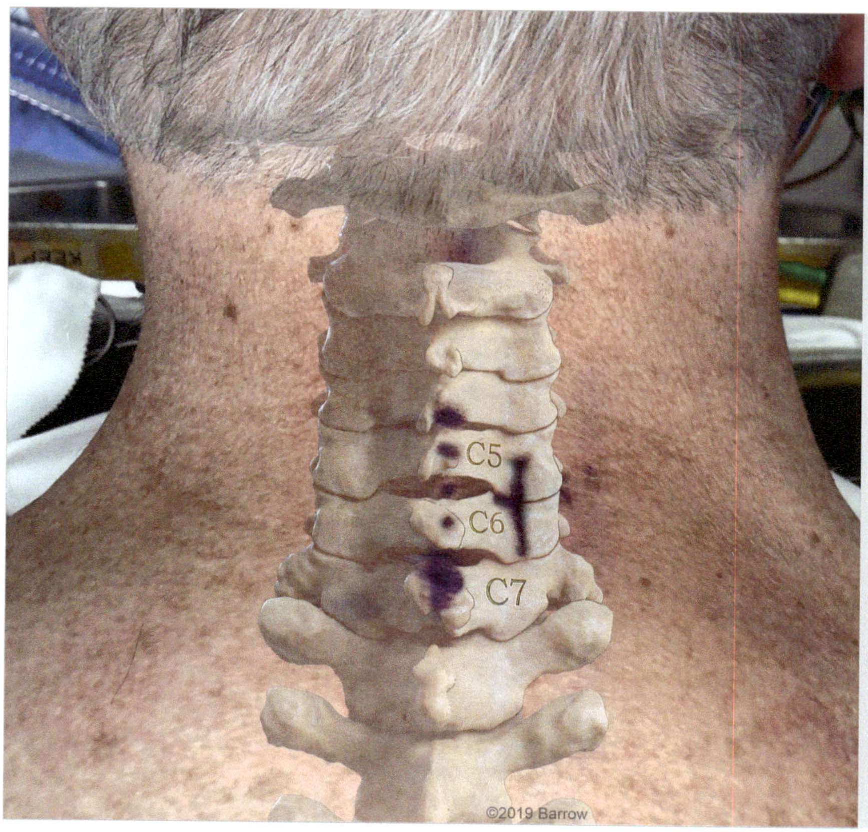

Fig. 7.15 Planning the incision. The midline is marked by palpating the spinous processes as shown in this photograph by the dots in the midline. The spinous process of C7 (*vertebra prominens*) is readily palpated and marked (denoted in the image as a cross at inferior-most aspect of the markings). A 16-mm incision is planned 1.5 cm off the midline and over the top of the area confirmed by fluoroscopy. The surgeon's mind needs to begin to reconstruct the anatomy at depth at this point in the operation.

7.9 Localization

Admittedly, I find localization and positioning the minimal access port more harrowing in the cervical spine than in the lumbar spine. The consequences of having any instrument enter the spinal canal at this phase of the operation are dire, a topic that is covered in greater depth in Chapter 8 on the minimally invasive posterior cervical laminectomy. At the same time, I have confidence in my knowledge of the anatomy at depth. As long as I know where the midline is, I know I can safely dock laterally on the facet–lateral mass complex. Knowledge and certainty of the midline is imperative. Based on the anthropometric measurements reported by Panjabi et al,[11] the distance from the geometric center of the canal to the lateral aspect of the canal is approximately 12 mm. I know that with an incision planned 15 mm lateral to midline, I will safely dock onto bone, provided I do not overly converge.

All the prepping and draping are done around the fluoroscope. To optimize the operative flow, it is essential that I do not move the fluoroscope after the ideal image has been captured during the preoperative localization process. As mentioned in Section 7.7, Operating Room Setup and Workflow, I stand at the head of the bed facing the monitors of the fluoroscope (▶ Fig. 7.16) when I begin the operation. Thus, I am out of the way of the fluoroscope, and I am not craning my neck trying to look at the images while the radiology technologist intermittently and inadvertently irradiates parts of my body, which invariably get in the way when standing at the side of the patient. The fluoroscope monitors are at the foot of the bed, which allows me to look directly at the images and the operative site simultaneously. Because I do not move the fluoroscope after localization, I know that the first image I take will be the ideal image.

As I drape the patient, I also drape the fluoroscope into the field without altering either the height or the position of the operating table or the fluoroscope. The boom of the fluoroscope is the only exception. Release of the boom enables me to drape the X-ray tube and the image intensifier in a sterile manner. After draping, I pass a 20-gauge spinal needle through the planned incision I had marked earlier and onto the spine. Even though I am 1.5 cm lateral to midline, I still want the spinal needle to diverge slightly from the midline as I insert it. I may check a fluoroscopic image or two as I pass it onto the facet–lateral mass complex. Encountering the unmistakable firmness of bone with the tip of the spinal needle is a very reassuring and comforting feeling (▶ Fig. 7.17).

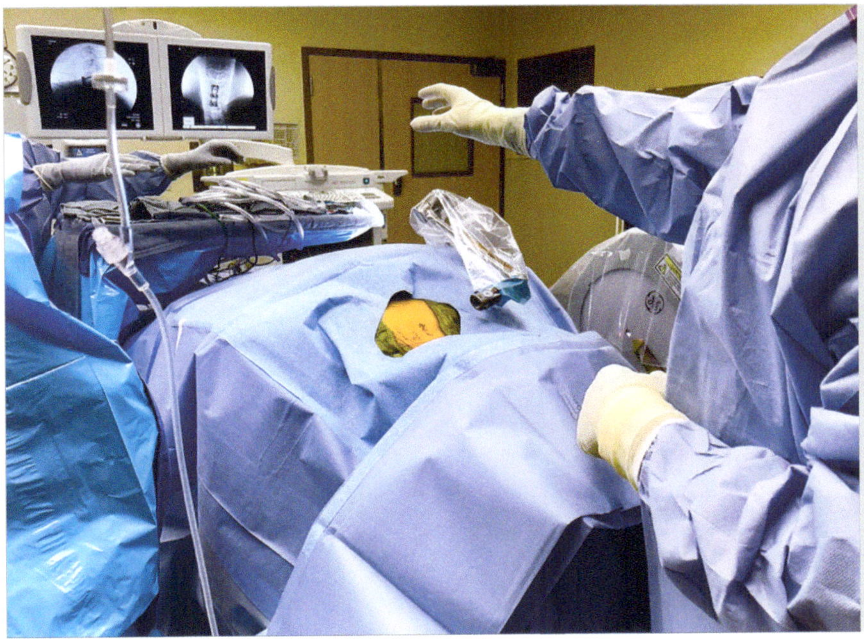

Fig. 7.16 Photograph of surgeon positioned at the head of the bed for the placement of the minimal access port. Standing at the head of the bed optimizes the ergonomics of positioning the access port while avoiding the path of the fluoroscope. With the fluoroscope monitors at the foot of the bed, the surgeon has a simultaneous, direct line of sight to the fluoroscopic images and the optimal working space.

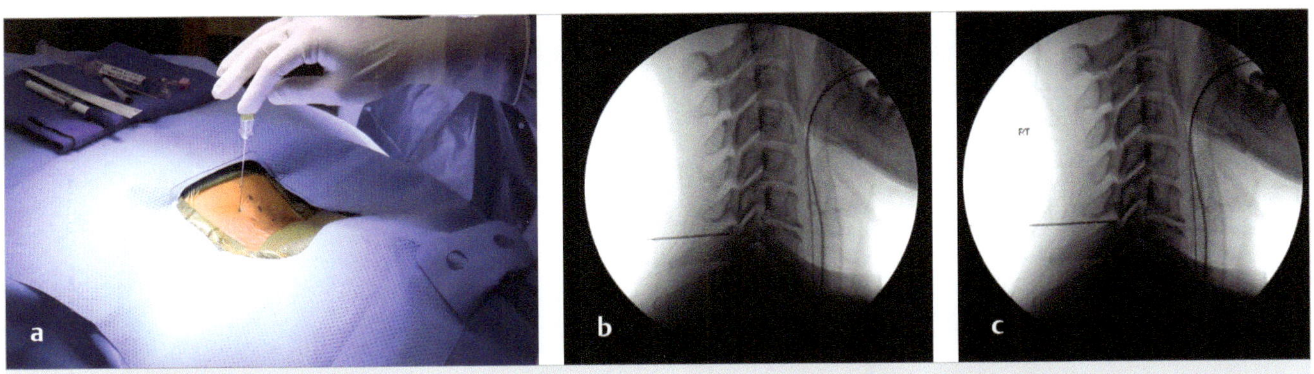

Fig. 7.17 Confirmation of the operative level. **(a)** Intraoperative photograph showing passage of the needle onto the lateral mass–facet lamina junction. The needle should always diverge from the midline and never converge onto it. **(b)** Lateral fluoroscopic image showing spinal needle localization. The needle passes along a divergent trajectory away from the canal and onto the facet–lateral mass complex. Note the ideal lateral image with alignment of facet joints in both images. The initial placement of the needle demonstrates a suboptimal trajectory. The needle is too low for an optimal trajectory as it is well below the disc space. **(c)** Lateral fluoroscopic image showing the tip of the spinal needle at the inferior aspect of the articular process and parallel to the disc space. The ideal incision will be centered around this entry point on the skin.

The trajectory of the needle must be parallel to the disc space of the segment to be operated upon, which ensures that the position of the incision will provide the optimal trajectory for the exposure (▶ Fig. 7.17c). The spinal needle insertion point may be adjusted rostrally or caudally to optimize the angle, and the incision may be adjusted from there. Once I have confirmed the level and optimized the trajectory, I remove the stylet and connect a syringe filled with a local anesthetic (a lidocaine/bupivacaine mixture that contains epinephrine). First, I pull the needle away from the bone, and then I begin to infiltrate the musculature as I pull the needle out. I then use a hypodermic needle to infiltrate the skin of the proposed incision.

Only after I am satisfied that I have confirmed the operative level and have an optimal trajectory onto the symptomatic nerve root will I re-mark the incision, precisely measuring it so that it will be 2 mm greater than the access port I will use. Although the anatomical basis for the minimally invasive approach discussed earlier indicates that 14 mm provides all the exposure needed for a decompression of the cervical nerve root, a 16-mm diameter provides more leeway. The larger 16-mm diameter is a good starting point early in your learning curve. As your experience grows, you should feel more comfortable employing a 14-mm-diameter access port, which is the diameter access port I use for all circumstances, whether to address bony foraminal compromise or removal of a disc extrusion. As discussed in Section 7.5, Anatomical Basis for the Minimally Invasive Approach, the anatomy of the cervical neural foramen does not mandate more surface area than that for a complete decompression of a cervical nerve root.

7.10 Incision and Securing the Access Port

I make the incision with a No. 15 blade and then use cautery to begin the dissection down to the cervical fascia. The posterior cervical fascial layer is substantially thicker than that in the lumbar or thoracic spine. Early in my experience I attempted to dilate through this fascial layer with the sequential dilators and found myself using an inordinate amount of downward force to get through the fascia and reach the spine. Sometimes the downward pressure would alter the position of the patient's neck or the skull clamp, giving me an unsettling feeling. I read several technique papers where the authors described using Metzenbaum scissors to create a corridor through the fascia and onto the spine. In my hands, such dissection seemed imprecise and inelegant, and it created troublesome bleeding. In light of this, I began to open the fascia precisely the same way that I do in open cases: with cautery. Working through the incision, a suction tip in one hand and cautery in the other, I dissect a linear path down onto the posterior cervical fascia. I make a precise fascial opening with direct visualization while simultaneously controlling any bleeding that may occur. An insulated cautery tip is essential to prevent inadvertent cautery of the skin while dissecting down to the fascia.

The posterior cervical fascia has an unmistakable toughness to it but when encountered by the tip of the cautery, it melts away. The paraspinal musculature lies immediately beneath the fascial layer and comes into view after vertically linear division of the fascia. It is only at this point that I begin to pass the sequential dilators. Although the posterior cervical fascia is tough and inhospitable to the dilators, offering stiff resistance to their passage, the paraspinal muscles are more docile and more welcoming. The magnitude of downward pressure for a dilator to reach the spine is substantially less with the fascia divided.

Recall that neither the operating table nor the fluoroscope has been moved since the initial preoperative localization with the spinal needle. Maintaining the fluoroscope and operating table position saves time as I pass the dilators sequentially onto the spine. Images appear instantly without having to again optimize the position for fluoroscopy. The result is an uninterrupted flow to the operation. Again, I emphasize the need for a perfect lateral image with the facets perfectly lined up to ensure the optimal placement of the access port.

The first dilator that I pass onto the spine is the most important one. An ideal trajectory onto the spine without convergence is critical. The target is the inferior articular process of the rostral vertebra; for example, for a C6 posterior cervical foraminotomy, the target is the inferior articular process of C5. Before I place the second dilator, I must feel the unmistakable tactile sensation of metal in contact with bone. It is essential to have the tip of the first dilator firmly up against the inferior articular process of the rostral vertebra. From there, the tactile sense of slipping down off the inferior articular process and back up upon it is a distinctive feeling that allows your mind to begin to reconstruct the anatomy at depth. The more familiar you become with this sensation, the more precise your position will be over the compressed nerve root with the minimal access port. Wanding in the lumbar spine allows for generous sweeping motions of the dilator onto the lamina that facilitates the exposure. In contrast, the extent of wanding for a posterior cervical foraminotomy is slipping on and off the inferior articular process. As I dilate with the subsequent dilators, I ensure that the tip of each dilator is firmly pushed down against the bone. Again, the key to positioning the access port is securing the first dilator in perfect position (▶ Fig. 7.18).

After passing the initial dilator onto the inferior articular process, it becomes increasingly more difficult to maintain the subsequent dilators against the bone. However, meticulous dilatation minimizes the amount of muscle that must be removed from the bone once the access port is in position. With each increase in the diameter of the dilator, there is a tendency for the dilator not to reach all the way to the bone. Although the smaller diameter dilators readily contact the lamina–facet junction illustrated in ▶ Fig. 7.18c, larger diameters tend to be further and further from the spine. As I review the sequential passage of dilators on the lateral fluoroscopic images, I note the position of the last dilator and study the image to determine if it has migrated off the spine. It is imperative to identify that separation and step back to where the dilator was on the bone. To a certain extent, migration of the minimal access port away from the spine is unavoidable. However, when the dilator is not well positioned against the lamina–facet junction, the surgeon might need to traverse a considerable amount of paraspinal muscle to reach the spine. Traversing a significant amount of paraspinal muscle translates into increased postoperative discomfort for the patient. Taking a step back and dilating again makes that postoperative discomfort altogether avoidable. Once the dilatation is complete, I select the length of the minimal access port and secure it into position (▶ Fig. 7.19).

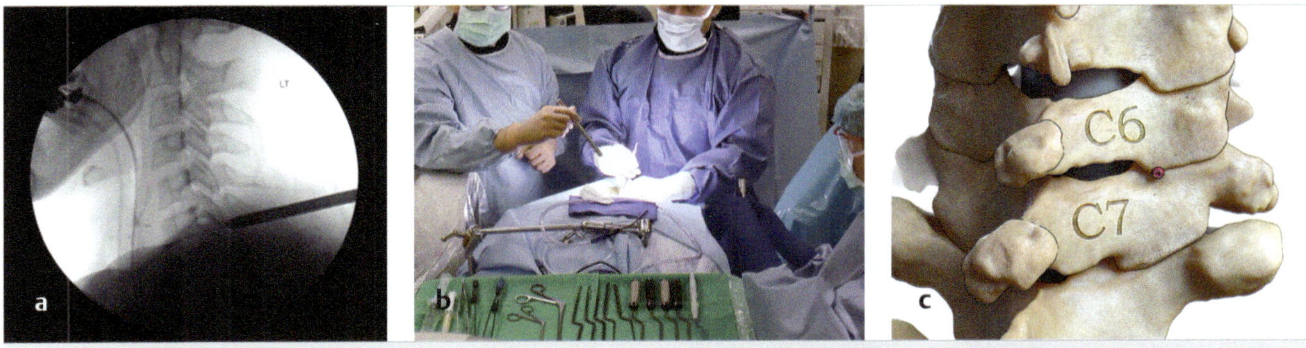

Fig. 7.18 Photographs and illustrations of positioning the first dilator. **(a)** Lateral fluoroscopic image demonstrating a dilator in position for a right C7 posterior cervical foraminotomy. Note the tip of the dilator is firmly in contact with the inferior articular process of C6. **(b)** Intraoperative photograph demonstrating sequential dilatation up to 14 mm to accommodate the access port. Note the surgeon working at the head of the bed with the fluoroscope in position. The line of sight of the surgeon is directly toward the fluoroscopy screens. **(c)** Illustration showing the ideal position of the first dilator. The magenta fiducial marks the ideal target for the first dilator at the junction of lamina and the facet.

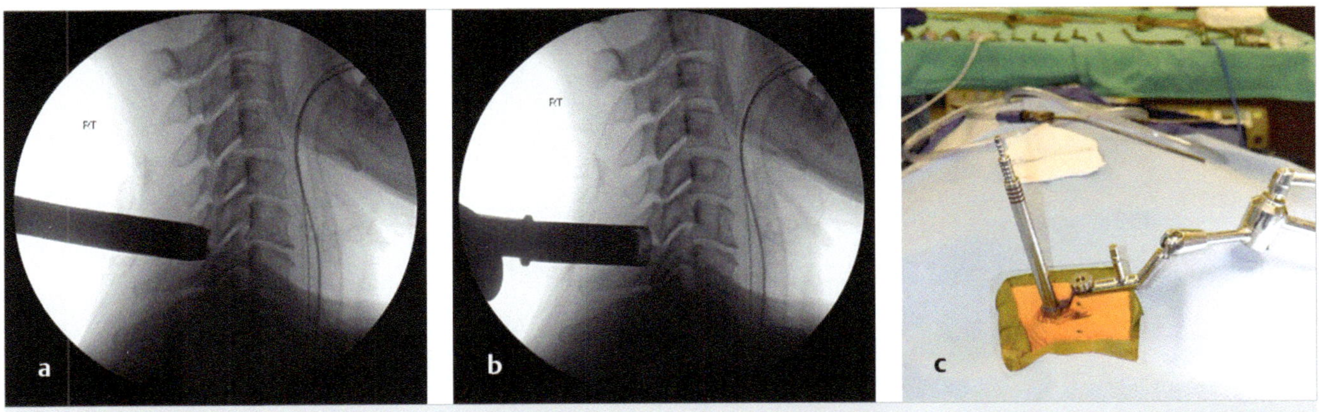

Fig. 7.19 Fluoroscopic and photographic images of ideal dilator positioning. **(a)** Lateral fluoroscopic image demonstrating the last dilator in the ideal position against the lamina–facet junction. **(b)** Lateral fluoroscopic image with the minimal access port in position. A small distance is now present from the lamina–facet junction to the spine. Downward pressure when securing the access port to the table-mounted arm minimizes that distance, and thereby muscle creep. **(c)** Intraoperative photograph with the minimal access port secured in position with the dilators still in place.

As I secure the access port to the table-mounted arm, I exert moderate downward pressure to minimize any upward migration of the minimal access port. A sustained downward pressure minimizes, if not eliminates, the muscle creeping into the operative field. With the minimal access port in position, I tighten all the joints of the table-mounted arm and obtain the final lateral fluoroscopic image. The radiology technician then rotates the fluoroscopic unit into an AP configuration for the final image. The final lateral and AP images remain on the screens for the duration of the operation. Those images serve as a valuable reference to maintain orientation throughout the case (▶ Fig. 7.20). I keep the fluoroscope in the room in case a need arises to reconfirm the level or reposition the access port. As the fluoroscope is rolled out of the operative field and the microscope is rolled in, I move from the head of the bed to the symptomatic side of the patient and begin to expose the bony anatomy (▶ Fig. 7.21).

7.11 Exposure

The first phase of the exposure under the microscope is discovery. The goal is to define the anatomy at depth. My mind begins the process of integrating the information of the AP and lateral fluoroscopic images with the information I gleaned from sounding the anatomy with the initial dilator. I must transpose all these data into a mental image of the anatomy and then superimpose that image onto the 14-mm-diameter access port at depth (▶ Fig. 7.22).

My objective during the discovery phase is to confirm the anatomy that I have already reconstructed in my mind's eye. I expect to identify the inferior articular process almost immediately upon peering down into the minimal access port and discharging one or two bursts of cautery. If not, I begin to make the adjustments that will center the access port over the relevant anatomy. As I peer into the access port through the microscope, I look for evidence of the facet–lateral mass complex. If I cannot directly visualize the bone of the lateral mass, I probe gently with the suction to confirm that, in fact, bone lies beneath the diameter encompassed by the port. Using an extended, bayoneted and protected cautery tip, I lightly touch the muscle on top of the bone at the outer lateral-most aspect of the field of view.

If I have been meticulous in my positioning, incision planning, measurements and dilatation, then I should immediately

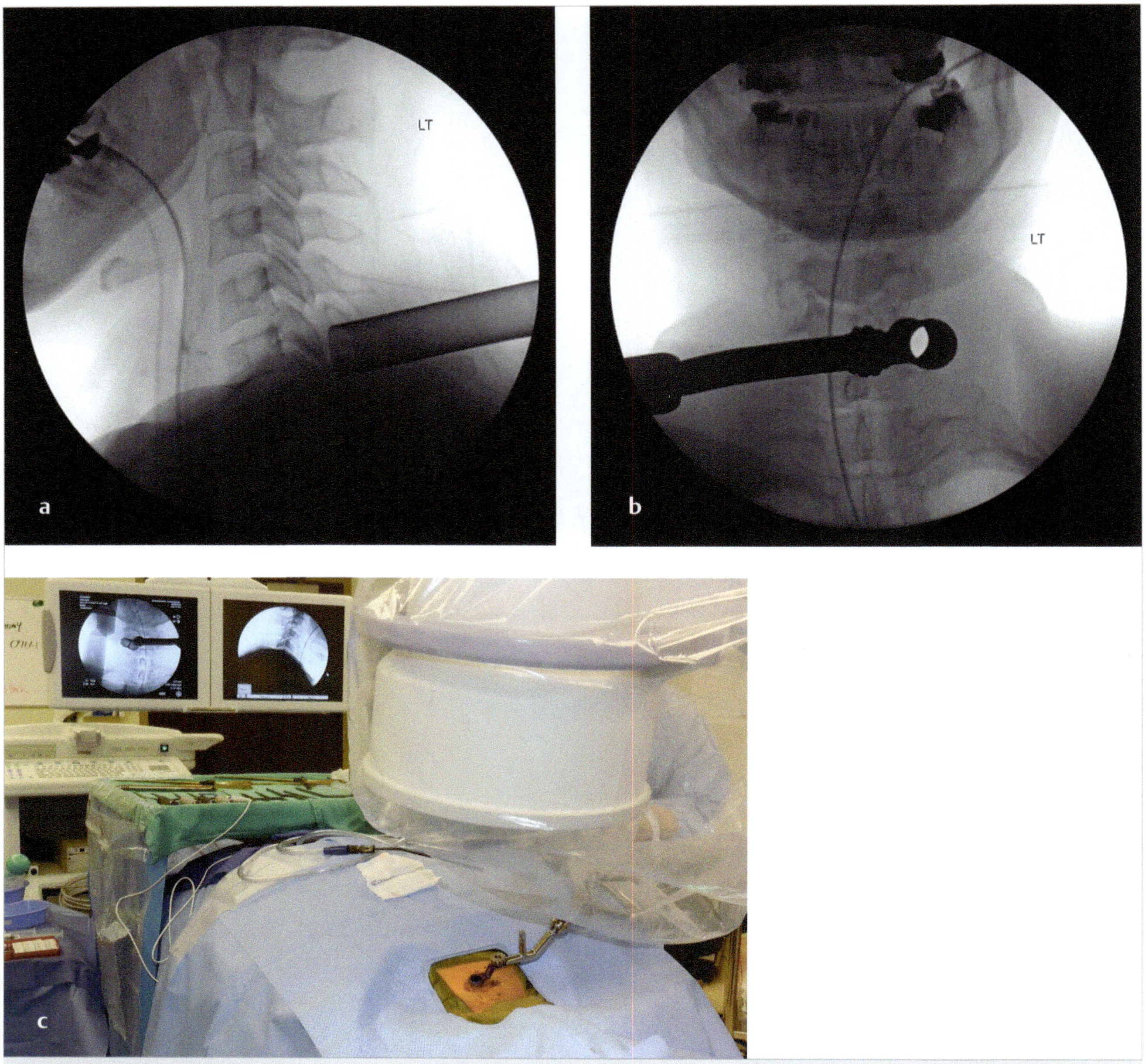

Fig. 7.20 Fluoroscopy for a right C7 posterior cervical foraminotomy. (a) Lateral fluoroscopic image showing the minimal access port parallel to the C6–7 disc space, which is a minimal distance from the facet–lamina junction. (b) Anteroposterior fluoroscopic image showing the minimal access port immediately over the midpedicular line, which provides ready access to the medial and lateral aspect of the cervical foramen. (c) Intraoperative photograph of the final fluoroscopic image being obtained before rolling the fluoroscope out of the operative field.

see the unmistakable ivory color of bone after lightly cauterizing a thin veil of muscle in the upper outer quadrant designated as quadrant I (▶ Fig. 7.23). I continue to probe gently with the suction to ensure the bone is directly beneath the paraspinal muscle and begin to sweep away the remaining strands of muscle with cautery, thereby exposing the confluence of the inferior articular process and the lateral rostral lamina. I completely expose the medial aspect of the rostral facet (quadrant II). I prefer to work at the rostral-most aspect of the exposure as I sweep away the muscle over the rostral lamina. I always avoid the use of cautery in the interlaminar space. Once the lateral aspect of the rostral lamina and the medial aspect of rostral facet are completely exposed, I return to the lateral and inferior quadrant (quadrant III) and proceed with the exposure of the caudal facet and lamina. Again, the exposure proceeds from lateral to medial. At all times during my dissection, I refrain from using cautery in the vicinity of the intralaminar space (quadrant IV). Instead, I always sweep toward it, and whatever soft tissue remains in that vicinity, I resect with a Kerrison rongeur (▶ Fig. 7.24). I avoid the temptation to pluck the strands of muscle with a pituitary rongeur, which tends only to pull more tissue into the field of view.

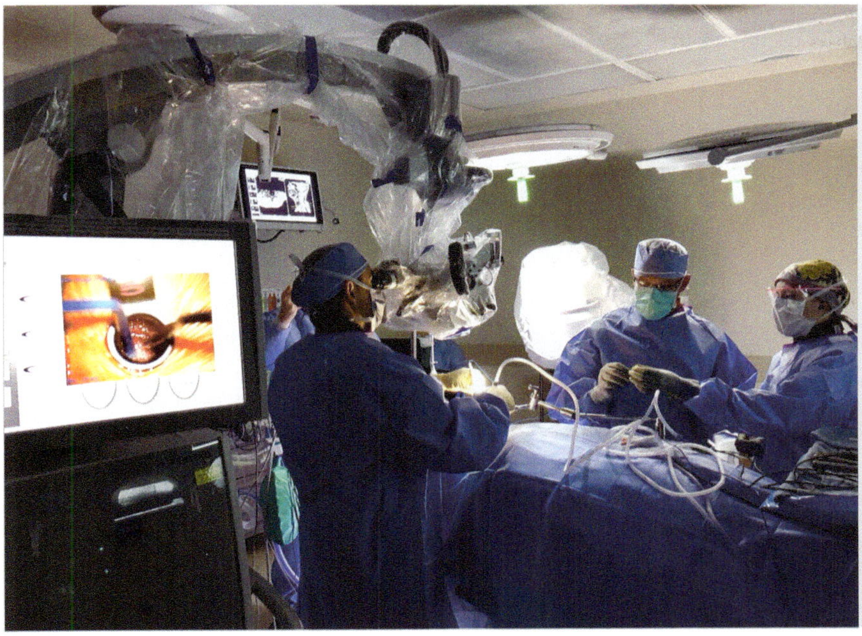

Fig. 7.21 Intraoperative photograph of the operating room setup. Once the final fluoroscopic image has been obtained and the minimal access port has been secured, the fluoroscope is rolled out of the operative field but remains available should the need for further fluoroscopy arise. The microscope, draped and ready on the symptomatic side of the patient, is rolled into position.

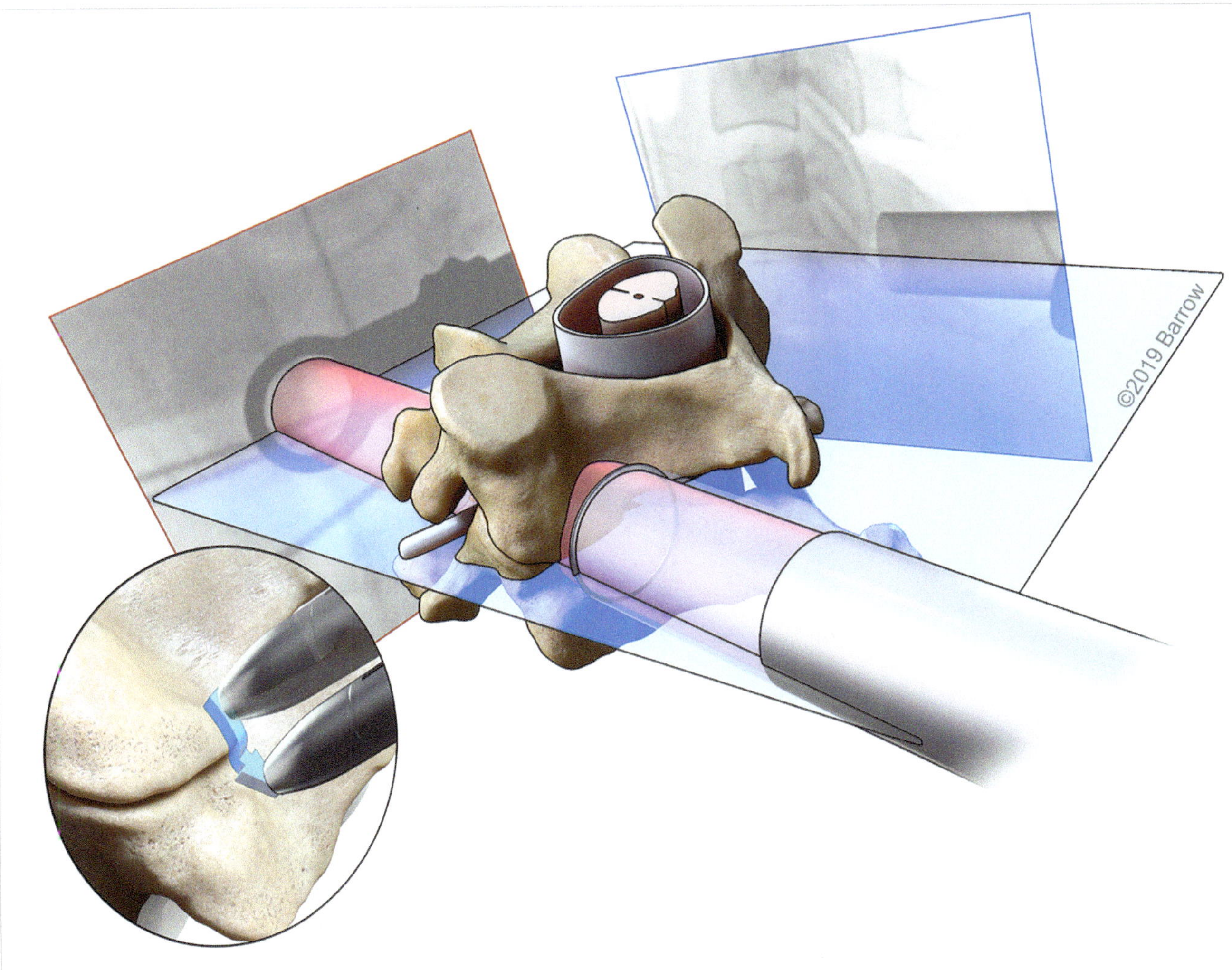

Fig. 7.22 Integration of the visual and tactile feedback through the 14-mm access port. Reconstruction of the anatomy at depth requires integration of the tactile feedback provided by the tip of the initial dilator slipping off the inferior articular process of the rostral vertebra and onto the superior articular process of the caudal vertebra (far left inset, magnified view) and the position of the access port based on the anteroposterior (outlined in *red*) and lateral (outlined in *blue*) fluoroscopic images. The integration of these visual and sensory inputs allows for anatomical certainty when exposing the anatomy.

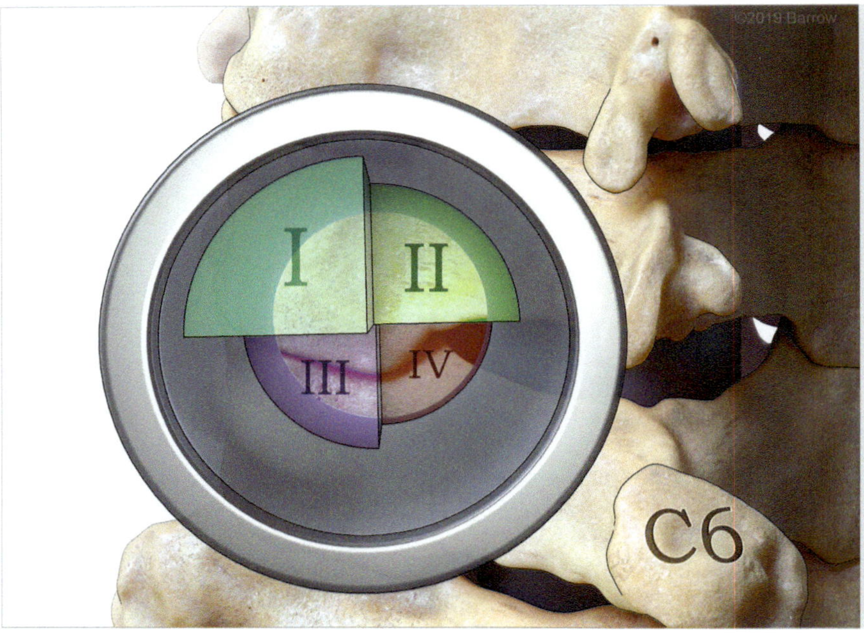

Fig. 7.23 Illustration of the sequence of exposure of the posterior cervical anatomy for a foraminotomy as seen through a 14-mm-diameter minimal access port. The safe quadrant to begin the exposure with cautery is in the upper and outer region of the diameter denoted as quadrant I. Upon exposing the bone of the inferior articular process in quadrant I, the dissection proceeds toward the medial aspect of the facet and lateral lamina, which is denoted as quadrant II. The dissection then resumes laterally to quadrant III and finally cautery sweeps away soft tissue over the lateral caudal lamina seen in quadrant IV.

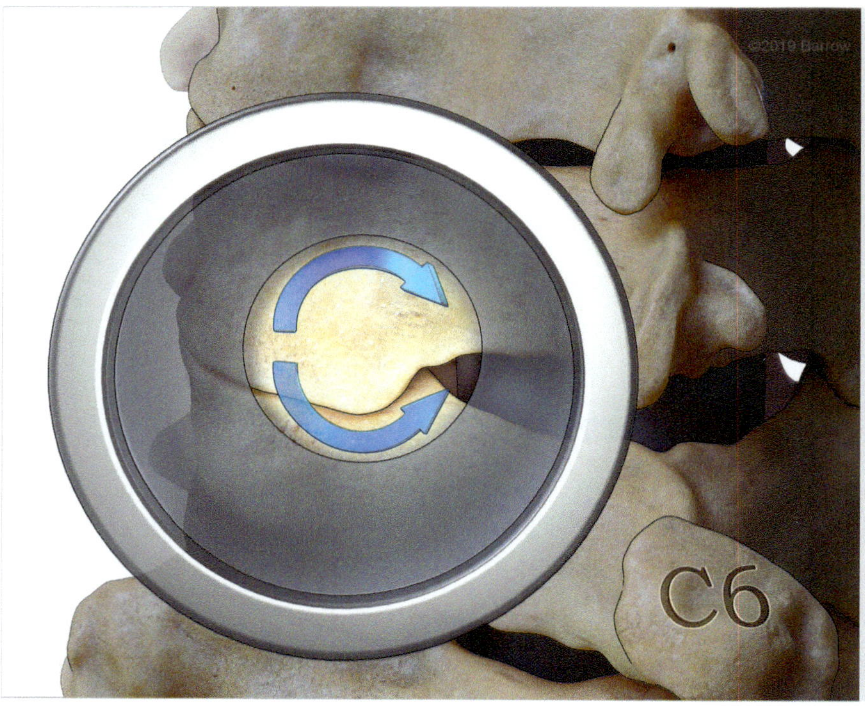

Fig. 7.24 The sequence of exposure using cautery. The *blue* arrows in the illustration demonstrate the safe use of cautery for exposure of the superior and inferior articular processes. The emphasis is on sweeping from the lateral aspect of the exposure over the inferior and superior articular processes and toward the interlaminar space. It is essential to refrain from the use of cautery in the vicinity of the intralaminar space.

7.12 Iterative Dilatation with Direct Visualization

At times, despite meticulous technique in the dilatation of the paraspinal musculature, the minimal access port resides a full centimeter over the spine with a column of paraspinal muscle fibers between the access port and the inferior articular process. The amount of muscle that would need to be removed in order to achieve adequate exposure of the requisite anatomy is far too much and would contribute to unnecessary postoperative patient discomfort. Removing that much muscle is also inconsistent with the principles of the preservation of the native spine and the minimal disruption of the anatomy. A preliminary exposure of the bony anatomy and secondary dilatation remedies such a circumstance (▶ Fig. 7.25).

The first step is to create a linear path onto the inferior articular process using cautery (▶ Fig. 7.25). Since the AP and lateral images demonstrate the position of the minimal access port over the midpedicular line, cautery may be used to create a

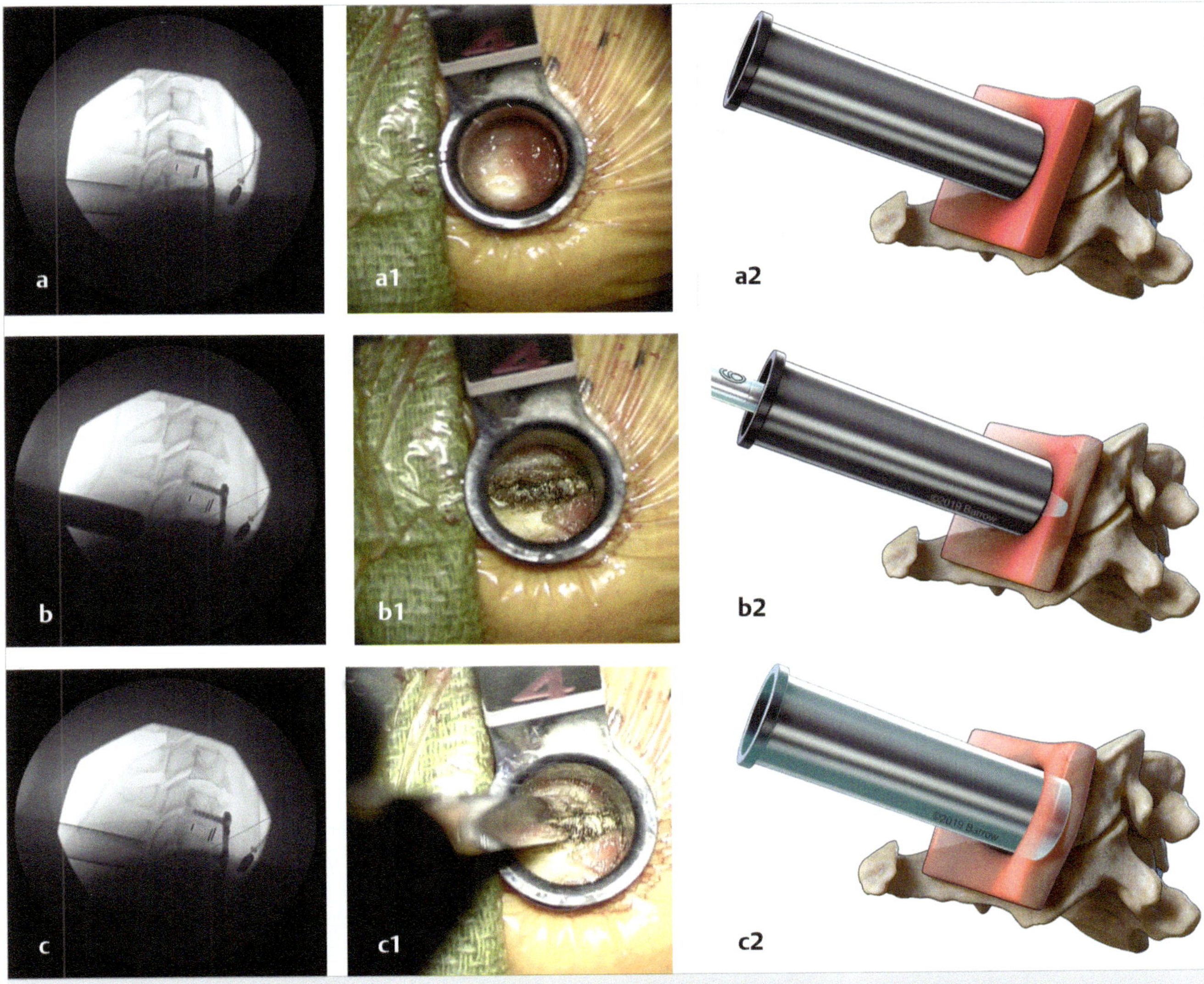

Fig. 7.25 Secondary dilatation to optimize the access port–cervical spine interface. **(a)** Lateral fluoroscopic image demonstrating a 14-mm access port positioned over a previous C5–6 and C6–7 anterior cervical discectomy and fusion in a patient with persistent C7 radiculopathy. The final position of the access port is 1 cm from the inferior articular process. **(a1)** Intraoperative photograph of the field of view through the access port with suboptimal dilatation. The image shows the paraspinal musculature overlying the posterior cervical anatomy. **(a2)** Illustration demonstrating the access port in position with 1 cm of paraspinal muscle (*red*) between the tip of the access port and the spine. **(b)** Lateral fluoroscopic image demonstrating the second dilatation. **(b1)** Intraoperative photograph after creating a narrow seam with cautery in the muscle to unveil the bone of the inferior articular process below. **(b2)** Illustration showing the initial dilator placed under direct visualization precisely onto the exposed inferior articular process after creating a seam in the overlying muscle. At this point, the access port is removed, and the sequential dilatation is repeated. **(c)** Lateral fluoroscopic image demonstrating the access port well positioned against cervical lamina and facet complex. **(c1)** Intraoperative photograph with the initial dilator in position. The 14-mm access port is removed, and the dilators are passed over the initial dilator. The final dilator may now displace the paraspinal muscle by dilating the seam that was created by the cautery. The same access port may now be secured onto the lamina and facet junction with minimal muscle creep. **(c2)** Illustration showing the final position of the access port just millimeters from the inferior articular process, sparing the paraspinal musculature.

narrow but direct path onto the inferior articular process until the unmistakable appearance of bone comes into view. Direct visualization of the inferior articular process through this narrow seam created in the column of muscle provides an opportunity for a secondary dilatation to optimize the interface of the access port and the facet–lamina junction. With the inferior articular process in my direct line of sight, I pass the first dilator and place it directly onto the inferior articular process and anchor it firmly into position. I will need to pass two more dilators to achieve the requisite 14-mm diameter, but I cannot do so with the microscope in position. So, I raise the microscope to a height that allows for a working zone to pass the dilators into the access port. For the time being, I am using the microscope as a light source, since I can no longer peer through the oculars at its current height. I pass the second dilator, knowing the position of the initial dilator with certainty. Before I pass the third dilator, I remove the access port altogether and pass the third dilator all the way down to the spine. I then place the

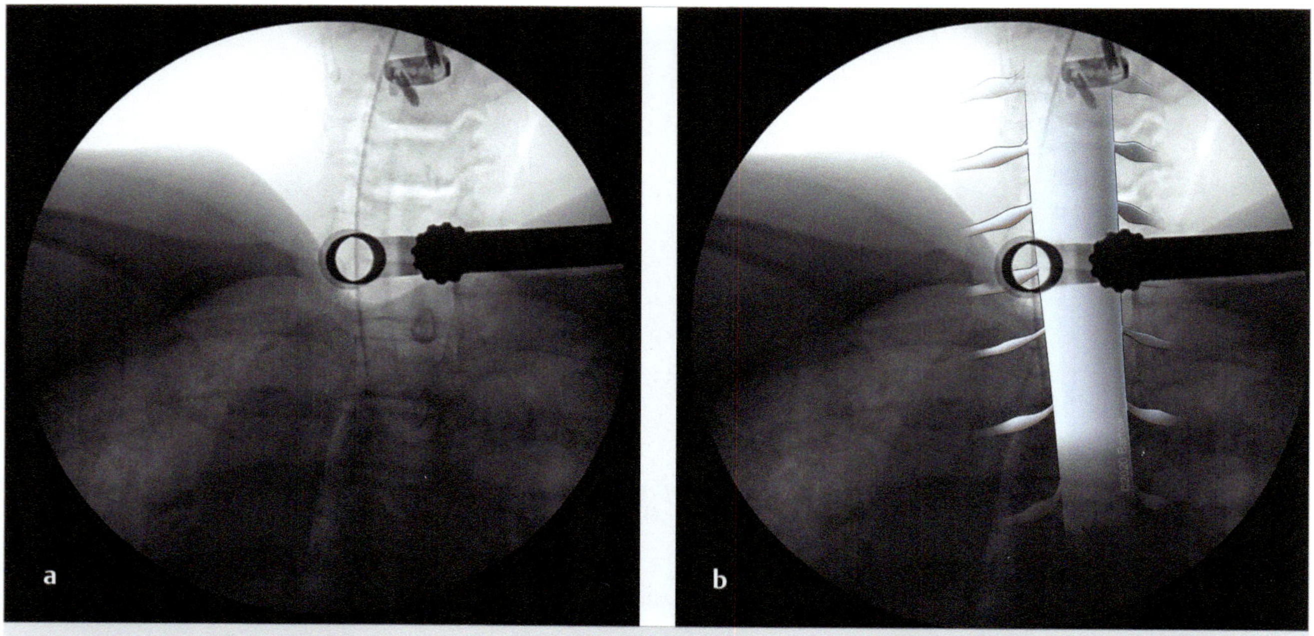

Fig. 7.26 Ideal position of the access port. (a) Oblique anteroposterior image in line with the trajectory of the access port (owl's eye view). This view is particularly helpful for determining the position of the field of view relative to the pedicle. (b) Superimposition of the neural anatomy over the fluoroscopic owl's eye view seen in a. Given the narrow field of view, reconstruction of the anatomy in the mind's eye is an essential component of working through the access port. This image captures what the surgeon needs to mentally reconstruct prior to beginning the exposure.

minimal access port back in position over the third dilator. I have now traversed that entire centimeter of paraspinal muscle without having had to resect a single strand of it. The minimal access port now has an optimal interface on the spine, with no muscle creeping into the field of view (▶ Fig. 7.26). Because I have repositioned the access port, I obtain a confirmatory lateral and AP fluoroscopic image before proceeding with the operation.

Iterative dilatation with direct visualization adds only a few minutes to the operation and two additional fluoroscopic images. It is a worthwhile investment in time that pays immediate dividends by decreasing the postoperative discomfort of the patient.

With an optimally placed minimal access port, I should be able to see the inferior articular process overriding the SAP, along with the rostral and caudal lamina. I begin to reconstruct the anatomy of the neural foramen in my mind's eye (Fig. 7.26). I envision where I anticipate the caudal pedicle to reside. Under ideal circumstances, the diameter of the access port should include the caudal pedicle at the inferior aspect of the exposure centered along the vertical axis of the diameter. ▶ Fig. 7.27 illustrates the ideal position with the face of a clock superimposed on the access port. The rostral pedicle resides at the 9 o'clock position, and the caudal pedicle at the 3 o'clock position. Achieving this positioning before I begin to drill the bone places the nerve root within the crosshairs of the minimal access port. The discovery phase of the operation is complete once the rostral and caudal lamina, the inferior articular process and the SAP come into view. It is imperative to ensure the optimal placement of the minimal access port at this point in the operation. If any adjustment of the minimal access port over the nerve root is needed, it should be done before drilling the articular processes and lamina to optimize the flow of the operation.

7.13 Decompression

7.13.1 Phase I: Drilling the Articular Processes and Lamina

A drill with a minimally invasive attachment is imperative, especially when working down a 14-mm-diameter access port. I prefer to use a diamond burr for drilling the bone in a posterior cervical foraminotomy for two reasons. First, a diamond burr remains stable over uneven surfaces. Therefore, regardless of the topography of the bone you are drilling, a diamond burr has less of a propensity to skip. Second, the bit itself becomes increasingly dull the closer it gets to the nerve root. The potential downside of a diamond burr is the heat that it generates. However, intermittent irrigation remedies that liability.

Drilling the lamina and the articular processes is a four-step process, again based on the quadrant system introduced in ▶ Fig. 7.23. An overview of the steps are as follows (Video 7.1):

- Step 1: Drill the inferior articular process of the rostral vertebra in quadrant I.
- Step 2: Drill the lateral aspect of the rostral lamina in quadrant II.
- Step 3: Drill the SAP in quadrant III.
- Step 4: Drill the lateral aspect of the caudal lamina in quadrant IV.

I begin with the superolateral aspect of the inferior articular process and drill this bone until I encounter the articular space of the facet joint (▶ Fig. 7.28a). From there, I extend my bone work medially into the rostral lamina (▶ Fig. 7.28b). I continue thinning the bone until I have identified the ligamentum flavum and perineural fat, which indicates that I have reached the

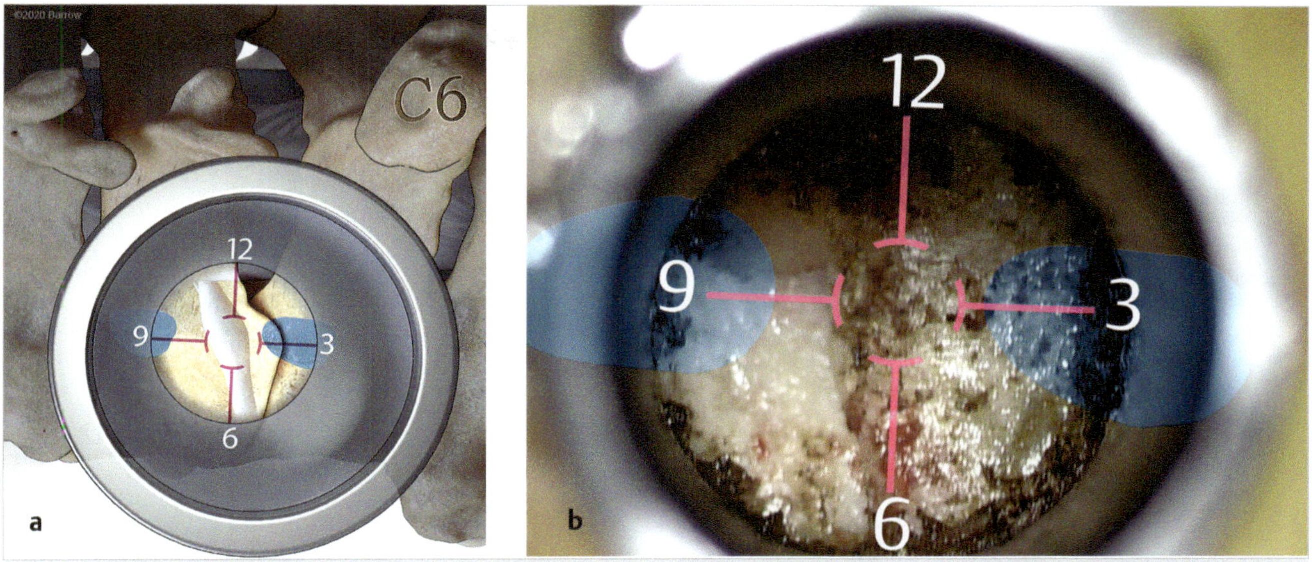

Fig. 7.27 Illustration of the ideal placement of a 14-mm-diameter minimal access port. **(a)** View of anatomy in surgical orientation through the access port over the top of the nerve root in a left C6 posterior cervical foraminotomy. The inferior aspect of the diameter should encompass the C6 pedicle (*shaded blue*) at the 3 o'clock position while the superior aspect of the access port should encompass the C5 pedicle (*shaded blue*) at the 9 o'clock position. With the access port in this position, a decompression from pedicle to pedicle can be reliably achieved. **(b)** Intraoperative photograph of a left C5–6 posterior cervical foraminotomy (surgeon's view) that corresponds to the illustration in **a**. The surgeon's mind must continue to reconstruct the anatomy at depth, "to see" the pedicles of C5 and C6 through the bone (*shaded blue*).

central canal. I continue to work medially rounding out the bone work toward the canal.

I completely drill the inferior articular process and rostral lamina within the field of view of the access port until the rising slope of the SAP comes fully into view. For the purpose of this example, the lamina and inferior articular process belong to C5 (▶ Fig. 7.28c). I use a straight curet to remove the articular cartilaginous layer of the SAP, and I expose the bone of the SAP of the rostral vertebra. I have found it important to remove the cartilaginous layer because it is an unfavorable surface for the interface with the tip of the drill. I then begin to drill the C6 SAP as shown in ▶ Fig. 7.28c. This bony structure requires the greatest amount of drilling in this operation. It is helpful to be mindful of the sloping geometry of the SAP when drilling. Keeping this geometry in mind allows for safe and efficient drilling of the SAP, which resides immediately over the cervical nerve root. The rostral-most aspect of the SAP is the thinnest and the closest to the foramen, whereas the caudal-most aspect of the SAP is the thickest (▶ Fig. 7.29).

As I drill the SAP, I am looking for a change in the color of the bone from a stark white to a pinkish hue. That subtle color change is an indication that I am coming increasingly closer to the nerve root and the epidural veins that surround it. Keeping the sloping geometry of the SAP in mind, I drill the SAP as evenly as possible. Invariably, an opening in the bone will occur, signaling that I must transition from the drill to a small forward-angled curet and Kerrison rongeur. I am beginning to unveil the nerve root. The fourth and final step in the drilling involves the lateral aspect of the lamina. I drill the laminar bone down to the thickness of a shrimp shell, which indicates that I have reached the lateral aspect of the central canal. I remove any remaining lamina and extend the foraminotomy to the central canal using a forward-angled curet and Kerrison rongeur.

En Bloc Removal of Medial SAP and Lamina

An alternative to drilling the entire SAP and lateral lamina in a sequential fashion is to perform an en bloc removal of the bone segment. ▶ Fig. 7.30 shows that by focusing the drilling on the perimeter of the access port, one can essentially combine steps 3 and 4. A well-positioned 14-mm access port demarcates the boundary of the bone work. Drilling at the point of disarticulation prevents the need to thin the entire SAP and lamina, which is time consuming. Instead, beginning in quadrant III and working toward quadrant IV, I drill to thin the perimeter of the SAP, which creates a breach large enough for a No. 1 Kerrison rongeur. Working from the breach, I carve a path through the thinned bone in the rostral direction, toward the rostral pedicle (C5 in this case) and, in the medial and caudal directions, toward the caudal pedicle (C6) and canal. I can then remove the entire section of the SAP and lateral lamina with a small forward-angled curet. The main advantage of this technique is efficiency. Instead of drilling the entire thickness and span of the SAP, which can take a considerable amount of time, focusing on the perimeter and disarticulating the SAP results in a significant time savings.

The bone work to enlarge the foramen is now complete, and I turn to my next objectives: confirmation of the rostral and caudal pedicles.

7.13.2 Phase II: Identifying the Rostral and Caudal Pedicles

When elevating the final leaflet of bone with a curet, I prefer to start laterally in the direction of the nerve root instead of medially in the direction of the central canal. I create an opening large enough for a No. 2 Kerrison rongeur using a combination

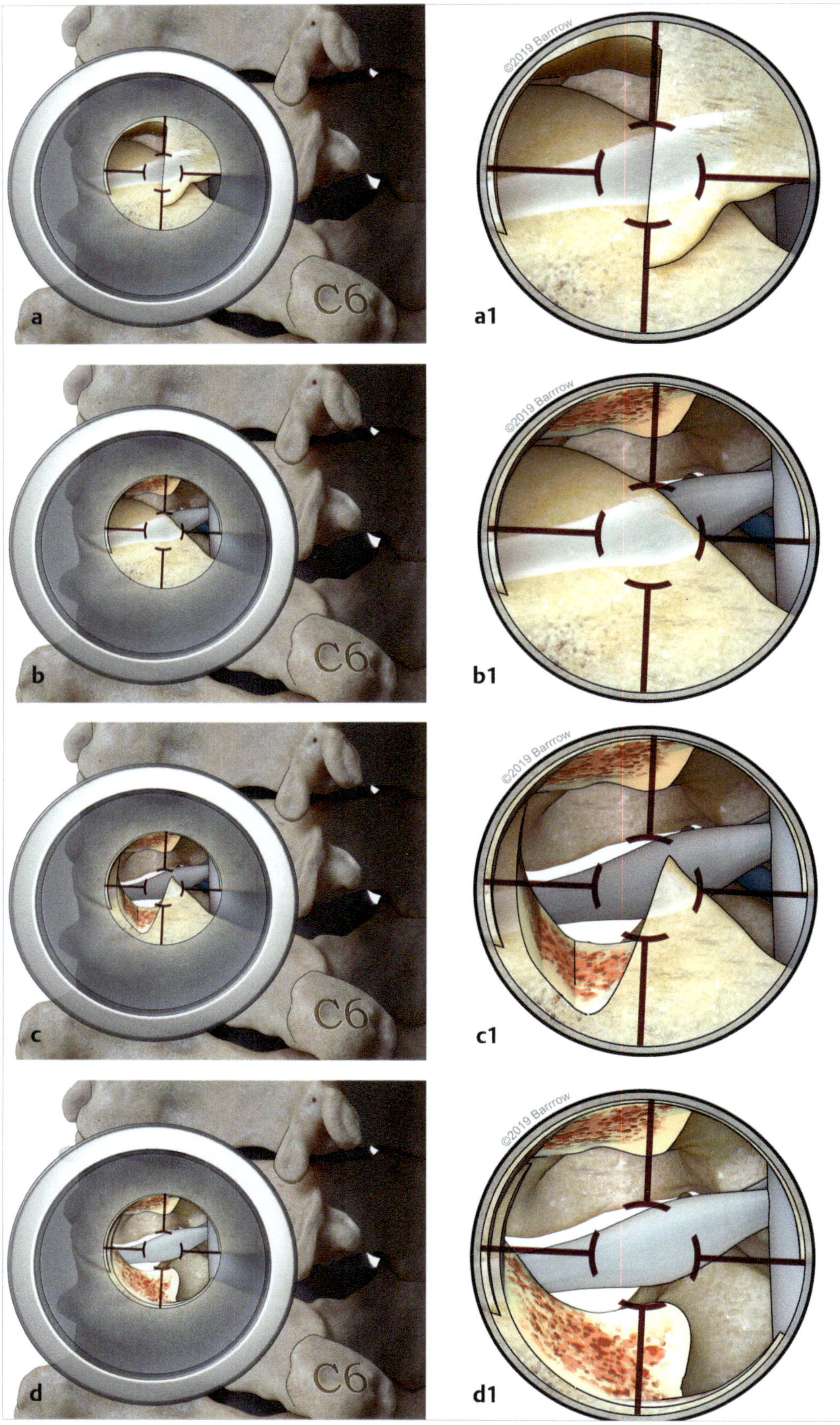

Fig. 7.28 Illustration demonstrating the sequence of drilling the bone in a posterior cervical foraminotomy. **(a)** Drilling begins in the superior and lateral aspect of the exposed inferior articular process and rostral lamina, in this case C5. **(a1)** Magnified microscopic view. **(b)** Once the superior articular process (SAP) is identified, the bone work is extended medially over the top of the lamina until the ligamentum flavum comes into view. At this point, the SAP of C6 comes clearly into view. The symptomatic nerve root is immediately behind the C6 SAP as shown. **(b1)** Magnified microscopic view. **(c)** The next target for drilling is the lateral aspect of the exposure, which is the SAP of the caudal vertebra, in this case C6. **(c1)** Magnified microscopic view. **(d)** The final part of the foramen to be drilled is the medial aspect of the rostral SAP and lamina, which in this case, belongs to C6. **(d1)** Magnified microscopic view.

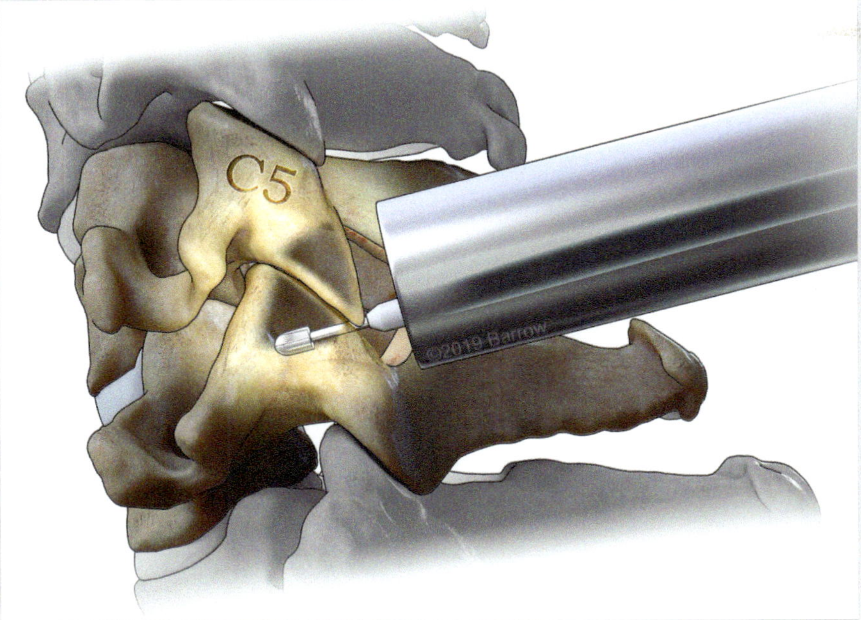

Fig. 7.29 Drilling the superior articular process (SAP). The illustration demonstrates the operation at step 3 for a C6 foraminotomy. The rostral lateral lamina and inferior articular process of C5 have been removed. It is important to keep in mind the sloping geometry of the SAP when drilling. The SAP is thinnest at its rostral aspect and thickest at its caudal aspect. The objective is to decompress the nerve from pedicle to pedicle. As such, the SAP must be drilled down to the caudal pedicle.

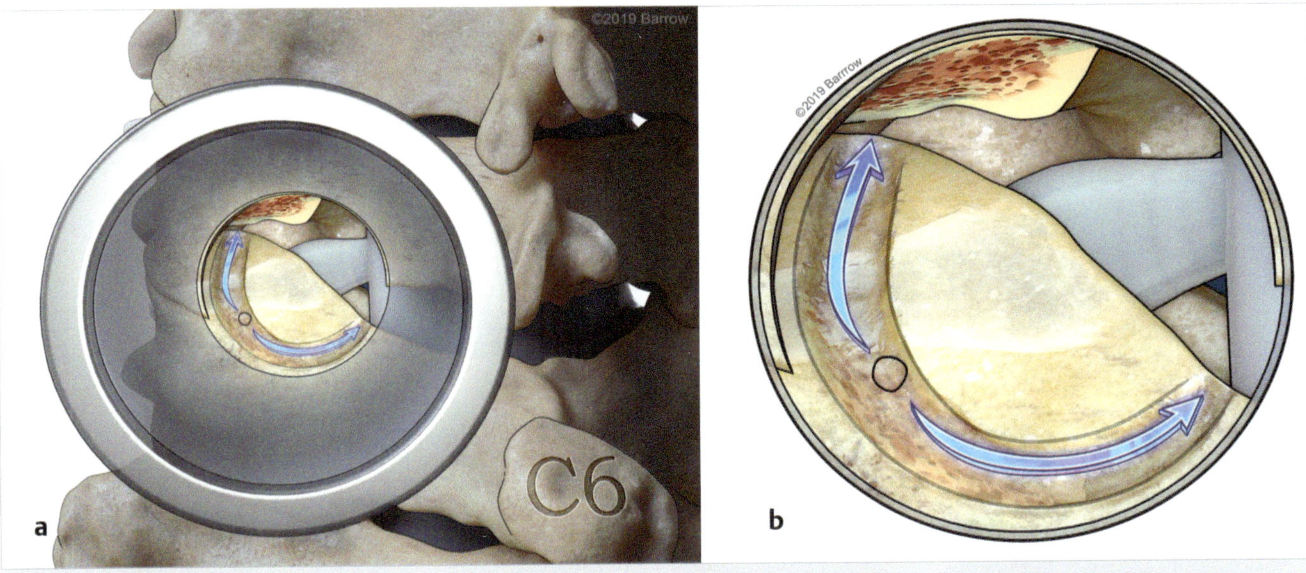

Fig. 7.30 Illustration of completing the removal of the superior articular process (SAP). **(a)** Surgical view of a left C5–6 posterior cervical foraminotomy. The inferior articular process and lateral lamina of C5 have been completely drilled. The SAP has been thinned, and a breach has been created. The use of a forward-angled curet ensures the safe passage of a No. 1 Kerrison rongeur, which is used to remove the remainder of the SAP. **(b)** Enlarged microscopic view through the 14-mm access port. The arrows indicate the path of the No. 1 Kerrison rongeur working around the perimeter of the bone from the breach.

of a small forward-angled curet and a No. 1 Kerrison rongeur. When the footplate of the No. 2 Kerrison fits into the preliminary bone work, I can safely and efficiently begin to enlarge the foraminotomy. As I do, it is no surprise to encounter vigorous epidural venous bleeding. The engorged epidural veins do not require much more than slight contact with an instrument to open up and flood the operative field. Liquid gel foam and a very light pressure with a ½ × ½-inch cottonoid is all that is needed to control the bleeding. You should anticipate that venous bleeding will recur throughout the remainder of the decompression. In short order, your scrub technician will become accustomed to the repetitive routine of liquid gel foam and cottonoid.

Once I have drilled all the bone on the SAP and removed any remaining bone with the Kerrison rongeur, I can identify and skeletonize the caudal pedicle. Skeletonizing the caudal pedicle ensures optimal decompression of the nerve root.

I have found the safest way to identify the pedicle is with a small right-angle nerve hook, which I place into the exposed foramen just under the nerve root and rotate downward. By probing in this manner, the pedicle becomes obvious. At times, I have found that I have actually already drilled the superior

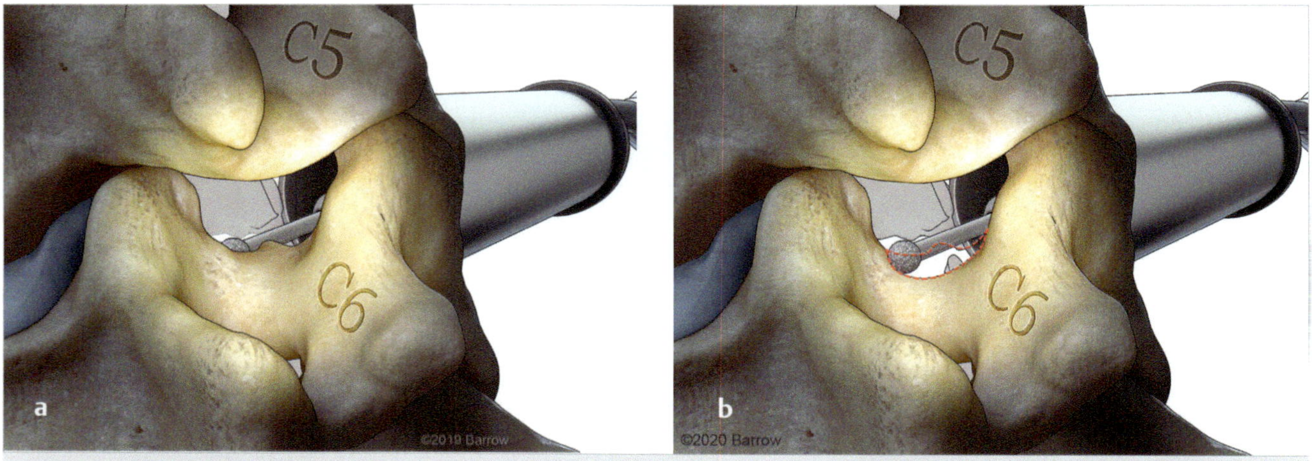

Fig. 7.31 Illustration of a left C6 pediculotomy. **(a)** View from the vantage point of looking back into the cervical foramen from anterior to posterior. The minimal access port is in position, and the drill bit can be seen beginning to work on the superior aspect of the C6 pedicle. **(b)** A completed C6 pediculotomy. The *red* line indicates the initial level of the pedicle.

aspect of the pedicle when I did my preliminary bone work. Other times, I find that there is more SAP bone to drill in order to reach the caudal pedicle. Because the nerve root to be decompressed courses over this pedicle, it is imperative to clearly identify it. Once I have a sense where the pedicle resides, I focus the remainder of my bone work on ensuring easy passage of a nerve hook medially to the pedicle, lateral to the pedicle and over the top of the pedicle.

Pediculotomy

In Webb and coworkers' 2002 article, Dr. John Jane describes the cervical pediculotomy technique in great detail.[12] A few years later, in Jagannathan and colleagues'[13] series of 162 posterior cervical foraminotomies, Dr. Jane mentions a cervical pediculotomy as an adjunct to a foraminotomy. Both articles are essential reading to achieve a mastery of this operation. Once I studied these publications, I incorporated Dr. Jane's indications and technique into the posterior cervical foraminotomies where the disc height was particularly collapsed. An inherent limitation to the posterior cervical foraminotomy is the inability to restore the disc height. Therefore, a collapsed disc space in a cervical segment has a compromised rostrocaudal dimension. However, removing the superior aspect of the pedicle creates a few precious additional millimeters for the nerve root and thereby adds to the rostrocaudal dimension. Because this pediculotomy may require additional drilling with the nerve root exposed, I take special precautions to protect it.

In those circumstances when I intend to remove the superior aspect of the cervical pedicle, I keep the lateral aspect of the lamina intact to protect the spinal cord. I place a small piece of thrombin-soaked gel foam over the top of the nerve root and then carefully drill down the superior aspect of the pedicle. Again, the diamond burr, which has been dulled from the drilling thus far in the operation, is ideal for this particular task. The inherent design of the burr, especially when it has been slightly dulled, makes it less likely to jump than a cutting burr might when it contacts an uneven edge. The focus is drilling within the pedicle itself to prevent any inadvertent contact with the surrounding neural structures. As the superior aspect of the pedicle is flattened so that it is flush with the vertebral body, a straight curet may be used to fold in the walls of the pedicle (▶ Fig. 7.31, ▶ Fig. 7.32).

The exposure of the caudal pedicle makes the boundaries of the neural foramen come into focus. The rostral pedicle is 12 mm away at most. To enlarge the foramen, I pass the footplate of a No. 2 Kerrison rongeur over the pedicle in the lateral direction and out the foramen. Then, I continue with the Kerrison medially to the pedicle to remove a few more millimeters of bone and further free the cervical nerve root. I now turn my attention to the rostral pedicle and ensure that I can palpate it with a nerve hook or small forward-angled curet. One potential pitfall of this procedure is leaving a part of the SAP within the superomedial aspect of the foramen. Working up to the rostral pedicle prevents leaving any residual SAP while simultaneously ensuring a pedicle-to-pedicle decompression.

The final bone work that I perform is medial. As mentioned in Section 7.13.1, Phase I: Drilling the Articular Processes and Lamina, even though the laminar bone over the lateral aspect of the spinal cord has been drilled, I have left it in place up to this point to protect the spinal cord during decompression of the nerve root. However, before completing the operation, it is imperative to ensure that there is no laminar bone on top of the nerve root as it comes off the spinal cord. The mistakes that I made early in my career with this procedure were caused by not taking the decompression medially enough. Any laminar bone left on top of the nerve root essentially pins an otherwise decompressed nerve root at the point of the residual lamina. Thus, removing the lateral aspect of the rostral and caudal lamina exposes the lateral aspect of the spinal cord and thereby completes the decompression (▶ Fig. 7.33).

Final Systems Check

As part of a final systems check, I ensure that I have identified the boundaries of the foramen, specifically the rostral and caudal pedicles and the lateral boundary of the canal. I further ensure that a nerve hook can freely pass medially and laterally

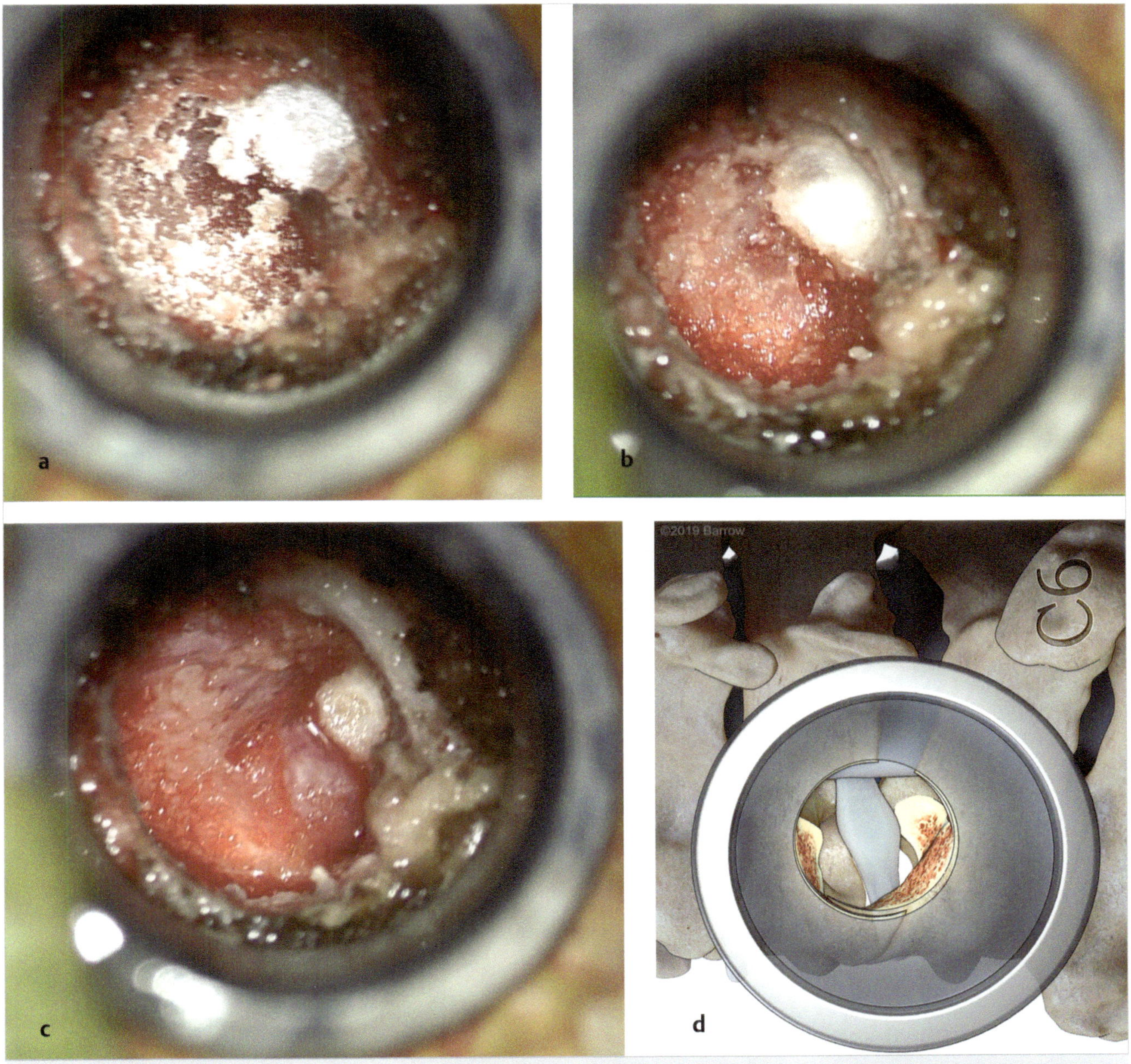

Fig. 7.32 Pediculotomy of the caudal pedicle in a C6 foraminotomy. Surgical view of a left C6 foraminotomy where the superior aspect of the C6 pedicle is flattened flush with the C6 vertebral body to increase the rostrocaudal dimension of the foramen by a few millimeters. **(a)** Intraoperative photograph showing preliminary drilling of the C6 pedicle. **(b)** Drilling within the pedicle is the safest method of flattening the pedicle while minimizing risk to the nerve root. **(c)** A completed posterior cervical foraminotomy with a pediculotomy. The pedicle has been flattened flush with the vertebral body. The C6 nerve root has been decompressed from pedicle to pedicle. **(d)** An illustration of a pediculotomy performed at C6.

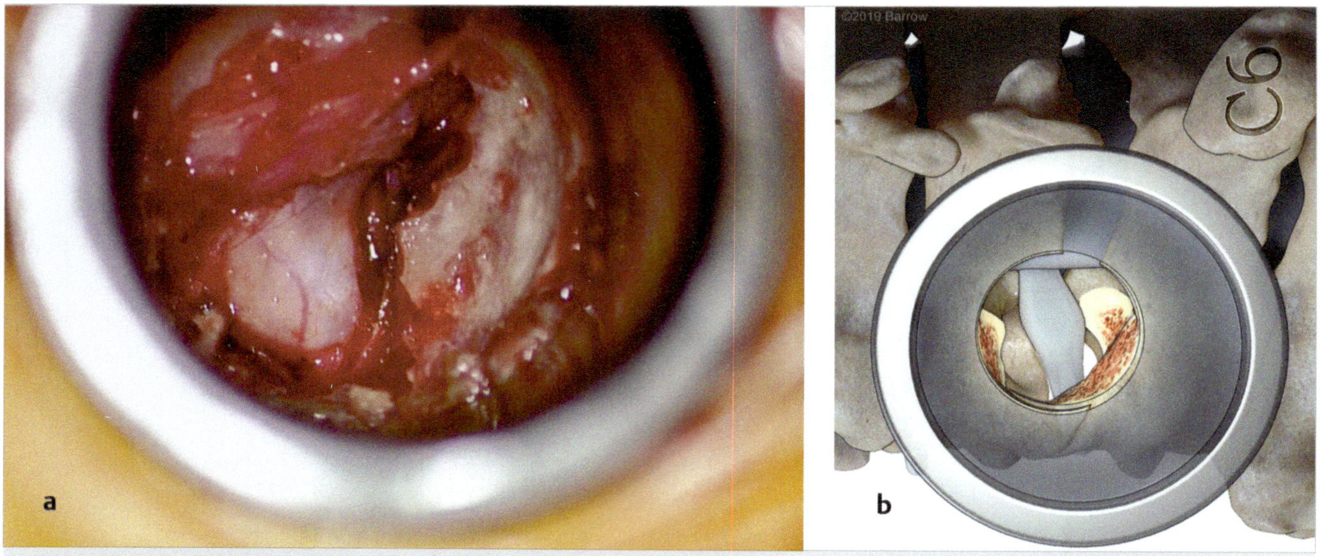

Fig. 7.33 A completed posterior cervical foraminotomy. **(a)** Intraoperative photograph showing complete decompression of the cervical nerve root from pedicle to pedicle. The nerve was revealed to remove a disc herniation. The ligamentum flavum was removed up to the shoulder of the nerve root. **(b)** Illustration of the decompression accomplished in the intraoperative photograph.

to the pedicle. My preference is to pass a No. 2 Kerrison medially to the pedicle parallel to the canal and laterally to the rostral and caudal pedicles. With the systems check complete, I have accomplished the goals of the operation.

7.14 Posterior Cervical Microdiscectomy

The following section covers a foraminotomy for the purposes of performing a microdiscectomy. When a patient has a lateral disc herniation in the absence of any significant spondylosis, the operation of choice is a posterior cervical foraminotomy with discectomy. It eliminates any concern for adjacent segment degeneration, risk of pseudarthrosis and implant-associated issues. The younger the patient, the truer this statement becomes.

Although the vast majority of the content in the preceding pages applies to both a microdiscectomy and foraminal stenosis, there are some subtle modifications that I make when the primary intent is to remove a soft disc herniation. The first modification is to center the minimal access port immediately over the disc herniation instead of the pedicle. At times, a disc herniation can be medial to the pedicle, in line with the pedicle or lateral to the pedicle. The center of the access port, or rather the cross hairs, should be focused on the disc herniation instead of the pedicle (▶ Fig. 7.34). Thus, for microdiscectomies, the long axis of the diameter of the tubular retractor should be in line with the disc herniation instead of the pedicle.

For disc herniations medial to the pedicle, more bone work needs to be done medial to the pedicle, and less bone work needs to be done lateral to the pedicle. However, it is still helpful to identify the boundaries of the neural foramen and feel confident with the course of the nerve root. For posterior cervical microdiscectomies, partial pediculotomies (Section 7.13.2, Phase II: Identifying the Rostral and Caudal Pedicles) are tremendously helpful. Removing the superior and medial aspects of the pedicle minimizes any traction on the nerve root and provides a corridor to the disc without any significant contact with the spinal cord.[12]

I perform a medial laminoforaminotomy to visualize the lateral dura of the spinal cord. Removal of the ligamentum flavum is another distinction from a simple cervical foraminotomy. Elevating the fibers of the ligamentum flavum unveils the epidural veins on top of the nerve root and spinal cord. I have found the epidural veins to be especially prominent at the axilla of the nerve root and spinal cord. Addressing these veins requires equal parts bipolar cautery, liquid hemostatic foam and patience. Achieving hemostasis allows me to identify the dura over the spinal cord and the nerve root. The disc herniation then becomes evident. At times, the nerve root can be distorted because of the disc herniation in front of it. The nerve root can also be displaced in the rostral direction by the disc herniation. If the anatomy is not entirely clear, it is a good investment in time to extend the bone work and the exposure until the anatomy lies clearly before you. The caudal pedicle is the guiding North Star of this operation. Any disorientation can be quickly dispelled by identifying the pedicle and confirming the anatomy from there.

A right-angle nerve hook is the ideal instrument for mobilizing the nerve root for the purposes of a discectomy. Sliding the nerve hook alongside the pedicle and sweeping it beneath the nerve root establishes a plane between the nerve root and the disc herniation. I prefer to establish a plane beneath the nerve root with the right-angle nerve hook from the medial border of the pedicle to the lateral border. Again, these maneuvers can be met with significant epidural bleeding, which should be countered with liquid hemostatic foam, micro cottonoids and light pressure applied with the suction tip. I develop a plane between the nerve root and the disc herniation, so I can begin to retract

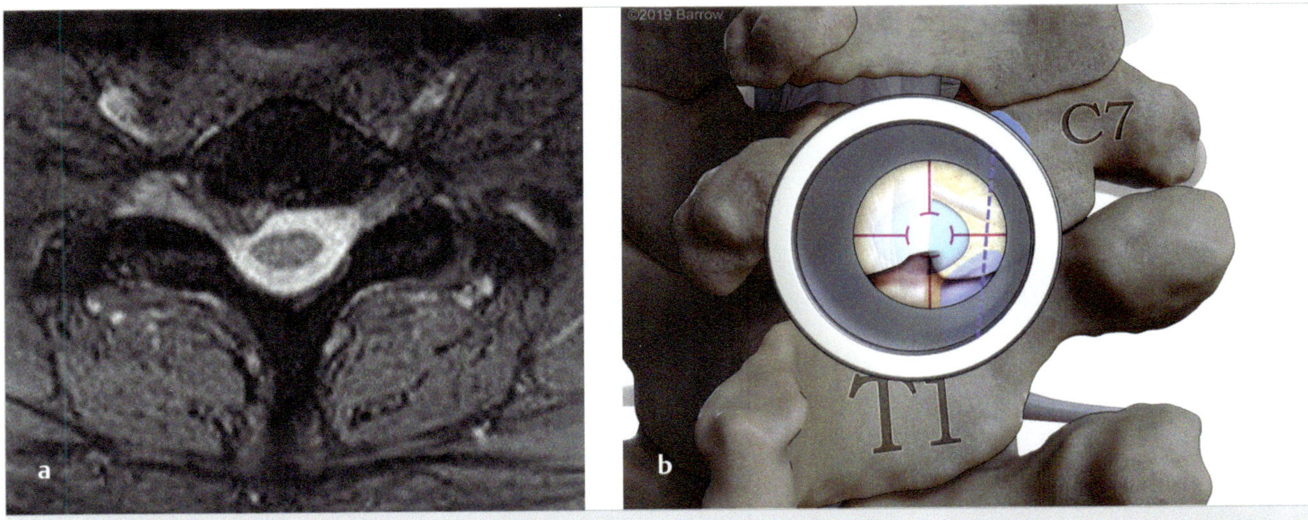

Fig. 7.34 Posterior cervical foraminotomy with discectomy. **(a)** Axial T2-weighted magnetic resonance imaging of the cervical spine showing a disc herniation at C7–T1. The disc herniation in this particular case is medial to the pedicle. Therefore, the minimal access port needs to be medial to the pedicle as well. **(b)** The illustration demonstrates the cross hairs of the minimal access port over the disc herniation instead of the pedicle (denoted in *blue*).

the nerve root in the rostral direction and further expose the disc herniation. At times, the disc is a free fragment and is easily removed with a micropituitary rongeur. Other times, it is a contained fragment, and I will need a No. 11 blade to open the annulus to retrieve it (Video 7.1).

Wielding a No. 11 blade through a 14-mm access port with the nerve root and spinal cord exposed has its potential challenges. Similar to a lumbar microdiscectomy, it is imperative to distinctly identify the nerve root and spinal cord. Once these two structures are unequivocally identified, I retract the nerve root in the rostral direction with either the right-angle nerve hook or small Penfield dissector (▶ Fig. 7.35). I never apply traction to the spinal cord, nor is any traction necessary because even a disc herniation medial to the pedicle is still lateral to the spinal cord. Retracting the nerve root in the rostral direction brings the disc herniation into clear view and keeps the nerve root out of harm's way. If a free disc fragment does not unveil itself, I will use a No. 11 blade to make a small annulotomy. I then begin to deliver the disc herniation through the annulotomy with either a right-angle nerve hook or a micropituitary rongeur. In my experience, the discectomy work in the posterior cervical spine is analogous to that of a lumbar microdiscectomy. At times I find myself retrieving one large satisfying fragment of the herniation with a pituitary rongeur and, thus, find the nerve root completely decompressed. Other times, I find myself endlessly plucking impossibly small fragments of disc to accomplish the decompression. Regardless of the size of the fragment or fragments removed, I continue with the discectomy until the nerve root rests within the foramen without any displacement.

7.15 Systems Check

A final systems check ensures adequate decompression of the nerve root. Similar to what I presented in Chapter 2, I zoom out to the lowest magnification of the microscope, step away from the operative field and take a moment to reexamine the sagittal and axial MRIs. I then compare my review of the images in my mind with what I saw during surgery. I return to the operative field, zoom back in and examine the extent of the decompression. I pass the right-angle nerve hook over the top of the nerve root, beneath the nerve root and medial and lateral to the pedicle. I ensure that I have not left a fragment of disc behind. The absence of any persistent compression of the nerve root signals the conclusion of the operation.

7.16 Closure

When I remove the minimal access port, I do so slowly, with a right-angled bipolar in one hand and suction in the other. I am preparing for a potential deluge. More often than not, there are small bleeding vessels that need nothing more than a touch of the cautery tip. After a few bursts of cautery, the minimal access port is out, and there is not so much as one drop of blood coming from the wound.

On occasion, vigorous bleeding may be encountered, and thus, it is essential to be prepared for it. I ask my assistant to loosen the table-mounted arm and slowly pull the minimal access port upward. The vigorous bleeding is typically due to a small arterial branch to the muscle that may have been divided during the dilatation. When this situation occurs, it is unmistakable. Should it happen, it is imperative to identify both sides of the vessel and cauterize them. If in fact it is an arterial branch to the muscle, liquid hemostatic foam and tamponade will not work to stop the bleeding. Pulling the tubular retractor out too quickly can complicate matters because it is difficult to slip the access port back into its previous track amidst the bleeding. The most proficient way to address the bleeding is to slowly remove the access port in a controlled manner, stopping each time bleeding is encountered to achieve hemostasis. Simply securing the retractor in its current position halts the bleeding and provides time to identify and cauterize the bleeding vessel.

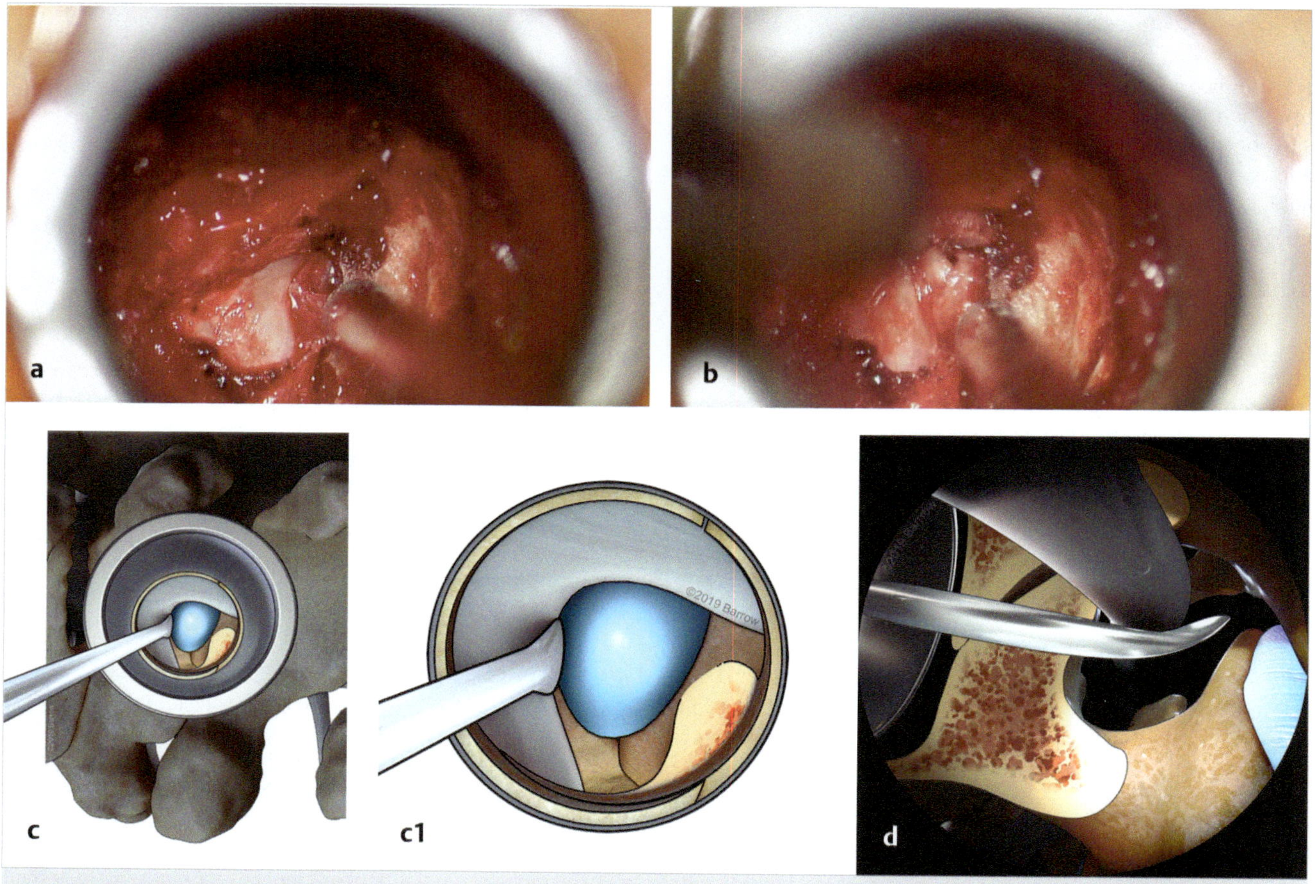

Fig. 7.35 Posterior cervical microdiscectomy. **(a)** Intraoperative photograph showing a C7–T1 microdiscectomy. The nerve root has been exposed and the T1 pedicle has been flattened to facilitate access to the disc space. A small suction tip hovers over the pedicle of T1. **(b)** Intraoperative photograph showing retraction of the nerve root and exposure of the disc extrusion. The epidural veins have been cauterized, the cervical nerve root has been completely exposed and the interface between the nerve root and disc extrusion is defined. A small Penfield dissector can then be used to retract the nerve root in the rostral direction to reveal the disc extrusion. A free fragment is readily retrieved at this point whereas a contained fragment requires an annulotomy with a No. 11 blade. **(c)** An illustration of the photograph in **b** showing the bone work centralized over the top of the disc herniation and the retraction of the nerve root. **(c1)** Magnified microscopic view. **(d)** A view from within the cervical canal looking out of the cervical foramen with the nerve root retracted. This illustration demonstrates how removal of the superior aspect of the pedicle creates a larger working channel to complete the microdiscectomy.

As I remove the access port, I sometimes encounter a vein that causes torrential bleeding. At least, it appears to be so under the operating microscope. The process of dilating through the muscle has the capacity to stretch a vein until it tears. You will not recognize the disruption of the vein initially because the minimal access port will tamponade the bleeding. It is only after you remove the access port that the bleeding occurs. This possibility is all the more reason to remove the minimal access port slowly, much slower than removing the equivalent access port in the lumbar spine surgery. Removing the minimal access port too quickly closes the door on the opportunity to clearly identify and cauterize a torn vein. In my experience, when bleeding is from a vein, it is seldom divided in half like arterial branches, which would be a straightforward situation to handle with bipolar cautery sealing either end. Instead, I have found that the side of the vein tends to be interrupted, which is a more challenging scenario to handle. With a suction tip in one hand and a right angle bipolar in the other, I take the time to identify the course of the vein and cauterize the length of it. Intermittently putting upward pressure on the minimal access port unveils the bleeding and helps identify the vein. Blindly cauterizing along the previous tract of the access port is an exercise in futility.

I remove the minimal access port and then infiltrate the incision once again with a lidocaine–bupivacaine mixture. I use size 0 polyglactin 910 (Vicryl, Ethicon US, LLC, Somerville, NJ) on a UR-6 needle to close the fascia. At best, two or three sutures are feasible within a 16-mm incision. I then use 2.0 polyglactin on an X-1 needle to bring together the subcutaneous tissue and, if needed, 4.0 polyglactin on an RB-1 needle to bring together the skin edges. I apply a liquid adhesive and wound-closure adhesive strips, a small Telfa bandage (KPR US, LLC, Dublin, OH) and a lidocaine dressing over the wound. I position the patient supine on a gurney, remove the skull clamp and infiltrate the pin sites with local anesthetic.

7.17 Postoperative Course

A vast majority of patients go home an hour or so after the operation. Most patients report more discomfort from the pin sites on their heads than from the incision in their necks. In addition to pain medication, muscle relaxants are a valuable adjunct. I obtain flexion, extension, AP and lateral radiographs at the first postoperative visit to rule out instability and to evaluate the foraminotomy (▶ Fig. 7.36). If the patient is asymptomatic, I release them to activity as tolerated. I impose no restrictions or limitations after 30 days, even in the most active of patients. After all, I am not awaiting an arthrodesis to form across a segment or incorporation of bone into the interface of an arthroplasty device. In the rare circumstance of persistent radicular symptoms, further imaging is needed and consideration of an anterior approach with fusion or arthroplasty is warranted. Admittedly, early in my learning curve, there were patients who required additional anterior surgery for persistent radicular symptoms after what I considered to be a successful foraminotomy. Failure is always the best teacher, and it was listening to these patients and studying the postoperative imaging that gave me an opportunity to evaluate and then improve my technique. The multiplanar images on a CT scan in particular were of tremendous value. The coronal and sagittal reconstructions invariably revealed suboptimal bone work. More often than not, I would find a residual medial component of the SAP within the foramen or an incomplete pedicle-to-pedicle decompression. These cases unveiled my blind spots, improved my systems checks and allowed me to evolve my technique. In my current practice, after a pedicle-to-pedicle decompression in a well-selected patient, persistent symptoms are exceedingly rare.

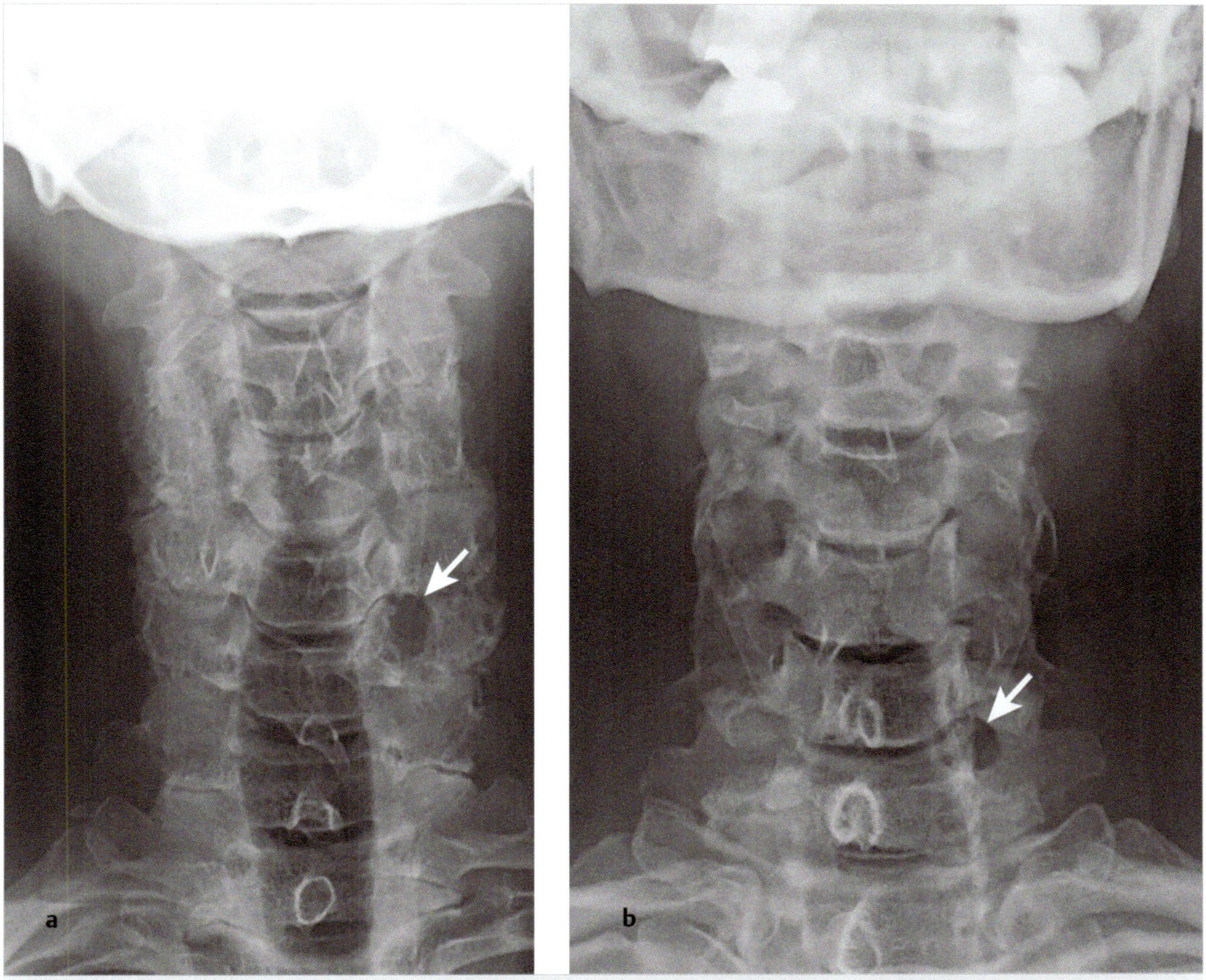

Fig. 7.36 Postoperative images of posterior cervical foraminotomies. **(a)** Postoperative anteroposterior (AP) radiograph of a patient who presented with a left C6 radiculopathy. At the time of presentation, he requested arthroplasty and was adamantly opposed to a fusion. Given the degree of facet arthropathy seen on AP, he was not a candidate for arthroplasty. If an anterior approach was selected, it would have required a fusion. A pedicle-to-pedicle foraminotomy as seen on the radiograph *(arrow)* completely alleviated his radiculopathy. **(b)** Postoperative AP radiograph of a police officer who underwent a left C7 foraminotomy *(arrow)*. He returned to unrestricted, full duty within 3 weeks of surgery.

7.18 Illustrative Cases

The following section presents various case illustrations where the minimally invasive posterior cervical foraminotomy was the operation of choice for the management of a unilateral radiculopathy in a variety of clinical circumstances. I present the clinical history, radiologic studies and neurologic examination along with the rationale for selecting a posterior over an anterior approach.

7.18.1 Case Illustration 1: Nonadjacent Segment Radiculopathy after a Two-Level Fusion

Clinical History

A 59-year-old left-hand–dominant retired firefighter presented with a 6-week history of left radicular arm pain. The patient had surgical history significant for an uncomplicated C3–4 and C4–5 ACDF 11 years prior with complete resolution of symptoms. The patient had been referred to physical therapy and had undergone chiropractic manipulations, cervical traction and epidural injection therapy without resolution of his symptoms. At the time of presentation, the patient had a neck disability index (NDI) of 46 and a visual analog scale (VAS) arm score of 65 mm.

Neurologic Examination

The patient demonstrated significant atrophy of the left triceps on visual inspection. A motor examination by confrontation demonstrated 4-/5 strength in the left triceps compared to 5/5 on the right. The remaining muscle groups in the left and the right were 5/5. Lower extremity reflexes were normal, but upper extremity reflexes were blunted. The patient had a positive Spurling sign on the left and positive shoulder abduction sign. The sensory examination was intact for pinprick and light touch. Electromyelography confirmed a left C7 radiculopathy.

Radiologic Studies

AP and lateral radiographs showed the cervical plate in position from C3 to C5 (▶ Fig. 7.37). Mild spondylosis was present at C5–6 and C6–7.

MRI of the cervical spine (▶ Fig. 7.38) showed a lateral disc osteophyte complex at C6–7 compressing the left C7 nerve root. There was no central stenosis or foraminal stenosis at C5–6.

Surgical Decision Making

A unilateral symptomatic nerve compression syndrome at a nonadjacent segment presents a unique circumstance when considering the optimal surgical strategy for this patient. An anterior approach at C6–7 with either arthrodesis or arthroplasty is a reliable option that would adequately address the patient's symptoms. However, it would be problematic to fuse a segment and strand the C5–6 segment in between two moment arms (a C3–5 arthrodesis and C6–7 arthrodesis). The patient has mild spondylosis, making arthroplasty an option. Motion preservation would nullify the concern of fusing a segment nonadjacent to a fusion, but at 59 years of age, the patient is at the upper age limit of an ideal arthroplasty candidate. The absence of spinal cord compression and unilateral symptoms is

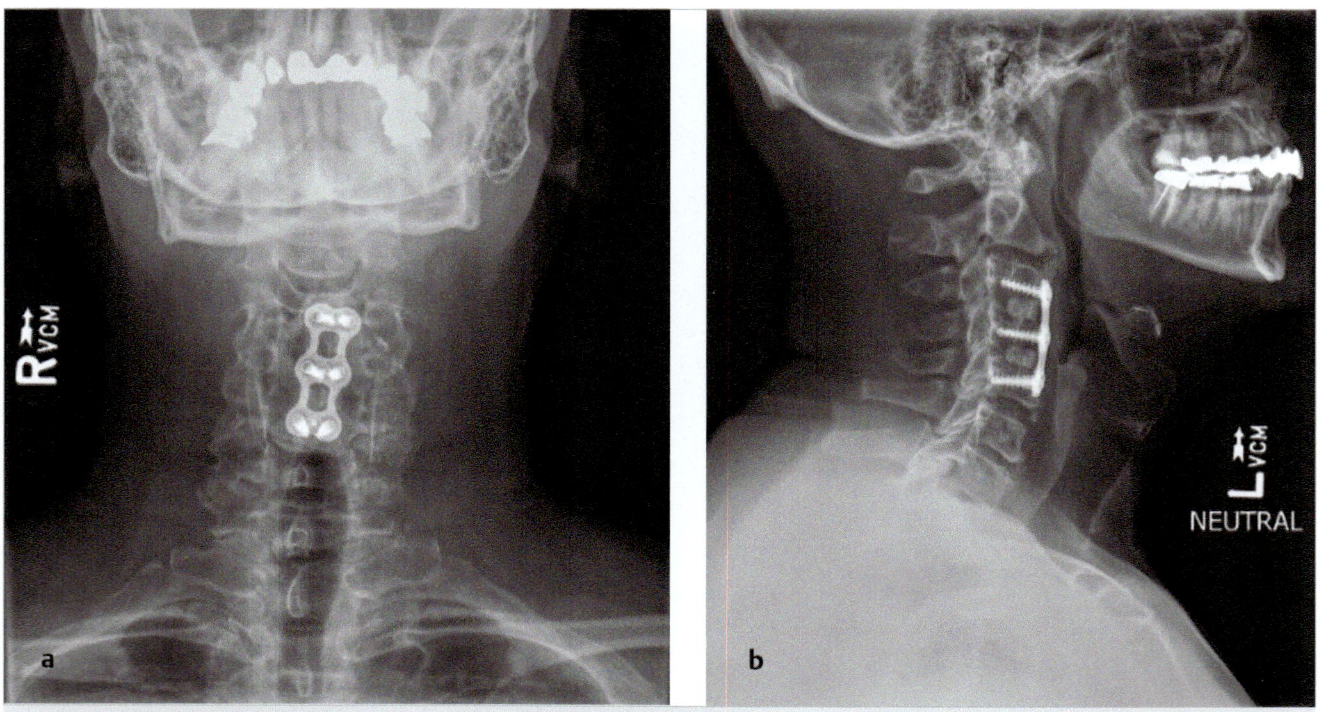

Fig. 7.37 Radiographs showing cervical radiculopathy after cervical fusion at a nonadjacent segment. **(a)** Lateral and **(b)** anteroposterior studies show a C3–4, C4–5 instrumented cervical fusion. The patient presented with a left C7 radiculopathy secondary to a disc–osteophyte complex at the C6–7 segment.

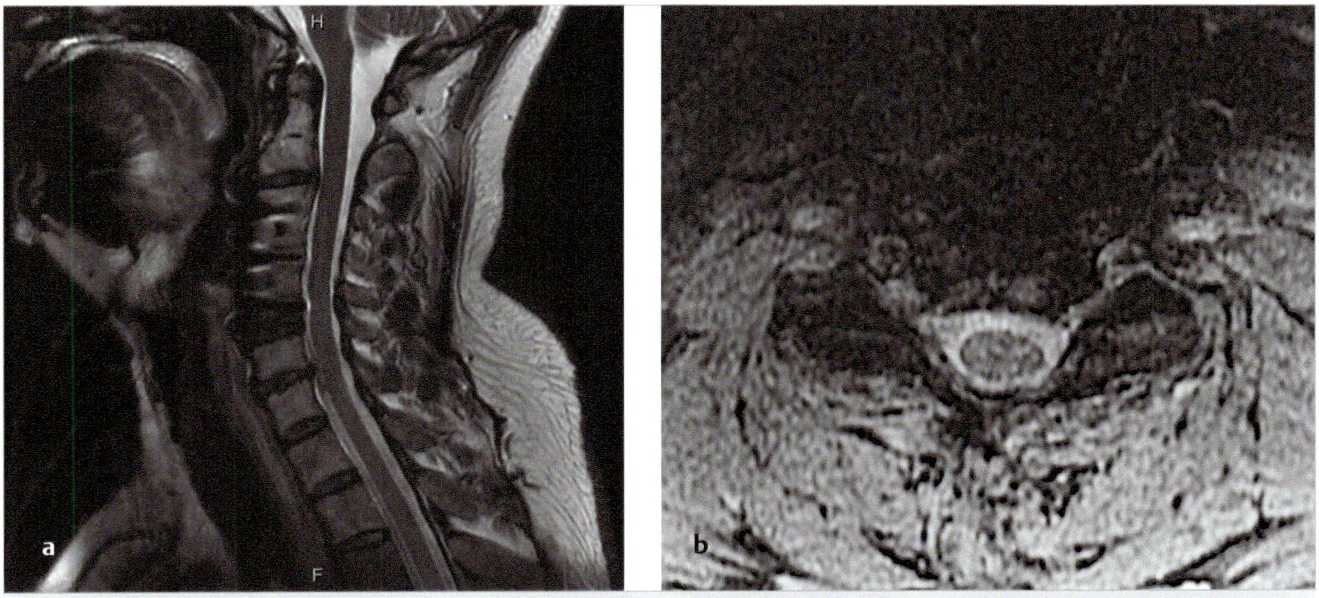

Fig. 7.38 Magnetic resonance imaging (MRI) showing cervical radiculopathy at a nonadjacent segment. **(a)** Sagittal T2-weighted MRI of the cervical spine shows the expected artifact of the instrumentation at C3–4 and C4–5. The C5–6 segment does not demonstrate any significant degeneration. There is no central stenosis at the C5–6 level or neural foraminal compromise. At C6–7, a disc–osteophyte complex eccentric to the left is compressing the C7 nerve root. **(b)** Axial T2-weighted MRI of the C6–7 segment shows foraminal compromise of the left C7 neural foramen.

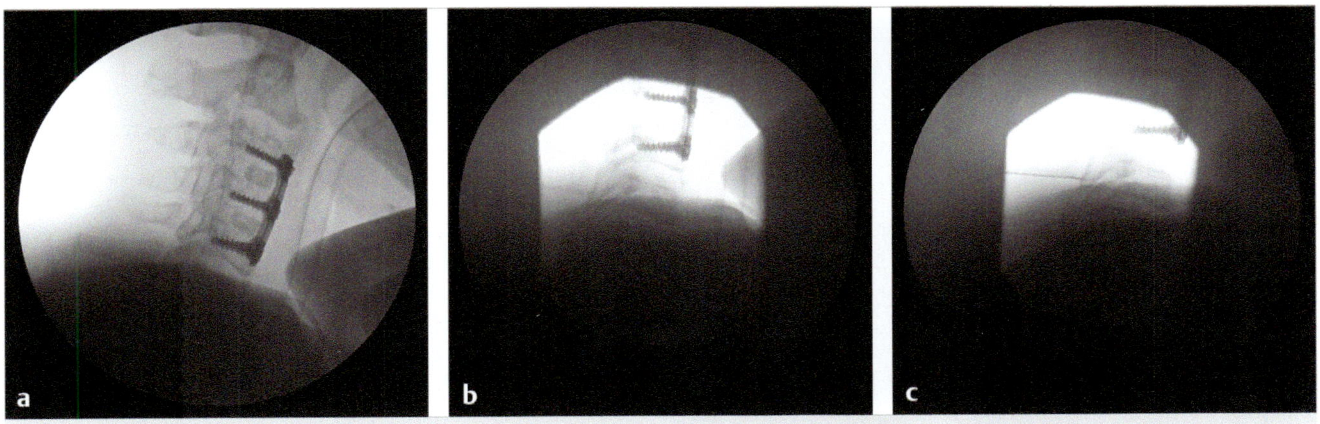

Fig. 7.39 Fluoroscopic sequence for localization of a C7 posterior cervical foraminotomy. **(a)** Lateral fluoroscopic image demonstrating an anterior cervical plate spanning C3–C5. Visualization of the symptomatic C6–7 level requires collimation. The inferior aspect of the plate assists in confirmation of the level. **(b)** Lateral fluoroscopic image with the C6–7 level in ideal alignment. **(c)** Confirmation of the C6–7 level to confirm incision and trajectory. In this image, the spinal needle is in contact with the inferior articular process, which is the target of the first dilator.

especially well suited to a posterior cervical foraminotomy. Although it is important to inform the patient that this procedure does not prevent further degeneration from occurring and that additional surgery from an anterior approach may eventually become necessary, it will alleviate the nerve root compression syndrome without the need for instrumentation, implants or arthrodesis. I felt that the ideal management for this patient, given the unique anatomical circumstances in this case, would be a minimally invasive motion-preserving posterior cervical foraminotomy.

Surgical Technique

The patient was positioned prone on chest rolls with his head stabilized in a skull clamp. With the bed in reverse Trendelenburg position and the shoulders taped down to optimize visualization of the C6–7 level, the incision was planned by using a Kelly clamp on the skin 1.5 cm off the midline and 16 mm in length. After the patient was prepped and draped, a 20-gauge spinal needle confirmed the planned incision and trajectory (▶ Fig. 7.39).

Working from the head of the bed, I made the incision as planned and dissected down to the posterior cervical fascia. I used cautery to divide the fascia and passed the first dilator onto the inferior articular process of C6, which I confirmed with a lateral fluoroscopic image. I proceeded with sequential dilatation to a 14-mm diameter and secured the minimal access port parallel to the disc space. I confirmed the ideal placement of the minimal access port on AP, lateral and owl's eye views of the fluoroscopic images before bringing in the operating microscope (▶ Fig. 7.40).

The foraminotomy was performed using the four-step method described in Section 7.13.1, Phase I: Drilling the Articular Processes and Lamina. Upon completion of the bone work, a pedicle-to-pedicle decompression was confirmed, and the decompression was extended until a No. 2 Kerrison rongeur could be passed both lateral and medial to the C7 pedicle.

Postoperative Course

The patient was discharged 1.5 hours after the surgery with significant relief in his symptoms. At the 1-month follow-up visit,

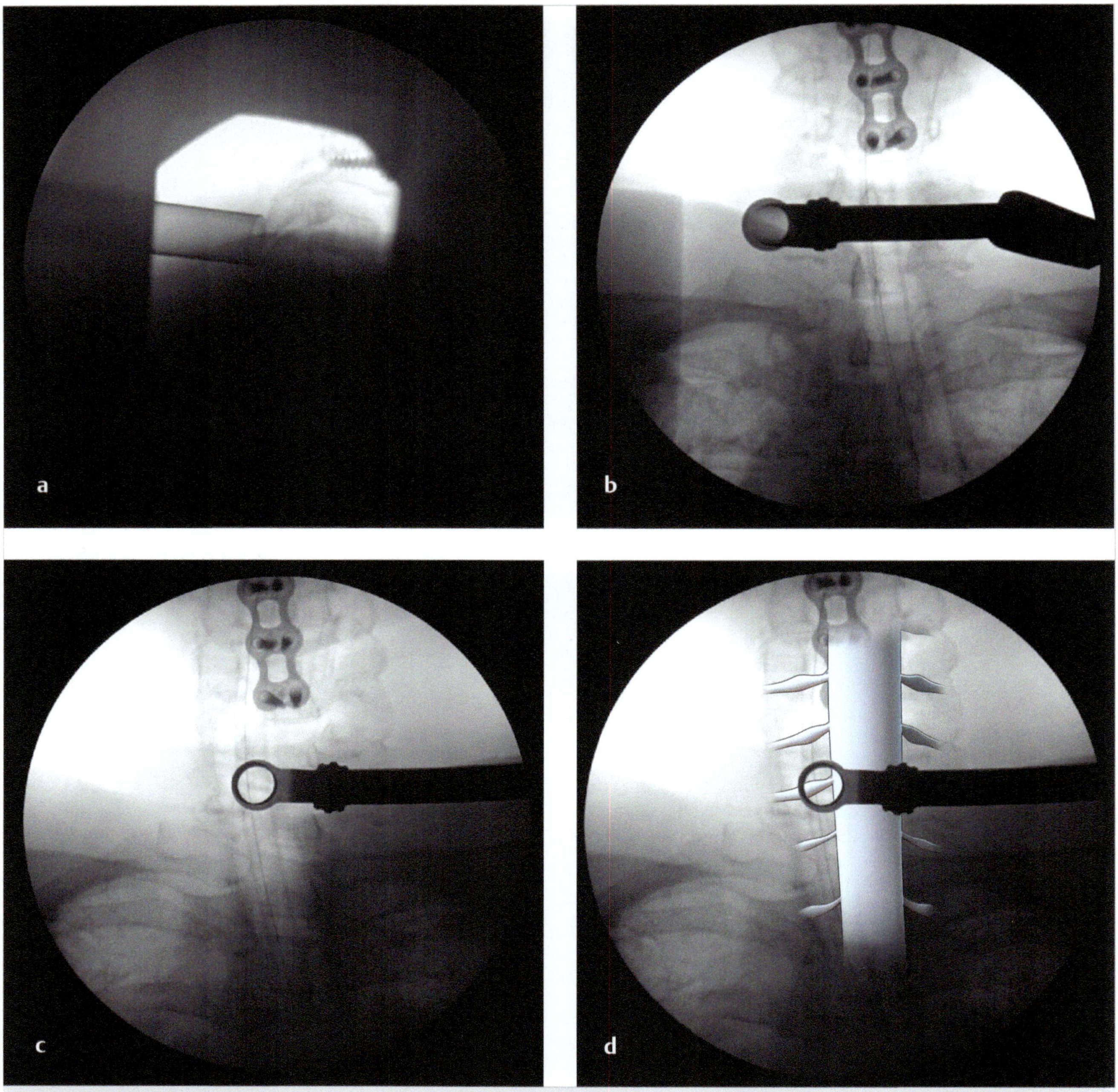

Fig. 7.40 Securing the access port in a left C7 posterior cervical foraminotomy. **(a)** Lateral fluoroscopic image showing a 14-mm × 6-cm minimal access port in close apposition to the inferior articular process of C6 after a second dilatation as described in Section 7.12, Iterative Dilatation with Direct Visualization. **(b)** Anteroposterior fluoroscopic image with the access port over the top of the C6–7 segment. **(c)** Owl's eye view demonstrating the access port with the C7 pedicle and nerve root in the field of view. **(d)** Superimposition of the neural structures onto the fluoroscopic image in **c.**

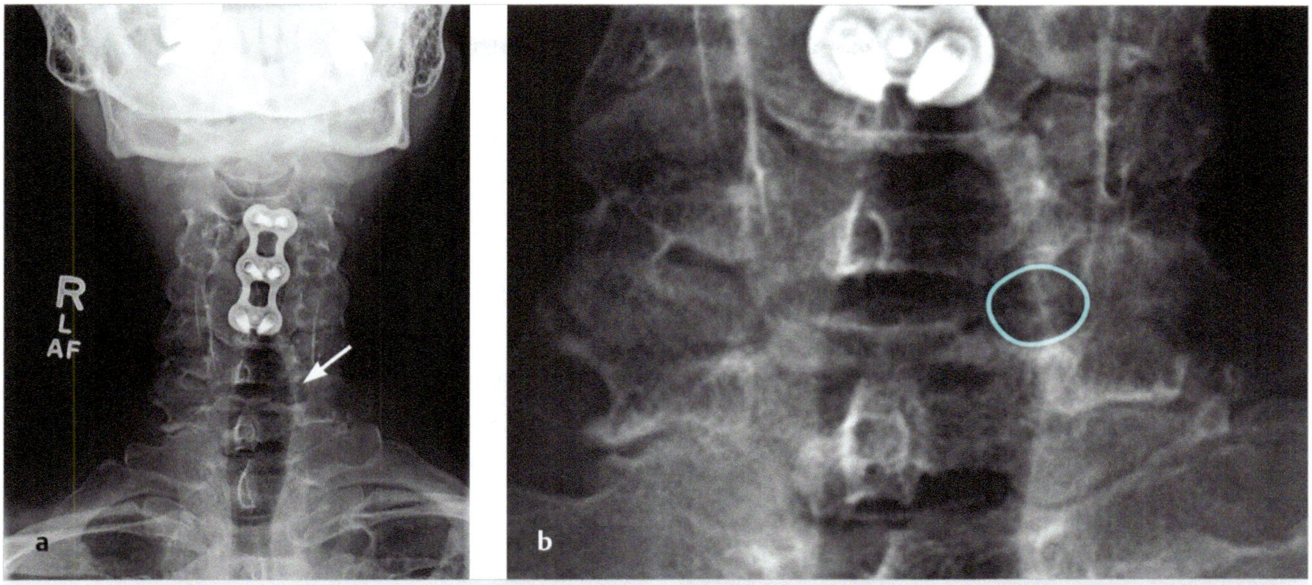

Fig. 7.41 Postoperative C7 posterior cervical foraminotomy. **(a)** Anteroposterior (AP) radiograph showing the posterior cervical foraminotomy at C7 on the left (*arrow*). **(b)** Magnified AP view of foraminotomy shown in **a** (*turquoise circle*).

he reported an NDI of 7 (decreased from 46) and a VAS (arm) score of 10 mm (decreased from 65). He was off all narcotic pain medication. He reported taking only an occasional anti-inflammatory medication. The postoperative AP radiographic image shows the foraminotomy at C7 on the left. No instability on flexion–extension radiographic studies was noted (▶ Fig. 7.41).

7.18.2 Case Illustration 2: Persistent Radiculopathy after Arthroplasty

Clinical History

A 40-year-old left-hand–dominant woman presented for an additional opinion regarding persistent left radicular arm pain after undergoing a C6–7 arthroplasty at an outside facility. One year before the patient developed left radicular arm pain, she had experienced a low-energy trauma. The left radicular arm pain was refractory to exhaustive nonoperative treatments, and therefore, she decided to undergo cervical arthroplasty. However, she did not have meaningful relief of her radicular symptoms after arthroplasty. Her primary surgeon recommended an additional arthroplasty at the C5–6 segment to address her persistent symptoms. The patient presented to clinic with a relatively low NDI of 23 but a high VAS (arm) score of 78 mm.

Neurologic Examination

On examination, the patient did not demonstrate any focal weakness in the biceps or triceps on the left or the right. Both were 5/5 on examination by confrontation. The patient had a decrease in pinprick and light touch limited to the left index finger, which she reported as unchanged from her arthoplasty operation. The biceps and triceps reflexes were absent bilaterally. The patient had a positive Spurling sign, with the point of maximal pain intensity residing in left trapezius and radiating through the arm into the dorsum of the hand.

Radiologic Studies

The artifact from her arthroplasty device limited meaningful interpretation of the MRI (▶ Fig. 7.42). Axial images are not shown because of the degree of artifact. Plain radiographs show a well-centered keel-based device with no evidence of implant failure and mild spondylosis at C5–6. Despite the neutral position of the cervical spine, the patient had a focal segmental kyphosis at the C6–7 level, possibly due to the persistent radiculopathy.

The inability to glean any insight from the patient's postoperative MRI studies prompted a review of her preoperative studies before she had undergone cervical arthroplasty (▶ Fig. 7.43). These studies showed a disc extrusion at C6–7 to the left and mild spondylosis at C5–6, without any significant foraminal narrowing on the left.

Surgical Decision Making

The patient did not have a clear-cut C6 or C7 nerve root compression syndrome. The absence of motor weakness and a sensory examination that did not offer compelling evidence of one cervical nerve root over the other complicated surgical decision making. The patient may have been persistently symptomatic from compression of the C7 nerve root or newly symptomatic from compression of the C6 nerve root. The surgical options included another arthroplasty to be performed at C5–6, as recommended by her primary surgeon, or reconsideration of the C6–7 level as the possible persistent source of the radiculopathy. The latter consideration could be managed by a revision using an anterior or a posterior approach. Revising an anterior keel-based arthroplasty device is not without its perils. Furthermore, the arthroplasty device is in an ideal position in the AP dimension, and if C6-7 were the surgical target, a posterior approach would be preferred. To guide the decision-making process, a selective nerve root block at C7 was performed. The

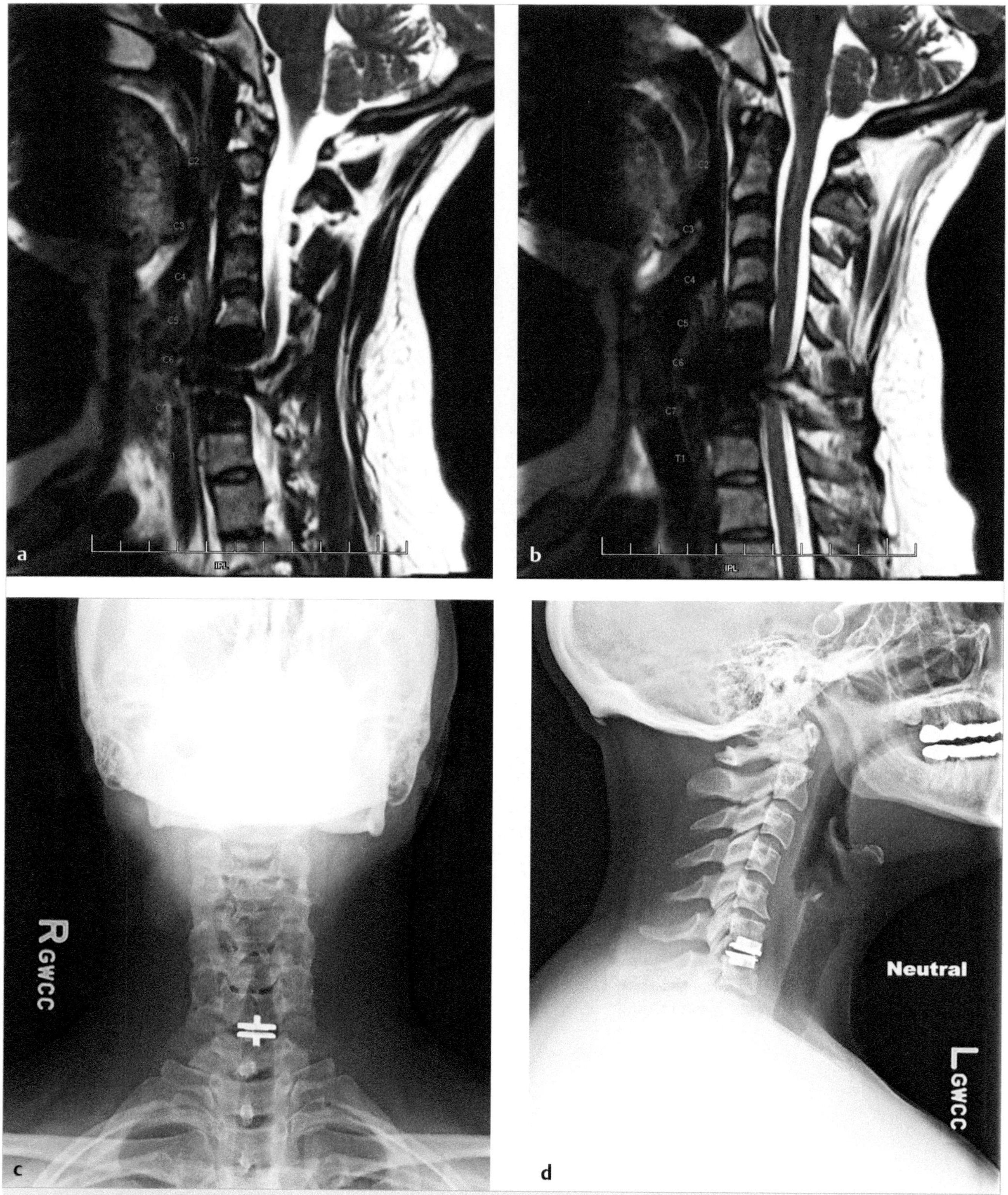

Fig. 7.42 Persistent radiculopathy after cervical arthroplasty. T2-weighted magnetic resonance imaging **(a)** parasagittal and **(b)** midsagittal views. Both of these images show the artifact created by the chromium cobalt arthroplasty device, which limits the ability to interpret the images. **(c)** Plain radiograph showing well-centered keel-based arthroplasty device without implant-related complication. **(d)** Neutral lateral plain radiograph shows the implant in position but not in a lordotic position. The patient had positive sagittal balance likely related to the persistent cervical radiculopathy.

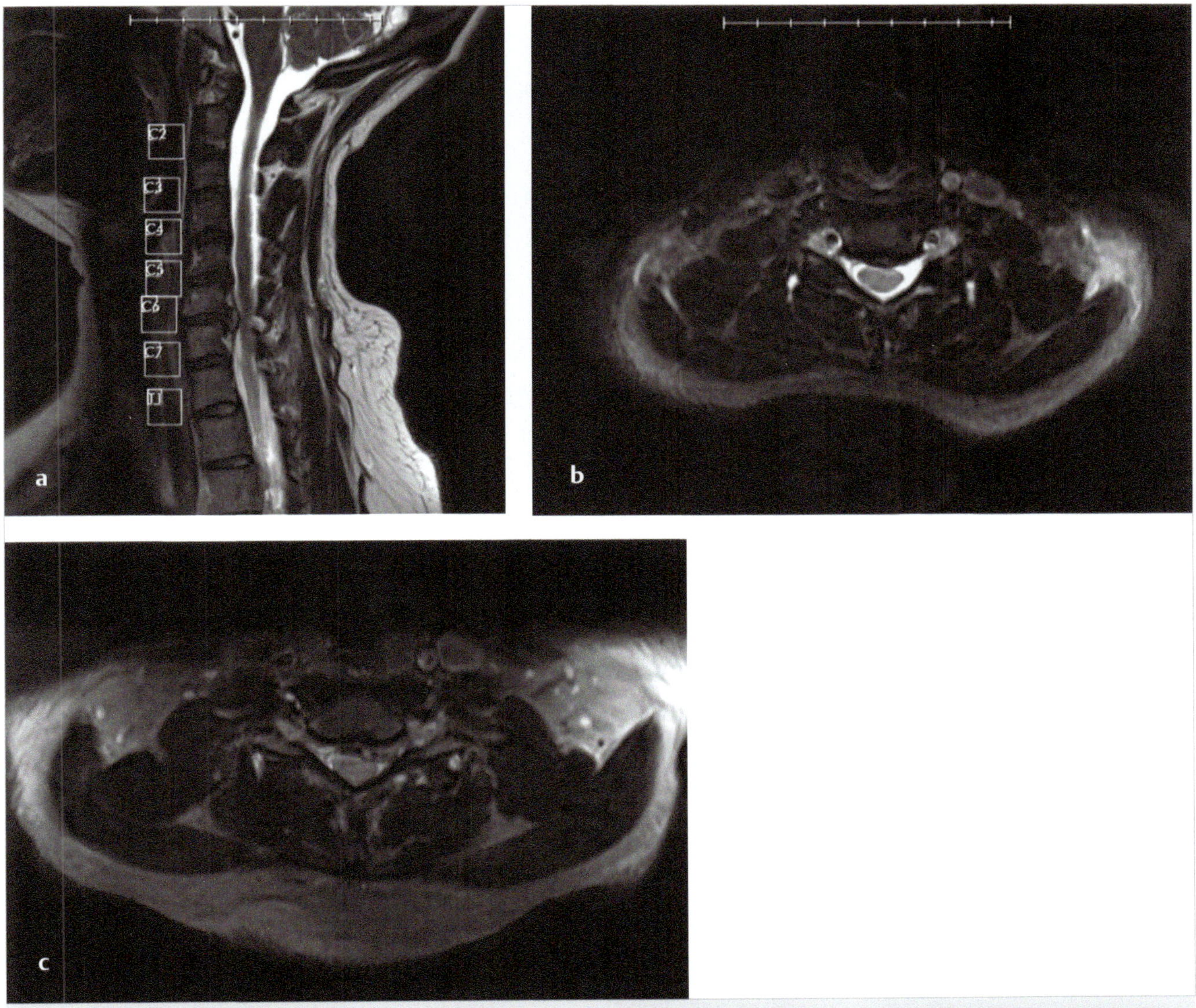

Fig. 7.43 Magnetic resonance imaging (MRI) of the cervical spine before cervical arthroplasty. **(a)** Sagittal T2-weighted MRI shows a disc extrusion at C6–7. **(b)** Axial T2-weighted MRI through C5–6 shows a widely patent C6 neural foramen. **(c)** Axial T2-weighted MRI through C6–7 demonstrates a disc extrusion compressing the C7 nerve root.

patient reported substantial but temporary symptom relief; therefore, a C7 posterior cervical foraminotomy was recommended.

Surgical Technique

With the patient in a skull clamp and positioned prone on chest rolls in the reverse Trendelenburg position, I planned the incision with the help of lateral fluoroscopy. The incision was marked (1.5 cm off the midline and 16 mm in length), and the patient was prepped and draped. The inferior articular process of C6 was the target for the spinal needle and the first dilator. A 14-mm × 5-cm minimal access port was secured to the table-mounted frame once lateral, AP and owl's eye fluoroscopic images showed the ideal placement of the access port (▸ Fig. 7.44). The four-step method of drilling the inferior articular process and lamina of C6 and the SAP and lamina of C7 was then performed. The C7 nerve root was widely decompressed from pedicle to pedicle and then mobilized to retrieve any residual disc fragment within the foramen.

Postoperative Course

The patient was discharged 2 hours after surgery with substantial relief of her left radicular symptoms. At 1 month, the patient reported a 95% improvement in her overall symptoms. Her NDI was 9 (preoperative, 23) and her VAS (arm) score was 0 mm (preoperative, 78 mm). Postoperative radiographs demonstrated the pedicle-to-pedicle foraminotomy on the AP image and an improvement in her sagittal balance on the lateral radiograph (▸ Fig. 7.45).

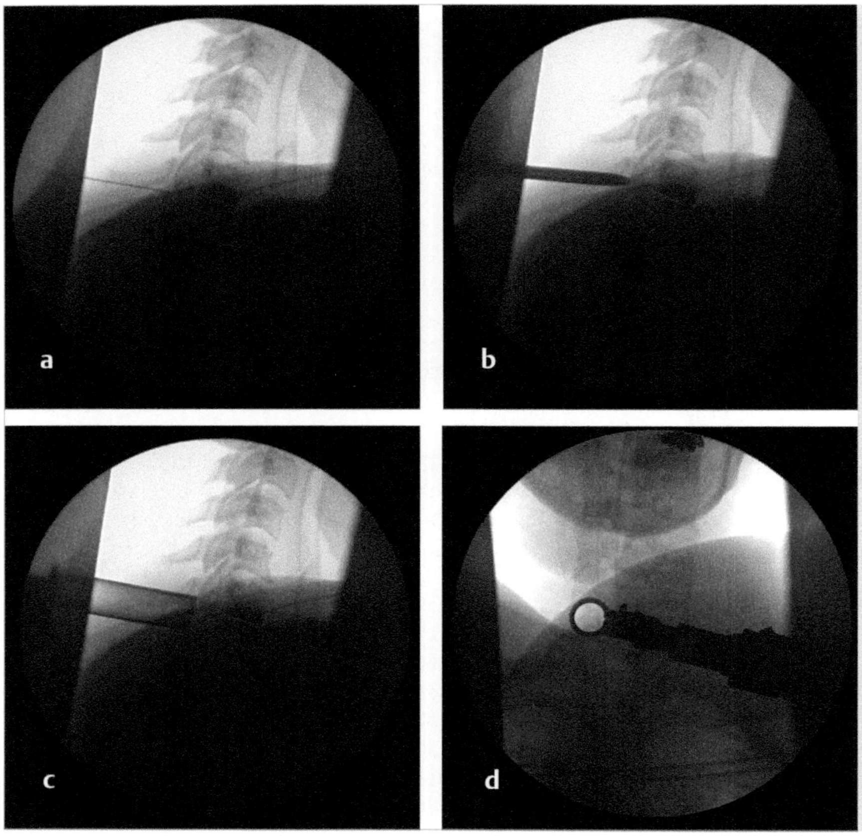

Fig. 7.44 Fluoroscopic sequence for the management of a persistent radiculopathy after cervical arthroplasty. **(a)** Lateral fluoroscopic image showing localization with a 20-gauge spinal needle. **(b)** Initial dilator in position on the inferior articular process of C6. **(c)** Lateral fluoroscopic image demonstrating a 14-mm access port in position parallel to the disc space. **(d)** Owl's eye view through the access port showing the placement of the field of view over the top of the foramen.

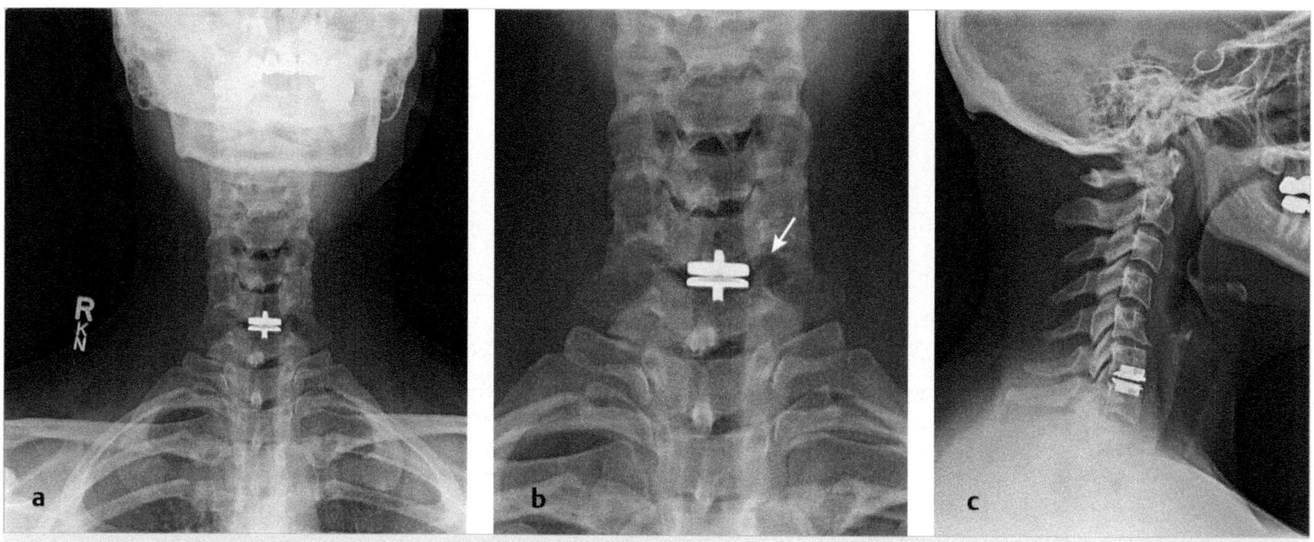

Fig. 7.45 Postoperative radiographs after posterior cervical foraminotomy for persistent radiculopathy after arthroplasty. **(a)** Anteroposterior image shows the bone work performed for the foraminotomy. **(b)** Magnified view of the bone work at the C7 neural foramen on the left (*arrow*). Less than 50% of the facet joint was removed. **(c)** Lateral radiograph shows an improvement in the sagittal balance and the segmental lordosis at C6–7 when compared to the preoperative study.

7.18.3 Case Illustrations on the Ideal Posterior Cervical Foraminotomy and Discectomy Candidate

Instead of describing a single-case illustration dedicated to cervical disc herniation, I believe this section would be of greater value to the reader to review those anatomical circumstances where patients are ideal candidates for posterior cervical microdiscectomies and circumstances where I would be more confident with an anterior approach. Thus, I juxtapose a more compact case illustration of two patients suited for posterior cervical microdiscectomy with two patients in which I applied the anterior approach. All four of these patients presented with unilateral radiculopathy referable to a single level. The common denominator in the ideal posterior cervical microdiscectomy patient is the acute presentation of a unilateral radiculopathy without the disc extrusion contacting or displacing the spinal cord. The following case illustrations emphasize these unique radiographic findings, which guided the surgical decision making.

The first case is that of a 54-year-old right-hand–dominant man who presented with a 3-week history of incapacitating arm pain after a sneeze. His symptoms were refractory to injection therapy, physical therapy and cervical traction. A motor examination was notable for profound weakness in the right abductor pollicis brevis, the adductor pollicis and the abductor digiti minimi muscles (2/5). The patient had paresthesias and decreased pinprick and light touch feeling on the palmar and dorsal aspects of the fourth and fifth digits. His symptoms were incompatible with his work as a journalist. MRI of the cervical spine (▶ Fig. 7.46) demonstrated a disc extrusion at C7–T1. The axial T2-weighted MRI at C7–T1 showed a disc extrusion on the right, without contact with the spinal cord. The absence of spinal cord compression and the foraminal location of the disc extrusion made the patient especially well suited for a posterior cervical foraminotomy with microdiscectomy. The operative video that accompanies this chapter demonstrates the annulotomy and removal of the disc extrusion (Video 7.1). Although the patient recovered all his strength in his dominant hand, he continued to experience decreased sensation in the fourth and fifth digits. His radicular pain completely resolved.

The second case is that of a 41-year-old right-hand–dominant woman who presented with right C7 radicular symptoms of 2 months' duration that occurred after beginning a new exercise regimen with a personal trainer. After exhaustive nonoperative measures, she presented with right triceps weakness (4/5), a positive Spurling sign and a positive shoulder abduction sign. Similar to the previous case, the MRI demonstrated a disc extrusion in contact with the C7 nerve root but not the spinal cord (▶ Fig. 7.47). The disc extrusion was medial to the pedicle. The patient underwent a successful foraminotomy and discectomy.

The following two case illustrations describe circumstances where the patients presented with acute disc herniations causing a unilateral cervical radiculopathy similar to the two previous cases, but the location and configuration of the disc extrusion prompted an anterior instead of a posterior approach.

The next case is that of a 48-year-old right-hand–dominant woman who presented after a motor vehicle accident with an acute radiculopathy. On examination, she did not demonstrate any evidence of myelopathy, no Lhermitte sign and no hyperreflexia. She had a classic left C6 nerve root compression syndrome with decreased sensation over the C6 dermatome, absent left biceps reflex and left biceps weakness. There was no evidence of myelomalacia on the sagittal T2-weighted MRI, but the location of the disc extrusion displaced and rotated the spinal cord at the C5–6 segment, which prompted a comprehensive anterior approach (▶ Fig. 7.48). My concern was that an attempt to retrieve a disc fragment in contact with the ventral

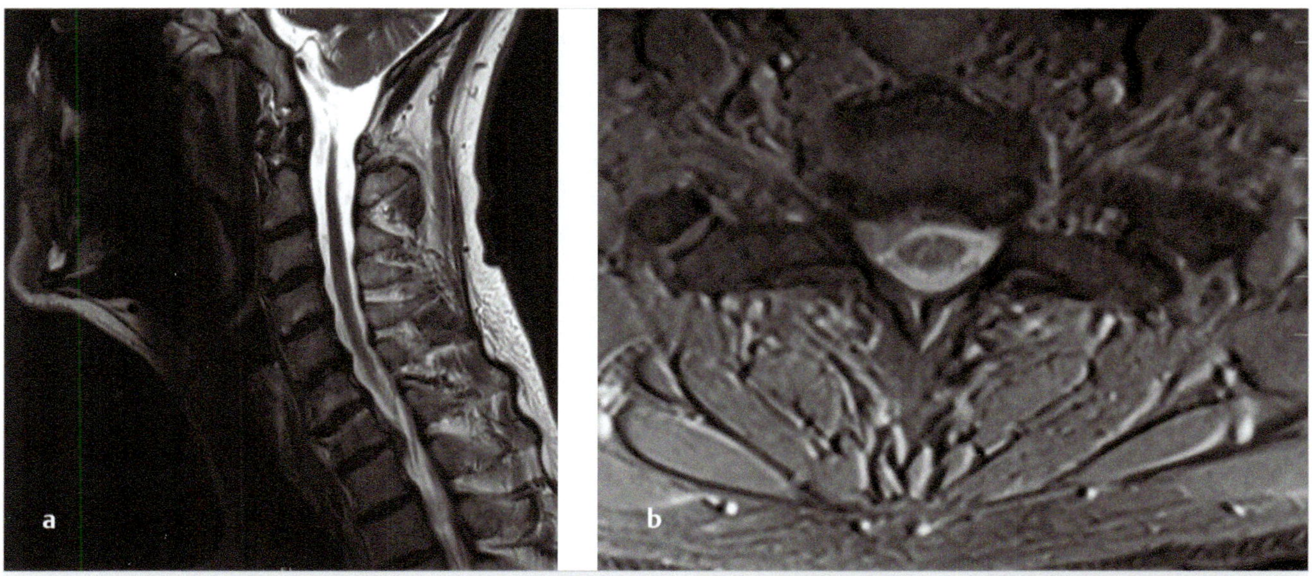

Fig. 7.46 Magnetic resonance imaging (MRI) showing unilateral, right eighth cervical nerve radiculopathy from a C7–T1 disc extrusion. **(a)** Parasagittal T2-weighted MRI of the cervical spine shows a disc extrusion at C7–T1. **(b)** Axial T2-weighted MRI at C7–T1. The disc extrusion is on the right, without contacting the spinal cord. The absence of spinal cord compression and the foraminal location of the disc extrusion lends itself particularly well to a posterior cervical foraminotomy. The patient in this case underwent an uncomplicated microdiscectomy with complete resolution of his radicular symptoms, an increase in his hand strength, but persistently decreased sensation in his fourth and fifth fingers.

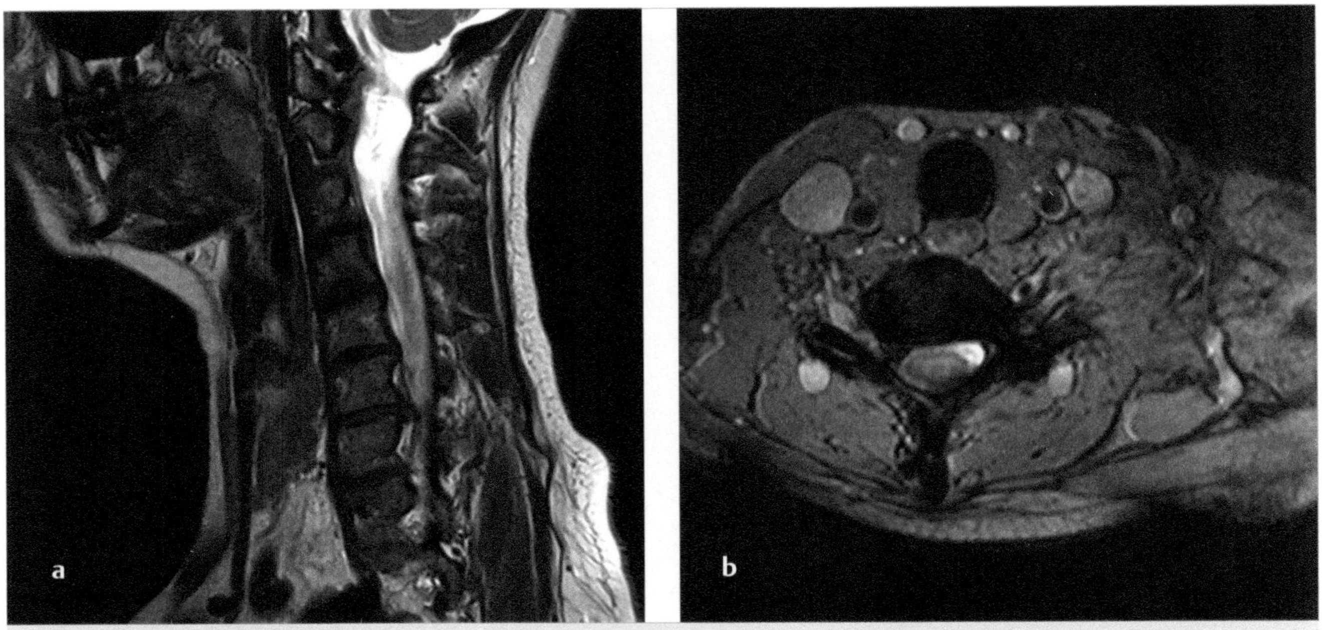

Fig. 7.47 Magnetic resonance imaging (MRI) showing unilateral, right C7 radiculopathy from a C6–7 disc extrusion. **(a)** Parasagittal T2-weighted MRI of the cervical spine shows a disc extrusion at C6–7. **(b)** Axial T2-weighted MRI at C6–7. Similar to ▶ Fig. 7.41, the disc extrusion is on the right and has no contact with the spinal cord. A posterior cervical foraminotomy with discectomy allowed for the complete decompression of the nerve root and alleviation of the symptoms.

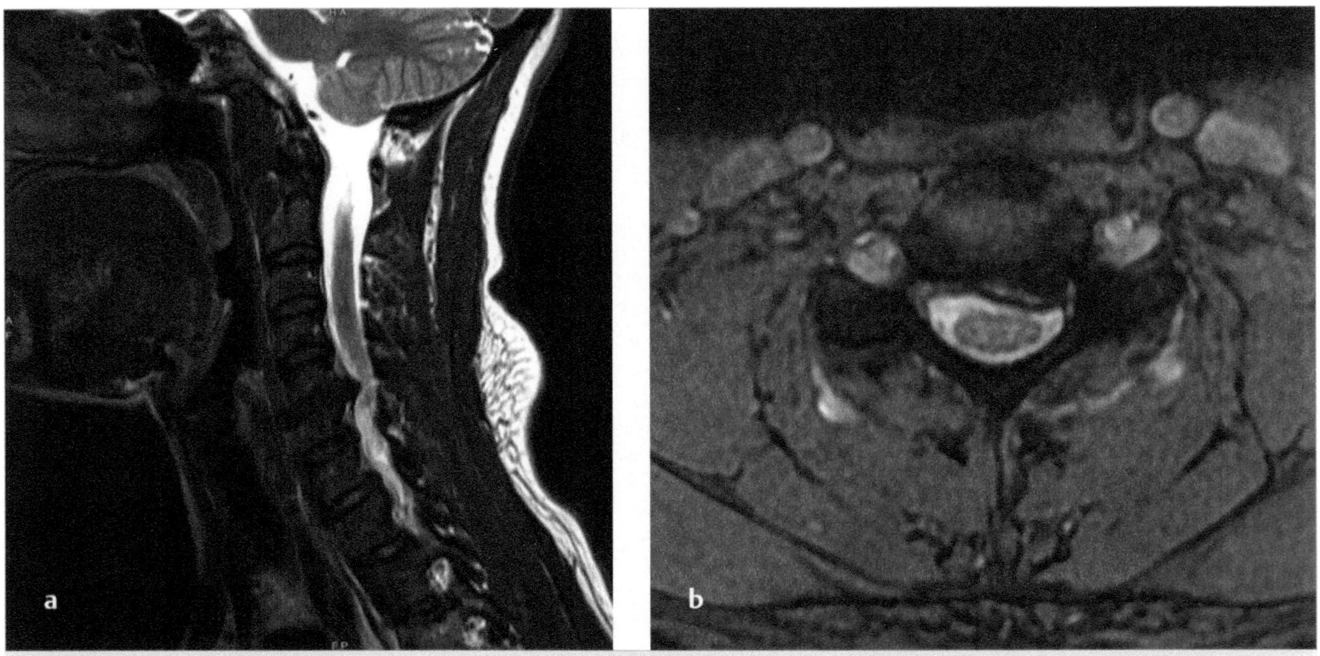

Fig. 7.48 Magnetic resonance imaging (MRI) showing a disc herniation with both central canal and nerve root compression causing cervical radiculopathy. **(a)** Sagittal T2-weighted MRI of the cervical spine shows the disc extrusion at C5–6 in contact with the spinal cord. **(b)** Axial T2-weighted MRI of the cervical spine at the C5–6 level shows the herniation in contact with the spinal cord and displacement of the cord. The concern with the retrieval of such a disc extrusion is traction on the spinal cord.

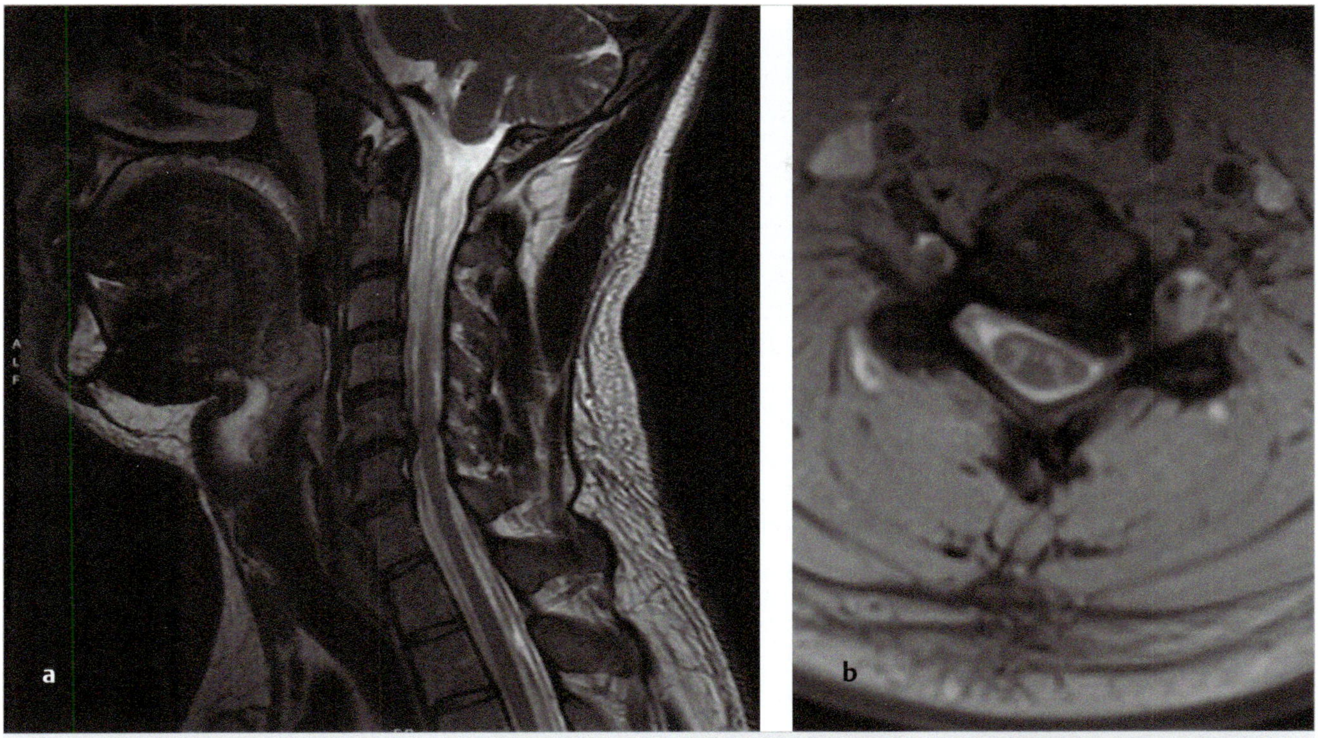

Fig. 7.49 Magnetic resonance imaging (MRI) showing a disc herniation with both central canal and nerve root compression, which caused cervical radiculopathy. **(a)** Sagittal T2-weighted MRI of the cervical spine shows the disc extrusion at C5–6 in contact with the spinal cord. **(b)** Axial T2-weighted MRI of the cervical spine at the C5–6 level demonstrating disc extrusion in the central canal more than in the foramen. The patient underwent arthroplasty, with resolution of his symptoms.

aspect of the spinal cord would require traction on the cervical spinal cord, which should never be done. Unlike in the previous two cases, the disc extrusion was not limited to the foramen. The patient had significant clinical improvement in both her symptoms and neurological status after a C5–6 ACDF.

The final case of this series is of a 41-year-old, right-hand–dominant, semiprofessional hockey player who presented after he was checked into the boards of the skating arena. He described instantaneous left-side neck and trapezius pain, along with left radicular arm pain. After 6 weeks of persistent symptoms despite epidural injections and physical therapy, he sought a surgical evaluation. ▶ Fig. 7.49 demonstrates a disc extrusion that was more in the canal than it was in the foramen. The same concern for traction on the spinal cord prompted an anterior approach for decompression and the placement of an arthroplasty device.

7.19 Conclusions

The Baudelaire quote that began this chapter bears repeating at its closure: "He who sees through an open window, sees less than he who looks through a closed window." The "closed window," or rather the minimally invasive window that we look through to perform these procedures, requires the surgeon's mind to reconstruct the surrounding anatomy more so than if the anatomy of the cervical segment were laid out before us. Our field of view may only be 14 mm, but the skill set developed in the reconstruction of the anatomy at depth has enabled the surgeon to acquire the anatomical certainty of the pedicle, the spinal cord, the nerve root, the dimensions of these structures and the dimensions of the foramen.

In the end, the benefit of the paramedian transmuscular technique with a 14-mm-diameter access port is to equalize the difference between the posterior cervical approaches and the well-tolerated anterior approach. The introduction of the minimally invasive principles has allayed, to some extent, the concern put forth by Aldrich in 1990 regarding the trend in anterior versus posterior cervical approaches. The minimally invasive spine surgeon has a procedure that is now routinely performed in the outpatient setting with minimal disruption of the posterior cervical musculature and a Caspar ratio of nearly 1. The ability to address unilateral cervical radiculopathies at one and two levels that precludes the need for instrumentation, whether for motion preservation or arthrodesis, is invaluable. The minimally invasive posterior cervical foraminotomy is especially indispensable for the management of patients with a history of single-level or multilevel fusions presenting with a unilateral radiculopathy at an adjacent segment. A posterior approach precludes the need to remove a cervical plate, which at times may span multiple levels and fuse yet another segment. The posterior cervical foraminotomy is the ideal approach for the management of persistent cervical radiculopathies after anterior approaches. Finally, it is a particularly ideal procedure for an acute foraminal cervical disc extrusion that does not contact the spinal cord.

As seen from the case illustrations, the capacity to treat an array of unilateral cervical radiculopathies with a variety of clinical circumstances places the minimally invasive posterior cervical foraminotomy in a unique role within the armamentarium of the minimally invasive spine surgeon. Similar to the experience gained from the minimally invasive microdiscectomy, which lays the foundation for the lumbar laminectomy, the experience gained from posterior cervical foraminotomies builds the experience and confidence to converge the access port medially and decompress the central canal. It should be no surprise to the reader that the minimally invasive posterior cervical laminectomy is the next chapter in this Primer.

References

[1] Tumialán LM, Ponton RP, Gluf WM. Management of unilateral cervical radiculopathy in the military: the cost effectiveness of posterior cervical foraminotomy compared with anterior cervical discectomy and fusion. Neurosurg Focus. 2010; 28(5):E17

[2] Aldrich F. Posterolateral microdisectomy for cervical monoradiculopathy caused by posterolateral soft cervical disc sequestration. J Neurosurg. 1990; 72(3):370–377

[3] Roh SW, Kim DH, Cardoso AC, Fessler RG. Endoscopic foraminotomy using MED system in cadaveric specimens. Spine. 2000; 25(2):260–264

[4] Adamson TE. Microendoscopic posterior cervical laminoforaminotomy for unilateral radiculopathy: results of a new technique in 100 cases. J Neurosurg. 2001; 95(1) Suppl:51–57

[5] Mixter WJ, Barr J. Rupture of the intervertebral disc with involvement of the spinal canal. N Engl J Med. 1934; 211:210–215

[6] Love JG, Camp JD. Root pain resulting from intra-spinal protrusion of intervertebral disks: diagnosis and surgical treatment. JBJS. 1937; 19(3)

[7] Semmes RE, Murphey F. The syndrome of unilateral rupture of the sixth cervical intervertebral disk with compression of the seventh cervical nerve root with compression of the seventh cervical nerve root: a report of four cases with symptoms and simulating coronary disease. JAMA. 1943; 121(15): 1209–1214

[8] Spurling RG, Scoville WB. Lateral rupture of the cervical intervertebral disc: a common cause of shoulder and arm pain. Surg Gynecol Obstet. 1944; 78: 350–358

[9] Frykholm R. Deformities of dural pouches and strictures of dural sheaths in the cervical region producing nerve-root compression; a contribution to the etiology and operative treatment of brachial neuralgia. J Neurosurg. 1947; 4 (5):403–413

[10] Barakat M, Hussein Y. Anatomical study of the cervical nerve roots for posterior foraminotomy: cadaveric study. Eur Spine J. 2012; 21(7):1383–1388

[11] Panjabi MM, Duranceau J, Goel V, Oxland T, Takata K. Cervical human vertebrae. Quantitative three-dimensional anatomy of the middle and lower regions. Spine. 1991;16(8):861-869

[12] Webb KM, Kaptain G, Sheehan J, Jane JA, Sr. Pediculotomy as an adjunct to posterior cervical hemilaminectomy, foraminotomy, and discectomy. Neurosurg Focus. 2002; 12(1):E10

[13] Jagannathan J, Sherman JH, Szabo T, Shaffrey CI, Jane JA. The posterior cervical foraminotomy in the treatment of cervical disc/osteophyte disease: a single-surgeon experience with a minimum of 5 years' clinical and radiographic follow-up. J Neurosurg Spine. 2009; 10(4):347–356

8 Minimally Invasive Posterior Cervical Laminectomy

Abstract

Dorsal compression of the cervical spinal cord at a single segment is a rare circumstance in clinical practice. As such, the minimally invasive posterior cervical laminectomy is the least commonly performed procedure described in this book. However, when that particular circumstance arises, there is no better management strategy than decompression using minimally invasive techniques. A paramedian approach through a limited access corridor spares the interruption of the intricate insertion pattern of the posterior cervical musculature and avoids exposure of the midline and the associated devascularization of the paraspinal muscles related to that exposure. Instead, a minimal access port secured after dilating through a focal corridor and placed immediately over the area of dorsal compression allows for the removal of that compression with the preservation of the spinous process, the contralateral lamina and the motion of the segment. The current chapter presents the anatomical basis, operating room setup and surgical technique for this procedure. The chapter ends with clinical circumstances where the minimally invasive posterior cervical laminectomy was applied for the management of patients with single-segment dorsal compression of the cervical spinal cord. Although not commonly performed, the minimally invasive posterior cervical laminectomy has a role in the management of degenerative, neoplastic and infectious pathologies that afflict the cervical spine.

Keywords: access corridor, decompression, laminectomy, midline approach, paramedian approach, paraspinal muscles, spinal anatomy, stenosis

Sometimes seeing everything just gets in the way.

Chris Lynch

8.1 Introduction

Conventional wisdom encourages us to identify the strengths and limitations of any particular procedure, whether minimally invasive or open. The decision to employ one surgical approach over another involves careful consideration of both the strengths and limitations of each individual approach in the context of the anatomical constraints. That statement holds as true when considering a costotransversectomy transpedicular approach versus a thoracotomy for decompression of the spinal cord to address ventral compression as it does when we consider the topic of this current chapter, a minimally invasive posterior cervical laminectomy.

The strength of any minimally invasive approach is a focused exposure of the requisite anatomy through a corridor that minimally disrupts the surrounding musculature. Cervical degenerative pathology of the central canal, however, is seldom a single-level entity. The very nature of the pathology tends to involve multiple levels that also raise the specter of alignment and sagittal balance. Furthermore, the musculature of the posterior cervical spine is complex. The intricate array of muscular insertions and multiple layers of crossing fibers are distinct from the longitudinal and compartmentalized arrangement of muscles in the lumbar spine. The inevitable consequence is that creating multiple corridors to traverse the cervical musculature and reach the spine in the absence of a focused field will be significantly disruptive. Multiple levels of decompression accomplished with a minimally invasive approach would inevitably lead to substantial postoperative discomfort to the patient and long hours in the operating room for the surgeon. Minimally invasive decompression of multiple levels in the lumbar spine is one thing, but minimally invasive decompression of multiple levels in the cervical spine is entirely another.

My experience in clinical practice has led to the observation that patients who present with cervical stenosis with myelopathy caused predominantly by a posterior component typically have multiple levels of involvement. The root cause of the problem in these patients tends to be a congenitally narrow canal in the context of multiple levels of degeneration with disc osteophyte formation. If the compression is primarily posterior, definitive management entails a wide decompression and, at times, an instrumented fusion if the patient is trending into kyphosis. Laminoplasty remains an option for those patients with preservation of cervical lordosis. However, laminoplasty is also currently outside the realm of a minimally invasive approach.

Despite the desire by many, including me, to address multiple levels of cervical stenosis with a minimally invasive approach, no such procedure has reliably achieved all the goals that can be so readily accomplished by a definitive midline open operation. One reason is that minimally invasive approaches are trajectory dependent. In the lumbar spine, an instrumented decompression and fusion may be accomplished from the same general trajectory. Pedicle screws converge onto the spine 15 to 25 degrees from the point of the incision, and the decompression requires convergence of 20 to 30 degrees *in the same direction*. For decompression and instrumentation of the cervical spine, these trajectories are divergent. The trajectory for placement of a lateral mass screw is entirely the opposite of the trajectory needed for a central decompression. Over the years, the divergent trajectory conundrum for instrumentation and decompression in the cervical spine has been an insurmountable Gordian knot for minimally invasive spine surgeons to unravel (▶ Fig. 8.1).

In the end, it is difficult to conceive a minimally invasive procedure that can offer both trajectories for decompression and instrumentation from one incision and thereby accomplish the goals of the operation in a circumstance that requires multiple levels of decompression. Even if we were to consider laminoplasty, a multilevel minimally invasive laminoplasty would have its own set of challenges. Finally, the nature and complexity of the posterior cervical musculature create a difficult circumstance for any multilevel minimally invasive solution. Although it pains me to write these words, the reality is that the anatomy of the posterior cervical spine is a circumstance where the clinical utility of a minimally invasive approach for posterior multilevel cervical stenosis with our current techniques is limited, at least at the time of this writing. Perhaps, in the years to come, the Gordian knot will be disentangled by a reader of this Primer.

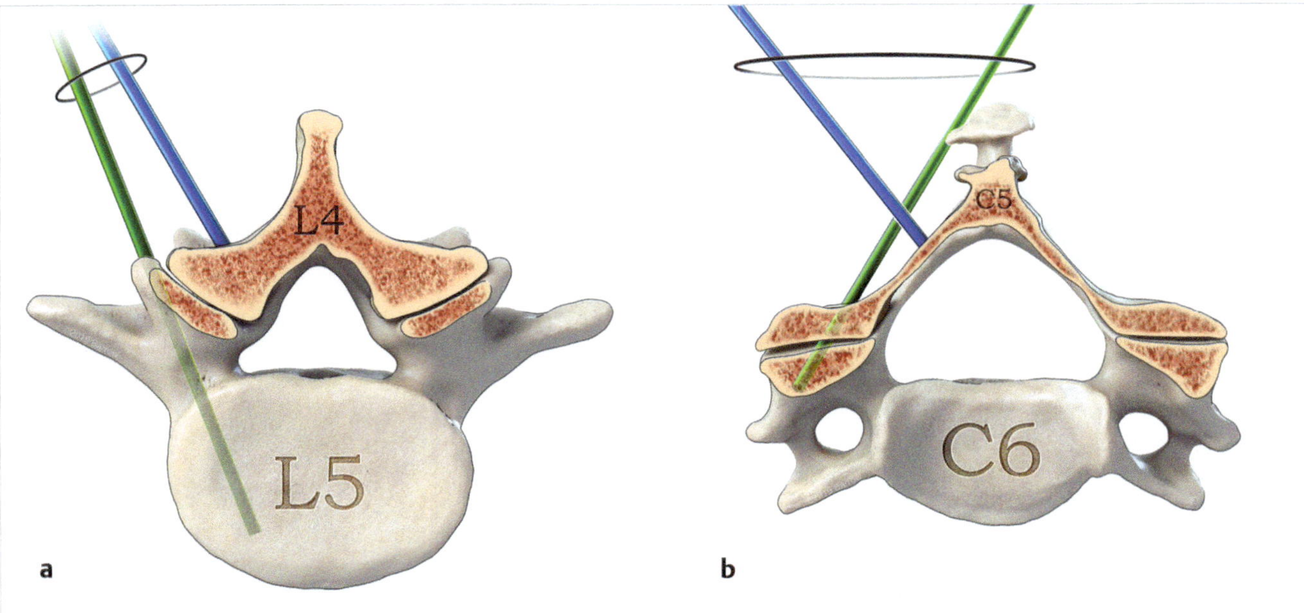

Fig. 8.1 The distinct trajectories for decompression and instrumentation in the lumbar and cervical spine. **(a)** Illustration of an axial view at L4–5. The trajectories for decompression (*blue trajectory*) and instrumentation (*green trajectory*) converge onto the spine. Working through trajectories that converge toward the pedicle and the lamina, instrumentation and decompression may be accomplished with minimal disruption of the anatomy. **(b)** Illustration of an axial view of the cervical spine at C5–6. The trajectory for decompression (*blue trajectory*) converges onto the cervical lamina, whereas the trajectory for instrumentation (*green trajectory*) diverges from the lamina for a trajectory that allows instrumentation into the lateral mass.

On the other hand, a midline incision with wide exposure of the cervical lamina and lateral masses affords the surgeon the greatest capacity to safely decompress and, if need be, instrument the spine. Therefore, it would make little sense in a patient with a congenitally narrow canal and multiple levels of stenosis due to posterior compression from C3 to C6 with myelomalacia to attempt a minimally invasive procedure. It is not the incapacity to perform such a procedure. Rather, as mentioned above, the unique anatomical elements of the posterior cervical spine do not allow such a procedure to play to the strengths of a minimally invasive approach.

At times, patients present specifically requesting a minimally invasive procedure (▶ Fig. 8.2). Other times, elderly patients with comorbidities present needing a comprehensive operation with a well-intended referring physician recommending minimally invasive surgery. In both of these circumstances, it is essential to be mindful of the goals that need to be accomplished by the operation and determine whether those goals can be met through a focused minimally invasive approach. If not, proceeding with a minimally invasive option would be ill-advised and likely lead to incomplete relief, potential complications and the need for more surgery. Taking the time to counsel patients who have an understandable preference for a minimally invasive motion-preserving approach is an investment in your clinical time and the patient's overall well-being. In the circumstance of the elderly patient with comorbidities, keep in mind that if that particular patient is not healthy enough for the appropriate operation, then they certainly are not healthy enough for the wrong one.

On occasion, cervical stenosis with dorsal compression of the spinal cord occurs focally at one segment. Such circumstances present an opportunity to apply the minimally invasive approach. Much in the same way that a minimally invasive approach is more of a liability than an asset for multilevel cervical exposures, the tables are completely reversed for a traditional midline exposure for focal compression. The strength of a midline approach is the capacity to widely expose multiple levels of the spine for both decompression and possible instrumentation. However, for focal dorsal compression of the spinal cord, that wide exposure now becomes more of a liability than an asset. Just as I would never consider a minimally invasive approach for a patient with multiple levels of cervical stenosis, it would be difficult for me to conceive of a midline approach for such a focal single-level entity in the cervical spine. Open posterior exposures themselves come at the cost of considerable disruption and devascularization of the posterior musculature.

Furthermore, the very nature of a midline approach results in disruption of the posterior tension band and the potential for postoperative progressive kyphosis. The morbidity and discomfort introduce the question of whether or not such exposure is truly needed for a single level of stenosis. After all, the majority of the exposure is the unavoidable consequence of having to reach the anatomy with conventional retractors. Therein lies the weakness of a midline approach: the need for such an extensive subperiosteal dissection of the muscle insertions off of the spinous process and lamina and the sacrifice of the posterior tension band to see a limited amount of the anatomy. Couple this with the use of self-retaining retractors that compromise the blood flow to the muscles and the skin, and it would be difficult to argue an open approach for single-level compression. As already identified throughout this Primer,

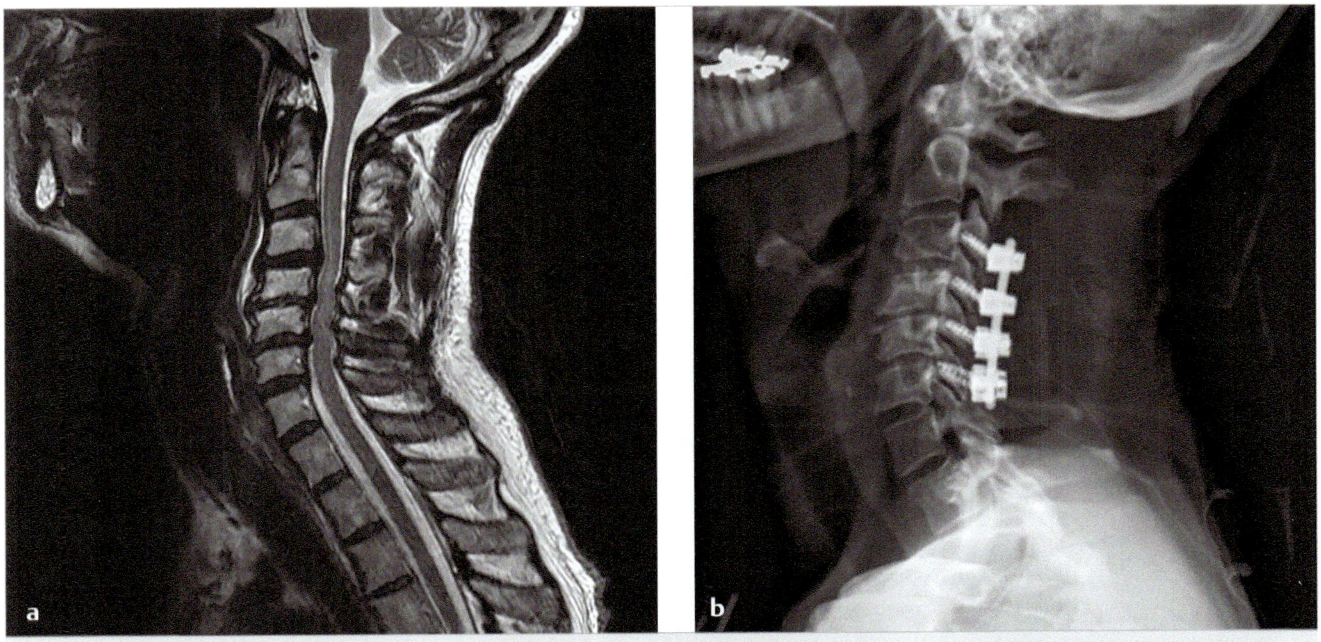

Fig. 8.2 Multilevel cervical stenosis in a congenitally narrow canal. **(a)** Sagittal T2-weighted magnetic resonance imaging of the cervical spine demonstrating a congenitally narrow canal. This patient presented interested in minimally invasive options only. A neurologic examination demonstrated brisk hyperreflexia in all four extremities, positive Hoffman's sign bilaterally, positive Babinski's sign bilaterally, positive Romberg's sign and lack of ability to walk in a tandem gait. **(b)** After extensive counseling regarding the limits of minimally invasive surgery and the natural history of myelopathy, the patient underwent a C3–6 laminectomy and lateral mass fusion. Cervical laminoplasty from C3–6 or a three-level anterior cervical discectomy and fusion would have been another perfectly reasonable option. However, there was no posterior minimally invasive option that would offer a comprehensive solution to this anatomical circumstance.

open procedures do not utilize the entire field of exposure. The fact of the matter is that surgeons work through a fraction of an open exposure to accomplish the goals of the operation (► Fig. 8.3).

Throughout this Primer, a theme that continues to arise is what I have referred to as the Caspar ratio, which is the ratio of the surgical target to the surgical exposure. From that standpoint, minimally invasive approaches are highly efficient techniques for the simple reason that almost every millimeter of exposure is utilized to perform a procedure. On the other hand, midline open procedures, by their very nature, are not as efficient. In the occasional circumstance where there is focal dorsal compression of the cervical spinal cord, a wide exposure is not only unnecessary but also becomes burdensome. I believe that Mr. Chris Lynch captured the essence of minimally invasive posterior cervical surgery versus its open equivalent for a single-level entity by making the statement that began this chapter, "Sometimes seeing everything just gets in the way." The minimally invasive cervical laminectomy is the embodiment of that statement and a perfect illustration of the Caspar ratio (► Fig. 8.4).

What I hope to convince the reader of in this chapter is that for focal dorsal compression of the cervical spinal cord, a wide exposure through a traditional midline approach is not only cumbersome, but also unnecessary. Since only a fraction of the open exposure is used to accomplish the goals of the operation, a focused exposure of the affected level is not only preferable but also ideal. Although focal single-level dorsal compression of the spinal cord may be rare, I suggest to the reader that the one approach that readily accomplishes the goals of decompression most effectively and efficiently is a minimally invasive one.

8.2 A Unique Clinical Circumstance

As mentioned in the Introduction, cervical stenosis with only dorsal compression tends to be a multilevel entity, and decompression of a single level or two is seldom the clinical circumstance for any one patient. Nonetheless, these circumstances do occur. The cause may be a degenerative, neoplastic, hemorrhagic or an infectious process. All of these scenarios are presented in the case illustrations at the end of this chapter. When such a patient presents, a mind prepared with a minimally invasive perspective sees a straightforward approach that precludes the need for exposure of the spinous process, disruption of the posterior tension band and devascularization of the paraspinal muscles. Louis Pasteur's adage rings especially true in this circumstance, "Fortune favors the prepared mind." The management of these focal lesions with minimally invasive approaches is more straightforward for the surgeon and better tolerated by the patient than its open counterpart.

Analogous to the lumbar spine, where the microdiscectomy serves as the platform from which to step into the lumbar laminectomy, the prerequisite for the minimally invasive posterior cervical laminectomy is mastery of the posterior cervical foraminotomy described in Chapter 7. Once you have established

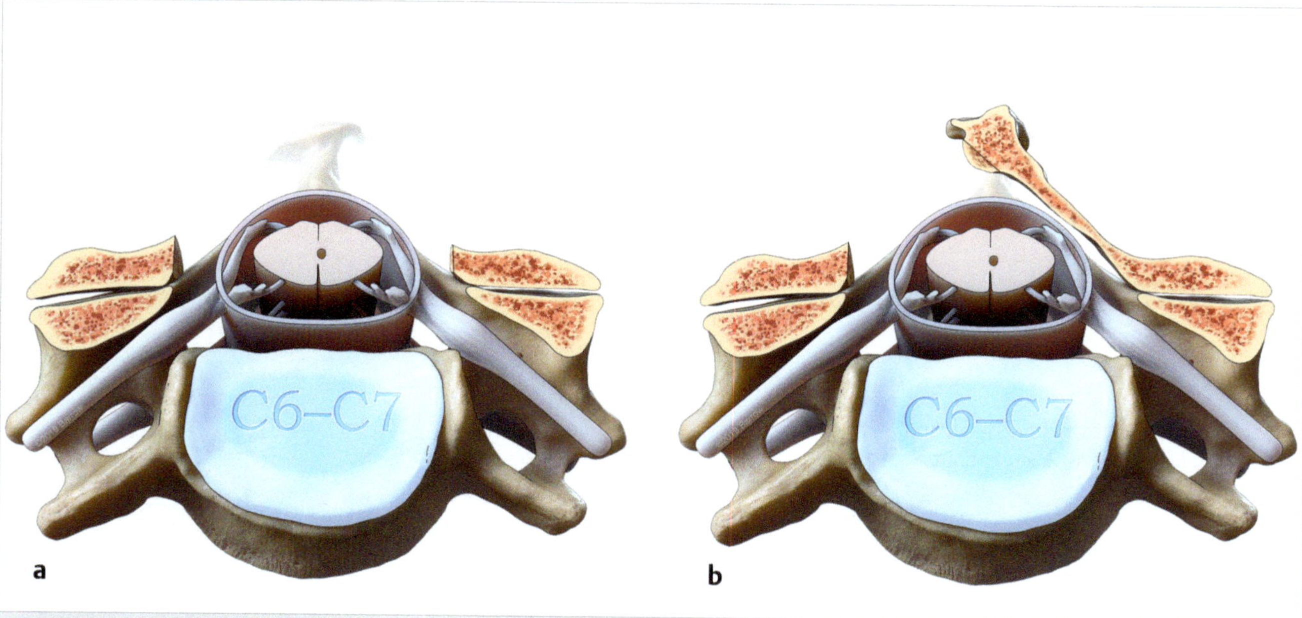

Fig. 8.3 Comparison of single-level cervical laminectomies. **(a)** Midline open cervical laminectomy at C6–7. In order to accomplish the exposure for this procedure, the spinous process needs to be removed, which compromises the posterior tension band. A wide subperiosteal dissection of the paraspinal musculature from its insertions is needed to complete the exposure. The surgical exposure far exceeds the surgical target to visualize all of the requisite anatomy for the operation. **(b)** A minimally invasive operation uses a 14-mm access port to expose the requisite anatomy. The spinous process is preserved and so is the posterior tension band. A focal area of exposure precludes the need for extensive subperiosteal dissection of the paraspinal muscles and does not compromise access to the surgical target or the objective to decompress the spinal cord.

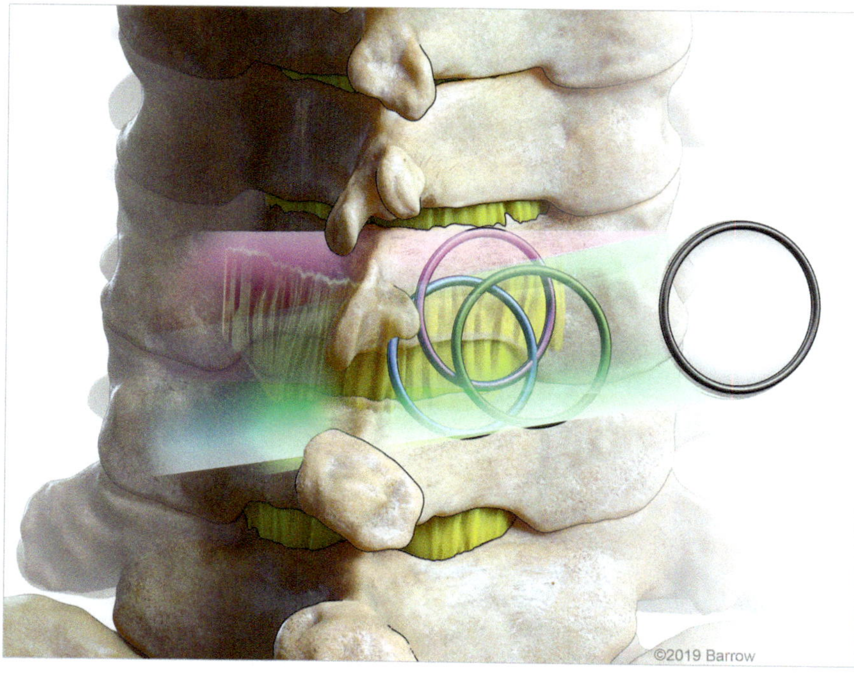

Fig. 8.4 The Caspar ratio in the minimally invasive posterior cervical laminectomy. The use of a 14-mm access port placed in three distinct positions on the posterior cervical lamina allows for the complete exposure of the surgical target through the incision. As a result, the exposure of the surgical target is considerably greater than the size of the incision. Similar to that of the lumbar laminectomy, the ratio of the surgical target to surgical exposure is greater than 1.

facility with the exposure and poise with the approach, you will confidently be able to turn the trajectory of the access port from the foramen of the cervical nerve root onto the lamina to decompress the cervical spinal cord.

8.3 Cervical Interlaminar Measurements

When I first began turning my dilators medially onto the lamina for minimally invasive cervical laminectomies, the greatest concern I had was the inadvertent passage of the initial dilator through the interlaminar space and into the spinal canal. After all, a minimally invasive posterior cervical laminectomy was distinct from a posterior cervical foraminotomy. The final target for the field of view was immediately over the central canal where the interlaminar spaces widened. For a posterior cervical foraminotomy, the target was over the nerve root and, therefore, lateral to the canal where the lamina converged. I found that passing dilators onto the lateral cervical spine was less harrowing for me than dilating over the central canal itself. Although there is always a concern for the potential passage of a dilator into the canal, the trajectory for a posterior cervical foraminotomy places the dilator in an area of the cervical spine where the laminae converge to form the articulation of the facets. The convergence of the lamina decreases the interlaminar space and thereby the theoretical risk of passage of a dilator into the canal (▶ Fig. 8.5).

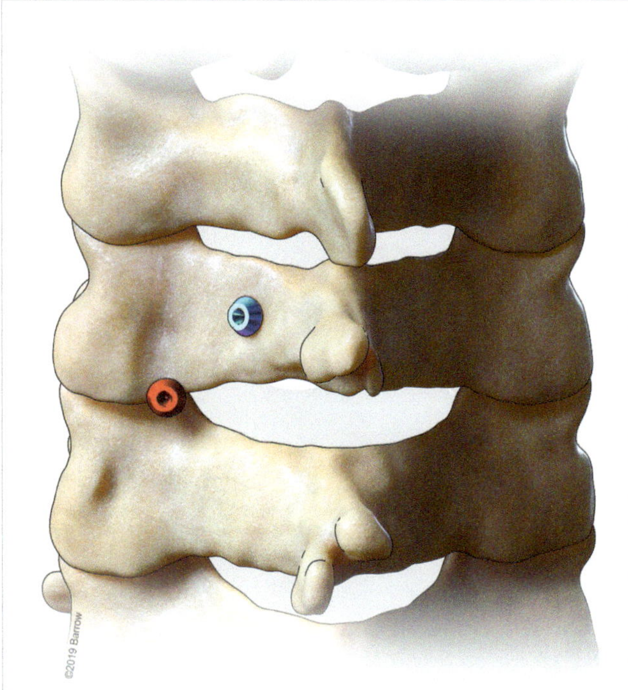

Fig. 8.5 Illustration of the posterior cervical spine. The *red* fiducial is the target for a minimally invasive posterior cervical foraminotomy. The convergence of the lamina at the junction of the lateral lamina and facet for the posterior cervical foraminotomy target decreases the interlaminar space and thereby the risk of passage of a dilator into the canal. The *blue* fiducial is the target for a minimally invasive cervical laminectomy. There is a considerable increase in the interlaminar space toward the midline, which increases the potential risk of passage into the canal when attempting to dock dilators onto the lamina. That risk is proportional to the diameter of the dilator relative to the interbody space.

Dilating with a medial trajectory onto the cervical lamina, on the other hand, has always been more irksome for me. As the tip of the dilator ventures from the lamina–facet junction toward the midline, in preparation for a midline decompression, the laminae diverge, thus creating the interlaminar space. Passage of a dilator into the canal all of sudden becomes a possibility. Intuitively, I reasoned that the interlaminar space only increases when proceeding from the rostral levels to the caudal ones. That interlaminar space increases even more when a patient is positioned in flexion, but by how much?

To allay my concerns and increase my understanding of the anatomy, I once again turned to the literature to review the various anthropometric studies that reported the dimensions of the cervical spine. In particular, I sought the measurements of the cervical interlaminar spaces and the effect that flexion had on the measurement. I felt that a greater understanding of the interlaminar measurements would make the dilatation process for a posterior cervical laminectomy less vexing. Furthermore, the knowledge would allow me to establish the theoretical risk of passage into the canal by juxtaposing the diameters of the dilators I was using to the cervical interlaminar dimensions. Understanding the interlaminar dimensions relative to the dilator diameter would replace concern with confidence as I dilated onto the cervical lamina. However, as I sifted through the various publications, I found a glaring hole in the reported measurements; there were no reported measurements for the cervical interlaminar spaces.

The various published studies reported on the dimensions within each cervical vertebral body but not the relation of one lamina relative to another. The common denominator in these publications was that they were written before the rise of minimally invasive techniques. In an open approach, knowledge of the interlaminar dimension is not essential. Dissection proceeds from the spinous process to the lamina with direct visualization. Direct visualization of the bony anatomy allows the interlaminar space to be identified and safely avoided. However, in a minimally invasive approach, knowledge of the interlaminar measurements has an increased relevance. A dilator needs to find its way directly onto the lamina without visualization of the midline structures. Equally important, the dilator needs to exert downward pressure onto the lamina to optimize the interface of the minimal access port with the lamina and prevent muscle creep. All the while, the interlaminar space remains unseen and thus susceptible to a potential passage of the initial dilator if not optimally positioned immediately over the lamina. I recognized that the risk of passage into the canal would be proportional to the size of the dilator relative to the interlaminar space. I knew the diameters of the various dilators; what I needed to find out was the dimensions of the interlaminar space.

Using eight cervical cadaveric specimens, my biomechanics team and I measured the distance between the cervical lamina in the neutral, flexed and extended positions of the cervical spine. The interlaminar distances that we measured are reported in ▶ Table 8.1.

Table 8.1 Cervical interlaminar distances in the neutral, extended and flexed positions

Level	Neutral (mm)	Extension (mm)	Flexion (mm)
C2–C3	6.6±1.7	6.0±1.6	7.6±1.6
C3–C4	4.8±1.3	4.0±1.6	6.7±1.7
C4–C5	3.8±1.0	3.0±1.2	6.0±1.2
C5–C6	5.0±1.5	4.0±1.2	7.1±1.4
C6–C7	5.3±1.8	4.5±1.4	7.7±1.6
C7–T1	4.8±1.7	4.4±1.8	6.2±1.4

Table 8.2 Diameters of the various dilators in commercially available minimally invasive dilator sets

Dilator number	Medtronic (mm)	Depuy-Synthes (mm)	Globus (mm)	Stryker (mm)
1	5.3	3.0	2	6
2	9.4	10	5	10.75
3	12.8	13	8	12.75
4	14.6	16	12	14.75
5	16.8	19	15	16.75
6	18.8	22	18	18.75
7	20.8	25	22	20.75
8	22.8	28		24.75
9	24.8			

Using these values, I generated a visual interpretation of the effect of flexion and extension on the interlaminar space (▶ Fig. 8.6).

I then collected the various diameters of various commercially available dilators and placed them into ▶ Table 8.2. Juxtaposing these two tables provided me with the theoretical risk of passage into the canal during the dilatation process.

There were several observations that I made looking at the data in ▶ Table 8.1. The first observation is that a Kirschner wire, with a diameter of 0.9 to 1.5 mm, would have the greatest risk of passage into the canal. Conventional wisdom among minimally invasive circles had already convinced me to forgo the use of this wire in any minimally invasive approach years ago. The knowledge of the interlaminar measurements only served to reinforce that principle. The second observation was that in certain positions of the cervical spine, specifically flexion, the first dilator, and in some instances the second (depending on the system), could enter the canal. The interlaminar distances range from 3.8 to 6.6 mm in the neutral position. In flexion, the interlaminar distance increases by several millimeters, up to 7.68 at C6–7, one of the most common levels requiring surgical intervention.[1] Therefore, the unthinkable consequence of passing a dilator through the interlaminar space was a theoretical possibility when considering the interlaminar space relative to the diameter of the first dilator (▶ Fig. 8.7).

The cervical interlaminar measurements in ▶ Table 8.1 create a crucial framework for the dilatation phase of a posterior cervical laminectomy. The first dilator needs to begin its trajectory over the top of the foramen, similar to that of a posterior cervical foraminotomy. Placing that first dilator where the laminae converge, rather than diverge, decreases, if not eliminates, the risk of passage into the spinal canal. It is important to note that, based on the measurements in ▶ Table 8.1, the diameter of the first dilator in all of the commercially available systems has the theoretical risk of passage into the canal when the neck is flexed. The sequence of dilatation, therefore, proceeds from the top of the foramen with the smallest diameter dilator, where the interlaminar distance is narrowest. With each sequential dilator, the angle may converge increasingly onto the lamina. By the third dilator, the risk of passage into the canal becomes almost an anatomical impossibility and downward pressure against the lamina may be safely applied to optimize the lamina–access-port interface.

Before I measured the cervical interlaminar space, I passed the dilators onto the lamina with hesitation and avoided downward pressure against the lamina out of concern for passage into the canal, which resulted in suboptimal exposure and excessive muscle creep. The outcome was a suboptimal interface of the minimal access port with the lamina, and the need arose for excessive muscle resection to reach the cervical lamina. The additional muscle resection resulted in unnecessary postoperative discomfort for the patient.

I found that once I had studied the dimensions of the cervical interlaminar space relative to the diameters of the dilators, I was confidently able to establish an ideal corridor onto the requisite lamina. In this circumstance, knowledge is the true organ of sight, as quoted in the beginning of Chapter 2. Even though I could not see the interlaminar space, the knowledge of the interlaminar measurements relative to the diameter of the dilators transformed the dilatation phase of the operation. The certainty of the exact diameters of the dilators relative to the cervical interlaminar measurements is the first step in establishing this confidence. Mastery of the measurements and diameters in ▶ Table 8.1 and ▶ Table 8.2 and integrating them into the dilation process allow your mind to reconstruct the anatomy at depth. Knowledge of these values allows you to safely navigate the unexposed and unseen interlaminar space and dilate onto the cervical lamina for a minimally invasive cervical laminectomy.

8.4 Anatomical Basis

Understanding the interlaminar distance enables one to have confidence in the placement of the dilators onto the lamina but does not establish the anatomical basis for the operation. The anatomical basis for a minimally invasive cervical laminectomy becomes readily clear when the dimensions of the cervical canal and the lamina are examined. Panjabi and colleagues measured these dimensions in 12 fresh autopsy specimens (8 males and 4 females).[2] The mean measurements reported in Panjabi and colleagues' paper truly provide an understanding of the cervical dimensions in the average patient (▶ Table 8.3).

The two most important dimensions for a minimally invasive cervical laminectomy are spinal canal width (SCW) and spinal canal depth. ▶ Table 8.3 provides these dimensions for each cervical vertebra, and ▶ Fig. 8.8 provides a visual interpretation of that data.

The average SCW among the most commonly operated lamina (C5, C6 and C7) is approximately 25 mm. The hemilamina of

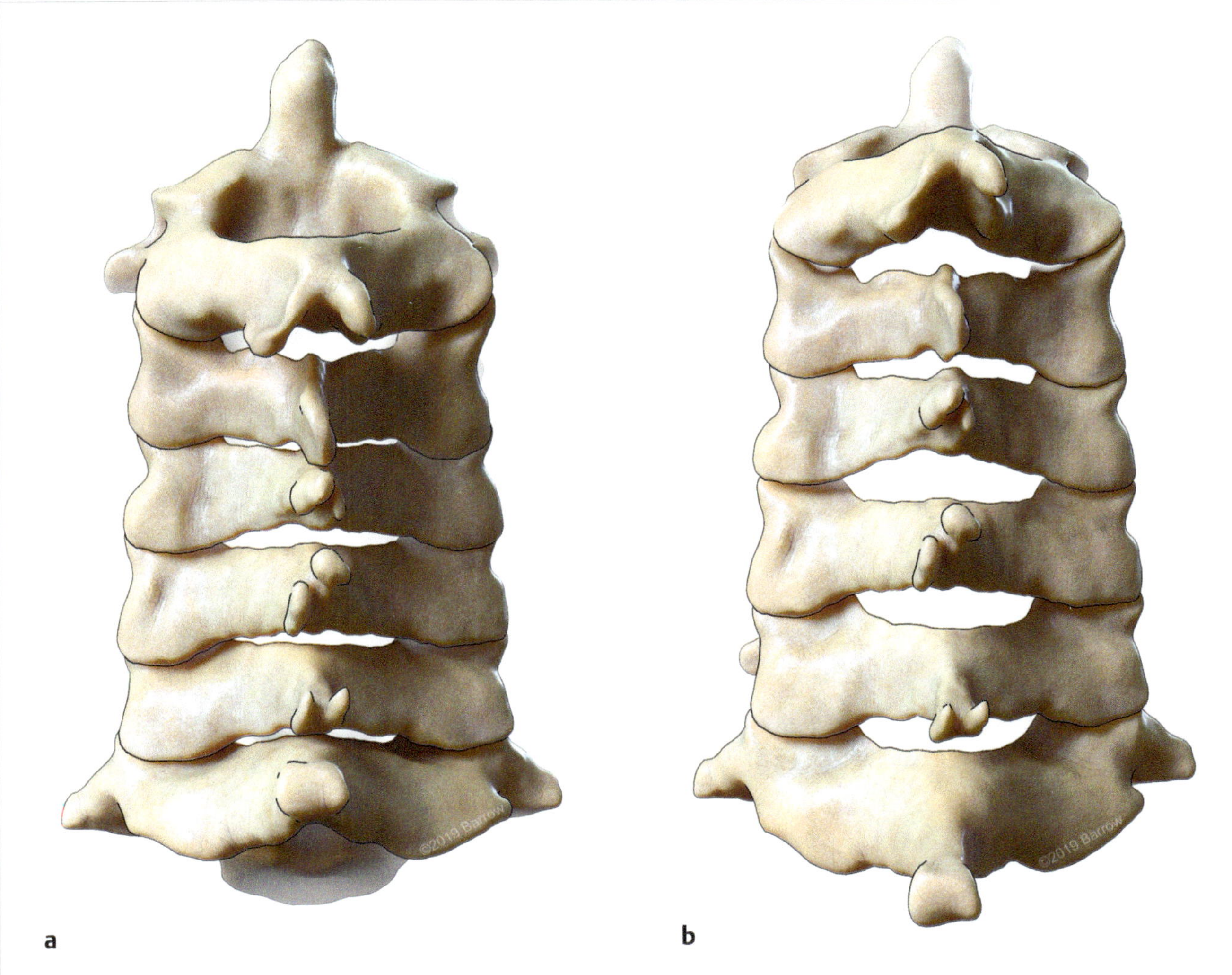

Fig. 8.6 The cervical interlaminar distances in extension and flexion. (a) Posterior view of the cervical spine in extension. The interlaminar distance decreases to a value as small as 3 mm at C4–5 with the majority of the distances being in the 4-mm range. (b) Posterior view of the spine in flexion. The interlaminar space can open to a distance of up to 7.7 mm at C6–7. In flexion, all of the interlaminar measurements are larger than the smallest dilator in any of the commercially available minimally invasive dilator sets.

the cervical spine from lateral mass to the spinous process measures approximately 13 mm throughout the cervical spine. With that number in mind, it becomes readily conceivable how a 14-mm field of view that converges onto the cervical lamina allows for access to the entire width of the canal in the three positions demonstrated in ▶ Fig. 8.9.

8.5 Operating Room Setup

The operating room setup is identical to the posterior cervical foraminotomy (▶ Fig. 8.10). As mentioned in Chapter 7, the fluoroscope and microscope are positioned to optimize the transitions. I position the fluoroscope opposite the side of the approach and the microscope on the same side of the approach. I prepare my colleagues in anesthesia for a crowded space at the head of the bed (▶ Fig. 8.11). Additional room is needed at the head for both the anesthesiologist to have access to the airway and for me to have access to the posterior cervical spine, which requires the operating table to be shifted further away from the anesthesia circuit and more into the middle of the room. As meddlesome as this seems initially, I have found that my anesthesia colleagues welcome this warmly over having the patient in the seated position. Similar to the posterior cervical foraminotomy, the clamp for the table-mounted arm resides at the level of the elbow opposite the side of the approach.

8.6 Skull Clamp and Positioning

As described in Chapter 7, the skull clamp needs to have good purchase into the cranium to provide the stability needed for the operation while avoiding the temporalis muscle, which will invariably cause postoperative discomfort for the patient. The

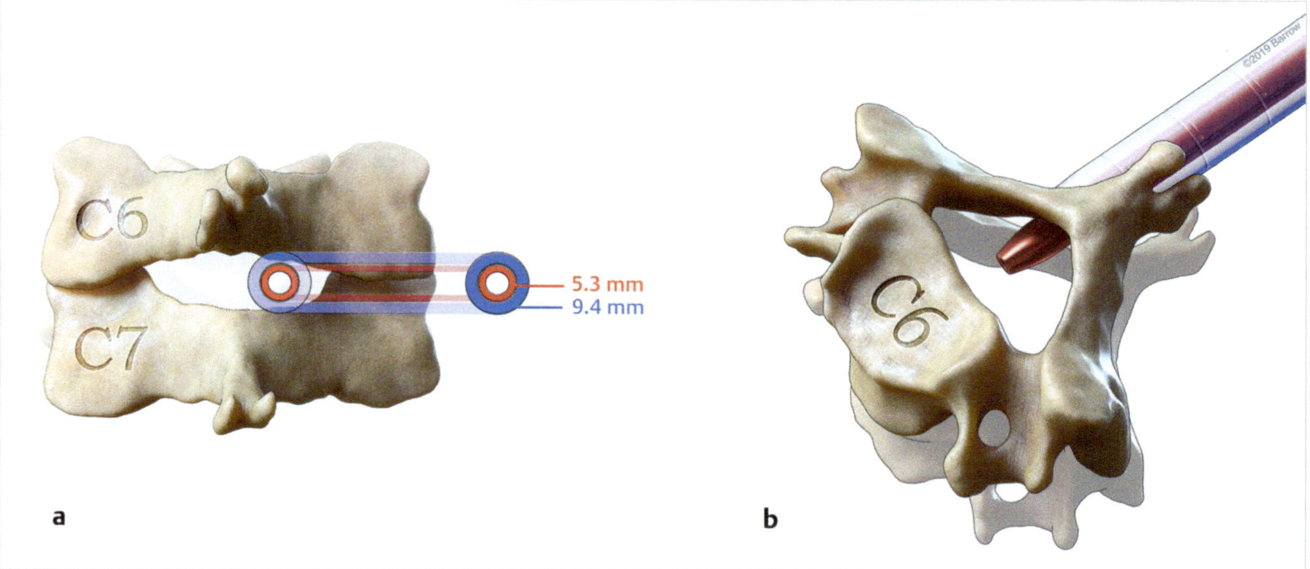

Fig. 8.7 The theoretical risk of passage of a dilator through the canal. **(a)** Posterior view of the cervical spine at C6–7 in flexion. With an average measurement of 7.68 mm in flexion at C6–7, a dilator with a diameter of 5.3 mm, the smallest diameter in my preferred set, has the theoretical risk of passing into the canal. **(b)** Superior oblique view of the dilators demonstrating the unthinkable entry of the initial dilator into the canal.

ideal position, therefore, is to have all the pins at the superior temporal line above the temporalis muscle. One pin will be in line with the tragus; the other will have the two pins on either side of the tragus (▶ Fig. 8.12). I apply 60 pounds of pressure onto the skull clamp after confirming optimal positioning of the pins and have the patient rolled onto chest rolls. It is crucial that my team roll the patient into the center of the operating table so that the components of the skull clamp system do not obstruct the anteroposterior (AP) image. As I hold the patient's head in a neutral position, my assistant secures the articulating arm and locks the system into position.

When positioning a patient, it is worth revisiting the effect that capital flexion has on the interlaminar spaces of the cervical spine. After completion of the anthropometric measurement study on the cervical interlaminar spaces that I described in Section 8.3, Cervical Interlaminar Measurements, I have refrained from ever positioning a patient in flexion for a posterior cervical laminectomy. As demonstrated in ▶ Table 8.1 and seen in ▶ Fig. 8.6, flexion increases the interlaminar space to an average distance of 7.7 mm, a distance that exceeds the diameter of the initial diameters in every commercially available minimally invasive dilator set. Keeping the patient in the neutral position keeps the interlaminar distance hovering around 5 mm, which is a safer distance with which to dilate onto the cervical lamina.

8.7 Localization

With the patient positioned on chest rolls and the skull clamp anchored to the bed with the articulating arm, I have the microscope draped on the side of the approach as the fluoroscopic technician rolls the fluoroscope into position for an image. I palpate the spinous processes in order to mark the midline and then approximate an incision 2 cm lateral to midline over the symptomatic segment, which is slightly more lateral than a posterior cervical foraminotomy to facilitate convergence. I base my approximation on the prominent spinous process of C7, and I count up from there, fully recognizing that fluoroscopic confirmation is needed to finalize the incision. Distinct from lumbar operations where I do not obtain preoperative images, in the cervical spine, I obtain a lateral image and leave the fluoroscope in position once the ideal patient position is achieved. I confirm the planned incision with a blunt probe on the skin and another lateral fluoroscopic image and make any necessary adjustments before prepping and draping the surgical site.

With all the sterile drapes placed, I pass a spinal needle onto the facet in the exact same manner that I would for a posterior cervical foraminotomy. Even though this is a laminectomy that requires converging onto the lamina and spinous process, I still diverge the spinal needle for localization to eliminate the risk of interlaminar passage of the spinal needle into the canal (▶ Fig. 8.13). Once I have confirmed my level, I remove the stylet and slowly pull back the spinal needle as I inject a local anesthetic mixture (lidocaine with epinephrine and bupivacaine).

My preferred diameter for a minimal access port in cervical laminectomies is 14 mm, which is based on the distance from the lateral canal to the spinous process (~13 mm). Using the entry point of the spinal needle as the center mark, I measure a 16-mm incision in preparation for the 14-mm minimal access port. I then infiltrate the skin incision with some more local anesthetic before making the incision with a No. 15 blade. As in a posterior foraminotomy, I divide the fascia with cautery. Holding a suction in one hand and cautery with a protected tip in the other allows me to directly visualize the division of the fascia. The key difference between the foraminotomy and laminectomy occurs at this point (▶ Fig. 8.14). I begin to converge toward the midline with the fascial opening, whereas in a foraminotomy I proceed straight onto the foramen. Keep in mind,

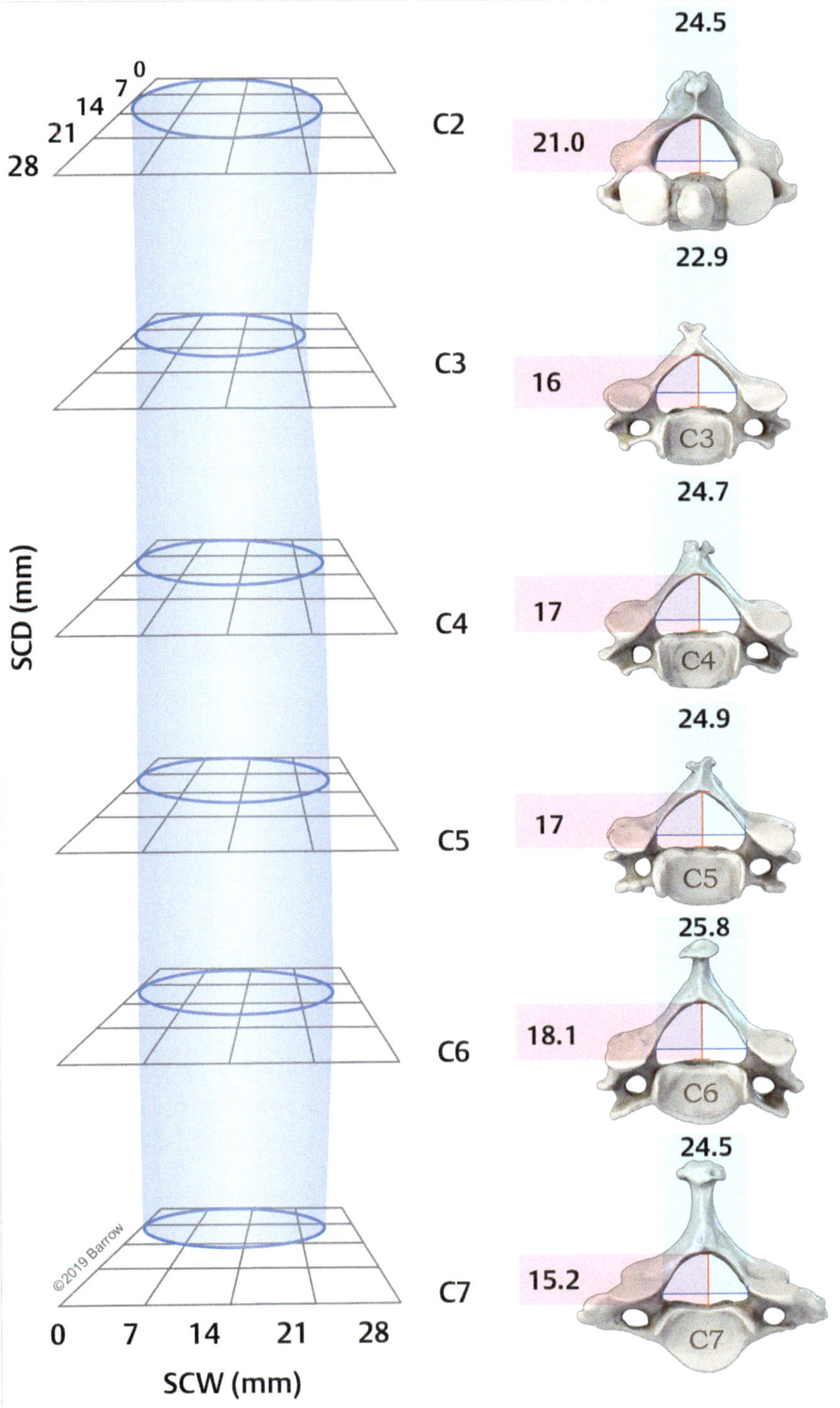

Fig. 8.8 Dimensional analysis of the cervical spine, giving the spinal canal depth (SCD) and spinal canal width (SCW) in millimeters.

Table 8.3 Cervical canal width and depth as reported by Panjabi et al[2]

	C2	C3	C4	C5	C6	C7
SCW (mm)	24.5	22.9	24.7	24.9	25.8	24.5
SCD (mm)	21.0	16	17	17	18.1	15.2

Abbreviations: SCD, spinal canal depth; SCW, spinal canal width.

the starting point for the laminectomy is 2 cm from the midline to optimize the trajectory onto the lamina and access the midline. For this reason, convergence needs to begin with the fascial opening. I begin the fascial opening medial to the skin incision and proceed obliquely through the fascia until I reach the muscle layer. Once I see the muscle past the fascial opening, I begin with the dilators.

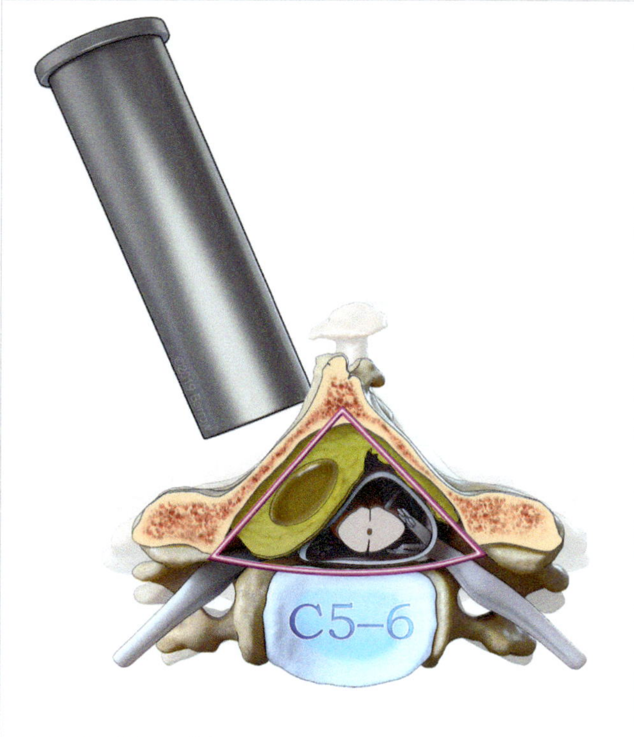

Fig. 8.9 Anatomical basis for a minimally invasive posterior cervical laminectomy. Illustration demonstrating a 14-mm access port that converges over the top of the C6 lamina in a patient with a facet cyst causing unilateral dorsal compression of the spinal cord. The magenta triangle represents the area of the spinal canal.

When I pass the first dilator onto the spine, my target is the inferior articular process (IAP) of the rostral segment (▶ Fig. 8.15). I want to feel the drop-off from the IAP onto the superior articular process (SAP). The sensation of the drop-off from the IAP onto the SAP tells me exactly where I am on the lateral cervical spine. The convergence onto the lamina begins with the second dilator. I begin the convergence by wanding in a rostral and medial direction onto the lamina (▶ Fig. 8.16). The knowledge of the interlaminar distances and the dilators becomes exceedingly valuable for the third dilator, which is now at a diameter where the risk of translaminar passage is almost absent based on the interlaminar measurements.

It is essential to continue to feel the unmistakable tactile sensation of metal against bone throughout the dilatation process. Maintaining downward pressure with the larger dilators up against the laminar bone minimizes the muscle that needs to be swept away with cautery in order to reach the lamina. If at any time I have lost that feeling, I begin again from the first dilator. We are all inherently more cautious in the posterior cervical spine with downward pressure onto the lamina than in the lumbar spine. That caution makes a suboptimal dilatation a greater risk than perhaps the interlaminar passage of a dilator. However, the result is too much muscle creep instead of the interlaminar passage of a dilator. Having to traverse several centimeters of posterior cervical musculature to reach the lamina does not harness the true advantage of a minimally invasive approach. A suboptimal dilatation of the access port up against the lamina results in the need for excessive disruption of the posterior musculature and causes significant discomfort to the patient. One of the main benefits of the minimally invasive approach has been lost. If you cannot readily palpate the cervical lamina with the suction tip using light downward pressure once the access port is in position, you have a suboptimal dilatation. Either start over beginning with the first dilator or apply the iterative dilatation process described in Chapter 7 and reviewed in the section below. Regardless, be meticulous about downward pressure keeping the tip of each dilator firmly against the lamina as the diameters increase and converge.

After securing the minimal access port into position, I evaluate the fluoroscopic image. I am especially critical of the AP image (▶ Fig. 8.17). If I do not feel that I have converged adequately, I keep the fluoroscope ready for another AP image as I loosen the table-mounted arm and converge a few more degrees while maintaining downward pressure. I secure the retractor arm and obtain another fluoroscopic image. Once I am satisfied with the position of the minimal access port, I bring in the operating microscope.

8.7.1 Iterative Dilatation with Direct Visualization

As described in Chapter 7, an option for repositioning the minimal access port when I have identified a suboptimal interface of the access port with the lamina facet complex in a posterior cervical foraminotomy is to create a linear window through the paraspinal musculature, directly expose the lamina and dock the initial dilator onto the target with direct visualization. In doing so, I have the utmost confidence in my position, and subsequent dilators displace the muscle and optimize the interface of the access port with the lamina facet complex. Should I find a thick wall of muscle that keeps me from seeing the lamina, I apply the same technique. Similar to the procedure in a posterior cervical foraminotomy, I use cautery to cleave a plane directly onto the cervical lamina. Once I can see the unmistakable ivory of the cervical lamina, I pass the initial dilator with direct visualization and secure it onto the lamina. I remove the access port and begin the dilatation process again with the absolute certainty of my position. That certainty provides me with the confidence to apply downward pressure and optimize an interface against the lamina that has very little muscle creep. The iterative dilatation with direct visualization allows me to harness one of the strengths of minimally invasive approaches: preservation of the posterior paraspinal musculature.

8.7.2 Exposure of the Lamina

It is worthwhile at this point to consider the exposure of the lamina in an open laminectomy and contrast that with a minimally invasive exposure. In an open technique, exposure begins by first identifying the tips of the spinous processes and then revealing the entire spinous process before descending onto the

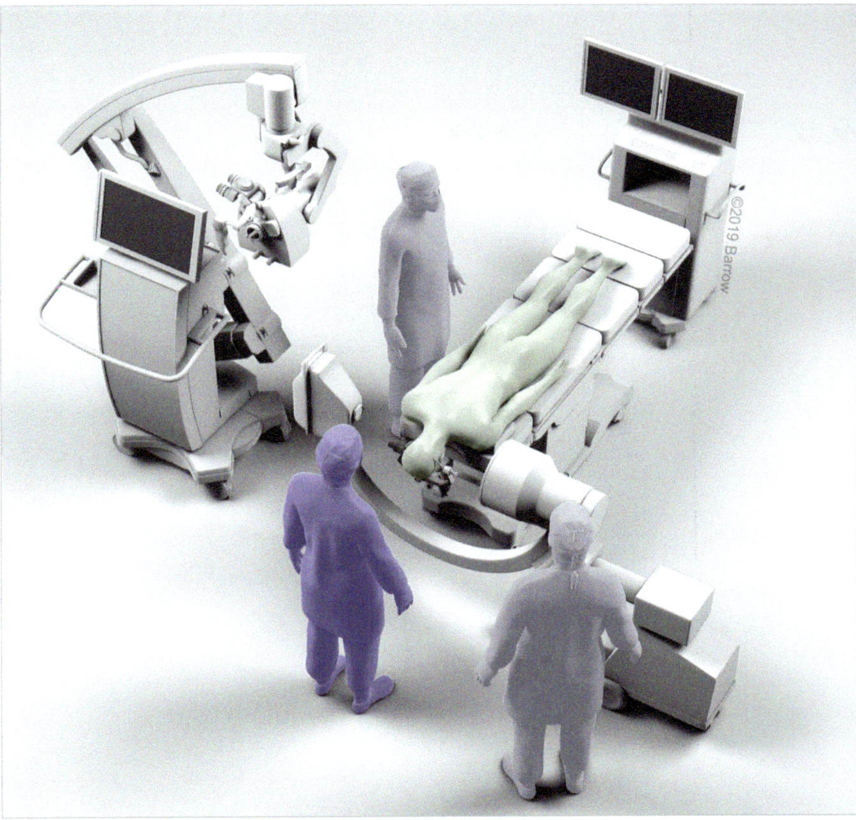

Fig. 8.10 Operating room setup. The patient is positioned on a standard operating table on chest rolls with the table reversed to allow for easy passage of the fluoroscopic unit. The base of the fluoroscope is positioned opposite the microscope. The fluoroscopic monitors are positioned at the foot of the bed to allow for a direct line of sight when passing the dilators. The surgeon (*dark blue*) stands at the head of the bed for the incision and dilation with a direct line of sight onto the monitors. The anesthesiologist is also at the head of the bed but off to the side (*light blue*). The scrub technician sets up their Mayo stand in a manner that facilitates handing instruments to the surgeon at the head of the table.

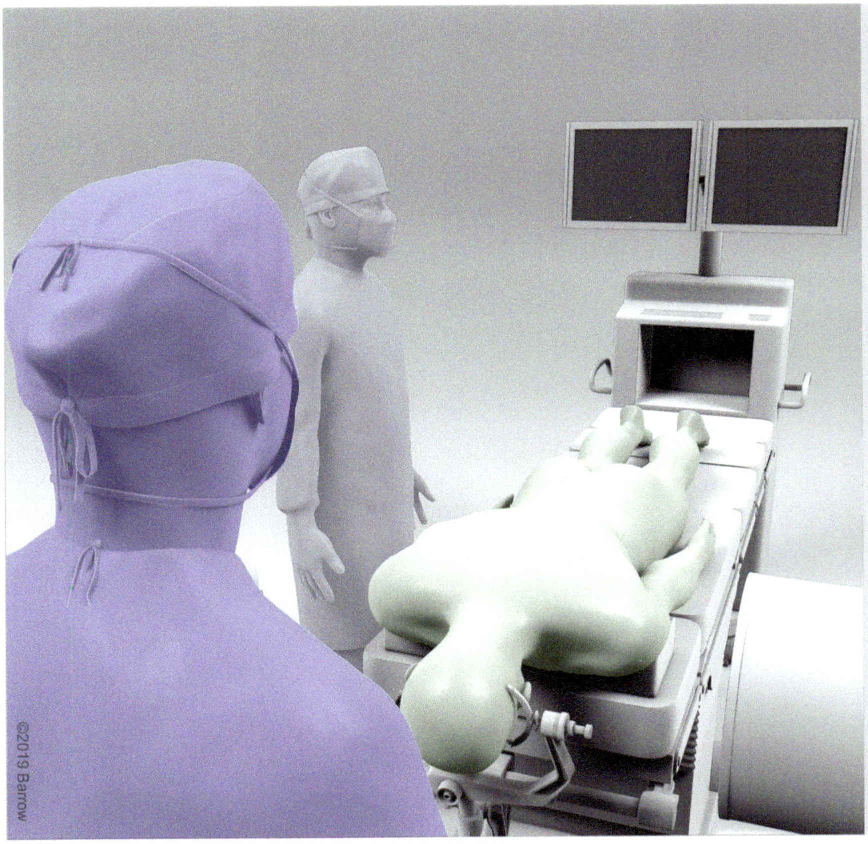

Fig. 8.11 Over the shoulder view of the operating room setup. Illustration demonstrating where the surgeon stands for docking of the access port. In this manner, the line of sight on the fluoroscopic monitors has been optimized. Working at the head of the bed is also the ideal ergonomic position for the surgeon to position the access port.

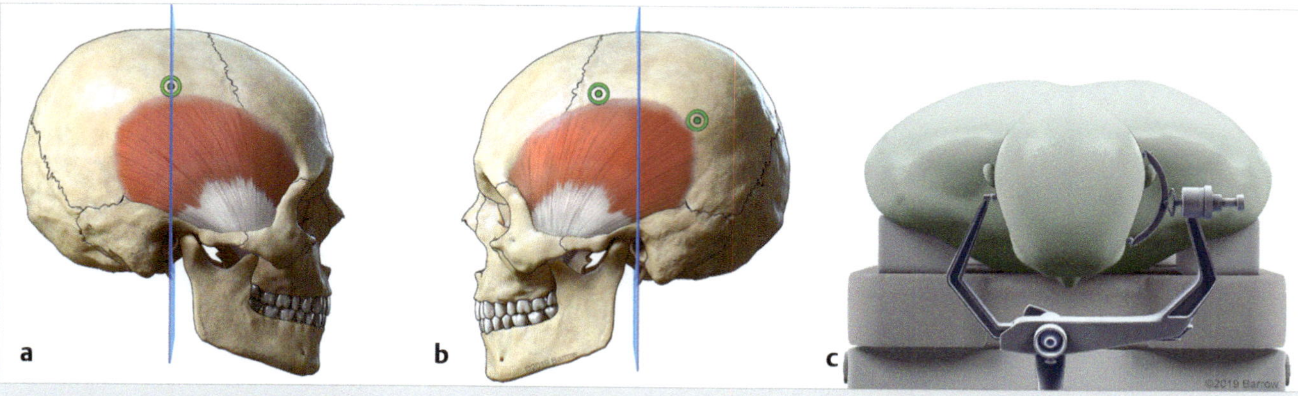

Fig. 8.12 Illustrations of positioning the patient's head in a skull clamp. **(a)** Location of the temporalis muscle relative to the ideal position for the pin sites. Avoiding the temporalis muscle prevents any postoperative discomfort from the pins piercing the temporalis muscle. **(b)** The ideal placement is on either side of the tragus for the two-pin arm and in line with the tragus with the one-pin arm above the temporalis and into the superior temporal line. **(c)** Head-on view of skull clamp positioning.

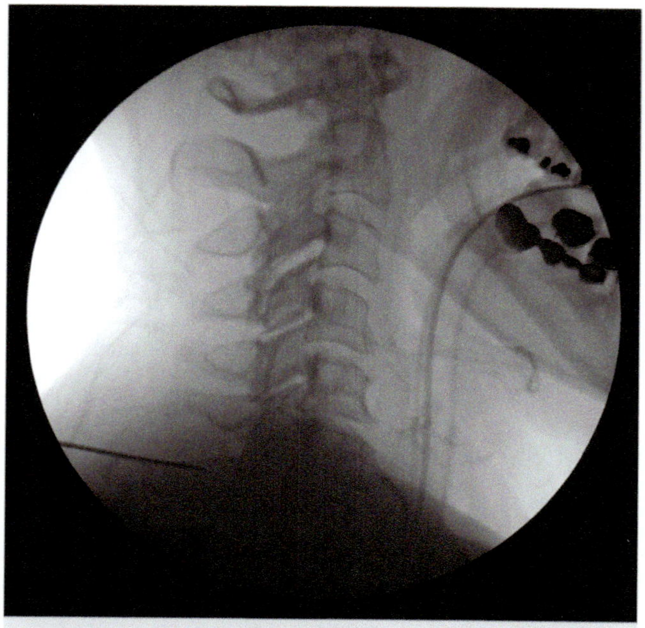

Fig. 8.13 Needle localization and confirmation of the cervical segment. Lateral fluoroscopic image with the spinal needle in position for localization of the segment and planning the incision for a C6–7 laminectomy.

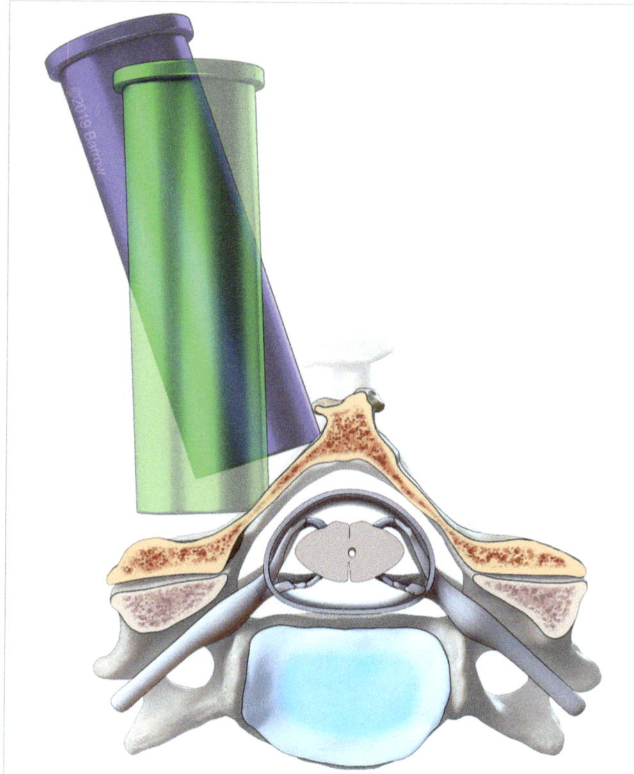

Fig. 8.14 Laminectomy versus foraminotomy. Illustration demonstrating the difference between the straighter trajectory of a foraminotomy (*emerald green*) and converging trajectory of a laminectomy (*cobalt blue*).

lamina using a subperiosteal dissection. Finally, exposure of the facet lateral mass complex completes the exposure. This particular sequence of exposure for an open approach is logical, orienting and safe.

In a minimally invasive cervical laminectomy, the sequence of exposure is almost exactly the opposite. The first target to expose is the medial facet. It is the medial facet that becomes the orienting structure instead of the tips of the spinous processes. The junction of the medial facet blending into the lamina is the next target, which will guide your exposure of the lamina to the base of the spinous process. In a similar but opposite manner, the sequence of exposure is logical and safe, but it does have the potential to be disorienting. After securing a minimal access port, it would be ill-advised to attempt to begin the exposure in the middle of the field of view without the absolute anatomical certainty of precisely where the lamina

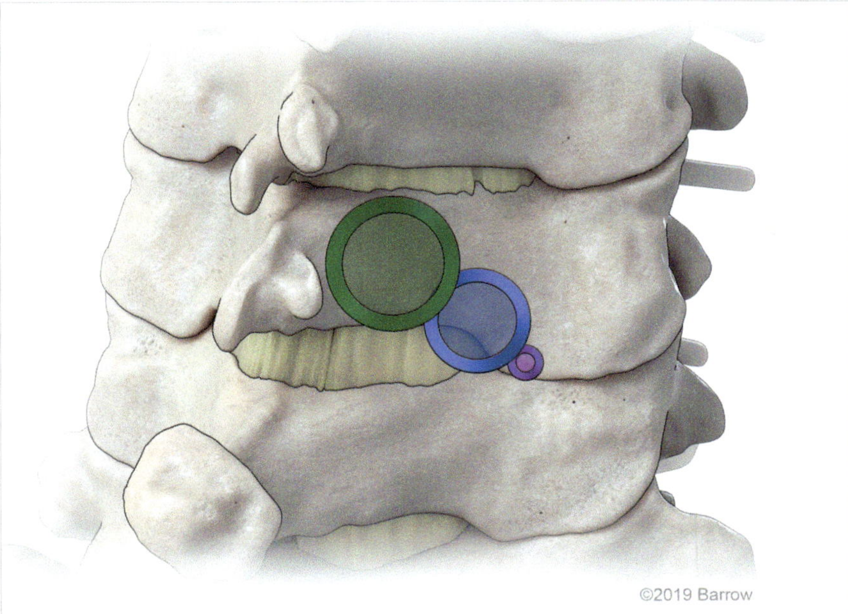

Fig. 8.15 Sequential convergence of the dilators. Illustration demonstrating the sequential convergence onto the spine with the increasing diameters of the dilators. With each increasing diameter, the wanding proceeds in both a medial and a rostral trajectory.

resides. The key to transitioning to a minimally invasive exposure is becoming as familiar with the medial facet for the basis of your orientation as you are with the tips of the spinous processes in midline approaches. That is why the posterior cervical foraminotomy is the vehicle to accomplish this familiarity. Converging in the medial direction onto the lamina from the familiarity developed through posterior cervical foraminotomies is not too far off a bridge to cross.

With the minimal access port in position, the place to begin the exposure is in the superior and lateral quadrant of the diameter of the port, which is similar to the exposure for a posterior cervical foraminotomy. My first objective is to expose the medial aspect of the IAP of the superior segment. That last sentence can be confusing, and perhaps, a better way to phrase it is in the context of a clinical scenario. In a C6–7 decompression, I would begin with exposure of the medial facet of C6 (the superior segment; ▶ Fig. 8.18). Once I see the indisputable ivory of the exposed facet, I gently probe with the suction in one hand confirming the presence of the lamina and sweep away the muscle with cautery held in the other hand. If I have any concern about the presence of the lamina where I intend to cauterize, I use a forward-angled curet to confirm its presence. I do this by passing a straight curet into the location where I distinctly see the exposed lamina and sweep it beneath the muscle to confirm the lamina underneath. In doing so, I can peel back the muscle and directly see the lamina below as I expose it. I now continue to sweep back the muscle with cautery confident that lamina resides below.

The exposure proceeds until I have reached the base of the spinous process. Additional fluoroscopy throughout this process offers little added value because nothing replaces the direct visualization of the lamina rising steeply into the sloping spinous process. However, if there is a question regarding the position of the minimal access port, an additional image may be of value.

Visualizing the lamina blending into the spinous process allows me to turn to the superior articular surface of the caudal facet, in this case, C7. I am meticulous to avoid the interlaminar space by staying at the caudal aspect of the exposure. If I am unable to confidently expose the caudal lamina, I leave the third and fourth quadrants (▶ Fig. 8.18) untouched until I remove the IAP and rostral lamina, which will unveil those structures. With the exposure complete, the final step before beginning the bone work is to rotate the bed slightly away from myself. That rotation optimizes access to the contralateral lamina on the underside of the spinous process (▶ Fig. 8.19).

8.8 Anatomy of the Cervical Ligamentum Flavum

Rahmani and colleagues[3] published one of the most comprehensive analyses of the cervical ligamentum flavum, and I would consider their work as mandatory reading for any posterior cervical surgery. The authors provide the dimensions of the ligamentum flavum at each segment of the cervical spine, which is of tremendous value for decompression of a segment. As in a lumbar laminectomy, I target the insertion points of the ligamentum flavum on the cervical lamina. ▶ Fig. 8.20 demonstrates the insertion points from the underside of the lamina. The laminar bone work that I perform needs to encompass just slightly beyond these insertion points so that I may release the ligamentum flavum in an en bloc manner, just as I did in the lumbar spine.

8.9 Drilling the Cervical Lamina

Although I use a diamond burr for posterior cervical foraminotomies, the amount of bone that needs to be drilled for a laminectomy is substantially more. A diamond burr is still an

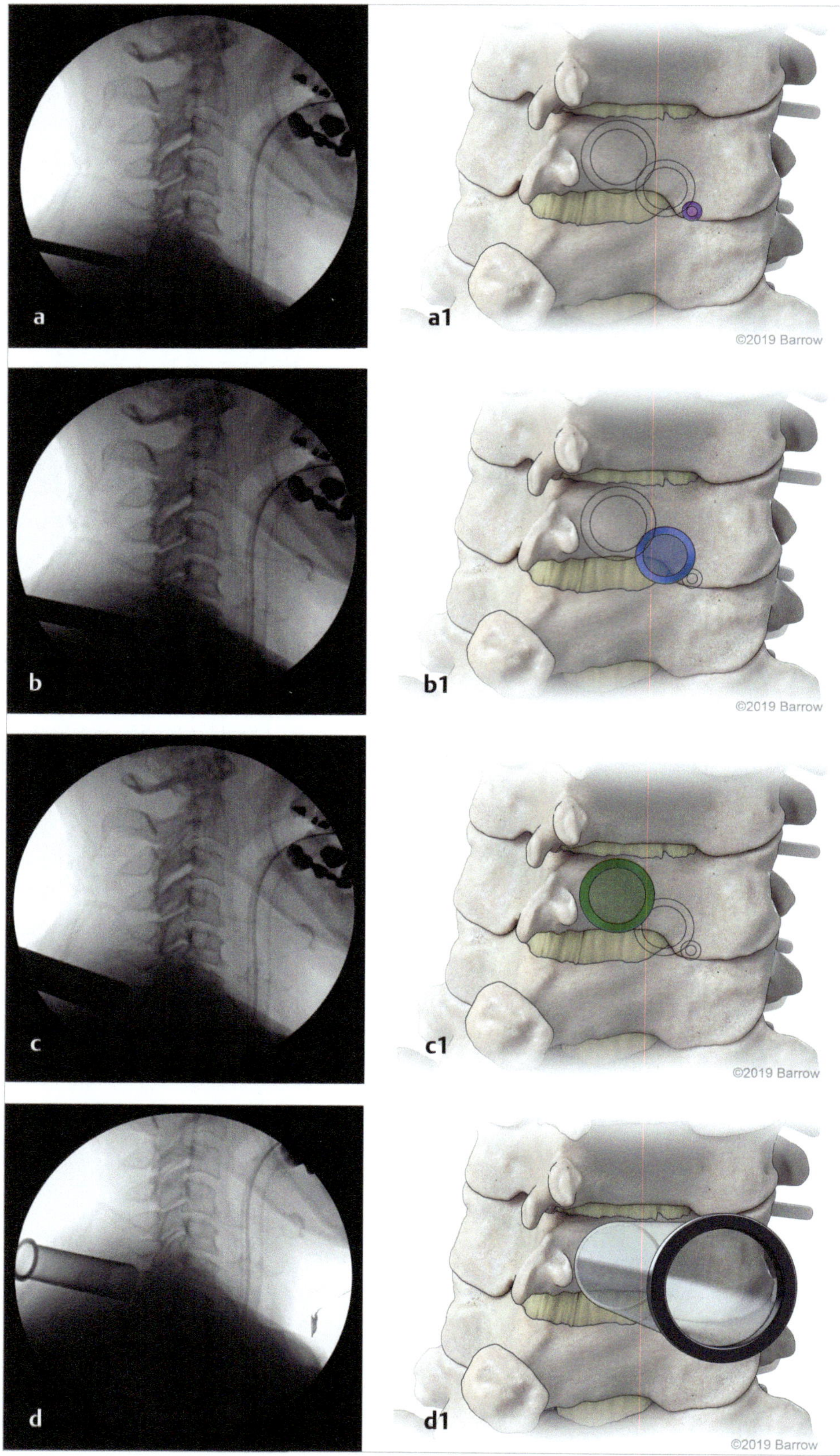

Fig. 8.16 A sequence of lateral fluoroscopic images juxtaposed with the sequential convergence toward the midline with increasing diameters. **(a)** The first dilator is docked in the same position as in a foraminotomy. **(a1)** Corresponding illustration shows the location of the initial dilator on the cervical spine. **(b)** The subsequent dilators begin to converge toward the medial spine as the dilator diameter increases. **(b1)** Corresponding illustration shows the location of the second dilator on the cervical spine. **(c)** Medial convergence against the spinous process. **(c1)** Corresponding illustration shows the location of the third dilator on the cervical spine. **(d)** Minimal access port in position with convergence onto the lamina. Convergence on the lamina is demonstrated by the open appearance of ring at the base or top of the access port. A flattened ring suggests a straight trajectory. **(d1)** Corresponding illustration shows the convergence of the access port onto the lamina.

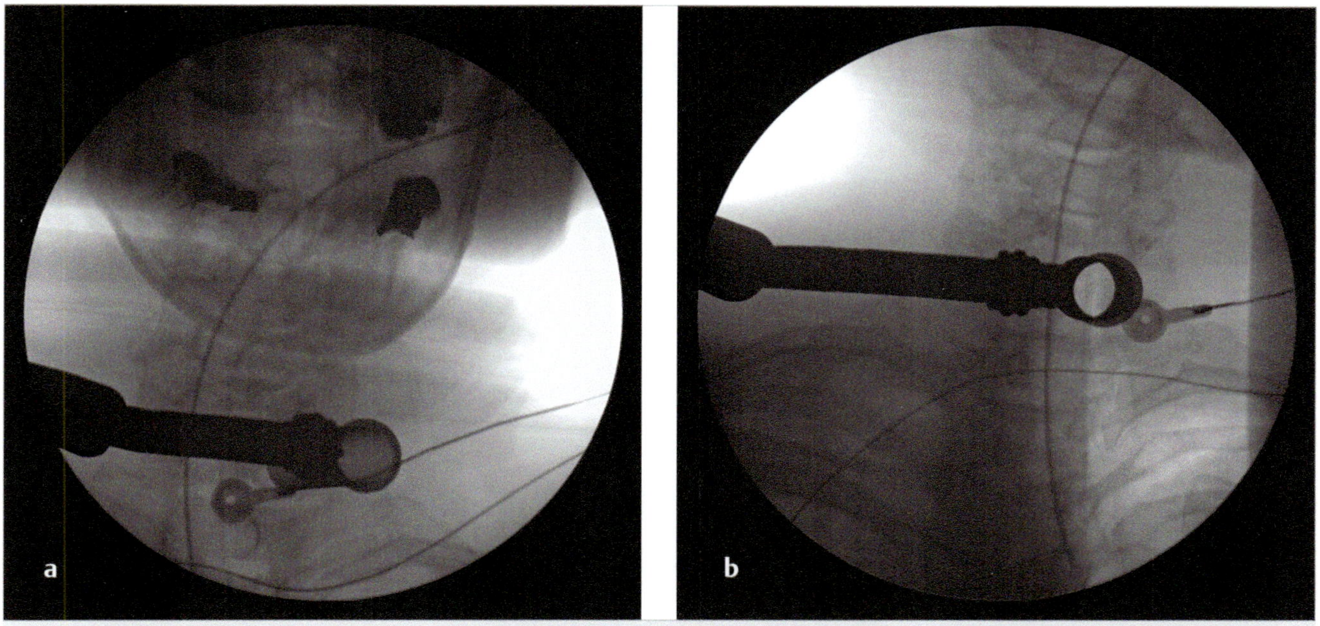

Fig. 8.17 Convergence of the access port over the lamina. **(a)** True anteroposterior (AP) fluoroscopic image demonstrating the convergence onto the lamina–spinous process junction. **(b)** Oblique AP image demonstrating a view in line with the diameter of the minimal access port. This oblique view reveals that the interface of the access port is apposed against the lamina.

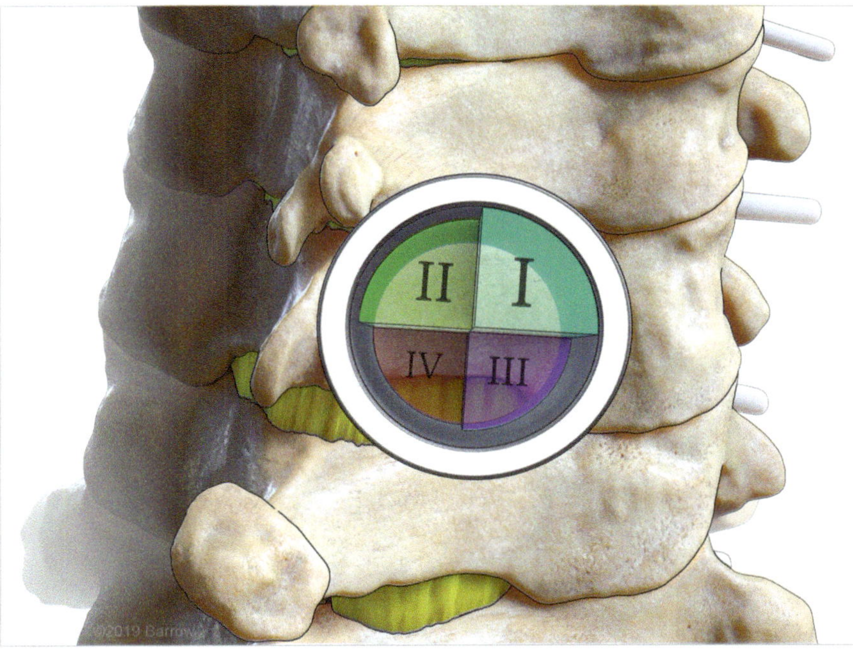

Fig. 8.18 Sequence of cervical lamina exposure. Illustration of a 14-mm access port over the C6 lamina. The safest location for the exposure is the superior and lateral quadrant of the field of view (quadrant I). From there, the exposure proceeds sequentially into quadrants II (superior and medial), III (inferior and lateral) and then IV (inferior and medial).

option, but my preference has evolved into a cutting burr for a cervical laminectomy. I begin drilling from lateral to medial in quadrants I and II (▶ Fig. 8.18) to thin the bone to a shrimp-shell thickness. Once the ligamentum flavum begins to come into view, I focus on thinning the remaining lamina to the same depth. The 14-mm diameter is a useful guide to the amount of bone work that I have accomplished. My goal is to erase all of the laminar bone in my field of view. The insertion of the ligamentum flavum should be in that field of view, and working beyond the insertion facilitates its resection, similar to the technique performed for the lumbar laminectomy (▶ Fig. 8.21).

The final step with the access port in the initial position is drilling the underside of the spinous process and contralateral lamina, analogous again to the lumbar laminectomy technique (▶ Fig. 8.22).

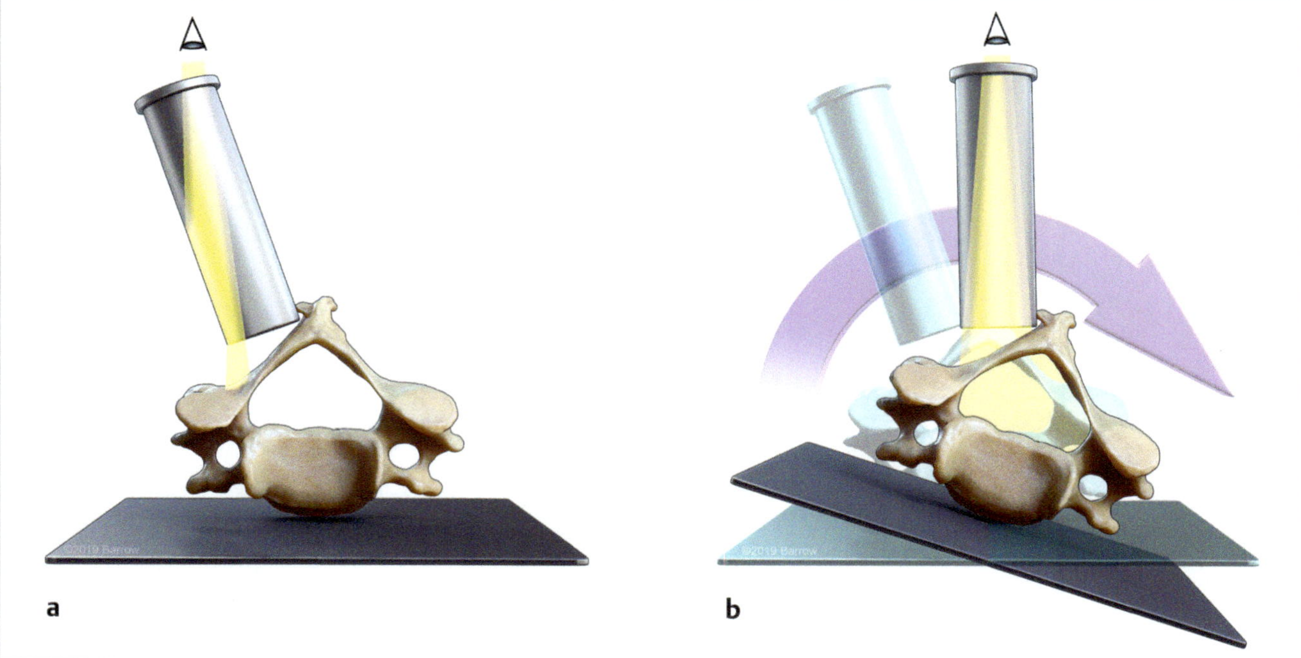

Fig. 8.19 Position for a minimally invasive posterior cervical laminectomy optimized by rotation of the bed. **(a)** Conceptual axial view of the cervical spine showing a suboptimal line of sight onto the lamina. **(b)** Rotation of the bed optimizes the line of sight and working corridor to allow for complete decompression of the segment.

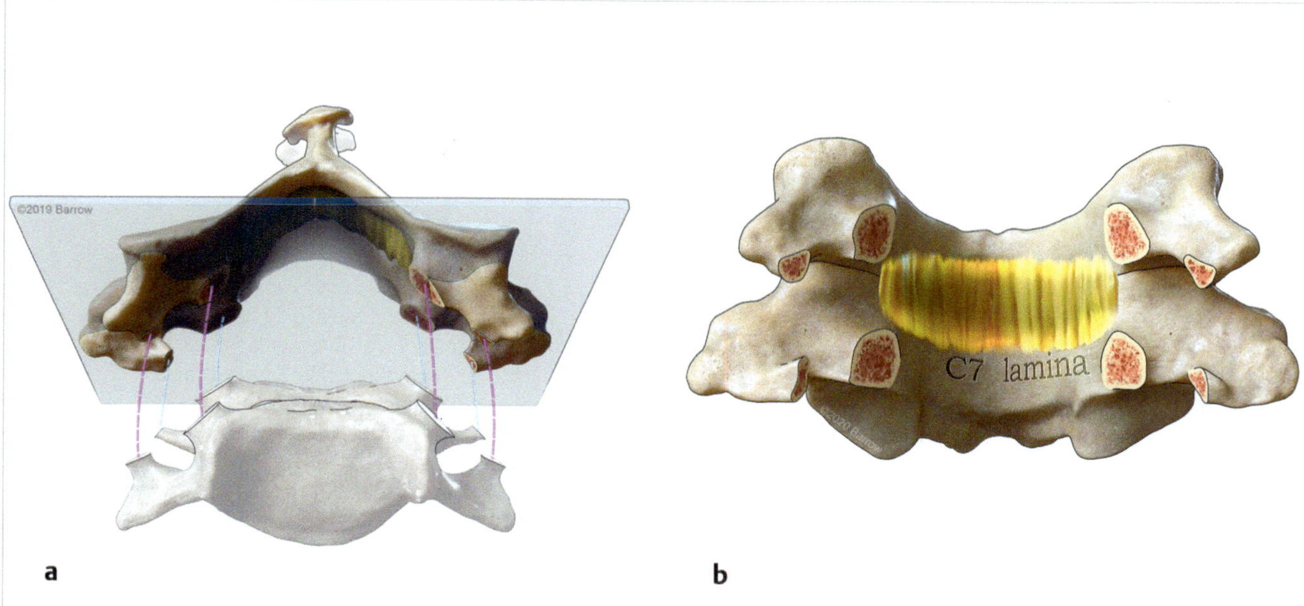

Fig. 8.20 Anatomy of the ligamentum flavum. **(a)** Axial view of the cervical spine demonstrating the cut plane to orient the reader for the image in **b.** **(b)** A view of the cervical lamina from within the canal to appreciate the insertion points for the ligamentum flavum into the lamina. Understanding these insertion points is tremendously valuable when decompressing a segment. The insertion points of the ligamentum flavum are the limits of the laminar bone work.

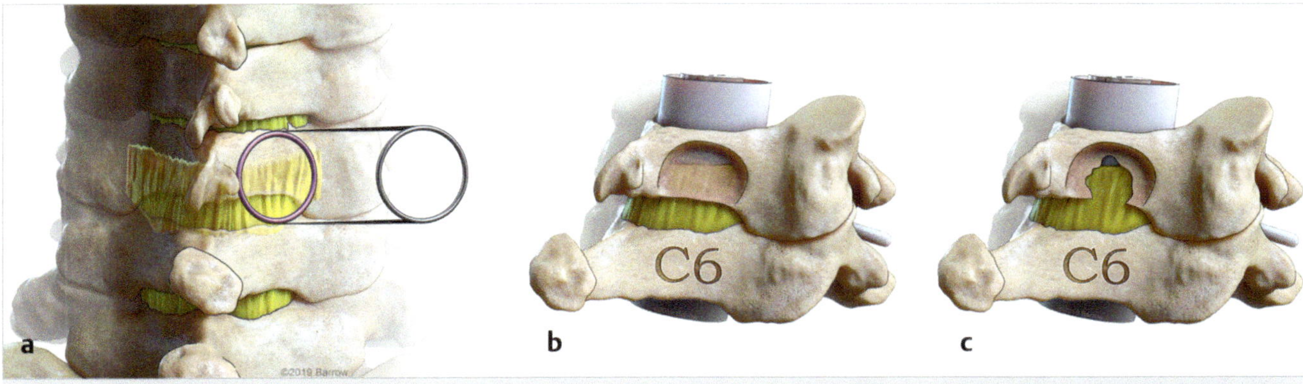

Fig. 8.21 Thinning of the cervical lamina and exposure of the ligamentum flavum. **(a)** Posterior view of the cervical spine indicating the position of the port (*magenta ring*). **(b)** Posterior view of the cervical lamina thinned to a shrimp-shell thickness for the entire field of view. **(c)** Removal of the thinned bone up to the insertion point on the underside of the lamina. The process of exposing the ligamentum flavum in the cervical spine is analogous to the lumbar laminectomy.

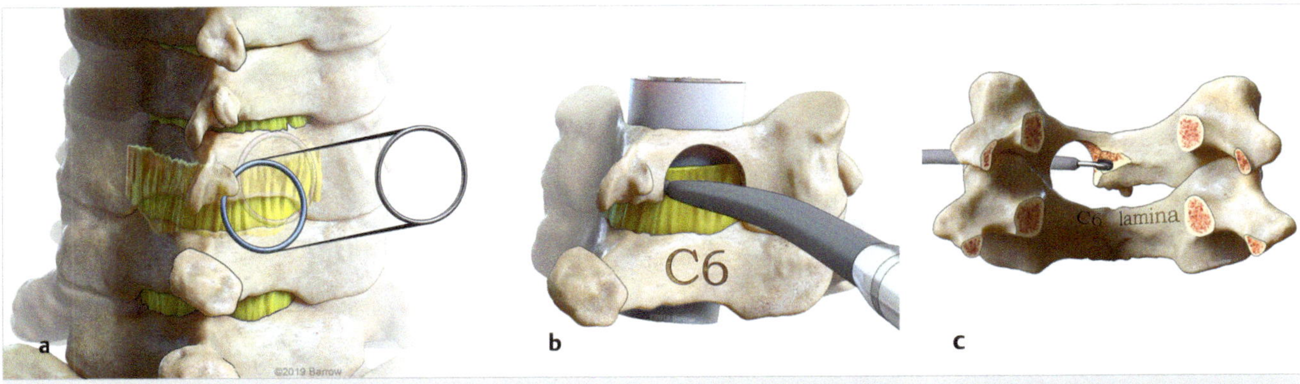

Fig. 8.22 Drilling the contralateral lamina. **(a)** Posterior view of the cervical spine indicating the position of the port (*turquoise ring*) to access the contralateral lamina. **(b)** With the entire cervical lamina in the initial field of view drilled, the attention turns to the underside of the contralateral lamina as demonstrated in this figure. **(c)** A view from within the canal, looking at the underside of the spinous process and contralateral lamina.

If this exposure affords access to the caudal lamina, then I drill that lamina down at this time. If I do not yet have an exposure to the caudal lamina, I complete the work in the current position of the access port. Specifically, I release the ligamentum flavum from its rostral and lateral insertions before shifting the access port into the second position. With the ligamentum flavum released but still on top of the spinal cord, I shift the access port over the caudal lamina. I ensure that the exposures are overlapping by at least 50% so that I can continue the decompression that I have already begun.

Now that the access port has been repositioned, the process starts anew with drilling the caudal lamina down to beyond the ligamentum flavum insertion, which will complete the central decompression (▶ Fig. 8.23). Drilling down to a shrimp-shell thickness allows the safe use of a Kerrison rongeur or a forward-angled curet to finish the decompression on top of the dura. Depending on the nature of the pathology, angling the access port further up or down remains an option. Working beyond the insertion of the ligamentum flavum allows for the elevation of the ligamentum flavum and its en bloc removal.

The final position of the access port is over the cervical foramen to decompress the lateral aspect of the spinal cord and the exiting nerve root (▶ Fig. 8.24). I place the final dilator into the access port, loosen the table-mounted arm and straighten the trajectory so that the field of view is more like what I would have for a posterior cervical foraminotomy. The bed rotates back into the neutral position after I have repositioned the access port. The familiar position of a posterior cervical foraminotomy allows for completion of the decompression over the nerve root and the lateral aspect of the spinal cord. I have accomplished the goals of the operation with the entire spinal cord decompressed and the exiting nerve root free.

8.9.1 Hemostasis and Closure

Prior to closing the incision, I perform my final systems check. I reassess the fluoroscopic image, review the magnetic resonance image (MRI), and then peer down the microscope one last time. When I feel that I have accomplished all of the goals of the operation, I begin to remove the access port. Similar to that in the posterior cervical foraminotomy, I do this very slowly with

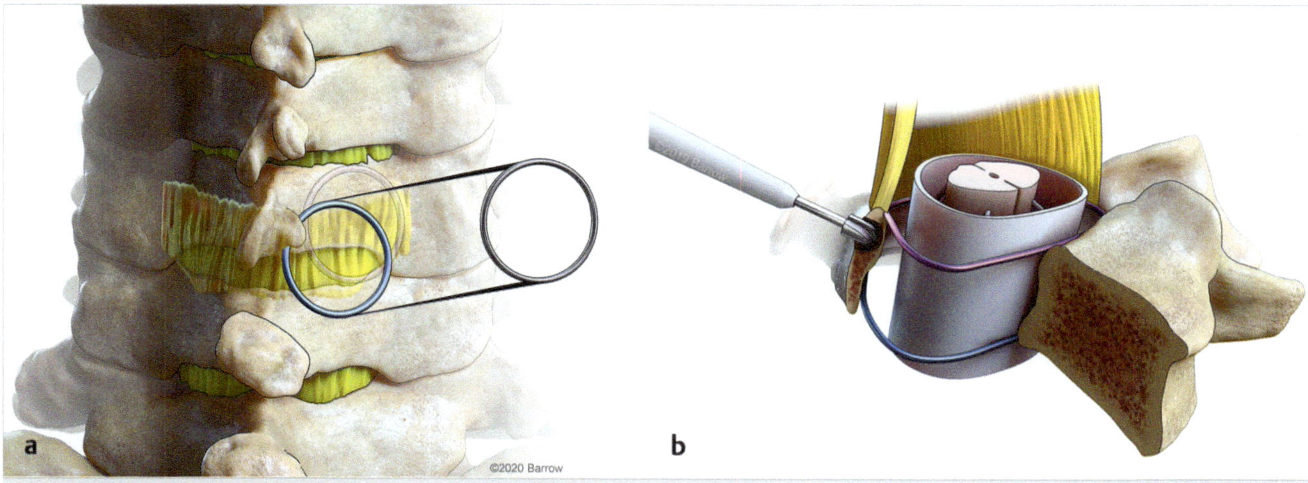

Fig. 8.23 Drilling the caudal insertion of the ligamentum flavum. **(a)** The position of the access port (*turquoise ring*) remains in the second position. **(b)** Illustration demonstrating drilling the caudal cervical lamina distal to the insertion. The magenta ring represents the smaller diameter of the canal; therefore, the drill works beyond the magenta ring to minimize injury to the neural elements. The canal widens distally, as can be seen in the turquoise ring. The rings in this image represent canal diameters and not the position of the access port.

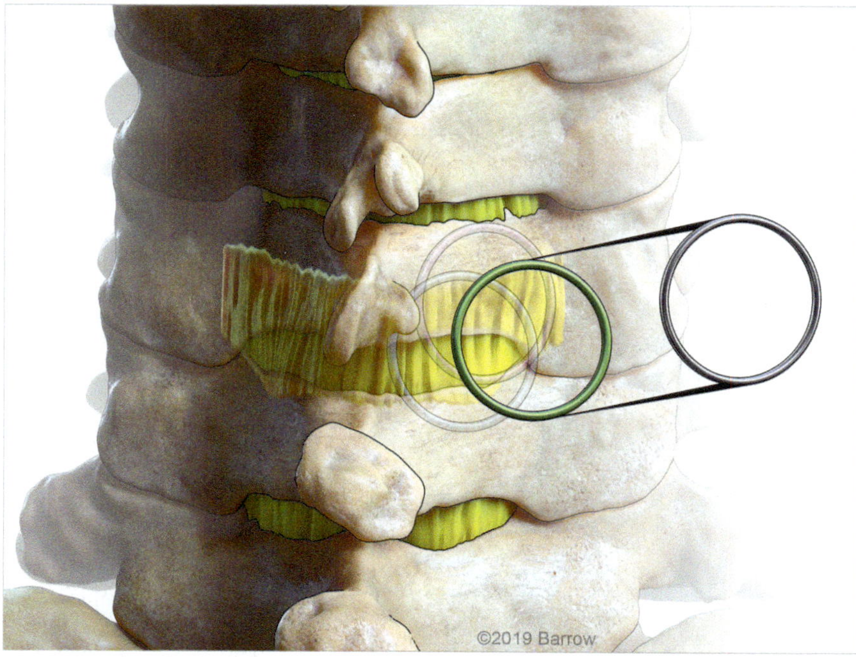

Fig. 8.24 Drilling ipsilateral lamina and medial facet. Posterior view of the cervical spine indicating the final position of the port (*emerald ring*) for completion of the laminectomy.

direct vision of the muscle as the access port slides out. For the most part, the minimal access port can be removed with nothing more than an occasional touch of cautery along the walls of the exposure. On occasion, an arterial vessel bleeds, and it is imperative to cauterize both sides of the vessel where it has been divided by the dilatation process. A right-angled bipolar cautery is incredibly adept at accomplishing this task. Although bleeding muscular arterial branches may be relatively straightforward to handle, their venous counterparts may present a challenge. It has been my observation that veins in the path of the minimal access may stretch and tear along the side of the vein, whereas small muscular arteries tear end to end. Therefore, cauterization of these veins may require some additional time and attention. The bleeding at times may be vigorous, and using the minimal access port to tamponade the bleeding is essential to adequately visualize the source. Recognizing that the bleeding may be from the side of the vein expedites hemostasis. The entire length of the vein will need to be cauterized.

After removal of the minimal access port, I inject the skin and soft tissues once again with a mixture of 1% lidocaine with epinephrine and bupivacaine. A size 0 polyglactin 910 suture on a UR-6 needle is the best for grabbing either side of the fascia for closing. Two or three sutures reapproximate the fascia. A 2-0 polyglactin suture on an X-1 needle is used to reapproximate the subcutaneous layer and a 4-0 polyglactin suture on an RB-1 needle brings together the skin edges. I apply a liquid adhesive to the skin and then Steri-Strips (3M Company, Maplewood, MN). A small Telfa dressing (KPR U.S., LLC, Dublin, OH) covers the Steri-Strips (3M Company) and a lidocaine patch covers the entire surgical site. With the dressing in place, the operation is complete. I place the patient supine on the transfer gurney, remove the skull clamp and infiltrate the pin sites with a lidocaine/bupivacaine mixture.

8.10 Case Illustrations

Focal compression of the spinal cord at a single level is unusual enough of a clinical circumstance that case illustrations are almost necessary to demonstrate the selection process and the application of the surgical technique. The three following cases are examples of my successes with the minimally invasive posterior cervical laminectomy. Nonetheless, failure is perhaps the best teacher, and those failures have come in my attempts to achieve multiple levels of decompression in a single operation. In those cases, although the clinical outcome was acceptable, the process was not. Time under anesthesia, blood loss and postoperative course are all part of the equation. If a minimal access procedure cannot be performed more expeditiously, with less blood loss and less postoperative discomfort, it warrants careful consideration of whether or not to employ such a technique.

At the beginning of this chapter, I emphasized the importance of a focused area of compression as part of the criteria for considering a posterior minimal access approach to the cervical spine. In the report by Dahdaleh and colleagues[4] on the minimal-access cervical laminectomy, Dr. Fessler writes that the average number of levels decompressed was 2.2, with a range of one to four levels. Dr. Fessler's experience demonstrates the reach of this technique. As surgeons, we are all shaped by our experiences in caring for patients. It has been that experience that has limited the number of levels that I would consider for a minimally invasive procedure to two. Simply put, in my practice I have not been able to demonstrate a benefit to multilevel cervical decompressions performed in a minimally invasive manner that have been advantageous to both the patient, most importantly, and the surgeon, secondarily. It is important to recognize that the lack of benefit of multiple levels of decompression in my hands may reflect more on the surgeon than on the technique.

The following case illustrations demonstrate the management of single-level focal compression of the cervical spinal cord with a minimally invasive cervical laminectomy.

8.10.1 Case 1: Cervical Myelopathy Secondary to a C3–4 Facet Cyst

Clinical History and Neurologic Findings

A 68-year-old right-hand-dominant man presented with progressive gait disturbance and decreased manual dexterity. He had gone from fully ambulatory to walking with a walker in a matter of weeks. On physical examination, the patient arrived ambulating with the assistance of a walker but with trouble holding onto the walker because of decreased manual dexterity. The patient was briskly hyperreflexic on neurologic examination. He was positive for the Romberg sign. Strength was remarkably preserved in the proximal muscle groups of the upper extremities, but he demonstrated decreased manual dexterity in both hands.

Radiographic Studies

An MRI of the cervical spine demonstrated a facet cyst at C3–4 causing compression of the spinal cord. The sagittal T2-weighted MRI demonstrated a cyst emanating from the left C3–4 facet. The axial T2-weighted MRI demonstrated lateral displacement of the spinal cord (▶ Fig. 8.25). The lesion did not enhance with gadolinium. There was no previous history of a malignancy. Flexion and extension radiographs (not shown) did not demonstrate any evidence of abnormal motion.

Rationale for a Minimally Invasive Approach

The criteria for a minimally invasive cervical laminectomy described in the beginning of the chapter included no history of previous cervical laminectomy, only dorsal compression, only one or two segments affected, and no need for instrumentation.

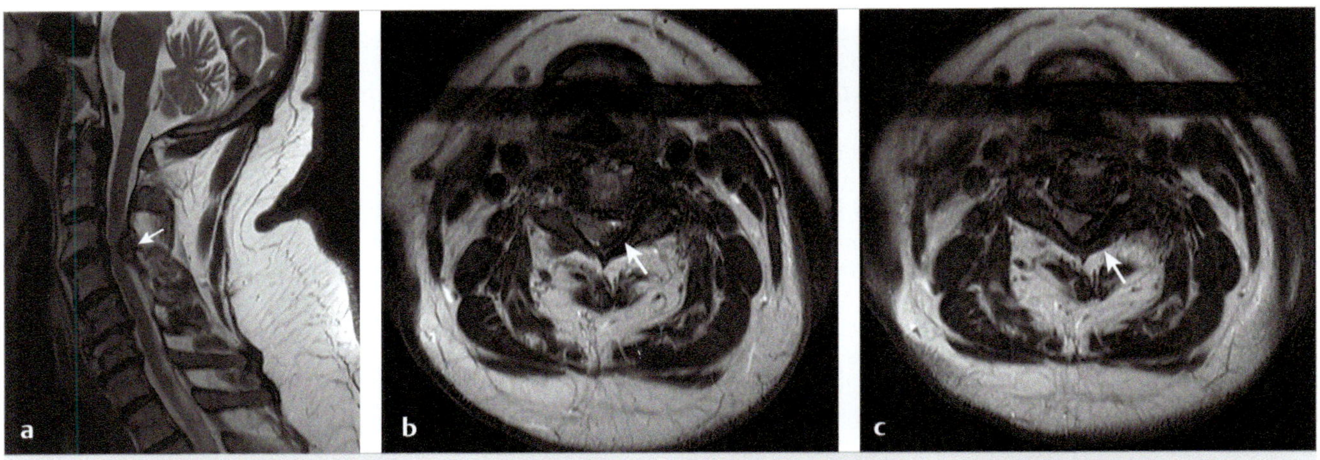

Fig. 8.25 Cervical spinal cord compression at C3–4. **(a)** Sagittal T2-weighted magnetic resonance imaging (MRI) demonstrating a focal dorsal compressive lesion (*arrow*) causing compression on the spinal cord. **(b,c)** Axial T2-weighted MRI sequences suggest a facet cyst (*arrows*) emanating from the left C3–4 facet.

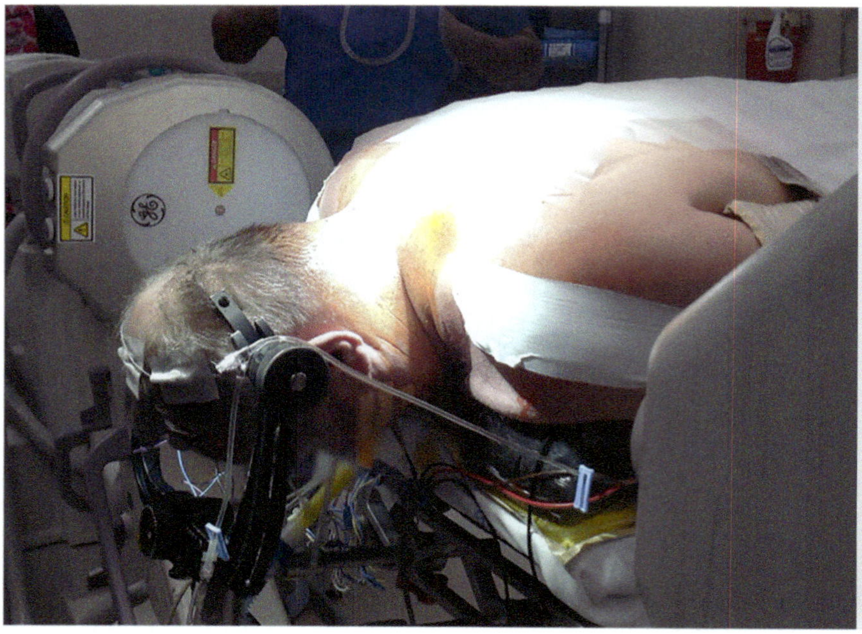

Fig. 8.26 Positioning for a cervical laminectomy. Intraoperative photograph of the patient positioned prone on chest rolls in a Mayfield head holder. The head is placed in some capital flexion and the shoulders taped down to facilitate visualization of the spine.

The sagittal and axial MRIs clearly demonstrate only dorsal compression of the spinal cord at a single segment, which makes this case ideal for a minimally invasive approach. A potential pitfall in this case is instability. The formation of a facet cyst suggests an abnormality at the level of the articulation of the facet. Instability may be one of the causes for the formation of the cyst, and it is essential to rule this out before proceeding with a simple decompression. With normal flexion and extension radiographs of this patient, all three criteria for a minimally invasive laminectomy are met. For the management of this patient, I recommended a minimally invasive C3 and partial C4 laminectomy with medial facetectomy and resection of facet cyst.

Intervention

I positioned the patient into a skull clamp, prone on chest rolls on the operating table. Since the facet cyst was on the left, the microscope was draped and ready on the left side of the prone patient, and the image intensifier of the fluoroscope was brought in from the right (▸ Fig. 8.26).

I began the localization with a protected Steinman pin on the skin to approximate the incision (▸ Fig. 8.27). I planned for an 18-mm skin incision in preparation for an expandable 16-mm minimal access port (▸ Fig. 8.28). Working from the head of the bed, I infiltrated the proposed incision area with a lidocaine and bupivacaine mixture and made the incision with a No. 15 blade. I opened the posterior cervical fascia with cautery just as I would if I were performing the operation in an open fashion. I made a generous opening in the fascia to visualize the posterior cervical musculature before beginning to dilate onto the lamina. I passed the first dilator onto the medial facet and lateral lamina until I encountered the unmistakable sensation of metal encountering laminar bone. Aware of the interlaminar space at C3–4, I refrained from a convergent trajectory.

After I sounded the anatomy with the first dilator, I confirmed the lamina-facet complex by feeling the drop-off where the tip of the dilator slips off the inferior aspect of the IAP and lands on the articular surface of the SAP. As I passed the second dilator, I began to converge onto the cervical lamina with the goal of having the medial aspect of the subsequent dilators encounter the spinous process laminar junction. I am aware that the increase in the diameter of these subsequent dilators continues to decrease, if not eliminate, the risk of passage into the spinal canal. With this in mind, I can confidently maintain downward pressure unto the lamina feeling the unmistakable sensation of metal against bone (▸ Fig. 8.29). As I performed

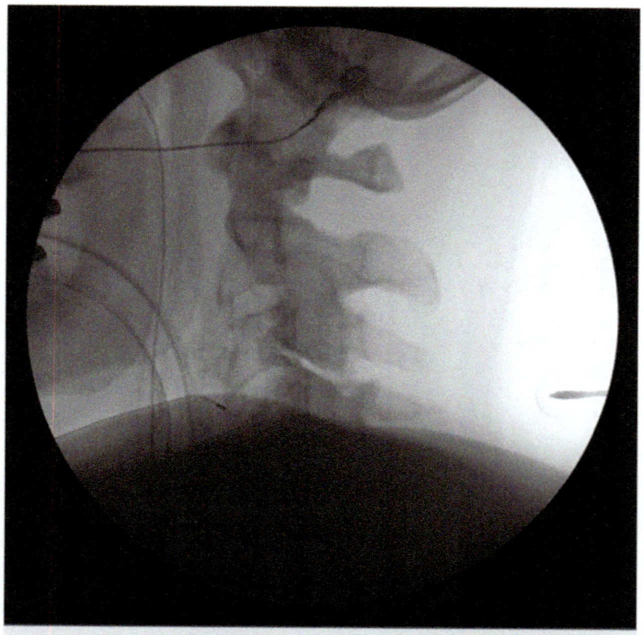

Fig. 8.27 Localization of the incision. Lateral fluoroscopic image demonstrating a protected Steinman pin to localize the level and plan the incision.

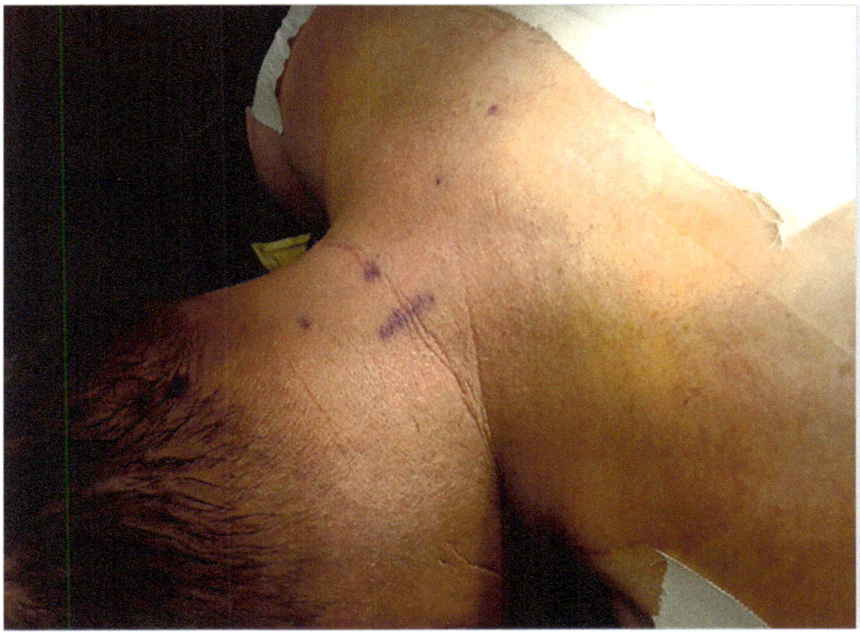

Fig. 8.28 Intraoperative photograph demonstrating the planned incision. The first step in planning the incision is marking the midline. This is accomplished by palpating and marking the spinous processes, as seen in this image with the dotted line. From there, an incision is planned 2-cm lateral to midline to allow for convergence onto the lamina.

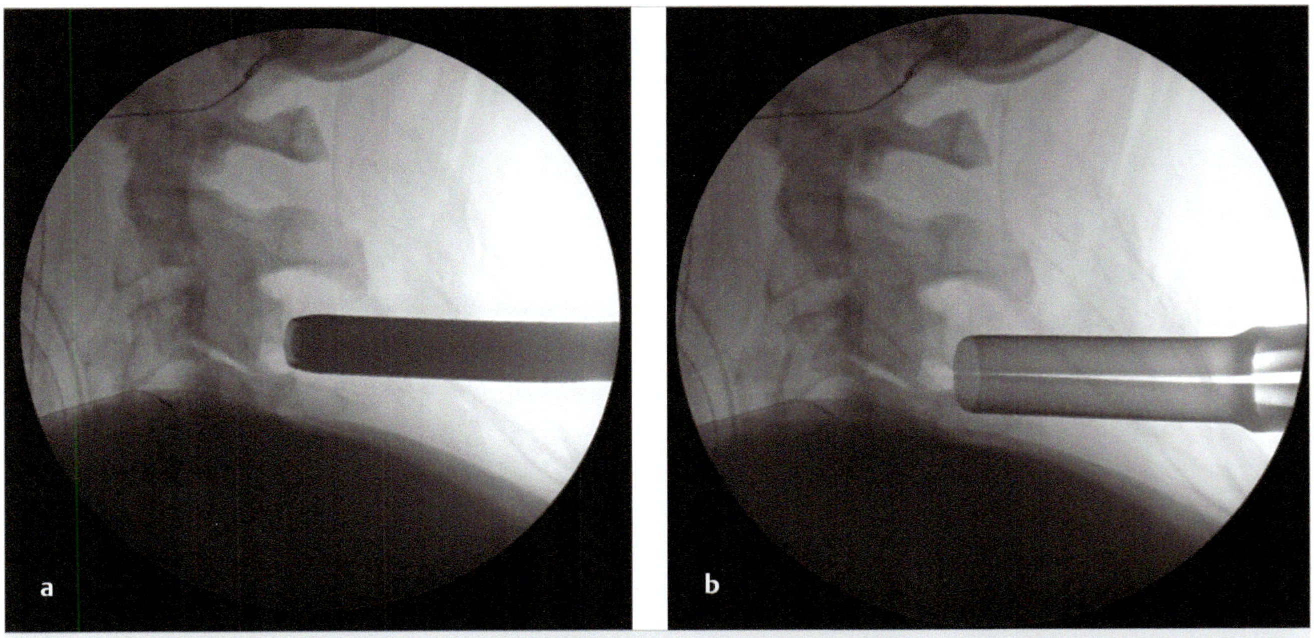

Fig. 8.29 Lateral fluoroscopic images demonstrating the positioning of the minimal access port. **(a)** Sequential dilators in position. **(b)** An expandable 16-mm minimal access port secured into position over the dilators.

this part of the dilatation, I continued my convergence toward the midline keeping in mind that the axial MRI demonstrates the facet cyst extending to midline.

After I secured the minimal access port into position, I obtained a final AP image to ensure I had the medial convergence needed for the operation (▶ Fig. 8.30). In my experience, these additional images have helped me to begin to reconstruct the anatomy at depth. Thus, I begin thinking about the anatomy relative to the diameter of the access port before the microscope is even in position (▶ Fig. 8.31).

Under the operating microscope, I exposed the laminae of C3 and C4. Regardless of how meticulous I was about my dilatation of the paraspinal muscles, there is always a cuff of muscle that requires removal with cautery. My objective is to see nothing but the lamina within the diameter of the access port. Once I exposed the laminae of C3 and C4, I drilled the lamina of C3 until I reached the ligamentum flavum. At the most lateral aspect of the exposure, I visualized the C3–C4 medial facet articulation. I drilled the C3 lamina until I reached the rostral aspect of the ligamentum flavum insertion. Once I had thinned

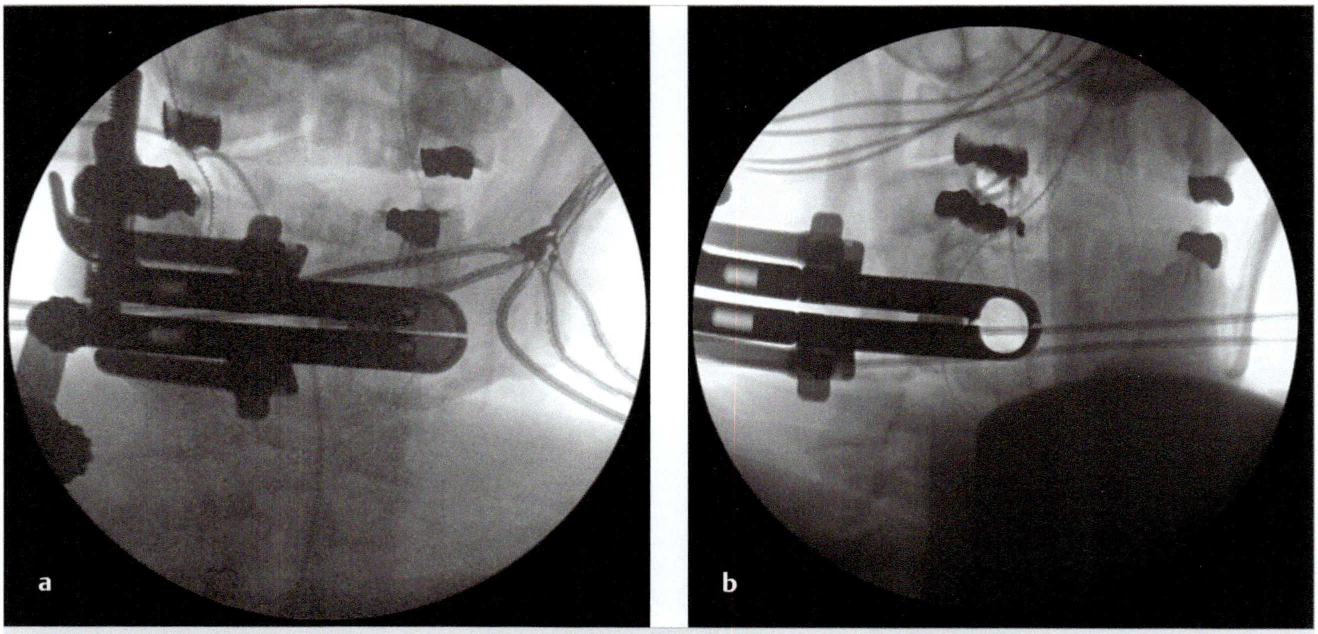

Fig. 8.30 Anteroposterior (AP) fluoroscopic images demonstrating the position of the access port. **(a)** True AP image demonstrating the convergence of the minimal access port. The odontoid process and the C1–C2 articulation can clearly be seen at the top of the image. **(b)** Oblique AP image (owl's eye view) focusing through the aperture of the minimal access port. The lateral masses of the cervical spine can be clearly visualized confirming the minimal access port is on the lamina.

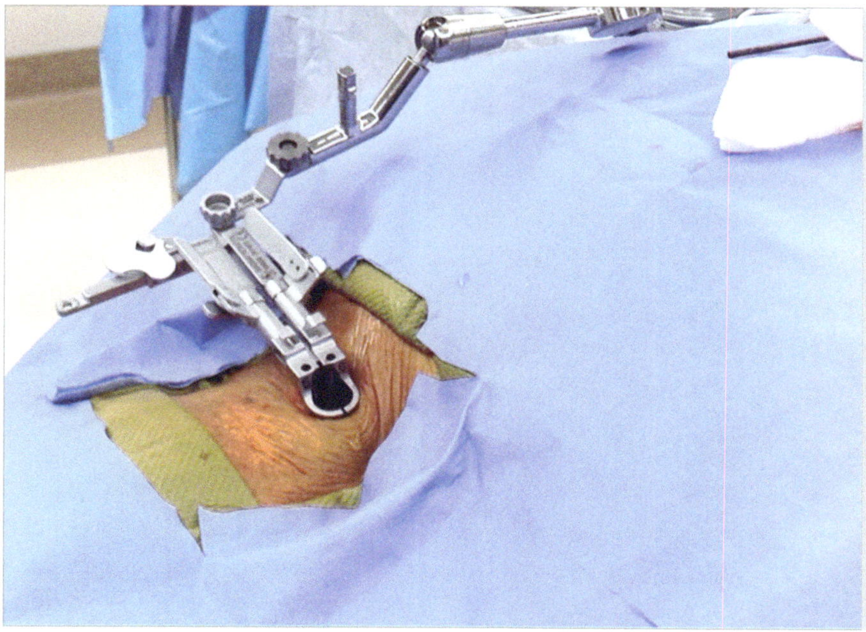

Fig. 8.31 Intraoperative photograph of the minimal access port in position after the final fluoroscopic images have been taken. The microscope is now rolled into position as the fluoroscope rolls out.

the lamina beyond the insertion point, I intentionally left the ligamentum flavum intact to protect the spinal cord and turned my attention to the C4 lamina. With the lamina thinned to a shrimp-shell thickness, I exposed the ligamentum flavum across the entire segment. Next, I exposed the spinal cord and released the ligamentum flavum from its insertion on the underside of the cervical lamina in the midline to ensure that I was beyond the facet cyst. The dura of the spinal cord came quickly into view, and I released the remaining ligamentum flavum from its medial and lateral insertion points. The operation then became a facet cyst operation, where the primary objective was to secure a perimeter around the facet cyst.

A review of the MRI demonstrated that the facet cyst causing the compression extended to the midline. It is imperative that the exposure reach the midline to ensure the ability to establish a perimeter around the facet cyst and ensure an adequate decompression. I proceeded to resect the ligamentum flavum around the facet cyst until I reached the medial facet. I then undercut the medial facet until it appeared that there was no longer any evidence of compression of the spinal cord. Upon completion of the decompression, I removed the minimal access port and closed the incision in a multilayered fashion as described in Section 8.9.1, Hemostasis and Closure (▸ Fig. 8.32).

Postoperative Course

The patient had an uneventful postoperative course and was discharged on the first postoperative day. He returned to clinic for his first postoperative appointment walking independently and with a marked improvement of his manual dexterity. On examination, the patient continued to demonstrate some mild hyperreflexia, and he was Romberg negative and capable of performing a tandem gait. A postoperative MRI obtained 2 years after his initial surgery for other cervical symptoms demonstrated a complete decompression of the spinal cord at C3–4 (▸ Fig. 8.33).

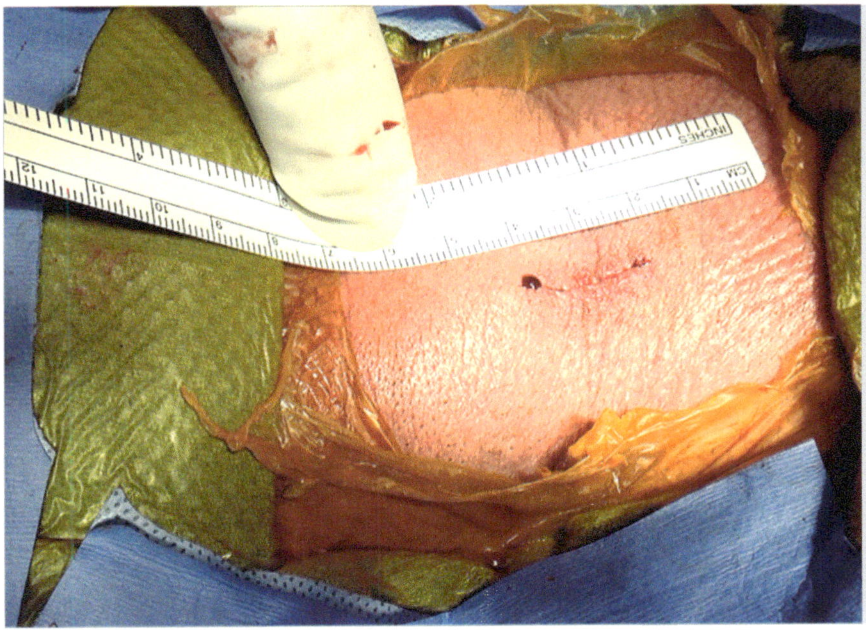

Fig. 8.32 Intraoperative picture of the skin incision after closure of a C3 and partial C4 laminectomy for resection of a facet cyst and decompression of the spinal cord.

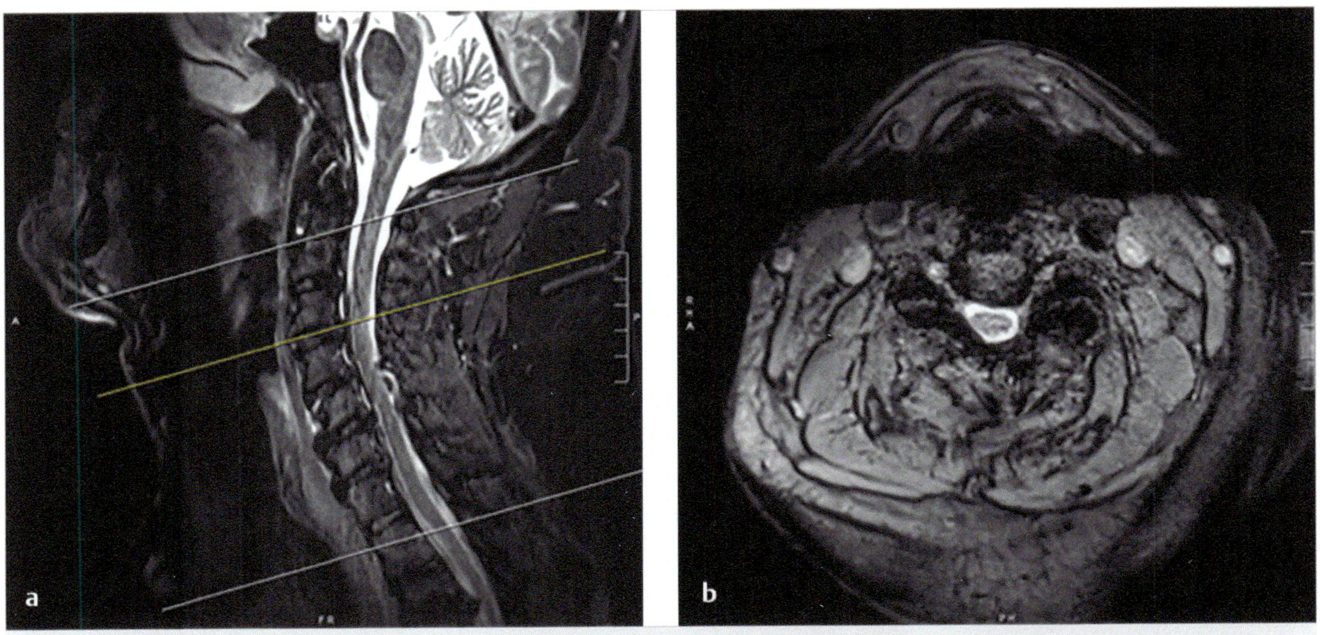

Fig. 8.33 Postoperative magnetic resonance imaging (MRI) of the cervical spine obtained 2 years after the facet cyst resection. **(a)** The sagittal T2-weighted MRI and **(b)** corresponding axial T2-weighted MRI show complete decompression of the spinal cord at the C3–4 segment (as demonstrated by the lines in **a**).

8.10.2 Case 2: Cervical Radiculopathy and Early Myelopathy Secondary to an Epidural Abscess

Clinical History and Neurologic Findings

A 55-year-old right-hand-dominant man presented to the emergency room with a 72-hour history of fever, shaking chills and incapacitating interscapular pain that radiated down his left arm. Within the last 24 hours, the patient had experienced a decrease in manual dexterity in his left hand and difficulty walking. The patient had a recent history of travel to Mexico, where he had sustained a significant laceration to this hand on a coral reef 1 week earlier. The hand wound appeared to be healing poorly at the time of his presentation. A neurologic examination demonstrated 4–/5 strength in the triceps on the left side. The patient had positive Hoffman's and Babinski's signs bilaterally. Strength was preserved in the lower extremities and the right upper extremity. He had difficulty with a tandem gait. His laboratory data revealed a white blood cell count of 13,500 cells/μL, erythrocyte sedimentation rate of 95 mm/h and a C-reactive protein level of 15.4 mg/L.

Radiographic Studies

MRI of the cervical spine obtained with and without gadolinium demonstrated a dorsal enhancing epidural mass eccentric to the left that was most consistent with an abscess that spanned C5 to T1 (▶ Fig. 8.34).

Rationale for a Minimally Invasive Approach

A sound argument can be made for a traditional midline incision with wide laminectomies for decompression of the spinal cord, which would completely decompress the spinal cord and address all levels of compression. In this case, the patient was a former professional football player and a currently active bodybuilder. As a result, the musculature of the posterior cervical spine was exceptionally well developed. I was concerned about a midline approach, dissecting off all of the musculature from their insertions and disrupting the posterior tension band, especially at the cervical–thoracic junction, in an active 55-year-old man. I could envision not only the immediate postoperative discomfort this approach would cause for the patient, but also the discomfort that would occur in the weeks to months to come. So instead, I considered the possibility of a minimally invasive approach, which would spare the midline elements and the posterior tension band and be less disruptive to the posterior cervical musculature. The patient had no need for instrumentation, and the compression was purely dorsal and off to one side. However, the abscess spanned from C5 to T1. The question became whether a complete decompression of the entire abscess was necessary to adequately treat the patient or if a focal decompression at the epicenter, which resided at C7–T1, would be adequate. After an extensive conversation with the patient, where I communicated that the greatest risk of surgery was the need to perform a more extensive debridement, I made the decision to proceed with a C7 laminectomy for decompression of the epidural abscess, which corresponded to the epicenter of the abscess.

Intervention

Similar to the cases already presented in the previous chapter and in this chapter, I positioned the patient prone on chest rolls, with his head in a skull clamp. The initial preoperative fluoroscopic image demonstrated what I had initially suspected in this former National Football League linebacker: there would be no visualization of C7–T1 on lateral fluoroscopic imaging (▶ Fig. 8.35a). Realizing this, I passed a spinal needle onto the C6–7 level (▶ Fig. 8.35b) and planned an incision relative to this reference point. In the absence of direct fluoroscopic visualization of the level, I had to rely more on the tactile skill set that I developed in posterior cervical foraminotomies to establish my location on the cervical spine. I was relying more on my experience sounding the anatomy and my knowledge of the anatomy at depth than what I could see on a lateral fluoroscopic image.

I made the incision over the top of the C7–T1 segment, opened the fascia widely with cautery and began the dilatation. With lateral fluoroscopic images over-penetrating the shoulder,

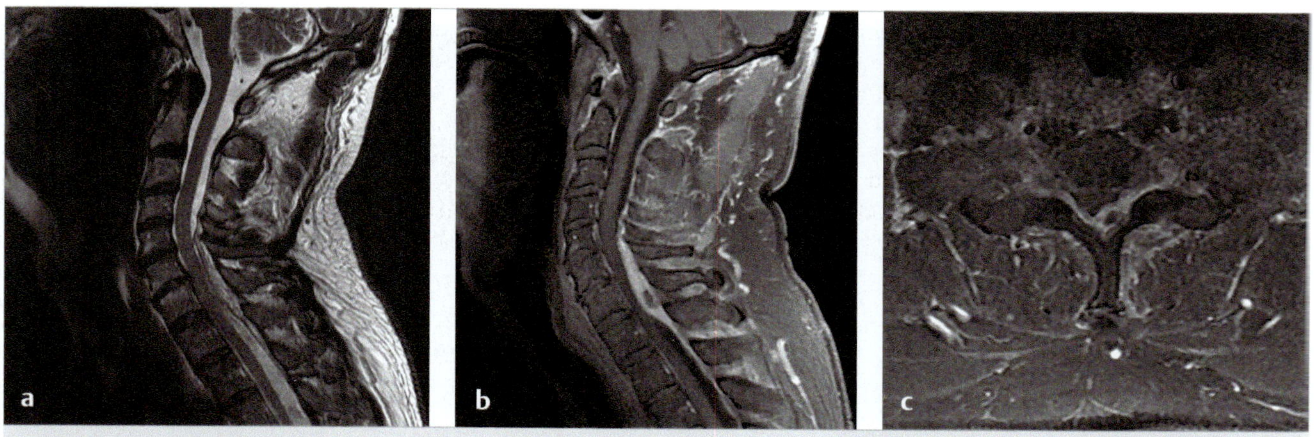

Fig. 8.34 Magnetic resonance imaging (MRI) of the cervical spine with and without gadolinium. **(a)** Sagittal T2-weighted MRI demonstrating an extra-axial mass with mass effect on the spinal cord extending from C5–6 to T1. **(b)** Gadolinium-enhanced sagittal T1-weighted MRI demonstrates dorsal enhancement from C5–6 to T1 with the epicenter of the presumed abscess at C7–T1, with absence of enhancement in the center of the abscess. **(c)** Gadolinium-enhanced axial T1-weighted MRI of the cervical spine demonstrating the mass effect on the spinal cord and the absence of enhancement in the center of the presumed abscess.

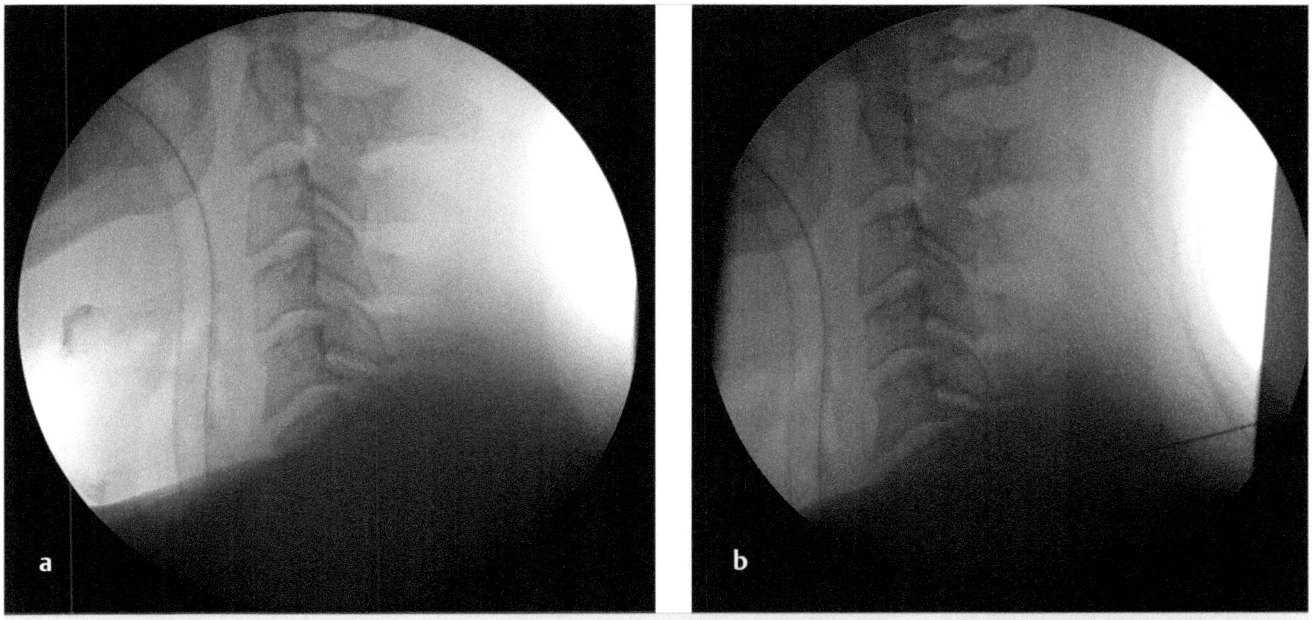

Fig. 8.35 **(a)** Preoperative lateral fluoroscopic image demonstrating that despite aggressively taping the shoulders down with maximum tension, the limit of visualization would be C5–6. The C7–T1 level would need to be confirmed with an anteroposterior fluoroscopic image. **(b)** Lateral fluoroscopic image showing a spinal needle passed onto the C6–7 level to serve as a reference point to dock the minimal access port and confirm the level.

I could approximate the C7–T1 segment relative to the C6–7 spinal needle. Remember, knowledge is the true organ of sight. I knew that once I had the tip of the first dilator onto the facet-lamina junction, I could confidently dilate and dock a minimal access port with my tactile sense of the anatomy. The unmistakable feeling of the metal dilator against the bone and the feeling of the drop-off from the IAP onto the SAP would replace what the fluoroscope could not reveal because of a muscular body habitus. Hence, I secured the minimal access port into position and then captured an AP image, which allowed me to confirm the level of C7–T1. Based on that image, I adjusted the minimal access port so that it converged more prominently onto the lamina (▶ Fig. 8.36). I was now ready to transition to the microscope.

Under the microscope, I began my exposure of the lamina in the superior and lateral aspect of the diameter. I swept away the remaining cuff of muscle off the bone and could clearly visualize the lamina of C7 and T1 (Video 8.1). I drilled the lamina of C7 and T1 until it was thinned to a shrimp-shell consistency and completed the laminectomy with a Kerrison number 2 rongeur. As I proceeded with the laminectomy, I encountered the abscess and released a large pocket of purulent fluid, which I collected and sent to be cultured. After debriding these pockets and obtaining the fluid for culture, I proceeded with extending the laminectomy in all directions. I encountered the phlegmon, which was adherent to the dura and did not allow for the development of a clear plane. I continued to debulk the phlegmon and decompress the dura using a right-angled ball-tipped probe passed beyond what I had already exposed. This debulking interrupted more of the phlegmon, with drainage of more purulent material. Once I was able to pass the ball-tipped probe freely in all directions, I used it to help reach beyond my exposure and irrigated the area copiously with hydrogen peroxide. With the spinal cord decompressed and the abscess drained, I removed my minimal access port and closed the incision in the usual fashion (see Section 8.9.1, Hemostasis and Closure).

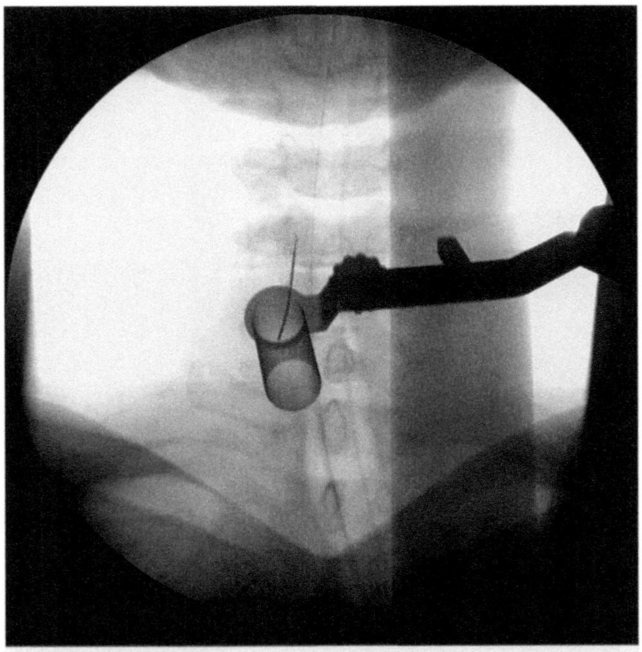

Fig. 8.36 Anteroposterior fluoroscopic image confirming the minimal access port at the C7–T1 level. Note the spinal needle is in position at C6–7. For the procedure, the minimal access port must converge medially toward the spinous process to achieve a midline decompression.

Postoperative Course

Immediately after the operation, the patient had complete resolution of his left radicular arm pain. On the first postoperative day, he was fully ambulatory with no evidence of myelopathy on the neurologic examination. The cultures grew *Salmonella* species; the patient was treated with an antibiotic course for 6 weeks. As so often happens with a patient who presents with an epidural abscess, he returned to society and was lost to follow-up. I was unsuccessful in my attempts to get him back to the clinic for postoperative imaging.

8.10.3 Case 3: Cervical Myelopathy Secondary to Hemorrhagic Metastatic Lesion

Clinical History and Neurologic Examination

A 58-year-old woman with a history of breast cancer diagnosed 4 years earlier and currently in remission presented with acute gait imbalance, unilateral loss of manual dexterity in her right hand and neck pain. Working as a school teacher, she had sudden onset of neck pain without antecedent trauma while teaching a class and was taken by ambulance to the hospital. On examination, she had a profoundly ataxic gait; she had a positive Romberg sign and was incapable of a tandem gait. She demonstrated 3 + patellar reflexes and sustained clonus in her lower extremities bilaterally. She also demonstrated a positive Hoffman sign. She was initially suspected of having vertebral artery dissection. However, MRI of the brain did not reveal evidence of restricted diffusion in the posterior circulation, and magnetic resonance angiography of the brain and cervical spine were within normal limits. MRI of the cervical spine demonstrated an extra-axial lesion causing spinal cord compression at C6–7 (▶ Fig. 8.37).

Rationale for a Minimally Invasive Approach

Once again, this case represents a unique clinical circumstance with a focal area of compression limited to one segment. Based on the criteria set forth in this chapter, a minimally invasive approach plays to the strengths of the posterior cervical laminectomy and is the ideal intervention. Furthermore, given the history of a malignancy, a minimally invasive approach allows for the use of radiation therapy almost immediately if indicated. Some consideration has to be given to the fact that this entity is likely an epidural hematoma, and the ability to achieve hemostasis through a small diameter of exposure may be an issue. However, after carefully weighing the risks and benefits, the decision was made to proceed with a minimal access approach based on the focal area of compression.

Intervention

With the patient positioned in a skull clamp, prone and on chest rolls and shoulders taped down to facilitate visualization of the C6–7 segment, the posterior cervical spine was prepped and draped. Similar to all the previous posterior cervical foraminotomy and laminectomy cases, an ample amount of room is created between the head of the bed and the anesthesia circuit to allow me to confirm the level and position of the access port. Since the presumptive hematoma was on the right, the microscope was draped and positioned on that side, and the fluoroscope was positioned with the image intensifier on the left.

I marked a 16-mm incision 2 cm from the midline approximating the incision based on the prominent spinous process of C7. I passed a spinal needle with absolutely no convergence directly onto the lateral mass of C6 (▶ Fig. 8.38).

With the level confirmed and an incision with an ideal trajectory onto the segment planned, I infiltrated the proposed trajectory with the usual lidocaine/epinephrine and bupivacaine

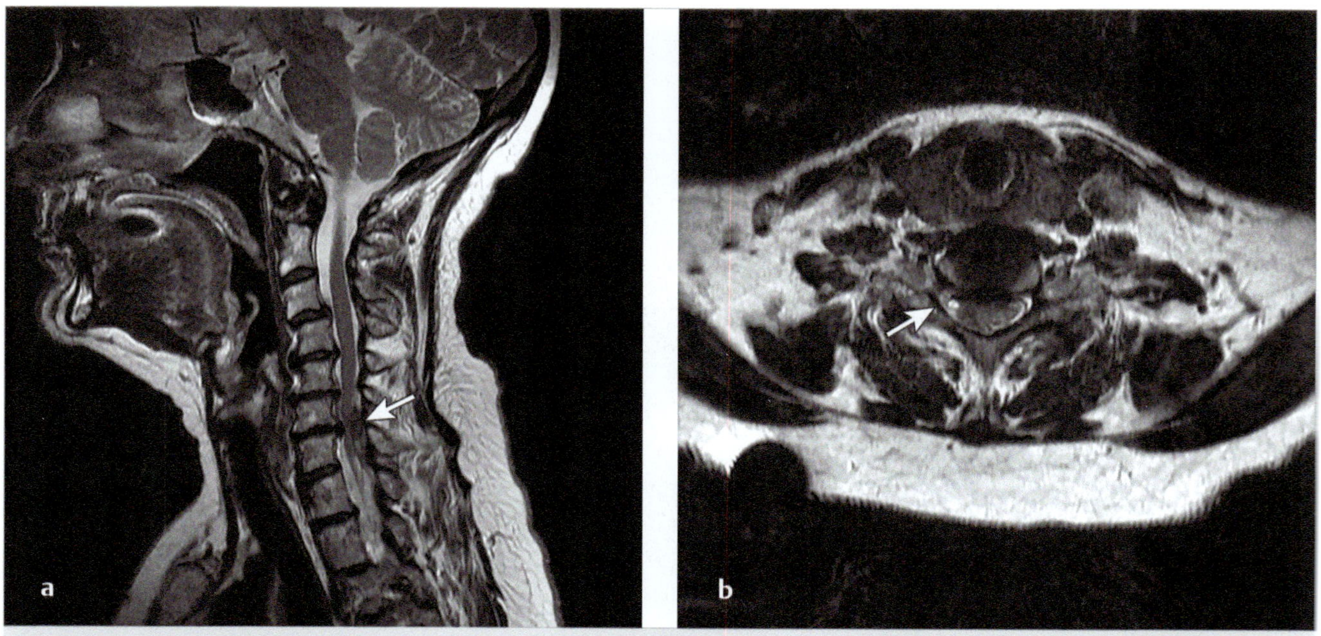

Fig. 8.37 Extradural lesion causing spinal cord compression. **(a)** Sagittal T2-weighted magnetic resonance imaging (MRI) demonstrating an extradural lesion (*arrow*) causing compression of the spinal cord. A preexisting disc osteophyte complex at C6–7 further compounds the stenosis that caused this extradural lesion. **(b)** Axial T2-weighted MRI demonstrating epidural lesion (*arrow*) off to the right causing compression of the spinal cord.

mixture. I marked a 16-mm incision in preparation for a 14-mm access port, infiltrated the skin of the incision and began the operation with a No. 15 blade. I then divided the fascia with a protected cautery tip until I could unequivocally visualize the paraspinal musculature. I made the fascial opening generous to minimize any resistance when dilating through the muscle on top of the lamina and then passed the first dilator (▸ Fig. 8.39). As described in the previous case illustrations, the importance of the first dilator is to safely dock onto the lamina–facet junction. There should be minimal convergence at this point. With each subsequent dilator, the diameter increases to a point that the risk of passage into the spinal canal becomes an impossibility. Therefore, increasing convergence up against the lamina with the larger diameter dilators can be achieved with comfort.

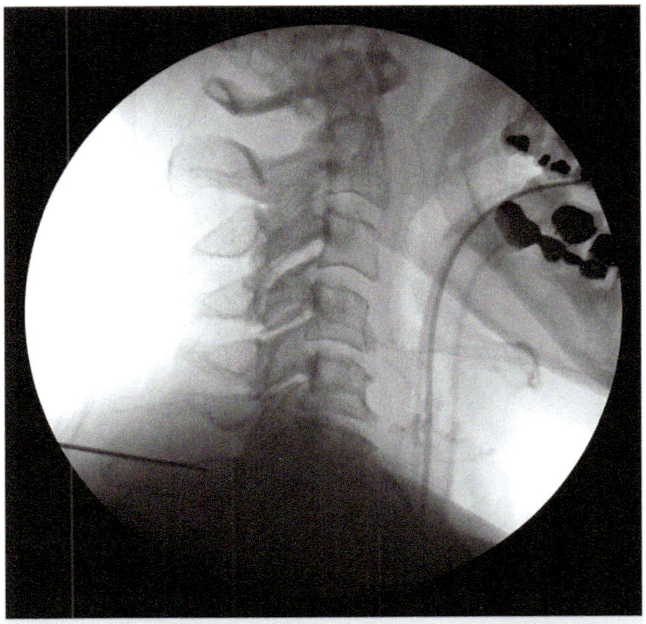

Fig. 8.38 Localization. Lateral fluoroscopic image demonstrating the spinal needle at the C6–7 segment. With the level confirmed, the incision may be marked and infiltrated with local anesthetic.

The minimal access port should have the greatest convergence that can be readily appreciated on the lateral fluoroscopic image, specifically the appearance of the diameter of the ring at the top of the port (▸ Fig. 8.39).

Before I bring in the operating microscope, I obtain an AP image to ensure an ideal converging trajectory onto the lamina (▸ Fig. 8.40).

With this AP image, I confirmed that the minimal access port was in the ideal position. I proceeded to the upper lateral aspect of the exposure with cautery and identified the lateral aspect of the lamina, which provided me with the foothold from which to sweep away what remains of the muscle overlying the lamina. Before even considering wielding the drill, I ensured that the entire lamina within the entire diameter of the minimal access port was exposed (Video 8.1).

In this case, I began drilling in the lateral aspect of the exposure, extending my bone work medially. As always, my goal was to thin the bone to a shrimp-shell thickness. The hematoma became immediately obvious as the Kerrison rongeur removed the remaining shell of bone over the spinal cord (Video 8.1). What is further demonstrated by the operative video is the range of the minimal access port. Once I had removed the entire diameter of the lamina within my field of view along with the epidural hematoma, it became evident that more hematoma remained outside the exposure. By replacing the final dilator and using it to angle the access port rostrally, I was able to expose more lamina, which I drilled to expose and complete the decompression (▸ Fig. 8.41). The abnormal tissue identified within the hematoma was sent to the pathology laboratory and was confirmed to be consistent with metastatic breast cancer.

Postoperative Course

The patient had complete resolution of her incapacitating neck pain immediately after the operation. Her gait imbalance resolved, and she was capable of tandem walking on the day of surgery. She experienced numbness and tingling in the right upper arm in a nondermatomal distribution, without radicular pain, which slowly resolved over the span of 2 weeks. She

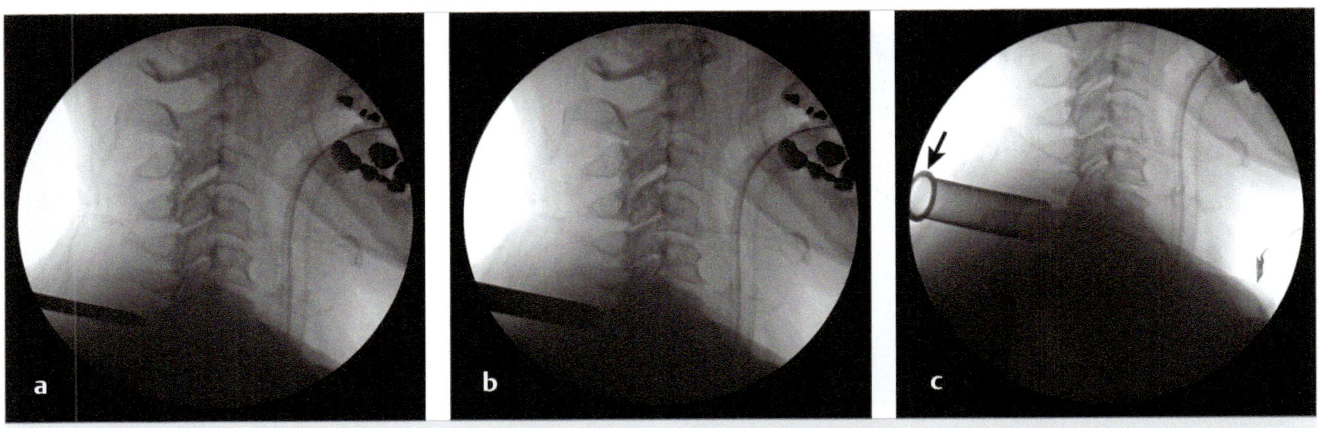

Fig. 8.39 Sequence of dilatation. (a) Lateral fluoroscopic image with the first dilator in position against the facet of C6. (b) Lateral fluoroscopic image with the third dilator in position. With each sequential dilator, more and more convergence onto the lamina may be safely accomplished. (c) Lateral fluoroscopic image with the 14-mm minimal access port in position. Note the degree of convergence as demonstrated by the diameter of the ring at the top of the port (*arrow*).

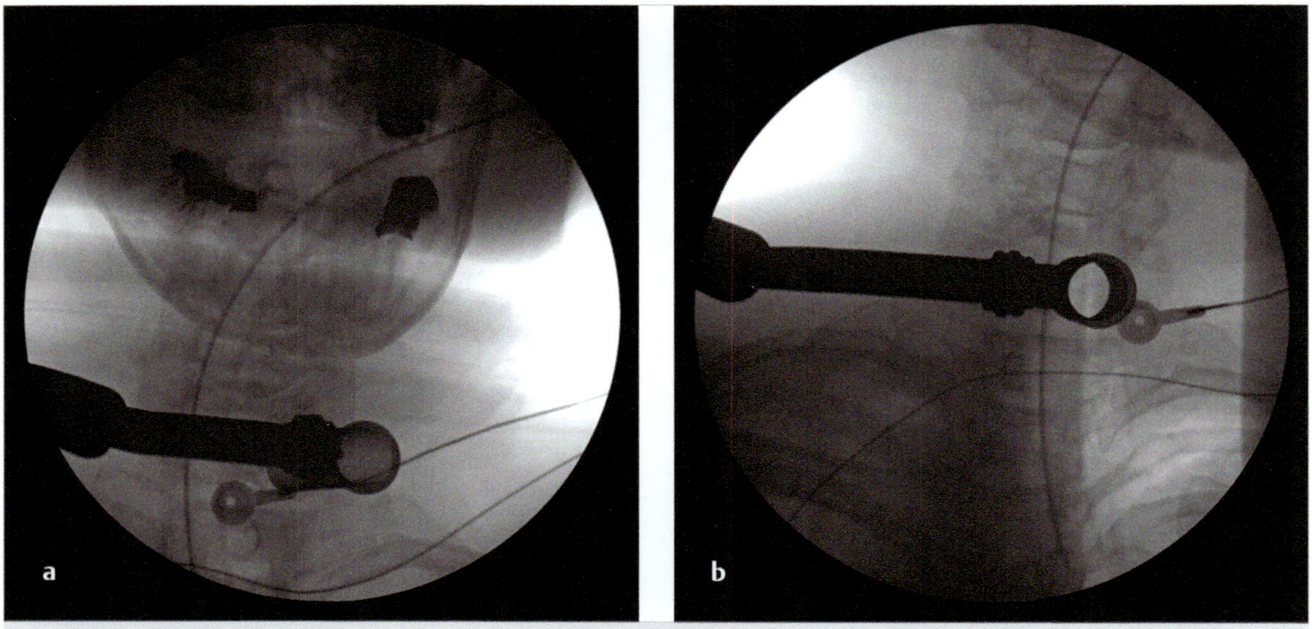

Fig. 8.40 Minimal access port in position. (a) True anteroposterior (AP) image demonstrating convergence onto the lamina of C6. (b) Oblique AP (owl's eye view) image with the trajectory of the fluoroscope down the minimal access port. This image demonstrates the access port up against the face of the C6 lamina.

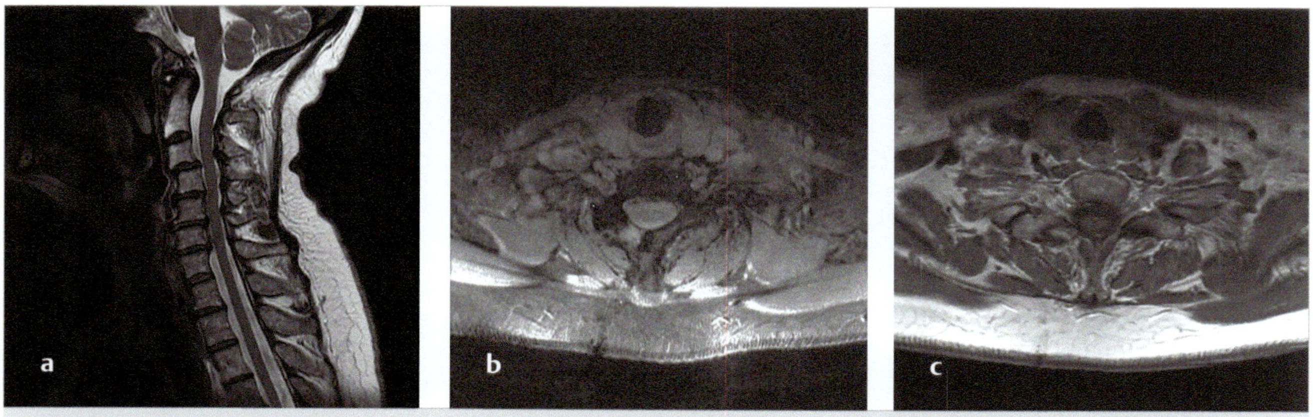

Fig. 8.41 Postoperative magnetic resonance imaging (MRI) 3 months after minimally invasive cervical laminectomy for epidural metastatic lesion. (a) Sagittal T2-weighted MRI demonstrating complete evacuation of the hemorrhagic metastatic lesion. (b) Axial T2-weighted MRI demonstrating the hemilaminectomy defect on the lamina at C6. (c) Axial T1-weighted MRI with gadolinium demonstrating no abnormal enhancement.

completed a full metastatic workup, which did not reveal metastatic disease elsewhere. After the pathology of the lesion was confirmed, the patient began radiation therapy 7 days after her surgery. She remained disease free at the 4-year follow-up after surgery.

8.11 Conclusion

Although uncommon, cervical stenosis with dorsal compression of the spinal cord that occurs focally at one segment represents a unique opportunity to benefit the patient by performing a minimally invasive technique. The three case illustrations demonstrate the successful application of working through a limited corridor onto the cervical spine that preserves the midline structures and posterior tension band to address compressive pathology on the cervical spinal cord. In each of these circumstances, a traditional midline laminectomy would have taken longer, disrupted the posterior tension band and required a significant amount of disruption and devascularization of the complex posterior cervical musculature. Even though no current clinical study supports minimally invasive techniques as a prevention for kyphosis, the potential risk of progressive kyphosis by disrupting the posterior tension band, especially at the cervicothoracic junction, is difficult to ignore. The minimally invasive posterior cervical laminectomy offers an elegant solution to these rare anatomical circumstances. On average, I perform two or three of these operations a year, and so the volume is not significant. In fact, the posterior cervical laminectomy is the least common minimally invasive procedure that I perform. But the benefit to the patient who presents with focal dorsal compression of the cervical spinal cord certainly is significant in the short term and the long term.

Chapter 7 and this chapter have focused on cervical minimally invasive techniques applied posteriorly. Chapter 9, Anterior Cervical Discectomy with Arthroplasty or Fusion, may initially seem out of place here, but after reading it, I hope the reader agrees that its presence in this Primer is mandatory. After all, the anterior cervical discectomy was the first minimally invasive spinal operation in the spine surgeon's armamentarium.

References

[1] Tumialán LM, Lehrman JN, Mulholland CB, de Andrada Pereira B, Newcomb AGUS, Kelly BP. Dimensional characterization of the human cervical interlaminar space as a guide for safe application of minimally invasive dilators. Oper Neurosurg. 2020 Mar 6. pii: opaa013. doi: 10.1093/ons/opaa013. [Epub ahead of print].

[2] Panjabi MM, Duranceau J, Goel V, Oxland T, Takata K. Cervical human vertebrae. Quantitative three-dimensional anatomy of the middle and lower regions. Spine. 1991; 16(8):861–869

[3] Rahmani MS, Terai H, Akhgar J, et al. Anatomical analysis of human ligamentum flavum in the cervical spine: special consideration to the attachments, coverage, and lateral extent. J Orthop Sci. 2017; 22(6):994-1000

[4] Dahdaleh NS, Wong AP, Smith ZA, Wong RH, Lam SK, Fessler RG. Microendoscopic decompression for cervical spondylotic myelopathy. Neurosurg Focus. 2013; 35(1):E8

9 Anterior Cervical Discectomy with Arthroplasty or Fusion

Abstract

The anterior approach to the cervical spine for discectomy followed by fusion or arthroplasty is the most consistent and durable of operations for management of a cervical radiculopathy or spinal cord compression. While this operation does not rely on a minimal access port for exposure of the cervical spine, it still adheres to the various principles of minimally invasive spinal surgery presented thus far in this Primer. The anatomical certainty of the dimensions of the vertebral bodies, uncovertebral joints and the foramen transversarium instills the confidence in the surgeon to complete a wide decompression while limiting the exposure to only the requisite anatomy needed for either arthrodesis or arthroplasty. The current chapter reviews the anatomical basis for an anterior cervical discectomy with fusion or arthroplasty. The focus of the anatomical basis is to understand the requisite exposure for an operation. A particular emphasis is placed on identifying the midline. From there, the chapter covers positioning of the patient and operating room setup before reviewing the operative technique for single- and multilevel fusions or arthroplasties. The principles of interbody fusion and anterior cervical plating will also be presented. Throughout the chapter, application of minimally invasive principles presented in the previous eight chapters is woven into the rationale and operative technique.

Keywords: anterior cervical spine, arthrodesis, arthroplasty, cervical plating, decompression, discectomy, foraminotomy, osteophyte, radiculopathy

Symmetry generally conveys an imprecise sense of harmonious or aesthetically pleasing proportionality and balance; such that it reflects beauty or perfection.

Euclid

9.1 Introduction

The question arose as to why I chose to include a chapter on the anterior cervical discectomy (ACD) in a primer on minimally invasive spinal surgery. After all, I was told by several of my colleagues, fellows and residents that this procedure is not a minimally invasive one. I respectfully disagree with that opinion. All of the principles of minimally invasive spinal surgery that I have presented thus far in this book also apply to the ACD. Anterior cervical approaches are no exception to Caspar's mandate to minimize the ratio of the surgical target to the surgical exposure. An anterior approach offers extensive exposure of the anatomy without disruption or devascularization of the musculature. Finally, an ACD allows for the comprehensive treatment of a single- or multilevel cervical pathology through a single modest incision. Therefore, the ACD represents the first minimally invasive operation successfully and routinely performed on the spine. Understandably, it has been hailed as the operation that saved spine surgery. From beginning to end, the ACD is a well-conceived and unfailingly reproducible procedure. Not including a chapter on the ACD would have left a glaring void in this Primer.

For the purposes of this Primer, therefore, I frame the operative technique presented in this chapter in the context of the minimally invasive tenets that I have described throughout this book. Similar to the microdiscectomy, laminectomy or transforaminal approaches, there are anatomical measurements that can help guide the procedure. For instance, when we consider the minimally invasive lumbar fusion, we now know that the distance between the pedicle of L4 and L5 is anywhere from 28 to 32 mm. That particular anatomical measurement is helpful in executing the procedure in a manner that limits the disruption of the native spine. I know there is no need to open an expandable minimally invasive access port beyond what the anatomy dictates. We have already discussed that overexpansion and overexposure do not help the procedure. In fact, they may hinder visualization because of muscle creep and may increase the postoperative discomfort the patient experiences.

In a similar manner, the immediate knowledge that the distance between the vertebral arteries is 24 to 29 mm throughout the cervical spine is helpful when performing a decompression with a lateral osteophyte causing a radiculopathy. Placing a half-inch by half-inch cottonoid that hardly fits into what is supposed to be a decompressed cervical disc space would suggest that only 12 to 14 mm of a decompression has been achieved, and if a reliable midline has been established, an additional 8 mm of the disc space may be safely exposed and the neural elements below may be more widely decompressed. Knowledge and application of such anatomical measurements is a characteristic of minimally invasive surgery. Throughout this Primer, I have discussed the importance of reconstructing the anatomy at depth in the mind's eye. It is that knowledge that helps me ensure an adequate decompression every time. Few things in spine surgery have the potential to be more useful than absolute certainty of the anatomical dimensions in a surgical procedure. That certitude is inherent to ensuring the reproducibility of a spinal procedure. In this chapter, I review the cervical dimensions of the vertebral body and use those measurements to frame the technique for decompression and instrumentation.

At the very core of the anterior cervical procedure is an appreciation of the symmetry provided by the uncinate processes. These gentle slopes on either side of the disc space reliably establish the midline and guide the placement of the arthroplasty device, in the case of motion preservation, or the interbody spacer as well as the midline placement of the anterior cervical plate, in the case of an arthrodesis. Whether performing an arthrodesis or arthroplasty, the principles of securing the midline remain the same. In this chapter, I focus on the anatomical basis of the procedure. In doing so, I have applied all of the principles of minimally invasive spine surgery that have been the basis for the other procedures presented in this book. I hope that the reader finds that this chapter on the ACD indeed fits seamlessly into this Primer.

9.2 Anatomical Basis

Knowledge of the three-dimensional anatomy of the cervical vertebral body is an absolute necessity for mastery of decompressions and instrumentation of the anterior cervical spine.

The surgeon must develop an intuitive understanding of the dimensions of the cervical vertebral bodies, including their heights, widths and depths, to achieve a command of the necessary exposure of the bony anatomy and decompression of the neural elements. Panjabi and colleagues offer a comprehensive quantitative three-dimensional analysis of the subaxial spine, and their paper is mandatory reading for surgeons striving to master anterior approaches.[1] I summarize some of the key elements of that analysis, but nothing replaces the in-depth understanding achieved by reading and rereading Panjabi's article (▶ Fig. 9.1 and ▶ Table 9.1).[1]

The height of each cervical vertebral body provides a sense of the rostrocaudal exposure needed for a single-level arthroplasty or a four-level ACD fusion (ACDF). This knowledge also helps in planning the length of the anterior cervical plate. The width of the vertebral body provides a sense of the medial-lateral exposure needed for placement of an interbody graft, arthroplasty device or anterior cervical plate. Knowledge of the distance between the foramen transversarium provides the confidence needed to achieve a wide decompression of the cervical nerve roots compressed by lateral spurs on the uncovertebral joints. This section presents a brief summary of the key dimensions of the cervical vertebral bodies to begin the process of making the dimensions of the cervical spine intuitive.

The average vertebral body height is roughly 11 mm, with C6 being the shortest at 10.9 mm and C7 being the tallest at

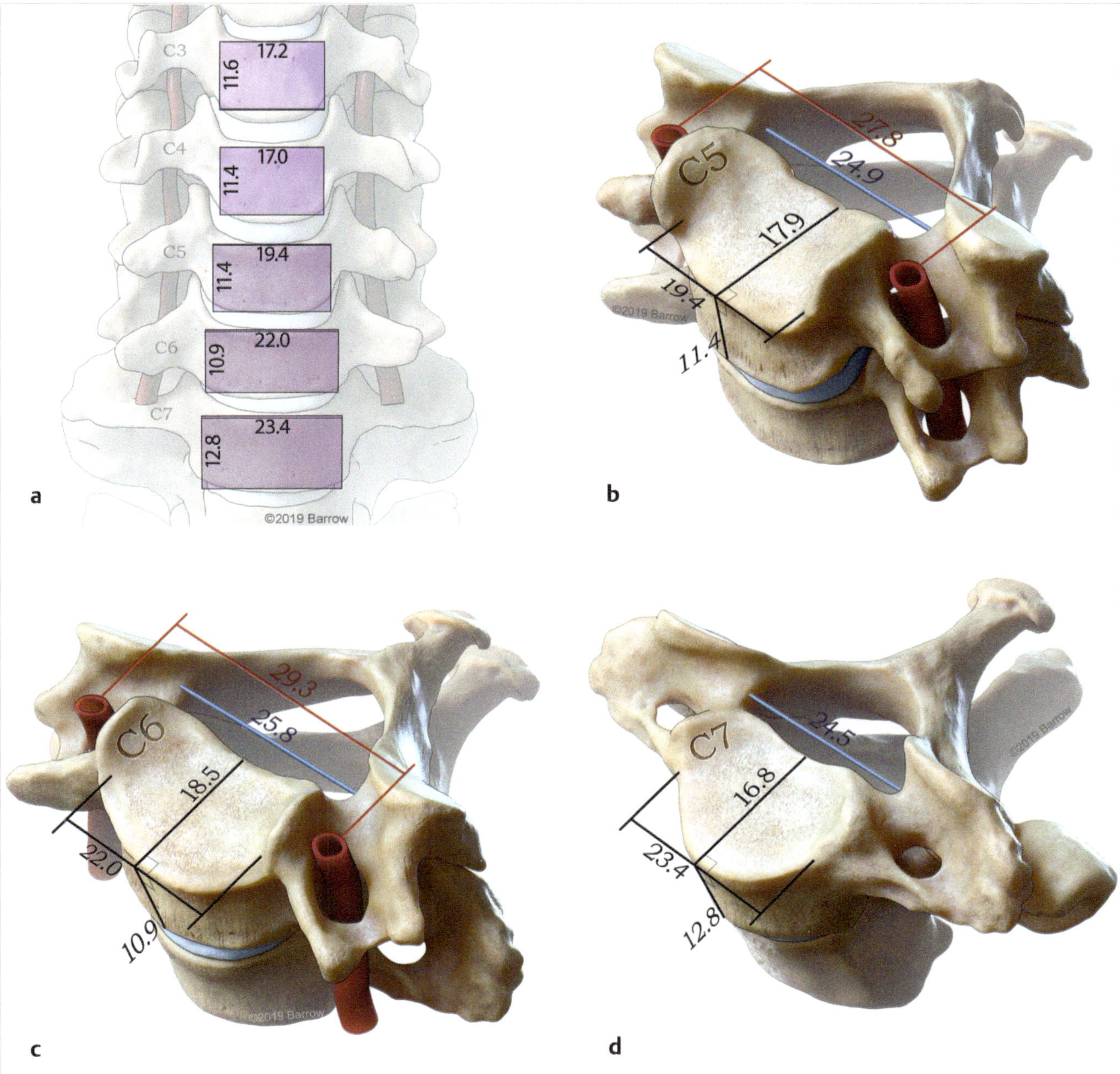

Fig. 9.1 Dimensions of the cervical spine in millimeters. **(a)** Anterior view of the cervical spine with the dimensions of each vertebral body height and width from C3 to C7. Superior oblique view demonstrating the dimensions of **(b)** C5, **(c)** C6 and **(d)** C7 vertebral body depth; the distance between the uncinate processes, the canal width and the distance between vertebral arteries as reported by Panjabi et al.[1]

12.8 mm. Understanding the height of a vertebral body helps prevent unnecessary exposure of a segment when performing a single-level ACDF. The disruption of the disc space during exposure may contribute to problems in an adjacent segment years or decades after an operation. An exposure of 5 mm above a disc space is just shy of the midportion of the vertebral body in just about every circumstance and is all that is needed for the rostral or caudal exposure in an operation. The anterior vertebral body width averages roughly 20 mm. That value becomes the minimum dimension needed for a medial-lateral exposure to accomplish a complete decompression. The spinal canal width is the distance from pedicle to pedicle and just shy of the foramen transversaria. An average of 25 mm from pedicle to pedicle provides an intuitive sense of the location of the vertebral arteries. Finally, vertebral body depth, which averages 16.7 mm across all segments and ranges from 15.6 to 18.5 mm, provides a sense of the depth of the interbody graft, arthroplasty device or vertebral body screw for anterior plate fixation.

Throughout this chapter, I place particular focus on the importance of completely exposing the uncinate processes during the discectomy phase of the operation. These gently sloping joints are the North Star for anterior approaches to the cervical spine. Whether for motion preservation or for arthrodesis, the uncovertebral joints, also known as the joints of Luschka, named after the German anatomist Herbert von Luschka, are the orienting structures whose complete exposure reliably allows the surgeon to establish the midline. Identifying and marking the geometric midline is the sine qua non of an adequate decompression, ideal positioning of an artificial disc or the orthogonal and midline placement of an anterior cervical plate (▸ Fig. 9.2).

The upslope of the uncovertebral joints is the lateral boundary of the decompression. On the other side of that lateral boundary courses the vertebral artery (▸ Fig. 9.3). Absolute certainty of the vertebral artery location provides you with the confidence to completely decompress a nerve root within its foramen. As mentioned previously, reconstruction of the anatomy at depth with anatomic measurements at your mental fingertips is a characteristic of minimally invasive surgery. The cadaveric analysis by Panjabi and colleagues provides a valuable reference regarding the canal width.[1] Vaccaro and colleagues

Table 9.1 Mean measurements of the cervical spine as reported by Panjabi et al[1]

Measurement	C2	C3	C4	C5	C6	C7	Mean
VB height, mm	–	11.6	11.4	11.4	10.9	12.8	11.6
Anterior VB width, mm	17.5	17.2	17.0	19.4	22.0	23.4	19.4
VB depth, mm	15.6	15.6	15.9	17.9	18.5	16.8	16.7
Spinal canal width, mm	24.5	22.9	24.7	24.9	25.8	24.5	24.5

Abbreviation: VB, vertebral body.
Notes: These average measurements are based on 12 fresh cadaver specimens (8 males and 4 females) with an average age of 46.3 years, average weight of 67.8 kg and average height of 167.8 cm (about 5 feet 5 inches). An average of the cervical vertebral body dimensions is provided to begin to build a foundation of an intuitive sense of the cervical spine at the time of surgery. There was little variability in the measurements (standard error range, 0.25–1.15 mm).

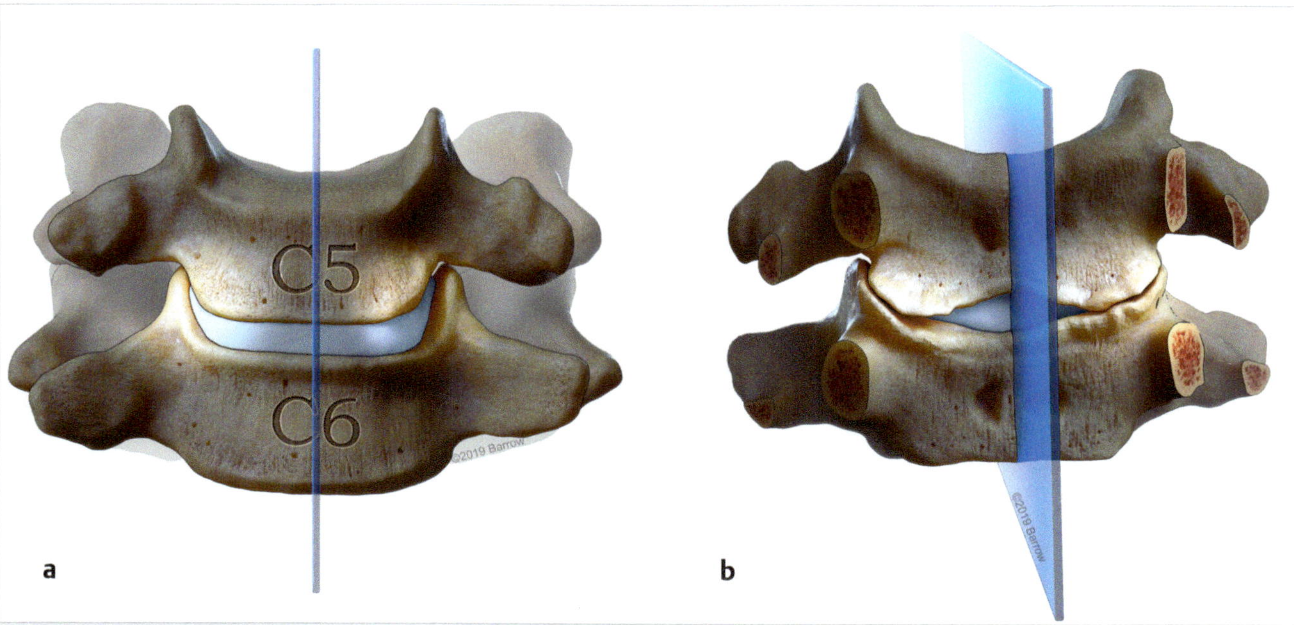

Fig. 9.2 The uncovertebral joints, or the joints of Luschka, are the North Star of the anterior cervical discectomy. **(a)** Anterior view of the cervical spine at C5–6 demonstrating how the midline may be identified with a complete exposure of the uncovertebral joints. The upward slope of the uncovertebral joints provides a proportional and balanced symmetry to the segment that allows the surgeon to identify and mark the midline. **(b)** Posterior view of the cervical spine demonstrating how, with the certainty of the midline, a surgeon may confidently decompress the foramen with removal of the uncovertebral spurs. These joints guide the extent of decompression and placement of the interbody graft or arthroplasty device.

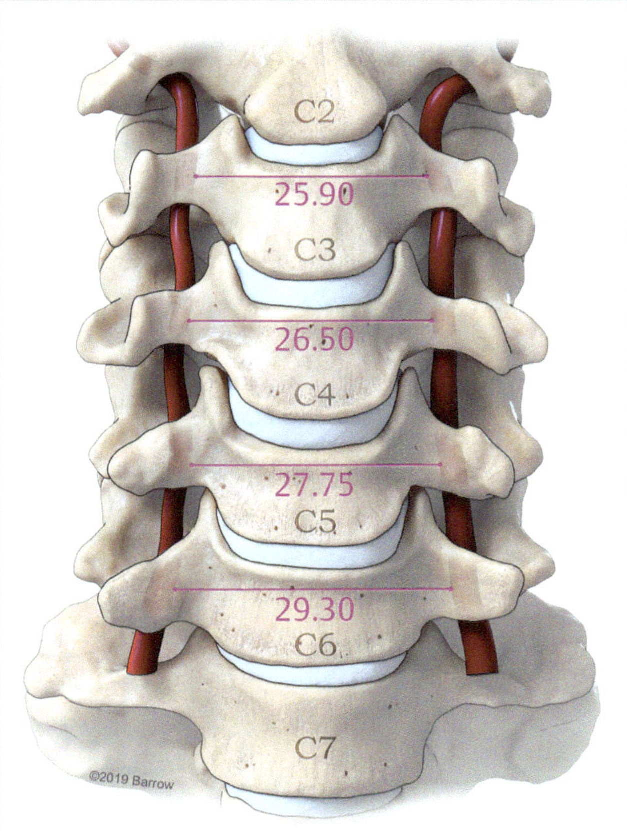

Fig. 9.3 Illustration of the anterior cervical spine with the distance between the vertebral arteries in millimeters listed from C3 to C6. Knowledge of the trend in the slopes of the uncovertebral joints, the distance between the uncovertebral joints, the distance between the vertebral arteries and the depth of the disc space collectively establish the anatomical basis of the anterior cervical discectomy. Understanding these dimensions from C3 to C7 helps ensure a consistent, reproducible decompression and guide placement of the interbody spacers, arthroplasty implants or anterior cervical plates.

corroborate Panjabi and colleagues' reported measurements with a radiographic analysis of axial computed tomography (CT) in which the authors measured the intervertebral artery distance throughout the subaxial spine. The range of the intervertebral artery distance is as high as 29 mm at C6 and as little as 25 mm at C3.[2] As will be discussed in the technique section of this chapter, these measurements, alongside those reported by Panjabi and colleagues, demonstrate the anatomical basis for at least a 20- to 22-mm decompression of the disc space in the majority of patients (▶ Fig. 9.2). It has become part of my preoperative routine to review the foramen transversaria by scrolling through the axial images at the level or levels that I intend to decompress and make note of any potential irregularity, such as an ectatic or tortuous vertebral artery.

9.3 Requisite Anatomy

Bringing together all of the anatomical measurements of the anterior cervical spine leads to a definition of the requisite anatomy for an anterior cervical operation. The mediolateral dimension of an exposure for any particular segment should be a minimum of 20 mm and up to 22 mm of the vertebral bodies. The rostral and caudal exposures should not exceed 5 mm above and below the disc space to mitigate the risk of adjacent segment degeneration. ▶ Fig. 9.4 illustrates the requisite anatomical unit needed for a single-level decompression with arthrodesis or arthroplasty. Logically, a multilevel surgery is the sum of the various requisite anatomical units in need of decompression, all of which should be exposed at the outset of the operation (▶ Fig. 9.5).

9.4 Operating Room Setup

The surgery is performed on a standard operating table that is reversed to shift the base away from the head of the bed. Configuring the operating table in this manner facilitates positioning the fluoroscopic unit. I position the patient's head in a Caspar head holder to maintain the position of the cervical spine in an ideal orthogonal position. A stable head makes for a stable cervical spine. Furthermore, the head holder achieves and captures

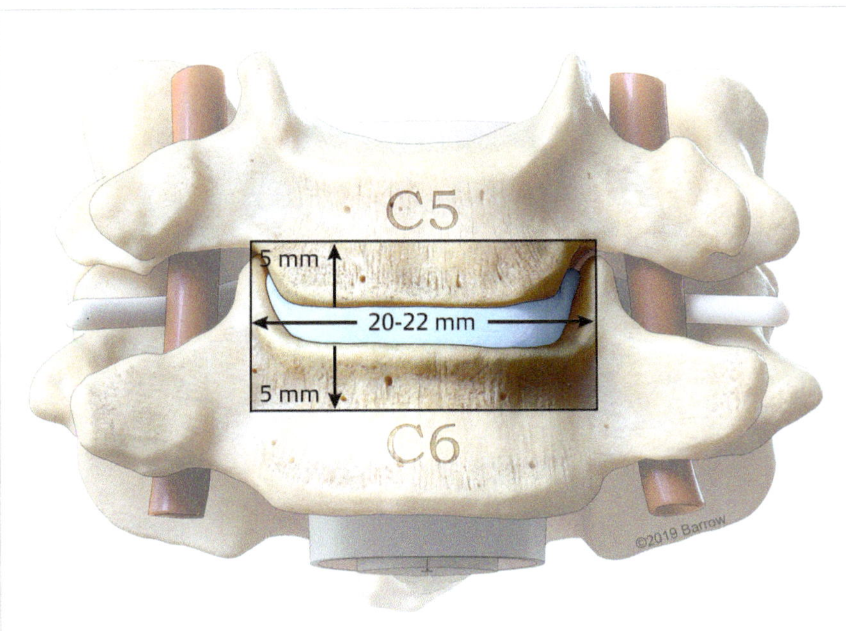

Fig. 9.4 Requisite anatomical unit for anterior cervical discectomy. Anterior view of the cervical spine with the requisite anatomy for a single-level C5–6 anterior cervical discectomy outlined by the box.

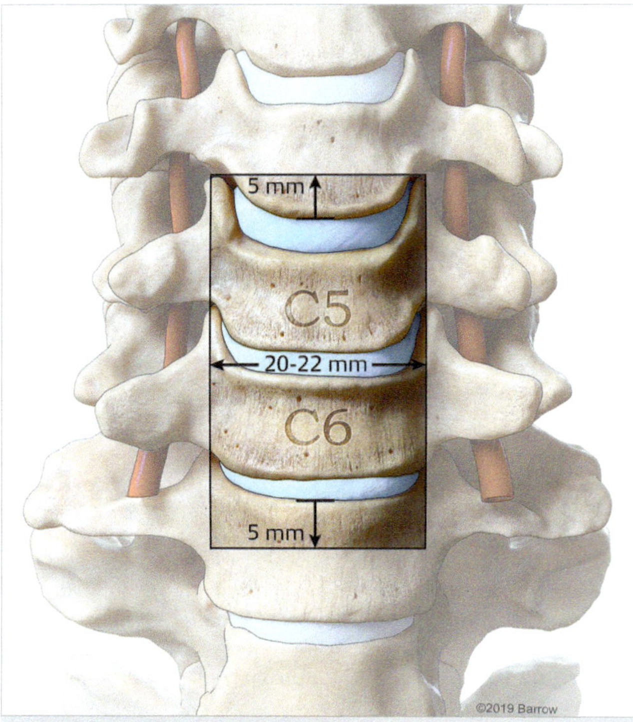

Fig. 9.5 The requisite anatomy for a three-level anterior cervical discectomy at C4–5, C5–6 and C6–7. The requisite anatomical unit defined in ▶ Fig. 9.4 is performed at each level to be decompressed. The extent of rostral and caudal exposure remains the same at 5 mm above and below the disc space, respectively. A mediolateral exposure of 20 to 22 mm should be accomplished at each segment.

the ideal lordotic position with the use of a bolster in the posterior cervical spine. In my estimation, the quest for the geometric midline of the cervical spine begins with positioning the patient. The stability added by the Caspar head holder is a valuable element in identifying and securing the midline. I discuss the merits of this contraption further in the patient positioning section.

The laterality of the approach needs to be determined so that the operating room staff know where to place the microscope and fluoroscope to set up the operating room properly. I prefer to approach the cervical spine opposite the side of the symptoms. For instance, if a patient presents with a left C6 radiculopathy secondary to a large disc herniation that is eccentric to the left, I use a right-sided approach. The rationale is that a right-sided approach provides a direct line of sight onto the contralateral aspect of the disc space and foramen. Applying that same rationale to right-sided symptoms would then prompt a left-sided approach. It is important to clearly communicate the laterality of the approach in advance to the operating room staff to enable them to efficiently set up the operating room. Admittedly, a complete decompression of the entire segment can be achieved from either side. However, I have found that approaching from the side opposite of the symptoms optimizes my visualization into the most symptomatic lateral recess.

The fluoroscope is positioned and remains in the operative field from the outset to optimize the flow of the operation before the patient is prepped and draped. Similar to the previous techniques mentioned in this Primer, the image intensifier of the fluoroscope is always positioned on the side opposite of the side of the incision, whereas the microscope stands ready to roll in on the same side of the incision and opposite of the image intensifier. I avoid any difficulty navigating the bases of the microscope and fluoroscope with this configuration (▶ Fig. 9.6).

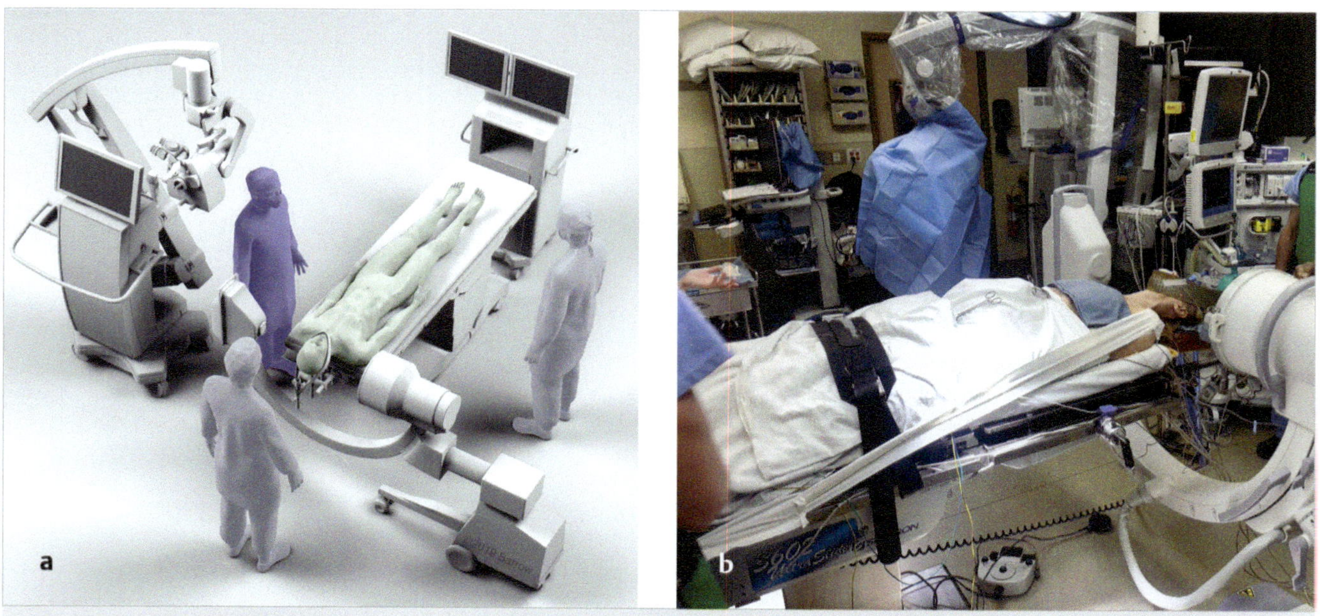

Fig. 9.6 Operating room setup for anterior cervical approaches. **(a)** Schematic illustration of a patient positioned for a left-sided approach. The surgeon stands on the side of the incision, and the microscope is draped and ready. The image intensifier of the fluoroscope is opposite the microscope. **(b)** Intraoperative photograph of a patient positioned for a right-sided approach. Note that the operating table has the base reversed to facilitate the positioning of the fluoroscope. The head of the patient is stabilized in a Caspar head holder. The fluoroscope is in position with the image intensifier opposite the side of the microscope, which stands draped and ready. The patient's shoulders are lightly taped down to optimize visualization. By convention, the pedal to the bipolar cautery is always placed on the floor at the head of the bed, and the drill pedal is placed more toward the foot of the bed, as seen in the photograph. Position of the pedals remains the same regardless of the laterality of the approach.

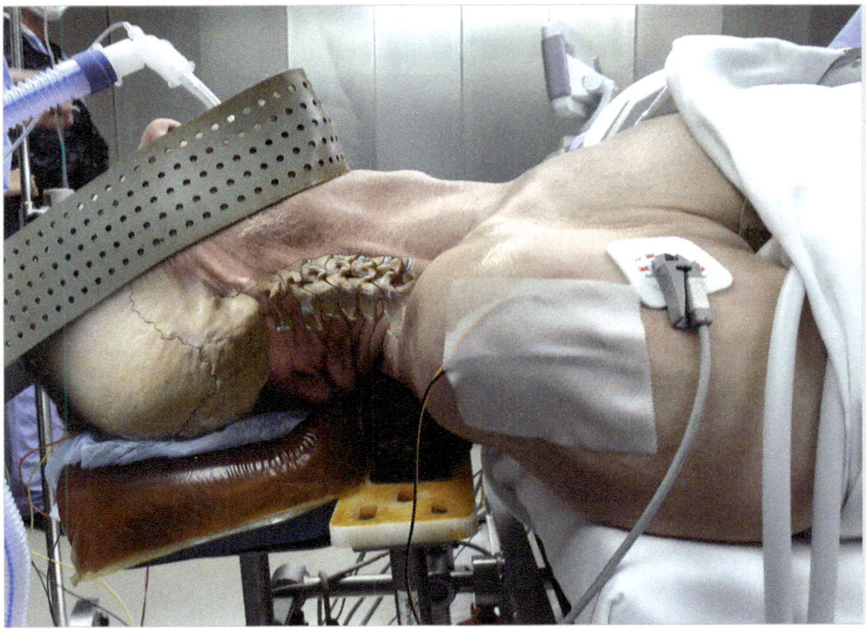

Fig. 9.7 Patient positioning with a Caspar head holder. This photograph shows a patient positioned for an anterior cervical discectomy and fusion in a Caspar head holder. A chin strap firmly secures the head and maintains a lordotic position by keeping upward tension on the chin. The head-holding device maintains the orthogonal position of the cervical spine throughout the operation. The bolster further maintains the lordotic position and acts as a counterforce when securing a graft or artificial disc. An illustration of the cervical spine has been superimposed onto the photograph to demonstrate how cervical lordosis is captured by the combination of the chin strap and the bolster.

9.5 Patient Positioning

When I first started in practice, I positioned the patient with nothing more than a bag of intravenous fluid behind the shoulder blades and the head positioned in a doughnut-shaped gel roll. The shoulders were taped down to facilitate exposure of the lower cervical levels. The problem I encountered with this positioning technique was that there was nothing to stabilize the head. If the head rotated during the operation, I found that it had an impact on putting the cervical plate in a perfectly midline and orthogonal position, or it affected the placement of an arthroplasty device. Maintaining the spine in a perfectly orthogonal position is a principle tenet of instrumentation of the spine at any level.

A stable head makes for a stable cervical spine, and therefore, some sort of head holder is ideal for stabilization of the head and cervical spine for anterior cervical approaches. The headpiece centers the patient's head on the operating table, the chinstrap captures and holds a midline orthogonal position and the shoulder bolster ensures a lordotic position for the neck. The bolster is helpful when tapping a tight-fitting graft into place, and it is particularly valuable as a counterforce when securing an artificial disc (▶ Fig. 9.7).

An adhesive spray is applied to the shoulders, which are then taped down onto the bed to facilitate visualization of the lower cervical segments. The fluoroscope, which has been parked above the head of the bed, rolls into position to facilitate planning the incision.

9.6 Planning the Incision

For a single-level operation, I plan the incision precisely over the disc space (▶ Fig. 9.8).

For a multilevel operation, I plan the incision over the top of the central vertebral body or disc space. For example, when performing a C5–6, C6–7 ACDF, I plan the incision over the top of the C6 vertebral body, which is the central point of the exposure (▶ Fig. 9.9). For a three-level ACDF, I plan the incision over the top of the central disc space. For example, for a C4–5, C5–6 and C6–7 ACDF, I plan the incision over the C5–6 disc space, which is the central point of the exposure (▶ Fig. 9.10).

Finally, for a four-level ACDF, I use the two-incision technique as described by Riew in Chin et al.[3] For example, for a C3–4, C4–5, C5–6 and C6–7 ACDF, I plan one smaller incision over the C4 vertebral body, which provides access to the disc spaces of C3–4 and C4–5, and a second longer incision over the C6 vertebral

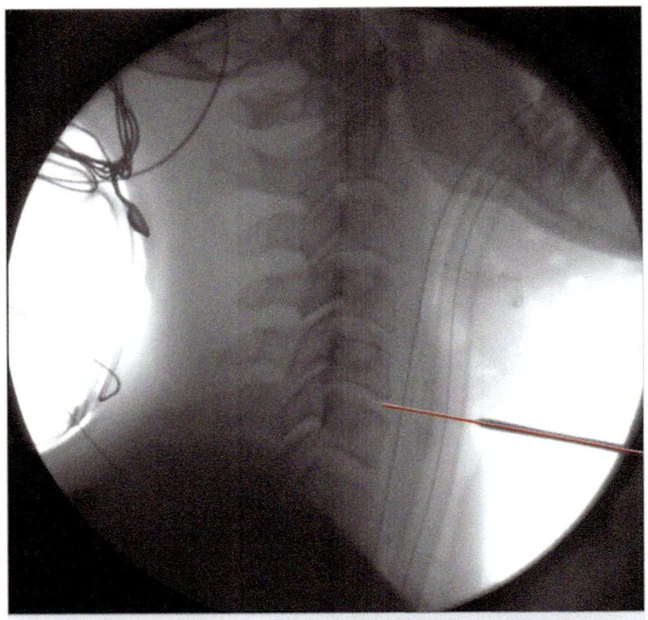

Fig. 9.8 Planning the incision for a single-level operation. This lateral fluoroscopic image shows a Steinman pin with a protective plastic cover pointing precisely to the disc space. In this case, it is pointing to the C5–6 disc space. If a neck crease is in the vicinity of the mark, it is aesthetically pleasing to the patient to plan the incision in the crease.

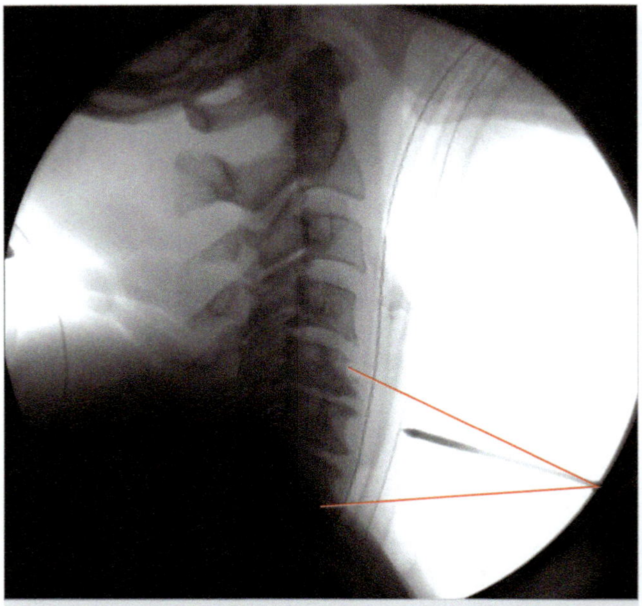

Fig. 9.9 Lateral fluoroscopic image used for planning an incision for a two-level anterior cervical discectomy and fusion. A Steinman pin with a protective plastic cover points to the C6 vertebral body, and the incision is marked. In this example, the pin has been placed in a neck crease and therefore in a slightly higher plane than at the midpoint of the C6 vertebral body. The C6 vertebral body is the center of the exposure; centering the incision there facilitates exposure to both the C5–6 and C6–7 levels (*red lines*).

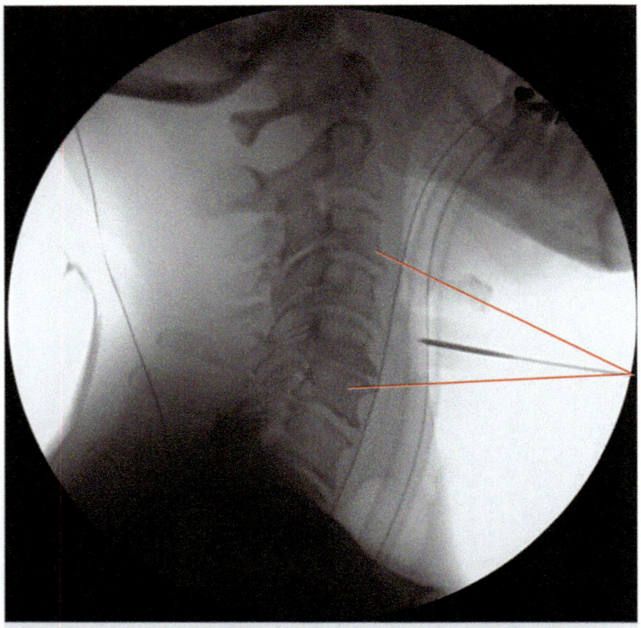

Fig. 9.10 Lateral fluoroscopic image used for planning a three-level anterior cervical discectomy and fusion at C3–4, C4–5 and C5–6. The Steinman pin marks the C4–5 segment, which is the central point of the exposure, making the C3–4 and C5–6 segments (*red lines*) roughly equidistant from the C4–5 disc space.

body, which provides access to the disc spaces of C5–6 and C6–7 (▶ Fig. 9.11). The two-incision technique is described in greater detail in Section 9.8, Operative Technique.

As mentioned earlier, I plan the incision on the side of the neck opposite the symptoms, which provides me an optimal view of the symptomatic lateral recess. I mark the incision by placing a protected Steinman pin perfectly vertical and alongside the sternocleidomastoid muscle. Vertical positioning of the Steinman pin for the fluoroscopic image is important to establish the trajectory of exposure. During the exposure, completing the dissection along the same trajectory of the vertically positioned Steinman pin almost guarantees the exposure of the intended level. One or two fluoroscopic images allow me to confirm an ideal location on the skin to plan the incision. I mark the ideal incision immediately over my intended target and then look for a prominent neck crease in the vicinity of this mark (▶ Fig. 9.12). If I am able to identify two neck creases, I use the higher one because rostral dissection is more restricting than caudal dissection. In the absence of an obvious neck crease, I use the initial mark.

After I mark the incision, I mark a prominent V in the sternal notch as a reference point for the midline (▶ Fig. 9.13). An electrocardiogram lead may be placed on the tip of the nose so that it may be palpated under the sterile drapes. The tip of the nose and the sternal notch become two reference points for the midline, which are of tremendous value when plating. I widely prep and drape the surgical site to include the midline and the V to provide as many visual cues as possible for establishing the midline.

9.7 Historical Vignette

The surgical approach to the anterior spine that I describe in the surgical technique section is known as the Smith–Robinson approach. The story of the evolution of that approach for management of cervical radiculopathy and myelopathy is worthy of a chapter, if not a book, of its own. Although outside the purview of this Primer, it would be impossible for me, given my insatiable penchant for the history of spinal procedures, not to include a comment or two on this topic. The hope is to nudge the reader into reviewing those original papers, both of which make for extraordinarily insightful reading and provide all of us with a greater appreciation of our origins and how far we have come.

The year 1958 was a remarkable year for the anterior cervical spine. Prior to that year, the management of cervical radiculopathy and myelopathy was limited to posterior approaches. Spine surgeons had long recognized the limitations of cervical laminectomies and foraminotomies and began exploring decompression of the spinal cord and nerve roots from an anterior approach, especially for midline compression of the spinal cord. Writing from Honolulu, Hawaii, Ralph Cloward published "Anterior Approach for Ruptured Cervical Disks" in the *Journal of Neurosurgery* in 1958, while the very same year, writing from Baltimore, Maryland, George W. Smith and Robert A. Robinson published "The Treatment of Certain Cervical-Spine Disorders by Anterior Removal of the Intervertebral Disc and Interbody Fusion" in the *Journal of Bone and Joint Surgery*.[4,5] The Cloward procedure involved a drill that reamed a hole within the disc

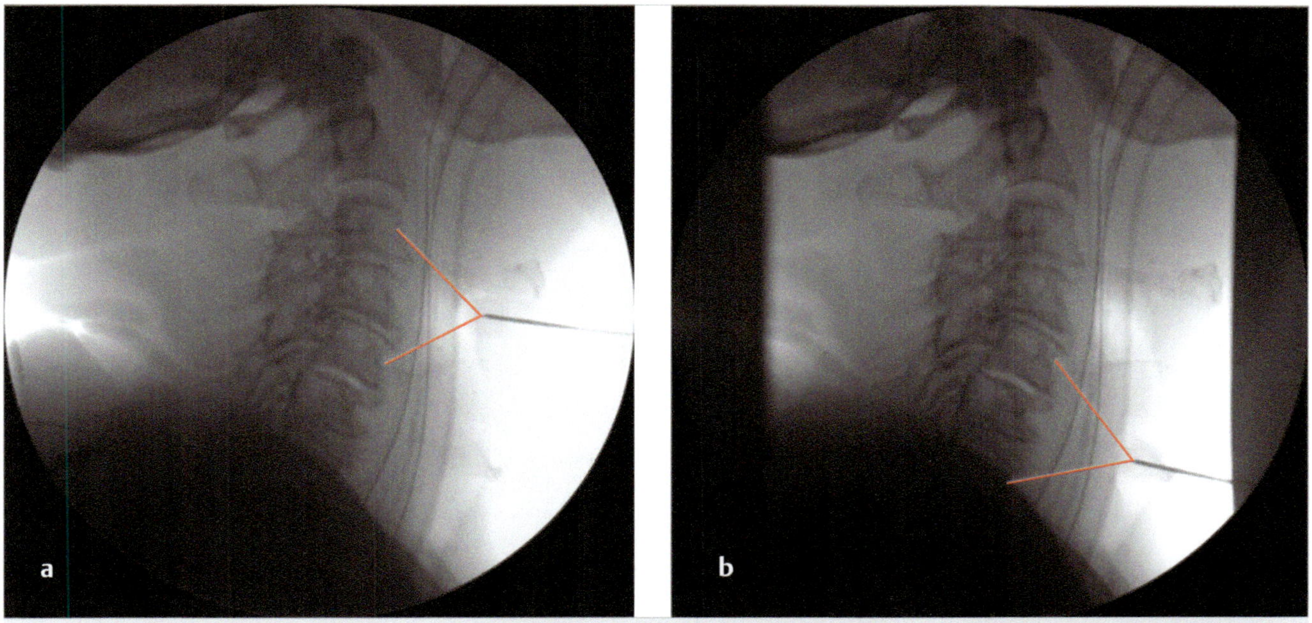

Fig. 9.11 Two-incision technique for a four-level (C3–4, C4–5, C5–6 and C6–7) anterior cervical discectomy and fusion. **(a)** Lateral fluoroscopic image used for planning the top two levels, C3–4 and C4–5 (*red lines* span C3, C4 and C5). The Steinman pin marks the C4 vertebral body. **(b)** The Steinman pin in this lateral fluoroscopic image points to the C6 vertebral body. The longer of the two incisions is marked at this level to access C5–6 and C6–7 (*red lines* span C5, C6 and C7).

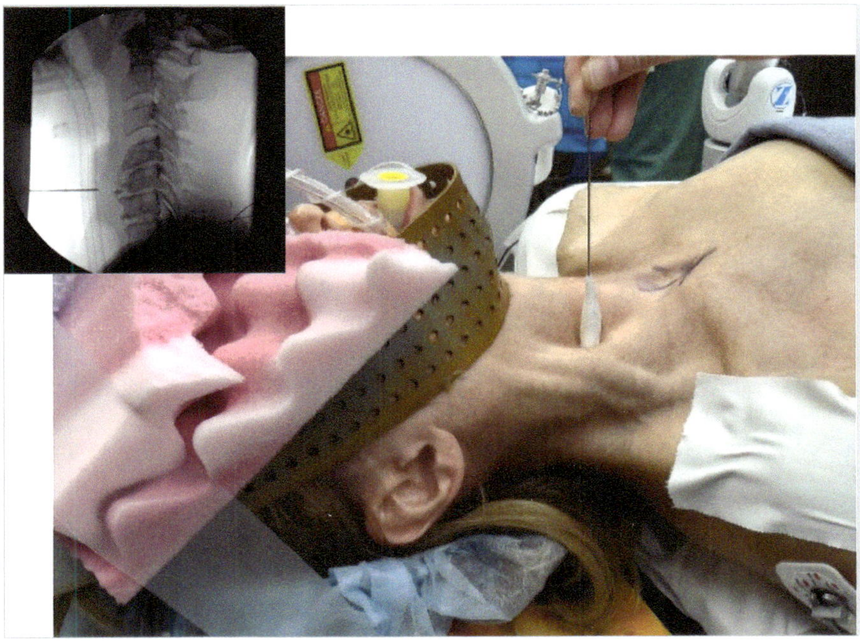

Fig. 9.12 Planning the incision for a C4–5, C5–6 anterior cervical discectomy and fusion. Photograph of a protected Steinman pin placed alongside the sternocleidomastoid muscle and over the top of the C5 vertebral body. Note that the Steinman pin is positioned vertically, which is the trajectory of the exposure. An exposure that proceeds along the vertical access of the marked incision assuredly lands on the C5 vertebral body.

space for the decompression and then placement of a bone dowel for fusion (▶ Fig. 9.14),[4] whereas the Smith–Robinson procedure was more in line with the procedure performed today: discectomy and placement of a shaped iliac crest autograft for interbody fusion (▶ Fig. 9.15).[5]

Surgeons had some understandable concerns about the risk involved in drilling with a large drill bit through the disc space and in the direction of the central canal, and the Cloward procedure gradually fell out of favor. The simplicity and reproducibility of the Smith and Robinson approach, on the other hand, allowed for much wider adoption. As a result, the anterior approach to the anterior cervical spine has become known as the Smith–Robinson approach and is the approach I describe in the next section. It is important to recognize that both the Cloward and Smith–Robinson techniques use the same avascular plane medial to the sternocleidomastoid muscle that allows

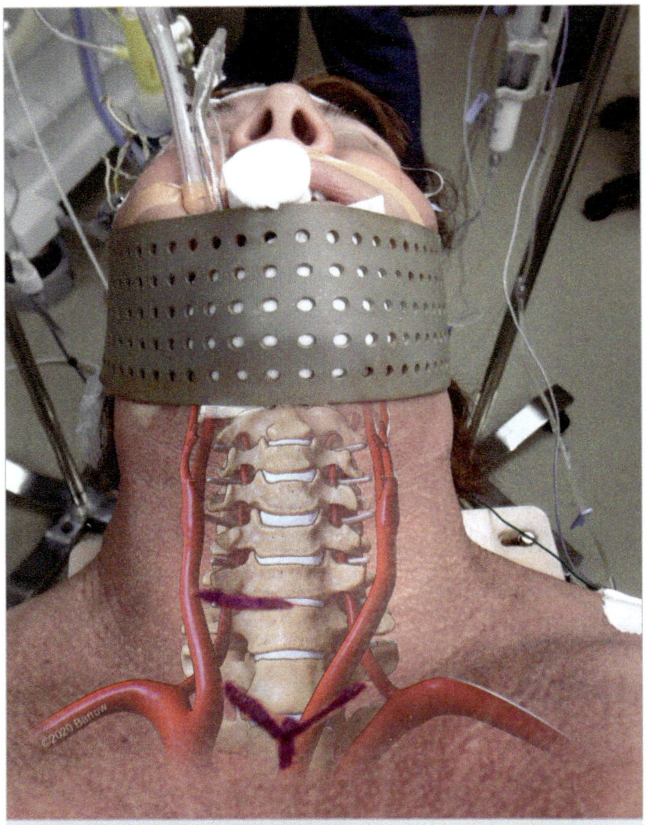

Fig. 9.13 Planning the incision and marking the sternal notch. This photograph demonstrates a patient positioned in the Caspar head holder for a C6–7 anterior cervical discectomy and fusion. The incision is marked with fluoroscopic guidance, and a prominent V is marked into the sternal notch. An illustration of the cervical spine has been superimposed onto the photograph to demonstrate the location of the C6–7 disc space relative to the incision as well as the vertebral arteries.

for a bloodless dissection onto the anterior cervical spine. From the standpoint of exposure, these two techniques are indistinguishable.

9.8 Operative Technique

In Jonathan Swift's novel *Gulliver's Travels*, the tiny men from the island of Lilliput tied down the hero, Lemuel Gulliver, with hundreds of tiny ropes, which were no more than threads to Gulliver. Although one rope of the Lilliputians could never hold the enormous Gulliver down, the combination of hundreds of tiny ropes made the giant their prisoner.[6] I oftentimes think of Swift's tale when I am exposing the anterior cervical spine. The exposure can be a painful struggle or an effortless joy; it depends on how much attention I direct toward freeing the tissue planes. The hundreds of tiny ropes holding me back from the cervical spine need only be identified and meticulously spread or divided. The exposure then becomes effortless and the surgery enjoyable. At the same time, whereas one of these tiny ropes alone could not hold me back, the combination of adhesions and fascial bands between the tissue planes can make me their prisoner. The operation then becomes laborious, the exposure becomes suboptimal and everything from the decompression to the plating becomes a struggle. Welcome to Lilliput.

With all of this in mind, the theme for exposure is to dissect the various tissue planes in a manner that allows for near effortless retraction of the esophagus and trachea medially and maximizes the exposure of the requisite anatomical unit(s). The more these tissue planes are identified and freed, the easier it becomes to visualize the requisite anatomy of the operation. Not doing so limits the retractor blades' capacity to expose the requisite anatomical unit. As illustrated in ▶ Fig. 9.4, the goal is exposure of the inferior 5 mm of the rostral vertebral body and exposure of the superior 5 mm of the caudal vertebral body

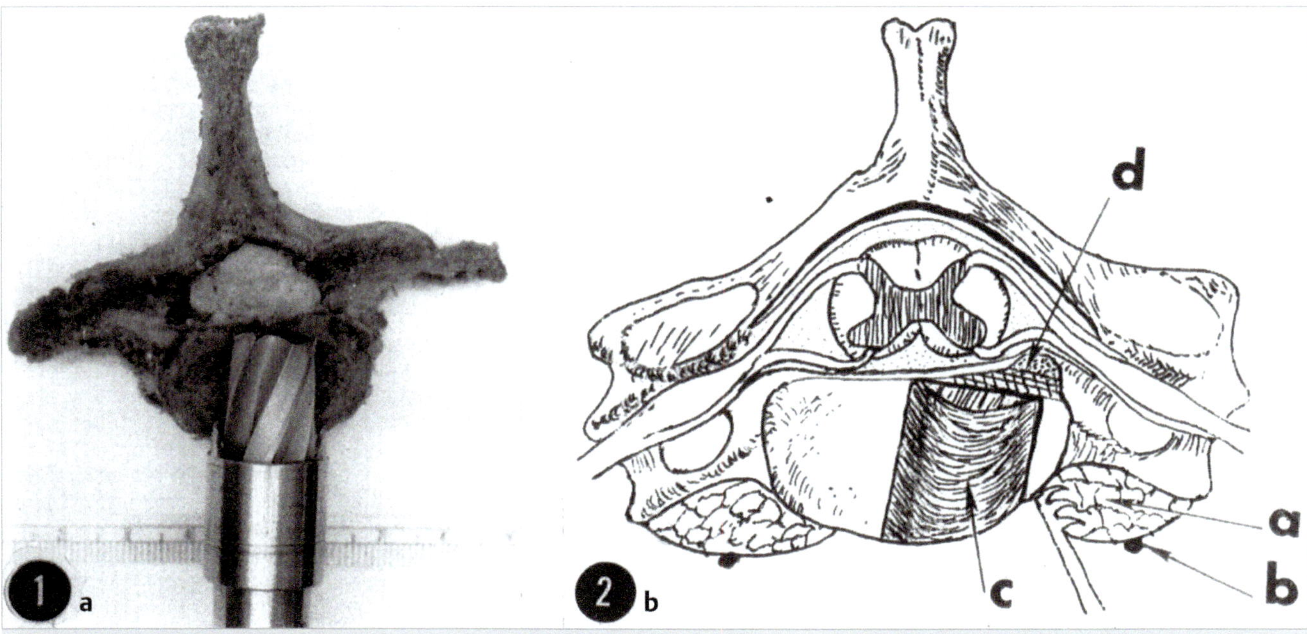

Fig. 9.14 Images from Cloward's landmark paper illustrating his anterior cervical technique. **(a)** Photograph of a cadaveric specimen with the drill in position within the disc space. **(b)** Cloward's illustration of his technique. (a, longus colli muscle; b, sympathetic chain ganglion; c, drill; d, osteophyte.) Cloward would fill the defect with a matching bone dowel harvested from the patient's iliac crest or from a cadaver bone bank.[4] (Reproduced with permission from Cloward RB. The anterior approach for removal of ruptured cervical disks. J Neurosurg. 1958; 15(6):602–617.)

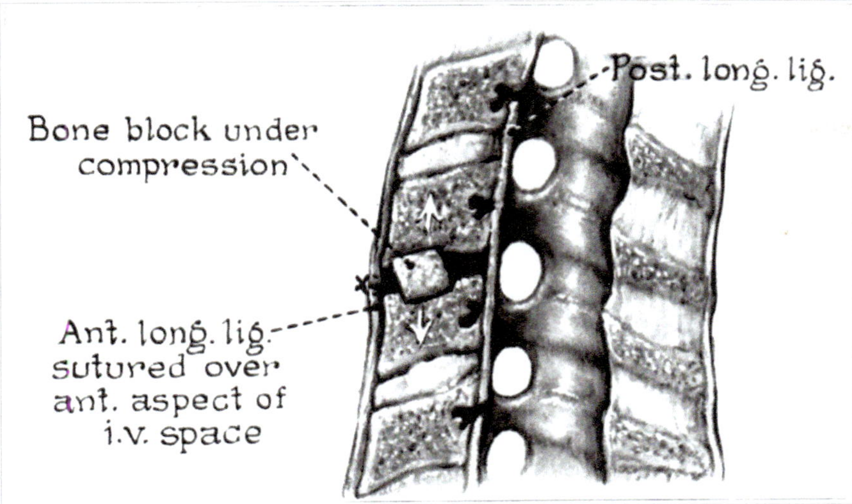

Fig. 9.15 The Smith–Robinson interbody graft technique after discectomy. Illustration from Smith and Robinson's landmark paper, which described discectomy, preparation of the end plates and placement of a structural autograft from the patient's anterior superior iliac spine. There is no description of division of the posterior longitudinal ligament in the manuscript.[5] Abbreviations: ant., anterior; i.v., intravenous; lig., ligament; long., longitudinal; post., posterior. (Reproduced with permission from Smith GW, Robinson RA. The treatment of certain cervical-spine disorders by anterior removal of the intervertebral disc and interbody fusion. J Bone Joint Surg Am. 1958; 40-A(3):607–624.)

along with a mediolateral exposure of 20 to 22 mm. By way of example, for a C5–6 ACDF, I expose the inferior half, approximately 5 mm, of the C5 vertebral body and the superior half (5 mm) of the C6 vertebral body. I mobilize the longus muscles and expose the 20 to 22 mm of the anterior vertebral bodies. An identical exposure is needed for arthroplasty. I always make a concerted effort not to expose a segment that is not being operated on to prevent a degenerative cascade from beginning.

All of the exposure that is needed for the entire operation, including plating, should be accomplished before placing the self-retaining cervical retractor blades or Caspar posts. Whether the operation is a single- or a four-level operation, completing the exposure of all the requisite anatomical units at the outset optimizes the flow of the operation. A potential pitfall is placing the Caspar posts into the vertebral bodies too early. The posts become a distraction and end up limiting the exposure. I complete the entire exposure for the decompression and the plating with Cloward handheld retractors between my assistant and myself before beginning the decompression of any segment. In that way, when I complete decompression and interbody graft placement for the final segment, there is no need for additional exposure. Instead, after the final interbody spacer is placed, I know that I can slide the cervical plate into position and fixate it to the anterior cervical spine. The work performed at the beginning of the operation should make plating the easiest part of the operation.

9.9 Exposure

For a single-level operation, I make an 18-mm transverse incision with a No. 15 blade within a neck crease. For a two-level operation, I typically plan a 20-mm transverse incision, and for a three-level operation, a 25-mm transverse incision. I perform a four-level operation with one small rostral transverse 20-mm incision and a second caudal transverse 30-mm incision. All incisions begin on the muscle and extend laterally over the sternocleidomastoid.

After I make the skin incision, I apply cautery using the "cut" setting and complete the division of the subcutaneous tissue and expose the platysma. I generously release the soft tissue superficial to the platysma in the rostral, caudal and medial directions. I position a small blunt Weitlaner self-retaining retractor with the handles directed away from me. Slightly opening the Weitlaner retractor places the platysma muscle on stretch. Now, with a pair of DeBakey forceps, I pick up the platysma at its most lateral point in the incision and begin spreading along the fibers of the platysma muscle in a rostrocaudal direction with Metzenbaum scissors until I enter the potential space beneath the platysma. The distinct divisions of the anatomy below the platysma make it obvious when I have entered the potential space. I am careful to keep the tips of the Metzenbaum scissors pointed up and closely adhered to the underside of the platysma. There may be a number of veins of various sizes and vulnerabilities immediately beneath this muscle layer. Keeping the scissor tips up and slowly spreading them prevents tearing one of the various veins that resides in this space.

With a plane of dissection below the platysma, I slide the Metzenbaum scissors underneath the thin veil of platysma, spread the scissors open and use cautery to divide the fibers of the platysma along the length of the incision. I use DeBakey forceps again to pick up each limb of the divided platysma and undermine it in the rostral, caudal and medial directions. These fascial adhesions and bands beneath platysma are what contribute to those Lilliputian ropes holding me back from an effortless exposure onto the cervical spine. With the platysma divided and undermined, I can deepen the position of the self-retaining Weitlaner retractor to beneath the divided platysma. The sternocleidomastoid muscle becomes clearly visible as the prominent muscle in the lateral aspect of the exposure when I open the Weitlaner retractor (▶ Fig. 9.16). The trachea and esophagus lie medial to the sternocleidomastoid muscle, whereas the carotid artery and jugular vein lie immediately below the muscle.

With minimal dissection, the corridor that leads directly onto the cervical spine becomes obvious when following the medial aspect of sternocleidomastoid muscle belly along the avascular plane. I use DeBakey forceps to lightly pull the sternocleidomastoid muscle laterally to reveal the medial fascial bands. The action of the Metzenbaum scissors is to spread those fascial bands and develop the avascular plane. With nothing more than spreading the blades of the scissors, the plane of dissection

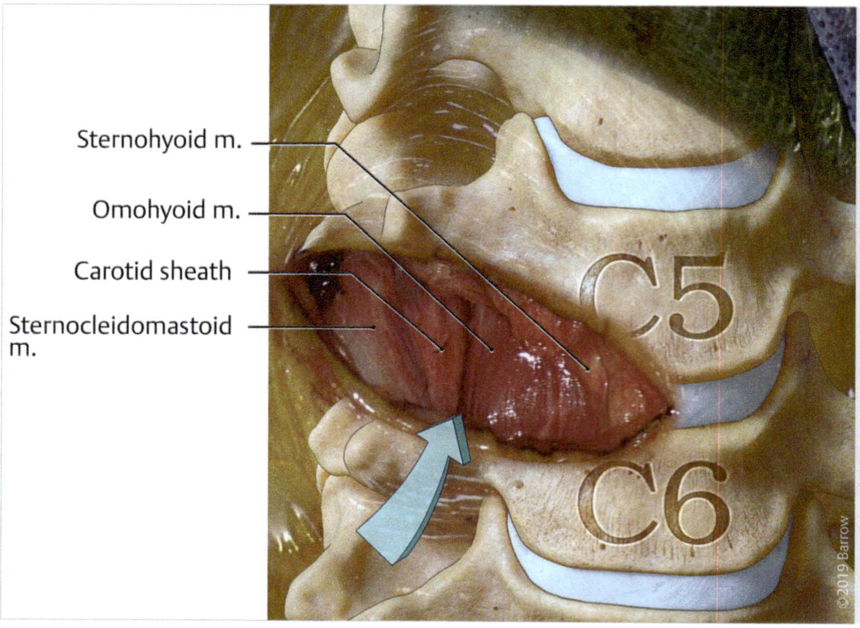

Fig. 9.16 Intraoperative photograph of the anterior cervical spine musculature in a right-sided approach, with a superimposed illustration of the cervical vertebrae involved. After division of the platysma, the sternocleidomastoid muscle is the prominent musculature in the lateral aspect of the exposure. Dissecting along the avascular plane (*arrow*) medial to the sternocleidomastoid muscle and carotid sheath leads directly to the precervical fascia on the anterior cervical spine. Abbreviation: m, muscle.

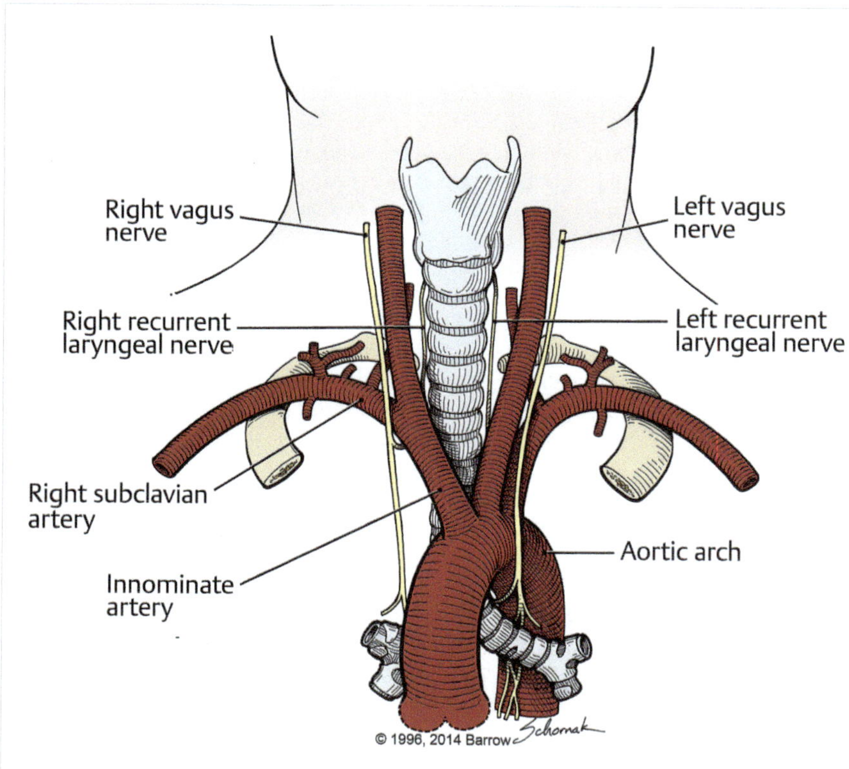

Fig. 9.17 Illustration of the vascular and nervous structures in an anterior cervical exposure. The recurrent laryngeal nerve on the left loops below the arch of the aorta, whereas on the right, the nerve loops beneath the subclavian. It has been hypothesized that the shorter, more oblique course on the right makes the recurrent laryngeal nerve more prone to a traction injury.

between the sternocleidomastoid laterally and the sternohyoid, sternothyroid and omohyoid muscles medially opens and leads directly to the prevertebral cervical fascia. I routinely use an index finger to confirm that the pulsing carotid artery is lateral to my plane of dissection and the cartilaginous rings of the trachea are medial, precisely the same way Smith and Robinson described their approach in their 1958 landmark paper.[5]

9.10 Recurrent Laryngeal Nerve

Inspection of a right-sided exposure may reveal the recurrent laryngeal nerve (▶ Fig. 9.17). If so, it is a worthwhile endeavor to ensure that the nerve is safely mobilized and that no traction will be upon it when the self-retaining retractors are in place. If I do not see the recurrent laryngeal nerve, I make no attempt to search for it. The literature on the incidence, cause and prevention of injury to recurrent laryngeal nerves is voluminous. There are several studies that suggest a left-sided approach decreases the incidence of such an injury.[7,8] However, that body of literature has been countered with an equal body that does not support this hypothesis.[9,10] Regardless of the side of the approach, deflating the endotracheal cuff after the retractors are in position and reinflating it to less than 20 mm Hg, as recommended by Apfelbaum and colleagues, is a worthwhile routine to incorporate into your technique.[11]

9.11 Exposure of the Requisite Anatomical Unit

At this point, I pass Cloward handheld retractors into the dissected plane and onto the prevertebral cervical fascia, and I begin to retract the trachea and esophagus as I bluntly dissect my way to the cervical spine with Kittner dissectors. Smith and Robinson described this part of the operation with the following sentence: "The anterior longitudinal ligament glistens over the mid-line of the vertebral bodies even through the prevertebral fascia. It clearly marks the mid-line."[5] That statement is as true today as it was in 1958 and is something I always keep in mind as I begin to identify the midline.

With my assistant retracting medially, I use two Kittner dissectors to bluntly dissect in opposite directions in the rostrocaudal plane against the anterior cervical spine. My goal is to separate the prevertebral cervical fascia without sharp dissection and visualize the glistening anterior longitudinal ligament on the cervical vertebral bodies and disc spaces. Before bluntly dissecting, I inspect the area for traversing veins on the top of the prevertebral cervical fascia. Although these veins are small, they are capable of causing bleeding that can become quite a nuisance during the exposure. To eliminate the risk of tearing these veins, I find it worthwhile to cauterize them and then sharply divide them over the segment to be operated on before proceeding with blunt dissection of the rostrocaudal plane using Kittner dissectors.

Because I have proceeded along the vertical path in line with the Steinman pin that I used to plan my incision, I will reliably reach my intended target. I do not use a spinal needle to confirm the level. Instead, I place a Kittner on the disc space to confirm the location with a fluoroscopic image. I long ago abandoned the practice of using a spinal needle to puncture the presumptive disc space on the off chance that I am off by a level. There is literature to suggest that puncturing an unaffected disc level begins the degenerative cascade that ushers in adjacent segment degeneration.[12] So instead of a spinal needle, I hold the Kittner on the disc space, remove the handheld Cloward retractor, since it is not radiolucent, and bring in the fluoroscope as the operating table rises to the predetermined fluoroscopic height. A lateral fluoroscopic image confirms that I am at the correct level (▶ Fig. 9.18). In the event that I am off by a level, there is no consequence since the annulus has not been punctured; there has not been a disruption in the prevertebral cervical fascia, nor have I used cautery up to this point. I merely extend my dissection either up or down to the correct level by freeing the various fascial bands medial to the sternocleidomastoid muscle. It is only after I have confirmed the correct level

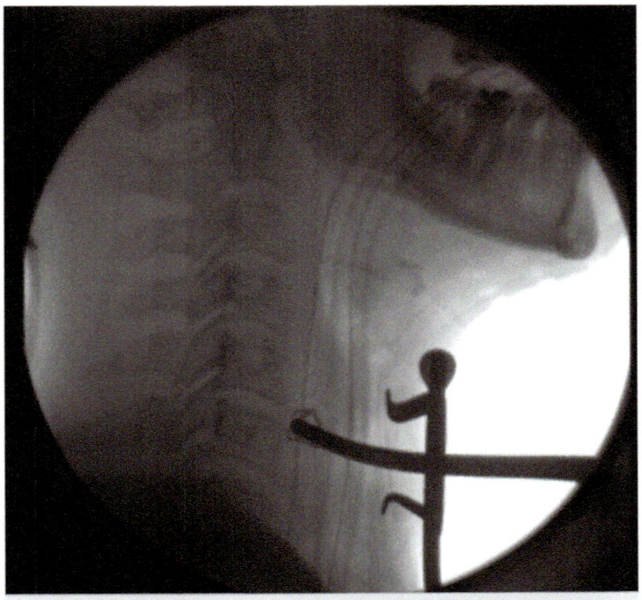

Fig. 9.18 Confirmation of the C5–6 level for cervical arthroplasty. Lateral fluoroscopic image demonstrating confirmation of the C5–6 level. Instead of using a spinal needle, a Kittner is placed over the top of the segment and a fluoroscopic image taken to confirm the operative segment.

that I make a preliminary mark above and below the disc space into the vertebral bodies with cautery and return to completing the exposure.

With the segment confirmed, I return to using the handheld Cloward retractors and ensure that I have bluntly dissected through the prevertebral cervical fascia. The longus colli muscles become readily evident on either side of the disc space. Those vertical columns of muscle provide me with my first opportunity to establish the midline. I hold the Cloward handheld retractor so that I am holding back the soft tissue above the longus colli without actually retracting the longus colli. The objective is to prevent any distortion of the muscular columns. My assistant does likewise on their side. I then visualize the two columns of longus colli muscle coursing over the segment (▶ Fig. 9.19). The midpoint between longus colli pillars is a very close approximation of the midline of the spine. I cauterize a vertical line into the vertebral body just above the disc space and then mark it with a purple marking pen. I do not use black ink, because it is indistinguishable from the anatomy that encountered the tip of the cautery. That purple mark is evaluated again later relative to the exposed uncovertebral joints to further confirm the midline.

With the midline marked, I now expose the lateral aspects of the vertebral bodies by releasing and elevating the medial aspect of the longus colli muscle with cautery. I strive to develop a cuff that the retractor blades can capture with their hooked configuration. Principles that I have embraced in minimally invasive spine surgery are applicable at this point. A measurement that should be at the forefront on every spine surgeon's mind is the distance between the vertebral arteries, which varies from 24 to 29 mm throughout the cervical spine. Anatomical studies have established that the intervertebral

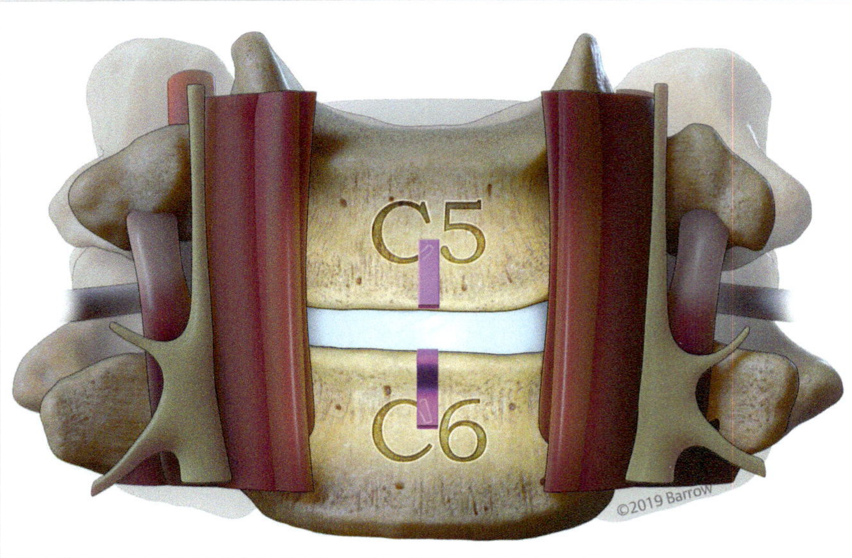

Fig. 9.19 Preliminary midline mark based on the longus colli muscles. Illustration demonstrating the course of the longus colli muscles. The sympathetic chain ganglia course on the lateral aspects of the longus colli as illustrated. Before mobilizing the longus colli from the vertebral bodies, a preliminary mark is made in the midline with cautery and marked with purple ink.

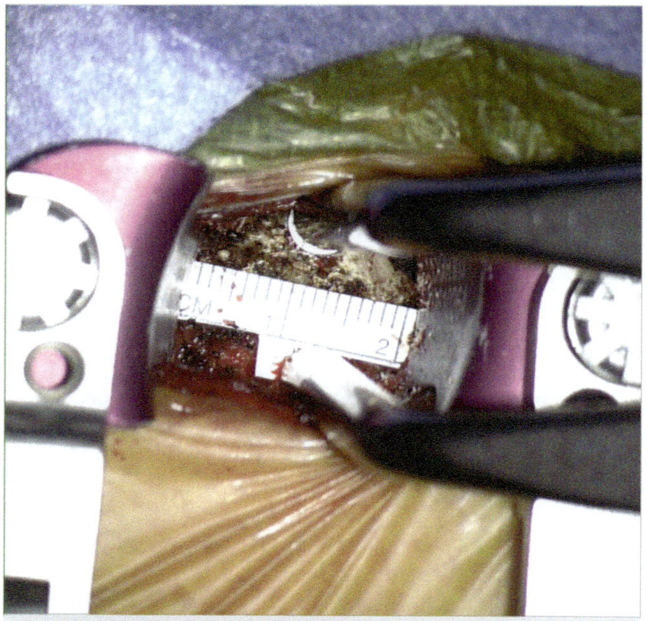

Fig. 9.20 Requisite anatomical unit exposure. Intraoperative photograph of the requisite anatomical unit for a C4–5 anterior cervical decompression and fusion. Note that 22 mm has been exposed in the transverse dimension along with 5 mm above and below the disc space. A ruler cut to 22 mm confirms the transverse dimension.

artery distance is the least at C3 and the greatest at C6.[2] Therefore, exposing up to 22 mm of the transverse dimension of the vertebral bodies is a safe, if not necessary, distance to expose the disc space for an adequate decompression of a cervical segment. If 22 mm of exposure is not accomplished at the time of the initial dissection, it will not be accomplished after the self-retaining retractors are placed. I am cognizant of the sympathetic chain ganglia that course in the lateral aspect of the longus colli and keep my dissection at the interface of the medial muscle belly of the longus colli and lateral vertebral body.

Incorporating yet another element of minimally invasive spinal surgery that we have routinely used in the various other procedures presented in this Primer is helpful in developing the cuff on the longus colli muscle for the eventual hooked blades of the retractors. The larger of the two minimally invasive suction retractors is ideal for this component of the procedure. The minimally invasive suction retractor lifts the insertion point of the longus colli muscle and allows for cautery to dissect the medial insertion off the vertebral body to complete the lateral exposure while simultaneously eliminating the smoke created from the cautery. The cuff that is created can engage and hold the retractor blade.

To ensure the same operation every time, I have the scrub technician trim a plastic ruler to 22 mm, which should fit easily within the exposure. Once I have 22 mm of the disc space exposed, I complete the exposure by exposing the inferior half of the rostral vertebral body to a distance of 5 mm and the superior half of the caudal body to a distance of 5 mm. I extend my dissection 22 mm in the medial-lateral dimension at both levels. Reaching those dimensions, I am now confident that I have the exposure I need for an optimal decompression, interbody graft placement, fixating a cervical plate or placing an arthroplasty device. I repeat the exposure process just described for every segment that I intend to operate on before I place the blades for the self-retaining retractors and secure the Caspar pin posts (▶ Fig. 9.20).

I prefer to perform the exposure for the entire operation and place the first set of Caspar distraction posts under loupe magnification and headlight illumination. I begin a preliminary discectomy and keep the loupes and headlight on until the disc has been almost completely removed and the posterior aspect of the disc space is seen, at which point I bring in the operating microscope. My operating room team knows that, after the Caspar posts are in, it is only a matter of minutes before I ask my team to roll the microscope into position (▶ Fig. 9.21).

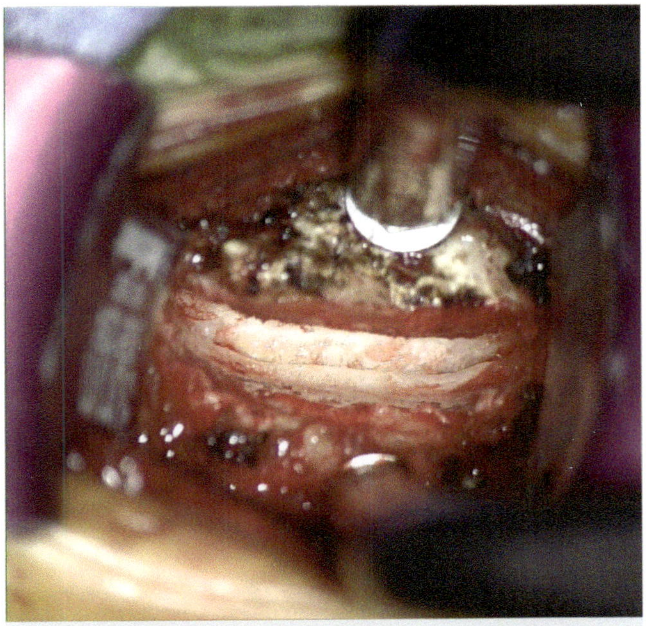

Fig. 9.21 Requisite exposure for an anterior cervical discectomy. The knowledge that the intervertebral artery distance is 24 to 29 mm would indicate that 22 mm of exposure is a safe distance to mobilize the longus colli muscles and expose the disc space. In this intraoperative photograph, the Caspar posts are in position, and the discectomy has been completed to expose the uncovertebral joints.

9.12 Exposures for Multilevel Anterior Cervical Discectomy and Fusion

The natural tendency when performing a multilevel ACDF is to expose the first segment and then extend either upward or downward from there. That was my routine for years until I stumbled onto a manuscript written by Riew and colleagues, who used two incisions to perform a four-level operation.[3] The crux of their manuscript is essentially to have two operative sites above the skin and connect them below the skin and platysma, thereby reducing the amount of exposure and retraction on the esophagus and trachea. The elements of that concept may be applied to a single incision for two- and three-level ACDFs. Instead of exposing one level and then working up or down, I remove the handheld Cloward retractors altogether and begin the dissection anew. The principle is to expose the segments as a series of "silos," as if each silo were a single-level procedure, and then connect the exposures into one.

With no retractors in the surgical site holding open the previous exposure, I begin descending down the avascular plane medial to the sternocleidomastoid as if my only intent were to expose the level above or below. Once I am onto the prevertebral cervical fascia, I again use Kittners for blunt dissection and invariably connect to the previous exposure. At this point, I identify those fascial bands holding me back from a continuous exposure and divide them. I now have a continuous exposure between the two disc spaces. If I am performing a three-level surgery, then I repeat the process.

What I have found using this technique is that, in the end, it is faster than extending the exposure from the first level. Furthermore, I am more readily able to identify that it is either the platysma holding me up or a fascial band here or there. Connecting three different silos of exposure (in the case of a three-level ACDF) offers an exposure that is vastly superior and almost tension free compared to the exposure that I accomplish by extension from the first level I expose to the third level. In my experience, attempting to extend the exposure with the self-retaining retractors in position blurs the anatomy and hides the very bands that need to be identified and divided. In the end, whether it is a single- or four-level operation, I perform all of the exposures level by level sequentially connecting these silos of exposure until all of the operative levels have been exposed to a width of 22 mm. By adhering to this principle, I am certain that, before I place the self-retaining retractors in position, no further exposure will be needed during the plating phase of the operation.

9.13 Table-Mounted Arm for Self-Retaining Retractor: A Minimally Invasive Surgery Modification

When I was in training, I watched my attendings attempt to anchor the cervical retractor using a Ray-tech sponge and a Kelly clamp, with minimal effectiveness. For years after my training, I did the same—behavioral mimicry. The objective of wrapping these sponges and using these clamps was to create stability, but all these attempts fell short. More often than not, as a resident, I found myself holding the retractor in position to optimize the exposure. The self-retaining cervical retractor represents yet another opportunity to steal a page out of the minimally invasive surgery playbook. By anchoring the cervical self-retaining retractor onto the table-mounted arm, the same table-mounted arm that we use for all of the minimal access ports we work with, all the frustration that comes with using the cervical retractor evaporates. This opportunity presented itself when various types of connectors to the self-retaining cervical retractor became available that allowed the cervical retractor to be anchored onto the table-mounted arm used for minimally invasive approaches. Connecting the cervical self-retaining retractor now fixates the retractor into position and, if needed, allows repositioning with added stability to capture and expose the ideal midline position (▶ Fig. 9.22).

Although I have found the simple use of this minimally invasive table-mounted arm invaluable, it does not take away from the fact that the key component for the self-retaining cervical retractor is the mobilization of the longus colli muscles and the soft-tissue planes. An adequate cuff of longus colli muscle is necessary for the retractor blade to properly engage the edge of the muscle and proficiently retract it. The benefit of having the retractor anchored to the table-mounted frame is that it prevents the temptation to overly open the retractor. Doing so only dislodges the retractor blade from the underside of the longus colli muscle and compromises the exposure. I am careful when I open the retractor to ensure the cuff of the longus colli muscle stays within the confines of the curved aspect of the cervical retractor blade. Downward pressure on the retractor helps

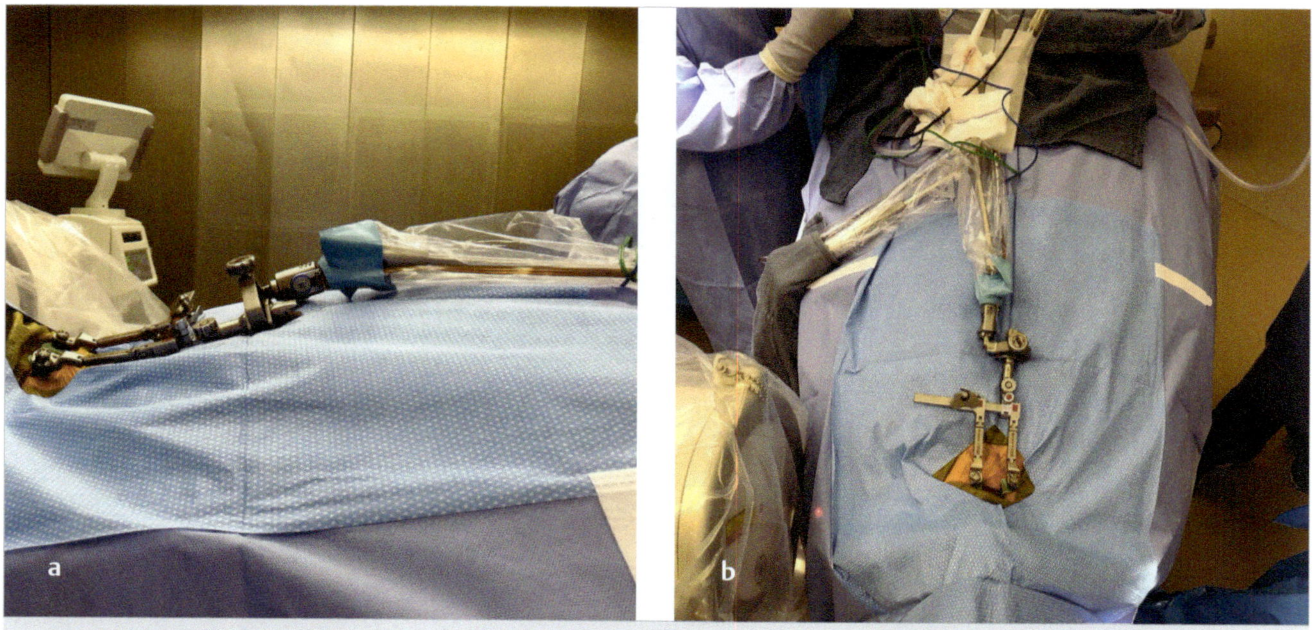

Fig. 9.22 Application of the table-mounted minimally invasive retractor arm for cervical surgery. The adapter configures onto the cervical retractor and allows the retractor arm to capture the ideal placement of the exposure. **(a)** Photograph taken from the right side of the patient demonstrating the pneumatic arm holding the self-retaining cervical retractor. **(b)** Photograph taken from the head of the bed demonstrating a pneumatic arm holding the cervical retractor in the midline.

maintain its position as I open the blades. But as careful as I am, at times I go one click too far and lose the contact of the muscle on the retractor blade. The mobilized longus colli then flops itself into the lateral aspect of my exposure. Salvaging this without removing the blade is difficult, almost futile. It is a mistake to accept such a field of view. Instead, it is a worthwhile investment in time to simply start over with reengaging the longus colli and positioning the retractor. I apply one less click the second time around.

9.14 Caspar Distraction Posts

Now that the self-retaining retractor is in position, the anesthesiologist raises the bed once again to fluoroscopic height, and I secure the Caspar posts into the vertebral bodies with fluoroscopic guidance. I use my preliminary midline marks as my guide to place the posts in the midline. Based on my 5-mm approximation from the disc space, I place the awl or Caspar post at what I perceive to be 1 to 2 mm shy of the midportion of the vertebral body. A fluoroscopic image confirms the correct position. By doing so, I accomplish one of my ancillary objectives: to cause as little disruption to the adjacent segment as possible. If I am performing arthroplasty with a keel-based device, placement of the post three-quarters of the way from the disc space will be necessary to have room for the keel cut. However, non-keel-based arthroplasty devices allow me to remain shy of the midportion of the vertebral body and therefore have become my preferred implant.

Inserting the Caspar posts into the hard, cortical bone of a vertebral body can be a challenge. An awl or a smaller pitched plate holding the screws can create a pilot hole for the Caspar post. In my mind, creating a small starter hole in the vertebral body is a more rational approach than holding a Caspar post and tapping it with a mallet. I have always been concerned about transmitting the energy of the mallet tap onto the spinal cord, which is already under compression by an osteophyte. Instead, once I have created the pilot hole, the Caspar post screws into the vertebral body without resistance.

There are two sizes of Caspar posts, 12 and 14 mm. Using the dimensions from Panjabi et al[1] as my basis, I use 12-mm posts in women and 14-mm posts in men. Once the posts are secured into position, their appearance on fluoroscopy also becomes a helpful reference point for deciding the length of the cervical screws or the depth of the interbody space or arthroplasty device. These topics are discussed in greater detail in Section 9.22, Interbody Graft Placement, and Section 9.23, Sizing the Interbody Spacer.

I use a fluoroscopic image or two to confirm the location on the vertebral body and set the trajectory for ideal placement of the Caspar posts. First and foremost, I want to ensure that the posts are perfectly perpendicular to the posterior aspect of the vertebral body and, second, that they are a safe distance from the adjacent segment (▶ Fig. 9.23). Since the consensus distance has been demonstrated to be less than 5 mm, I attempt to place my posts just shy of the midpoint of the vertebral body for fusions.[13,14] For a keel-based arthroplasty, the posts need to be positioned a safe distance from the keel cuts. ▶ Fig. 9.24 demonstrates the need to be well beyond the midportion of the vertebral body to accommodate the keel of the arthroplasty device.

In many circumstances, patients have focal kyphosis at the segment of cervical spondylosis (▶ Fig. 9.25). The most effective manner to address the kyphosis is to ensure that the posts are completely perpendicular to the back wall of the vertebral body

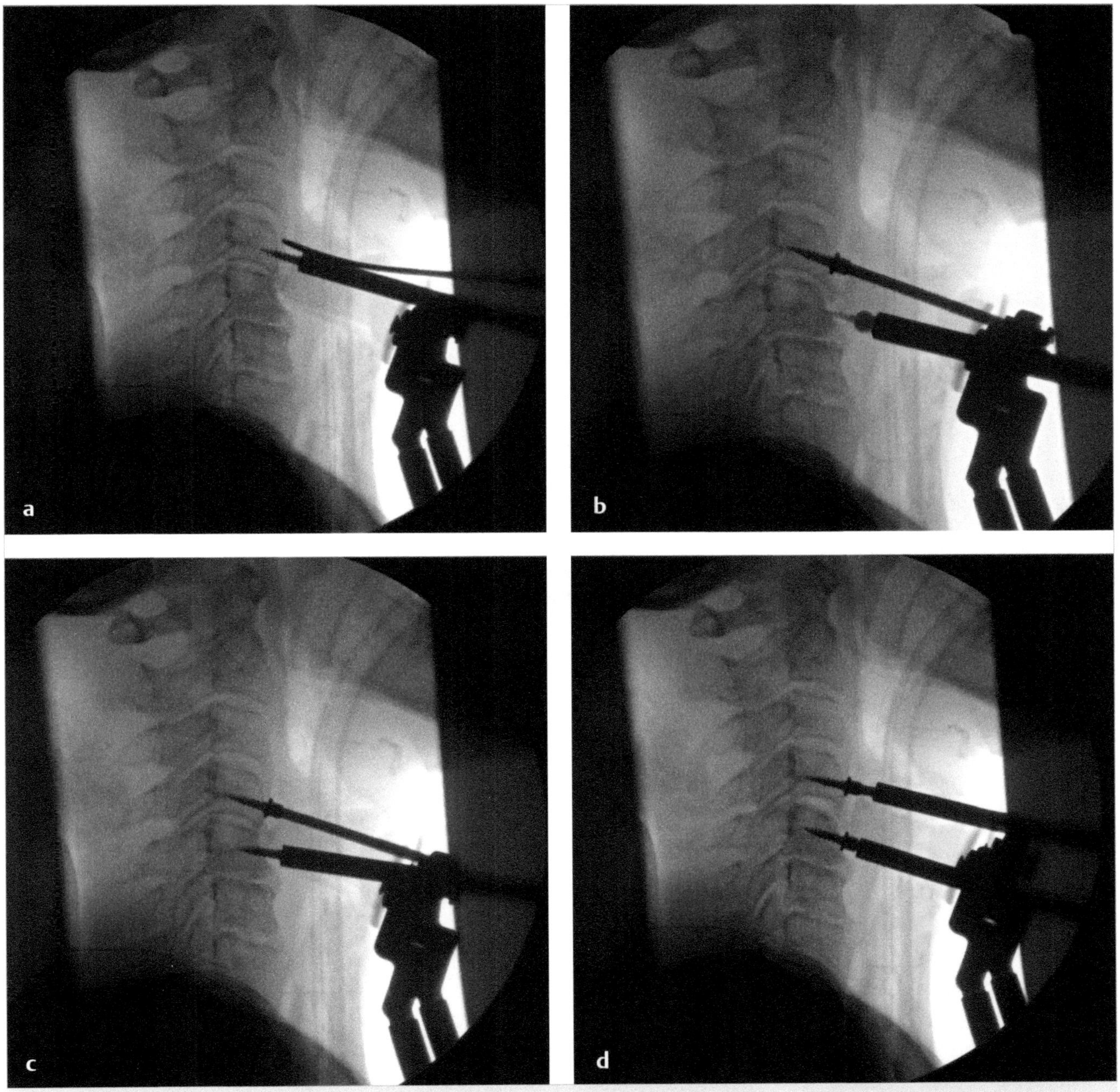

Fig. 9.23 Placement of the Caspar posts in a C4–5, C5–6 and C6–7 anterior cervical discectomy and fusion. **(a)** Lateral fluoroscopic image demonstrating placement of a Caspar post into the C4 vertebral body. A fluoroscopic image guides the trajectory perpendicular to the posterior wall of C4. **(b)** Lateral fluoroscopic image demonstrating use of a small caliber plate-holding pin to create a pilot hole into C5 with **(c)** subsequent placement of the Caspar post. An awl, available in the majority of sets, would accomplish the same objective. The Caspar posts are placed shy of the mid vertebral body to prevent any disruption at the adjacent segments. Note the convergence of the Caspar post in this fluoroscopic image. **(d)** Distraction of the disc space to restore the segmental lordosis. Note that the Caspar posts are now parallel to each other with distraction.

so that the posts reverse the kyphosis when they are distracted, and a more lordotic geometry of the segment is captured for the arthrodesis. Again, it bears repeating that, for cervical fusions, I make every effort to maintain the distance away from the adjacent segment to minimize the risk of causing adjacent segment degeneration. I have already alluded to the minimum distance from the adjacent disc space being 5 mm, a value that I qualify in Section 9.25, Cervical Plating.

In order to pass the Caspar post distractor over the post, Penfield nos. 3 and 1 dissectors are helpful to prevent the soft tissue from getting caught as the distractor slips over the posts. At times, because the focal kyphosis is so pronounced, the posts converge so greatly that placement of the distractor becomes untenable without separating the posts into a parallel alignment. For these circumstances, I place a handheld Cloward retractor between the posts and turn it enough to alter the

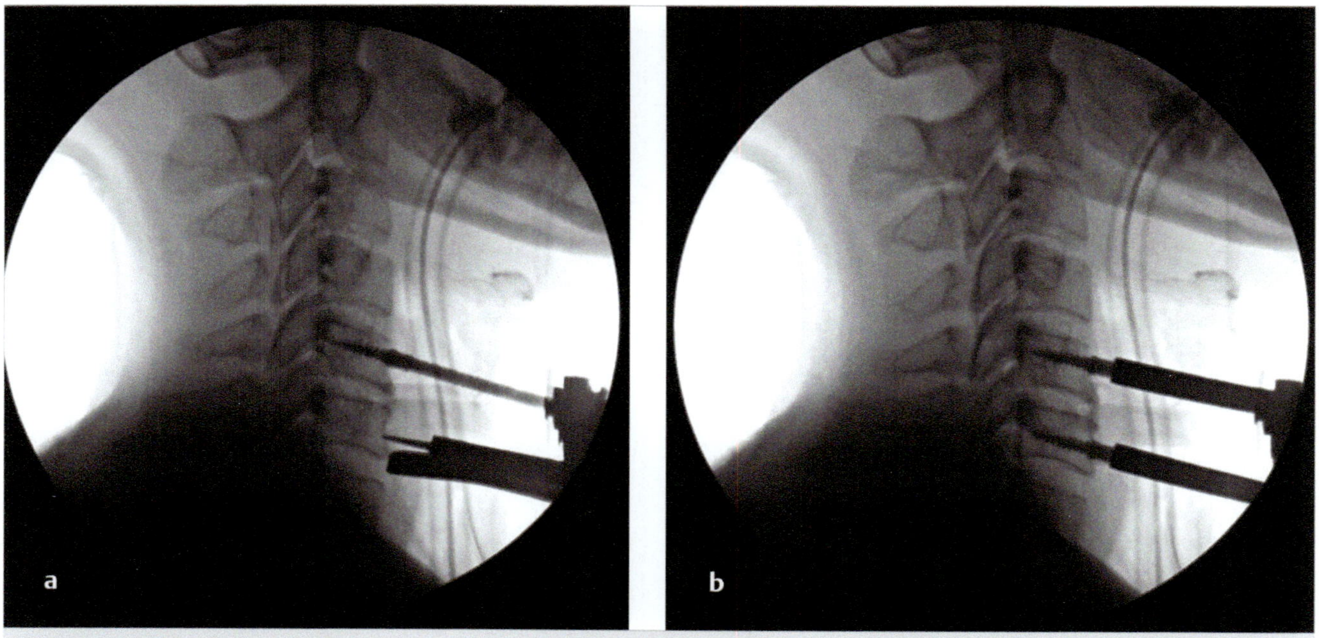

Fig. 9.24 Caspar posts for a keel-based arthroplasty device. **(a)** Placement of the Caspar post is at the three-quarter mark of the vertebral body. This fluoroscopic image demonstrates the use of an awl to pilot the hole into the vertebral body. **(b)** In this lateral fluoroscopic image, the Caspar posts are three-quarters of the distance from the disc space to allow for the keel cuts.

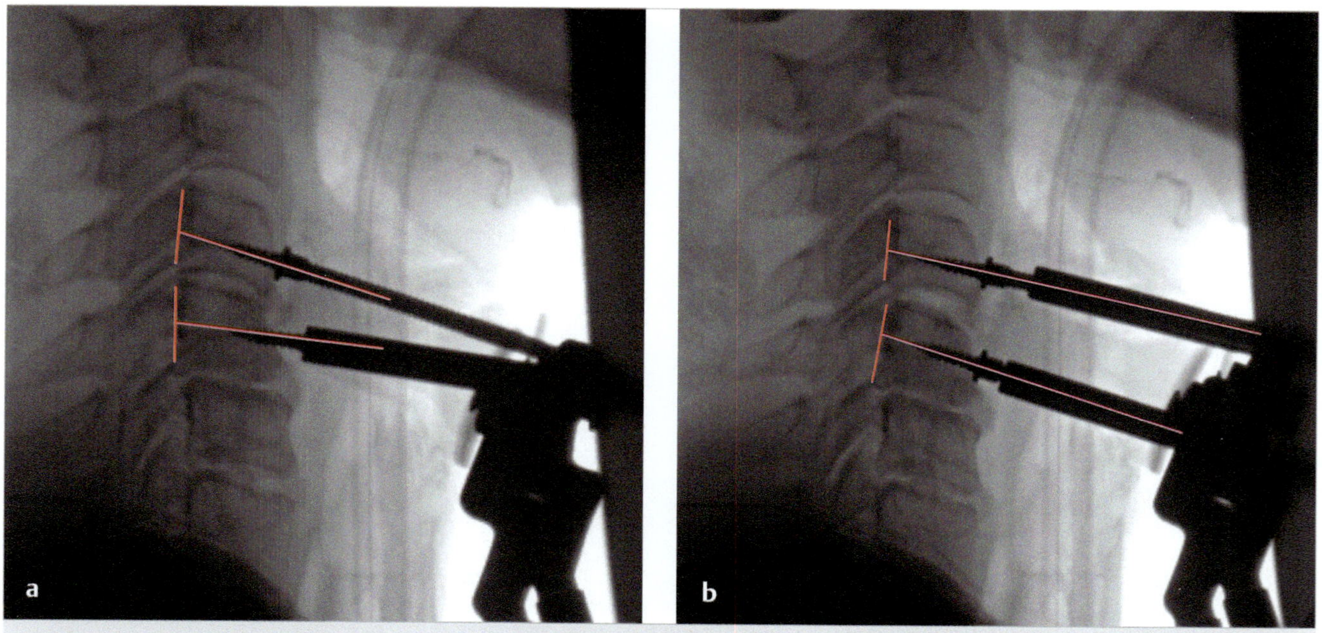

Fig. 9.25 Correction of segmental kyphosis with perpendicular placement of the Caspar posts. **(a)** Magnified lateral fluoroscopic image of the patient seen in ▶ Fig. 9.24. The Caspar posts are converging (*red lines*), which indicates kyphosis at the segment. **(b)** Lateral fluoroscopic image showing the distraction of the Caspar posts and subsequent restoration of disc height and segmental lordosis, with the Caspar posts perpendicular (*red lines*) to the posterior wall of the vertebral body.

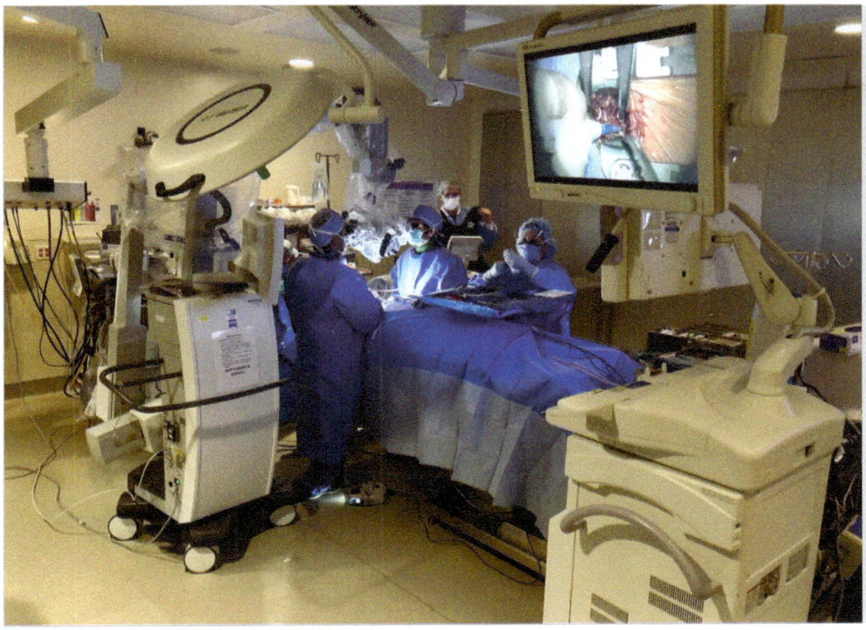

Fig. 9.26 Operating room setup. Once the surgeon is working under the microscope, the fluoroscope is positioned at the head of the bed so that when the decompression is complete, it may be brought back immediately into position for placement of the interbody graft, artificial disc or cervical plate.

convergent trajectories to parallel. The post distractor may now slide into position; using Penfields, hold back any soft tissue that may get in the way. At times, closing the mediolateral cervical retractor just a click or two takes just enough tension off the rostral aspect of the exposure to facilitate passage of the Caspar post distractor onto the posts. I distract the posts with a click or two to reverse the kyphosis and open the disc space and begin the discectomy. The fluoroscope rolls to the head of the bed as the microscope rolls into position for the decompression phase of the operation (▶ Fig. 9.26).

9.15 Discectomy for Fusion: Two Distinct Approaches for Two Distinct Patterns of Degeneration

I approach a soft disc herniation in younger patients with a completely different mindset than for an older patient with advanced spondylosis and osteophytes that cause either radiculopathy or myelopathy. In anterior cervical approaches, different pathologies require slightly different techniques.

The two patients in ▶ Fig. 9.27 illustrate the point of varying techniques depending on the degree of spondylosis. The magnetic resonance imaging (MRI) of the 41-year-old patient in ▶ Fig. 9.27a shows a soft disc herniation at C5–6. She has no spondylosis, and if it were not for her midline disc herniation, a posterior cervical foraminotomy with discectomy would have been preferred. The MRI of the 68-year-old patient in ▶ Fig. 9.27b shows obvious spondylosis at C5–6 and C6–7. Her symptoms are a result of disc collapse, osteophyte formation and loss of her cervical lordosis that collectively occurred as a result of her spondylosis. Since the origin of the pathology in both of these patients is distinct, the technique I employ to handle them is equally distinct.

9.16 Discectomy for Soft Disc Herniation

The principles that guide the management of a soft disc herniation in the absence of spondylosis are minimal distraction of the Caspar posts and minimal use of the drill. Once I have confirmed the level, exposed the requisite anatomical unit, placed the self-retaining retractors and secured the Caspar posts, I distract the disc space only to the point to restore the cervical lordosis and then begin the discectomy. In a patient without significant spondylosis, the less I distract the Caspar posts, the better it is for the patient. I use a No. 11 blade to make a shallow transverse incision on the annulus of the disc for a distance of approximately 20 mm. Next, I use pituitary rongeurs and begin to remove the disc material to create a working space to accommodate other instruments. With the majority of the disc removed, I begin to level the concavity of the rostral end plate to create a suitable surface for arthrodesis and optimize visualization of and access to the posterior longitudinal ligament (PLL). It is important to note that I level out the end plate for arthrodesis but not for arthroplasty. For motion preservation, the approach is different. I make every effort to maintain the concavity of the end plate so as to appropriately seat the arthroplasty device. Arthroplasty has its nuances, and therefore a section of this chapter is devoted to it.

The rationale behind the removal of the concavity of the end plate is to optimize the line of sight onto the back of the disc space and thereby maximize the decompression. The combination of a drill and Kerrison rongeurs together accomplishes this task. I use a No. 2 Kerrison rongeur to level off the anterior lip of the concavity on the underside of the rostral end plate and a drill to level the posterior aspect of the disc space (▶ Fig. 9.28).

With the preliminary discectomy completed and the concavity of the rostral vertebral body removed, the next objective is preparation of the end plates. The ideal environment for an

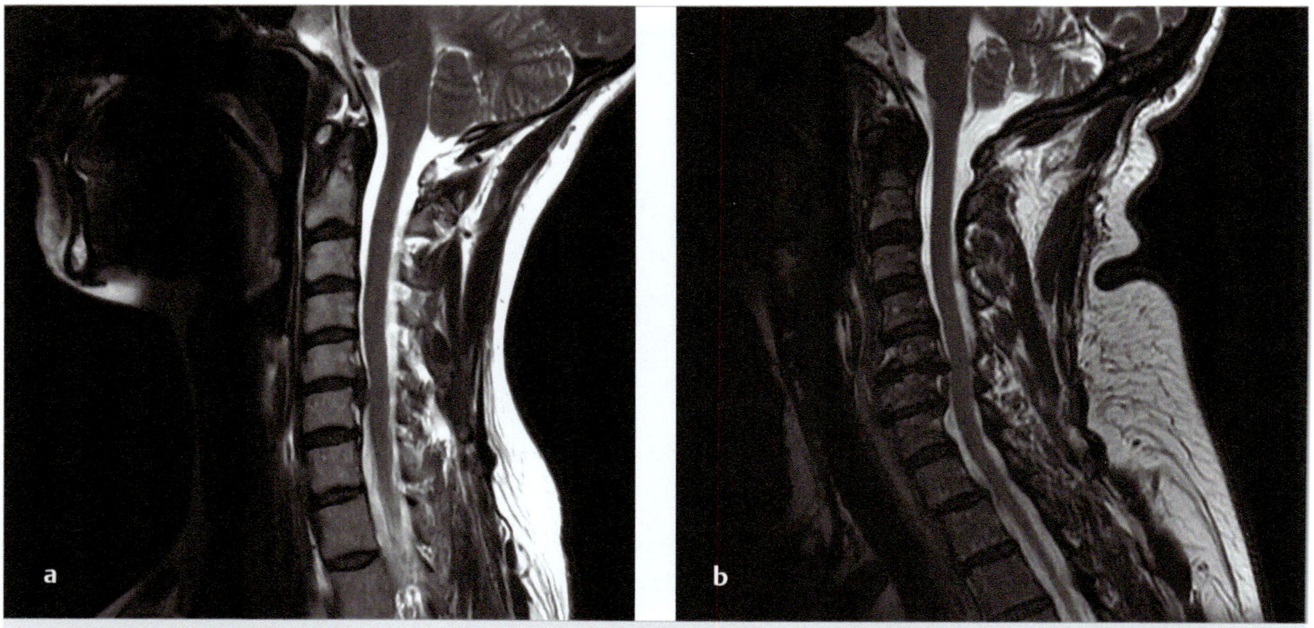

Fig. 9.27 Anterior cervical discectomies with and without spondylosis. Sagittal T2-weighted magnetic resonance imaging (MRI) of the cervical spine demonstrating two distinct anatomic scenarios. (a) Sagittal MRI of a 41-year-old patient demonstrates an acute disc herniation without any significant spondylosis. (b) Sagittal MRI of a 68-year-old patient demonstrating advanced cervical spondylosis. The approach to these two clinical scenarios is a variation on a theme to decompress the neural elements.

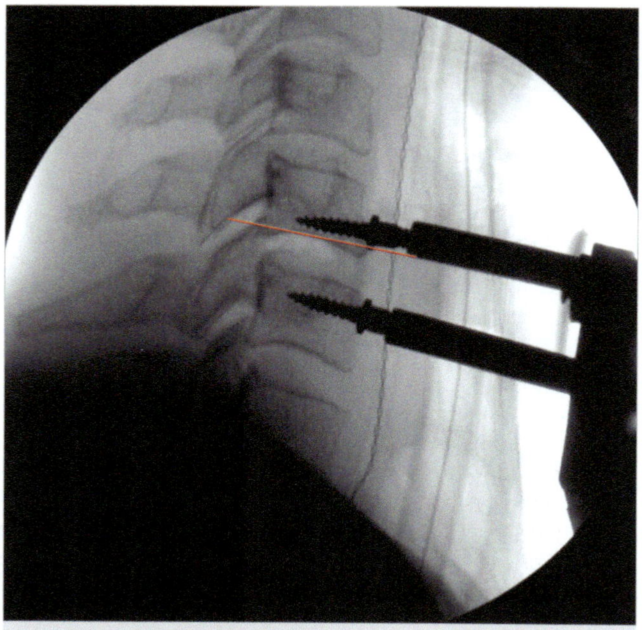

Fig. 9.28 Preparing the end plate for arthrodesis. Lateral fluoroscopic image showing the concavity on the underside of the rostral end plate. The *red line* marks the proposed removal of bone to flatten the concavity and create an ideal surface for arthrodesis.

arthrodesis requires removal of the cartilaginous end plates and exposure of the bleeding cortical bone of the end plates. I prefer to prepare the end plates at this point in the procedure, before the neural elements are exposed. Cervical bayoneted Karlin curets, forward straight and backward straight, are ideal for this purpose. These curets are very effective at scraping the cartilage off the end plate to expose the cortical bone of the end plate, and their bayoneted configuration allows for an optimal line of sight while working within the disc space. There is an unmistakable sound and feeling of metal scraping against cortical bone, which must be heard and felt to ensure adequate preparation of the end plate. As mentioned in Chapter 4, the unmistakable sound of metal scraping against bone is the "sound of fusion." The entire end plate must be prepared, but I focus especially on that area of the end plate where the graft will reside at the completion of the procedure. I remove the fragments of the cartilage from the end plates with a pituitary or a Kerrison rongeur.

9.17 Decompression of the Spinal Cord and Nerve Roots

The longus colli muscles are, for the most part, a reliable marker of the midline. But at times, these vertical columns of muscle are susceptible to asymmetry and, therefore, may potentially mislead the surgeon as to the location of the midline mark. The uncovertebral joints, on the other hand, always accurately indicate the location of the midline. For that reason, I use those joints for the final confirmation of the midline under the operating microscope. Complete exposure of the uncovertebral joints is performed with the small Karlin curets (forward straight 000 and 0000) and forward-angled microcurets that can slip between the lateral aspect of the joint and remove the cartilaginous end plate. Complete exposure of both uncovertebral joints makes the midline plainly obvious. When exposing these sloping joints of Luschka, I should be able to unequivocally visualize the rise of the joint on the left and the right side in the same field of view. I have a ruler cut to exactly 22 mm to place into the disc space and assess my exposure. Once both the uncovertebral joints are visualized, I zoom out the microscope and position it directly in line with disc space to eliminate parallax and re-mark the midline first with cautery and then again with a marking pen. These final marks now become the most reliable markers for the midline that I will use as my reference as I plate the spine or insert the arthroplasty device (▶ Fig. 9.29).

With the midline marked, the next objective is decompression of the segment. In the case of a soft disc herniation, I now expose the posterior annulus (Video 9.1). In the absence of any significant spondylosis, I seldom see a need for further use of a drill at this point in the operation. A forward-angled cervical micro-curet may pass within a plane that I have created between the posterior annulus and the posterior aspect of the vertebral body. A Kerrison No. 1 or 2 now passes into that plane behind the posterior inferior aspect of the vertebral body above and below to resect the posterior annulus. Any disc herniation becomes evident and retrievable with this maneuver. The combination of a blunt-tipped nerve hook and pituitary rongeur is all that is needed to deliver it. Careful review of the axial MRI indicates where to focus one's attention. The PLL is now all that remains between the surgeon and the dura of the cervical spinal cord.

9.18 Division and Resection of the Posterior Longitudinal Ligament

The PLL may be either as thin as a layer of velum behind the posterior annulus, easily divided and resected, or as thick as leather, requiring meticulous dissection. Regardless of the thickness of the PLL, its greatest vulnerability lies on the lateral aspects, whereas its greatest strength is in the center. A strategy that focuses on the flank is the most efficient manner to establish a plane between the PLL and the dura to safely resect the PLL. My preferred instrument for this task is the smallest available micro forward-angled cervical curet. I begin by zooming in the microscope to its highest magnification. I then place the curet in the lateralmost aspect of the disc space and rotate it behind the caudal vertebral body. The expectation is that the tip of the curet finds the weakness within the PLL and slides beneath it. It may take a few attempts to find the plane between the ligament and the dura. If I do not have success at the caudal vertebral body, I sweep laterally beneath the rostral body. Once I hook the PLL and catch a glimpse of the unmistakable bluish-white sheen of the dura, I elevate the PLL with the curet and slide the footplate of a No. 1 or, if the space allows, a No. 2 Kerrison beneath it to begin its division.

That first bite of the PLL with a No. 1 or No. 2 Kerrison secures a corridor into the plane between the dura and the PLL. I now use a No. 2 Kerrison to complete the resection. Instead of cutting straight across the PLL with the Kerrison rongeur, I employ a technique for this procedure that is akin to rolling up a rug. I carefully slide the footplate of the No. 2 Kerrison under the PLL and then turn it obliquely into the underside of the rostral vertebral body. My objective is to secure bone and ligament into the jaws of the Kerrison as it bites (▶ Fig. 9.30, Video 9.1). I then do the same on the caudal vertebral body. I alternate back and forth from the rostral to the caudal vertebral body making oblique bites until I reach the uncovertebral joint. I make it a point throughout this process to stay away from the midpoint of the PLL. I have found that cutting the PLL down the middle of the disc space makes it more difficult to achieve a complete resection of the PLL. The focus is to resect the ligament and osteophyte (when present) by undercutting the rostral and caudal vertebral bodies. Once I reach the contralateral uncovertebral joint, the PLL has essentially been rolled up like a rug, and one final bite with a Kerrison into the uncovertebral joint is all that is needed to complete the resection. I should now be admiring the unmistakable bluish-white sheen of the dura of a widely decompressed cervical spinal cord and nerve roots. Under the microscope, I can appreciate the decompressed neural elements pulsating below the translucent dura. A No. 2 Kerrison completes the job on the ipsilateral side, where at most two or three bites with the Kerrison are all that is needed.

9.19 Systems Check Under the Operating Microscope

My final systems check is to ensure I have accomplished an adequate decompression every time. I check the measurement of my decompression under low magnification of the microscope. The high magnification used for the PLL resection alters one's perspective of the extent of decompression achieved. Time and time again, it is under low magnification that I identify an inadequate amount of decompression, typically on the ipsilateral side. I prefer to pass a blunt-tipped nerve hook into the lateral recesses to ensure there is no residual disc material and no compromise of the foramen. I also pass the instrument posterior to the rostral and caudal vertebral bodies to ensure there are no free fragments of disc material. With the systems check complete, I proceed to sizing the interbody graft and plating or trial placement of an artificial disc.

9.20 Discectomy and Osteophyte Removal for Spondylosis

The approach for a patient who presents with advanced spondylosis and is symptomatic due to the presence of disc osteophyte complexes impinging the cervical nerve root in the foramen or the canal is as different from a soft disc herniation as night is from day. In order to achieve a complete decompression of the segment, I need to adopt a completely different mindset. The generous distraction of the Caspar posts and generous use of drill are the principles that guide management of the spondylotic cervical spine. Although I use a drill sparingly in a patient with a soft disc herniation, in a patient with advanced spondylosis and disc osteophyte complexes, the discectomy and osteophytectomy are, at times, performed almost exclusively with the drill. The pathology in these circumstances is the osteophyte, not the disc. For a patient with advanced cervical spondylosis to improve, it is the osteophytes more than the disc that must be removed.

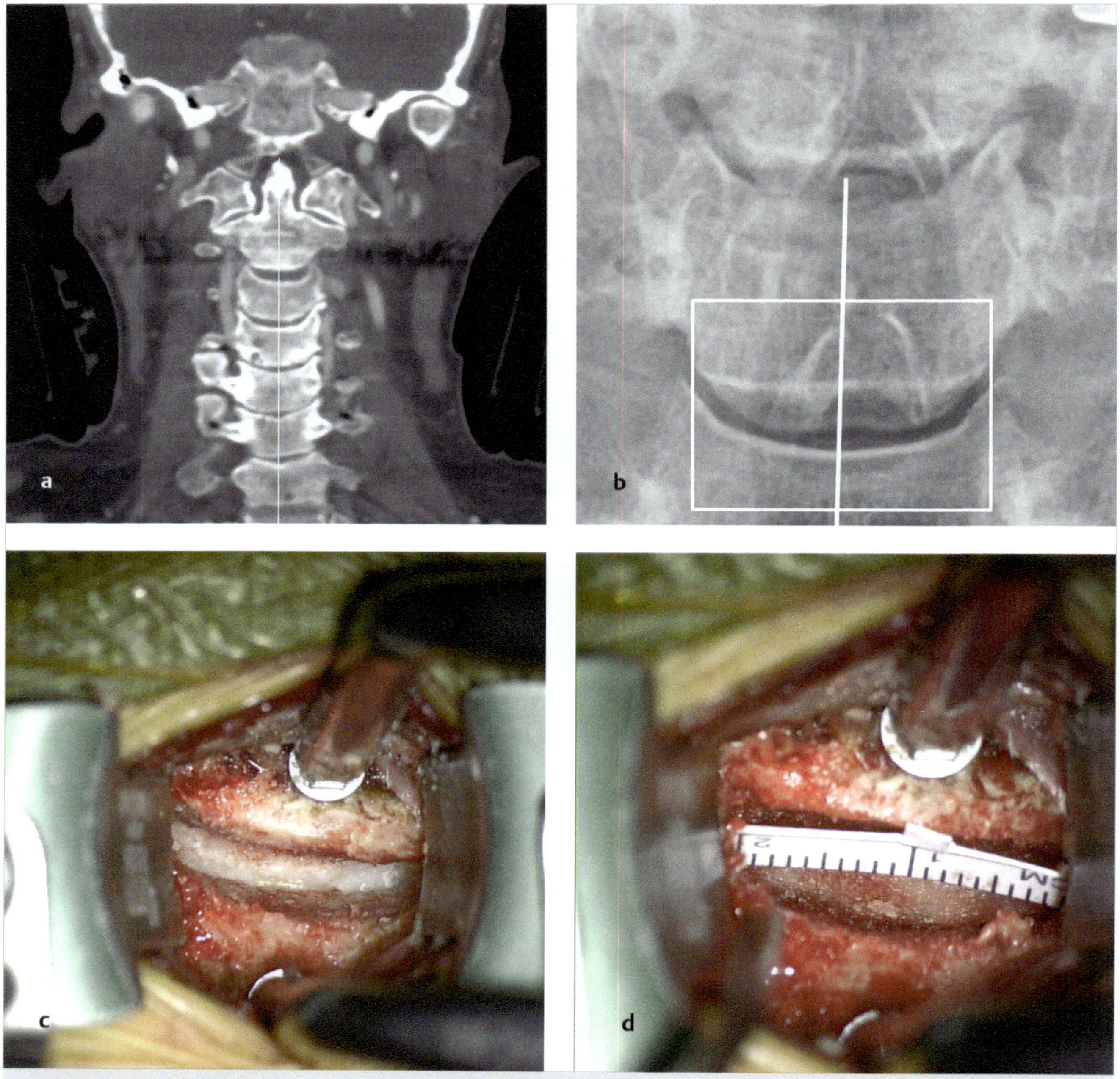

Fig. 9.29 Uncovertebral joints unveiling the geometric midline. **(a)** Coronal reconstruction of a cervical computed tomography. The center of the disc space is equidistant from the uncovertebral joints. Identifying the unequivocal rise of these joints is a reliable method to mark the midline. **(b)** Plain anteroposterior radiograph demonstrating the requisite anatomy for a single-level anterior cervical decompression (ACD). Only 5 mm of the rostral and caudal vertebral bodies need to be exposed. As seen in the radiograph, the uncovertebral joints are the essential reference points to establish the midline. **(c)** Intraoperative photograph of a C5–6 ACD and fusion. Cervical retractor blades engage the cuff of the longus colli to expose 22 mm of the disc space. Caspar posts and post distractor are in position to distract disc space. **(d)** A ruler cut to 22 mm confirming adequate decompression of the disc space.

Advanced spondylosis with osteophytic formation walks hand in hand with a loss of disc height and segmental kyphosis. It stands to reason, therefore, that the key to addressing this pathology is to reverse the focal segmental kyphosis that has occurred at each of these segments and then distract the disc space. Nonetheless, I have found that, in most circumstances, distraction of the disc space is inadequate for access to the posterior aspect of the disc space, which is so essential for the removal of the osteophytes. Drilling a parallel channel to the back of the disc space creates an optimal working corridor to access and resect the osteophyte and decompress the neural elements. In the end, it is the trumpet shape created out of the posterior aspect of the disc space that ensures an adequate decompression (▶ Fig. 9.31).

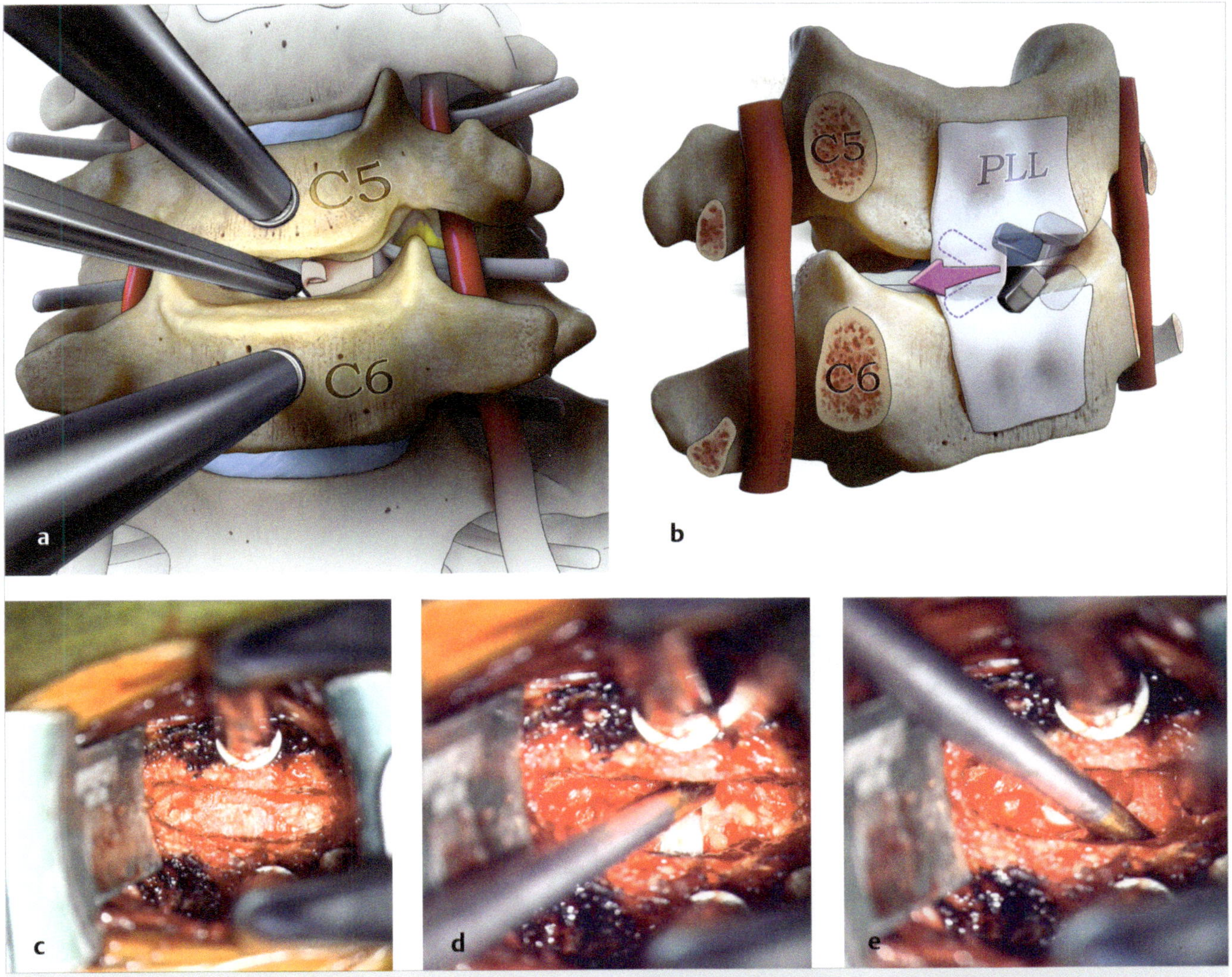

Fig. 9.30 Resection of the posterior longitudinal ligament (PLL) at C5–6. **(a)** Anterior view of the cervical spine demonstrating the principle of alternating rostral and caudal actions with the Kerrison rongeur for a complete resection of the PLL at the level of the disc space. **(b)** A posterior view of the cervical spine with the posterior elements removed to demonstrate the actions of the Kerrison rongeur from within the canal. **(c)** Intraoperative photograph demonstrating the exposure of the PLL. **(d)** A No. 2 Kerrison rongeur removing the osteophyte and PLL with a rostral bite. **(e)** A No. 2 Kerrison rongeur removing the osteophyte and PLL with a caudal bite.

By way of example, ▶ Fig. 9.31 shows a lateral radiograph of a patient with spondylosis and radiculopathy. As seen on the radiograph, the C5–6 and C6–7 segments have the unmistakable appearance of disc collapse and segmental kyphosis at those two levels.

After the exposure of the operative levels, the Caspar posts are secured into position perpendicular to the back wall of the vertebral body. The amount of kyphosis correction and disc height restoration that can be achieved by distraction is limited by the degree of spondylosis. Furthermore, distraction alone will not be enough to access the posterior osteophytes. Removal of several millimeters of the inferior and superior end plates will be necessary to create a working corridor in the posterior aspect of the disc space (▶ Fig. 9.32). I open the Caspar post distractor to capture whatever disc height restoration the disc space will allow. I remove whatever remains of the disc and begin to identify the uncovertebral joints to establish the midline. With the amount of drilling required for the decompression of this segment, it is crucial to identify the midline to maintain a safe distance from the vertebral arteries.

I use a drill to remove several millimeters of the inferior aspect of the rostral vertebral body and the superior aspect of the caudal vertebral body. Because of the distraction of the disc space, these parallel channels offer access to the posterior aspect of the disc space and, thereby, the osteophyte projecting into the spinal canal.

9.21 Minimally Invasive Surgery Drill Attachments for Removal of the Posterior Osteophytes

It is worthwhile at this point to discuss yet another page lifted out of the minimally invasive surgery playbook in the context

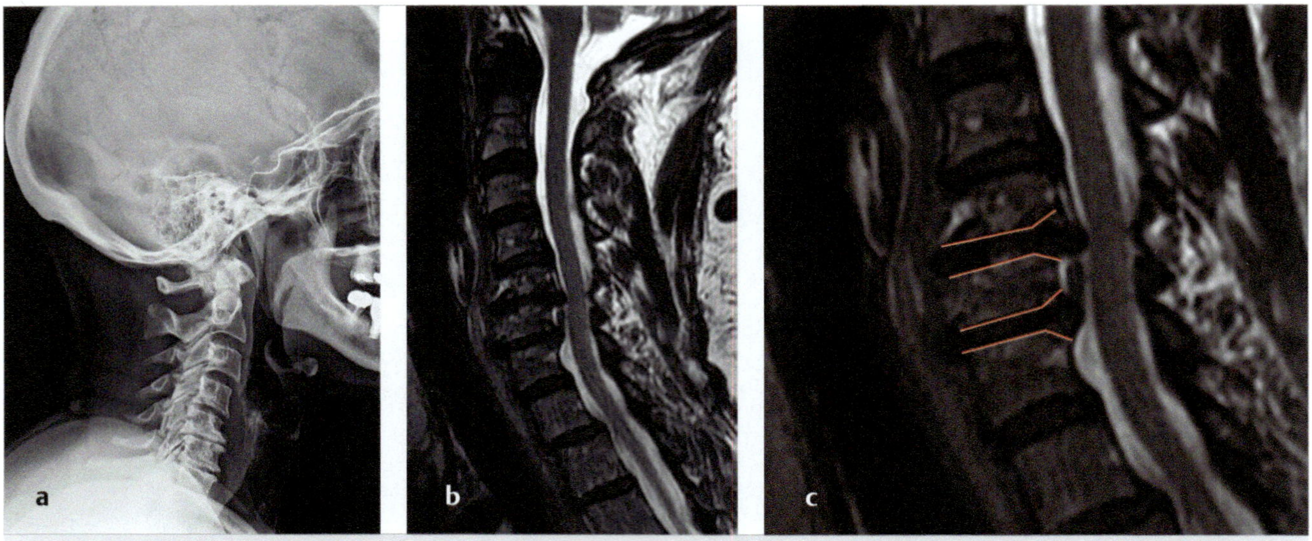

Fig. 9.31 Advanced cervical spondylosis C5–6 and C6–7. **(a)** Lateral radiograph demonstrating advanced cervical spondylosis at C5–6 and C6–7. At both of these segments, there is advanced disc collapse, osteophyte formation and loss of the segmental lordosis. The anterior projection of the osteophyte is an indication of the extent of the posterior osteophyte. **(b)** Sagittal T2-weighted magnetic resonance imaging showing the central stenosis from the disc osteophyte formation. Restoration of the disc height and lordosis along with decompression of the spinal cord and nerve roots are the surgical objectives of the operation. Complete removal of the posterior osteophyte is necessary to accomplish these objectives. **(c)** The concept of removal of the posterior osteophyte is illustrated. Trumpet-shaped (*red lines*) decompressions reach above the rostral and caudal aspects of the osteophytes. The approach to the management of this patient is completely distinct from a patient with a soft disc herniation.

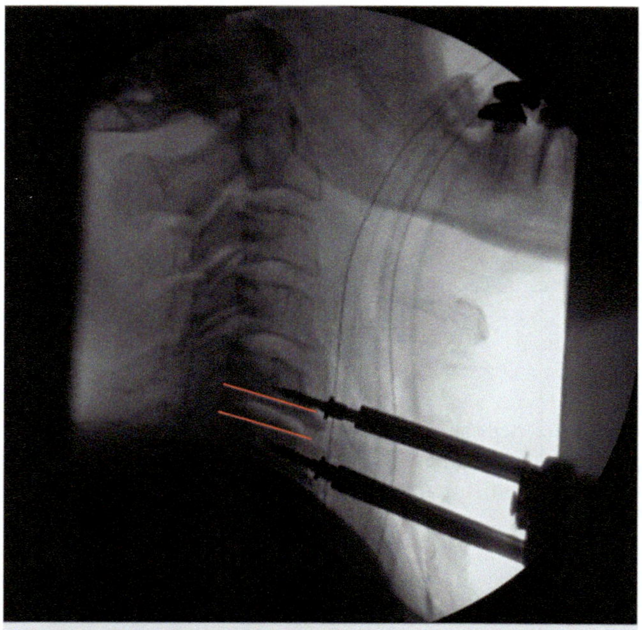

Fig. 9.32 Creation of a working corridor. Lateral fluoroscopic image with the *red lines* demarcating the proposed osteophyte removal. Despite distraction of the disc space with the Caspar disc space distractor, there is limited restoration of the disc height. A discectomy will not accomplish the goals of restoration of lordosis, disc height and decompression. Drilling a parallel channel provides a working corridor to access the posterior osteophyte compressing the spinal cord.

of the drill. As discussed earlier in this book, minimally invasive drill attachments have a gentle curve that allows for optimal visualization within a fixed diameter or expandable minimally invasive access port. In the case of an ACD, the working channel is analogous to a minimally invasive access port. Thus, the gently curved configuration allows access to the posterior aspect of the disc space without compromising the line of sight. Specifically, the tip of the drill is readily visible when drilling the bone at the posterior aspect of the disc space without obstruction from the hand holding the drill. All the while, the hand is in a stable and ergonomic position. I have adopted the use of minimally invasive drill attachments for all anterior cervical surgeries, which represents the evolution of the drill for spinal procedures.

Once the inferior and superior aspects of the vertebral bodies have been drilled parallel to the back of the disc space, a more oblique angle may be used for the last few millimeters of the vertebral body, which allows for a trajectory that reaches above the posterior osteophyte and allow for its complete resection. The shape that I am seeking to create with this trajectory is that of a trumpet (▶ Fig. 9.33). Drilling the posterior aspect of the disc space in this manner provides access above the posterior osteophyte on the rostral vertebral body and below the posterior osteophyte on the caudal vertebral body. A micro-curet is all that is needed to elevate the final leaflet of bone away from the neural elements and expose the PLL for resection.

The division of the PLL may be more challenging in advanced cases of spondylosis than a soft disc herniation without spondylosis. However, the strategy, mentioned earlier, remains the

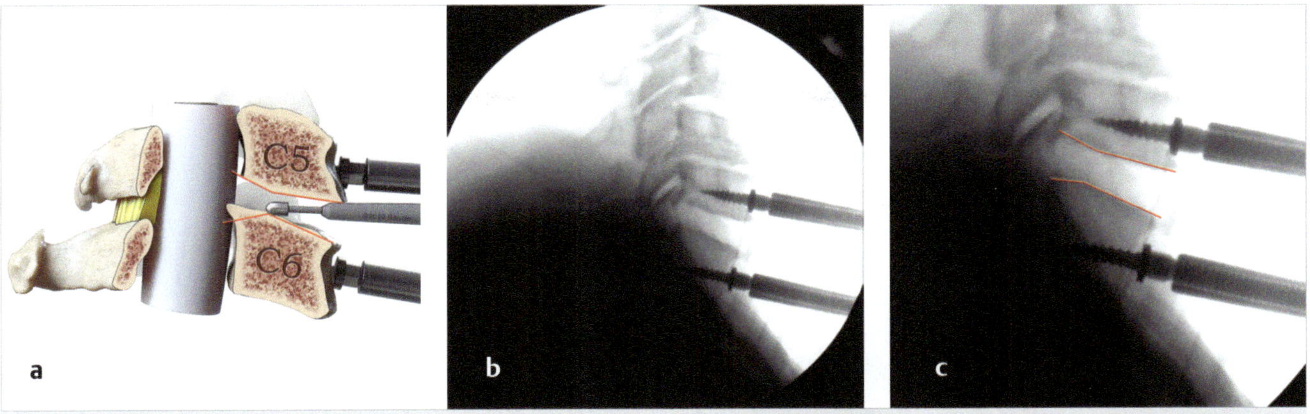

Fig. 9.33 Posterior osteophyte removal. **(a)** Illustration demonstrating the concept of removing the posterior osteophyte. In this illustration, the osteophyte on the inferior aspect of C5 has been removed and the process has begun at C6 with the minimally invasive drill (*red lines*). **(b)** Lateral fluoroscopic image demonstrating the removal of the posterior osteophyte and restoration of the disc height. **(c)** Magnified view of the lateral fluoroscopic image in **b** demonstrating the bone work in the shape of a trumpet (*red lines*).

same. I prefer a blunt-tipped nerve hook or micro-curet to probe for a weakness in the ligament in the lateral recess. Once the nerve hook or micro-curet finds its way behind the ligament, the footplate of a Kerrison finds its way into the opening and begins to divide the PLL.

With the initial opening made in the PLL, I continue to resect the posterior osteophyte above and below with oblique cuts undercutting the vertebral body while simultaneously resecting the PLL as previously described in Section 9.18, Division and Resection of the Posterior Longitudinal Ligament. When I have resected the PLL from the inferior and superior aspects of the vertebral bodies, I extend the decompression into the cervical foramen on the left and the right. At times, vigorous bleeding may be encountered with the final lateral action of the Kerrison rongeur. It is essential to recognize that the posterior aspect of the vertebral body and the vertebral artery are on two different planes. The source of the bleeding is unlikely to be arterial and instead originates from the epidural venous plexus. Although the bleeding may be vigorous, the combination of a hemostatic agent, ½ × ½ cottonoid and light pressure from the tip of the suction readily controls it (▶ Fig. 9.34). Free passage of a Kerrison No. 2 out the cervical foramen and the visual confirmation of a pulsatile spinal cord beneath the dura indicate the decompression of the segment is complete. The next phase of the operation is the placement of the interbody.

9.22 Interbody Graft Placement

Over the years, I have employed cortical grafts, cortical cancellous grafts, metallic grafts and polyetheretherketone (PEEK) grafts. If the cortical end plates are adequately prepared, I have found that all of these grafts work equally well to accomplish an arthrodesis across the segment. It was the occasional cortical graft that "pistoned" into an end plate or the cortical cancellous graft that mysteriously dissolved over time within the disc space that began my gradual shift away from a cadaveric allograft. I drifted toward PEEK implants, which were unresorbable. However, the more recent studies on surface technology informed me that osteoblasts prefer the crevices on the titanium interbody surface created by 3D printing more so than the smooth surface of PEEK.[15] So I migrated toward these 3D printed metal implants. I drifted back toward PEEK implants when further surface technology science concluded that it was not the PEEK but rather the smoothness of the PEEK that these fickle osteoblasts took issue with. Osteoblasts appear to be as perfectly content in porous PEEK as they are in the 3D printed clefts of a titanium implant.[16] In the final analysis, the literature has not identified one interbody type that is superior to another.[17] I can only conclude from my review of the remarkable history of cervical interbody spacers that the most important element in achieving an arthrodesis is not the type of interbody chosen but the craftsmanship performed on the surface of the end plates. Nothing replaces the complete removal of the cartilaginous end plates and preparation of the cortical end plate. Bleeding cortical bone on the end plates and a graft under compression are the components that optimize an environment for arthrodesis—nothing else.

The interbody devices I describe in this chapter will be PEEK and titanium. Although I am drawn to the science of surface technology, that is not the reason that I have chosen them. Instead, I wish to leverage the stability offered by an interbody spacer that will allow me to template the size of the cervical plate and predrill the holes. I discuss the use of a cervical template for plate fixation of the cervical spine in Section 9.25, Cervical Plating.

9.23 Sizing the Interbody Spacer

In the absence of trauma or ligamentous instability, the first step I take in sizing the graft is to assess the first normal level above or below the decompression level, which provides me a ballpark measurement for the ideal interbody size. It has never made any sense to me to insert a 9-mm-high spacer into a disc space that originally housed a 6-mm-high disc. The argument of restoration of foraminal height does not resonate with me because the foramina were never that large to begin with. After all, that is the purpose of the decompression. Furthermore, I have found that the larger the implant, the greater the stretch

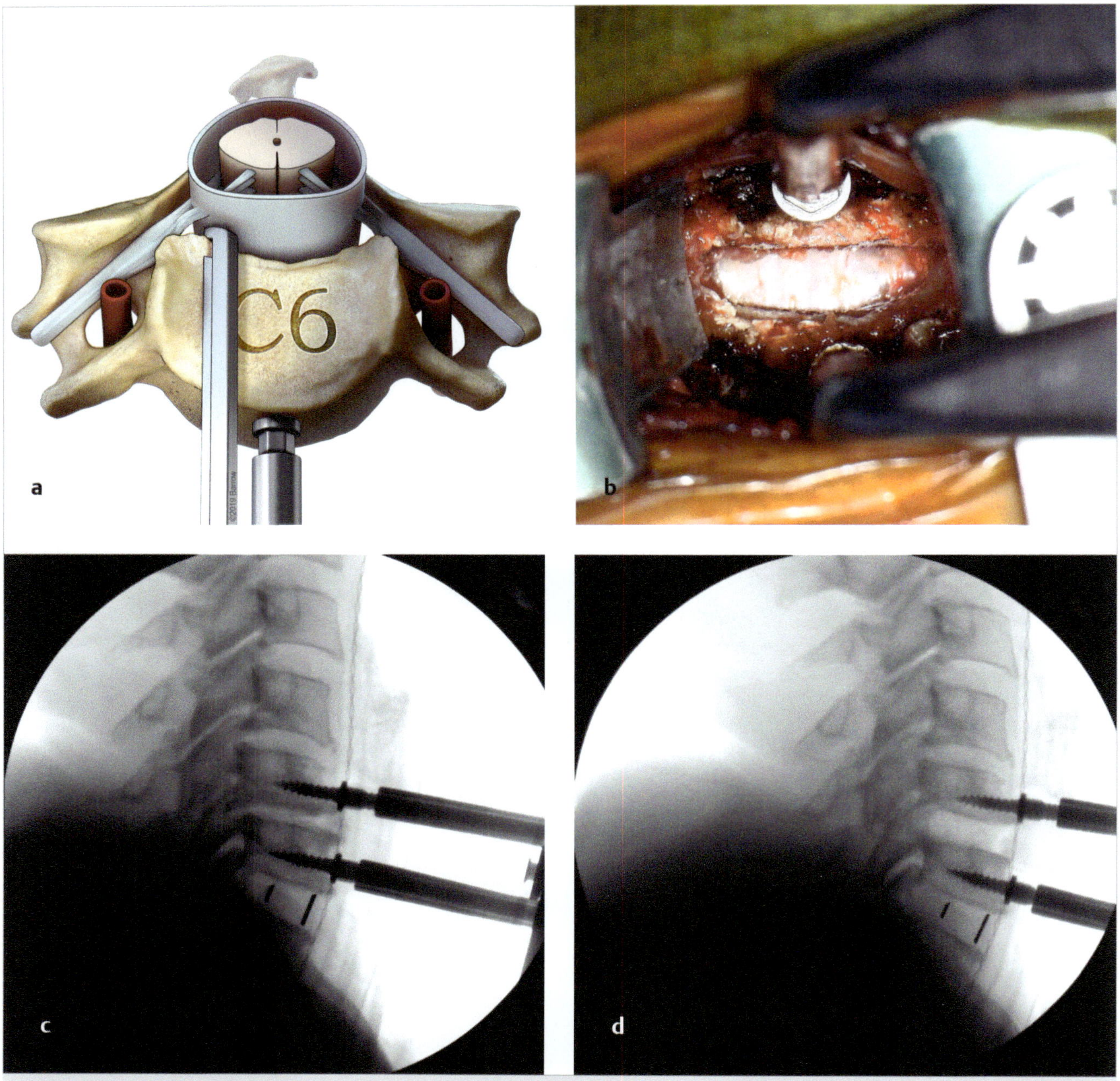

Fig. 9.34 Two-level anterior cervical discectomy and fusion for advanced cervical spondylosis. **(a)** Illustration demonstrating the final removal of the osteophyte with a Kerrison. Note that the posterior aspect of the vertebral body is in a different plane than the vertebral artery. Bleeding encountered during the lateral removal of the osteophyte originates from the epidural venous plexus. **(b)** Intraoperative photograph of a decompressed segment after resection of the posterior longitudinal ligament from uncovertebral joint to uncovertebral joint. **(c)** Lateral fluoroscopic image demonstrating interbody spacer in position at C6–7 and Caspar posts in position at C5–6 prior to decompression. **(d)** Lateral fluoroscopic image demonstrating completion of the decompression at C5–6.

of the surrounding musculature, ligaments and facet capsules, the greater the postoperative discomfort of the patient.

My goals, when it comes to the interbody, are simple: capture the height restored by the Caspar posts and restore the segmental lordosis with a tightly fitting lordotic interbody spacer that will reliably achieve an arthrodesis. With regard to optimizing an environment for arthrodesis, I strive to secure the widest and deepest interbody footprint that the anatomy allows. Furthermore, the larger the footprint, the more self-centering the interbody device becomes. The uncovertebral joints guide the implant into the anatomical midline. Knowing that my exposure is 20-mm wide, I favor the placement of an interbody graft with a width of 16 to 18 mm. The anatomical limitation of the graft is rarely the width. Instead, it is the depth. A guide for the depth may be determined with a quick glance at the Caspar post. For instance, in ▶ Fig. 9.35, the 12-mm posts indicate that there is ample room for a 14-mm-deep implant. Therefore, a 16 × 14-mm implant may be secured. In those circumstances

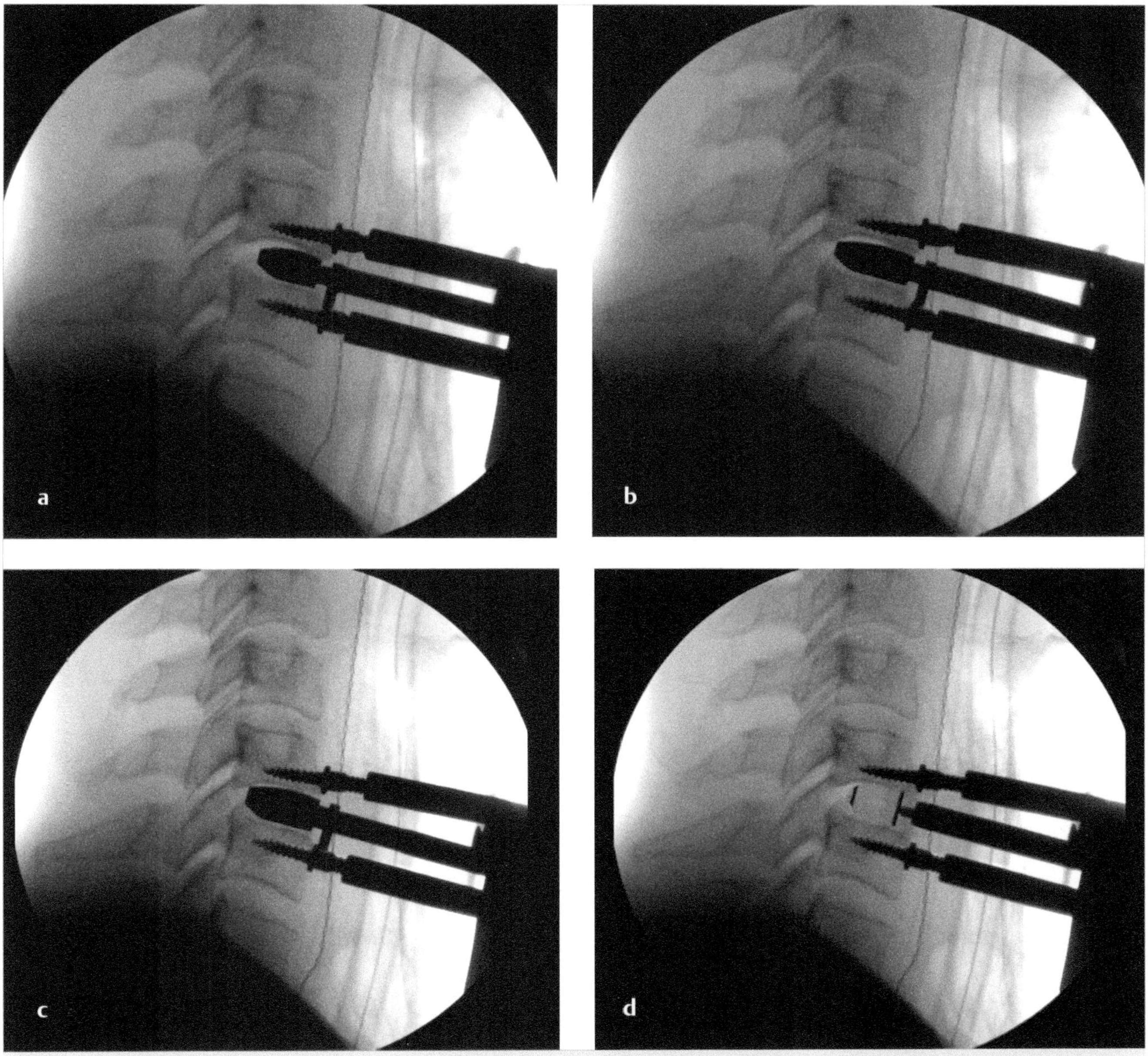

Fig. 9.35 Sizing the interbody spacer in an C4–5 anterior cervical discectomy and fusion for treatment of a soft disc herniation. **(a)** Lateral fluoroscopic image demonstrating a trial in position. The Caspar posts are 12 mm, a valuable reference point that allows the approximation of at least 5 mm to the posterior wall of the vertebral body. In this image, a 14 × 11 × 6-mm interbody trial appears too small in height and depth. **(b)** Lateral fluoroscopic image now with a 16 × 14 × 6-mm trial in position. The anterior aspect of the concavity prevents an optimal interface with the end plate. **(c)** Lateral fluoroscopic image with a 7-mm trial in position. The inferior and anterior aspect of the rostral vertebral body was flattened with a drill in order to optimize the interface with the trial. **(d)** A tight-fitting 16 × 14 × 7-mm polyetheretherketone interbody spacer secured into position.

where the 12-mm Caspar post is nearing the posterior vertebral body, an 11-mm-deep spacer may be all that the anatomy allows. It is essential to know the various dimensions of interbody graft options available regardless of the system you elect to use.

Once I select the ideal graft size, I pack it with morselized autograft collected from the drill shavings and morselized allograft and tap it into position. I take one or two fluoroscopic images to check the fit. I want to ensure that the graft is adequately recessed into the disc space. A well-fitting graft wedges into the disc space and does not advance despite a firm tap of the mallet. With a firm-fitting graft secured into position, I release the Caspar post distractor completely and give the graft one last tap with the mallet to ensure the graft is firmly secured into the disc space. If I am performing a multilevel operation, I remove the post from the level that no longer needs distraction, secure that post into the next vertebral body and begin work on the next level (▶ Fig. 9.36). I repeat the process until I have completed the decompression of all of the affected levels.

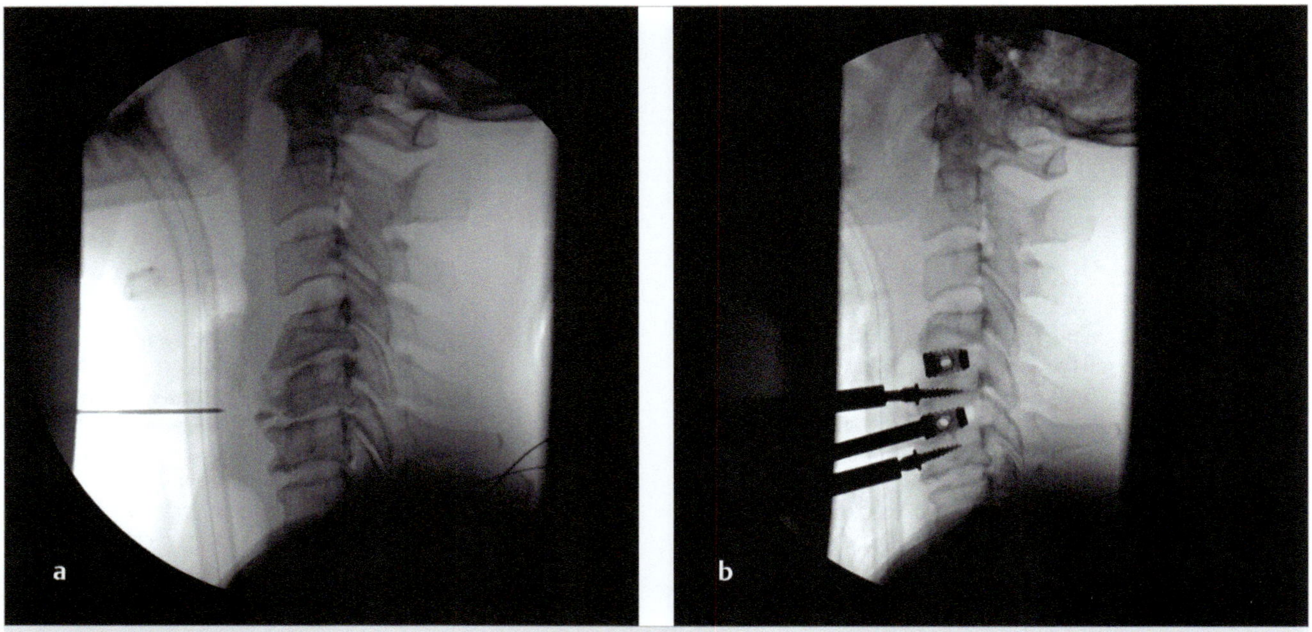

Fig. 9.36 Two-level anterior cervical discectomy and fusion for treatment of cervical spondylosis and radiculopathy. **(a)** Lateral fluoroscopic image demonstrating two levels of advanced cervical spondylosis at C4–5 and C5–6. **(b)** Lateral fluoroscopic image at the completion of the two-level cervical discectomy and placement of titanium interbody spacers.

9.24 Removal of the Caspar Posts

When interbody graft placement is complete, I remove the Caspar posts and fill the void in the vertebral body with bone wax. To facilitate removal of the Caspar post, I relax the tension on the mediolateral retractor, which eliminates the tension on the rostral and caudal aspects of the exposure. A Penfield dissector No. 1 or 3 may now be used to effortlessly hold back the soft tissues while the Caspar posts are removed, and bone wax is placed to seal off the bleeding from the vertebral body.

9.25 Cervical Plating

There is an intuitive sense in all our minds of how things should appear. The basis of that intuitive sense is symmetry. As mentioned at the beginning of this chapter, symmetry captures that intuitive sense in all of us and conveys "*an imprecise sense of harmonious or aesthetically pleasing proportionality and balance; such that it reflects beauty or perfection.*" Patients seldom comment about how well a plate is centered and how orthogonally it was placed. In their mind, that is what they expect. In the event of a tilted plate, the process is quite different. I always marvel at a patient looking at their cervical radiographs and watch their eyes studiously analyze the tilt of a plate on the postoperative anteroposterior (AP) radiograph. Then, after some thoughtful deliberation, that patient never hesitates to look at me and ask, "why is my plate tilted?"

Whether consciously or unconsciously, their eyes are looking for the same symmetry in their plate that they see in their skeletal anatomy. They are looking for that imprecise sense of the harmonious. Whether they recognize it or not, they are looking for an orthogonal plate in the midline. Such a plate conveys proportionality and balance. A tilted plate, on the other hand, disrupts the perfect symmetry of skeletal anatomy. It is not proportional. It is unbalanced.

While there is something intuitive and imprecise about recognizing symmetry, there is a precise definition of the term that can be demonstrated according to geometry. In the case of the cervical plate, the symmetry we as surgeons are striving for is to have equal parts of the vertebral body fall on either side of the long axis of the cervical plate, which, by definition, requires placement of an orthogonal midline plate.

There are no biomechanical studies that demonstrate that a midline plate is superior to a plate off of the midline or that an orthogonal plate is more structurally sound than one that is tilted. There are, however, inherent risks to a tilted plate depending on the degree of rotation. It is simply the anatomy that dictates that a multilevel cervical plate with a significant tilt may increase the risk of a potential injury to the vertebral artery from a screw securing the plate venturing too far off the midline. Over the span of several segments, the impact of a tilt forces the placement of screws increasingly lateral on the vertebral body. Lateral starting points in the vertebral body place those screws increasingly close to the foramen transversarium and, thereby, to the vertebral artery. There is also a concern with the purchase of the screws. A rotated plate has screws on two different planes of the vertebral body. While one screw may capture the harder cortical bone near the end plate, the second screw will purchase more in the center of the vertebral body and therefore purchase more in cancellous bone. Still, I have found no studies that demonstrate a biomechanical disadvantage to a tilted plate.

Few would dispute that another guiding principle of plating the anterior cervical spine is to secure a cervical plate that firmly stabilizes the segments for arthrodesis with the shortest plate possible. It is basic geometry that establishes that a 42.5-mm cervical plate that is tilted has a longer axis by several millimeters than that same plate placed perfectly orthogonally. Therefore, orthogonal placement of the cervical plate allows for the shortest plate to be secured.

There is an abundance of data that correlate the plate-to-disc distance with adjacent segment degeneration. The current body of literature has reached a consensus statement that the optimal distance from the cervical plate to the rostral adjacent disc space is 5 mm.[13,14] Distances that are less than this increase the risk for adjacent segment degeneration. With the current body of literature as our guide, I suggest that, when we strive to perform the perfect operation on the cervical spine of a patient, minimizing disruption of the uninvolved disc spaces, securing the shortest plate and maximizing the plate-to-disc distance are essential. When those principles are combined with the principles of a midline plate placement, the logical conclusion leads us to a midline orthogonally placed plate as the ideal for which to strive. The following paragraphs detail one approach for achieving this ideal.

9.26 Cervical Arthroplasty

The arthroplasty section at this point in this chapter is neither a misstep by the author nor an oversight by the editor. I recognize that the reader was undoubtedly expecting a description of the technique for placement of a midline orthogonal plate but instead has found a section on arthroplasty seemingly out of the blue. The reason for this is simple. It is your experience with performing cervical arthroplasty that leads to a better understanding of the anatomy of the cervical disc space, the uncovertebral joints and the midline. For cervical arthroplasty, the midline is crucial. Being off more than 2 mm from the midline may have a detrimental effect on the capacity of the artificial disc to function appropriately. It was cervical arthroplasty that gave me a true understanding of establishing the midline and thereby improving my ability to place a midline orthogonal plate. The sequence of reviewing arthroplasty before plating is essentially the story of my evolution as a surgeon operating on the cervical spine. It was only after I ventured into motion preservation that I found myself improving in all aspects of anterior cervical surgery.

9.27 Cervical Arthroplasty and Neurologic Outcome

I recall as a resident at a national meeting being mystified as I listened to a presentation on cervical arthroplasty. One of the data points reported was the neurologic success, specifically, improvement in strength and numbness of the region affected by the nerve root and resolution of the radicular symptoms.[18] One member of the audience stood up and questioned the data. His point was that the decompression component of the operation should be the same regardless of whether the surgeon is employing arthroplasty or arthrodesis. At the time, I had no experience with cervical arthroplasty, but it seemed to me that the inquisitive surgeon had a point. I could not conceive how these data regarding neurologic outcomes could be accurate. Over the ensuing years, report after published report began to demonstrate a consistent theme in arthroplasty patients with regard to improvement of neurologic outcomes regardless of the type of arthroplasty implant. Some data were statistically significant, while other data were not, but all of the reports echoed a consistent theme: there seemed to be a difference, albeit subtle, in neurologic outcomes with patients undergoing arthroplasty versus fusion. Arthroplasty demonstrated a clear advantage.[19,20,21] It was difficult for me to dismiss this data point.

This difference in neurologic outcomes circulated about my head as I began performing cervical arthroplasty, and then the answer became clear. In the end, I believe that it may have nothing to do with the device employed. It has everything to do with the extent of decompression in preparation for placement of the device. When I was performing arthroplasty procedures, whether I realized it or not, I was widening my decompression considerably to adequately expose the uncovertebral joints, unequivocally establish the midline and prepare for a larger trial and eventual prosthetic disc. My concern to create a wider exposure for a wider implant resulted in wider decompressions in arthroplasty cases that were more extensive than what I performed for arthrodesis.

The footprint of all cervical arthroplasty devices is wider than the typical interbody spacer for arthrodesis. Couple this with placing a device that occupies the entire disc space, and this knowledge influences the extent of the discectomy performed and drives a wider decompression. It is this wider decompression that must be performed for arthroplasty that may reconcile the data in the literature, where the cervical arthroplasty group had overall neurologic success (maintenance or improvement); success rates were high, exceeding 90% at all follow-up intervals, and were higher than those in the control arthrodesis group. In fact, at 24 months, the arthroplasty group's success rate was 92.8% compared with 84.3% in the control group. The overall rate of neurologic success in the investigational group was statistically significantly higher than the rate in the control group at both the 12- and 24-month follow-up intervals.[18]

One interpretation of these data is that motion preservation made a difference in the outcomes. Although that is a plausible explanation for the Neck Disability Index (NDI), it is difficult for me to explain how motion preservation can affect neurologic outcomes. My interpretation of the data is that neurologic outcomes in patients with radiculopathy are improved after wider decompressions. I believe this may be the most important lesson learned from the cervical arthroplasty data. It just might be the technique, not the device. Although surgeons deliberate the benefits of arthroplasty versus arthrodesis and the impact on adjacent segment degeneration, I place emphasis on the immediate outcome of surgery. That emphasis translates to having neurologic outcomes become equivalent in your arthrodesis and arthroplasty patients. The path to accomplishing this goal is performing the same decompression regardless of the implant used. There is no doubt in my mind that my experience with cervical arthroplasty made me more comfortable with decompressing further lateral than I had routinely performed with arthrodesis.

One of the guiding principles of arthroplasty is to place an implant with the largest footprint that the disc space can accommodate. The widest footprint accomplishes two objectives: it optimizes the device from a biomechanical standpoint and allows for the uncovertebral joints to center the device. I found that placing an implant with a wide footprint influenced my mindset as I approached the decompression. For instance, when I knew I would be placing a 17-mm implant for a trial, I would strive to have 1 to 2 mm on either side cleared of disc material. This situation equates to 21 mm of decompression needed, which is far more of a decompression than I would have accomplished for an arthrodesis, where I am preparing at times to place nothing more than a 14-mm-wide spacer.

In order to safely approach these wider decompressions, I return to the minimally invasive surgery mindset: knowledge of the anatomy at depth instills the confidence to see what cannot be directly seen and to connect what is known to what is unknown. Application of this principle for the cervical spine involves the certainty of the midline and the distance between the vertebral arteries. The midline is crucial for arthroplasty.

9.28 Arthroplasty Candidacy

The ideal arthroplasty patient should have very little if any spondylosis and normal motion of the affected level on flexion–extension radiographs. Arthroplasty should preserve motion, not restore motion that has been lost to spondylosis. My rule of thumb has been that the symptomatic segment should appear no different from the unaffected levels on a lateral radiograph. ▶ Fig. 9.37 shows a disc extrusion at C6–7 in a patient without significant spondylosis who benefited from cervical arthroplasty. By comparison, ▶ Fig. 9.38 shows a patient who specifically requested arthroplasty but had advanced spondylosis at the segment. The decision was made to proceed with arthrodesis.

9.29 Arthroplasty Technique

The principles of the arthroplasty technique include minimal distraction of the disc space with the Caspar posts and no use of the drill. If I find myself having to use a drill to remove an osteophyte, I reconsider the role of arthroplasty in that particular patient.

In a manner identical to that used in cervical arthrodesis, I position the patient on a reversed operating table in a Caspar head holder to ensure the stability of the head and neck throughout the procedure. Using the Smith–Robinson approach, I expose the same requisite anatomical unit for the segment as previously described. Placement of the Caspar posts needs to be tailored to the arthroplasty device that will be implanted. For keel-based devices, the Caspar posts need to be placed three-quarters of the way up or down the vertebral bodies. For non-keel-based devices, 5 mm above and below the disc space is more than adequate (▶ Fig. 9.39).

I perform a discectomy and extend my dissection laterally until I unequivocally visualize the rise in the slopes of the uncovertebral joints. I center the field of view of the microscope in line with the segment and thereby eliminate any parallax. When I have completely exposed and can fully visualize the uncovertebral joints, I have found that there is no need for an AP fluoroscopic image. An AP fluoroscopic image cluttered with retractors in place that will obscure the visualization of the midline seldom provides insight as to the location of the midline. When I have taken these AP images with the retractors in position, I spend half the time trying to convince myself that I know what I am looking at instead of focusing on the exposed anatomy before me. It has become my habit to forgo the AP image. Instead of relying on an image on a screen, I rely on the AP image before my eyes provided by a complete exposure of the anatomy. With the uncovertebral joints completely exposed, I cauterize a small midline mark on the rostral and caudal vertebral bodies in the midline and then mark them with a purple marking pen. Those marks guide the placement of the trial and the implant. I remove the cartilage from the end plates and expose cortical bleeding bone before placing the implant between the rostral and caudal end plates. I divide and resect the PLL and ensure both foramina are well decompressed.

The next step is the trial. The implant with the largest footprint that the disc space can accommodate is the guiding principle for the trial (▶ Fig. 9.40). There are now several cervical arthroplasty devices that have been approved by the U.S. Food and Drug Administration for implantation. There are nuances to the trial and placement of each of these devices. I refer the reader to the technique guides for these various implants and stress the importance of mentorship and training with the application of these devices. One thing is certain: mastering cervical arthroplasty will improve all aspects of the anterior cervical surgeries, including fixation of the cervical plate, which is described in the next section.

9.30 Cervical Plating Technique

Early in my career, I found the placement of an anterior cervical plate a daunting task. It became the part of the procedure that filled me with the greatest concern. My desire to place a perfectly orthogonal midline plate as an indication of the overall craftsmanship of the operation consumed me. I found myself placing an anterior cervical plate into position, with the plate-holding pins, and then obtaining an AP image in order to ensure a midline orthogonal placement. The AP image was always difficult to interpret with the retractors in position. As it turns out, early in my career, I was overly reliant upon the AP fluoroscopic image. In my mind, I felt I needed the AP to accomplish my goal of a midline orthogonal plate. I found myself chasing my tail with AP and lateral images going back and forth until I thought it was perfect. The following morning on rounds, my jaw would drop as I reviewed the standing AP image revealing a tilted plate that was off the midline for the entire world to see. Without fail, the patient would study their image at their post-operative appointment and ask me, "why is my plate tilted?"

I would defensively offer them an explanation that the angle of the plate was meaningless and what they could not see was the complete decompression that I had performed. It is the decompression that relieved them of their radiculopathy, not the plate or its placement. The patient would hesitantly nod, suppressing the look of disappointment. Inside my mind, I would cringe. I was disappointed too. The subconscious of the patient wanted what I wanted: that imprecise sense of the harmony that created proportionality and balance. The patient and I both wanted what the human eye effortlessly identifies as symmetry.

In the years after I finished my training, I went about searching for a technique that would efficiently ensure a balanced and

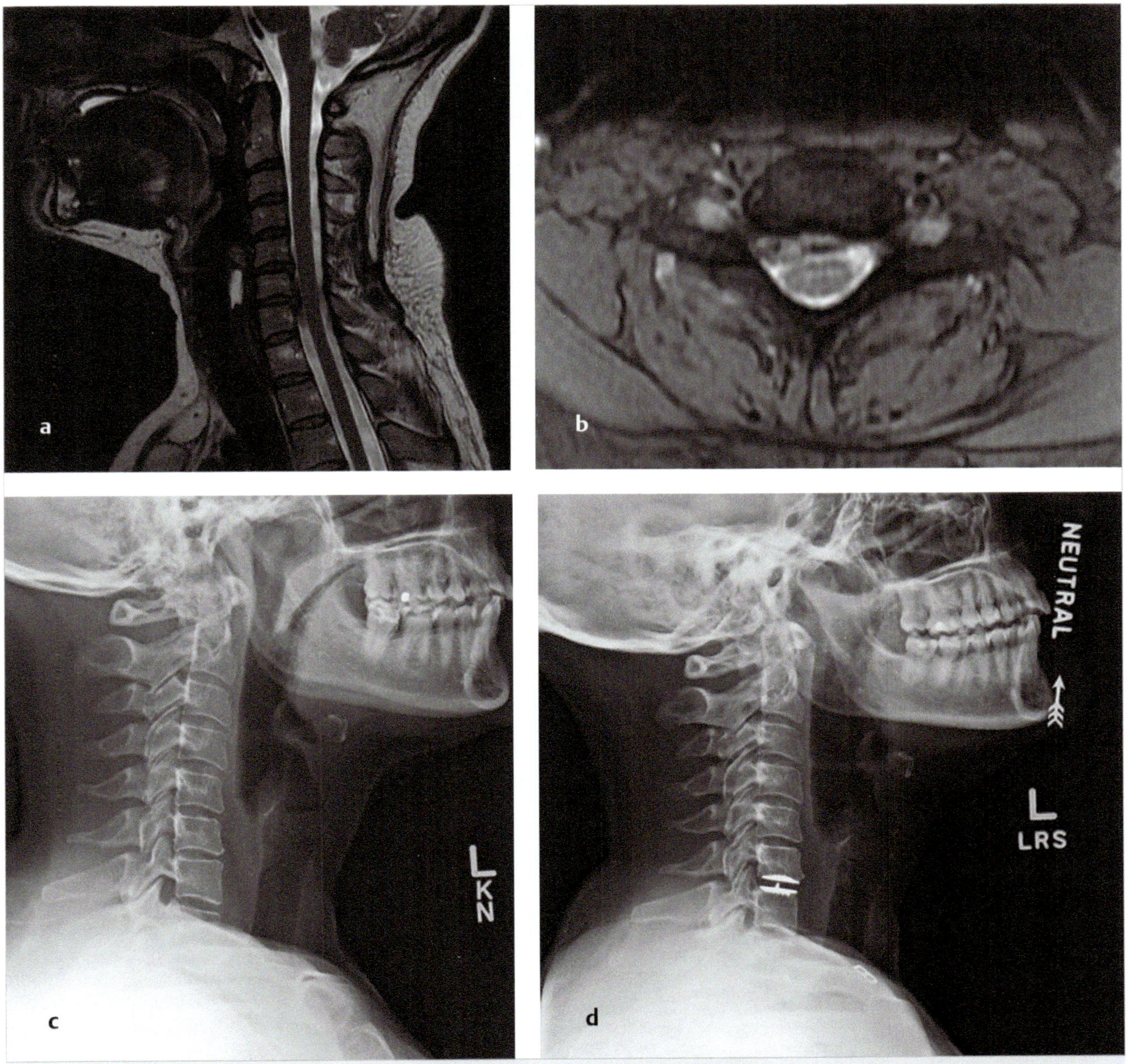

Fig. 9.37 Ideal arthroplasty candidate. **(a)** Sagittal T2-weighted magnetic resonance imaging (MRI) showing a disc extrusion at C6–7. There is no significant spondylosis of the disc space on MRI. **(b)** Axial T2-weighted MRI shows the disc extrusion with a central and foraminal component. No significant facet arthropathy is seen on the axial image. **(c)** Lateral radiograph shows preservation of the convexity of the disc space at C6–7 without osteophyte formation. There is mild loss of disc height. Note that the patient has a slightly positive sagittal vertical axis (SVA), likely from active radiculopathy. The patient had normal motion at C6–7 on flexion–extension radiographs (not shown). **(d)** Postoperative lateral radiograph after successful C6–7 arthroplasty. Note improvement of the SVA on the neutral radiograph.

proportional plate every time. Every surgeon has undoubtedly evolved their operative nuances that allow them to accomplish their surgical objectives. So, I readily acknowledge that there are several ways to accomplish the task of fixating a cervical plate to the spine. Regardless of the technique employed, there is an ideal to strive for. I have already presented the rationale in this chapter for an orthogonal midline placement as the shortest and safest plate. In addition, the current body of literature supports a minimum plate-to-disc distance of 5 mm to decrease the incidence of adjacent segment degeneration, especially at the rostral segment.[13,14] The following paragraphs detail just one surgeon's approach to accomplish these goals.

9.31 Three Principles

I have built my cervical plating technique upon three principles. The first is that the best visualization of the midline occurs before placing a cervical plate. The moment a plate rests upon

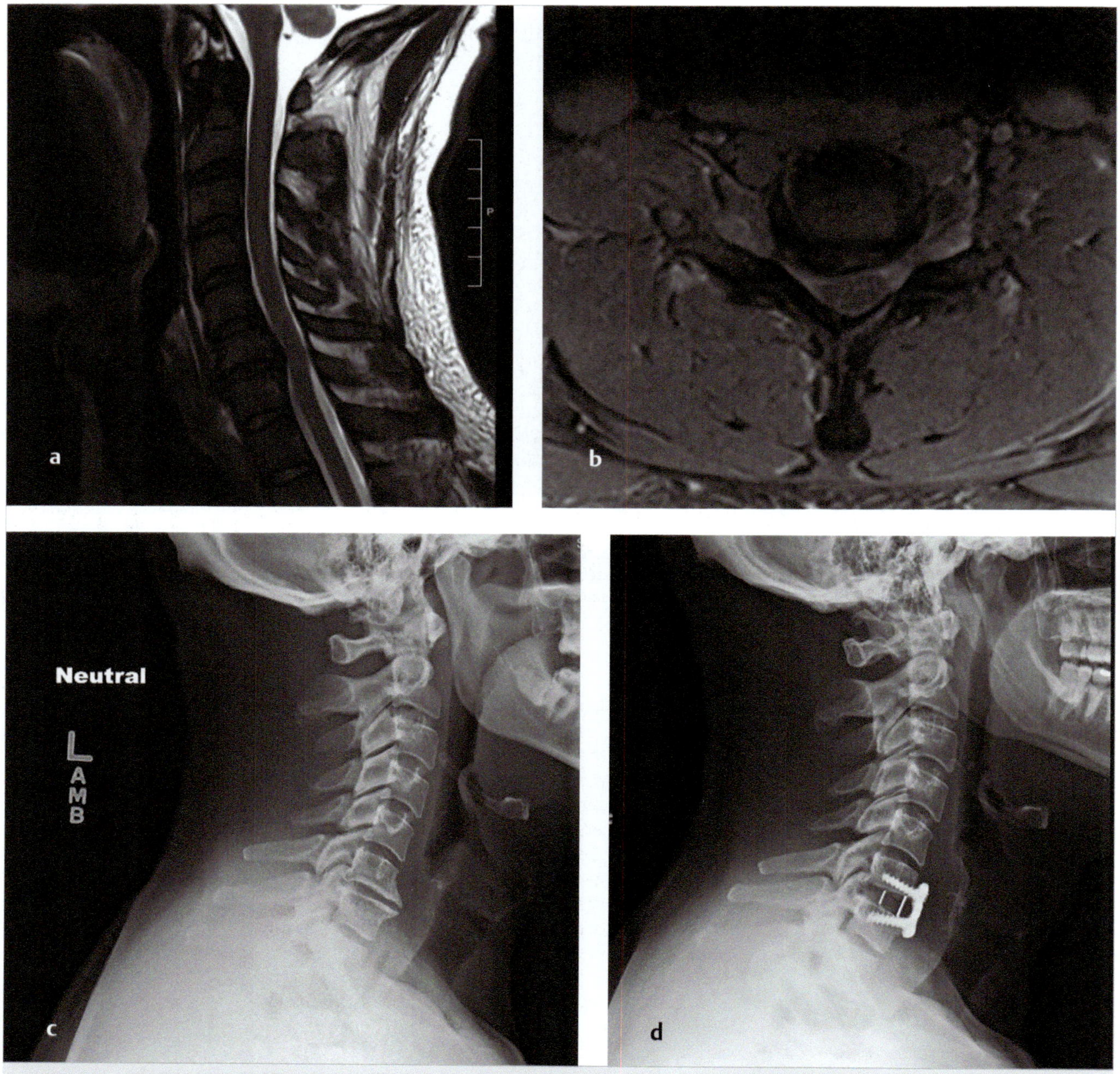

Fig. 9.38 Suboptimal arthroplasty candidate. (a) Sagittal T2-weighted magnetic resonance imaging (MRI) demonstrating a C6–7 disc osteophyte complex in contact with the ventral aspect of the spinal cord. (b) Axial T2-weighted MRI showing the disc osteophyte complex narrowing the C7 neural foramen. (c) Neutral lateral radiograph showing advanced spondylosis at C6–7. The absence of normal motion at the C6–7 level on flexion–extension studies (not shown) along with the loss of concavity on the underside of C6 and prominent osteophyte prompted the arthrodesis. (d) Lateral neutral radiograph demonstrating C6–7 anterior cervical discectomy and fusion.

the cervical vertebral bodies is the moment the midline becomes obscure. The second principle is that a screw always finds a hole that has been drilled. As spine surgeons, we know that one of the most difficult tasks to perform in spine surgery is to redirect a screw down an alternate path in the bone after one path has already been established. The final principle is that, in a well-performed anterior cervical decompression, the interbody is reliably in the midline. The question is how to harness all of these principles into facilitating the placement of a cervical plate and make the plating component the easiest and most enjoyable part of the operation. The following paragraphs will provide the answer to that question.

9.32 Exposure and the Midline

Earlier in this chapter, when I discussed the exposure of the cervical spine, I emphasized that the effortless placement of an anterior cervical plate at the end of the case begins upon

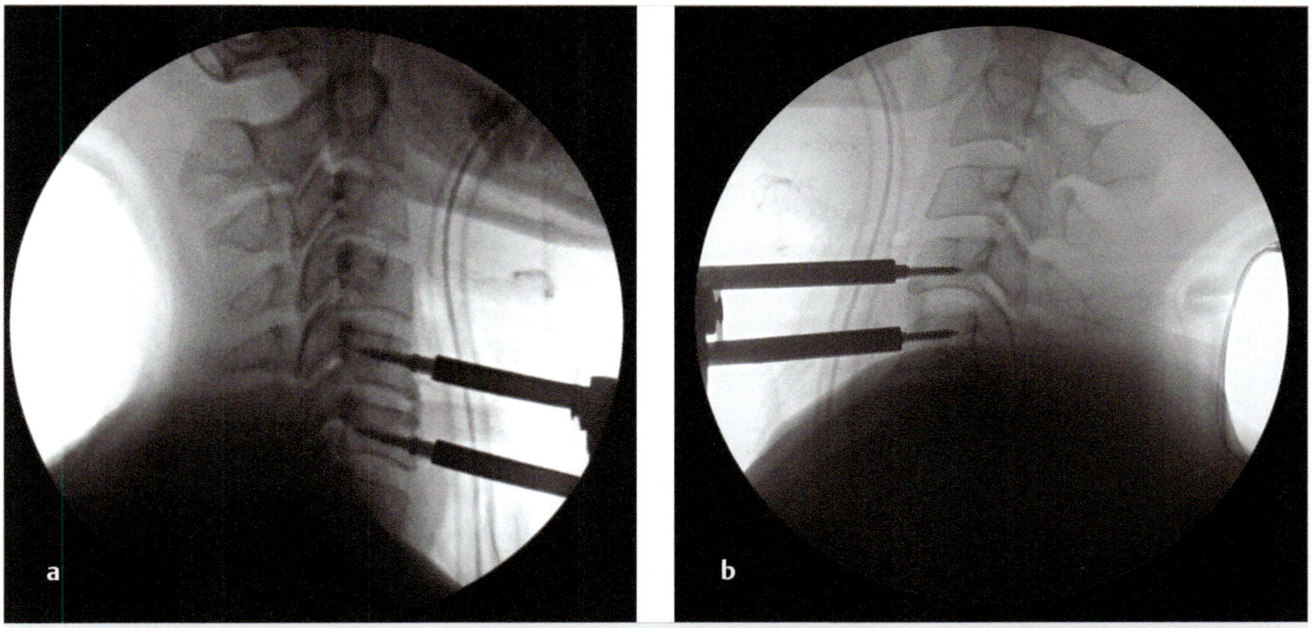

Fig. 9.39 Caspar posts for a keel-based arthroplasty device compared to a non-keel-based device. **(a)** Lateral fluoroscopic image showing the placement of the Caspar post is at the three-quarter mark of the vertebral body to allow for the keel cuts. **(b)** Lateral fluoroscopic image illustrating the difference in the placement of the Caspar posts for a non-keel-based device. In this arthroplasty case, the Caspar posts may be placed within 5 mm of the disc space, avoiding any disruption in the adjacent segment.

making the incision and appropriate exposure at the beginning of the case. Relaxing the tissue planes beneath the platysma as well as the fascial bands up and down the lateral border of the sternocleidomastoid is essential to prevent struggling with the passage of the plate onto the cervical spine. At a minimum, the inferior half of the rostral vertebral body and the superior aspect of the caudal vertebral body to be instrumented need to be exposed (▶ Fig. 9.4). One must be meticulous in the dissection not to disrupt the annulus or the ligamentous anatomy of the rostral and caudal adjacent segments to mitigate the risk of those segments degenerating. The time to ensure adequate exposure for an anterior cervical plate is before placement of the self-retaining retractors and beginning the discectomy. Discovering the need for additional exposure at the end of the case may require removal of the retractors and disruption of the workflow. The exposure is always best accomplished at the beginning.

Much has been written already within this chapter regarding the midline. Those same midline marks that will confidently guide the extent of decompression are also the beacons that will become the landing zone for a midline cervical plate. The first principle mentioned above was that the midline is never more evident than before the cervical plate rests upon the vertebral bodies. Therefore, before placement of the cervical plate, another assessment of the midline is worthwhile. If the technique recommended in the decompression and interbody placement section were employed, the anterior vertebral bodies would have their distinct purple midline marks demarcating the midline. Under the operating microscope, viewing the operative field in low magnification offers a superior perspective than at high magnification. However, it may be preferential at this point to view the entire field outside of the microscope, which would allow visualization of the "V" that was marked in the sternal notch and the entire neck to fall within the field of view. Such a view is far superior to obtaining an AP fluoroscopic image at this point.

9.33 Lateral Osteophytes

Once I have confirmed the midline, it is worthwhile to assess the topography of the anterior aspects of the vertebral bodies. Prominent osteophytes, especially those that are asymmetric, end up tilting the plate and compromise the plate–bone–screw interface. Preparing the anterior vertebral bodies for a plate has been referred to by many surgeons as "gardening," a term that I am not sure captures the essence of the procedure but which nonetheless continues to be used in this Primer, if only for historical purposes.

The most important component of gardening the cervical spine is to ensure that the lateral anterior osteophytes have been appropriately smoothed. The anterior osteophytes that reside in the midline are low-lying fruit and are readily drilled flat. Midline or paramedian osteophytes are seldom an issue when plating because they are so obviously in the way that they are the first thing you remove before attempting to lay down a plate. The anterior osteophytes that reside in the lateral margins of the vertebral bodies, however, are more treacherous. Because they are just out of the field of view, these lateral spurs have the greatest potential to be the most challenging when attempting to secure a plate. Over the years, the cervical plates with the greatest degree of tilt that I have placed have come as the consequence of these lateral osteophytes that I did not fully appreciate. These spurs led to an asymmetric rise on one side, which after fixation caused an unsightly tilt in a plate I had considered to be perfectly orthogonal.

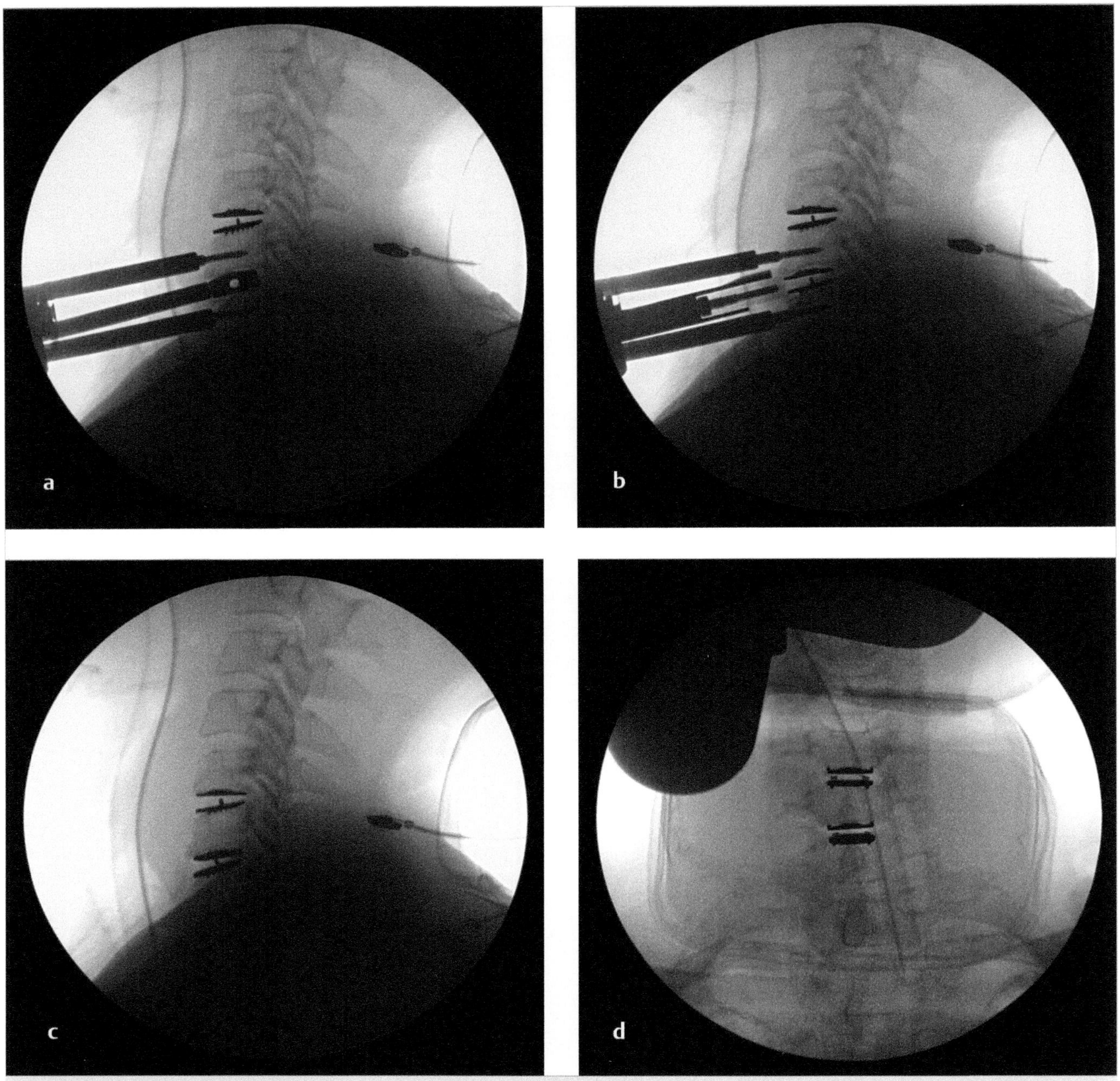

Fig. 9.40 Placement of the trial and implant in a C5–6 and C6–7 cervical arthroplasty. **(a)** Lateral fluoroscopic image of a trial in position for arthroplasty at the C6–7 segment. **(b)** Lateral fluoroscopic image showing the insertion of the device with a trajectory that creates a lordotic position for the implant. **(c)** Final lateral fluoroscopic image showing arthroplasty devices in a lordotic position. **(d)** Anteroposterior fluoroscopic image, taken at the completion of the procedure, showing midline placement of the devices.

In order to address these lateral osteophytes adequately, knowledge of the lateral dimension of the plate you intend to fixate should be at the forefront of your mind. Most cervical plates have a lateral dimension of approximately 18 mm or less. Regardless of the plate you select, you should be familiar with how much space you need to secure it onto the spine. Therefore, in order to facilitate the plating aspect of the operation, one must survey the lateral aspects of the vertebral bodies 10 mm lateral to the midline marks on either side. It is flattening the unrecognized and unseen osteophytes in the lateral margins that vastly facilitates fixation of the cervical plate. Addressing these osteophytes inadequately transforms what otherwise would be a pleasurable experience into an incredibly frustrating one.

At this point in the operation, I will open the self-retaining retractor a click or two more than where it was for the decompression. I then inspect the lateral margins of the anterior vertebral bodies by probing with a Penfield 4 or Penfield 1. In patients with advanced cervical spondylosis, these lateral osteophytes have the potential to be quite prominent. Typically, several bites with a large pituitary can readily level the osteophytes. Other times a drill will be needed with Cloward handheld retractors to protect the esophagus.

9.34 A Screw Hole Once Drilled in Bone...

I have found that one of the greatest challenges to plating is attempting to hold the plate in precisely the desired midline and orthogonal position and then drill a hole into the vertebral body to place a screw. The plate invariably moves or tilts or both. For this reason, the majority of anterior cervical plating systems have a plate-holding screw system as an option. Conceptually, this configuration is designed to hold the plate in position while holes are drilled for the screws that fixate the plate onto the vertebral bodies. The technique guides for these cervical plates typically recommend placing the plate into position and then securing the plate-holding pins. I have employed this technique in the past and have always marveled at how little I can see of the midline with the plate in position and how difficult it is to place a plate-holding pin into the desired position without moving the plate. As a result, the placement of my plate-holding pins did not end up where I intended them to be.

However, if we were to apply the first two principles that began this section into a technique, we could remedy the shortcomings just encountered. First, we would confirm the midline and then, second, place one of the plate-holding pins into position with the midline in plain view without the cervical plate in the way, which may be done on the rostral vertebral body precisely where one would like the plate to reside. Placement of the plate-holding screw without the plate obscuring the view is technically easier and more reliable than with the plate in position. Furthermore, one can secure the plate-holding screw close to the end plate and thereby ensure the plate-to-disc distance will be less than 5 mm. Once the screw is in three-quarters of the distance into the vertebral body, it is removed. I then drop the plate into position and apply the principle that a screw will always find a hole that has been drilled for it. With a minimal amount of probing, the screw will find its predrilled hole, and the plate will fall into its predetermined position. The main limitation of this technique is that it would be difficult to predrill a caudal hole since the distance between the holes is determined by the plate, not the disc space. I have tried on several occasions to approximate where the caudal hole would reside, and all of my attempts contributed more to destabilizing the plate than to its fixation. For this reason, when I employ this technique, I drill the caudal hole only after the plate is in position.

Once the plate is placed on top of the vertebral bodies and the plate-holding pin is secured into the rostral vertebral body, I can now rest assured that the cervical plate is in the midline. The next step is to ensure orthogonal placement of the plate.

9.35 Indexing off of the Interbody

I have observed time and time again that in patients with tilted off-center plates, whether placed by me or someone else, the interbody graft is perfectly in the midline. Furthermore, the interbody is squarely within the disc space. It has no tilt. This observation has prompted me to align the cervical plate in the same plane as the interbody graft. Most cervical plates have a window through the center that allows the surgeon to index off of the interbody. As part of a systems check, I confirm this alignment with the marks I created to establish midline. I align the plate with the marks and the interbody and then survey the entire anatomy from the marked "V" in the sternal notch to the head. Any adjustments at this point should be minor and are simply a judgment call by the surgeon. However, with all of these reference points, the proximity to the midline and orthogonal position is bound to be within millimeters with at most 1 or 2 degrees. With the plate aligned in this manner, I secure the caudal plate-holding pin and then proceed with drilling the holes for the placement of the vertebral body screws to fixate the plate.

9.36 Cervical Template: Single Level

Early in my practice, I found myself at times struggling with certain phases of the plating process, even with plate-holding pins, and still getting frustrated with the final position of the cervical plate. I asked myself what modifications I could do that would further streamline and facilitate my technique. What eluded me was a consistent and reproducible process that would ensure an orthogonal midline plate that would be less than 5 mm from the adjacent segment every time. At times, cases would go perfectly. The patient would have a wide decompression and a perfectly sized plate, centered and orthogonal. When these circumstances occurred, I considered myself a master incapable of faltering again. Soon afterward, I would find myself struggling with the placement of a plate and then cringing as I looked at the postoperative images, which showed a tilted plate for the entire world to see. After cases like these, I considered myself incompetent.

I sought to develop a technique that would ensure that every plate I placed would be perfect every time, regardless of the level, regardless of the degree of spondylosis and regardless of body habitus. I wanted to minimize any risk of adjacent segment degeneration. I wanted to give every patient who trusted me with their care the operation that I would want.

After refining my technique for securing the midline, based in large part on my arthroplasty experience, I focused on what I perceived to be the primary inadequacy of the technique: the capacity to firmly hold the plate in position in order to secure the screws. I observed that at the root of this inadequacy were the plate-holding pins. Plates that were in perfect position with the plate-holding pins would not always remain there. As the fixed-angle drill guide engaged into its hole within the cervical plate, the force of setting the guide and locking it into position would shift an otherwise well-positioned plate while the hapless plate-holding pins surrendered whatever purchase they had in the bone.

As I studied these pins, I acknowledged the small diameter of the screw and the limited length. A screw of this size could not reliably stabilize a plate against the forces created by the drill guides that are rotated onto and off of the plate. Too much was being asked of these modest plate-holding pins. Furthermore, I had become increasingly conscious of the adjacent segment and had begun lowering the location of the Caspar post in the vertebral body. The closer the Caspar post came to the end plate, the less undisrupted cortical bone was available for the plate-holding pin to engage. At times, the presence of a hole created by a Caspar post would compromise any fixation from the plate-holding pin at all. After briefly assessing the capacity of the longer plate-holding pins to accomplish the task, with limited success, I reconsidered my entire approach to plating the cervical spine.

In deconstructing the plating process, I considered what would be the ideal scenario: stabilization of a cervical plate onto the anatomical midline of the cervical spine that would not migrate when engaged with the drill guides. The ability to place the plate perfectly in line with the long axis of the spine, that is, orthogonal, should be facilitated. Fixed or variable-angle drill guides should be able to engage the plate and drill the screw hole without the risk of migration or tilt. In attempting to meet these criteria, I looked first toward the interbody spacer. I recognized time and time again on postoperative radiographs that, despite the location of my plates or the degree of the tilt I gave them, the interbody grafts were always in the midline and never tilted (▶ Fig. 9.41). To facilitate placement of the plate, I needed to harness the position of the midline provided to me by the interbody spacer. Instead of using plate-holding pins to hold a plate in the midline position, the question I asked myself was, how could I use the interbody spacer?

From there, I conceived the notion of a cervical template built on the three principles I presented earlier: the interbody graft is always in the midline, visualization of the midline is best before the cervical plate obscures the field, and a screw will always find a hole that was drilled for it. In order to harness the position of the interbody graft, I needed a method to engage the graft itself. For this, I turned to the use of a PEEK or titanium spacer, which allowed me to use the same hole that secures the inserter as an anchor for a template. A threaded shaft passes into the template and secures into the interbody spacer. Recognizing that an entire cervical plate obscures the view of the midline, I limited the template to only two of the holes that would correspond with the cervical plate. Before tightening the threaded shaft of the cervical template into the interbody spacer, it may be rotated on its axis into an orthogonal position. Having only a limited template optimizes the visualization and readily allows for confirmation of the midline. Once tightened, the fact that it is anchored into the interbody makes the template less susceptible to rotation when the fixed or variable-angle drill guide engages into the template holes (▶ Fig. 9.42). The anchor into the spacer disallows any lateral movement whatsoever.

The same geometry of the screw holes found on a cervical plate is present in the template, which allows a fixed-angle or variable-angle drill guide to engage the cervical template in exactly the same manner it engages a cervical plate. I now drill the holes through the template and then remove it. I then place the cervical plate that corresponds with the size of the template on top of the spine. Plating now becomes nothing more than lining up the cervical plate with the holes that have already been drilled and placing the screws (▶ Fig. 9.43). Embracing the principle that a screw always finds a hole that has been drilled for it allows for effortless fixation in the midline orthogonal position.

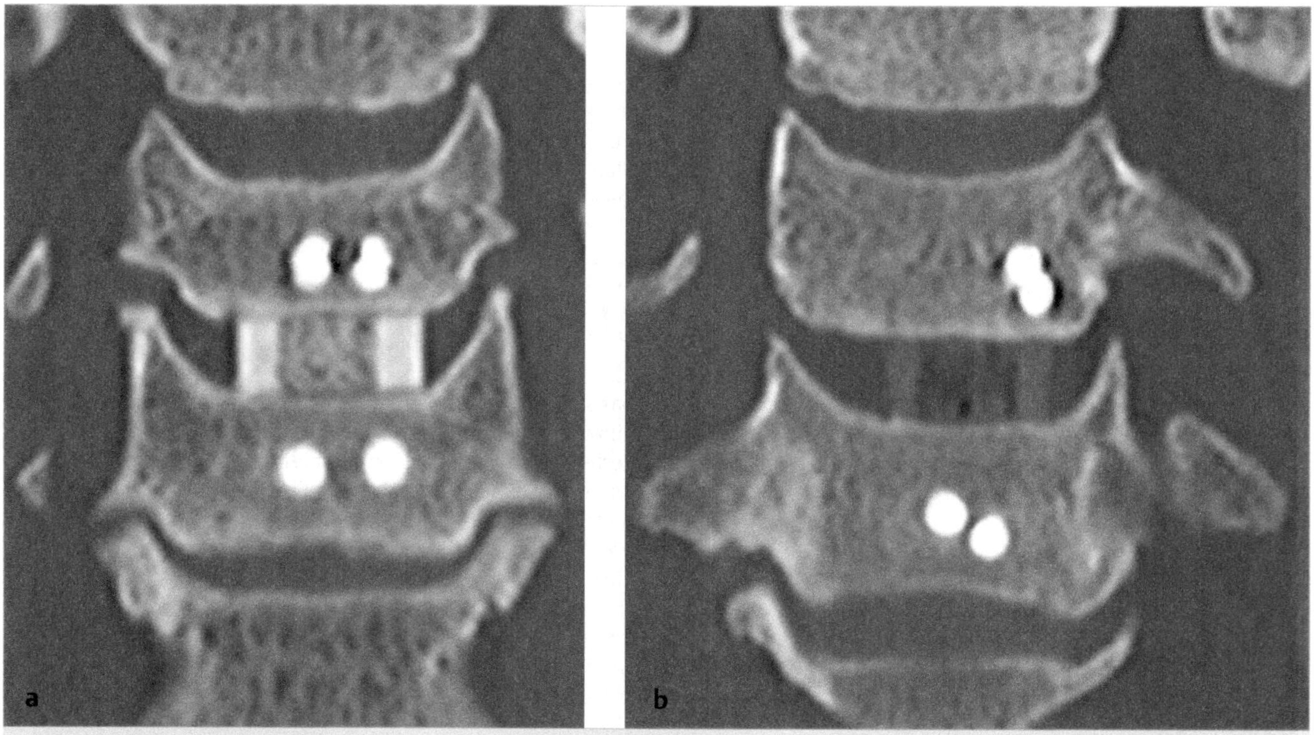

Fig. 9.41 Coronal computed tomography reconstruction demonstrating interbody spacers in the geometric midline of the disc space. **(a)** In this image of the coronal reconstruction, the cortical cancellous graft is in position precisely in the geometric midline. **(b)** Despite the midline placement of the polyetheretherketone interbody graft in this coronal reconstruction, the anterior cervical plate is considerably tilted off to the left. If the cervical plate were indexed off of the interbody device, the plate would have been both midline and orthogonal.

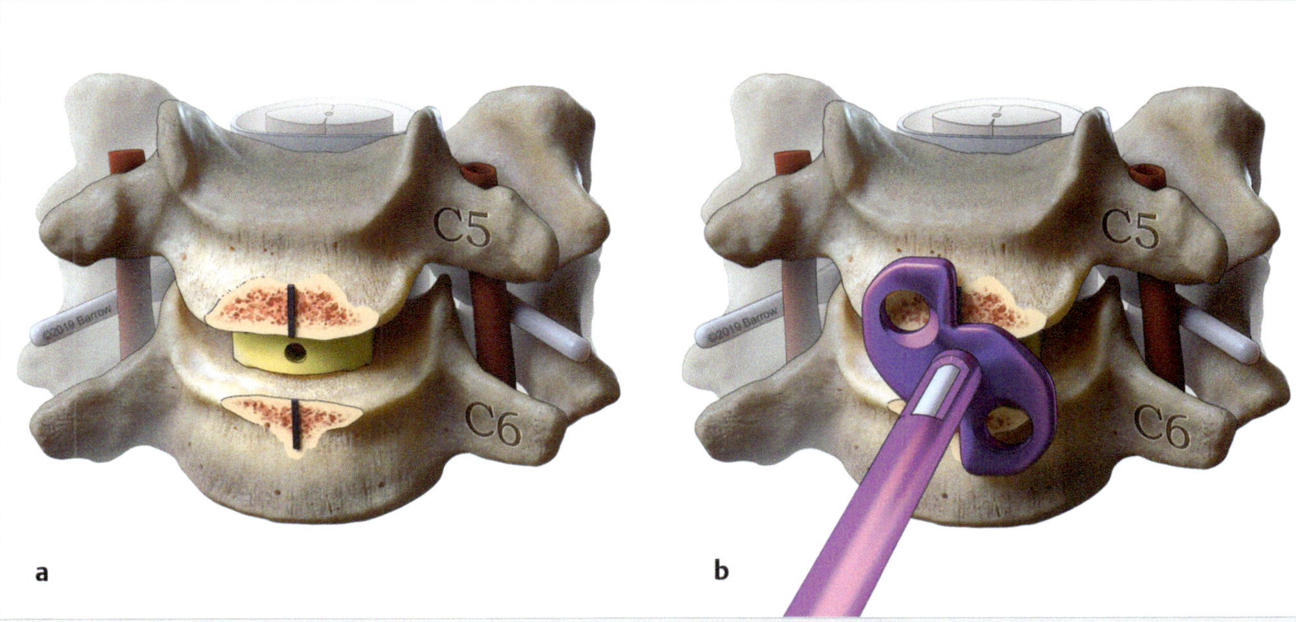

Fig. 9.42 Illustrations demonstrating the concept of the cervical template. **(a)** In a well-performed decompression, interbody spacers tend to find the midline because of the self-centering attributes of the uncovertebral joints. Midline marks made from the direct examination of the uncovertebral joints should fall in line with the inserter hole of the interbody spacer. **(b)** The template can firmly anchor into the interbody spacer assuring a midline position. Before tightening the template into position, it may be rotated into an orthogonal position in line with the long axis of the spine.

In practice, the single-level template has several advantages that further facilitate the placement of the cervical plate. The first is the capacity to size a single-level plate, preventing the need to go in and out of the surgical site with plates of various lengths attempting to select the appropriate size. The second more subtle advantage is the identification of lateral osteophytes. On several occasions, it was only after placement of the template that the extent and impact of a lateral osteophyte were identified. A lateral osteophyte becomes readily apparent when a struggle occurs attempting to secure the template into position. The template is easily rotated on its axis and the cause of the obstruction identified. The template is easily removed, the osteophyte flattened and the template repositioned. Having the template reveal a lateral disc osteophyte prevents the struggle that can occur when the entire cervical plate covers the vertebral bodies, preventing clear visualization of the obstruction. The third advantage is the capacity to confirm that the plate-to-disc distance is greater than 5 mm with either direct inspection or a lateral fluoroscopic image. Visual inspection alone reveals how the cervical plate will lay on the vertebral bodies and ensure the shortest plate possible for the segment.

The ability to engage the interbody is the main limitation of the template concept. At times, an interbody spacer has been recessed into a deep disc space, and the threaded shaft can no longer reach the center hole of the interbody spacer. The contrapositive is also true. An interbody spacer that cannot be recessed deeply enough will not allow for the template to firmly engage against the anterior aspect of the vertebral body. Under these circumstances, it may be more challenging to ensure an orthogonal position since the template can still rotate on its axis. Lateral movement, however, is still not possible with the template engaged into the interbody.

In my experience in a prospective observational cohort of 50 patients undergoing a single-level ACDF, the cervical template achieved a mean angle from the long axis of the spine of 2.4 (0.0–4.4) degrees, a mean distance from the midline of 1.3 (0.0–2.8) mm. Equally important, the mean distance from the plate ends to the adjacent segments above was 5.4 (4.6–6.2) mm, and the mean distance to the adjacent segments below was 5.1 (4.3–5.8) mm.[22] The template facilitated meeting the 5-mm plate-to-disc distance criteria to mitigate adjacent segment degeneration.

9.37 Cervical Template for Multilevel Cases

The geometric principle that two points define a line is the basis for the multilevel cervical template. A multilevel template allows two holes to be drilled in either the rostral or the caudal vertebral body, establishing a midline and orthogonal position for the plate. It has been my preference to apply the multilevel template to the most caudal vertebral body of the construct. The technique is similar to the single-level template, as it anchors into the interbody spacer. The main difference is that the two holes that will be drilled are at the same vertebral body. These two points, once established, prevent any significant tilt from occurring. In practice, even though I have predrilled both screw holes, I secure only one screw because placing both may elevate the plate off the rostral spine. Instead, I use one of the holes to secure the plate onto the cervical spine and then line up the plate with the interbody spacers above and below. I use the second hole that was drilled as a reference point and drill into one of the rostral vertebral bodies for the second screw to

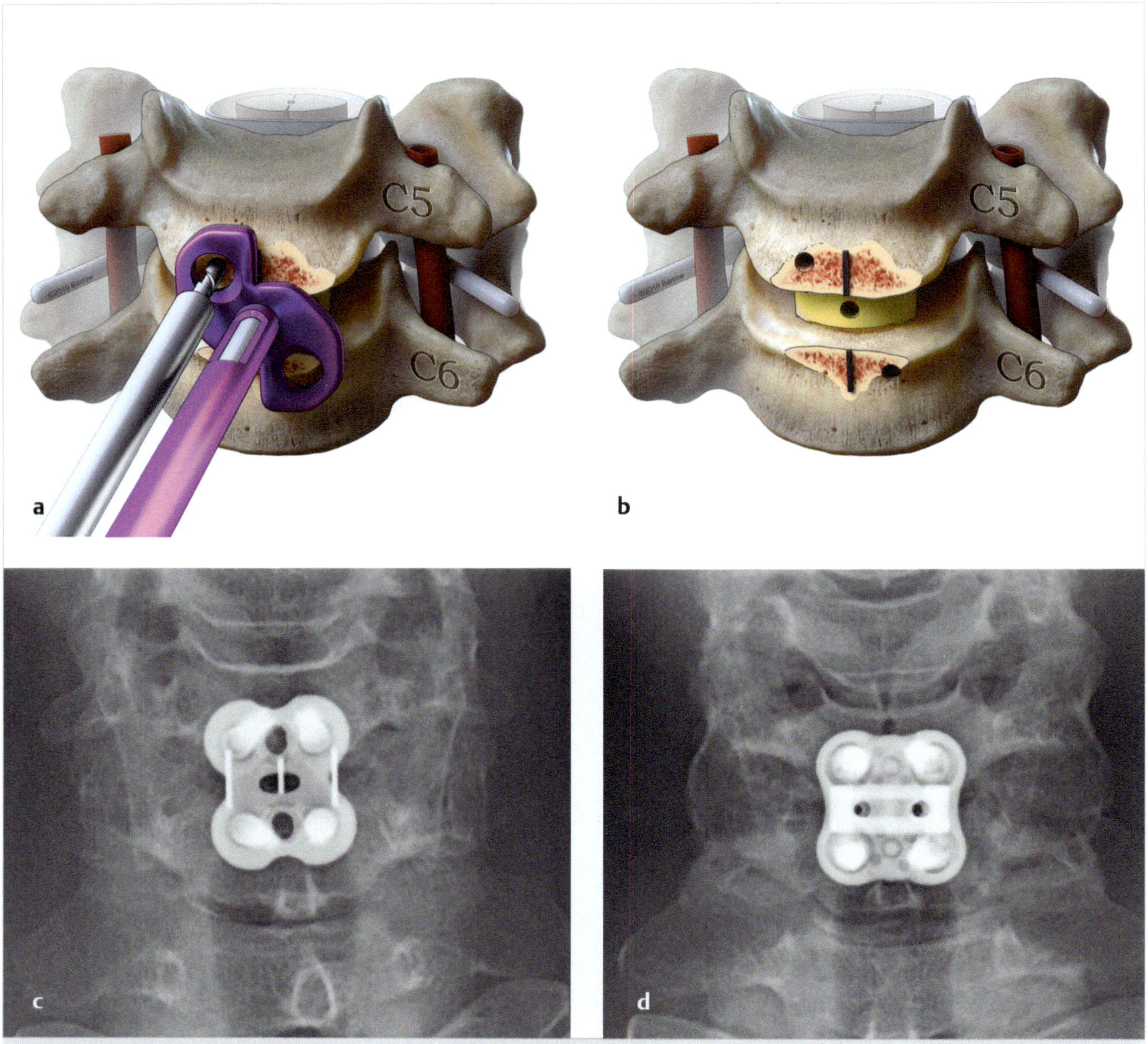

Fig. 9.43 Illustration demonstrating fixation of a cervical plate with a template. **(a)** With the template in position and aligned in the orthogonal position, the holes are drilled. **(b)** The template is removed, and the anterior cervical plate is placed over the top of the drilled holes. The cervical plate is then fixated to the spine. **(c)** Postoperative anteroposterior (AP) radiograph of a cervical template used with a polyetheretherketone interbody spacer for placement of an anterior cervical plate. **(d)** Postoperative AP radiograph of a cervical template used with a titanium interbody spacer for placement of an anterior cervical plate.

be placed. Once two distinct vertebral bodies have been drilled, the line has been defined, and I proceed with drilling and securing the remaining screws.

The main difference between the single-level and multilevel template is the inability to size the plate, which may require cervical plates to be passed in and out of the field. That feat is even more challenging in multilevel cases. Still, the multilevel template capitalizes on capturing midline and predrilling a hole that will be at least greater than 5 mm away from the adjacent segment. When the multilevel plate passes onto the spine, the screw finds its predrilled hole and one point of fixation is captured. The cervical plate is aligned using the various interbody spacers to ensure orthogonal placement (▶ Fig. 9.44).

With the plate aligned and points of fixation established, the final step is securing the plate onto the vertebral bodies. For this task, a combination of fixed and variable-angle screws creates an ideal environment for an arthrodesis to occur. Given its remarkable developmental history, it is worthwhile to review the biomechanics and rationale in such a construct.

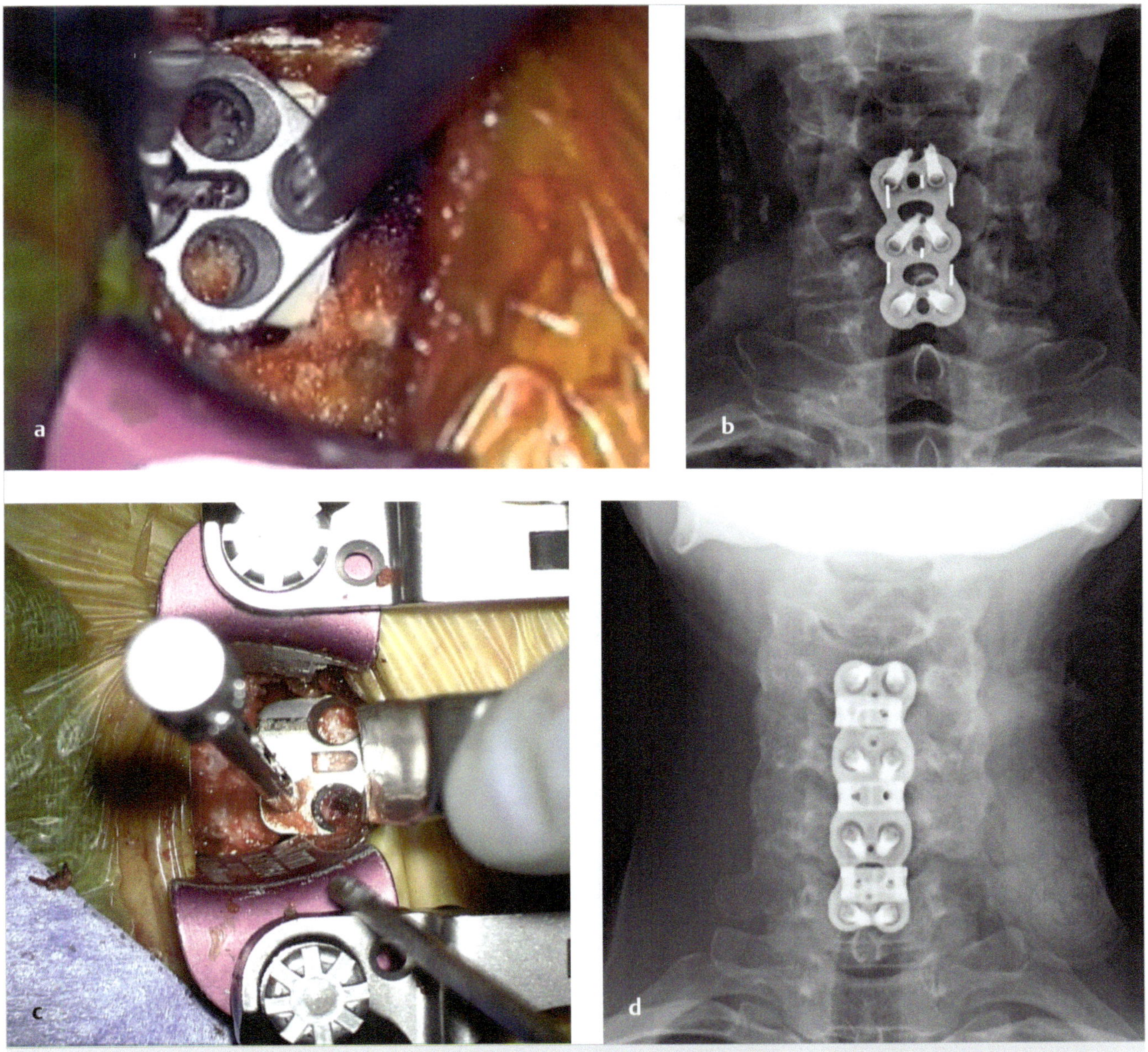

Fig. 9.44 Multilevel cervical template. Building on the principles of the single-level cervical template, the multilevel cervical template establishes the midline by securing two holes in the rostral or caudal vertebral bodies. These two points make a line that ensures orthogonal and midline placement of the cervical plate. **(a)** Intraoperative photograph of the multilevel cervical template secured into the interbody spacer of the rostral aspect of the construct. After the holes are drilled, the plate is placed, and one point of fixation is achieved. The caudal aspect of the plate is aligned with the guidance of the interbody spacer at the caudal aspect of the construct. The result is a midline plate in line with the long axis of the spine. **(b)** Anteroposterior (AP) radiograph showing a midline orthogonal plate. **(c)** A multilevel cervical template used in a three-level anterior cervical discectomy and fusion. The cervical template has been secured into a titanium interbody spacer. In this intraoperative photograph, the hole has been drilled into the caudal most vertebral body of the construct. **(d)** AP radiograph showing midline and orthogonal placement of the cervical plate.

9.38 Fixed versus Variable-Angle Screws

The origin of variable screws has a remarkable evolutionary tale of observation, trial and error. At its very core, the development of the screw–plate interface revolves around two concepts: Wolff's law and stress shielding.[23] Early in the history of instrumentation of the cervical spine, it seemed intuitive to place a rigid plate with rigid fixation onto the cervical spine, which held the cervical vertebrae immobile while the graft fused across the two vertebral bodies. After all, the pseudarthroses that occurred in noninstrumented fusions must have been due to the absence of fixation. Although such a concept works perfectly well in construction, where immobilization of two objects allows for an epoxy to dry or cement to solidify, remarkably, surgeons found this did not work in the human cervical spine. The observation was that screws and plates would break and the interbody graft would not reliably fuse between the vertebral bodies.[24] How could this be if what the interbody graft needed was immobilization for fusion to occur?

In afterthought, the answer was obvious. Surgeons were not waiting for epoxy or cement to dry. They were waiting for the biology of bone healing to occur. The presence of a rigidly fixated plate prevented the loading of the graft and, as a result, stopped the mechanotransduction needed for bone formation, which is a well-defined entity known as stress shielding.[25] A rigidly fixated plate protects the graft from any stress that would be loaded upon it. While this was ideal for construction, it was the antithesis of what was needed for arthrodesis to occur. Rigid fixation prevented an optimal environment for bone healing and growth. Our orthopaedic colleagues have incorporated prevention of stress shielding in many of their implants, which is best illustrated by the dynamic hip screw, which stabilizes a hip fracture while still allowing the fracture to be loaded by the weight of the patient and thereby heal with the advantage of the mechanotransduction empowering bone formation.

The German anatomist and surgeon Julius Wolff described these observations regarding bone physiology in the mid-19th century. Wolff made the simple observation that when a load on a particular bone increases, that bone will remodel itself over time to become stronger so that it may resist that load. The signal that conveys the need for remodeling is known as mechanotransduction, which translates the mechanical forces into the cellular cascades that remodel the bone. Wolff also observed that the inverse is also true, which explains why the early fixations with rigid plates on the cervical spine were prone to failure. If the load on a bone decreases, the stimulus for mechanotransduction also decreases. The absence of a signal to remodel bone favors increased turnover of bone and bone resorption. In the end, the bone becomes weaker. In the context of cervical fusion, if a rigidly fixated plate shields the interbody graft from loads that would otherwise trigger mechanotransduction, there is no signal to increase remodeling; as a result, the graft is not incorporated, becomes weaker and has the potential to resorb. The absence of an arthrodesis leads to the eventual metal fatigue, plate failure and screw breakage.[25]

One way to resolve this issue is with dynamic plates, where a mechanism is in place within the plate itself that allows for translation to occur and thereby load of the graft. Dynamic plates eliminate stress shielding. Another alternative is to examine the screw–plate interface in a rigid plate. As already demonstrated in the early experience with cervical plating, how a screw interfaces with a plate can stress shield the graft. An alteration of the geometry of the screw head may have the potential to change the way the screw interfaces with the plate. The rounded configuration of the variable-angle screw allows for the screw to interface with the plate but allows for a change in angulation of the screw within the plate so that the rostral vertebral body may still load the graft. Such a change in angle would otherwise be prevented by a fixed screw, which interfaces with the plate in a manner that locks the position of the screw at one angle.

As the stresses on the construct change, the variable-angle screw may slightly alter its angle within the plate and thereby load the graft. Benzel has called this entity "controlled subsidence."[25] Thus, it is at the plate–screw interface that an environment conducive to bone healing is created. By convention in my practice, I use fixed-angle screws only in the caudal vertebral body and variable-angle screws in all of the rostral segments. The fixed-angle screws anchor the plate, and the variable-angle screws allow for loading of the interbody grafts. I have had many residents and fellows ask why not use variable-angle screws at all segments. I always readily concede that the use of variable-angle screws throughout the entire construct is a perfectly viable option. However, I suggest that the use of fixed-angle screws throughout an entire construct is counter to our understanding of bone healing, and I would avoid such a construct.

9.39 Drill Guides and Craftsmanship

Another reason to strive for a perfectly placed midline and orthogonal plate is that it is indicative of the craftsmanship performed throughout the entire operation. Placement of the cervical screws into the plate should be in keeping with this theme.

I strive for the lateral image to have the appearance of one screw at each level. For this to happen, the screw holes in the plate need to line up on a perfect lateral image. The first step in this process is a perfect lateral fluoroscopic image. Crisp end plates and parallel facet joints of the level being operated upon are the prerequisites for such an image, which reinforces the importance of a reliable radiology technician. Viewing a lateral fluoroscopic image with the cervical plate pinned into position becomes yet another systems check to confirm orthogonality. If on a lateral fluoroscopic image where there are crisp end plates and parallel facet joints the screws holes do not line up, the plate must be tilted. You do not need an AP image to confirm this. In fact, I believe that an AP image adds to the confusion. If I see that the rostral and caudal screw holes in the plate do not line up on a lateral image, I reassess the position of the plate based on my landmarks and the interbody spacers.

Once the plate is in an orthogonal midline position, I use the fixed-angle drill guide to drill all the holes even though I am using variable-angle screws in the rostral vertebral bodies. The fixed-angle drill guide marries into the plate at one angle. For the particular cervical plate that I use, the fixed angle is 10 degrees in the rostral or caudal direction and 6 degrees medially. I have found it helpful for residents and fellows to engage the fixed-angle drill guide on the back table to grasp this concept and to experience the unmistakable tactile sensation of the drill guide engaging the plate. Once locked into position, there is very little movement of the guide. I can now ensure the same angle at every screw without so much as one fluoroscopic image. The result is all screws are in the same plane and parallel to one another with the distinct appearance of one screw per level on a lateral radiograph. The use of a fixed drill guide at the rostral level or levels is only for the trajectory. I still use variable-angle screws in these holes to allow for loading the interbody graft, but it is the fixed drill guide that makes these variable-angle screws line up in a symmetrical fashion (▶ Fig. 9.45).

At times, the guide will not lock into the plate when it is on the cervical spine. The cause is typically a bony prominence from an osteophyte preventing the nose of the guide from

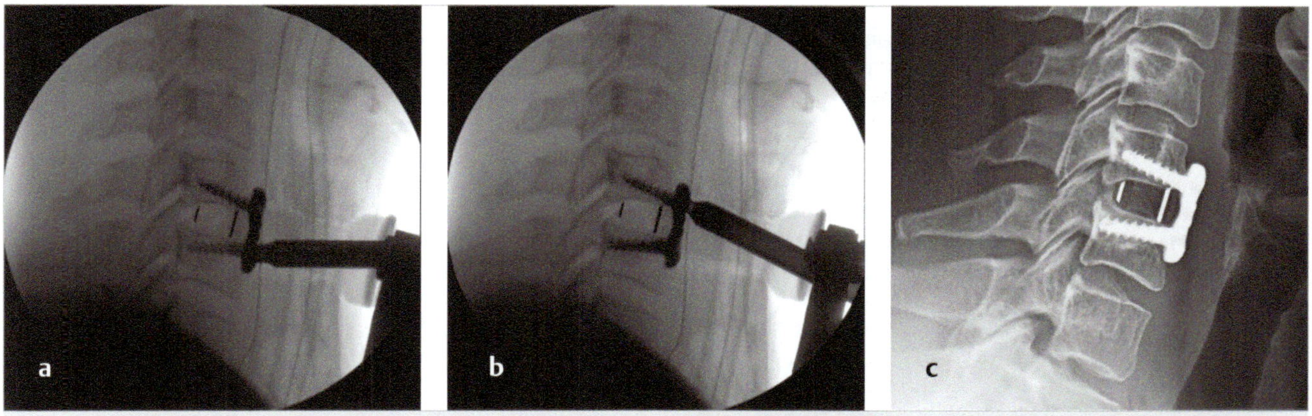

Fig. 9.45 Use of a fixed-angle drill guide for plate fixation. **(a)** Lateral radiographs demonstrating placement of an anterior cervical plate with the use of a fixed-angled drill guide at all screw holes. **(b)** When the fixed-angle drill guide marries into the cervical plate, the rostrocaudal angle and the angle of convergence will be the same for all screws. Variable-angle screws are still used at the rostral segment and fixed-angle screws at the caudal segment. **(c)** Postoperative lateral radiograph demonstrating coplanar placement of the screws.

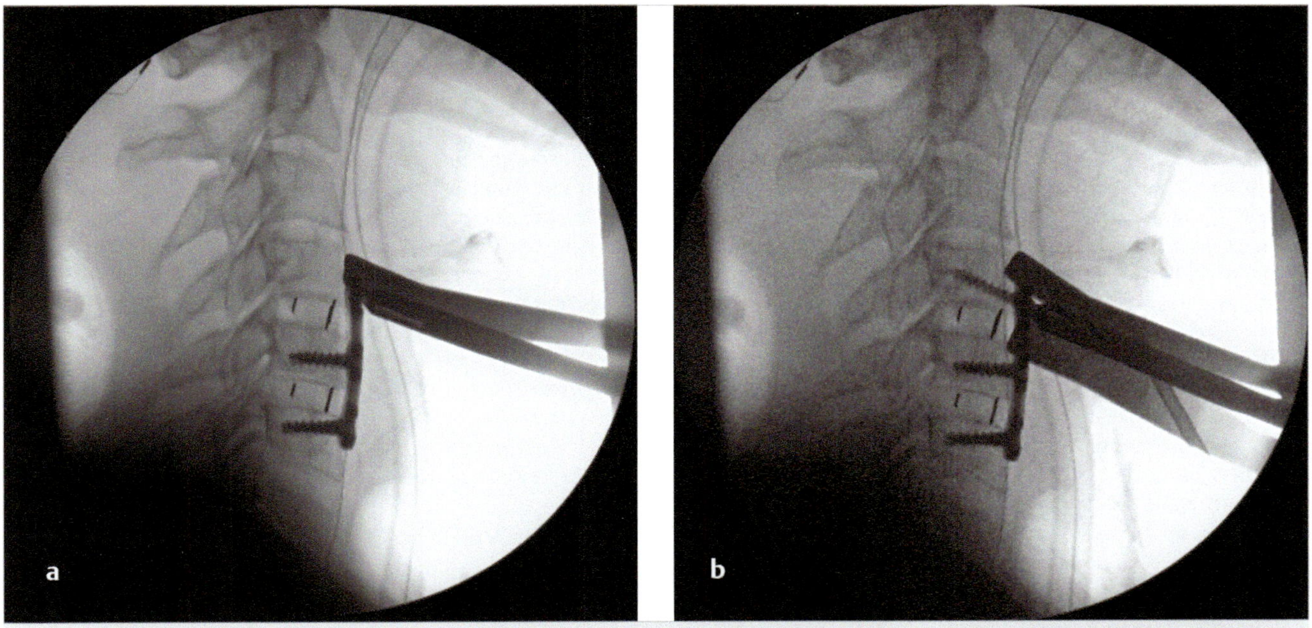

Fig. 9.46 Use of a variable-angle drill guide for fixation of the rostral screws. **(a)** Lateral fluoroscopic image where the circumstance arose that the 10 degrees of angulation allowed by the fixed-angle drill guide did not allow for the optimal trajectory into the vertebral body. **(b)** A variable-angle drill guide was used to set the optimal trajectory. This trajectory was matched for the ideal placement of the second screw to match the trajectory of the first screw.

advancing into the plate. A match head drill bit and a steady hand can drill out the bony prominence within the screw hole of the cervical plate to create a recess to allow the drill guide to lock into position. I have found that such precise drilling prevents the need to remove the plate from its ideal position in order to flatten the obstructive osteophyte.

9.40 Variable-Angle Drill Guide

On occasion, the size of the ideal plate for one particular segment is such that 10 degrees of angulation allowed by the fixed-angle guide in the rostrocaudal plane is inadequate to engage the bone. When I suspect this to be the case, I engage the fixed-angle drill guide and obtain a lateral fluoroscopic image. It becomes readily obvious if the angle afforded by the fixed-angle drill guide allows for an optimal trajectory into the vertebral body (▶ Fig. 9.46). If the trajectory is suboptimal, I need to use a variable-angle drill guide. The variable angle allows for up to 18 degrees of angulation in the rostrocaudal direction and can converge medially up to 17 degrees. It is important to keep in mind that too much of a medial convergence can result in the screws colliding within the vertebral body.

I can still recall one of my first operations where all that was left to complete it was to place one last screw in the top left corner of the plate. I remember encountering stiff resistance attempting to place that final screw. What I did not recognize was that I had set too much convergence on the medial trajectory. While the screw lined up in the lateral plane, the degree of convergence had the screws colliding with one another. I distinctly remember being mystified by my inability to advance the screw past the locking mechanism. After several wasted minutes of struggling, a quick AP fluoroscopic image answered the question: the left-side screw that I was attempting to place had encountered the overly converged right-side screw. Failure is the best teacher. It was the failure with that one last screw so many years ago that comes to mind every time I set a medial trajectory with a variable-angle drill guide. That episode also highlights the advantage of a fixed-angle drill guide, which sets the angle at 6 degrees of convergence in most systems.

Recognizing the perils of an overly converged trajectory, I am always more conscientious when I set the medial trajectory with a variable-angle drill guide. To ensure an adequate trajectory into the vertebral body, I typically set the rostrocaudal angle and obtain a lateral fluoroscopic image for the first screw. I then obtain a second fluoroscopic image for the second screw in order to match the trajectory (▶ Fig. 9.46).

9.41 Screw Length

I strive to place the longest screw that I can safely secure into each vertebral body. The optimal screw length is partly dependent on the trajectory and partly dependent on the size of the vertebral body. There are several visual cues readily available that indicate the ideal length of the screw. The preoperative measurements on an MRI or CT image can typically provide me with a sense of what length would be ideal for the patient. By convention, I select 12-mm Caspar posts for women and 14-mm posts for men. When I have a lateral fluoroscopic image of the posts in position, I will have my first frame of reference to decide what length of screw I can use. Screws typically come in increments of 2 mm, beginning at either 10 or 11 mm in length depending on the system.

I base my final decision for the length of the screw on the lateral fluoroscopic image with the guide in position. For the particular systems I use, I know the drill lengths when they are bottomed out within the drill guide. If there is any question regarding a safe length, a lateral fluoroscopic image with the hubbed drill guide allows me to reliably approximate the ideal length of the screw. A variable angle in a large vertebral body may allow for screw lengths as long as 19 mm (▶ Fig. 9.47).

9.42 Two-Incision Technique for a Four-Level ACDF

About six times a year, a patient presents to my clinic with an MRI and radiograph that resembles the images in ▶ Fig. 9.48. The patient's examination demonstrates overt signs of myelopathy. When these patients present, there is no question as to the role of surgery or the number of levels. The only question is whether the operation should be performed through an anterior approach, a posterior approach or a combination of the two. For the purposes of this section, we will assume the anterior approach is the surgery of choice.

Until I happened upon Chin et al,[3] in which Riew described the two-incision technique for the four-level ACDF, I have to admit that I did not look forward to these cases at all. For years, I struggled between an unsightly carotid incision and a long transverse incision for these four-level cases. I was never satisfied with these options, nor were my patients. The carotid endarterectomy type of incision was not aesthetically pleasing but provided generous exposure to the entire anterior cervical spine at all segments. However, the carotid incision was not in keeping with the tenet of the Caspar ratio that optimizes the surgical target to surgical exposure. One long transverse incision was more aesthetically pleasing, but even with relaxed tissue planes, the rostral and caudal poles of the exposure were difficult to reach, and fixation of the plate was quite a struggle. Either of these approaches resulted in prolonged dysphagia and sometimes permanent dysphagia. On one occasion, a patient required a temporary feeding tube. It was clear that I needed to find a better way to perform this operation. The ideal exposure would offer the extent of reach provided by a carotid endarterectomy type of exposure, with the aesthetics of a transverse incision and an overall decrease in dysphagia. One attempt at the two-incision technique for a four-level operation was all I needed to confirm that Chin and colleagues[3] had found a better technique for this operation.

Approaching a four-level ACDF with two incisions transforms the daunting task of a four-level ACDF into essentially two distinct two-level cervical operations that overlap only at the time of applying the anterior cervical plate. After my initial foray with the two-incision technique, I have never found a reason to consider any other approach. The two separate incisions vastly facilitate the exposure across all four segments, simplify passage of the cervical plate, optimize access and trajectory to the screw holes on the plate and expedite the entire procedure. The following section is a review of the two-incision technique. While I present the technique below, I invite the reader to go straight to the source and read Riew's original description in Chin et al.[3]

9.43 Planning the Incision for a Four-Level ACDF

I plan the two incisions with fluoroscopy as if the intention were to perform two distinct two-level ACDFs. I center each incision over the central vertebral body as shown in ▶ Fig. 9.49. By way of example, for a C3–4, C4–5, C5–6 and C6–7 ACDF, I center the first incision over C4 and the second incision over C6. The rostral incision is 20 mm in length, and the caudal incision is longer, 30 mm in length, to facilitate passage of the long cervical plate onto the spine (▶ Fig. 9.50).[3]

9.44 Surgical Technique

With the patient positioned and the incisions planned, I begin the operation at the rostral incision with the intent of exposing two requisite anatomical units. For clarity in the description of this technique, I use the C3–4, C4–5, C5–6 and C6–7 case described above. I divide the platysma, undermine the tissue planes and descend the avascular plane medial to the sternocleidomastoid muscle. Relaxing the various tissue planes is always important, but in a four-level ACDF, the importance becomes even more pronounced because of the extent of exposure that

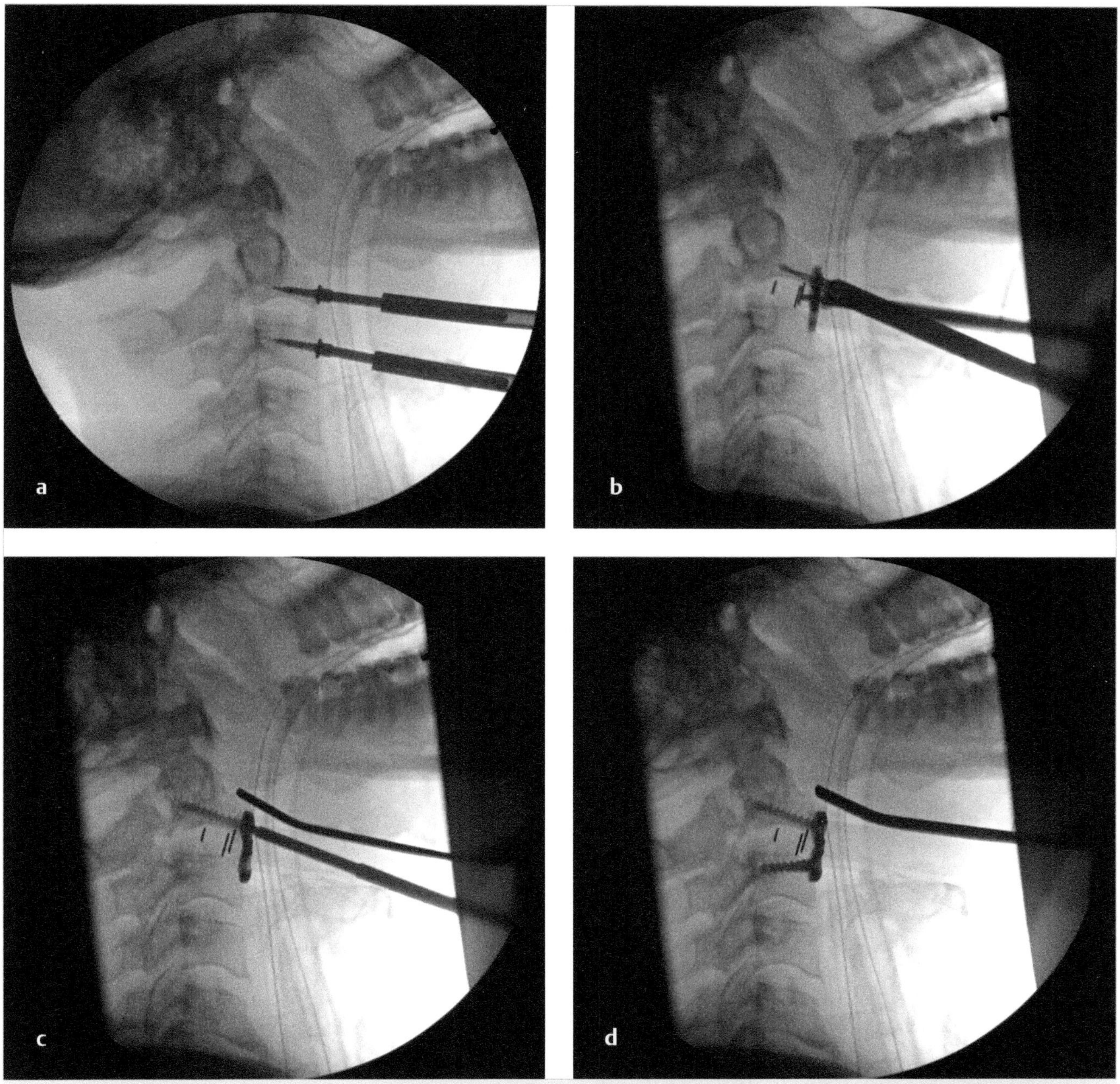

Fig. 9.47 Determination of the length of the cervical plate screw in the management of a Hangman fracture. (a) Lateral fluoroscopic image of the cervical spine with the Caspar posts in position. Knowing that the Caspar posts are 14 mm in length allows an early estimate regarding the length of the screw. (b) Lateral fluoroscopic image with the drill hubbed into the drill guide. Although the Caspar post allows for an approximation of the screw length, the trajectory of the screw also impacts the length. In this image, the trajectory of the screw is set, and the length of the drill guide is 11 mm. With the trajectory set, there appears to be more than 1 cm from the tip of the drill to the back wall of the vertebral body. A 19-mm screw was selected. (c) Lateral fluoroscopic image demonstrating placement of the 19-mm screw. Before locking the screw, an image is obtained to ensure ample distance to the back wall. (d) Lateral fluoroscopic image of the final construct demonstrating 19-mm screws at C2 and 15-mm screws at C3.

needs to be mobilized for placement of such a long anterior cervical plate. After confirming the level, I expose the requisite anatomical unit first for C3–4 and then begin anew along a more caudal plane of exposure medial to the sternocleidomastoid muscle and expose C4–5. I eliminate any fascial bands between these two exposures and confirm that I have exposed a transverse dimension of 22 mm from 5 mm above the C3–4 disc space to as much of the C5 vertebral body that I have access to from this exposure. I complete these two exposures using handheld Cloward retractors and confirm that no additional exposure will be needed at the time of plating by measuring the transverse and vertical dimensions of my exposure. No retractors are left in place in the first incision to avoid sustained retraction on the esophagus, and I turn my attention to the second incision.

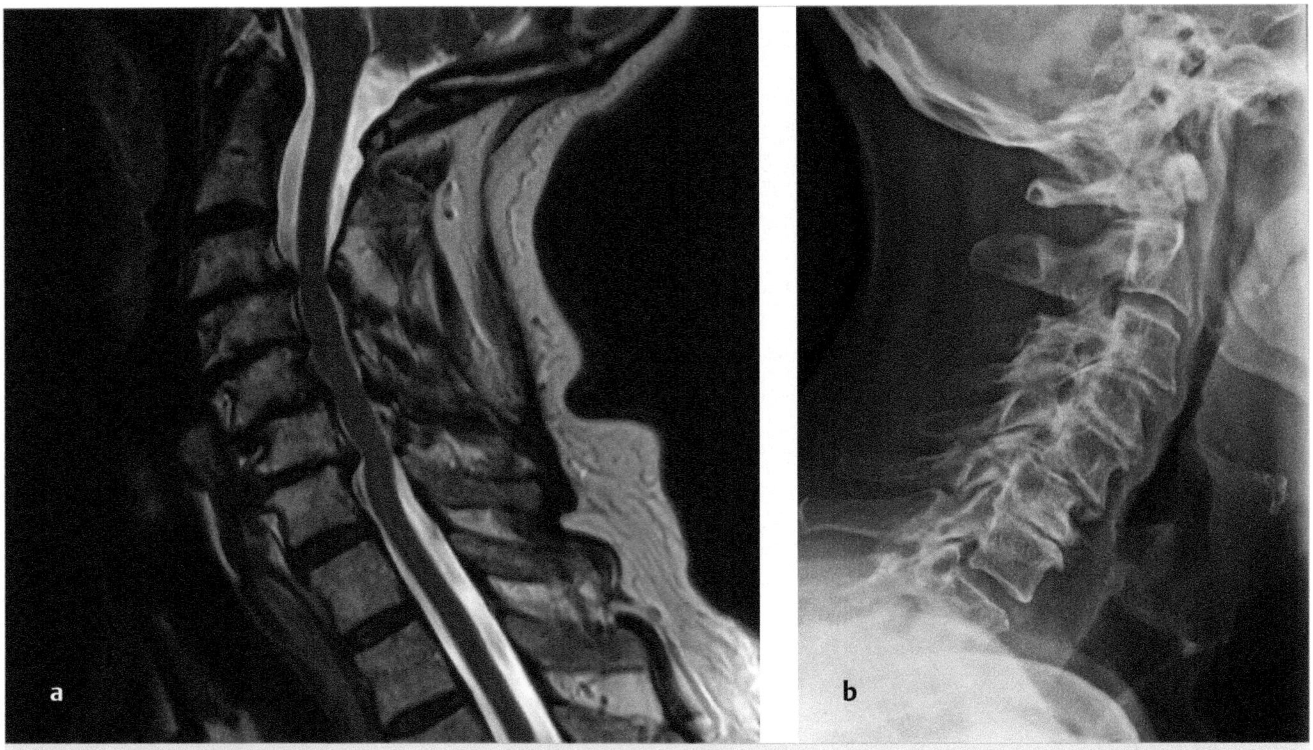

Fig. 9.48 Four levels of cervical spondylosis and stenosis. **(a)** Sagittal T2-weighted magnetic resonance imaging of a 58-year-old mechanic with four levels of advanced spondylosis and spinal cord compression. The patient presented with overt signs of myelopathy and was unable to work as a mechanic because of progressive loss of manual dexterity. **(b)** Lateral radiograph showing preservation of the C2–3 and C7–T1 disc space but advanced spondylosis at C3–4, C4–5, C5–6 and C6–7 with listhesis at C5–6. The only comprehensive anterior surgical solution for this patient was a four-level anterior cervical discectomy and fusion. A posterior operation and a combination of an anterior and posterior operation are equally viable options.

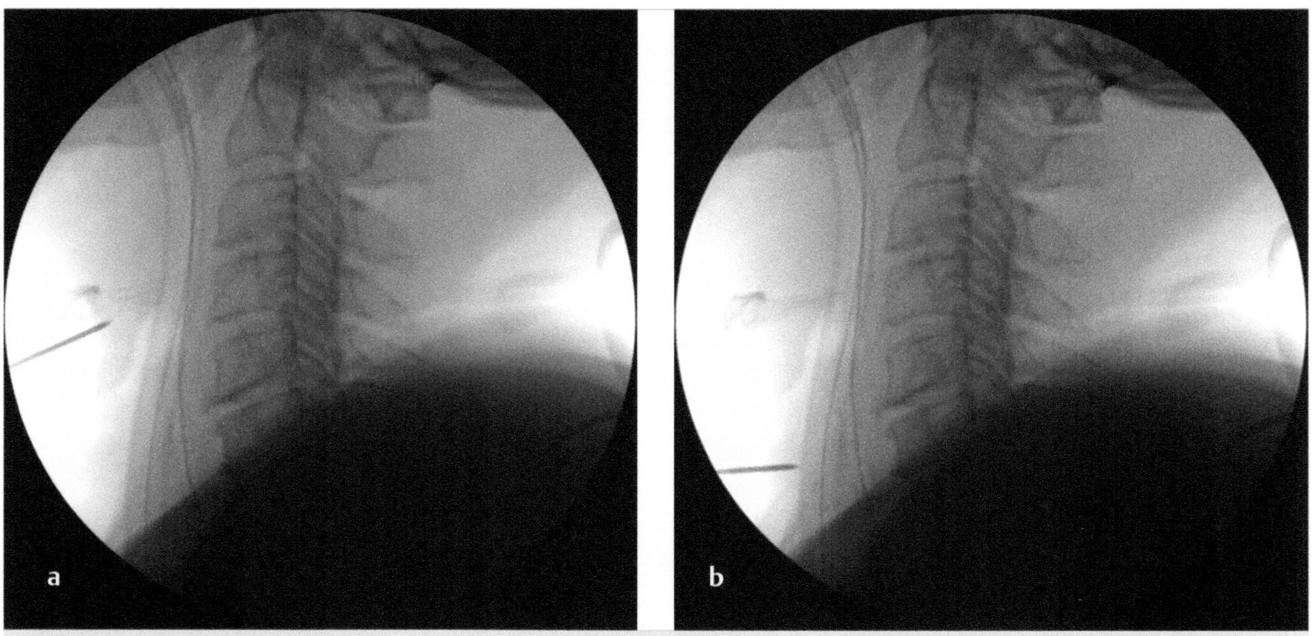

Fig. 9.49 Planning the two incisions for a four-level anterior cervical discectomy and fusion. **(a)** Lateral fluoroscopic image with a Steinman pin at the midpoint of the C4 vertebral body. An incision in that location provides access to the C3–4 and C4–5 segments. **(b)** Lateral fluoroscopic image with a Steinman pin at the midpoint of the C6 vertebral body. An incision in that location provides access to the C5–6 and C6–7 segments.

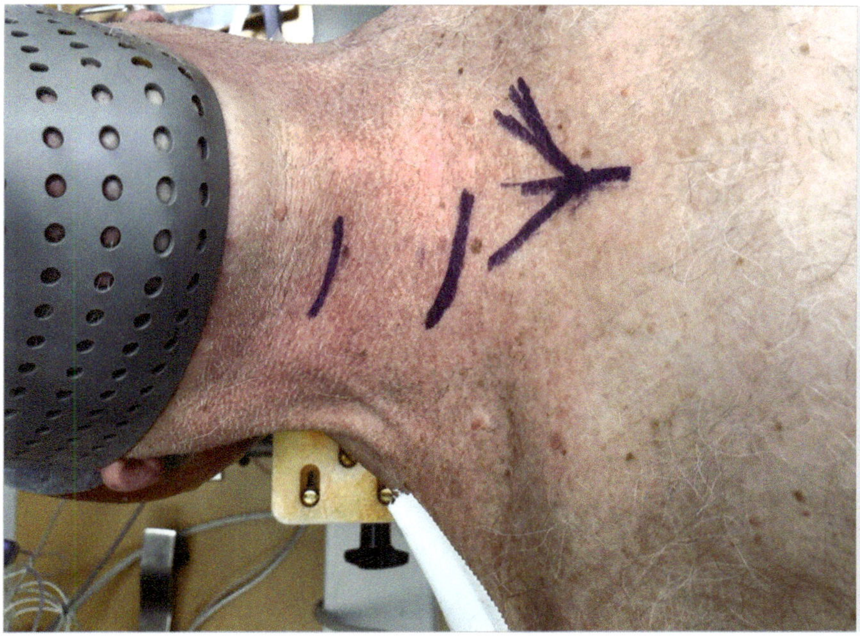

Fig. 9.50 Marking the incision for a four-level anterior cervical discectomy and fusion (ACDF). Photograph demonstrating the two incisions for a C3–4, C4–5, C5–6 and C6–7 ACDFs. The rostral incision is 20 to 25 mm in length, and the caudal incision is longer at 30 to 35 mm in length to facilitate passage of the long anterior cervical plate. Riew and colleagues recommend a minimum distance of 3 cm between the incisions.[3]

I begin the exposure of C5–6 and C6–7 as if I am doing an isolated two-level operation similar to the one I just performed at C3–4 and C4–5. After dividing the platysma, I descend the avascular plane medial to the sternocleidomastoid muscle and expose the requisite anatomical unit at C5–6 and then repeat at C6–7. When completing the exposure of the C5–6 segment, I encounter the caudal aspect of the initial exposure. I begin relaxing the tissue planes between these two exposures. Before I place the first set of self-retaining retractor blades to begin to decompress the first level, I confirm that I have access to 5 mm above the C3–4 disc space and 5 mm below the C6–7 disc space. I also confirm 22 mm of transverse exposure at each segment.

The self-retaining retractors are secured over the C3–4 segment, and Caspar posts are placed into the vertebral bodies of C3 and C4. By convention, I begin working within the first incision to complete the decompression and interbody spacer placement at C3–4 first and then remove the retractors altogether from that level leaving only the C4 Caspar post in place (▶ Fig. 9.51). All retraction on the esophagus at this level has now ceased. It is important to mark the geometric midline on C3 based on the uncovertebral joints, as discussed in Section 9.25, Cervical Plating. A prominent mark is one of the valuable guides that helps secure the plate into the midline. Then I turn to the C6–7 segment, placing the self-retaining retractors and Caspar posts in place to complete the decompression and interbody spacer at that segment (▶ Fig. 9.51). When complete, the Caspar post is removed from C7 but left in place at C6. Because the C6–7 is the caudal most segment, I use the two-level template at this time to place the two screw holes with a fixed-angled trajectory into C7 (Video 9.1). Bone wax or a liquid hemostatic agent controls any vertebral body bleeding. I mark the holes with a purple marking pen, to make them easy to locate when it becomes time to secure the plate.

I return to the rostral incision, replace the self-retaining retractors, place a Caspar post into C5 to complete the C4–5 ACDF and then remove the C4 Caspar post. Only C5–6 remains to be decompressed at this point. There is a Caspar post in C5 and C6 but through two different exposures. Logically, the caudal incision offers the greatest access to the C5–6 segment, and so the C5 Caspar post is removed from the rostral incision and immediately replaced into the same hole through the caudal incision. I have to accept the fact that the fit of the post is never as firm as when it was initially placed into C5.

One advantage of the two-incision technique is the absence of prolonged esophageal retraction from within one incision. The retractors are constantly being switched from one exposure to another as I systematically address each segment. However, perhaps the greatest advantage to the two-incision technique is the passage of the anterior cervical plate. With a long transverse incision, the passage of the plate is challenging, to say the least. In passing the plate, the inability to see where the plate encounters soft-tissue resistance and becomes hung up on an anterior osteophyte ridge from one of the vertebral bodies is its greatest liability. The two-incision technique eliminates any issue with visualization of the rostral segments as the plate passes onto the cervical spine. The long caudal incision affords the ability to pass a long plate. The rostral incision simultaneously allows for direct visualization of the plate and therefore the ability to guide the plate into the geometric midline of each segment as it is being passed from the caudal incision (▶ Fig. 9.52, Video 9.1).

There are two holes with a fixed-angled trajectory already drilled into C7 with the multilevel cervical template. These holes are based on the position of the interbody, which, almost by definition, places the plate in the midline. With confidence in the location of the screw holes, I place one fixed-angle screw into C7. I secure the C7 screw up to the plate without locking it into position and then turn my attention to the rostral exposure. I assess the length of the cervical plate with direct visualization or a lateral fluoroscopic image (▶ Fig. 9.53). The rostral aspect of the plate needs to be less than 5 mm away from the C2–3 disc space. If the plate is an appropriate length, I fixate it

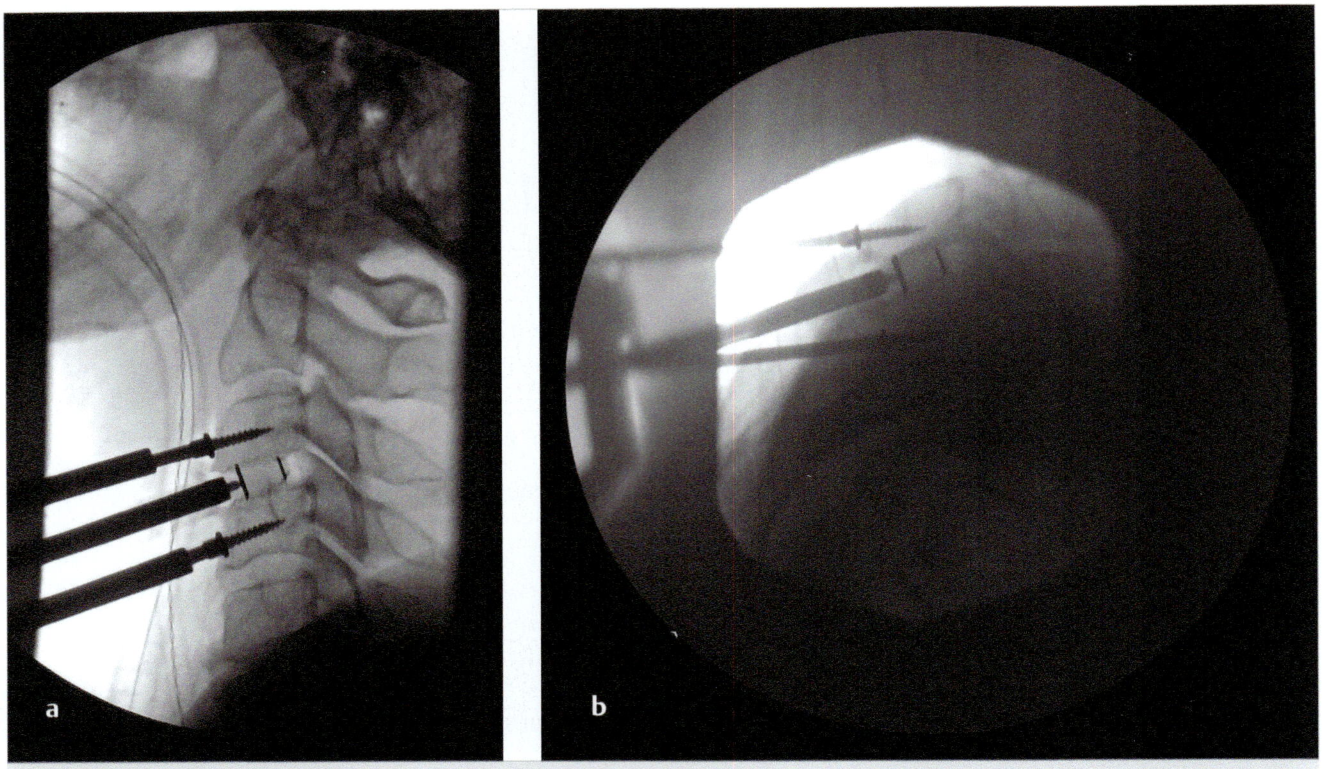

Fig. 9.51 The sequence of the decompression to minimize esophageal retraction. **(a)** Lateral fluoroscopic image showing C3–4 as the first level done in a four-level anterior cervical discectomy and fusion (ACDF). It is important to prominently mark the midline at C3 for the eventual cervical plate alignment in the midline. **(b)** Lateral fluoroscopic image showing C6–7 as the second level performed. Transitioning from exposure to exposure decreases the sustained esophageal retraction from one exposure and may translate into less dysphagia. Upon completion of the C6–7 ACDF, a multilevel template may be used to place fixed-angle screw holes that facilitate fixation of the cervical plate into the midline.

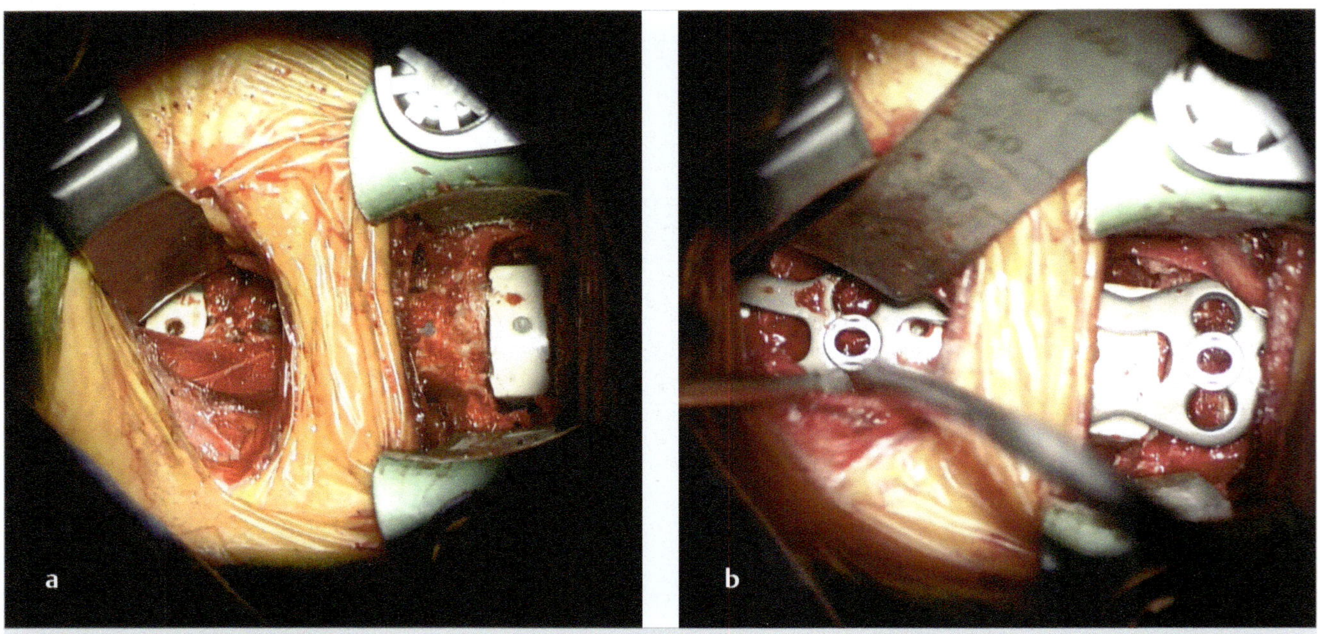

Fig. 9.52 Passage of a four-level plate using a two-incision technique. **(a)** Intraoperative photograph showing self-retaining retractors in position in the caudal incision over the top of the C5–6 segment and a handheld Cloward in the rostral incision exposing the C3–4 segment. **(b)** Intraoperative photograph of the passage of the long cervical plate. Working through the rostral incision allows the surgeon to guide the plate into position.

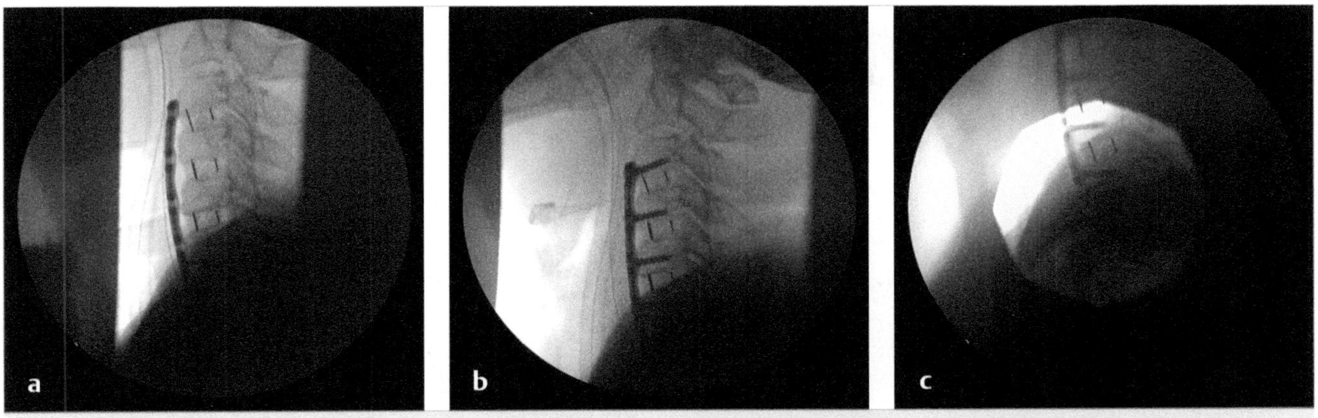

Fig. 9.53 Placement of a four-level anterior cervical plate. (a) Lateral fluoroscopic image with plate secured into only one screw hole in the C7 vertebral body in order to allow for rotation. Direct visual inspection at C3 demonstrates adequate coverage of the C3 vertebral body and less than 5 mm of a plate-to-disc distance. Note that there is no contact of the cervical plate with the C4 or C5 vertebral bodies. (b) Lateral fluoroscopic image with the anterior cervical plate secured into position. Note that the vertebral bodies were pulled up to the cervical plate with screw fixation, thereby restoring even more lordosis. (c) Coned-down view at C6–7 to confirm a plate-to-disc distance of 5 mm.

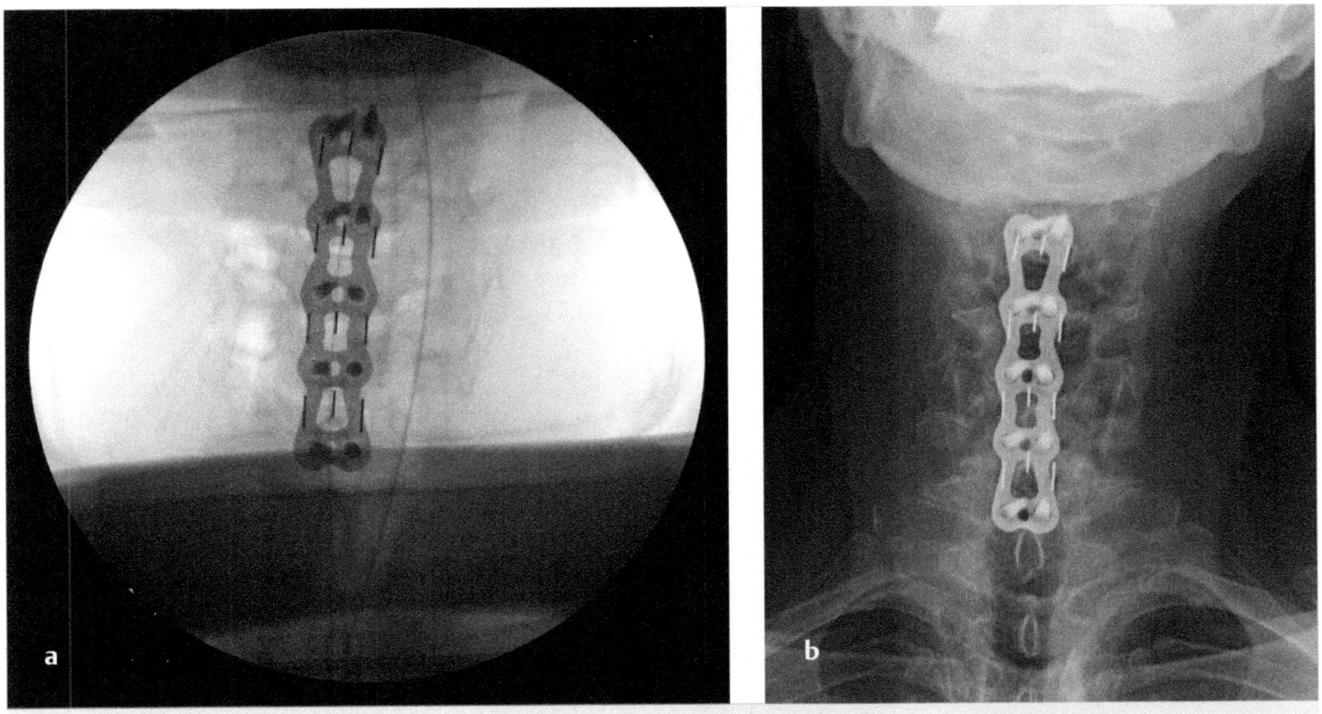

Fig. 9.54 Midline and orthogonal placement of a four-level anterior cervical plate. (a) Final anteroposterior (AP) fluoroscopic image of a four-level anterior cervical discectomy and fusion. When the cervical screw holes are indexed off of the interbody spacer at C7 using a template and the midline on C3 is prominently marked, a midline orthogonal plate can be achieved without the need for an AP fluoroscopic image. (b) AP radiograph 3 years after surgery. No additional posterior fixation was needed in this circumstance.

to the C3 vertebral body. The plate can still rotate with the C7 screw in position. I rotate the rostral aspect of the plate over the midline of C3 using the window within the plate to align it with the interbody and my midline mark and capture that position with a fixed- or variable-angle drill guide into C3. Once variable-angle screws are placed into C3, the plate is locked into a position. I have not found it useful to obtain an AP image at this point. Instead, I peer through the various windows of the cervical plate and should see the plate over the midline of the interbody spacer. I secure the plate at C4 and C5 through the rostral incision and C6 and C7 through the caudal incision. I ensure that I have locked the screws into the plate. I obtain the final AP and lateral fluoroscopic image before closure (▶ Fig. 9.54).

Part of the informed consent for a four-level ACDF should include a discussion regarding the potential for posterior instrumentation, especially in the context of a significantly

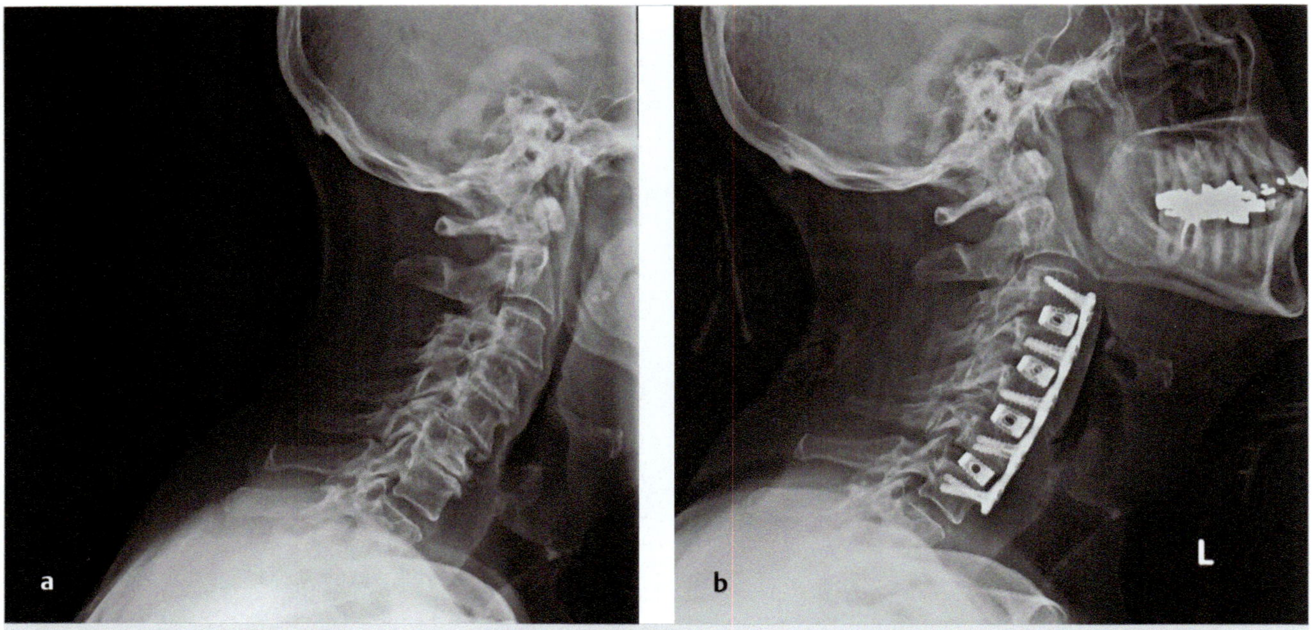

Fig. 9.55 Four-level anterior cervical discectomy with fusion in a patient with a positive sagittal vertical axis (SVA). Lateral radiographs of the patient shown in ► Fig. 9.48. **(a)** Preoperative study with multiple levels of degeneration and listhesis at C5–6. **(b)** Postoperative lateral radiograph that shows the decompression and restoration of disc height without significant improvement in the SVA. Such a patient needs to be monitored closely over time. This image was taken 12 months after surgery and shows evidence of arthrodesis in the four segments and no progression of the SVA. No additional surgery was required.

positive sagittal vertical axis (► Fig. 9.55). However, in the absence of a significant deformity, a four-level ACDF may be safely performed with close observation in the weeks and months afterward to determine whether posterior instrumentation is necessary (► Fig. 9.56). The literature has clearly demonstrated an increased incidence of pseudarthroses in multilevel cervical fusions, and so long-term follow-up for a minimum of 1 year is necessary for these patients.

My experience with the two-incision technique is consistent with the report by Chin and colleagues[3] regarding dysphagia. However, no formal objective assessment for dysphagia was used in the reported patients or in my series. From that standpoint, the two-incision technique remains worthy of continued study. The subjective assessment by the patients regarding the cosmesis of their incisions has been favorable (► Fig. 9.57).

9.45 Closure

Closure begins after the final AP fluoroscopic image. The self-retaining retractors are removed, and each level inspected for hemostasis with Cloward handheld retractors. In particular, I look for any bleeding along the longus colli muscles. I have had one symptomatic postoperative hematoma that required surgical evacuation the following day, and I will never forget it. At the time of exploration, I identified an arterial bleeder on the longus colli muscle undoubtedly caused by one of the self-retaining retractor blades. Since that event, I spend some time thoroughly examining those columns of muscle on either side of the vertebral body.

I seldom, if ever, leave a drain for a single- or two-level operation, unless it was performed due to trauma. On occasion, I may leave a drain for a three-level operation, based on my overall sense of hemostasis from the case. I always leave a fully fluted Jackson-Pratt drain for a four-level ACDF without being able to identify a logical argument to maintain such a dogmatic position on the matter.

I reapproximate the platysma and subcutaneous tissues with interrupted 3.0 polyglactin 910 sutures and bring the skin edges with interrupted 4.0 polyglactin sutures. Finally, I place a single Steri-Strip (3 M Company, Maplewood, MN) over the incision after the liquid adhesive has dried.

9.46 Postoperative Management

Single- and two-level ACDF and arthroplasty patients are not issued cervical collars, but three- and four-level ACDF patients are, and they are asked to wear them for the first postoperative month. Single- and two-level ACDF and arthroplasty patients are typically discharged the same day, whereas the three- and four-level ACDF patients are kept a minimum of 24 hours for observation and drain management, if applicable. All patients have some element of swallowing difficulty. I prepare all my arthrodesis patients to anticipate some element of posterior cervical discomfort proportional to the correction of disc height and alignment. Arthroplasty patients seldom experience that discomfort because there has been no significant change to the disc height in their operation.

I ask my patients to lift nothing heavier than 5 pounds for the first month. Clinical and radiographic assessments are made at 30, 90 and 180 days. I communicate to my patients the importance of radiographic follow-up until arthrodesis is seen across the segment, which can take up to a year in some patients (► Fig. 9.58).

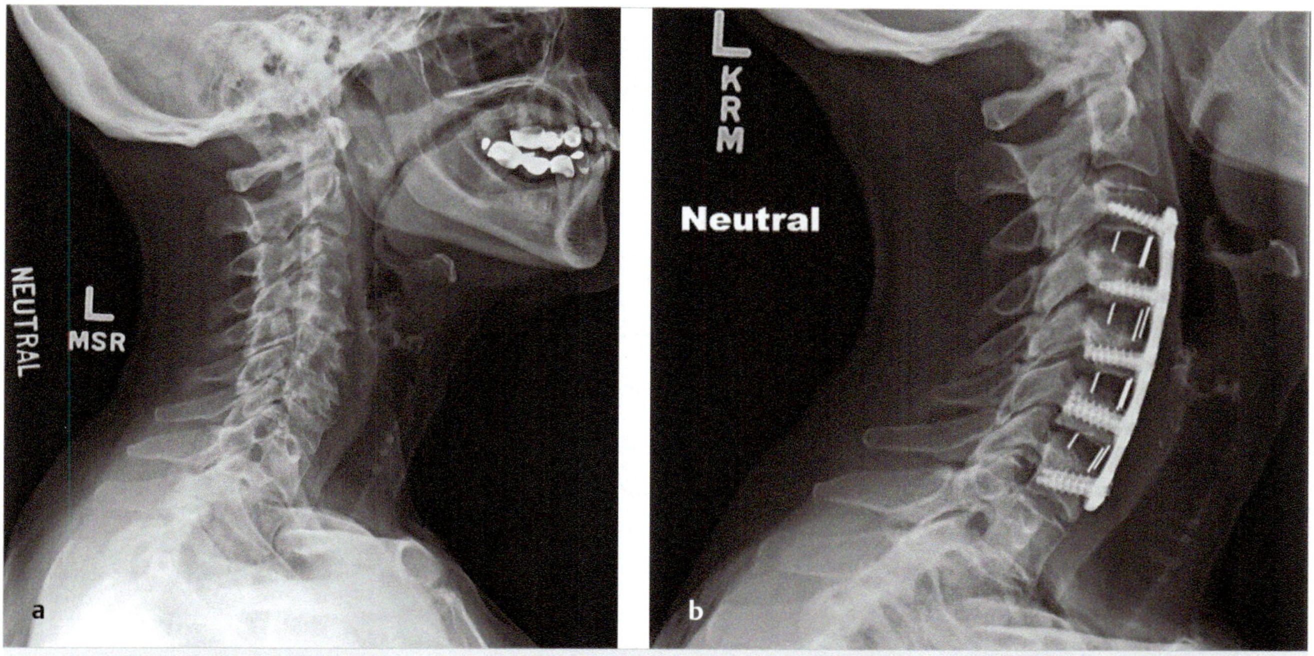

Fig. 9.56 Lateral radiographs of a patient with multiple levels of cervical spondylosis from C3 to C7 with myelopathy. **(a)** Preoperative lateral radiograph showing multiple levels of spondylosis with central cord syndrome that appeared after the patient fell. **(b)** Postoperative lateral radiograph showing the surgical management using a two-incision technique.

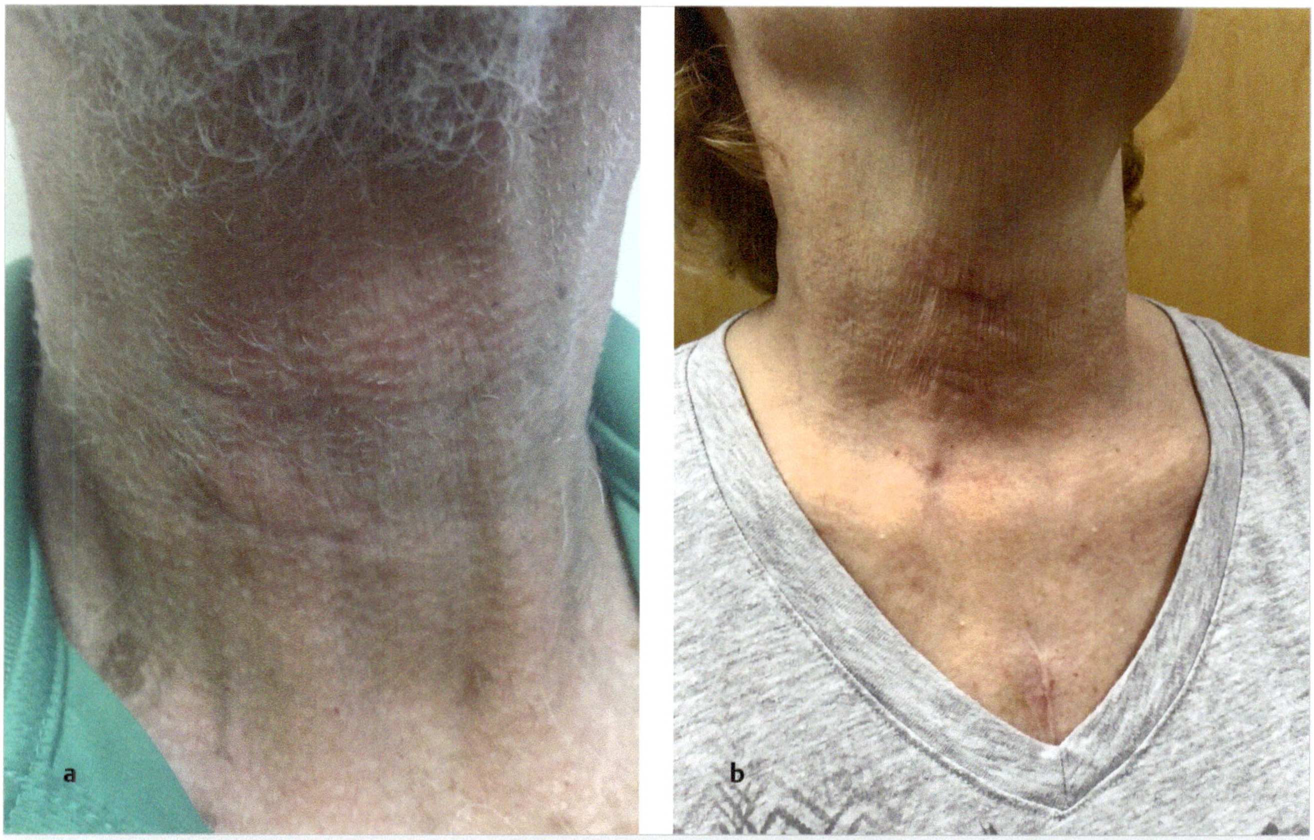

Fig. 9.57 The cosmesis of the two-incision technique. **(a,b)** Photographs of two patients who underwent the two-incision technique from C3 to C7.

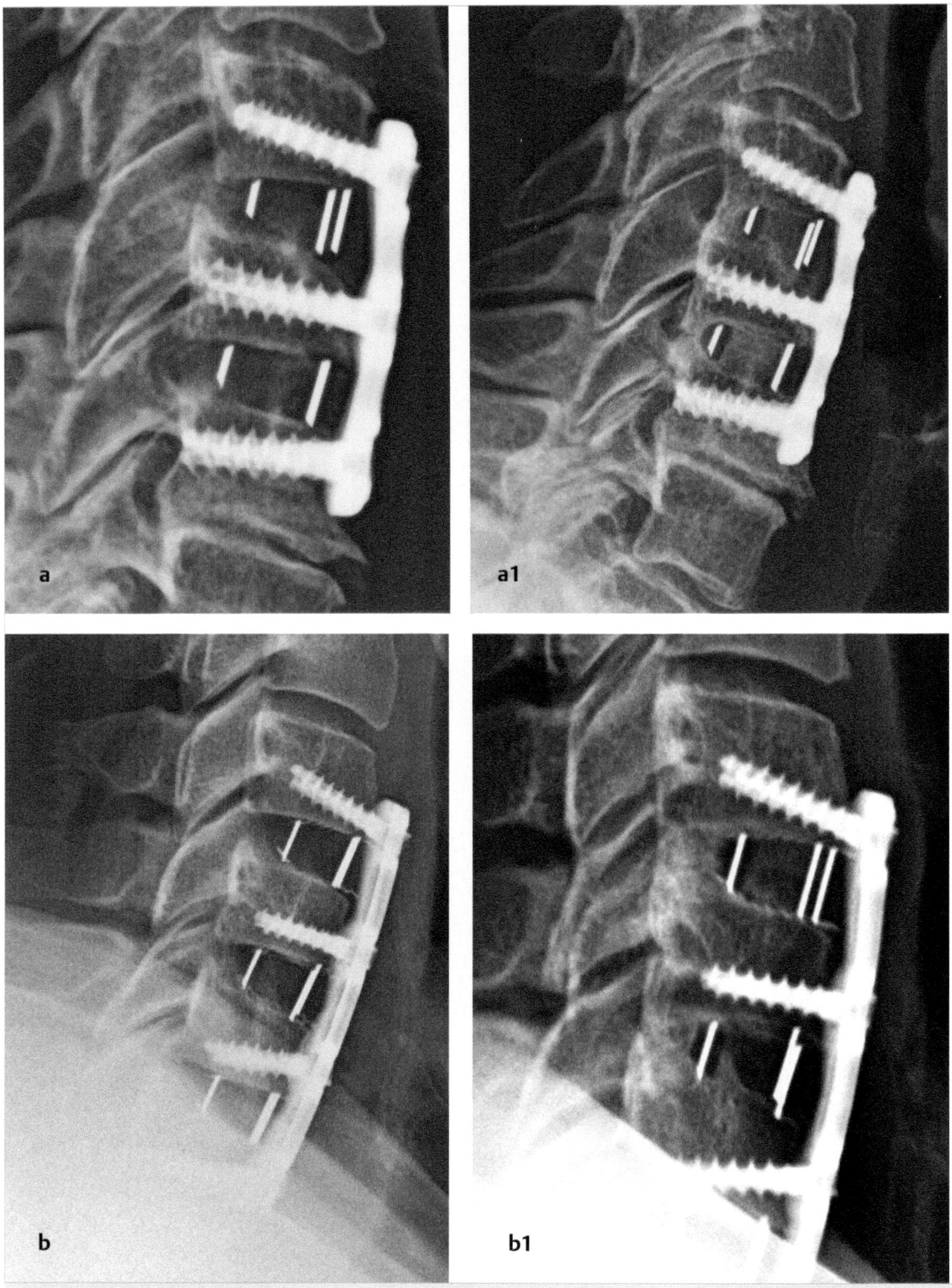

Fig. 9.58 Lateral radiographs for the assessment of an anterior cervical discectomy with fusion (ACDF). **(a)** Extent of arthrodesis for a C4–5 and C5–6 ACDF at the 30-day evaluation. **(a1)** Arthrodesis at the 1-year evaluation. Note the bridging bone across the segment both through the interbody spacer and posterior to it. **(b)** Extent of arthrodesis for a C4–5, C5–6 and C6–7 ACDF at the 30-day evaluation. Note the complete absence of bone posterior to the interbody. **(b1)** Extent of arthrodesis at the 6-month evaluation. Arthrodesis appears to be more robust posterior to the interbody than through it.

9.47 Complication Avoidance

Complications of ACDFs fall into three main categories: immediate, short term and long term.

9.47.1 Immediate Surgical Complication Avoidance

The immediate complications are those that are related to the exposure and the procedure itself. Recurrent laryngeal palsy, dysphagia, esophageal injury, vertebral artery injury, nerve root injury or spinal cord injury are the potential immediate surgical complication. A sizable body of literature exists regarding recurrent laryngeal nerve palsies, and I invite the reader to review those key references.[7,8,9,10,26] In my practice, I have found the greatest risk of a recurrent laryngeal nerve palsy happens in those patients with previous cervical surgery, especially with a right-sided approach, which is consistent with that reported in the literature.[27] No patient with previous cervical surgery undergoes an operation without one of my ear, nose and throat colleagues evaluating them with direct laryngoscopy to confirm medialization of the vocal cords. I have adhered to Apfelbaum and colleagues' recommendation to decrease the cuff pressure after the retractors are in position over the segment.[11,28]

Prevention of esophageal injury from the exposure comes with identification of the avascular plane and appropriate mobilization of the tissue planes. In patients with previous surgery, the dissection plane may be scarred. In those circumstances, I have found it valuable to stay lateral, identify the carotid sheath and bluntly dissect medially onto the spine. Fortunately, the risk to the esophagus remains exceptionally low at the time of surgery. Esophageal issues presenting in a delayed manner secondary to the hardware appears to be the greater risk.[29] The incidence of vertebral artery injury is also exceptionally low. The prevention of vertebral artery injury comes with meticulous identification of the midline and review of the axial images to rule out an ectatic or tortuous vessel.[30]

9.47.2 Short-Term Complication Avoidance

Inadequate decompression of a segment manifesting as persistent radiculopathy presents within the 30-day postoperative window. Complete exposure of the requisite anatomical unit and its complete decompression are the central tenets to prevention. A posterior cervical foraminotomy is one strategy for the management of this entity.

Hardware-related issues may begin to surface in the short-term period. A cervical screw that escapes past its locking mechanism falls into this category. Recognizing and monitoring these screw pullouts is important to prevent a potential esophageal injury (▶ Fig. 9.59). An esophageal study is valuable to demonstrate to the patient and oneself that the screw is a safe distance from the esophagus. Prevention of a screw pullout happens at the time of placement of the plate. Ensure that the necessary bone work has been completed to allow the plate to rest flush across all segments of the cervical spine so that when the screws are placed there is no significant vector force acting to pull out the screw.

The concern with screw pullout would also suggest incomplete immobilization of the segment that may lead to a pseudarthrosis.

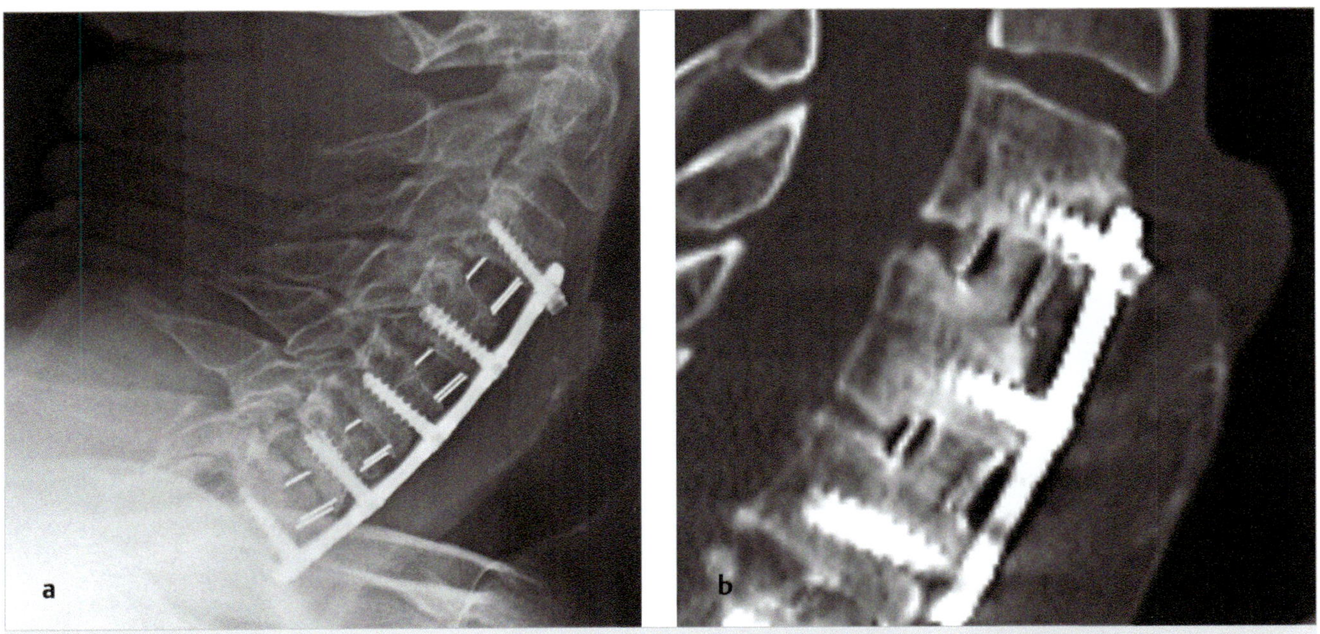

Fig. 9.59 Screw pullout after anterior cervical discectomy and fusion (ACDF). **(a)** Lateral radiograph of a patient who underwent a four-level ACDF. At the time of surgery, the fluoroscopic image and direct visualization confirmed the screw was past the locking mechanism. At 30 days, the top screws had pulled out past their locking mechanisms. Arthrodesis still occurred across the C3–4 segment, which was confirmed by computed tomography 1 year later. **(b)** The screw did not pull out any farther on subsequent radiographic follow-up. An esophageal study demonstrated that the screw was a safe distance from the esophagus.

9.47.3 Long-Term Complication Avoidance

Pseudoarthrosis and adjacent segment degeneration are the two leading long-term complications. Smoking cessation is a must for patients to optimize an environment conducive to arthrodesis. No graft material or implant surface technology will ever replace the meticulous preparation of the cortical end plate and the craftsmanship of securing a tight-fitting graft that embraces the principle of Wolff's law. From a statistical standpoint, a pseudoarthrosis is bound to occur. Management with posterior lateral mass fixation reliably achieves an arthrodesis across the segment (▶ Fig. 9.60).

Minimizing any disruption of the adjacent segments and maximizing the plate-to-disc distance mitigates the risk of adjacent segment degeneration. Refraining from using a spinal

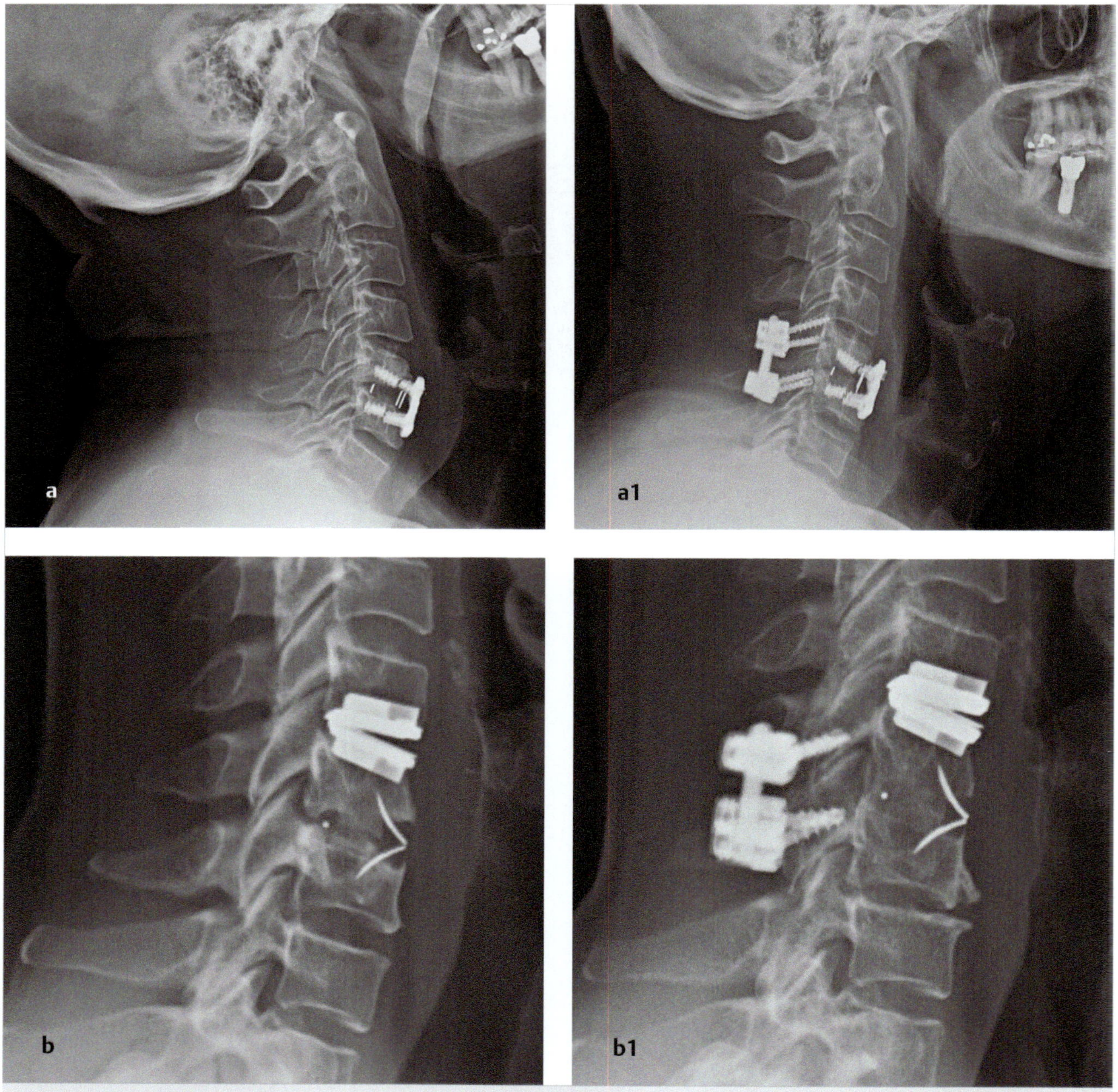

Fig. 9.60 Management of pseudarthrosis. **(a)** Active smoker who presented with an acute disc herniation at C5–6 underwent a C5–6 anterior cervical discectomy and fusion and was then lost to follow-up. The patient returned 2 years after surgery with a lateral radiograph **(a1)** showing all four screws had fractured within the vertebral body. The patient was managed with lateral mass fixation into C5 and C6 but was then lost to follow-up again. **(b)** A patient who presented with increasing neck pain 1 year after surgery performed at another institution. Lateral radiograph shows a hybrid construct with an artificial disc at C4–5 and an integrated interbody device at C5–6 that resulted in a pseudoarthrosis. A lucency can be clearly seen through the implant. **(b1)** The patient was managed with lateral mass fixation and, at 6 months, demonstrated radiographic union across the previously unfused segment.

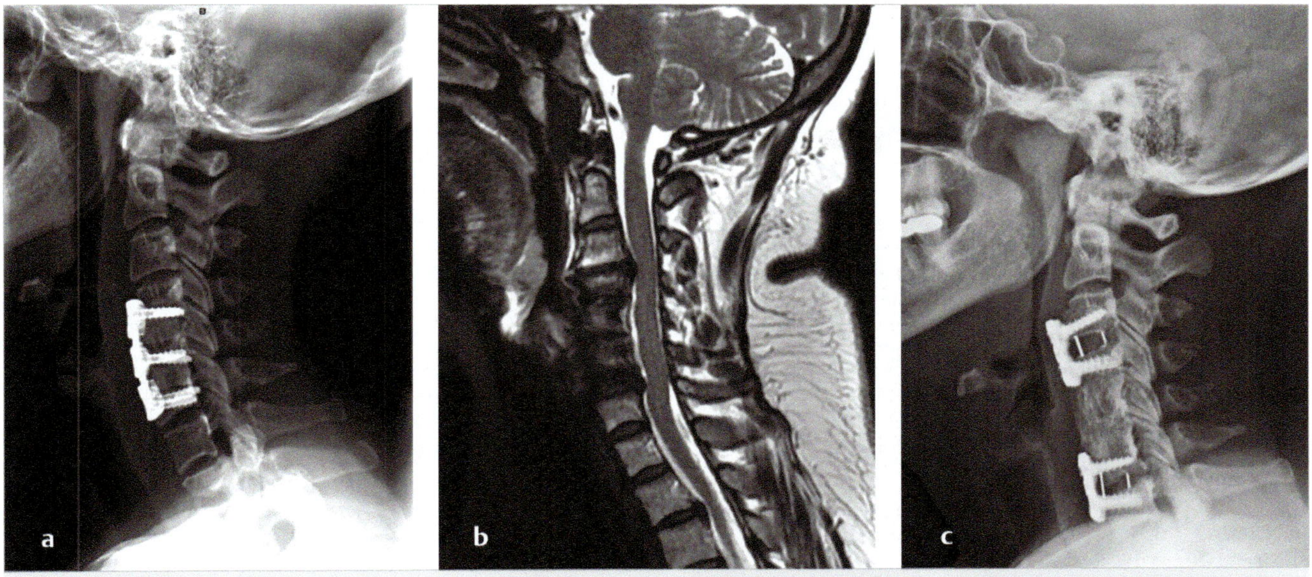

Fig. 9.61 Plate-to-disc distance (PDD) and adjacent segment degeneration. **(a)** Immediate postoperative lateral radiograph after a C4–5 and C5–6 anterior cervical discectomy and fusion (ACDF) performed at another facility. The PDD was 3 mm rostral and 1 mm caudal. Nine years later, the patient presented with cervical myelopathy. **(b)** The sagittal T2-weighted magnetic resonance imaging demonstrated spinal cord compression at the adjacent segments. **(c)** The patient required explantation of the plate and ACDF at the levels above and below, which was performed with a two-incision technique.

needle for localization, in the event the level is off by one, and limiting the exposure to 5 mm above and below the disc space are instrumental in preventing the degeneration of the adjacent segment.[12] Whenever appropriate, consider arthroplasty, which has demonstrated an association with a decreased incidence of adjacent segment degeneration. If arthrodesis is necessary, maintaining a minimum distance of 5 mm from the plate to the adjacent segment creates an environment that decreases the risk of adjacent segment degeneration (▶ Fig. 9.61).[13]

9.48 Conclusion

The ACD for fusion or motion preservation remains one of the most reliable surgical procedures in the spine surgeon's armamentarium. Well-conceived and consistently reproducible, this procedure can comprehensively address degenerative, traumatic and neoplastic conditions of the subaxial spine. Germane to this Primer, the ACD may be considered the first spine procedure to abide by the Caspar ratio, where the surgical exposure does not exceed the surgical target. By that benchmark alone, this procedure meets the criteria for a minimally invasive procedure. Unlike the other procedures in this Primer, the anterior approach did not evolve into a minimally invasive technique; rather, it was conceived as such from the outset. The elegant approach that navigates the cervical anatomy onto the spine is inherently minimally invasive. At the same time, the various open surgical approaches of the lumbar and cervical spine that did evolve into minimally invasive ones offer several techniques and nuances that further refine and facilitate the ACD. Incorporating these minimally invasive principles has been a particular focus of this chapter. Use of the minimally invasive retractor arm to stabilize the cervical retractor, the use of a minimally invasive drill attachment and reconstruction of the anatomy at depth in the mind's eye are three such examples. Thus, it is my hope that the reader has found this chapter relevant to this Primer.

As this chapter comes to a close, the various skill sets that you have developed across the procedures in the preceding chapters will come into play for the final chapters on management of metastatic lesions of the thoracic and lumbar spine and management of intradural extramedullary lesions.

References

[1] Panjabi MM, Duranceau J, Goel V, Oxland T, Takata K. Cervical human vertebrae. Quantitative three-dimensional anatomy of the middle and lower regions. Spine. 1991; 16(8):861–869

[2] Vaccaro AR, Ring D, Scuderi G, Garfin SR. Vertebral artery location in relation to the vertebral body as determined by two-dimensional computed tomography evaluation. Spine. 1994; 19(23):2637–2641

[3] Chin KR, Ricchetti ET, Yu WD, Riew KD. Less exposure surgery for multilevel anterior cervical fusion using 2 transverse incisions. J Neurosurg Spine. 2012; 17(3):194–198

[4] Cloward RB. The anterior approach for removal of ruptured cervical disks. J Neurosurg. 1958; 15(6):602–617

[5] Smith GW, Robinson RA. The treatment of certain cervical-spine disorders by anterior removal of the intervertebral disc and interbody fusion. J Bone Joint Surg Am. 1958; 40-A(3):607–624

[6] Swift J. Gulliver's Travels. New York, NY: Harper; 1950

[7] Jung A, Schramm J. How to reduce recurrent laryngeal nerve palsy in anterior cervical spine surgery: a prospective observational study. Neurosurgery. 2010; 67(1):10–15, discussion 15

[8] Jung A, Schramm J, Lehnerdt K, Herberhold C. Recurrent laryngeal nerve palsy during anterior cervical spine surgery: a prospective study. J Neurosurg Spine. 2005; 2(2):123–127

[9] Audu P, Artz G, Scheid S, et al. Recurrent laryngeal nerve palsy after anterior cervical spine surgery: the impact of endotracheal tube cuff deflation, reinflation, and pressure adjustment. Anesthesiology. 2006; 105(5):898–901

[10] Haller JM, Iwanik M, Shen FH. Clinically relevant anatomy of recurrent laryngeal nerve. Spine. 2012; 37(2):97–100

[11] Apfelbaum RI, Kriskovich MD, Haller JR. On the incidence, cause, and prevention of recurrent laryngeal nerve palsies during anterior cervical spine surgery. Spine. 2000; 25(22):2906–2912

[12] Nassr A, Lee JY, Bashir RS, et al. Does incorrect level needle localization during anterior cervical discectomy and fusion lead to accelerated disc degeneration? Spine. 2009; 34(2):189–192

[13] Kim HJ, Kelly MP, Ely CG, Dettori JR, Riew KD. The risk of adjacent-level ossification development after surgery in the cervical spine: are there factors that affect the risk? A systematic review. Spine. 2012; 37(22) Suppl:S65–S74

[14] Lee DH, Lee JS, Yi JS, Cho W, Zebala LP, Riew KD. Anterior cervical plating technique to prevent adjacent-level ossification development. Spine J. 2013; 13(7):823–829

[15] Olivares-Navarrete R, Gittens RA, Schneider JM, et al. Osteoblasts exhibit a more differentiated phenotype and increased bone morphogenetic protein production on titanium alloy substrates than on poly-ether-ether-ketone. Spine J. 2012; 12(3):265–272

[16] Torstrick FB, Lin ASP, Potter D, et al. Porous PEEK improves the bone-implant interface compared to plasma-sprayed titanium coating on PEEK. Biomaterials. 2018; 185:106–116

[17] Kersten RF, van Gaalen SM, de Gast A, Öner FC. Polyetheretherketone (PEEK) cages in cervical applications: a systematic review. Spine J. 2015; 15(6): 1446–1460

[18] Mummaneni PV, Burkus JK, Haid RW, Traynelis VC, Zdeblick TA. Clinical and radiographic analysis of cervical disc arthroplasty compared with allograft fusion: a randomized controlled clinical trial. J Neurosurg Spine. 2007; 6(3): 198–209

[19] Coric D, Nunley PD, Guyer RD, et al. Prospective, randomized, multicenter study of cervical arthroplasty: 269 patients from the Kineflex|C artificial disc investigational device exemption study with a minimum 2-year follow-up: clinical article. J Neurosurg Spine. 2011; 15(4):348–358

[20] Sasso RC, Smucker JD, Hacker RJ, Heller JG. Clinical outcomes of BRYAN cervical disc arthroplasty: a prospective, randomized, controlled, multicenter trial with 24-month follow-up. J Spinal Disord Tech. 2007; 20(7):481–491

[21] Murrey D, Janssen M, Delamarter R, et al. Results of the prospective, randomized, controlled multicenter Food and Drug Administration investigational device exemption study of the ProDisc-C total disc replacement versus anterior discectomy and fusion for the treatment of 1-level symptomatic cervical disc disease. Spine J. 2009; 9(4):275–286

[22] Tumialán LM. Cervical template to optimize the plate-to-disc distance in instrumented anterior cervical discectomies and fusions: instrumentation assessment. Oper Neurosurg (Hagerstown). 2019; 17(1):43–51

[23] Wolff J. The Law of Bone Remodelling. Berlin: Springer-Verlag; 1986

[24] Lowery GL, McDonough RF. The significance of hardware failure in anterior cervical plate fixation. Patients with 2- to 7-year follow-up. Spine. 1998; 23 (2):181–186, discussion 186–187

[25] Benzel E, Steimetz M. Benzel's Spine Surgery: Techniques, Complication Avoidance and Management. 4th ed. Philadelphia, PA: Elsevier; 2017

[26] Kilburg C, Sullivan HG, Mathiason MA. Effect of approach side during anterior cervical discectomy and fusion on the incidence of recurrent laryngeal nerve injury. J Neurosurg Spine. 2006; 4(4):273–277

[27] Erwood MS, Walters BC, Connolly TM, et al. Voice and swallowing outcomes following reoperative anterior cervical discectomy and fusion with a 2-team surgical approach. J Neurosurg Spine. 2018; 28(2):140–148

[28] Kriskovich MD, Apfelbaum RI, Haller JR. Vocal fold paralysis after anterior cervical spine surgery: incidence, mechanism, and prevention of injury. Laryngoscope. 2000; 110(9):1467–1473

[29] Halani SH, Baum GR, Riley JP, et al. Esophageal perforation after anterior cervical spine surgery: a systematic review of the literature. J Neurosurg Spine. 2016; 25(3):285–291

[30] Neo M, Fujibayashi S, Miyata M, Takemoto M, Nakamura T. Vertebral artery injury during cervical spine surgery: a survey of more than 5600 operations. Spine. 2008; 33(7):779–785

10 Minimally Invasive Decompressions for Metastatic Spinal Disease

Abstract

Up to 40% of cancer patients develop spinal metastases through the course of their battle against the disease. As many as 10% of those patients present with epidural spinal cord compression, some with neurologic deficits.[1] The objective of this chapter is to present the anatomical basis, rationale and surgical technique for minimally invasive management of metastatic disease to the spine of those patients. The principles of separation surgery are presented since they form the basis for minimally invasive decompressions. A particular focus of this chapter is the localization of lesions in the thoracic spine using fluoroscopy, computer-assisted navigation and preoperative embolization. Unlike previous chapters where a standard technique was presented and then applied to a variety of cases, no standard technique is given for the simple reason that metastatic disease to the spine is such a heterogeneous entity. Therefore, cases are presented, and the technique is described to address the specifics of that particular case. The expectation is that in covering a variety of clinical circumstances, the resulting overlap prepares the reader for the diversity of radiographic and clinical presentations that await them in their future practice.

Keywords: epidural, metastases, minimally invasive, neurologic deficit, radiation, separation surgery, thoracic

True vision is the art of seeing what is invisible to others.

Jonathan Swift

10.1 Introduction

It is inconceivable to have a comprehensive chapter on the management of metastatic spinal disease buried within a minimally invasive primer. In the realm of oncological spine surgery, metastatic disease to the spine is a complex topic with varying and passionate opinions with regard to its management. Fortunately, the work from the Spine Oncology Study Group (SOSG) has provided the necessary framework to assess the stability of the spine in the context of metastatic disease.[2] The development of the Spinal Instability in Neoplastic Disease Scale (SINS), the work product of the SOSG, reliably determines when a simple decompression is appropriate or when stabilization is required in addition to decompression.[2,3,4,5] The work of the SOSG is mandatory reading for any spine surgeon managing metastatic diseases of the spine, whether that management is minimally invasive or otherwise.

The body of the literature that has arisen regarding "separation surgery" followed by adjuvant stereotactic radiosurgery to achieve local disease control for metastatic disease to the spine continues to build a compelling argument for less invasive surgical strategies.[6,7,8,9] Separation surgery fits hand in glove with minimally invasive approaches for metastatic disease to the spine. The philosophy is to expose the patient to less risk of surgery by making the objective of surgery a separation of the lesion from the spinal cord instead of complete resection of the lesion. What remains is a radiosurgery target.

With the SINS classification system as our framework and separation surgery as our surgical stratagem, the concession I need from the reader for this chapter is this: we have presumed that in each instance discussed in the upcoming pages a simple decompression is the path forward for the patient's care. Without that concession, the reader and I will become mired in the complexities of biomechanics, tumor volumes, surgical approaches and the like. Decompression of the spinal cord with minimally invasive techniques is the focus of this chapter, not biomechanics. Again, it is the seminal work of SOSG that formed the basis for the decision to proceed with simple decompressions in each case presented in this chapter. By no means does this circumstance dismiss the importance of instrumented decompressions and fusion, which has a well-established role in the treatment of metastatic spinal disease, and they are procedures I routinely perform more often than not for management of this disease entity. However, at times, patients present with unilateral epidural compression in a stable spine with neurologic or impending neurologic deficits. That patient category is the focus of this chapter. For that reason, uninstrumented decompressions are the focus of the case illustrations. Equally important is the presentation of patients who are not candidates for uninstrumented minimally invasive separation surgery.

The very nature of this topic almost mandates that the chapter be constructed around case illustrations that, in turn, become the framework of explaining the technique. Unlike previous chapters in this text, where case illustrations were reviewed at the end of each chapter, this chapter places them front and center. I readily concede that each of these clinical scenarios may have several perfectly viable management strategies that include instrumented fusions, corpectomy, and anterior and posterior reconstructions. Several readers may not necessarily agree with the management strategy employed. Again, I emphasize that it is not the objective of this chapter to have a comprehensive review of these various options. Instead, the aim of this chapter is to review the technique of a minimally invasive decompression of thoracic metastatic lesions. Therefore, the technique selected for the management of each patient for this chapter is an uninstrumented decompression, which may include simple laminectomy, transpedicular decompression or both, depending on the location of the lesion. One statement that should stir little, if any, controversy is that spinal cord compression from a metastatic lesion in a patient with a progressive neurologic deficit is a surgical disease regardless of responsiveness to chemotherapeutic agents or radiation.[9]

The application of minimally invasive techniques for management of metastatic disease of the thoracic spine should come at a time when you have achieved mastery with minimally invasive decompressions of the lumbar spine. I have emphasized the thoracic spine in this chapter for two reasons. The first is that the vast majority of our experience with minimally invasive techniques originates in the lumbar spine. The degenerative processes of the aging spine that benefit from surgical intervention do not present with adequate frequency in the thoracic spine to achieve the same degree of comfort in that region of the spine. However, translating that lumbar skillset to decompression of metastatic lesions in the thoracic spine, while adding a level of complexity, can be relatively straightforward. As with any minimally invasive technique, a more refined understanding of the three-dimensional anatomy of the thoracic spine is essential.

Second, while metastatic lesions may occur throughout the entire spine, a review of my experience suggests that symptomatic spinal cord compression requiring surgical intervention occurs with greater frequency in the thoracic spine than in either the cervical or lumbar regions. The greater surface area of this region undoubtedly results in a higher statistical probability that a lesion will surface within one of the 12 thoracic vertebrae, more so than the lumbar or cervical regions. The literature has corroborated what I have found in my clinical practice. The various reviews in the literature report the thoracic spine as the most common site of metastasis, up to 70% of the time, followed by the lumbar spine representing 20% and the cervical spine with 10%.[10,11]

As you proceed with minimally invasive approaches in the thoracic spine, keep in mind the distinct topography of the thoracic spine when compared to the lumbar spine. While the anatomical regions are distinct, there are more similarities than differences. Understanding those unique elements of the thoracic landscape is a key component for the application of these techniques and successful decompression of the spinal cord due to metastatic disease.

In this chapter, the clinical cases are central to the surgical technique, and as such, they are discussed in great detail. Unlike the relative uniformity of the laminectomy or microdiscectomy, every metastatic lesion is truly unique. As a result, it is impossible to present one standard approach for the management of this clinical entity. Instead, I have selected several case illustrations, with the hope that the variations between them cover minimally invasive surgical management in greater depth than presenting a standard surgical technique section could.

Finally, before embarking on this topic, I cannot emphasize enough the importance of a multidisciplinary approach. In the absence of a neurologic emergency, it is imperative to have a clear line of communication with both the radiation and medical oncologists before determining a plan of care. An inextricable component of any treatment plan is knowledge of the underlying primary neoplasm. Understanding the biology of that primary neoplasm in the context of a patient who may have a single metastatic lesion or multiple lesions helps define and guide the role of surgical management. Furthermore, the knowledge that a neoplasm is exquisitely responsive to radiation or chemotherapy may further influence the role or the extent of surgery. Incorporating the aforementioned allows you to harness the advantages of minimally invasive techniques so they work in conjunction with radiation and chemotherapy in order to optimize the outcome for the patient. The presence of a metastatic lesion or lesions in the spine does not always equate to surgery. The vast majority of patients I see will not need an operation at all. The absence of a neurologic deficit provides you with the gift of time; take full advantage of it. Communicate with your colleagues in radiation and medical oncology and listen to their thoughts on the matter. Over the years, I have found it of tremendous value to know what my colleagues have in mind for the patient and how surgery fits into that plan of care.

10.2 Rationale

As already mentioned several times throughout this text, a smaller paramedian incision with a table-mounted access port that offers a focused exposure in lieu of a longer incision with self-retaining retractors allows for optimal blood flow to the muscles and skin edge during the procedure and limits the amount of tissue necrosis that may occur after the procedure. Therefore, a minimally invasive paramedian approach creates an ideal environment for healing in a patient population that may already be challenged with nourishment and facing further challenges to healing a wound through radiation and chemotherapy. The ability to begin adjuvant therapies almost immediately after a minimally invasive decompression without significant concern for wound healing may be far and above the greatest advantage of this approach.

In writing this chapter, I reviewed the patterns of spinal cord compression in the management of metastatic disease to the spine in my practice over the last 10 years. Patients who present with spinal cord compression from a lesion in the epidural space off to one side are ideal candidates for a paramedian minimally invasive resection. At times, the metastatic disease appears to originate from the vertebral body and then extend into the pedicle. From the pedicle, the disease expands into the epidural space, causing compression of the spinal cord off to one side. At other times, the lesion seems to originate in the epidural space but still cause compression predominantly on one side. Such laterality lends itself exceptionally well to a minimally invasive approach, where the lateral recess, epidural space and pedicle may all be readily accessed. A minimally invasive approach spares the posterior tension band and the spinous process, which is a biomechanical asset, provided no metastatic disease is present within the posterior tension band and the spinous processes. If the spinous processes are involved, this asset all of sudden becomes a liability. Careful consideration should be given to a traditional midline open approach if the procedure is not simply a palliative one.

Patients who present with circumferential compression of the spinal cord need a different strategy. ▶ Fig. 10.1 describes a 52-year-old woman 4 years after an initial diagnosis of colon cancer, who presented with circumferential compression of the spinal cord at T9. Her oncologist referred her for minimally invasive separation surgery, but the pattern of compression did not lend itself to such an approach. She underwent a midline costotransversectomy approach to the T9 body for corpectomy, placement of cage and posterolateral instrumentation from T6–T11 (▶ Fig. 10.2).

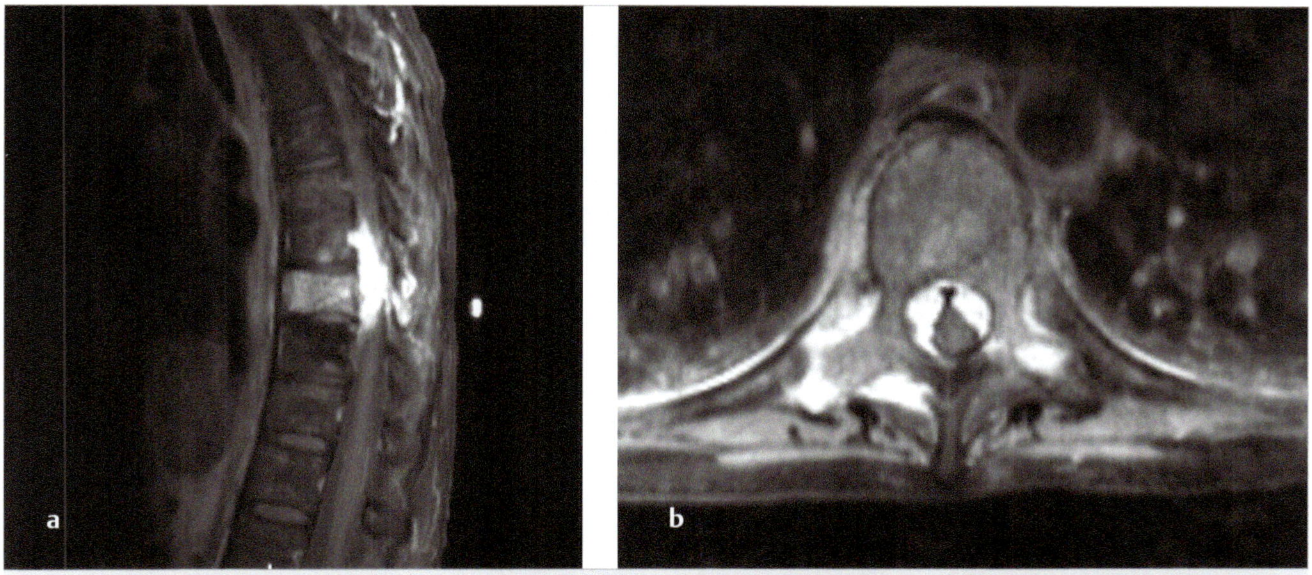

Fig. 10.1 Metastatic colon cancer to the thoracic spine. (a) Sagittal gadolinium-enhanced T1-weighted magnetic resonance imaging (MRI) showing a ventral lesion emanating from the T9 vertebral body. (b) Axial gadolinium-enhanced T1-weighted MRI showing the concentrated compression of the spinal cord. The patient underwent a costotransversectomy approach for a T9 corpectomy, placement of an interbody cage and instrumentation from T6 to T11.

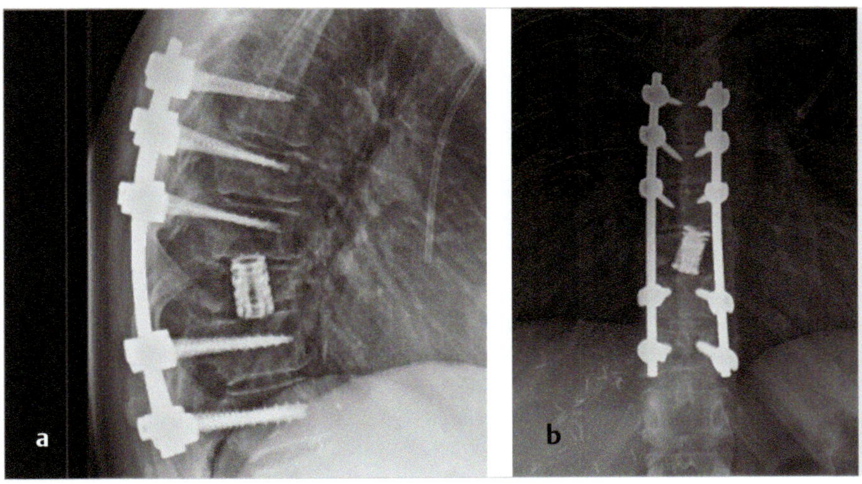

Fig. 10.2 Surgical management of metastatic colon cancer to the thoracic spine. (a) Lateral radiograph demonstrating an instrumented fusion from T6 to T11 with cage placement after T9 corpectomy. (b) Anteroposterior image of the construct.

For all minimally invasive decompressive separation surgeries, I use an expandable minimal access port, which allows simultaneous exposure of the medial and lateral structures during the decompression. I have found that a greater area of exposure is also helpful when obtaining hemostasis which, in the metastatic tumor resections, is no small task. Rare is the occasion where I can find an 18-mm diameter adequate for the work I need to accomplish in the decompression of a metastatic lesion, so much so that I have not included a fixed diameter minimal access port among the cases in this chapter. The cases I performed with fixed diameter access ports were part of my learning curve that convinced me to use an expandable access port. I feel that the advantages offered by an expandable access port far outweigh the liability of a few more millimeters to the incision.

10.3 Operating Room Setup

10.3.1 Patient Positioning and Localization

Before considering the operating room setup, one must consider the methods of identifying the level on which to operate. Localization in the thoracic spine is no small feat for traditional midline approaches. For minimally invasive surgery, the margin of error is even smaller; however, there is an element to metastatic disease that allows for a liability to be harnessed as an asset. Specifically, lytic lesions to the bone, which are readily identifiable on computed tomography (CT) images, all of a sudden introduce the capacity to use computer-assisted navigation for localization. One of the first things I look for in the management of metastatic disease in the spine is whether the disease has altered the architecture of the pedicle, vertebral body, transverse process or some other bony prominence in such a manner that allows for localization. If there is a distinct alteration at the level of the compression, I use computer-assisted navigation to localize, dock, secure my access port and accomplish the decompression. Localization by navigation has the added benefit of decreasing radiation exposure. The application of image guidance has vastly increased my efficiency in localization and has also alleviated almost all my anxiety about the level on which I am operating. However, if I am unequivocally unable to detect some unique identifier on the bony anatomy, I employ fluoroscopy. Localization by fluoroscopy is always confirmed in the anteroposterior (AP) and lateral views counting up from the sacrum. It is invaluable to have some preoperative study that demonstrates 5 non–rib-bearing vertebrae, whether by CT or conventional AP radiography.

Regardless of the method used for localization, all patients are positioned on a Jackson table. No Wilson frame is used for the simple reason that the gears from the frame can be seen on AP fluoroscopic images. Those same gears create scatter on the intraoperative CT images. Thus, the Wilson frame may obscure visualization of the bony anatomy during either fluoroscopy or computer-assisted navigation.

For lesions at T5 and below, I bring the patient's arms forward on arms boards. For lesions at T4 and above, the arms are tucked, allowing me better proximity to the operative field.

10.3.2 Computer-Assisted Navigation for Localization

With computer-assisted navigation, I obtain an AP fluoroscopic image with a Kirschner wire laid on the surface of the skin over the pedicles of T12 and a second AP image with a Kirschner wire over the pedicles of the vertebral body within a segment or two of the level of compression. As the field of view can typically cover 6 to 7 levels, one only needs to be in the approximate vicinity. By way of example, if I am operating on T3, I attempt to localize over the top of T5. I mark the spinous process of T5 based on one or two AP images counting from the 12th vertebral body, and identified as such by being above the last non–rib-bearing vertebrae. The steep slope of the thoracic spinous process creates the potential to be off by a level. Typically, it is the spinous process of the level above that is seen at the levels of the pedicles; that is, at the pedicles of T5, the spinous process of T4 is seen on AP imaging.

After the thoracic spine is prepped widely, I make a small incision over the top of the spinous process. The incision is just large enough to pass the navigation reference stem and clamp onto the spinous process. To optimize the clamp–spinous-process interface, I place the clamp at a slight angle, mimicking the slope of the stem and spinous process. I then anchor the reference frame onto the clamp and complete an intraoperative CT scan. After the images are loaded into the computer-assisted navigation system, I localize by identifying the abnormality of the bony architecture and then proceed with dilating up to a 22-mm diameter and anchoring an expandable minimal access port, which I discuss further in the second case illustration.

10.3.3 Localization with Fluoroscopy

Counting up from the sacrum with AP and lateral images is the most reliable method to localize a level in the midthoracic spine up to T4. The process is tedious, but it is the most reliable manner to unequivocally localize a level for the midthoracic and lower thoracic levels. AP images of the cervicothoracic junction at the correct angle reliably identify T1. From there, marking the pedicles and counting downward is a reliable method to localize. Unequivocal confirmation of T1 on AP imaging is necessary for this method to work. If body habitus permits, counting down from C2 is advisable. I use this method to confirm the upper thoracic spine levels, specifically T1, T2 and T3.

10.4 Surgical Technique

10.4.1 Case Illustration 1: Metastatic Non-Small-Cell Adenocarcinoma of the Lung at T9

Clinical History and Neurologic Examination

The patient is a 47-year-old, right-hand–dominant man who presented to the emergency room with a history of left flank pain for several months, difficulty walking for 3 days and overflow incontinence for the past 24 hours. Review of systems was positive for a chronic cough of several weeks' duration. On examination, the patient was found to be myelopathic in the lower extremities, with 3+patellar tendon reflexes, sustained clonus in the Achilles tendon and upward pointing toes, and normal reflexes, sensation and strength in the upper extremities. Proprioception and epicritic sensation were both diminished in the lower extremities, but the strength of the individual muscle groups was intact by confrontation. There was no distinct sensory dissociation level in the thoracic dermatomes.

Radiographic Evaluation

The patient was found to have a 2.9-cm lung lesion with pleural effusion on CT of the chest for evaluation of his cough. Metastatic disease was also identified in his liver. Further analysis of the CT demonstrated widely metastatic disease to the cervical, thoracic and lumbar spine, encompassing the entire vertebral body of C3 (resulting in a pathological fracture), the left transverse process of T7, the pedicle and transverse process of T9 on the left, the spinous processes of L1 and L2 and the lateral aspect of the vertebral body at L4 and L5. A subsequent magnetic resonance imaging (MRI) of the cervical, thoracic and lumbar spine demonstrated that the pathological fracture at C3 (not shown) and the lesion of T9 (▶ Fig. 10.3) were the only lesions causing spinal cord compression. There was no evidence of metastatic disease to the brain. Subsequent biopsy demonstrated this lesion to be non-small-cell adenocarcinoma of the lung.

Clinical Decision-Making

This patient presented with widely metastatic disease symptomatic of compression of the spinal cord in the thoracic spine

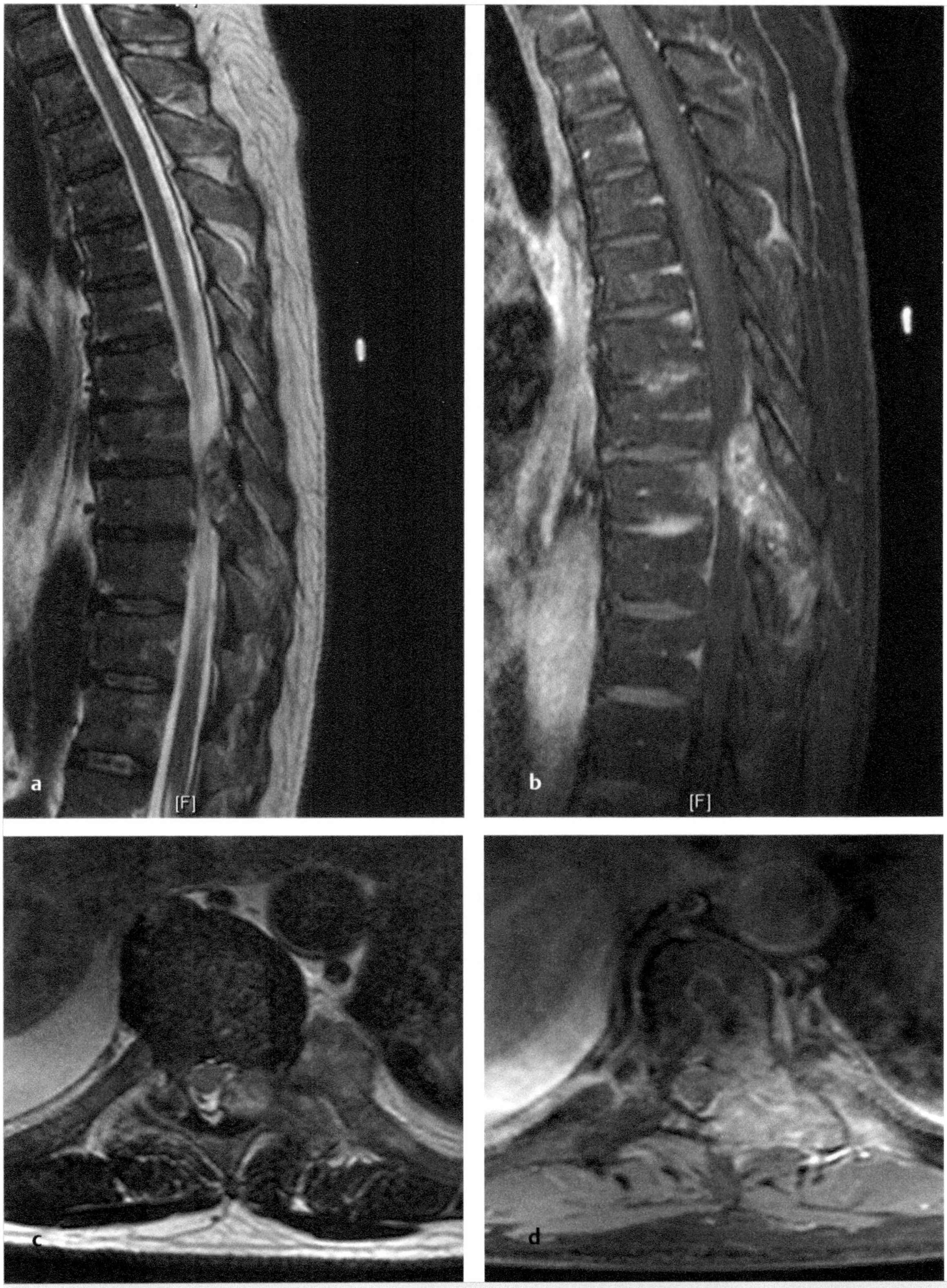

Fig. 10.3 Magnetic resonance imaging (MRI) of the thoracic spine with and without gadolinium demonstrating metastatic disease to T9 level. **(a)** Sagittal T2-weighted MRI demonstrating dorsal and lateral compression of the spinal cord at T9. **(b)** Sagittal T1-weighted MRI with gadolinium demonstrating the enhancement pattern consistent with metastatic disease. **(c)** Axial T2-weighted MRI demonstrating the involvement of the left lateral aspect of the lamina, the left pedicle of T9 and the left T9 transverse process. **(d)** Axial T1-weighted MRI with gadolinium demonstrating the enhancement pattern again consistent with metastatic disease.

and imminent instability in the cervical spine. The biopsy of the lesion in the lung established the histological diagnosis of non-small-cell adenocarcinoma. A multidisciplinary discussion with medical and radiation oncology delineated a plan of care. It was recognized that the patient had an advanced metastatic process with a life expectancy of 1 year, depending on his response to chemotherapy. Before beginning a comprehensive chemotherapeutic and radiation regimen, there was universal agreement that symptomatic compression of the spinal cord needed to be addressed to preserve his neurologic function. The patient had experienced a decline in his ambulatory status and had also begun to demonstrate signs of urinary retention. The central theme of this patient's management at this point was to preserve ambulatory status as well as bowel and bladder function, fully recognizing that surgical management was not curative. The goal of any surgical procedure is for decompression of the neural elements without delaying adjuvant therapies.

The T9 lesion was the most likely cause of his presenting symptoms, since he was asymptomatic in his upper extremities but symptomatic in his lower extremities. However, concern for the stability of the cervical spine in the context of a pathological fracture at C3 and the need to position the patient prone for a thoracic decompression prompted a C3 corpectomy with C2–4 arthrodesis.

The location and configuration of the lesion at the T9 level favored a minimally invasive approach. The compression originated from the left lamina and extended into the pedicle. There was involvement of the transverse process and rib head. Given the unique configuration of the metastatic lesion around the spinal cord, I recommended a minimally invasive hemilaminectomy, transpedicular decompression with partial costotransversectomy. ▶ Fig. 10.4 demonstrates the conceptual surgical strategy with the access port.

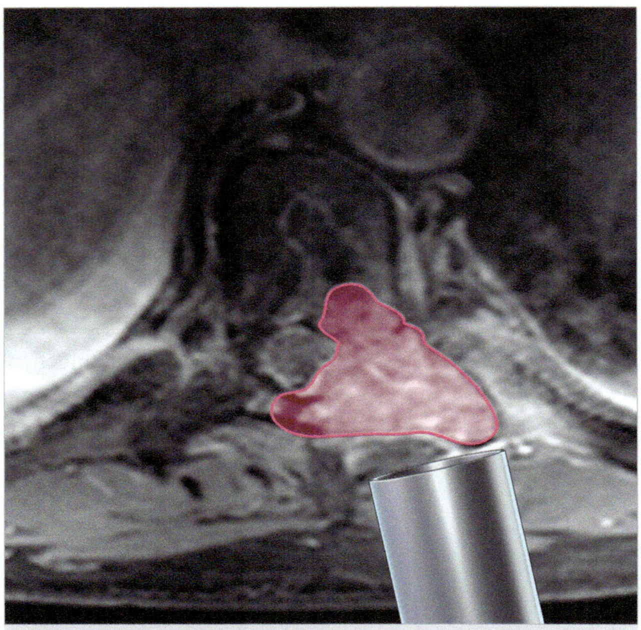

Fig. 10.4 Surgical plan for a minimally invasive decompression of the spinal cord. The *magenta*-shaded area represents the target of the decompression. The configuration of the lesion within the T9 level lends itself especially well to a minimally invasive approach.

Intervention

The patient was positioned prone on a Jackson table. Since this lesion was at T9, the arms were brought forward on arm boards. I used fluoroscopy for localization of the level. A preoperative lumbar radiograph confirmed 5 non–rib-bearing vertebral bodies. A preoperative AP radiograph of the thoracic spine demonstrated the lesion within the pedicle (▶ Fig. 10.5). Recognizing this phenomenon is one of those tremendously helpful findings on a radiograph that can help in the localization process at the time of surgery, the key element of which is actually making the observation. As mentioned throughout this chapter, localization in the thoracic spine is an unforgiving endeavor. For a minimally invasive approach, it is even more so.

Localization

Any localization for a level in the thoracic spine should be a systematic process utilizing both AP and lateral imaging that allows confirmation of the level counting from the sacrum upward (after 5 non–rib-bearing vertebrae have been confirmed). I localize the level in two phases. The first is a preliminary preoperative localization, where I confirm the level with a series of spinal needles and then mark the entry points for those spinal needles, so that I may repeat the process efficiently after draping the patient.

Before the patient is prepped and draped for the actual surgery, I prep him widely for the purpose of localization, but I do not drape the patient. The prepped area includes the lumbar and thoracic spine. I put on a pair of sterile gloves and have at my immediate disposal 5 spinal needles, both 18 and 20 gauge. I begin by palpating the anterior superior iliac spine and the

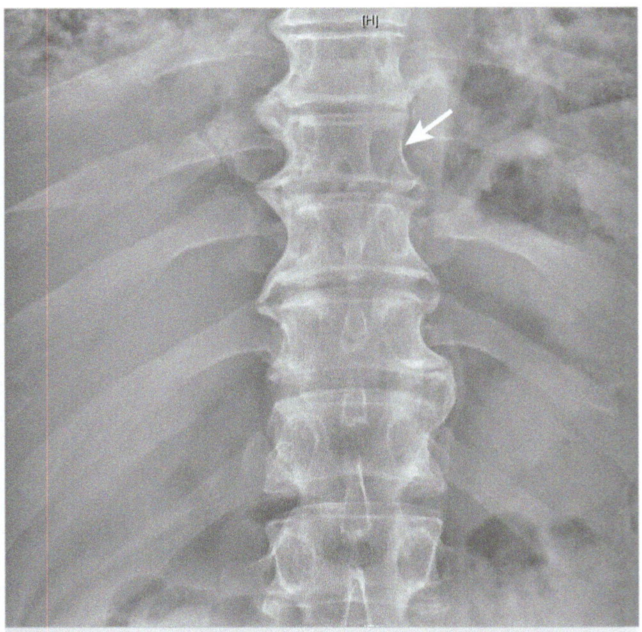

Fig. 10.5 Preoperative anteroposterior (AP) thoracic radiograph demonstrating the absence of a pedicle at T9 on the left (*white arrow*) which is indicative of the lesion. The L1 vertebral body is clearly visible as the first non–rib-bearing vertebral body. AP and lateral lumbar spine radiographs confirmed the presence of 5 non–rib-bearing vertebral bodies in the lumbar spine.

interspinous process space. This location places me at L4–5 or L3–4. I pass a spinal needle 2 cm off the midline onto the lateral aspect of the lamina–facet complex. Since the lesion is on the left, the localizing spinal needles are all placed on the right except for the spinal needle intended to identify T9. From there, I palpate the interspinous process space, and after every three levels, I pass another spinal needle. My first objective is to confirm T12. After the placement of three spinal needles, I obtain a lateral fluoroscopic image to confirm the current position of the needles. In this case, the first lateral image demonstrated that my first needle was at S1, and the second needle was pointing to the pedicle of L3 (▶ Fig. 10.6a). I then have the fluoroscopic technician roll the fluoroscope toward the head, while keeping the L3 spinal needle in the field of view, which allows me to confirm the spinal needle in position at T12. I adjust the needle at T12 so that it is precisely parallel to the pedicle of T12 (▶ Fig. 10.6b). Having the needle in this position makes it easier to confirm AP images. I obtain an AP image (not shown) to confirm that I am at the first rib-bearing vertebra. In this manner, I confirmed my spinal needle at T12 on AP and lateral imaging.

I repeat the process of sliding the fluoroscope toward the head, moving the T12 spinal needle to the bottom of the field of view and allowing me to visualize T9. I now pass a spinal needle onto T9, keeping in mind that this segment is riddled with metastatic disease. The needle has the potential to pass right through the diseased bone. As I pass the needle, I may take intermittent images with the fluoroscope until I feel that I have reached the spine or can see that I am at the level of the spine. Once I have confirmed my level at T9 on an AP image, I have completed my preoperative localization. I plan an incision 3 cm off the midline over the T9 level, which is 3.0 cm in length, and mark all the entry points of the needles for a second confirmation when the area is prepped and draped.

After prepping and draping the entire lumbar and thoracic spine, I begin by placing the spinal needles into their previous locations and reconfirming the levels with both AP and lateral fluoroscopic images. This step is part of a check and balance system to ensure the highest degree of certainty that after making the incision and exposing the anatomy, the lesion resides well within my grasp. The spinal needles are all kept in position to guide docking of the minimal access port. ▶ Fig. 10.6c demonstrates a lateral fluoroscopic image where the spinal needle is in position while the dilation of the muscle is taking place. ▶ Fig. 10.6d illustrates an AP fluoroscopic image where the expandable minimal access port is in position on the side of the lesion (left), and the spinal needle remains in position on the opposite side of the lesion pointing to T12. Even after the access port is in position, I leave the spinal needles in position until I have directly visualized the lesion, lest reconfirmation of the level is needed. It is after I have begun the resection of the lesion that I remove the spinal needles. The thoracic spine can be a lonely region if you find yourself at the wrong level. A meticulous, systematic and redundant approach minimizes, but never eliminates, such risk.

Exposure

With the level confirmed, I plan the incision 3.0 cm off the midline for a total length of 3.0 cm. My target for this procedure is the T9 transverse process, which provides me with a reliable corridor to both the lateral aspect of the central canal and the pedicle. As will be shown in Chapter 11, Minimally Invasive Resection of Intradural Extramedullary Lesions within the Thoracic Spine, there is a unique topography to the thoracic spine compared to the lumbar spine. The thoracic transverse process projects in the posterior plane, whereas the lumbar transverse process projects in the lateral plane. The posterior projection of this bony prominence makes it an ideal target for dilatation (▶ Fig. 10.7).

After making the incision with a No. 15 blade and opening the fascia with cautery, I carefully pass the first dilator onto the T9 vertebra. In metastatic disease of the spine, I have encountered circumstances where the dilator finds its way quite easily through the diseased bone. I prefer to palpate the transverse process directly and assess the stability of that bony prominence before dilating over the top of it. If I do not appreciate solid intact bone, I shift my position onto such a surface that I know for certain can withstand the downward pressure of dilatation. For successful dilatation and positioning of the minimal access port, intact lamina, facet or transverse process is essential. I confirm my docking position purely by sounding the anatomy with the first dilator. There is an unmistakable feeling of the tip of the dilator interfacing with the intact bone that you become familiar with in your minimally invasive experience in the lumbar and cervical spine. In this particular circumstance, the transverse process was intact and a suitable target to dilate onto for positioning the retractor.

With the minimal access port in position, I bring in the operating microscope and begin the exposure. Again, I am cautious with my use of the cautery. With a suction in one hand, I curiously and cautiously probe the surface of the bone to ensure its integrity before the tip of the cautery dares brush away the muscle. A transverse process, facet or lamina riddled with metastatic disease has the potential to melt away under the tip of the cautery. Keeping this in mind, I use short bursts of cautery until I achieve direct visualization, and tactile feedback instills in me the confidence that the bone is intact.

I embrace the principle of working from known normal anatomy to uncertain abnormal anatomy, just as I would if I were performing a revision operation. My goal is to expose a perimeter of intact lamina, facet and transverse process either above or below the affected area. At the same time, I make every effort to identify those areas weakened by metastatic disease and remain aware of the vulnerable spinal cord that lies beneath these areas. A careful review of the axial T1-weighted MRI with gadolinium guides me to locate the lesion (▶ Fig. 10.3). In this case, I identified and exposed intact bone on the lamina of T8 and intentionally avoided the T9 lamina, given its appearance on MRI.

Decompression

As I begin my decompression, my first objective is to identify the dura of the spinal cord in a region where there is no compression (Video 10.1). The compression on the spinal cord at T9 originates from the lateral structures, specifically the lamina, pedicle and transverse process. My intention is to identify the spinal cord in the midline above the lesion and work down toward the lesion. With the spinal cord and the metastatic lesion in full view, I extend the decompression into the lateral recess before finally addressing the pedicle.

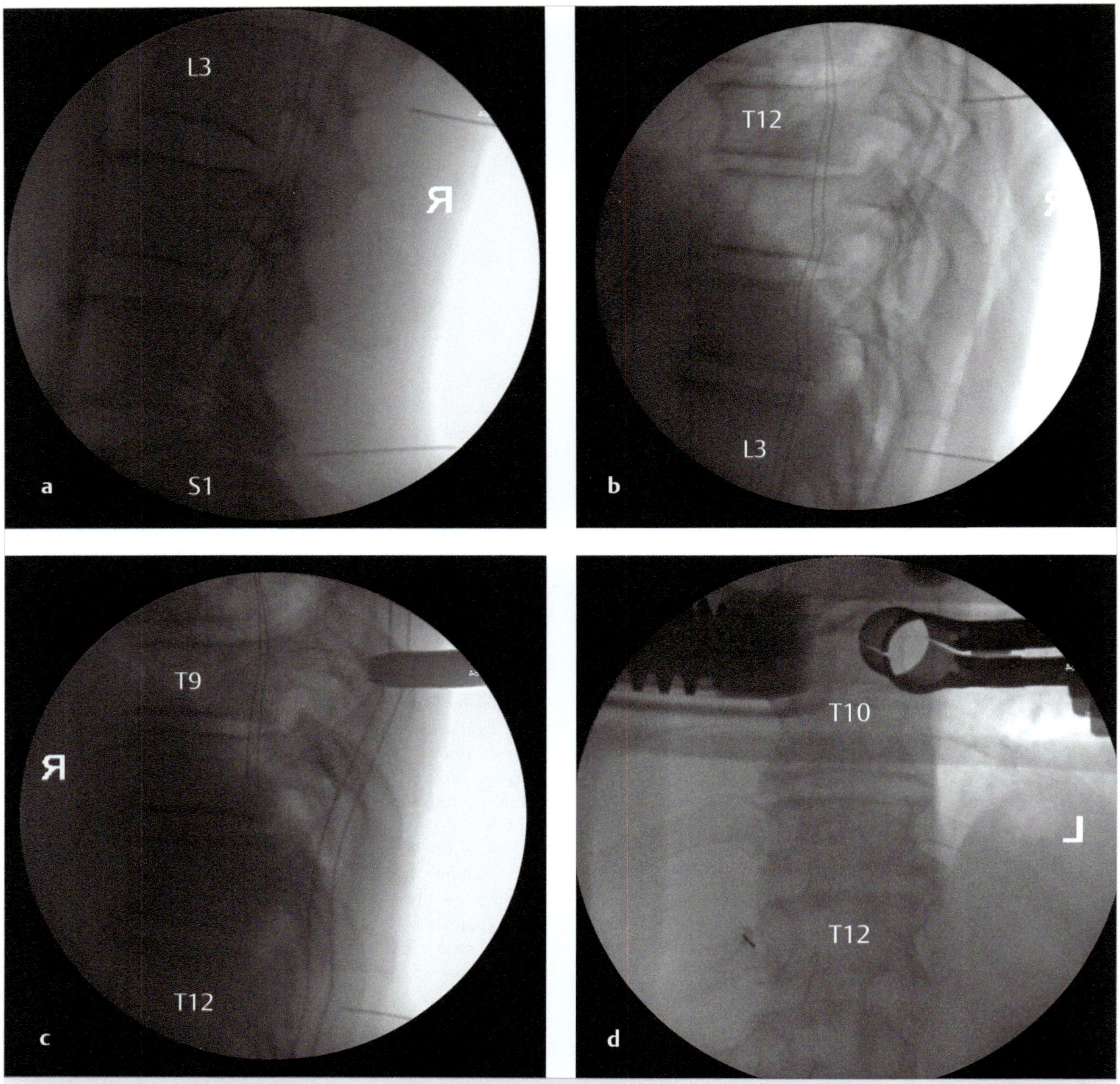

Fig. 10.6 Localization of the level in the thoracic spine. **(a)** Lateral fluoroscopic image demonstrating a spinal needle pointing to S1 and L3. **(b)** Lateral fluoroscopic image with the L3 pedicle at the bottom of the field of view, so that a spinal needle pointing to T12 may now be seen. **(c)** Lateral fluoroscopic image with the T12 vertebral body now at the bottom of the field of view, so that the T9 vertebral body and pedicle may be visualized. In this image, the second dilator is in position. **(d)** Anteroposterior fluoroscopic image demonstrating the spinal needle pointing to the right T12 pedicle and the minimal access port over the top of the T9 pedicle, which is the site of the lesion.

I begin with a laminectomy at T8, where I know I will find unaffected spinal cord. As demonstrated in the operative video, I drill down the lamina of T8 to the level of the ligamentum flavum and then resect the ligamentum (Video 10.1). I now have full visualization of the spinal cord in the midline. Working from rostral to caudal, I establish a plane between the dura of the spinal cord and the lesion with a right-angled, ball-tipped probe. With the plane established, I begin to resect the lamina of T9 with a forward-angled curet or Kerrison punch and continue working until the central canal has been cleared of metastatic disease. Because of the disease within the bone, a drill may be more of a liability than an asset for this component of the decompression. Once I have completed the preliminary decompression of the central canal, I work my way laterally.

Transpedicular Decompression

The next target is the lateral anatomy. Aware of the tumor within the transverse process and pedicle with some extension into the vertebral body, I begin the resection of the lesion in this

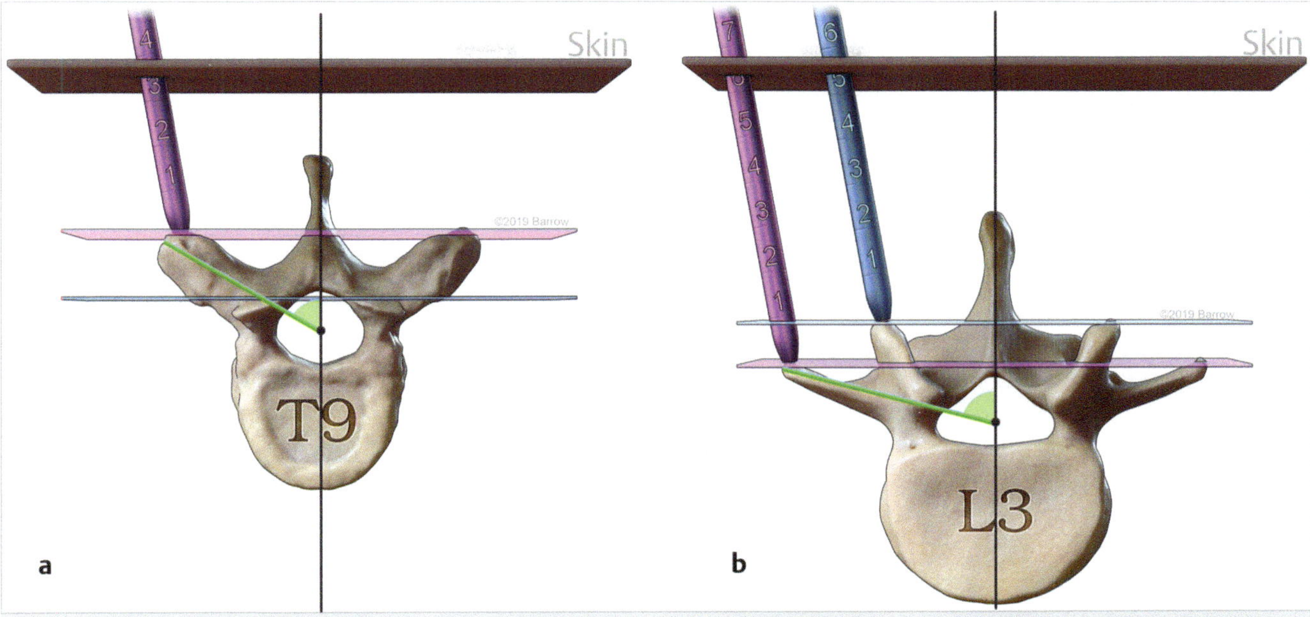

Fig. 10.7 Projection of the thoracic spine transverse processes. These illustrations demonstrate the topographic differences in the projection of the transverse process in the thoracic and lumbar spine. **(a)** Axial view of the T9 vertebra demonstrating the posterior projection of the transverse process. The posterior projection of the transverse process makes it an ideal target for the first dilator. **(b)** Axial view of the L3 vertebra showing the lateral projection of the transverse process. Note the laterality of the transverse process in L3 compared to the posterior projection of the process in T9.

area by first identifying the medial wall of the pedicle and then its superior and inferior aspects. Once I have the boundaries of the pedicle identified, I proceed with drilling into the pedicle. Despite the metastatic disease occupying a significant portion of the pedicle, in this particular circumstance, there was a considerable amount of viable bone that required drilling. Working primarily with the tip of the drill within the pedicle, I proceed with essentially coring out the pedicle until its walls have been thinned to the point that a pituitary rongeur may be used to remove what remains of the pedicle wall. Alternatively, an Epstein curet can begin to infold the walls of the pedicle. The T9 nerve root comes into full view and remains visible throughout this process. The transpedicular decompression continues into the vertebral body until it becomes evident that no further metastatic disease is visible. A final review of the gadolinium-enhanced MRI helps me decide how much further to proceed into the vertebral body.

After visual inspection demonstrates the absence of any further compression of the spinal cord from the tumor within the vertebral body, the area may be sealed off with bone wax or another hemostatic agent. As I am performing this component of the procedure, I always keep in mind that what I am doing is palliative. By no means is it intended to be curative. As mentioned at the beginning of this chapter, long-term survival is more a product of primary malignancy type and response to adjuvant therapy rather than from cytoreductive surgery on the spine. This patient has widely metastatic disease throughout the spine. Removing every last cell of the tumor within the vertebral body makes no difference in survival. On the other hand, if I remove too much of the vertebral body, I run the risk of making this segment unstable and in need of further surgery. The goal of the operation was the preservation of neurologic function, with the expectation that this intervention would improve the patient's quality of life. Separation of the tumor from the spinal cord with subsequent stereotactic radiosurgery, as reported by Laufer et al,[8] offers local disease control.

Upon completion of the decompression, I spend a great deal of time working on hemostasis. I cover all of the bleeding bone surfaces generously with bone wax and spend a great deal of time cauterizing the soft tissues. Resection of metastatic disease to the spine is the one circumstance in minimally invasive approaches where I routinely use a drain. I tunnel out a single limb of a Hemovac drain (Zimmer Technology, Inc., Warsaw, IN) and begin the closure in a multilayer fashion.

Postoperative Course

The patient recovered well from both the cervical corpectomy and fusion and the thoracic decompression. The drain was removed on the first postoperative day. The postoperative MRI demonstrated complete decompression of the spinal cord (▶ Fig. 10.8). By postoperative day 2, the patient was ambulating independently with the resolution of urinary retention symptoms and marked improvement in his gait. He was discharged on postoperative day 2 and began radiation therapy of the cervical, thoracic and lumbar spine on postoperative day 5. He completed radiation therapy and continued with chemotherapy without any wound healing issues. The patient succumbed to the progression of metastatic disease 16 months after his initial diagnosis. He maintained bowel and bladder function as well as ambulatory status until he entered hospice care 15 months after his diagnosis.

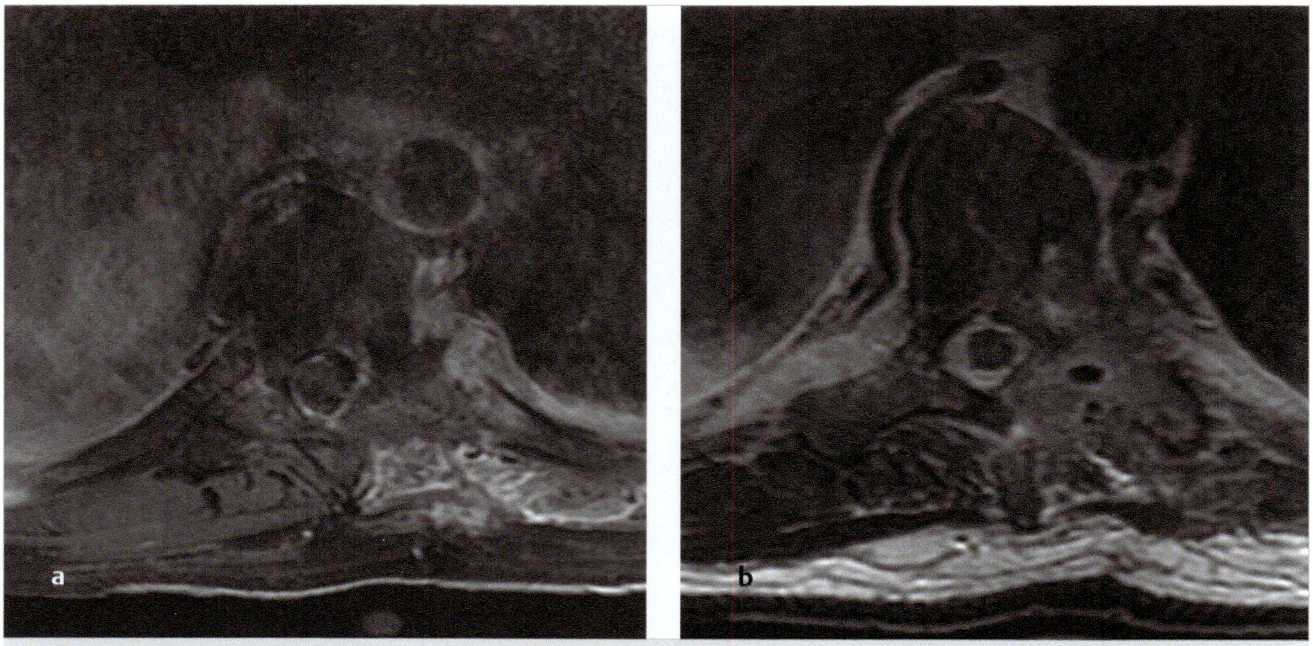

Fig. 10.8 Postoperative magnetic resonance imaging (MRI) with and without gadolinium demonstrating the extent of the decompression achieved with a minimally invasive decompression. **(a)** Postoperative axial T2-weighted MRI no longer showing the compression on the spinal cord. **(b)** Postoperative axial T1-weighted MRI with gadolinium demonstrating the extent of resection of the contrast-enhanced tumor. When compared to ▶ Fig. 10.3d the area of enhancement from the pedicle, lamina and within the vertebral body has been removed.

10.4.2 Case Illustration 2: Localization with Image Guidance for Resection of Metastatic Lesion

The liability of metastatic disease distorting the vertebral body and the pedicle can be harnessed in the form of an asset for the purpose of localization using image guidance. The previous case demonstrated the systematic but tedious process of localization with fluoroscopy. The following case demonstrates the localization and decompression of the spinal cord with computer-assisted navigation. Localization remains one of the challenges in relation to the management of any lesion in the thoracic spine, but especially in the upper thoracic spine. When a characteristic distortion of the vertebral anatomy occurs, computer-assisted navigation can streamline the localization process and guide the extent of resection. If this technology is available at your institution, it is a viable and reliable alternative to localization with fluoroscopy.

Clinical History and Neurologic Examination

A 78-year-old man, who was diagnosed with small cell lung cancer diagnosed 6 months earlier, presented with a precipitous decline in ambulatory function. On examination, the patient demonstrated normal motor, sensation and reflexes in the upper extremities. In the lower extremities, the patient possessed 3/5 strength in the proximal and distal muscle groups. The patient had a clear sensory dissociation level at the nipple line. A reflex examination demonstrated sustained clonus and upgoing toes bilaterally. While he had declining ambulatory function over the past week, he remained independently ambulatory up until 48 hours before admission. At the time of presentation, he was incapable of unassisted four-step ambulation.

Radiographic Evaluation

MRI of the thoracic spine (▶ Fig. 10.9) demonstrated the involvement of the vertebral body of T3. There was an element of ventral compression from the metastatic lesion within the vertebral body, but the majority of the compression originated from the dorsal epidural lesion eccentric to the right. The patient was also found to have lesions in the lower thoracic spine and upper lumbar spine without compression of the neural elements. This T3 metastasis was the first evidence of metastatic disease in the spine. An MRI of the brain with and without gadolinium demonstrated two lesions in the right frontal lobe, each measuring less than 1 cm in diameter (not shown).

Clinical Decision-Making

The definitive procedure, in this case, would be a T3 corpectomy. Anterior or lateral approaches are less viable options in the upper thoracic spine. Performing a thoracotomy in this elderly gentleman, who is already 6 months into a known diagnosis of metastatic small cell lung cancer and known metastatic disease in the brain, introduces a significant amount of morbidity. Therefore, a posterior approach is the most palatable. The definitive posterior approach in this circumstance is a costotransversectomy and transpedicular corpectomy with reconstruction of the anterior column as well as posterior instrumentation from the lower cervical spine to the midthoracic spine.

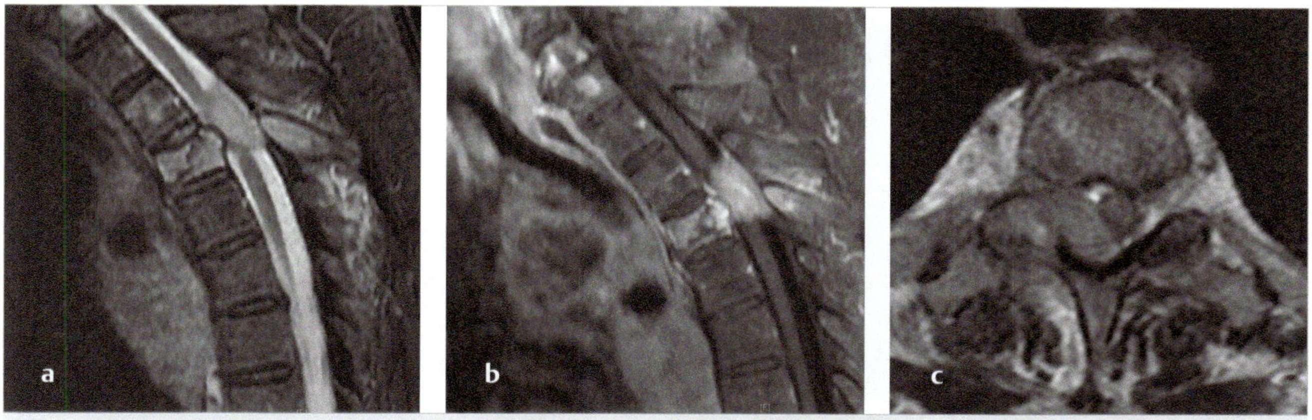

Fig. 10.9 Preoperative magnetic resonance imaging (MRI) of the thoracic spine showing a T3 lesion with predominantly dorsal epidural compression from the metastatic lesion on the right side, which also clearly involves the vertebral body. **(a)** Sagittal T2-weighted MRI with dorsal epidural compression. **(b)** Sagittal T1-weighted MRI with gadolinium demonstrating the enhancement of the lesion within the vertebral body and the dorsal epidural space. **(c)** Axial T2-weighted MRI revealing the spinal cord compression predominantly from the right, with mass effect on the spinal cord (axial T1-weighted MRI with gadolinium had a motion artifact).

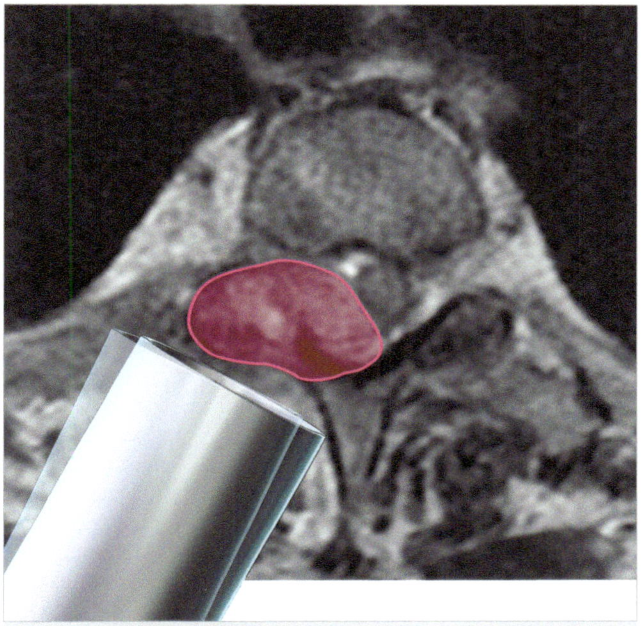

Fig. 10.10 Anatomical basis for minimally invasive decompressive separation surgery. The lesion (denoted in *magenta shading*) appears to have grown from the vertebral body into the right pedicle. From the right pedicle, it has extended into the epidural space on the right, displacing the spinal cord. Unilateral compression plays to the strength of a minimally invasive approach. A minimal access port has been superimposed onto the axial magnetic resonance image in this figure. When positioned in the two trajectories illustrated, the access port provides access to the entire span of the lesion.

Because the patient's projected life expectancy was less than 1 year, and the disease was spreading through the thoracic and lumbar spine, the goal of the operation was to return the patient to independent 4-point gait ambulation. A careful review of the CT demonstrated that less than 25% of the vertebral body of T3 was occupied with metastatic disease. With this situation in mind, another option would be separation surgery with decompression of the spinal cord compression and stereotactic radiosurgery. Up until this point, no radiation therapy had been administered to the spine. Although a pathological fracture of T3 is present, the cause of his neurologic deficit originated from the epidural compression. A minimally invasive approach would allow for decompression of the spinal cord with the removal of the epidural component of the metastasis only. Soon after, he could begin radiation therapy. ▶ Fig. 10.10 demonstrates the conceptual surgical strategy with a minimal access port.

Intervention

The patient was positioned on a Jackson table. Since the lesion was at T3, I secured the patient's arms at his side, which allowed me a greater reach to the upper thoracic spine than if the arms were brought forward. Review of the sagittal CT reconstruction demonstrated a characteristic appearance to the pedicle and vertebral body of T3, which made it distinct from the other levels (▶ Fig. 10.11). Given this appearance, image guidance was a plausible alternative to fluoroscopic localization.

Despite the plan to use image guidance, some preliminary fluoroscopy would still be needed to approximate the location of the reference frame. Ideally, I would place the reference frame at T5. With the patient positioned, I approximated the T5 level by laying down Steinman pins on the skin and obtaining only AP fluoroscopic images, counting up from T12. I do not confirm the AP and lateral planes because the location of the reference frame only needs to be approximated. In other words, while I want it precisely at T5, it can be off by a level, preferably at T6 instead of T4. I accomplish the precise localization of the level with computer-assisted navigation to identify that characteristic appearance of the pedicle and vertebral body.

Localization

After I approximated the T5 level with AP fluoroscopy, I marked the level, prepped and draped the area, and began with a small incision over the spinous process of T5. I secured a reference frame into position and then proceeded with bringing in the intraoperative CT scanner. Once I completed the registration of

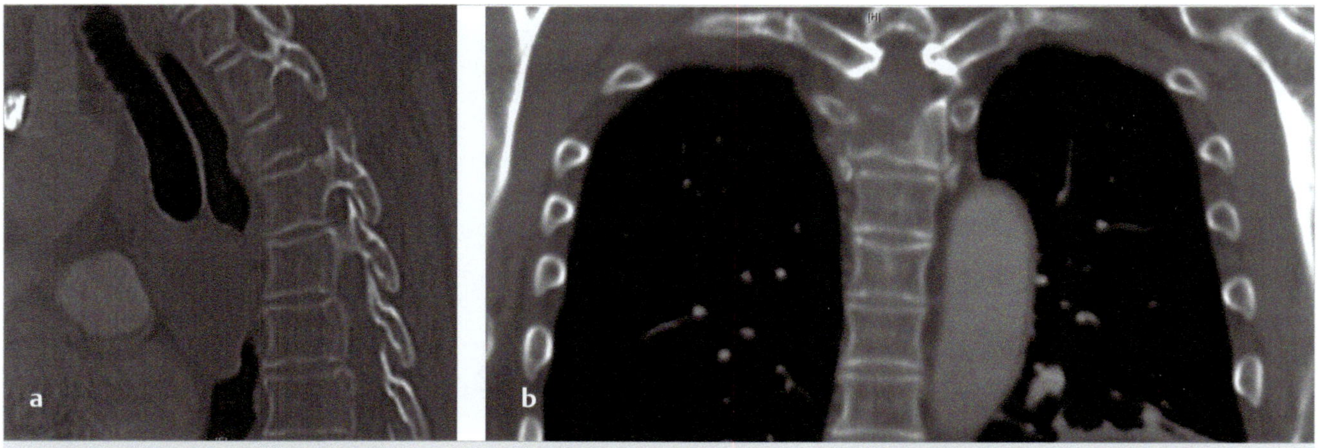

Fig. 10.11 Lytic involvement on computed tomography (CT). **(a)** Sagittal CT reconstruction demonstrating the involvement of the posterior aspect of the vertebral body and pedicle of T3. This characteristic appearance may be readily identified with image guidance. **(b)** Coronal reconstruction again demonstrating the lytic component on the right lateral aspect of the vertebral body.

the instruments, I used a trajectory view with the navigation pointer to confirm the level (▶ Fig. 10.12).

The characteristic appearance of the pedicle allows me to confirm the level and then plan the incision with an ideal trajectory. I plan a 3.0-cm incision 2.5 cm off the midline immediately over the pedicle of T3. After making the incision, I open the fascia with cautery 25% larger than the skin incision. As mentioned in the previous case, it would be ill-advised to begin dilating over the top of diseased bone. Instead, I target the lamina of the segment above or below as an anchor point for my dilatation. In this case, I confirmed an intact T2 lamina on the preoperative CT image and then again with the navigation system. I was able to palpate onto the T2 lamina and, with guidance from navigation, confirm intact lamina, which is yet another advantage of using navigation: the capacity to avoid diseased bone (▶ Fig. 10.13).

Decompression

With an expandable minimal access port in position, I begin first by exposing the unaffected lamina of T2 and then work my way onto the diseased lamina of T3 (Video 10.2). Despite the appearance on CT and MRI, the outer cortex of the lamina was remarkably preserved. In this circumstance, the lesion was predominantly within the canal off to the right (▶ Fig. 10.9, ▶ Fig. 10.10). My initial focus was on ensuring an adequate midline decompression. To that end, I drilled at the base of the spinous process and undercut the contralateral lamina. I continued to drill the lamina to a shrimp shell thickness. At such a thickness, the ligamentum flavum may be appreciated beneath. A forward-angled curet establishes a plane over the top of the ligamentum flavum, and a Kerrison rongeur removes what remains of the lamina. I extend the resection of bone until I reach the insertion of the ligamentum flavum above the level of the lesion. I then begin resecting the ligamentum flavum with a Kerrison rongeur and directly visualize the spinal cord. I have now secured a normal, unaffected area of the spinal canal from which I can begin to approach the lesion, which is an important point that bears repeating. If upon completion of the laminectomy and resection of the ligamentum flavum, I found myself within the metastatic lesion and unable to see the spinal cord, I would immediately stop and shift my work to the level above or below in order to identify normal anatomy and then work back toward the lesion. Working within the lesion without knowing exactly where the spinal cord resides adds unnecessary risk to the procedure and causes anxiety to the surgeon. It is imperative when resecting a metastatic lesion that causes compression of the spinal cord to identify the unaffected spinal cord first and develop a plane in between the lesion and the spinal cord. Identifying the lesion–spinal cord interface allows for safe cauterization of the lesion, and thereby an element of hemostasis, as you proceed with your resection.

Once I have identified the spinal cord and established a plane between the lesion and the cord, I alternate cauterization and resection. A right-angled bipolar is of tremendous value for this component of the procedure. I turn down the energy of the bipolar and use short bursts with the tips in the plane between the spinal cord and the lesion. Resection of the metastatic lesion can be met with significant blood loss. The intermittent cauterization technique mitigates the blood loss but does not eliminate it. Ultrasonic aspirators are another viable option. After cauterization, forward-angled curets can free up and even deliver the lesion. In this case, I continue the resection out into the left lateral recess, until I feel I have accomplished the decompression (Video 10.2). I use the navigation to assess my extent of resection. While helpful, nothing confirms the extent of decompression like direct visual inspection of the spinal cord itself. The goal involves the separation of the tumor from the spinal cord, so that stereotactic radiosurgery can achieve local disease control.

As mentioned in the first case, I routinely tunnel out a single limb of a Hemovac drain in all metastatic resections. After visual inspection of the area for hemostasis, I close the minimal access port and slowly remove it, obtaining hemostasis as I proceed with its removal. I closed the incision in a multilayered fashion, using a size 0 polyglactin 910 suture on a UR-6 needle for the fascia, a 2–0 polyglactin 910 suture on an X-1 needle for the subcutaneous layer and 4–0 polyglactin 910 on an RB-1

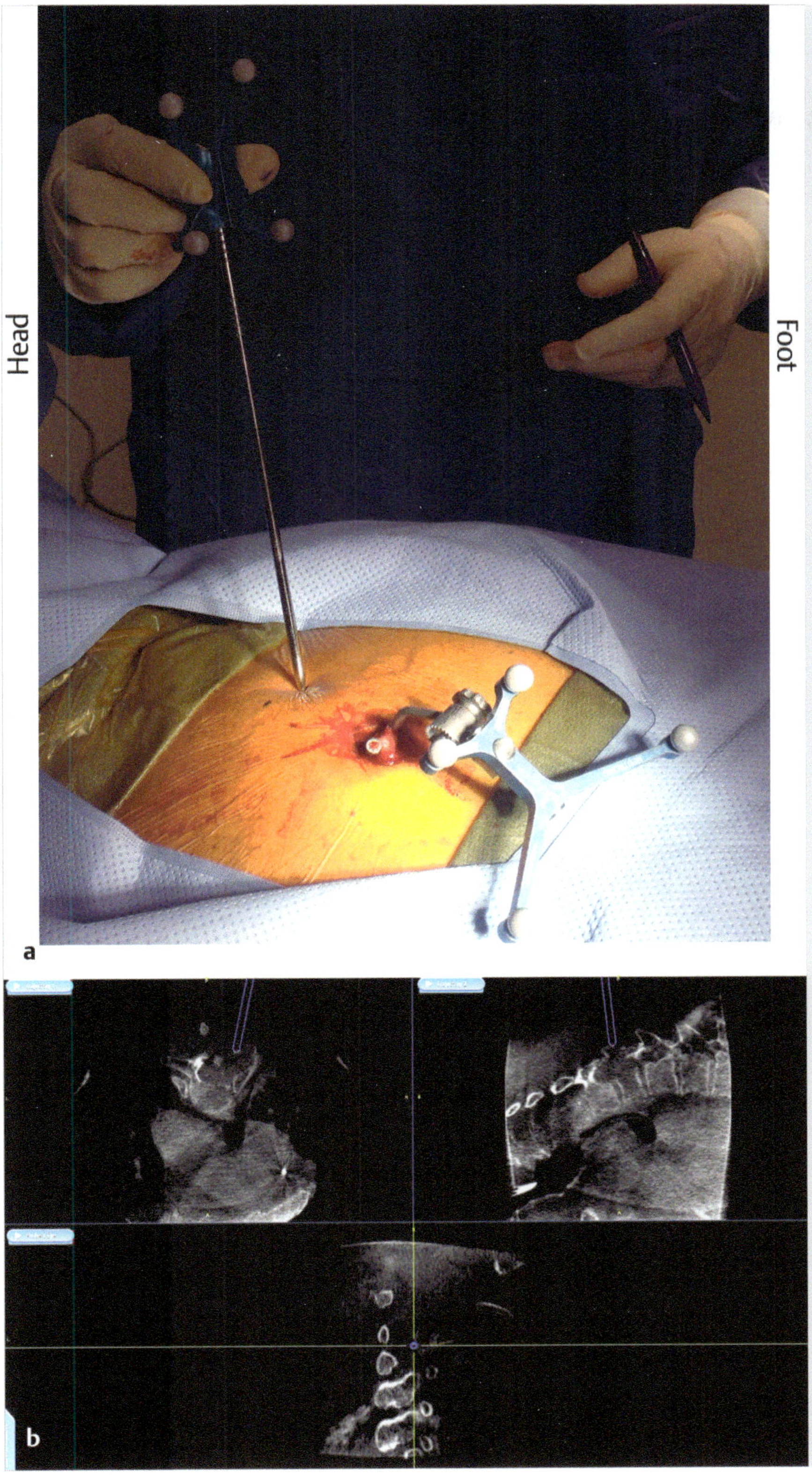

Fig. 10.12 Localization of the lesion with computer-assisted navigation. (a) Intraoperative photograph demonstrating localization of the T3 lesion for decompression. The reference frame has been secured at T5. The patient's head is to the surgeon's right (left side of image). (b) Screen capture image demonstrating localization of the level by identification of the distorted pedicle. Navigation assists with the planning of the incision.

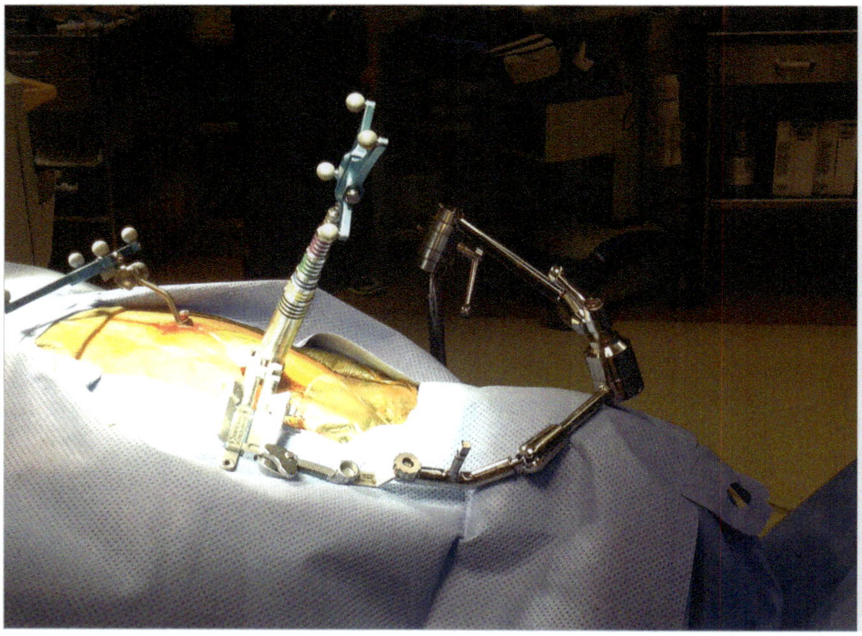

Fig. 10.13 Intraoperative photograph demonstrating an expandable minimal access port positioned with the guidance from the navigation system.

needle for the subcuticular layer. I secure the drain in position with a silk suture. Finally, I remove the reference frame and close that incision.

Postoperative Course

The patient had an uncomplicated postoperative course. The drain was removed on the first postoperative day. By postoperative day 2, the patient returned to four-step ambulatory function with minimal assistance. He began hypofractionated, stereotactic radiation therapy to the vertebral body of T3 and various other lesions in the spine on postoperative day 3, which was also his date of discharge. Two weeks after radiation therapy, the patient returned to independent ambulatory function. Despite the early commencement of radiation therapy, there was no delay in healing of the wound. A surveillance MRI 6 months after surgery demonstrated control of local metastatic disease at T3, without any evidence of spinal cord compression (▶ Fig. 10.14). The patient maintained full ambulatory function until the progression of his disease led to a precipitous decline of his pulmonary function and prompted a transfer to hospice care. The patient expired 14 months after his minimally invasive decompression surgery and 20 months after his initial diagnosis.

10.4.3 Case Illustration 3: Metastatic Testicular Cancer to the Thoracic Spine

In the previous two examples, I reviewed two forms of localization: fluoroscopy and computer-assisted navigation. In this example, I present the use of embolization using Onyx to facilitate not only the resection of the lesion but also assist in the localization of the lesion.

Clinical History and Neurologic Examination

A 37-year-old man diagnosed with testicular cancer at the age of 25 presented now with widely metastatic disease to the lungs, liver, and thoracic and lumbar spine. The patient had a known metastatic lesion of the T10 vertebral body, which was diagnosed 15 months prior, without canal compromise. At that point in time, the patient's chief complaint was pain; he had no neurologic complaints. The patient underwent external beam radiation to the thoracic spine which led to the alleviation of his symptoms. Over the past several months, the patient had been experiencing increasing right flank pain and difficulty walking. A neurologic examination demonstrated a T10 dissociation level, 3 + patellar reflexes and sustained clonus in the lower extremities. He possessed 4/5 strength in the proximal and distal muscle groups of the lower extremities but was capable of only limited four-step ambulation with the assistance of a walker. The patient denied experiencing any bowel or bladder issues.

Radiographic Evaluation

Thoracic spine MRI with gadolinium demonstrated a destructive lesion centered in the right T10 pedicle, extending into the canal and displacing the spinal cord to the left with resultant mass effect on the cord. The lesion also extended into the vertebral body and the transverse process of T10 (▶ Fig. 10.15, ▶ Fig. 10.16).

Clinical Decision-Making

The patient's prognosis for long-term survival was poor. After a discussion with the radiation and medical oncologist, it was felt that the realistic life expectancy of this patient was less than 6 months. In my mind, such a poor prognosis eliminated any possibility of corpectomy and instrumentation in this patient,

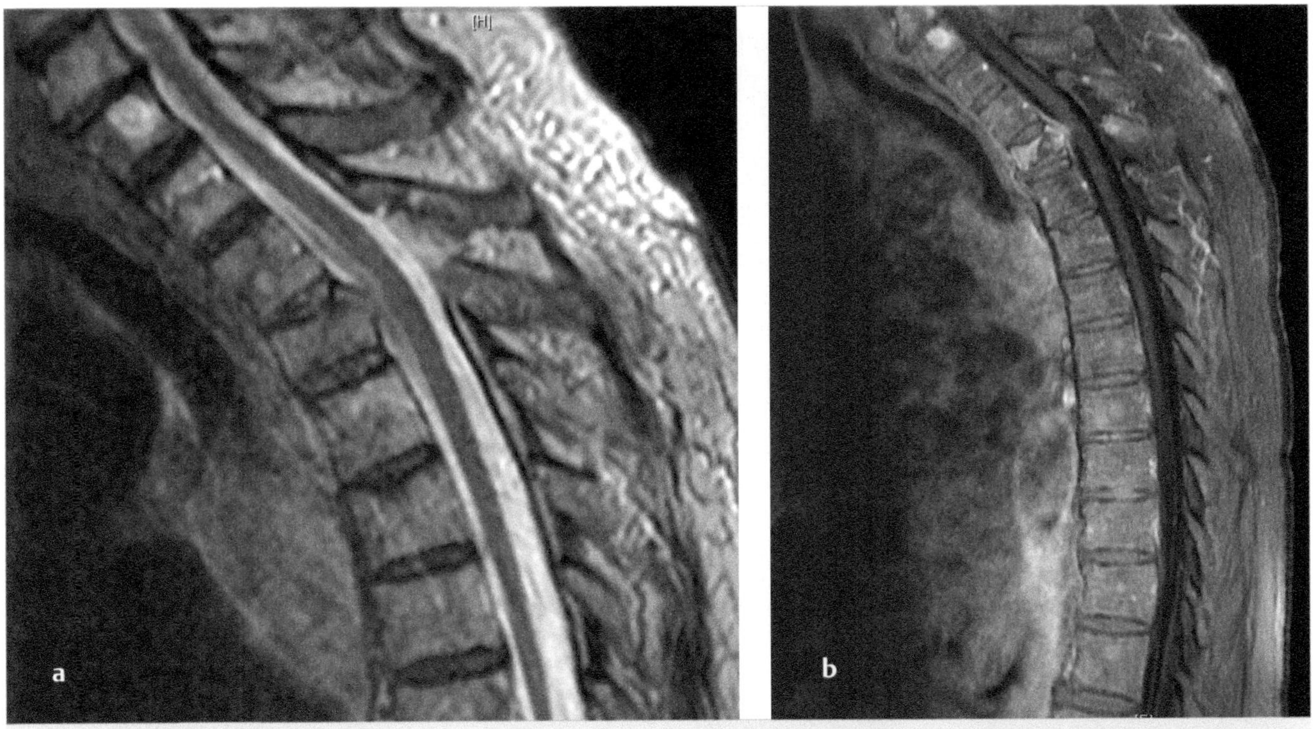

Fig. 10.14 Postoperative magnetic resonance imaging (MRI) of the thoracic spine. **(a)** Sagittal T2-weighted MRI demonstrating decompression of the spinal cord with complete removal of the dorsal compression. **(b)** Sagittal T1-weighted MRI with gadolinium showing persistent enhancement of the vertebral body of T3, but the removal of the dorsal enhancement of the spinal cord. The spinal cord was successfully decompressed, and the patient regained independent ambulatory function.

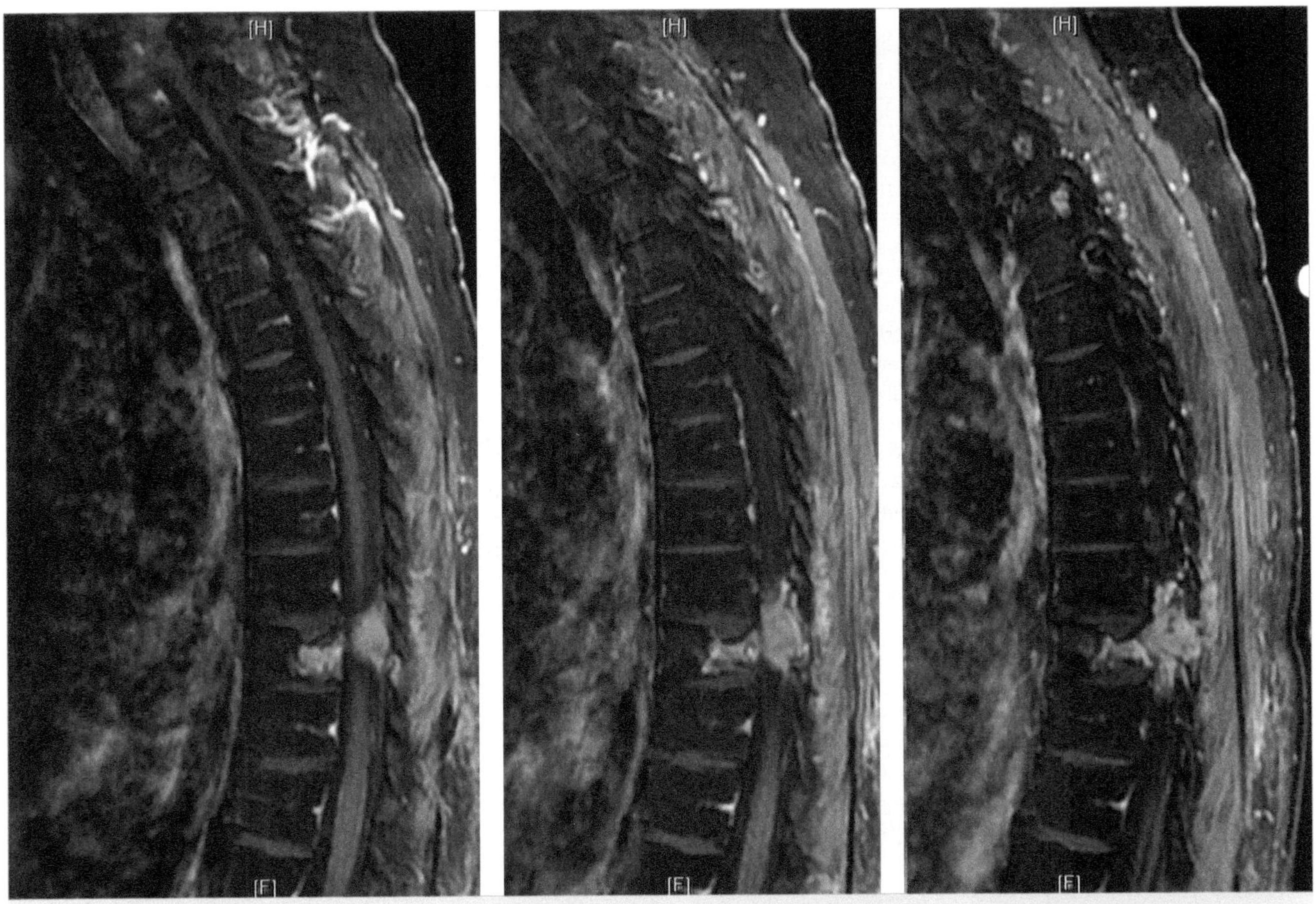

Fig. 10.15 Sagittal T1-weighted magnetic resonance imaging (MRI) of the thoracic spine with gadolinium. This series of sagittal MRIs demonstrates the epidural lesion within the vertebral body of T10, extending through the pedicle and into the epidural space.

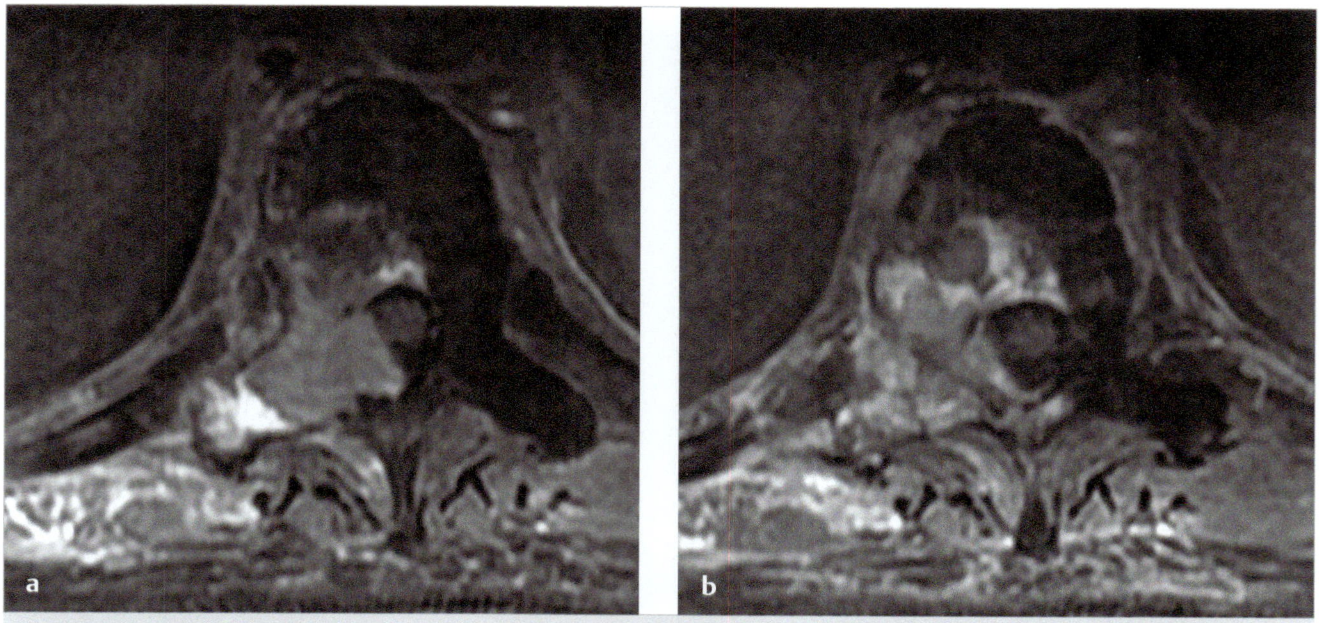

Fig. 10.16 Axial T1-weighted magnetic resonance imaging (MRI) with gadolinium. These two axial images demonstrate the involvement of the pedicle, vertebral body and transverse process. **(a)** MRI showing the mass effect on the spinal cord and the absence of involvement on the left. **(b)** The heterogeneity of the signal within the pedicle and the vertebral body was suspicious for a highly vascular lesion, prompting an angiogram for preoperative embolization.

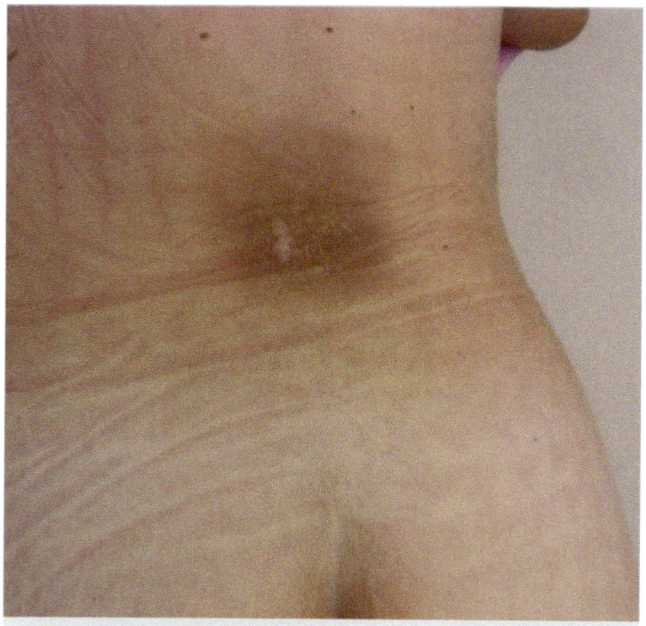

Fig. 10.17 Photograph of the patient with radiation dermatitis in the vicinity of the proposed surgical site. In this particular patient, a midline open approach through this irradiated area would present a significant challenge healing.

which would result in lengthy hospitalization and recovery. Furthermore, the patient had already undergone radiation to the spine previously and had persistent radiation dermatitis in the vicinity of the possible surgical site (▶ Fig. 10.17). An incision traversing this area would contribute to the risk of delayed wound healing and potential infection.

The goal of any surgical intervention would be palliative decompression of the spinal cord to restore and preserve neurologic function for this patient for as long as possible. The patient wanted to be home with his family and not in the hospital or in a rehabilitation facility. Any surgical intervention needed to include that objective as part of the calculus. Incorporating all these factors into the decision-making process led me to offer the patient a minimally invasive right transpedicular decompression of the T10 segment. Such an approach could decompress the neural elements through a small paramedian incision and optimize an environment for healing the wound in a previously irradiated area (▶ Fig. 10.18).

Localization

Before proceeding with surgery, preoperative angiography and embolization were performed to mitigate blood loss from the resection. With the patient positioned prone on a Jackson table and the arms brought forward, I began the process of localizing in the same manner that I had described in the first case illustration. More by accident than by design, the embolization had the unintended consequence of facilitating the localization for placement of the expandable minimal access port (▶ Fig. 10.19). I still used the identical process of preoperative fluoroscopic confirmation in the AP and lateral planes, counting up from the sacrum, but once I confirmed the level of the cast of the embolization material on the fluoroscopic image, I became vastly more efficient in the planning of my incision and docking of the expandable minimal access port.

Decompression

Similar to the first case illustration, the compression of the spinal cord originates from the lateral aspect of the canal and

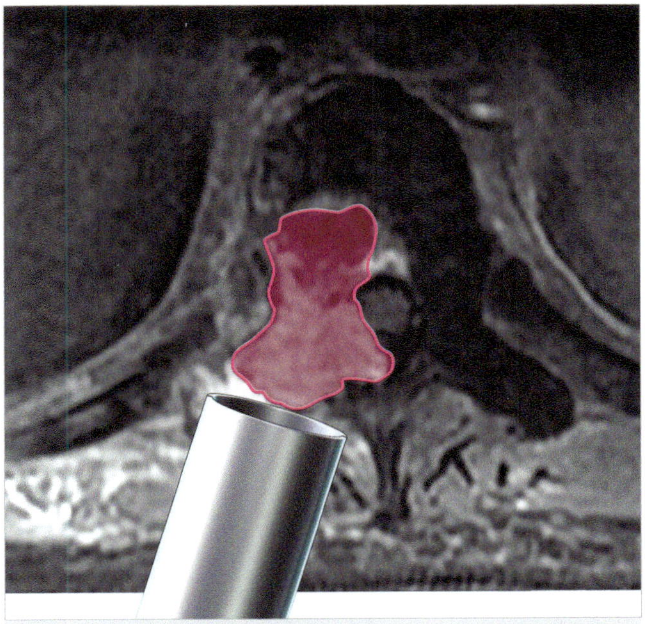

Fig. 10.18 Preoperative planning for the decompression of T10. Axial T1-weighted magnetic resonance imaging of the thoracic spine demonstrating the planned transpedicular decompression with laminectomy. Magenta shading shows the outline of the metastatic tumor compressing the spinal cord.

vertebral body (Video 10.3). Therefore, the approach would be a transpedicular one to access the pedicle and vertebral body and hemilaminectomy (▶ Fig. 10.18). As always, the posteriorly projecting transverse process is our North Star in the thoracic spine. The first step after securing the expandable minimal access port and bringing in the operating microscope is exposure of the transverse process. The transverse process leads us to the facet, lamina and base of the spinous process. I keep in mind, as I proceed with the exposure, that the bone is riddled with metastatic disease and I need to take care not to place excessive pressure on a bony prominence, which may not tolerate that kind of force and unexpectedly give way. I keep this vulnerability in mind from the moment I begin dilating and throughout the exposure. Before starting to drill, I confirm that I have all the exposure I need to complete the decompression.

As demonstrated in the operative video, the outer cortex of the lamina and transverse process were remarkably well preserved in this patient despite the metastatic disease that lay beneath them (Video 10.3). In the earlier chapters, I had described the technique of initially drilling laterally and identifying the lateral aspect of the canal before working medial toward the spinal cord. In the case of distorted anatomy, such as metastatic disease, working laterally in the transverse process and pedicle would place me in the thick of abnormal anatomy. Finding my bearings and maintaining my orientation would be difficult from a lateral position. My strategy, in this case, was to abide by the age-old adage of spine surgery, which advises us to identify the normal and work toward the abnormal. Therefore, I performed the laminectomy, identified the spinal cord and then worked from lateral to medial. In this circumstance, a laminectomy would be the safest and most efficient strategy and prevent disorientation.

With the patient rotated away from me, I drilled the junction of the lamina and spinous process until I reached the ligamentum flavum. I widened my bone work for a generous midline decompression and then removed the ligamentum flavum. As I extended my bone work laterally, the metastatic lesion came into view. I worked to develop a plane between the metastatic lesion and the spinal cord. Knowing the limits of the spinal canal and having direct visualization of the spinal cord, I was able to remove the diseased pars interarticularis and transverse process and work toward the transpedicular approach. Despite the embolization, the lesion remained highly vascular. Intermittent coagulation with right-angle bipolar cautery was essential as I proceeded with the resection. Once I could see the lateral aspect of the spinal cord, the boundaries of the pedicle came into view. I then proceeded with drilling down the pedicle and entering the vertebral body to decompress the ventral aspect of the spinal cord.

Upon completion of my decompression, I was able to visualize the entire posterior, lateral and ventral aspects of the right side of the spinal cord through my exposure. The objective of separating the spinal cord from the lesion had been achieved. Having removed the lateral aspect of the vertebral body, I poured methyl methacrylate into the void to prevent an asymmetric collapse, which also had the added benefit of sealing bleeding cancellous bone from the vertebral body. Meticulous hemostasis is imperative before closure. Sealing bleeding from the bone with bone wax and identifying soft tissue bleeding as well as residual metastatic disease are best managed by resection rather than cauterization. I find it remarkable how the absence of bleeding is a reliable marker for the extent of resection of a metastatic lesion. Regardless of how satisfied I am with the hemostasis, I always use a Hemovac drain in the resection of all metastatic lesions because of my concern for postoperative bleeding in cancer patients. It is always easier to remove a drain the following day than take the patient back to surgery for evacuation of a postoperative hematoma.

Closure

I placed the tip of the Hemovac drain into the void created by the transpedicular approach and secured it into position at the skin surface with a silk suture. I then begin the closure in a multilayered fashion, as described earlier in this chapter.

Postoperative Course

The patient was ambulatory with a walker on the day of surgery and reported complete alleviation of his incapacitating flank pain. Postoperative MRI demonstrated a well decompressed spinal cord (▶ Fig. 10.20). The drain was removed on the first postoperative day. He was discharged on postoperative day 2 and continued with adjuvant therapy. Two weeks after surgery, he was seen in clinic ambulating independently and had normal bowel and bladder function. Seven months after surgery, the patient went into multisystem organ failure and succumbed to a progression of his disease.

10.4.4 Case Illustration 4: Metastatic Breast Cancer

Thus far in this chapter, I have demonstrated multiple cases of metastatic disease successfully managed with minimally

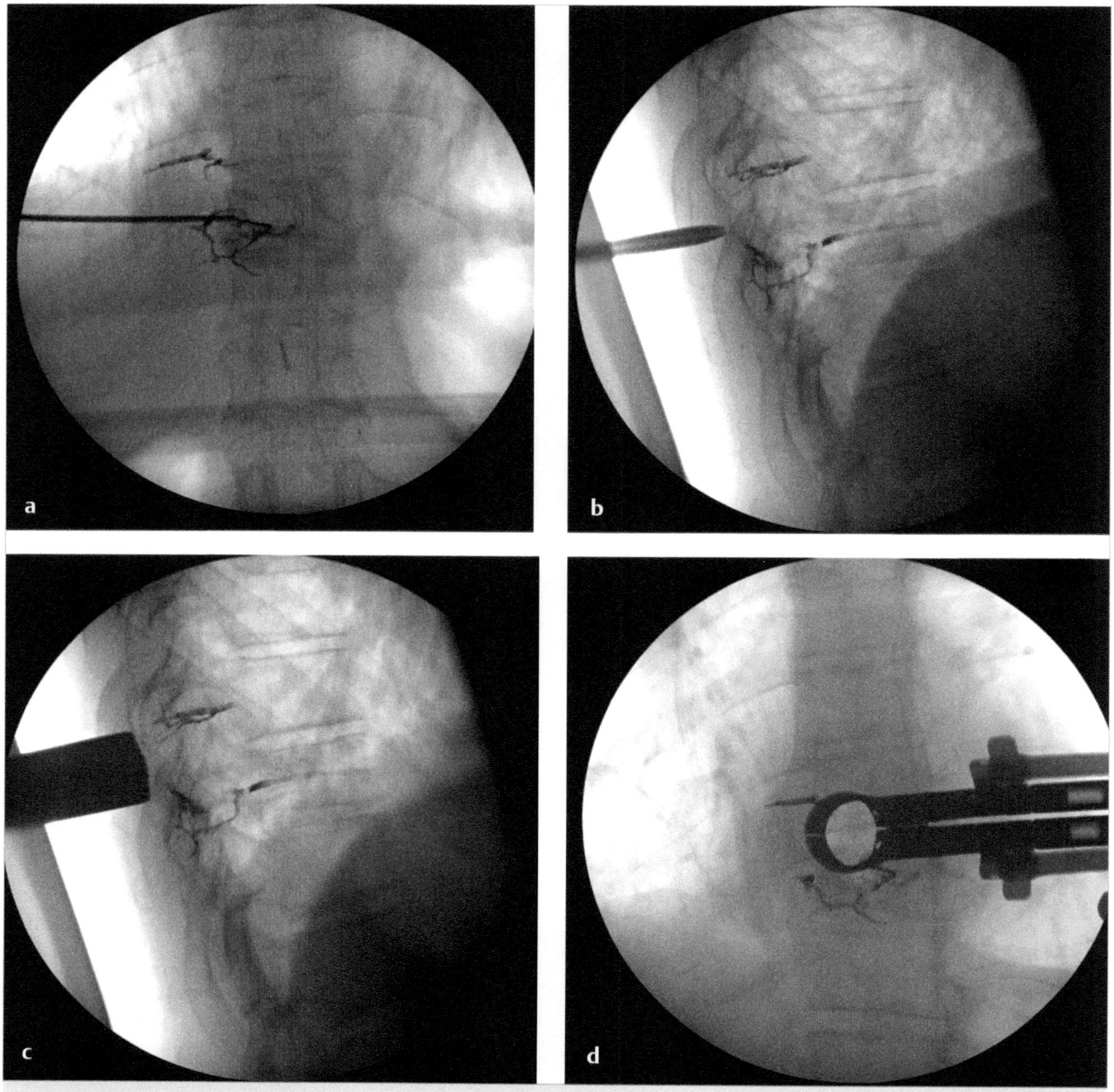

Fig. 10.19 Embolization of the metastatic tumor. **(a)** Anteroposterior (AP) fluoroscopic image demonstrating the embolic material within the radicular arteries feeding the lesion. With a spinal needle at T12, the pedicle of T10 is confirmed. The embolic material then becomes a reference point for localization. **(b)** Lateral fluoroscopic image demonstrating the first dilator at the level of the T10 pedicle. The embolic material has become the sole reference point for securing the minimal access port. **(c)** Lateral fluoroscopic image demonstrating the minimal access port in position. **(d)** Owl's eye AP view demonstrating the minimal access port overtop the T10 pedicle.

invasive approaches. However, not all metastatic lesions are amenable to minimally invasive resections. It is essential to recognize the limitations of minimally invasive approaches so that these techniques may be applied appropriately for patient care. The following example is one of those circumstances. The patient was sent to me by one of my colleagues in radiation oncology for the explicit purpose of undergoing a minimally invasive procedure so that radiation could begin quickly. However, after reviewing the images and the clinical history, I felt that a minimally invasive approach was not in the best interests of the patient. For this reason, a case of metastatic breast cancer to the spine managed with a traditional midline open approach has found its way into this Primer. Knowing when not to use minimally invasive techniques is as equally valuable as knowing how to use them.

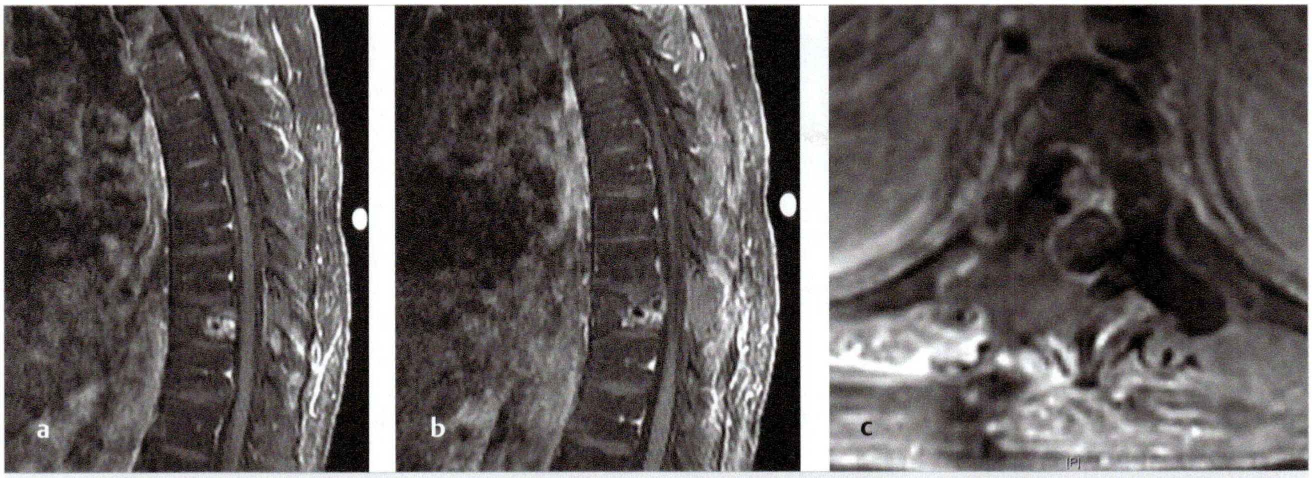

Fig. 10.20 Postoperative magnetic resonance imaging (MRI) of the thoracic spine. **(a)** Sagittal T1-weighted MRI of the thoracic spine demonstrating the ventral and dorsal decompression of the spinal cord. **(b)** Sagittal T1-weighted MRI of the thoracic spine with gadolinium. The areas of hypodensity represent the methyl methacrylate. **(c)** Axial T1-weighted MRI with gadolinium demonstrating the removal of the enhancement around the spinal cord.

Clinical History and Neurologic Examination

A 41-year-old woman diagnosed with infiltrating ductal cell carcinoma 5 years earlier presented to her oncologist with increasing back pain after a low-energy motor vehicle accident. The patient was in remission after bilateral mastectomies, chemotherapy and radiation. One year earlier, she had a negative positron emission tomography (PET) study. On examination, the patient was independently ambulatory but reported an unsteady gait. She demonstrated 5/5 strength throughout all muscle groups of the lower extremities, intact sensation on pinprick and light touch examinations, as well as proprioception. She had 3 + patellar reflexes and sustained clonus in both lower extremities. However, tandem gait was significantly altered. She had a negative Romberg test.

Radiographic Studies

MRI of the thoracic spine demonstrated a large epidural lesion centered at the T6 level, which extended from the midvertebral body of T5 to the superior aspect of T7 (▶ Fig. 10.21). The rostrocaudal dimension of the epidural lesion was 4.1 cm. The lesion involved the entire spinous process. The sagittal T1-weighted MRI with gadolinium shows a pattern of enhancement from the base and extending into the tip of the spinous process (▶ Fig. 10.21b). No other metastatic lesions were identified in the brain, cervical or lumbar spine on surveillance MRI of the neuroaxis.

Clinical Decision-Making

In this case, the patient had a solitary metastatic lesion, which was seen, after 5 years of quiescent disease, on T1-weighted MRI with gadolinium (▶ Fig. 10.21b). The axial MRI showed the epidural lesion extending into the entire spinous process. A minimally invasive approach can decompress the central canal and remove all of the epidural compression. The theoretical limit for a minimally invasive approach with access port fully open and the blades fully angled is 4.5 cm, but with such an approach, I will not be able to remove the entire spinous process. Without evidence of metastatic disease elsewhere, the goal of any surgical resection should be complete resection of the lesion. I would not view this procedure as palliative. Therefore, I would feel obligated to achieve a gross total resection.

The advantage of a minimally invasive approach, sparing the posterior tension band and the posterior elements, in this particular case is a liability. The very nature of a paramedian approach prevents the resection of the spinous process, which is riddled with disease. The best option for this patient is a traditional midline exposure, with the complete removal of the spinous process, followed by a laminectomy and the removal of the epidural metastatic lesion. The patient underwent this procedure and demonstrated improvement in her hyperreflexia and tandem gait. Postoperative MRI demonstrated wide decompression of the spinal cord (▶ Fig. 10.22). She underwent radiation therapy to the area 21 days after surgery and made a full recovery. Unfortunately, 2 years after decompression of the thoracic spine and 7 years after her initial diagnosis, she was found to have metastases in the brain. There had been no local recurrence of tumor in the thoracic spine.

10.4.5 Case Illustration 5: Metastatic Prostate Cancer to the Lumbar Spine

Thus far in this chapter, I have emphasized the thoracic spine for two reasons. First, on the basis of my experience over the years, I have found that the vast majority of metastatic disease presents in the thoracic spine. Second, we achieve a great familiarity with the lumbar spine in the management of degenerative diseases. The limited pathology that we manage in the thoracic spine limits our familiarity with the topography and anatomy of the thoracic spine. The focus of this chapter has been the unique anatomical aspects of the thoracic spine that make it distinct from the lumbar spine, which is further discussed in Chapter 11, Minimally Invasive Resection of

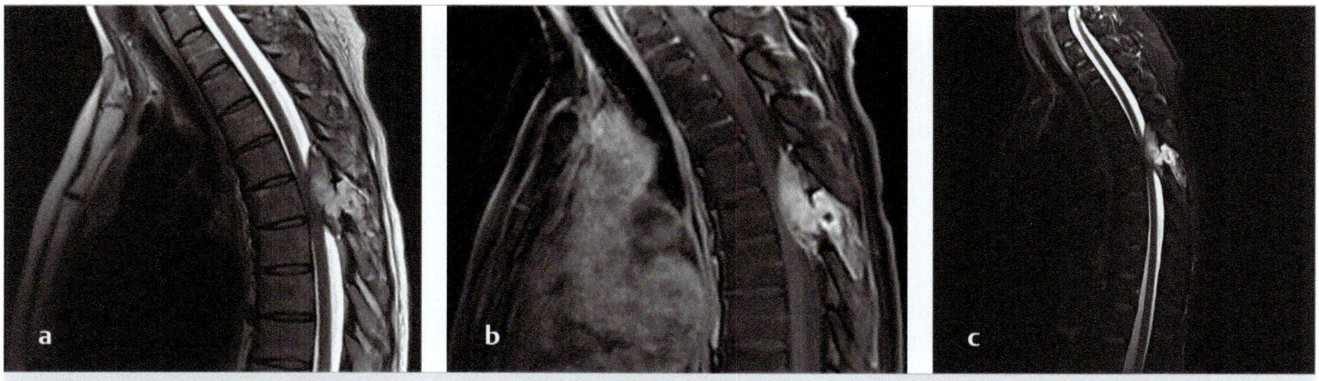

Fig. 10.21 Magnetic resonance imaging (MRI) of the thoracic spine with and without gadolinium. (a) Sagittal T2-weighted MRI demonstrating a dorsal epidural lesion at the T5, causing compression of the spinal cord. Increased signal intensity is seen within the spinous process. (b) Sagittal T1-weighted MRI with gadolinium demonstrating enhancement of the epidural lesion and enhancement of the spinous process. (c) Sagittal fluid-attenuated inversion recovery MRI with increased signal extending along the entire spinous process.

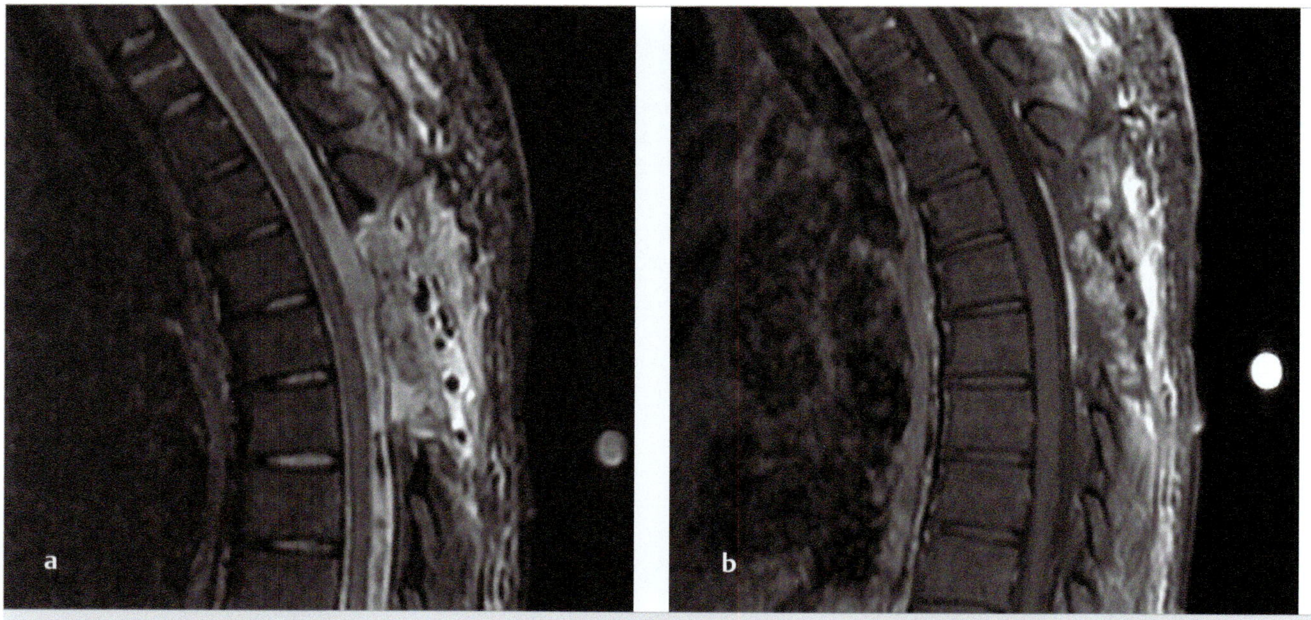

Fig. 10.22 Postoperative magnetic resonance imaging (MRI) after midline laminectomy and resection of the epidural lesion. (a) Sagittal T2-weighted MRI demonstrating a gross total resection of the epidural lesion and the affected spinous process. (b) Sagittal T1-weighted MRI with gadolinium does not exhibit any evidence of enhancement in the vicinity of the resection.

Intradural Extramedullary Lesions within the Thoracic Spine. However, I feel as if there would be a glaring omission in this chapter if a lumbar case were not presented. A review of my experience in the management of metastatic disease of the spine over the years reveals that metastatic disease presents three times more often in the thoracic spine than in the lumbar spine. However, the lumbar spine is not immune to metastatic disease, and the final case illustration reviews the management of a metastatic lesion in the lumbar spine.

Clinical History and Neurologic Examination

A 70-year-old man presented with a known history of prostate cancer. He presented with a 6-week history of progressively worsening axial back pain, 2-week history of difficulty walking and a 1-day history of urinary incontinence. An examination was difficult because of the degree of bilateral radicular leg pain. He was nonambulatory because of the symptoms in the lower extremities, but an examination by confrontation when supine demonstrated 4/5 strength throughout all muscle groups of the lower extremities bilaterally. He had an asymmetrical nondermatomal sensory loss in the lower extremities. A Foley catheter had been placed at the time of admission. The patient had decreased rectal tone, but the bulbocavernosus reflex was present.

Radiographic Evaluation

MRI of the lumbar spine demonstrated a lesion dorsal to the cauda equina causing compression. Gadolinium-enhanced MRI demonstrated a heterogeneously enhancing lesion flattening the thecal sac (▸ Fig. 10.23).

Clinical Decision-Making

This patient presented with early cauda equina syndrome secondary to a dorsal metastatic lesion causing compression of the neural elements. Urgent decompression of the cauda equina is indicated for this patient. The absence of facet involvement suggests the risk of instability from a simple decompression is low. Although a histologic diagnosis still needs to be made, this lesion likely represents metastatic prostate cancer. The possibility of a second primary cannot be entirely dismissed. Regardless, postoperative radiation is an element of the adjuvant therapy; consequently, wound healing and the timing of radiation therapy become part of the decision-making process. The need for urgent decompression, given the current neurologic deficits, prompted a minimally invasive approach at L3, the epicenter of the lesion, with the extension of the decompression spanning from L2 to L5. An expandable minimal access port would be able to accomplish this exposure (▸ Fig. 10.24).

Intervention

The Wilson frame was not used in the previous cases because of the thoracic location of the lesion. Returning to the lumbar spine allows for the return of the Wilson frame as well. The patient was positioned prone on a Jackson table atop a Wilson frame. The L3 segment was approximated with palpation of the bony landmarks. A 30-mm incision was planned 25-mm from the midline to converge adequately onto the spine for the decompression. The incision was made with a No. 15 blade and cautery to divide the fascia widely. The concern for the integrity of the lamina prompted me to palpate the lamina before probing for it with the dilator. Metastatic prostate cancer tends to be an osteoblastic process, which should make the integrity of the lamina less of a concern, but the possibility of a secondary metastatic process could not be entirely dismissed. Therefore, I approached this phase of the operation carefully to ensure the integrity of the lamina. With the integrity of the lamina confirmed, I dilated up to 22 mm diameter and used an expandable minimal access port that enabled me to access both the epicenter of the lesion and the epidural enhancement down to L5 (▸ Fig. 10.25).

Similar to performing a minimally invasive lumbar laminectomy for degenerative stenosis, I began the exposure of the lamina laterally and worked medially. In this circumstance, I identified the lamina riddled with metastatic disease almost immediately. I worked laterally to the lamina that was infiltrated with the disease, choosing to identify and work within normal anatomy as much as possible. With a preliminary orientation of the anatomical landscape, I rotated the operating table away from myself to access the contralateral corridor and achieve a wide decompression. I first worked to identify the insertion of the ligamentum flavum, and then the metastatic lesion quickly came into view. At this point, I worked to identify the thecal sac, so that I could establish a plane between the lesion and the dura. Developing this interface, I worked to resect the entire metastatic lesion that was causing compression of the thecal sac. As I worked and identified further compression, I continued to open and angulate the blades of the expandable minimal access port until I had achieved decompression of the entire dura (Fig. 10.26). I also wanted to be confident that I had encompassed the entirety of the gadolinium enhancement within my exposure, and so I reassessed the sagittal T1-weighted MRI with gadolinium relative to my exposure. I reminded myself that the goal of the procedure was to decompress the neural elements and confirm a histological diagnosis, but I was striving to be as cytoreductive as possible with this operation. I extended the decompression rostrally and caudally until all I encountered was normal tissue (▸ Fig. 10.26). I spent a great deal of time ensuring hemostasis before removing the access port. As with all metastatic lesions, a Hemovac drain was tunneled in, and the incision was closed with a multilayered closure, as previously described.

Postoperative Course

The patient was ambulatory the day following surgery. The Foley catheter was removed on the first postoperative day, and he demonstrated normal bowel and bladder function. His bilateral radicular leg pain resolved. On postoperative day 2, he was discharged and began radiation to the lumbar spine on the third postoperative day. Two years after the operation, the patient remains fully ambulatory with preservation of bowel and bladder function. Despite presenting with widely metastatic disease, he responded well to radiation therapy and continues on an androgen suppressive regimen. Postoperative MRI at 6 months demonstrated a well-decompressed lumbar spine (▸ Fig. 10.27).

10.5 Minimally Invasive Anterior Column Reconstruction

Notably absent in this chapter are those cases where the metastatic disease has resulted in instability, as determined by the SINS classification scheme.[2] Metastatic disease with instability or imminent instability requires instrumentation in addition to decompression. Combining the minimally invasive decompressions with percutaneous instrumentation for stabilization is the logical next step. At times, the involvement of the metastatic diseases requires a corpectomy and reconstruction of the anterior column (▸ Fig. 10.28). These circumstances are still in the realm of the minimally invasive precinct. However, I have not included those cases in this chapter because it would be disingenuous as an author to describe a technique that I have performed more in cadavers than in patients. Not every patient who presents with circumferential compression of the spinal

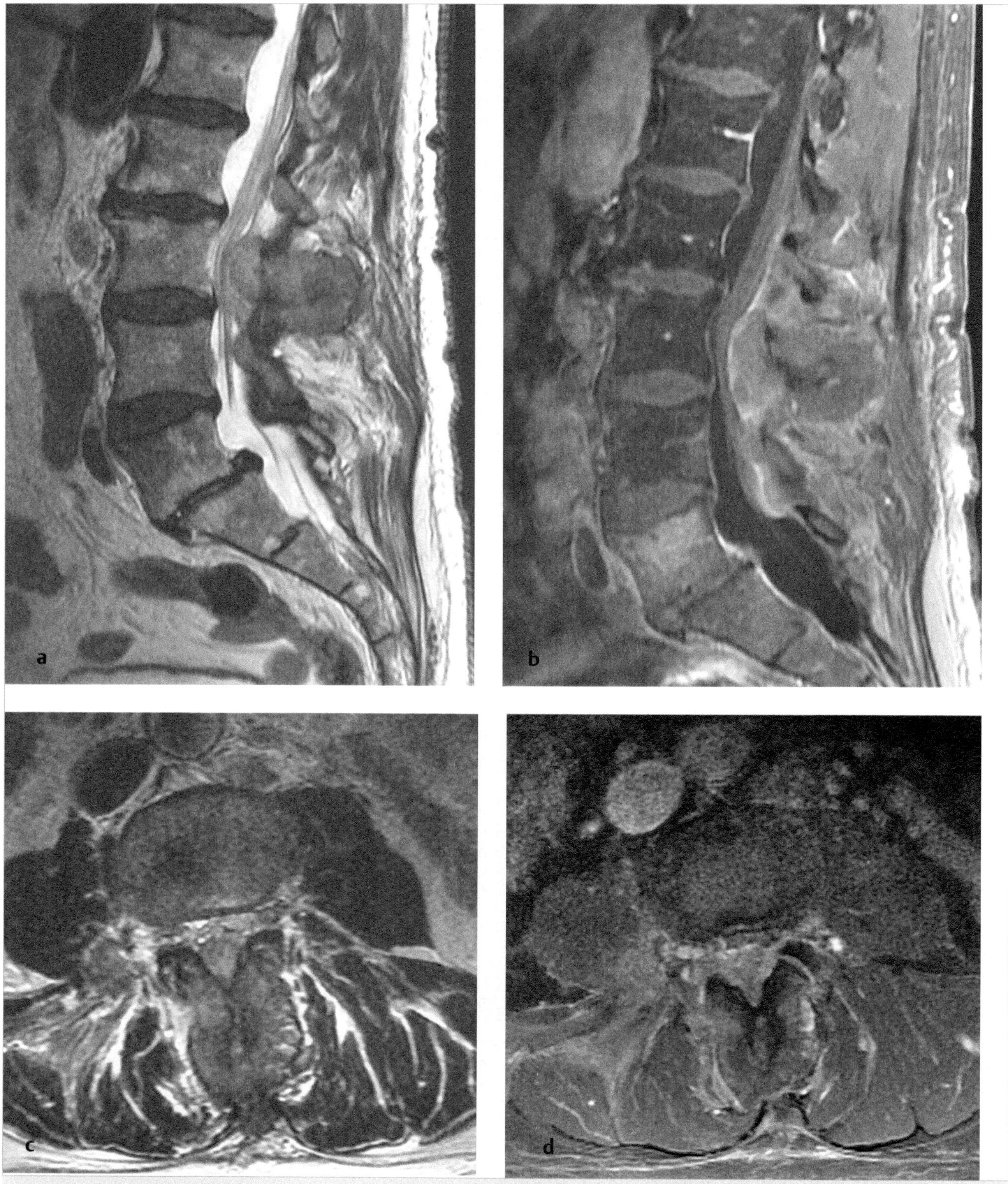

Fig. 10.23 Metastatic prostate lesion compressing the cauda equina. **(a)** Sagittal T2-weighted magnetic resonance imaging (MRI) demonstrating a lesion at the level of L3, causing compression of the cauda equina. **(b)** Sagittal T1-weighted MRI with gadolinium demonstrating the epicenter of the lesion at L3 but the extension of enhancement down to L5. **(c)** Axial T2-weighted MRI demonstrating the flattening of the cauda equina. **(d)** Axial T1-weighted MRI with gadolinium demonstrating the enhancement pattern of the lesion, primarily dorsal but slightly eccentric to the right. It is the recognition of this laterality that prompts a right-sided approach when considering which side to employ for a minimally invasive approach.

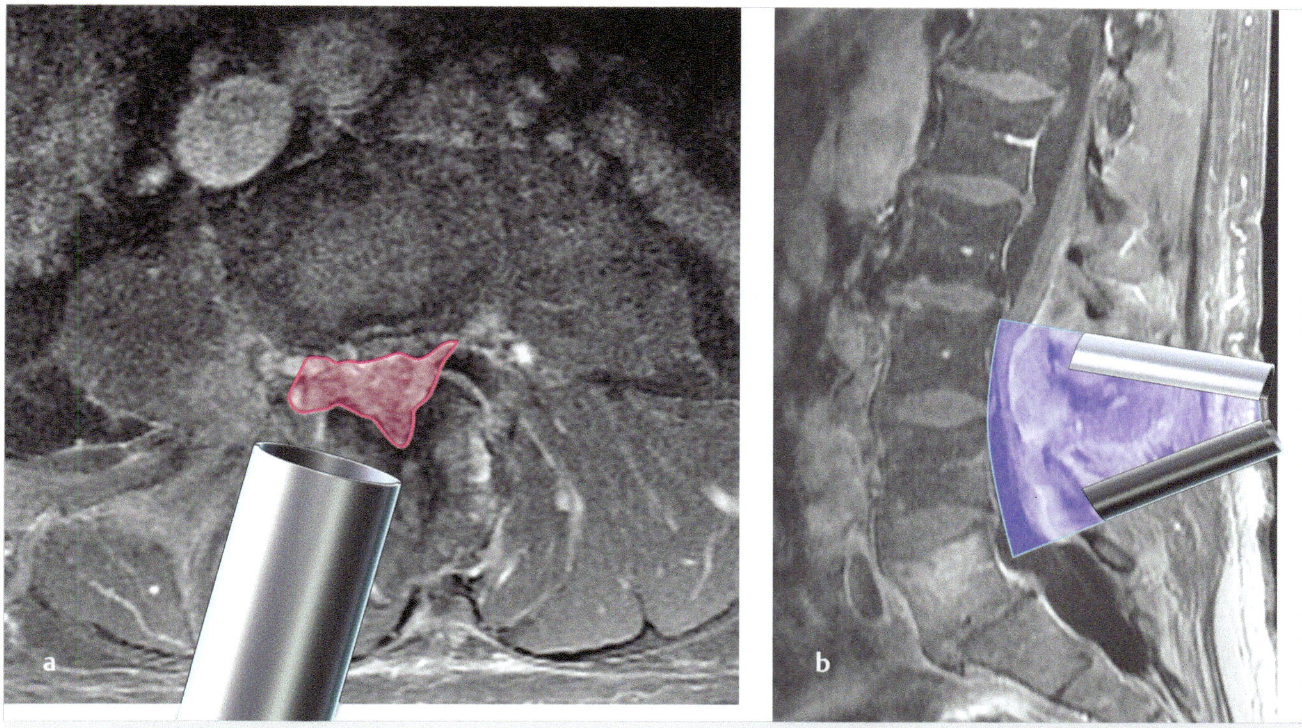

Fig. 10.24 Surgical plan for resection of a metastatic lesion. **(a)** Axial T1-weighted magnetic resonance imaging (MRI) with gadolinium outlining the metastatic lesion (*magenta*). Even though primarily midline and dorsal, the lesion is slightly eccentric to the right. This laterality suggests that a minimally invasive approach from the right side would be preferred. **(b)** The range that needs to be spanned by the exposure (*lavender*); therefore, the minimal access port is demonstrated on the sagittal T1-weighted MRI with gadolinium. A fixed-diameter port could potentially cover the area with multiple adjustments. An expandable minimal access port could cover the area of interest all at once.

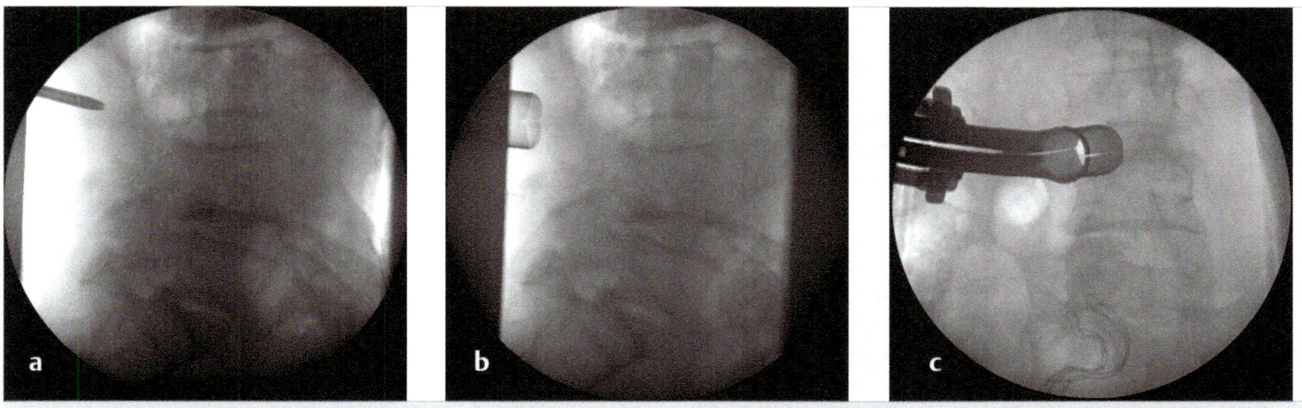

Fig. 10.25 Placement of minimal access port. **(a)** Lateral fluoroscopic image demonstrating the initial dilator up against the lamina after directly palpating the lamina to ensure its integrity. **(b)** Lateral fluoroscopic image demonstrating the expandable minimal access port in position. **(c)** Anteroposterior-oblique view with the minimum access port on the lamina of L3. This view represents the rotation of the patient on the operating table.

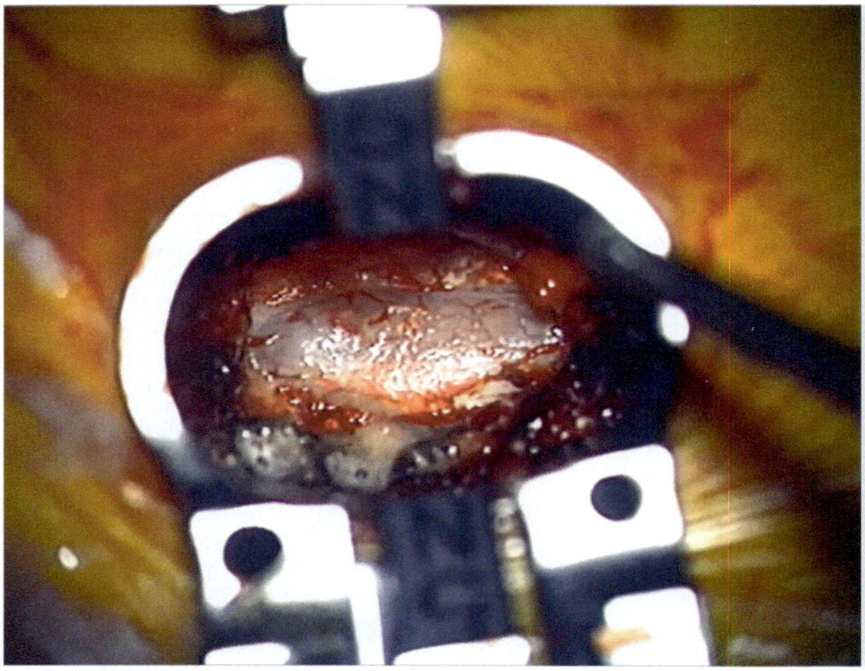

Fig. 10.26 Intraoperative photograph of the decompression. With the bed angled 15 degrees away from the surgeon, a complete decompression of the thecal sac is readily achievable. Progressive angulation of the blades allows for extending the area of decompression and resection.

cord is a candidate for a minimally invasive approach. If the spinous process and lamina are involved, as in case illustration 4 in this chapter (▶ Fig. 10.21), then a midline approach is necessary. I have found that it is the pattern and location of the metastatic disease that has limited the volume of these cases in my practice. Since my experience has been limited more to cadaveric specimens than living patients, I have not achieved a skill set where I feel that I can claim mastery of the technique. I am limited in this final section to describing where I am in the development.

A minimally invasive transpedicular decompression with the reconstruction of the anterior column is a technically demanding procedure, and it is an operation that should be entertained only after mastery of the open costotransversectomy approach as well as mastery of the various minimally invasive techniques described in this Primer. A high volume of open anterior column reconstruction procedures needs to have been performed before entertaining the minimally invasive approach to accomplish the same goals. I have adhered to the minimally invasive principle that any minimally invasive procedure needs to be indistinguishable from its open counterpart. Therefore, a minimally invasive version of the operation seen in ▶ Fig. 10.28 and ▶ Fig. 10.29 is performed with bilateral expandable minimal access ports secured over the affected segment. A costotransversectomy approach on one side and transpedicular approach on the other for a complete circumferential decompression of the spinal cord appear identical to the decompression in ▶ Fig. 10.28 and ▶ Fig. 10.29. Percutaneous fixation above and below limits plays to the strength of percutaneous technology, limits the extent of exposure and shortens time to healing. Confidence in such a technique is derived from a combination of performing these open operations and becoming increasingly comfortable with the minimally invasive transpedicular approach performed for decompression. The minimally invasive decompressions described in this chapter represent the first step in that direction. Uniting those minimally invasive decompressions with open anterior column reconstruction experiences lays the necessary foundation for a synthesis of those two skill sets to combine as one minimally invasive approach. Throughout this Primer, I have emphasized the importance of stepwise progression, beginning with simple decompressions and then proceeding with instrumentation. In this circumstance, such a stepwise progression is even more essential to establish the firm footing needed for successful minimally invasive reconstruction of the anterior column in metastatic disease. The last two figures in this chapter must seem entirely out of place to the reader in a book dedicated to minimally invasive approaches to the spine. However, they are an accurate representation of where I am in the year 2020. In the coming years, I intend to make those photographs an anachronism.

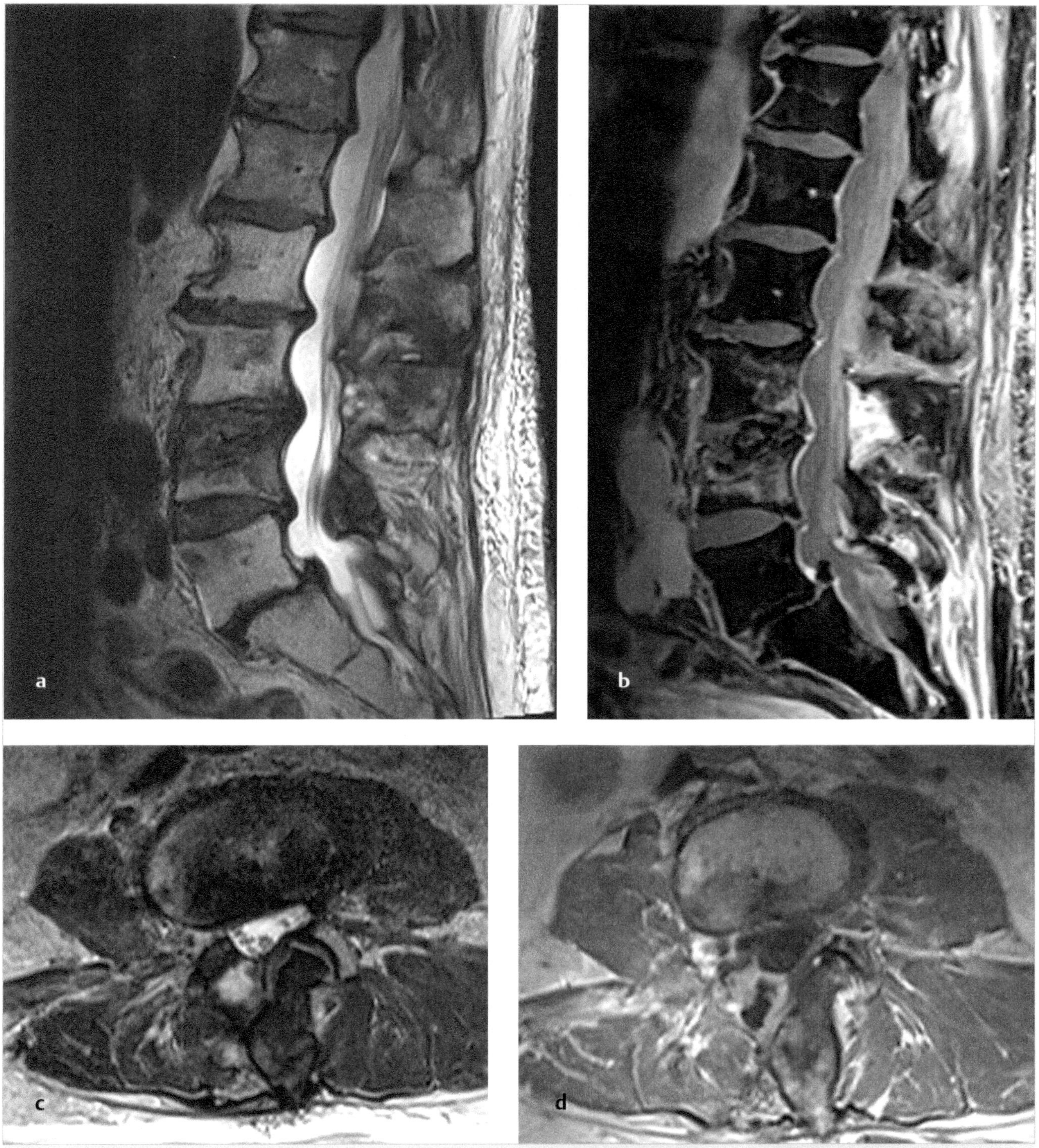

Fig. 10.27 Postoperative magnetic resonance imaging (MRI). **(a)** Sagittal T2-weighted MRI demonstrating complete decompression of the cauda equina at the L3 level. **(b)** Sagittal T1-weighted MRI with gadolinium demonstrating complete resection of an epidural metastatic lesion. **(c)** Axial T2-weighted MRI with complete decompression of the cauda equina. The right laminotomy defect may be appreciated. **(d)** Axial T1-weighted MRI with gadolinium again, demonstrating the absence of enhancement in the resection bed.

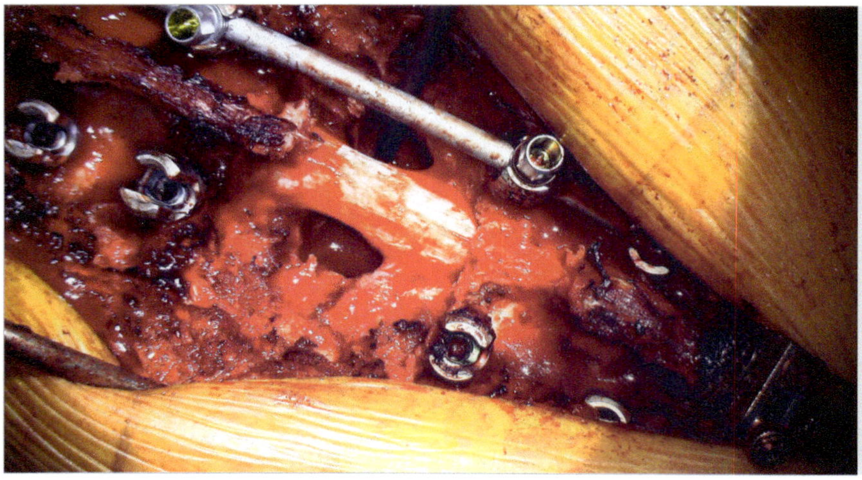

Fig. 10.28 Intraoperative photograph of a costotransversectomy approach to accomplish a T9 corpectomy for the management of metastatic colon cancer, with instability and circumferential decompression of the spinal cord. Not all separation surgery is minimally invasive.

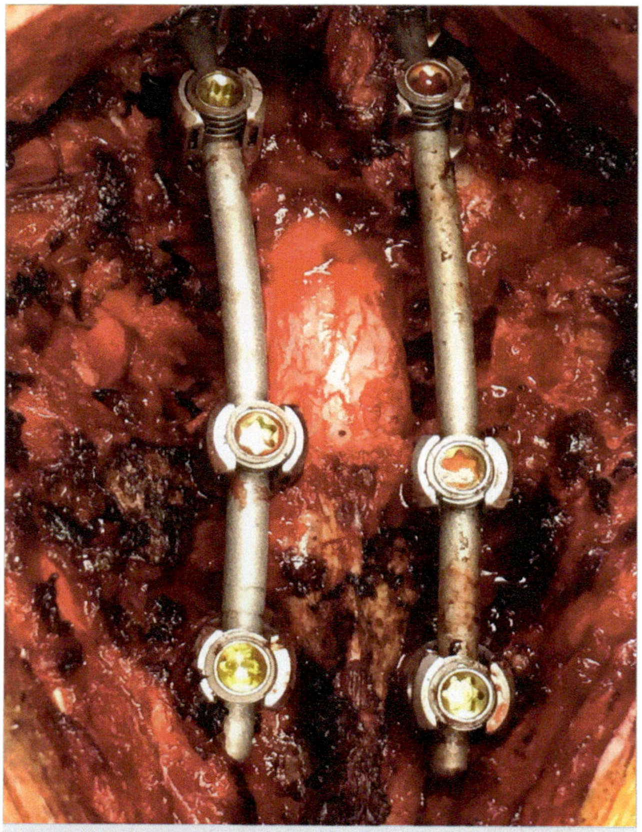

Fig. 10.29 Management of metastatic breast cancer. Intraoperative photograph showing circumferential decompression of the spinal cord in a 47-year-old woman with metastatic disease up to T7. The patient underwent a costotransversectomy approach for corpectomy with cage placement and T5–T9 instrumentation. It is my vision to transform that procedure into a minimally invasive one in the years to come.

10.6 Conclusion

The epidemiology of spinal metastases is staggering. Up to 40% of cancer patients develop spinal metastases during their battle against cancer. As many as 10% of those patients present with epidural spinal cord compression, some with neurologic deficit.[1] As the population increases and cancer treatments keep the disease at bay longer, we, as spine surgeons, can only expect to encounter more of these patients. The modest hope I have for this chapter is that its content prepares the reader for the occasion when a patient enters his or her professional life with metastatic spinal disease, compression of the spinal cord and a neurologic deficit. To remove the compression of the spinal cord and restore or preserve function of that person with metastatic spinal cancer preserves the person's dignity. Although the natural history and the progression of every cancer vary considerably, the natural history of a neurologic deficit does not. Some patients may live only months after a diagnosis of metastatic disease; others may live years. Regardless of life expectancy, every effort should be made to preserve the dignity that bowel and bladder function and ambulatory status offer all of us. Once a patient has lost bowel and bladder function, or the ability to walk, the capacity to restore those functions is a tall order under any circumstance. These deficits may represent an irreversible event and have a catastrophic impact on the outlook of life for that patient.

Spinal cord compression due to metastatic disease in the context of a progressive neurologic deficit is a surgical disease. A minimally invasive decompression of the spinal cord can preserve or restore neurologic function, and with it, the patient's dignity. There is a growing body of literature on separation surgery followed by stereotactic radiosurgery to achieve local disease control for spinal metastases, and the philosophy of that approach fits hand in glove with the minimally invasive decompression techniques described in this chapter.[6,7,8]

A small incision without compromising the blood flow to the skin and muscles, due to the use of a muscle retractor, further allows for the implementation of either chemotherapy or radiation therapy in a timely fashion, typically days after the operation. Minimally invasive decompression of the cervical, thoracic and lumbar spine for spinal cord compression from metastatic disease is, therefore, an invaluable weapon in the spine surgeon's arsenal to help our patients with their battle against cancer.

Facility with minimally invasive approaches and exposures in the thoracic spine allows for a natural progression to the point where the surgeon begins to consider opening the dura and addressing the pathology within. As this chapter comes to a close, I again invoke the importance of stepwise progression as an introduction to Chapter 11, Minimally Invasive Resection of Intradural Extramedullary Lesions within the Thoracic Spine. Mastery of the topography of the thoracic spine creates comfort in the minimally invasive exposure, access and resection of intradural extramedullary lesions.

References

[1] Quraishi NA, Gokaslan ZL, Boriani S. The surgical management of metastatic epidural compression of the spinal cord. J Bone Joint Surg Br. 2010; 92(8):1054–1060

[2] Fisher CG, DiPaola CP, Ryken TC, et al. A novel classification system for spinal instability in neoplastic disease: an evidence-based approach and expert consensus from the Spine Oncology Study Group. Spine. 2010; 35(22):E1221–E1229

[3] Fisher CG, Versteeg AL, Schouten R, et al. Reliability of the spinal instability neoplastic scale among radiologists: an assessment of instability secondary to spinal metastases. AJR Am J Roentgenol. 2014; 203(4):869–874

[4] Fisher CG, Schouten R, Versteeg AL, et al. Reliability of the Spinal Instability Neoplastic Score (SINS) among radiation oncologists: an assessment of instability secondary to spinal metastases. Radiat Oncol. 2014; 9:69

[5] Fourney DR, Frangou EM, Ryken TC, et al. Spinal instability neoplastic score: an analysis of reliability and validity from the spine oncology study group. J Clin Oncol. 2011; 29(22):3072–3077

[6] Zuckerman SL, Laufer I, Sahgal A, et al. When less is more: the indications for MIS techniques and separation surgery in metastatic spine disease. Spine. 2016; 41 Suppl 20:S246–S253

[7] Moussazadeh N, Laufer I, Yamada Y, Bilsky MH. Separation surgery for spinal metastases: effect of spinal radiosurgery on surgical treatment goals. Cancer Contr. 2014; 21(2):168–174

[8] Laufer I, Iorgulescu JB, Chapman T, et al. Local disease control for spinal metastases following "separation surgery" and adjuvant hypofractionated or high-dose single-fraction stereotactic radiosurgery: outcome analysis in 186 patients. J Neurosurg Spine. 2013; 18(3):207–214

[9] Barzilai O, Laufer I, Robin A, Xu R, Yamada Y, Bilsky MH. Hybrid therapy for metastatic epidural spinal cord compression: technique for separation surgery and spine radiosurgery. Oper Neurosurg (Hagerstown). 2019; 16(3):310–318

[10] Klimo P, Jr, Kestle JR, Schmidt MH. Treatment of metastatic spinal epidural disease: a review of the literature. Neurosurg Focus. 2003; 15(5):E1

[11] Byrne TN. Spinal cord compression from epidural metastases. N Engl J Med. 1992; 327(9):614–619

11 Minimally Invasive Resection of Intradural Extramedullary Lesions within the Thoracic Spine

Abstract
A minimally invasive surgeon views the spinal canal in three dimensions, where the spinous process no longer presents a barrier to accessing the central canal. The paramedian transmuscular approaches applied to microdiscectomies, laminectomies and instrumented fusions have gradually converted the mind to the minimally invasive perspective. Preservation of the midline structures has been a constant theme among surgeons for decades that actually precedes the rise of modern minimally invasive techniques. The current platform of minimally invasive access ports has facilitated the preservation of the midline structures, which pioneering surgeons believed was an understated benefit for the patient. The management of intradural extramedullary lesions with minimally invasive techniques represents the culmination of a skill set that developed while managing the common degenerative pathologies of the cervical and lumbar spine. Intradural extramedullary lesions within the thoracic canal possess the key characteristics that lend themselves especially well to a minimally invasive approach. Whether it is a T11 meningioma or a T8–9 dural arteriovenous fistula, these lesions have laterality and limited dimensions. Laterality allows for a midline sparing hemilaminectomy approach. A maximum dimension of 25 mm for a thoracic lesion allows an expandable minimal access port to readily encompass such a lesion in a manner that optimizes the Caspar ratio. This chapter presents the anatomical basis and surgical technique for a minimally invasive resection of intradural extramedullary lesions in the thoracic spine. The chapter ends with case illustrations demonstrating the application of the minimally invasive approach.

Keywords: extramedullary, intradural, laminectomy, meningioma, minimally invasive, schwannoma, spinal dural arteriovenous fistula, thoracic

You cannot depend on your eyes when your imagination is out of focus.

Mark Twain

11.1 Introduction

It dawned on me that I was looking at the spine through a distinctive minimally invasive lens when a colleague of mine asked me to review magnetic resonance imaging (MRI) of a thoracic spine. The study demonstrated a plum-sized enhancing intradural extramedullary lesion severely compressing the spinal cord in the lower thoracic spine. By this time in my career, I had converted my practice almost entirely to minimally invasive approaches. I felt comfortable with the instruments and confident with the exposures that I was able to achieve using the various minimally invasive access options. As I looked at the MRI, I began to envision how I would access the lesion with a paramedian minimal access approach. I was familiar enough with the anatomy that I could visualize an exposure with the rostrocaudal dimension of 28 to 30 mm. I knew that angling the blades of the access port would provide me with an additional 5 to 7 mm of rostrocaudal exposure. I could imagine exposing the midline of the canal by a combination of mediolateral blades and rotation of the bed. Undercutting the spinous process and contralateral lamina would provide me access to the contralateral recess. All these techniques are similar to those used in accomplishing those same objectives when working on a medial decompression for a minimally invasive transforaminal lumbar interbody fusion or a lumbar laminectomy. The only difference was that I was in a different region of the spine, and there was more work to do once the dura was exposed. I recognized that while the canal dimensions and interpedicular distances are unique in the thoracic spine, the experience with the management of extradural metastatic disease in the thoracic spine that I described in Chapter 10 provided me the familiarity with the thoracic landscape to feel confident with accomplishing the necessary exposures.

I snapped out of my trance when my colleague asked me for a hand. When he mentioned a midline approach, I plainly remember asking, "Why not a minimally invasive one?" Up until that time, I had never performed a resection of an intradural extramedullary lesion through a minimally invasive approach. But I could not find a compelling reason why we should not.

Yet another learning curve presented itself with this approach. However, the learning curve was distinct from the initial learning curve of minimally invasive spine surgery. Instead of developing new skills working with bayoneted instruments in the access port and becoming accustomed to new perspectives for maintaining orientation, this learning curve built upon the skill set that I had already refined by the microdiscectomies, laminectomies, cervical foraminotomies and instrumented lumbar fusions that I had performed over the years. I soon discovered the nuances of positioning the access port, the exposure of the spinal cord and the closure of the dura. As these cases began to accumulate and my experience continued to grow, I recognized that the operation reaches a point, specifically when the dura is open and the lesion exposed, where it becomes indistinguishable from an open midline operation. In certain circumstances, the operation actually becomes easier. A focused and highly efficient exposure fosters that facility. In the end, whether the exposure is through a midline approach or a minimally invasive one, you will employ the identical microsurgical techniques to remove the lesion from the spinal cord.

Time and again in this book, I referenced the concept of the efficiency of the exposure in minimally invasive approaches, a relationship that I have referred to as the Caspar ratio. In its most elemental form, the Caspar ratio translates into the percentage of the surgical target relative to the surgical exposure. I hope that I have been able to convince the reader at this point in this Primer that minimally invasive exposure is highly efficient, utilizing a higher proportion of the surgical exposure relative to the surgical target than its open counterpart.

The resection of an intradural extramedullary lesion is the quintessential example of the Caspar ratio. The skill of precise placement of the minimal access port directly over the lesion and the proficiency in securing every millimeter of exposure afforded by the minimal access port are of even greater importance in the management of intradural extramedullary lesions than in any other procedure that I have described earlier. It is essential to recognize that acquiring these skills does not require the management of dozens of intradural extramedullary lesions. Instead, those proficiencies develop with every microdiscectomy, laminectomy and instrumented lumbar fusion that you perform minimally invasively. Management of thoracic metastatic lesions further refines that skill set. These are the cases where your mind will effortlessly connect the lines of what cannot be seen to the limited exposure that you can see. Synthesis of these images inside of your mind, built on the experience of managing the characteristic pathology of the lumbar and cervical spine, is what you will harness to perform minimally invasive resections of intradural extramedullary lesions in the thoracic, lumbar or even cervical spine. The management of intradural extramedullary lesions through minimally invasive techniques is the zenith of a highly developed skill set. It is only after mastery of the various other minimally invasive procedures in the lumbar, thoracic and cervical spine presented in the earlier chapters that you should endeavor on this approach.

As will be discussed in the coming pages, master surgeons of yesteryear described the resection of intradural extramedullary lesions with preservation of the midline structures decades ago.[1,2,3] You need not jump immediately to a paramedian transmuscular approach through a minimal access port. There is tremendous value in performing resections of intradural extramedullary lesions with a midline incision but with preservation of the midline structures, as described by Yaşargil[3] and Seeger.[1] Understanding the amount of access to the entire canal through a hemilaminectomy exposure with the preservation of the spinous process is a component of the stepwise progression to a purely minimally invasive approach. It is important to recognize that these lesions have all of the characteristics that lend themselves exceptionally well to a minimal access resection. The very nature of a spherical lesion growing within a canal gives it laterality. The lesion always displaces the spinal cord to one side as it occupies the majority of the other side of the canal. The dimensions of the thoracic canal impose an upper limit of 25 mm in any dimension. The combination of laterality and limited dimensions plays to the strength of the minimally invasive approach.

It has been several years since that initial resection of a thoracic meningioma through an expandable minimal access port. The experience that I have gained through the management of the subsequent 26 intradural extramedullary lesions that I have encountered has led me to manage practically all of them using minimally invasive techniques. I have reached a point where my mind has a difficult time conceiving another manner to perform these operations. As mentioned time and again in this Primer, the mind once enlightened cannot again become dark.

In this chapter, I present the anatomical basis and then describe the technique for the resection of intradural extramedullary pathology using a minimally invasive approach. I highlight some of the subtle differences with the use of the minimal access port, along with the difference in the approach and bone work. At the end of the chapter, I provide case illustrations where intradural extramedullary pathology, including meningiomas and dural arteriovenous (AV) fistulas, are managed with minimally invasive techniques. However, it would be difficult not to begin the chapter with the remarkable history of a paramedian technique that would eventually evolve into the minimally invasive technique described in this chapter.

11.2 Historical Perspective

Concern for the stability of the spinal column after resection of spinal tumors has been on the mind of spine surgeons for decades. It was the unease caused by the potential risk of progressive kyphosis and scoliosis in the years and decades of life that followed the resection that prompted a few pioneering surgeons to ask themselves whether a complete laminectomy was, in fact, necessary to resect intradural lesions. Similar to the surgeons who did not view the spinous process as an obstruction for the management of lumbar stenosis, Seeger and colleagues[1] and Yaşargil and colleagues[3] viewed the lesion within the dura accessible without disruption of the posterior tension band or even sacrifice of the spinous process. The postoperative thoracic kyphosis they saw in their early patients drove these surgeons to explore surgeries that preserved the midline structures. The logical question was whether the same operation could be accomplished with less disruption of the native spine. The rational answer was a unilateral hemilaminectomy approach with preservation of the midline elements.[1,2,3] But could such a limited exposure provide the surgeon with the requisite anatomy needed for complete resection of an intradural extramedullary lesion?

Despite this text supposedly being a modern-day primer on minimally invasive spinal surgery, the techniques that I describe in the following pages were routinely used by surgeons over 35 years ago. Although the retractors used to access the spine may be different, the techniques are surprisingly the same. In fact, the figure in the wonderful manuscript by Yaşargil and colleagues[3] on unilateral hemilaminectomy for resection of spinal tumors could easily replace some of the figures created for this chapter (▶ Fig. 11.1).[3] The same could be said for the illustrations in the manuscript by Eggert and colleagues (▶ Fig. 11.2).[2]

Dr. Wolfgang Seeger[1] also championed this technique for intradural pathology, reserving full laminectomies for intradural intramedullary lesions. Again, with the exception of the retractors used then and the minimal access ports used now, there is essentially no difference between the approach described in this chapter and Seeger's approach three decades ago (▶ Fig. 11.2).

The common theme among all of these surgeons is consistent with the common theme that resonates through this book: preservation of the midline elements. Poletti[4] and Lin[5] saw no reason to remove the spinous process and disrupt the posterior tension band for a lumbar laminectomy; likewise, Seeger[1] and Yaşargil[3] did not view the spinous process as an obstruction to the central canal for resection of a tumor. It is this philosophy of accessing pathology within the spinal canal with minimal disruption to the native spine itself that culminated in Dr. Richard Fessler and colleagues's publication in 2006, where they reported their experience with the resection of intradural

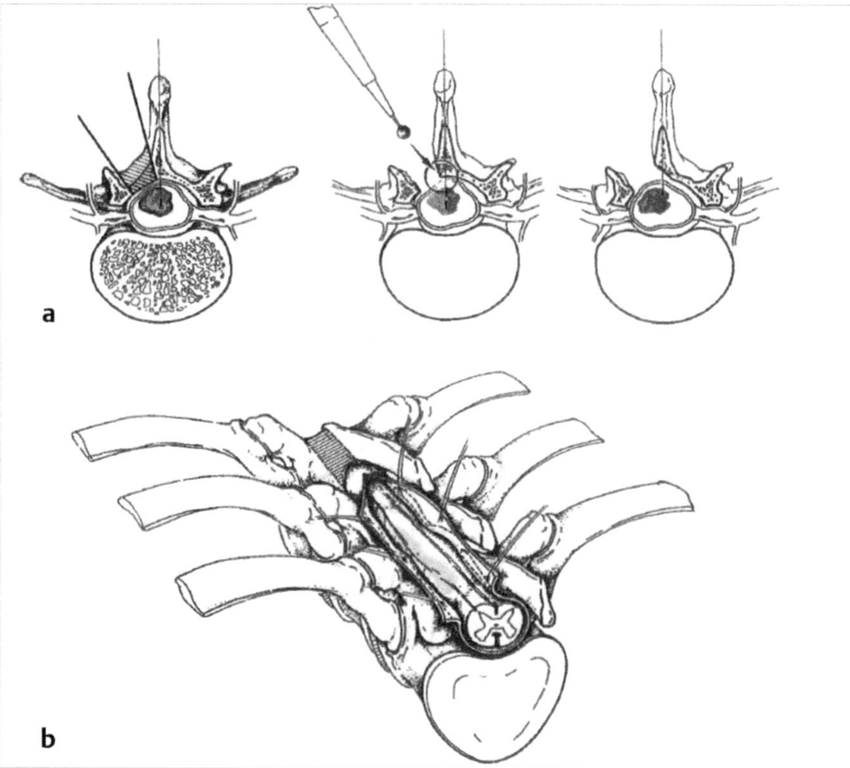

Fig. 11.1 A figure from Yaşargil et al[3] on the use of unilateral hemilaminectomy for the resection of intradural extramedullary lesions. The technique described by Yaşargil[3] is indistinguishable from the techniques described decades later by modern-day minimally invasive spine surgeons. Access to the spine is the only difference. **(a)** Axial illustrations of the thoracic spine demonstrating the bone work described by Yaşargil.[3] Note the use of the drill to undercut the spinous process in the middle axial image in order to provide access to the contralateral recess. **(b)** Posterior view of the thoracic spine with a 15-degree rotation where multiple hemilaminectomies have been performed and the dura has been opened and tacked up with sutures. Note the preservation of the spinous processes at all levels. (Reproduced with permission from Yaşargil MG, Tranmer BI, Adamson TE, et al. Unilateral partial hemilaminectomy for the removal of extra- and intramedullary tumours and AVMs. Adv Tech Stand Neurosurg. 1991; 18:113–132.)

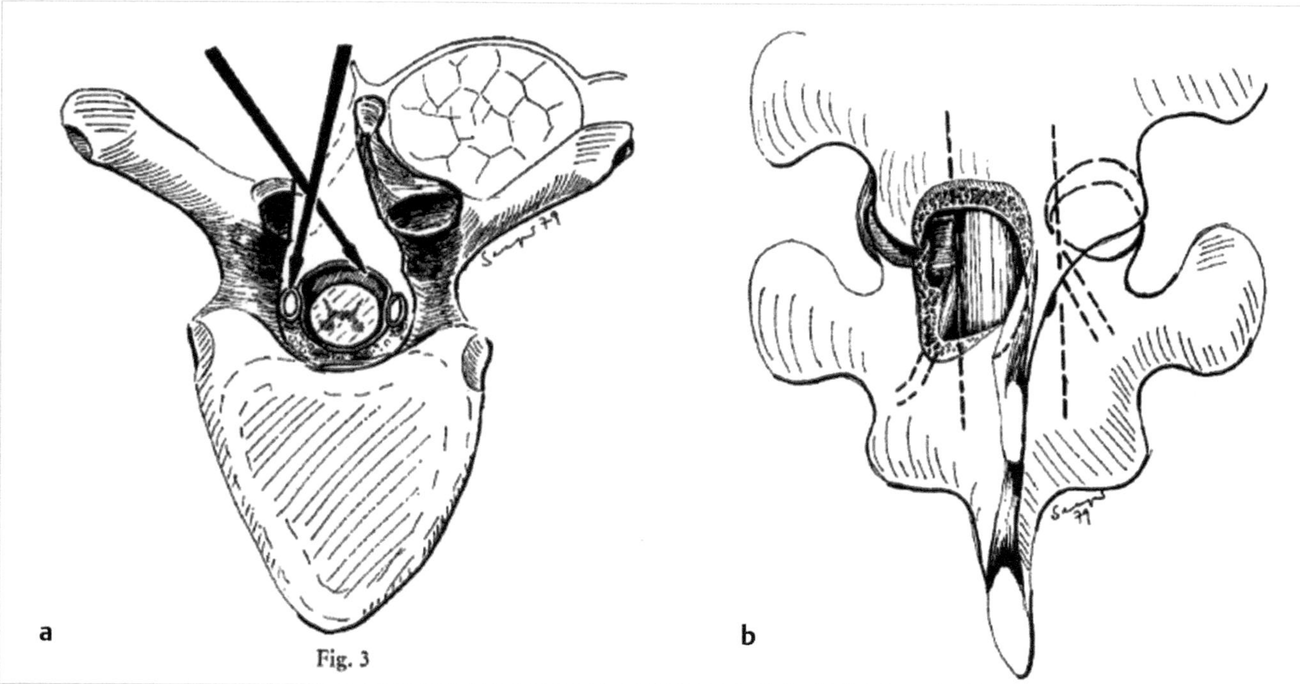

Fig. 11.2 Illustrations from the manuscript by Eggert and colleagues[2] demonstrate the use of hemilaminotomy for the management of intradural extramedullary lesions. **(a)** The trajectories shown in the figure (axial view of the spine) are indistinguishable from those used in a minimally invasive approach today. **(b)** This drawing shows a posterior view of the spine with a laminotomy used for resection of the lesion. The article was published in 1983, but the bone work demonstrated is as relevant today for minimally invasive approaches as it was over 30 years ago.[2] (Reproduced with permission from Eggert HR, Scheremet R, Seeger W, et al. Unilateral microsurgical approaches to extramedullary spinal tumours. Operative technique and results. Acta Neurochir (Wien). 1983; 67:245–253.)

extramedullary lesions using modern-day minimally invasive techniques.[6] Today, the minimally invasive resection of intradural extramedullary lesions has become routine in several centers around the country due in large part to the efforts of these pioneering surgeons.

11.3 Rationale for a Minimally Invasive Approach: An Observation

The first step for establishing the rationale for a minimally invasive approach for the resection of an intradural extramedullary lesion is a thoughtful analysis of the dimensions of the thoracic canal. Based on the anthropometric measurements of the thoracic spine by Panjabi and colleagues, the transverse dimension of the thoracic canal (the distance from pedicle to pedicle) is seldom more than 22 mm in the mid-to-upper thoracic spine (T1–T9) and seldom more than 24 mm in the lower thoracic spine (T10–12). The anteroposterior (AP) dimension tends to be more constant throughout the entire thoracic spine and ranges between 16 and 18 mm.[7] Unlike a metastatic lesion, which has a less predictable and more destructive growth pattern, an intradural extramedullary lesion has a more subtle presentation and more predictable growth pattern. There is an inherent limit that the lesion reaches within the thoracic canal before that patient becomes symptomatic. Therefore, the boundaries of the thoracic canal place an intrinsic limit on the dimensions of a thoracic intradural extramedullary lesion. Applying Panjabi's measurements, the limit of these lesions should be no greater than 20 mm in the AP and lateral dimension (▶ Fig. 11.3).[7] I tested that hypothesis with a dimensional analysis of 26 consecutive intradural extramedullary lesions.

Benign intradural extramedullary neoplasms that grow within the thoracic canal are indolent lesions with slow doubling times. The slow growth rate allows for a remarkable amount of accommodation by the spinal cord to take place. It is always astonishing to see these patients in clinic who present with only subtle neurologic findings when a lesion occupies their entire central canal. Early in my experience, I would peer at the axial T1-weighted gadolinium-enhanced MRI and look aghast at the thoracic spinal cord completely flattened into a ribbon by a tumor within the canal. Meanwhile, the patient would be *standing* alongside me, looking at the same image, asking me what I thought. It is these times that I can only but marvel at the resilience of the central nervous system (▶ Fig. 11.4).[7]

When patients become symptomatic, they have reached the tipping point of what their spinal cords can tolerate. At that point, neurologic symptoms begin to arise. Still, measurement of these lesions tends to be no more than 15 to 20 mm in any dimension, and the lesions typically have a remarkably spherical shape. A dimensional analysis of the 26 intradural extramedullary lesions identified the mean dimensions of 18.6 mm (range, 10–25 mm) in the rostrocaudal dimension, 13.0 mm (range, 7–18 mm) in the lateral dimension and 13.6 mm (range, 9–17 mm) in the AP dimension. Three additional observations were made from that series. First, all lesions displaced the spinal cord to one side, which plays to the strength of a paramedian approach. Second, the fact that the rostrocaudal dimension is the only dimension not bound by the bony structures of the canal made it always the largest dimension of the lesion. However, that dimension still never exceeded 25 mm, which falls within the range accessible to a minimally invasive approach. Finally, no lesion remodeled the lamina, foramen or pedicles of

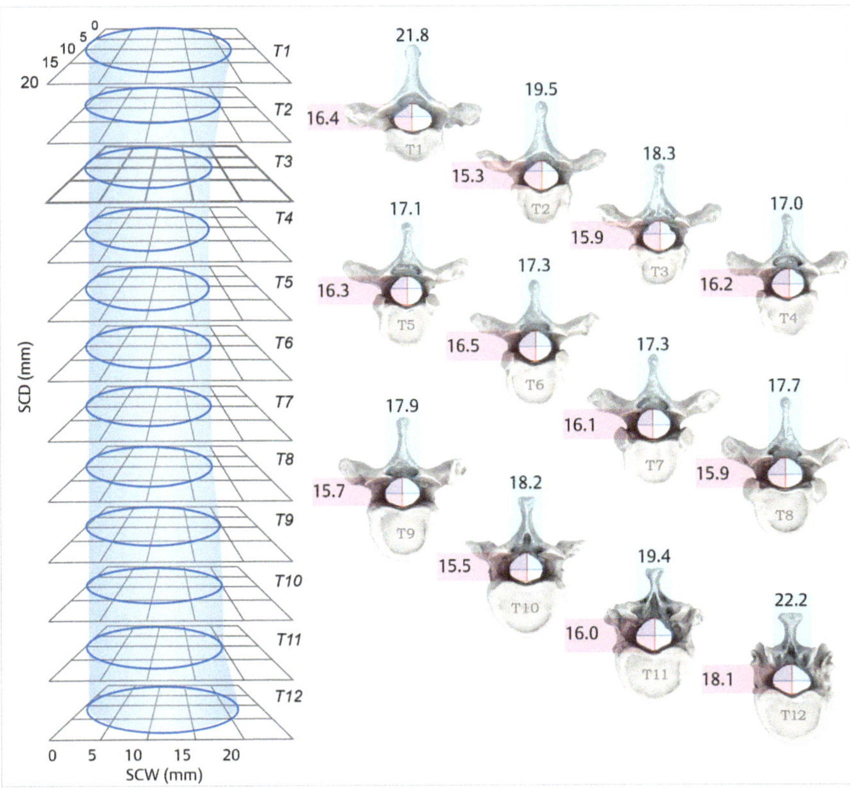

Fig. 11.3 Cross-sectional anatomy of the thoracic spine. Anteroposterior and lateral dimensions of the central canal in millimeters from T1 to T12. As patients tend to become symptomatic when an intradural extramedullary lesion reaches the boundaries of the thoracic canal, the dimensions of the canal define the dimensions of the lesion. Abbreviations: SCD, spinal canal depth; SCW, spinal canal width.

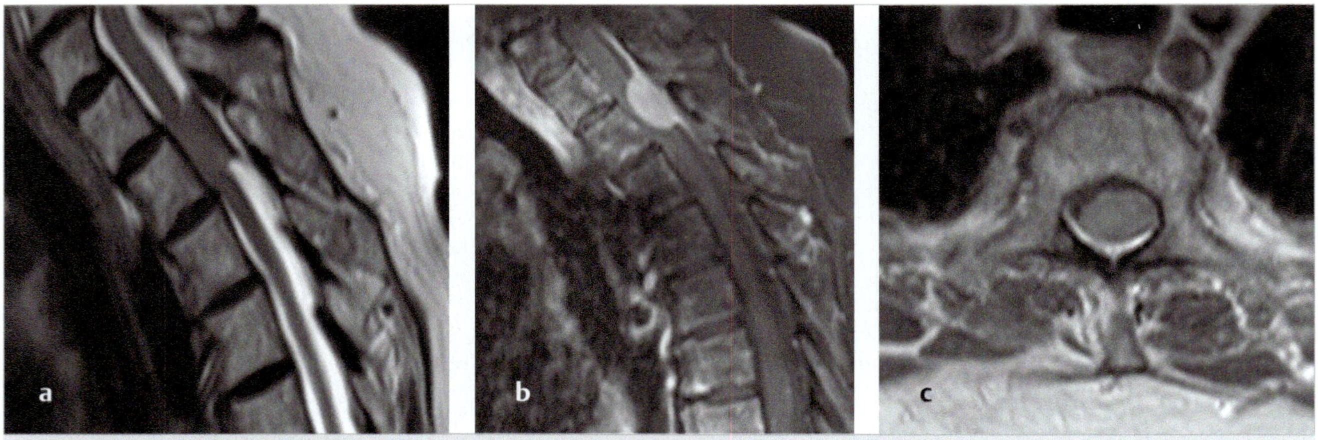

Fig. 11.4 Intradural extramedullary lesion at T3. This patient presented with a subtle gait disturbance and decreased proprioception but was otherwise intact. She was walking upward of 3 miles a day at the time of presentation. A neurologist discovered the lesion when evaluating the patient for an ill-defined neuropathy. **(a)** Sagittal T2-weighted magnetic resonance imaging (MRI) demonstrating an intradural extramedullary lesion at T3, remarkably without signal change abnormality on the spinal cord. **(b)** Sagittal T1-weighted MRI with gadolinium showing uniform enhancement of the lesion. **(c)** Axial T1-weighted MRI with gadolinium showing the lesion occupying almost the entire canal. The spinal cord can be seen flattened against the lateral aspect of the canal. Consistent with the observation that lesions become symptomatic when they approach the boundaries of the dimensions of the canal, this lesion measured 10 mm in the transverse dimension, 16 mm in the anteroposterior dimension and 20 mm in the rostrocaudal dimension. Those are consistent with the range of dimensions at T3 reported by Panjabi et al.[7] More importantly, those dimensions fall within the range of what may be safely resected through minimal access ports.

the central canal for expansion beyond the expected reported dimensions of the canal.[8] The dimensional analysis of these 26 lesions validated the prediction made earlier regarding the inherent dimensional limitation.

The first component in establishing a favorable Caspar ratio is defining the surgical target. The average dimensions from these 26 cases provide insight into the precise dimensions of any thoracic intradural extramedullary lesion. A near-spherical lesion in the thoracic canal with a maximum diameter of 20 mm that displaces the spinal cord to one side has all of the aspects that play to the strengths of a minimally invasive approach: focal and lateral. Defining the surgical exposure is the second component of the Caspar ratio that establishes the rationale for a minimally invasive unilateral approach to thoracic intradural extramedullary lesions.

When the average dimensions of a thoracic lesion, the average dimensions of the thoracic canal and the diameter of the minimal access port are superimposed one over another, the anatomical basis for a minimally invasive technique becomes self-evident. ▶ Fig. 11.5 brings together all of these measurements into one image, which firmly establishes the anatomical basis for such an approach.

11.4 Intradural Extramedullary Lesions of the Lumbar versus Thoracic Spine

There is a limitation to the minimally invasive approach with lesions in the lumbar spine. That limitation is due in part to the cauda equina being more accommodating than the spinal cord. The absence of the spinal cord provides lumbar lesions with the potential to grow larger in the rostrocaudal dimension before they become symptomatic. I have observed lesions in excess of 30 mm in the rostrocaudal dimensions in the lumbar spine only. Based on my experience, I have assigned a rostrocaudal limit for the exposure of 35 mm before the benefit of a minimally invasive approach I feel has been exhausted. Under these circumstances, a minimally invasive approach may become more of a liability than an asset when attempting to visualize the entire lesion at once.

Whether I manage a lesion through a minimally invasive paramedian approach or a traditional midline approach, it is imperative for me to visualize the rostral and caudal poles of the lesion simultaneously. Such visualization becomes a tall order once a lesion begins to exceed 30 mm and untenable after 35 mm (▶ Fig. 11.6). Although certainly possible, a limited exposure would result in the need for piecemeal resection, which is not a viable option with lesions such as myxopapillary ependymomas. If I encounter a lesion that I am not confident that I can visualize in its entirety through an expandable minimal access port, I forgo the paramedian transmuscular approach but still use a hemilaminectomy and spinous process-sparing approach as described by Yaşargil et al.[3] Having said that, I have found this situation to be a rare exception and limited to the lumbar spine. The growth pattern in the thoracic spine tends to be more predictable, and the rostrocaudal dimension is unlikely to exceed 25 mm.

11.5 Anatomical Considerations: Variations in the Lumbar and Thoracic Spine Topography

The majority of our experience in minimally invasive approaches occurs in the lumbar spine for the simple reason that degeneration of the spine that requires surgical intervention occurs predominantly in the lumbar region more so than

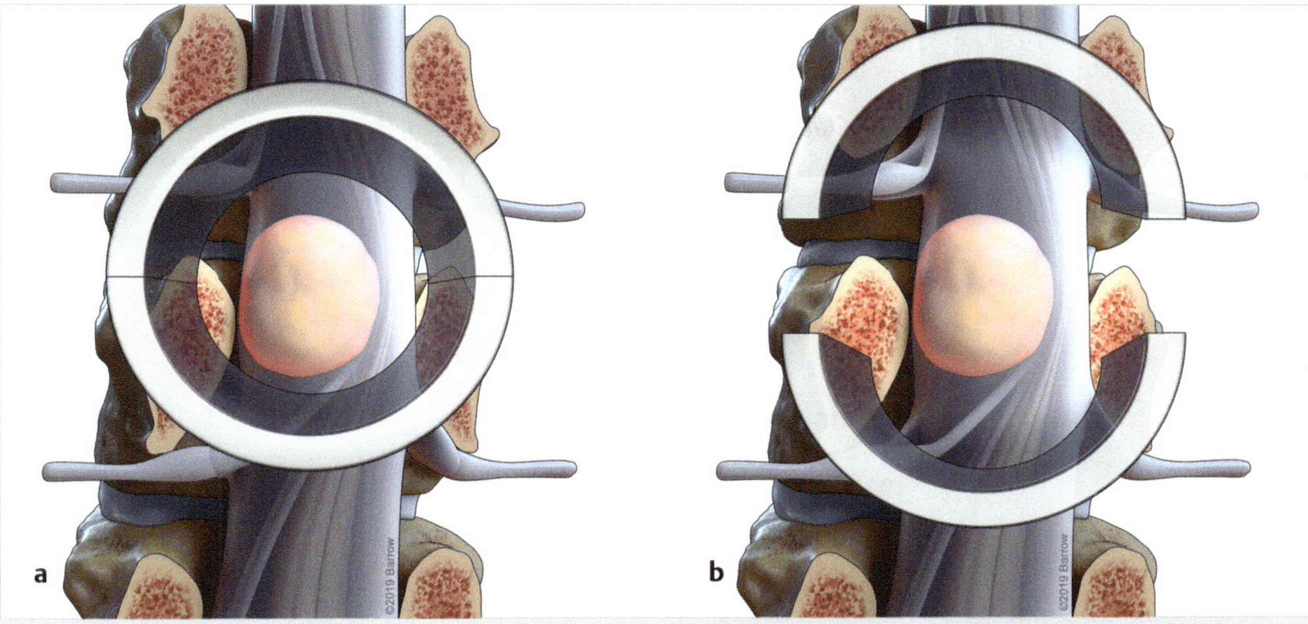

Fig. 11.5 Anatomical basis for a minimally invasive approach to intradural extramedullary lesion. Superimposing an expandable minimal access port over the intradural extramedullary lesion with the average measurements from the dimensional analysis of 26 lesions. **(a)** Illustration of an intradural extramedullary lesion with the following average dimensions: 18.6 mm in the rostrocaudal dimension, 13.0 mm in the lateral dimension and 13.6 mm in the anteroposterior dimension. As can be seen in this illustration, the lesion displaces the spinal cord to the right and occupies the left side of the canal. The laterality of the lesion plays to the strength of a minimally invasive approach. A 22-mm diameter minimal access port readily encompasses the entire lesion. **(b)** With a minimum expansion of the access port, 35-mm rostrocaudal exposure may be achieved, which is more than adequate to visualize the rostral and caudal poles of the lesion for resection.

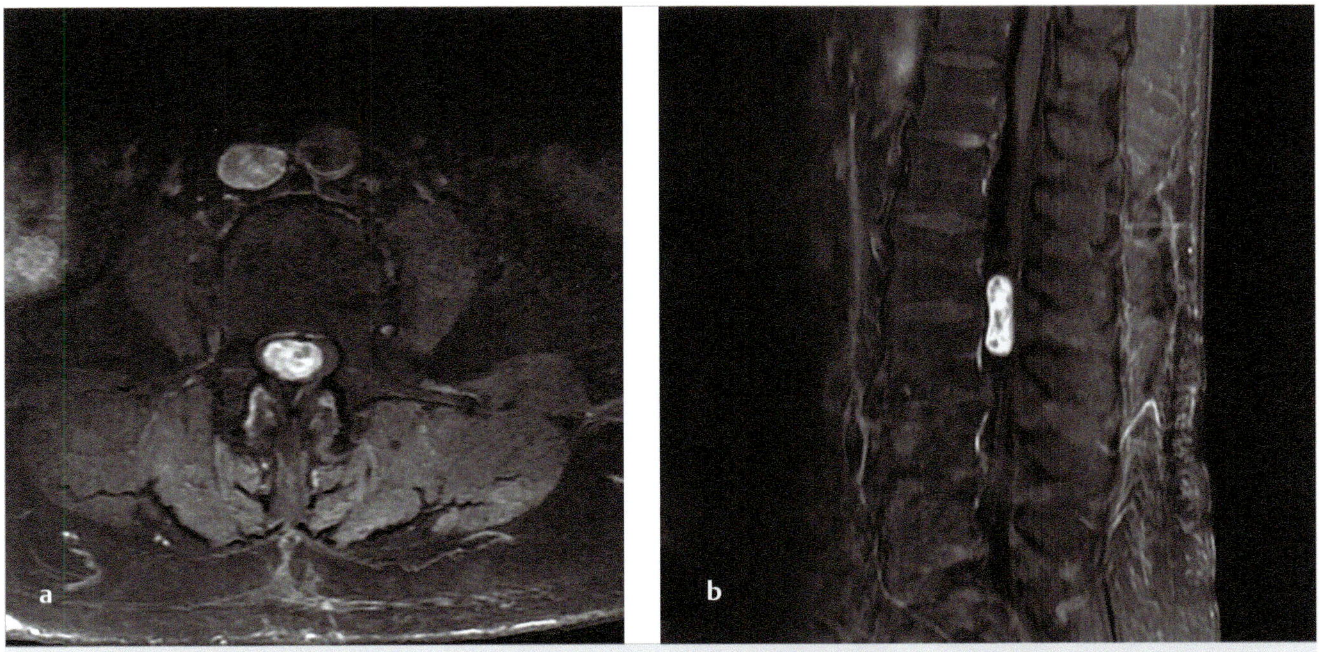

Fig. 11.6 Lumbar ependymoma. **(a)** Axial T1-weighted magnetic resonance imaging (MRI) with gadolinium enhancement demonstrating an intradural extramedullary lesion with an anteroposterior dimension of 11 mm and a transverse dimension of 14 mm consistent with the measurements in the thoracic spine. **(b)** Sagittal T1-weighted MRI with gadolinium enhancement demonstrating a rostrocaudal dimension of 31 mm. This lesion is approaching the upper limit of what may be safely resected through a minimally invasive approach; however, a paramedian, hemilaminectomy, spinous process sparing approach is still feasible.

the thoracic region. As a result, we achieve a great familiarity and sophisticated understanding with the subtleties of the lumbar spine anatomy. After a period of time, the subtle progression of the facets from their sagittal to coronal orientation, as we descend from the upper lumbar levels toward the sacrum, becomes intuitive.

Conversely, most of the intradural extramedullary lesions that we will manage in our careers occur in the thoracic spine. In the series by Seegar et al,[1] 152 of 256 intradural extramedullary lesions occurred in the thoracic spine. In the series by Yaşargil et al,[3] 141 of 250 occurred in the thoracic spine. Such ratios have been consistent with my experience with the management of these lesions, with 26 out of 35 intradural extramedullary lesions harbored in the thoracic spine. For this reason, the anatomy of the thoracic spine from a minimally invasive perspective is the focus of this chapter.

When turning your minimally invasive skill set to the thoracic spine, it is worthwhile to highlight the unique topography of the thoracic spine that distinguishes it from that of the lumbar spine. There are elements of the anatomy in this region that can be harnessed into an advantage in minimally invasive approaches. The transverse process of the thoracic spine is one of them. We begin our discussion of the anatomy with that bony prominence.

11.5.1 Thoracic Transverse Processes and Laminae

The lumbar spine transverse process projects more in the lateral projection than in the posterior projection (▸ Fig. 11.7). As a result, lumbar transverse processes have a small role in minimally invasive exposures and approaches, with the medial aspect of the lumbar transverse process limited to serving as a reference point for the pedicle screw insertion point. Instead, the lumbar facet joint is the main minimally invasive target in the lumbar spine. However, in the thoracic spine, the roles of these anatomical structures are reversed. The thoracic facet joint is not prominent enough to be palpable with the tip of a dilator or index finger in the thoracic spine. A review of the axial illustration in ▸ Fig. 11.7 demonstrates that it is recessed to the level of the lamina. The posteriorly projecting thoracic transverse process, however, is palpable and prominent. Therefore, the thoracic transverse process takes the place of the lumbar facet as the target for the initial dilator in minimally invasive approaches into the thoracic canal. This valuable prominence serves as a beacon for the location of the pedicle and the canal while assisting in docking the access port.

The transverse process in the thoracic spine projects more posteriorly than laterally. That orientation makes it a tremendously valuable target for minimally invasive approaches. After the incision and opening of the fascia, an index finger can immediately palpate the transverse process and use it to guide placement of the initial and subsequent dilator for the eventual placement of the minimal access port. Docking on the transverse process in the thoracic spine may be analogous to docking on the facet in the lumbar spine. It is a reliable and safe starting point for dilatation.

Another key difference between the lumbar and thoracic spine is the lamina. The thoracic lamina tends to be steeper than the lumbar lamina as it joins the spinous process. That steepness makes the corridor to work through narrower than

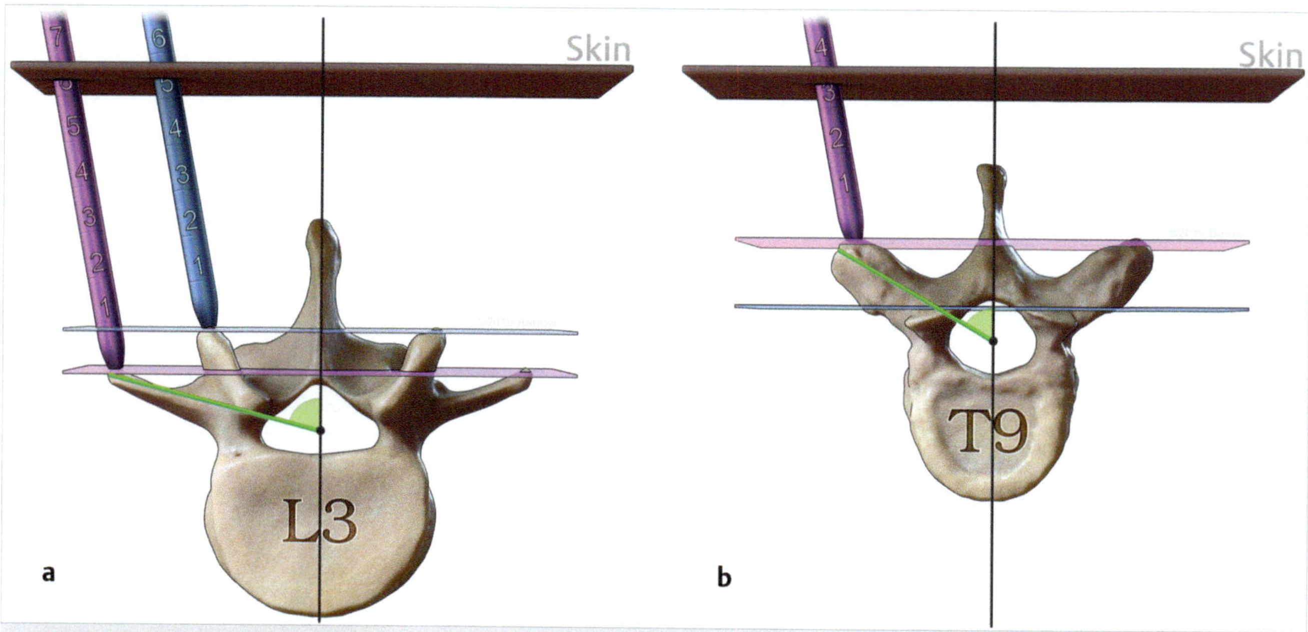

Fig. 11.7 The differences between the thoracic and lumbar facet joints and transverse processes. **(a)** In the lumbar spine, the transverse process serves as one of the three landmarks to identify the entry point for the pedicle, but it is not a landmark for docking the minimal access port. As the lumbar facet is at a shallower depth (*blue plane*) than the transverse process (*magenta plane*), it is readily palpable and an ideal target for the initial dilator. The angle of the projection as determined from the central canal to the tip of the transverse process is more obtuse than the angle in the thoracic spine (angle created by the *green line*). **(b)** In the thoracic spine, the more acute angle of projection of the transverse process (angle formed by the *green line)* makes it more prominent and in a higher plane (*magenta plane*). Therefore, in the thoracic spine, the transverse process is an ideal landmark for a docking target. The thoracic facet, on the other hand, is in a deeper plane (*blue plane*). The posterior projection and higher plane of projection are the unique attributes that make the thoracic transverse process an attractive prominence to target for initially dilating and securing a minimal access port.

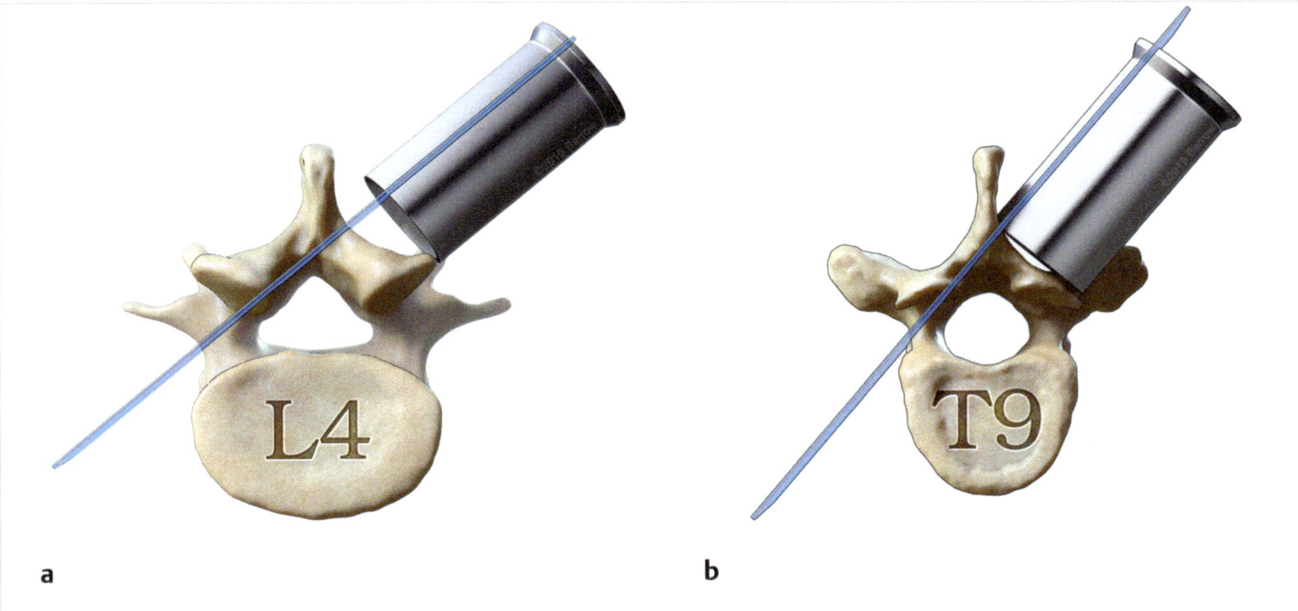

Fig. 11.8 Anatomy of the **(a)** lumbar and **(b)** thoracic spinous process and lamina. Compared to the lumbar spinous process and lamina working channel, the steeper thoracic spinous process and narrower lamina offer a more modest working corridor into the canal. However, that same steepness allows ready access to the entire canal by facilitating undercutting the lamina.

the lumbar spine laminar corridor (▶ Fig. 11.8). At the same time, the steepness of the thoracic lamina allows a better trajectory to readily undercut the spinous process and expose the midline of the thecal sac. The steeper lamina is an indication of the narrower canal in the thoracic spine and therefore a more constrained working area for intradural work. The canal may be enlarged to compensate for this constrained working channel by drilling down the medial aspect of the pedicle, a technique that I emphasize in the section on operative technique (see Section 11.9, Operative Technique).

11.6 Patient Positioning and Localization

Localization in the thoracic spine is a challenging endeavor under any circumstance; however, the stakes are significantly heightened when attempting an intradural lesion resection through a 30-mm incision. Being off by one level with localization changes the entire dynamics of the operation. Unlike an open procedure where the incision need only be extended in one direction or another and the relevant anatomy exposed, in a minimally invasive surgery case, the entire access port has to be removed, another incision planned or extended, sequential dilatation performed, the access port docked onto the appropriate level and another laminectomy performed. Midline open approaches in the thoracic spine are simply more forgiving. Although one always strives for correct identification of the thoracic level in any case, in minimally invasive approaches, there is no room for error. The segment has to be confirmed by counting upward from the sacrum for lower thoracic lesions or downward from the C7–T1 interspace for upper thoracic lesions. Distinct from destructive metastatic lesions in the thoracic spine, which can alter the vertebral body anatomy in a manner that allows for confirmation of the affected level on a fluoroscopic image or lends itself to identifying the altered bony anatomy on computer-assisted navigation, the anatomy of the vertebral bodies in these particular cases is not altered in the least bit. There is no identifiable characteristic appearance on either fluoroscopy or intraoperative computed tomography (CT).

In the operating room, only radiolucent tables are used to minimize any obstruction to seeing the bony anatomy. I avoid the use of standard operating tables and Wilson frames. The upper components of a Wilson frame have large circular gears, which can block visualization of the pedicles in an AP view. The base of a standard operating table prevents the free passage of the fluoroscope. My preference, as with all minimally invasive cases, is a Jackson table (or equivalent) with standard chest, hip and thigh pads. All of these components are radiolucent.

I confirm the localization of the level in two views, both AP and lateral. All patients have standard radiographs of the lumbar spine and confirmation of five non–rib-bearing vertebrae in the lumbar spine on the AP image. These radiographs also serve as a valuable reference in the operating room when looking at the fluoroscopic images.

For mid and lower thoracic cases, I localize twice counting upward from the sacrum. Prior to draping the patient for the actual surgery, I perform a preliminary localization with a series of spinal needles from the lumbosacral spine into the thoracic spine. For the first phase of level confirmation, I prep the entire lumbar and thoracic spine, not for surgery but for localization. I put on a pair of sterile gloves and approximate (by palpation) and mark the L4–5 segment. I employ five spinal needles, alternating an 18-gauge with a 20-gauge needle. Alternating the needles facilitates keeping track of them on AP and lateral imaging. I place the first spinal needle in the vicinity of the L4–5 facet. Depending on the level of the lesion, I pass two or three additional spinal needles in approximately 5-inch increments, docking them on the lateral aspect of the bony anatomy away from the canal. Lateral fluoroscopic images are then taken, and the levels of the spinal needles confirmed. The ideal position of the spinal needle is to have the tip of the needle pointing directly toward a pedicle, which is a position that minimizes any confusion on AP and lateral images. I strive to have the second spinal needle pointing directly toward the T12 pedicle and adjust it to ensure that I am pointing directly at the first rib-bearing vertebral body. Once I have adjusted the position of all the spinal needles to point directly toward the pedicle, I confirm the position with AP and lateral fluoroscopic images until I am satisfied that I am at the correct level. I mark the level and plan the incision 25 mm off the midline on the side of the lesion (more on that later). Then, I mark the entry points of all the spinal needles. Those marks are essential for the second phase of localization, where I repeat the entire process with the patient prepped and draped before I make an incision (▶ Fig. 11.9).

For the second phase of localization, I prep and drape the proposed incision along with the entire lumbar and thoracic spine once again. I use the previously marked entry points for the spinal needles to once again confirm the level of the incision in the AP and lateral planes. An incision is made only after I have verified the correct thoracic level with absolute certainty.

11.7 Planning the Incision: An Observation on the Location of the Lesion

Localization of the level is only the first component of planning the incision. The precision of planning an incision immediately over the lesion is the second component. Doing so involves an AP fluoroscopic image along with a thoughtful analysis of the exact location of the lesion within the thoracic segment. When only 35 mm of the spinal cord is exposed, the lesion must be precisely in the center of that exposure to optimize access to the lesion and closure of the dura. Review of the 26 intradural extramedullary lesions identifies a consistent position of the lesion relative to the disc space and the pedicle. The lesions in all of these cases, from T2–3 through T11–12, are consistently alongside the thoracic pedicle (▶ Fig. 11.10). The unfailing location, relative to the pedicle, reveals a great deal about the origin of the lesion and how it grows. ▶ Fig. 11.11 illustrates how a lesion that arises off a thoracic nerve root at the level of the thoracic pedicle grows into the exact location relative to the pedicle seen in all of the lesions in ▶ Fig. 11.10. Assuming a circumferential growth pattern, the majority of the lesion grows at the level of the pedicle. From there, the lesion either grows in a rostral direction toward the disc space or in the caudal direction toward the inferior aspect of the pedicle. The circumferential growth pattern extends into the canal and displaces the spinal cord to the opposite side (▶ Fig. 11.11). As seen in ▶ Fig. 11.10 and ▶ Fig. 11.11, the majority of the lesion resides immediately medial to the pedicle in every case. There is a pattern of the rostral component of the lesion reaching the disc space; however, on occasion, the lesion may grow in the caudal direction and occupy the level of the vertebral body. Therefore, the incision is planned relative to the center of the pedicle that corresponds to the center of the lesion (▶ Fig. 11.12). Bone work extends either rostrally or caudally from the pedicle, depending on the direction of the growth seen on the MRI. Understanding the origin and growth pattern also serves as the basis for the laminotomy work described below.

The final component of planning the incision involves considering the optimal angle that offers the ideal trajectory onto the

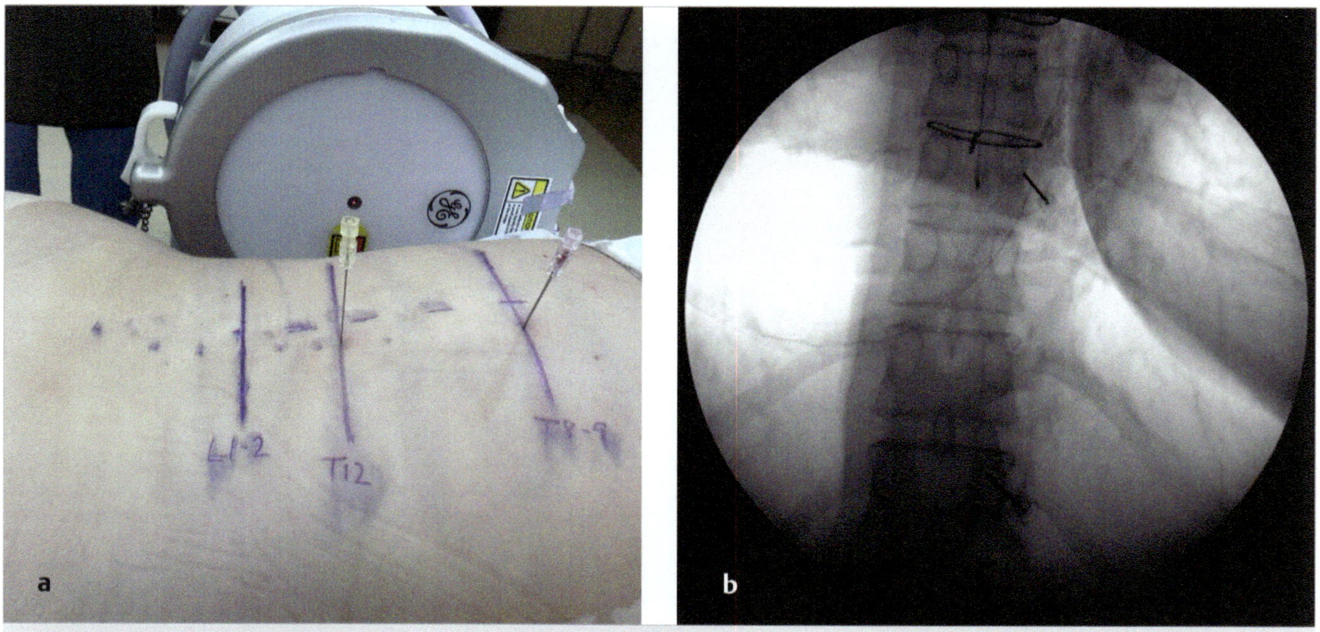

Fig. 11.9 Localization for resection of a T9 intradural extramedullary lesion. **(a)** Intraoperative photograph with spinal needles confirming T9 and T12 pedicles. The patient has been prepped but not draped for the localization process. The T12 pedicle was confirmed on both lateral and anteroposterior imaging. **(b)** Corresponding fluoroscopic image of the photograph in **a**. Note the spinal needle pointing directly toward the pedicle. The lesion is immediately medial to the pedicle of T9 on the right. The patient is prepped and draped again, and the localization process repeated.

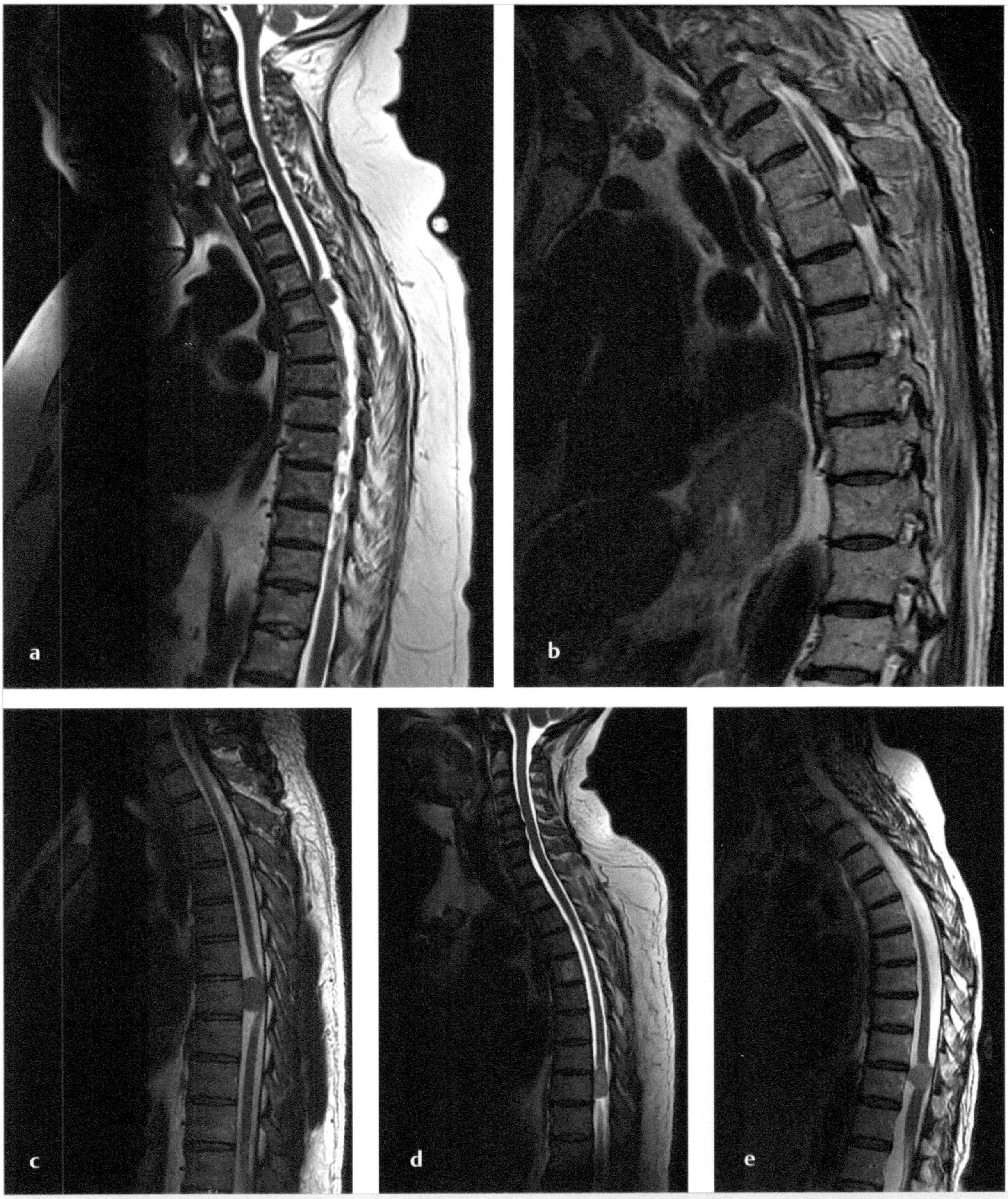

Fig. 11.10 Location of the lesion relative to the disc space. In planning the incision based on fluoroscopy, recognizing the consistent position of the lesion within the canal is essential for precisely locating the incision. **(a)** Sagittal T2-weighted magnetic resonance imaging (MRI) showing a lesion at the T2–3 disc space, with the majority of the lesion behind the vertebral body of T3. **(b)** Sagittal T2-weighted MRI showing a lesion at the T4–5 disc space with the majority of the lesion behind the vertebral body of T5. **(c)** Sagittal T2-weighted MRI showing a lesion at the T7–8 disc space with the majority of the lesion behind the vertebral body of T8. **(d)** Sagittal T2-weighted MRI showing a lesion at the T8–9 disc space with the majority of the lesion behind the vertebral body of T9. **(e)** Sagittal T2-weighted MRI showing a lesion at the T11–12 disc space with the majority of the lesion behind the vertebral body of T12. Note that in each of these circumstances, the lesion was found to be growing off a nerve root that was exiting beneath the pedicle of the caudal vertebral body. Therefore, the incision should be centered on the pedicle that corresponds with the lesion, as seen in ▶ Fig. 11.9.

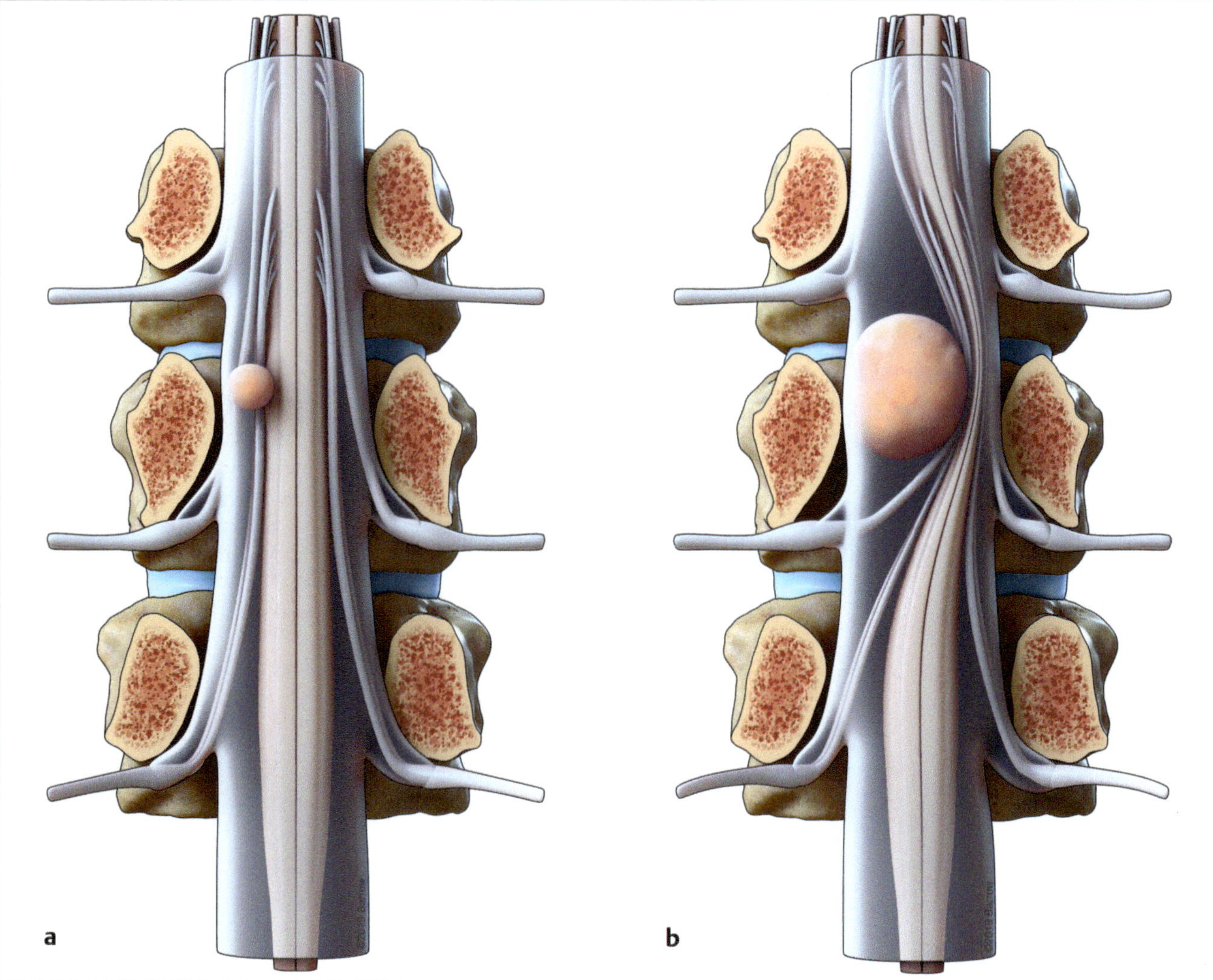

Fig. 11.11 Location of the lesion relative to the disc space and pedicle. Illustration of the proposed origin and growth pattern of intradural extramedullary lesions. (a) Illustration of the posterior view of the spine demonstrating a small lesion only millimeters in diameter and beginning at the level of the pedicle. (b) As the lesion grows in a circumferential pattern, it expands toward the disc space and down to the midpedicle. The hypothesis of this growth pattern is validated by the consistent location of all 26 intradural extramedullary lesions, which were confirmed to be schwannomas or meningiomas, as shown in ▶ Fig. 11.10.

thoracic lamina for exposure of the entire spinal cord. An incision planned too medial limits the angle of convergence onto the lamina and thereby curbs the exposure of the midline and contralateral aspect of the canal. An incision planned too lateral requires excessive convergence to reach the lamina, which limits access to the ipsilateral aspect of the thecal sac. An incision 25 to 30 mm off the midline offers an appropriate trajectory onto the thoracic lamina for access to the entire canal.

11.8 Minimally Invasive versus Midline Open Exposures

Throughout this book, I have emphasized that the fundamental tenet of minimally invasive spine surgery is to have the operation virtually indistinguishable from its traditional midline open counterpart. A minimally invasive resection of an intradural lesion is no different. A midline open approach of an intradural extramedullary lesion exposes approximately 25 to 30% of the posterior aspect of the thecal sac and spinal cord (▶ Fig. 11.13). In order to accomplish the equivalent amount of exposure of the thecal sac in a minimally invasive resection, a more lateral working channel is created. Undercutting the spinous process and contralateral lamina is the first step to expanding access to the central canal through the access port. Drilling down the pars interarticularis, facet and medial pedicle is the second step to expanding access to the canal. By taking these steps, there is no difference between the transverse dimension of bone work in a midline open approach or paramedian minimally invasive approach. The difference is the location of that bone work on the posterior thoracic spine. It goes without saying that a posterolateral approach has the added benefit of preserving the posterior elements and posterior tension band.

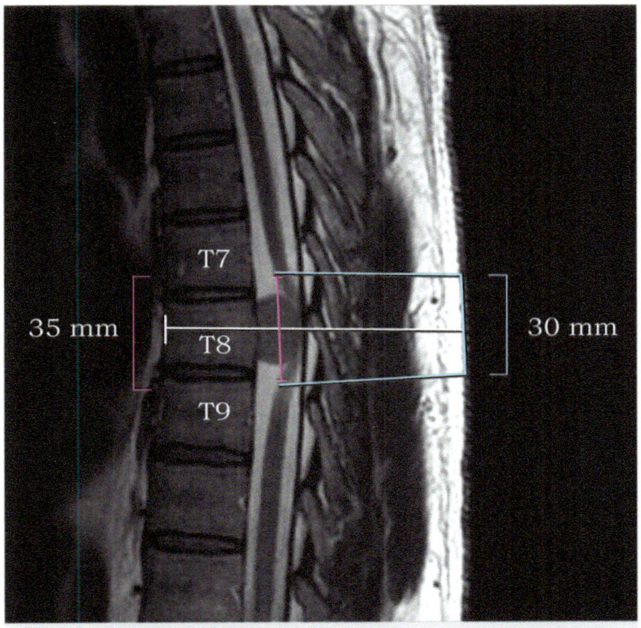

Fig. 11.12 Planning the incision. Sagittal T2-weighted thoracic spine magnetic resonance imaging showing an intradural extramedullary lesion at T8. Understanding the origin of the lesion and the growth pattern is the basis for centering the incision on the T8 pedicle (*white line*). A 30-mm incision (*blue line* at skin) centered on the pedicle (*white line*) allows for 35 mm of bony exposure (*magenta line*) when the blades of the access port are angled open.

Once the posterolateral bone work is completed, I have found that a generous exposure of the dura of the spinal cord is possible. This exposure is essential not only to access the lesion but to close the dura efficiently after resection. Similar to the bone work, there is no difference in the amount of dura exposed between minimally invasive and open approaches. There is only a difference in the location of the exposure, as illustrated in ▶ Fig. 11.13. The extent of exposure required further establishes my rationale for employing an expandable minimal access port.

11.9 Operative Technique

11.9.1 Final Marking of the Incision

Applying the understanding of the growth pattern of these lesions, and keeping in mind the importance of trajectory and localization strategies discussed above, the final element of planning the incision is marking a 30-mm incision precisely over the midpoint of the pedicle, which corresponds to the lesion and is 25 to 30 mm lateral to the midline (▶ Fig. 11.14). The origin of these lesions off a thoracic nerve root places the lesion immediately medial to the pedicle. Therefore, the pedicle that corresponds to the lesion is the "North Star" of this operation.

11.9.2 Docking the Minimal Access Port

Once I have confirmed the thoracic pedicle using the localization method described above, I make the incision but keep all of the spinal needles in place below the incision to confirm the

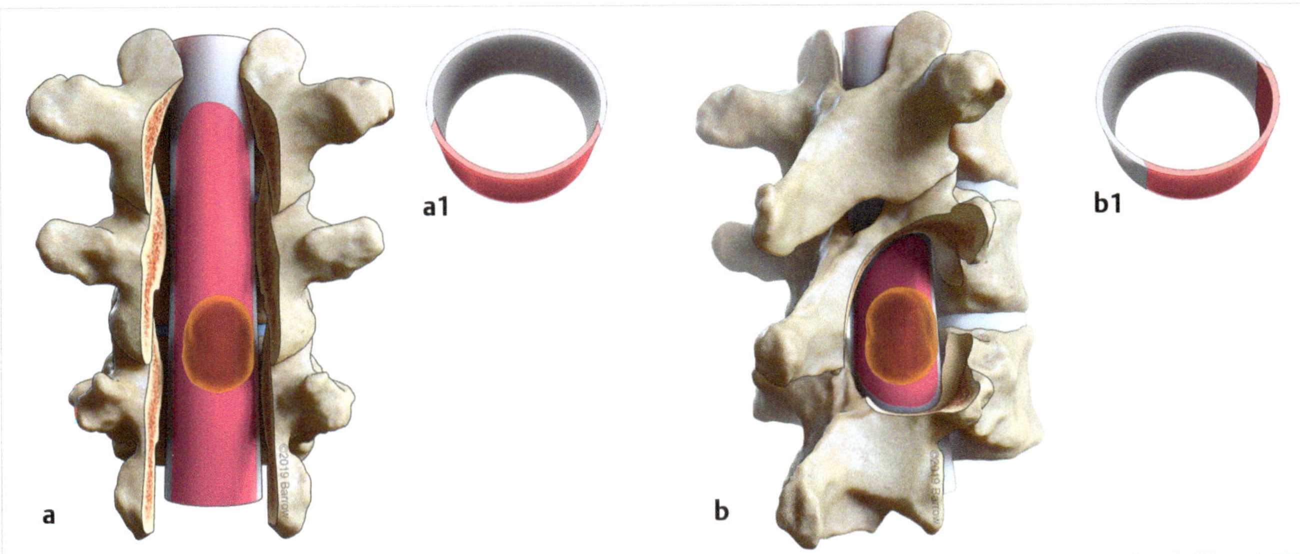

Fig. 11.13 Conceptual depiction of the exposure of the thoracic spinal cord comparing a midline open approach to a minimally invasive approach. **(a)** Traditional midline thoracic exposure with complete laminectomies for access to an intradural lesion. The access to the dura of the thoracic spinal cord is denoted by the dura highlighted in *fuchsia*; the lesion is ghosted in *orange*. **(a1)** A conceptual dural ring where the *fuchsia* corresponds with the amount of dura exposed through a midline approach. **(b)** Illustration of a minimal-access exposure with a lesion at the same level (ghosted in *orange*). Again, the access to the thoracic spinal cord is denoted by the dura highlighted in *fuchsia* and is exactly the same as the exposure accomplished with a midline approach. When the bed is rotated away from the surgeon, the operative exposure is centered immediately over the lesion. **(b1)** The conceptual dural ring has the same amount of exposure of the dural in a minimal access approach as in a traditional midline approach. The only difference between the two is the rostrocaudal exposure, which is overly generous with laminectomies above and below the lesion in a midline open approach, but limited and precise in the minimally invasive exposure.

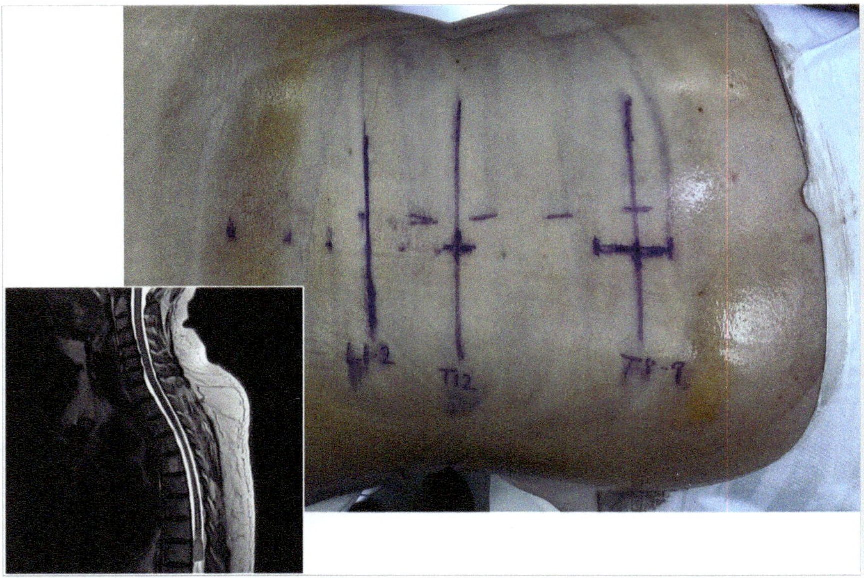

Fig. 11.14 A planned incision for resection of a T9 right-sided schwannoma (*inset*, T2-weighted magnetic resonance imaging). An incision 25 mm off the midline and 30 mm in length is planned immediately over the midpoint of the T9 pedicle. The entire lumbar and thoracic spine are prepped and draped to repeat the localization process. The spinal needle entry points for the L1–2 level and the T12 pedicle are marked for repositioning the spinal needles and reconfirming the T9 pedicle after all the sterile drapes are placed.

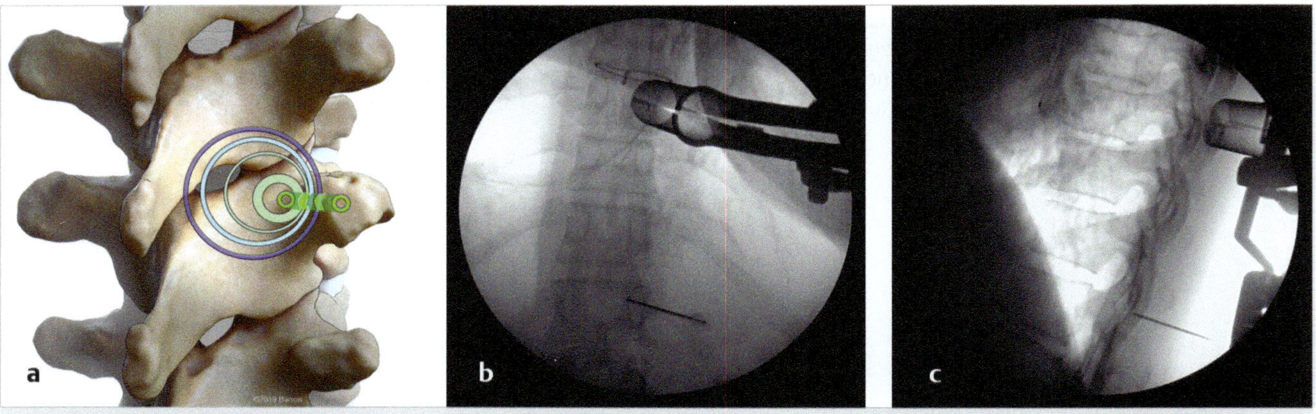

Fig. 11.15 Docking the minimal access port in the thoracic spine for resection of an intradural extramedullary lesion. **(a)** Illustration demonstrating the sequence of dilation with the transverse process as the initial target (*emerald ring*). The rings represent the increasing diameters of the dilators. Medial wanding (*emerald arrow*) from the transverse process onto the lamina with subsequent dilators encompasses the lamina. The larger diameter dilators (*green, aqua blue* and *purple*) then optimize an interface onto the spinous process, lamina and facet. **(b)** Anteroposterior fluoroscopic image of the minimal access port over the T9 pedicle. The spinal needle at T12 remains in position to confirm the T9 pedicle. **(c)** Lateral fluoroscopic image with the minimal access port centered immediately over the lesion.

position of the minimal access port. I do not remove these spinal needles until I directly see the lesion. If a circumstance arises where I need to reconfirm the level again, the spinal needles are already in place as reference points.

After infiltrating with a local anesthetic, I make the incision with a No. 15 blade and divide the fascia with cautery. Similar to the lumbar spine, when using an expandable minimal access port, I open the fascia 25% larger than the skin incision. A wider fascial opening allows the blades to open and angulate to the full 35 mm needed. The result is a larger area of exposure than the skin incision. With the fascia open, I sound out the bony anatomy with the first dilator. I begin palpating with the tip of the dilator to identify the transverse process that corresponds with the pedicle where the lesion resides. As discussed earlier, the thoracic transverse process projects more posterior than lateral. Once I palpate it with the tip of the dilator, I slide down the medial aspect of the transverse process and onto the lamina. It is essential to be medial to the transverse process when beginning to dilate in order to minimize the extent of muscle creep that can occur. The larger diameter dilators begin to engulf the transverse process in the lateral aspect of the diameter, as seen in ▶ Fig. 11.15. Upon reaching a 22-mm diameter, I secure the appropriate length with the expandable minimal access port in position. A converging trajectory ensures the medial aspect of the access port is at the confluence of the lamina and spinous process. With the ideal trajectory of approximately 15 to 20 degrees, I secure the access port onto the table-mounted arm. Final AP and lateral fluoroscopic images confirm the level and trajectory. As already mentioned, I keep the spinal needles that helped localize the lesion in place until the dura is opened and the lesion is directly visualized.

11.9.3 Exposure

With the expandable minimal access port in position, I bring in the operating microscope. Just like in the lumbar laminectomy, I rotate the bed away 15 degrees to allow for an optimal working angle onto the lesion. When peering through the microscope into the field of view for the first time, there should be elements of the thoracic lamina visualized. Because of the prominence of the transverse process and the depth of the valley created by the confluence of the thoracic lamina and spinous process, it is unavoidable to have some muscle in the field of view at the outset. I have firmly anchored the access port to the lamina so that after removal of the small cuff of muscle, a plane of dissection hopefully becomes evident as the access port opens.

The first step in exposure is to completely expose the lamina that corresponds to the level of the lesion. The confluence of the spinous process and lamina is identified first, and then cautery is used to wipe away the remaining soft tissue over the top of the lamina. Working laterally from the lamina leads directly to the transverse process at the level harboring the lesion, and from the transverse process, I proceed rostral and expose the facet. The complete exposure of the lamina, transverse process and facet allows for the mental reconstruction of the pedicle that corresponds to the lesion. In my mind's eye, I can see the medial aspect of the pedicle in the lateral aspect of my exposure that allows me to envision where the bulk of the lesion resides (▸ Fig. 11.16). I keep in mind the growth pattern of the lesion presented in Section 11.7, Planning the Incision: An Observation on the Location of the Lesion. More often than not, the lesion grows rostrally toward the disc space above the pedicle (▸ Fig. 11.10). At other times, it grows more in the caudal direction and resides behind the vertebral body (▸ Fig. 11.12). I tailor the 35 mm of the bony exposure to what I see on the MRI.

I always expose the entire hemilamina and transverse process at the level of the lesion. The variation comes with extending that exposure either rostrally or caudally. If the lesion extends to the disc space above, I expose the inferior half of the hemilamina above. If the lesion extends to the vertebral body, I expose the superior aspect of the hemilamina below. However, everything hinges on the exposure of the pedicle at the level of the lesion. I open the access port a click or two and then angle the blades either rostrally or caudally to help finish the exposure.

Prior to beginning any bone work, I ensure that I have all of the bone that I am going to drill exposed (▸ Fig. 11.17). An exposure 35 mm in the rostrocaudal dimension centered on the thoracic pedicle that corresponds to the lesion provides the necessary access to the spinal canal to resect the lesion and close the dura safely.

11.9.4 Bone Work

My strategy when it comes to the removal of the lamina in these thoracic cases is identical to my approach in a posterior cervical foraminotomy: drill the lateral aspect of the lamina first, identify the canal and then proceed medially to expose the spinal cord. Such an approach minimizes the risk of injury to the spinal cord. The second reason has to do with the placement of the medial–lateral retractor. As mentioned earlier, the transverse process in the thoracic spine projects posteriorly,

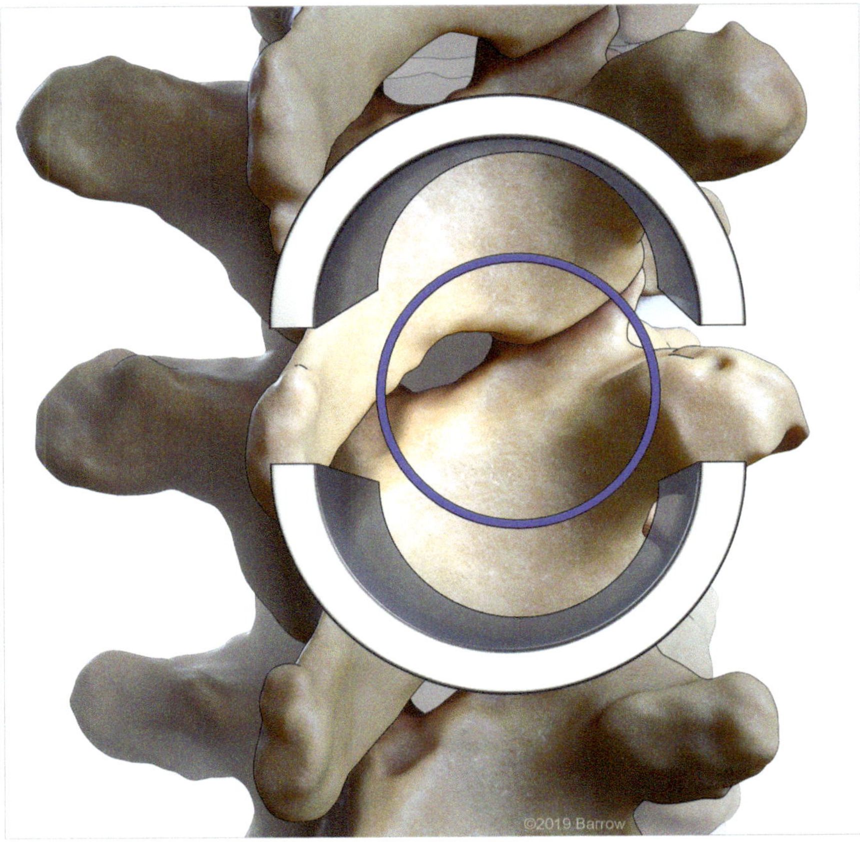

Fig. 11.16 Sequential exposure of the thoracic lamina, facet and transverse process. Illustration demonstrating the initial diameter of exposure of a 22-mm access port (*blue ring*) immediately over the pedicle that corresponds to the lesion. After exposure of the entire hemilamina that corresponds to the lesion, the exposure extends rostral to the inferior aspect of the lamina above. The expandable minimal access port is gradually opened to encompass a 35-mm exposure centered over the pedicle.

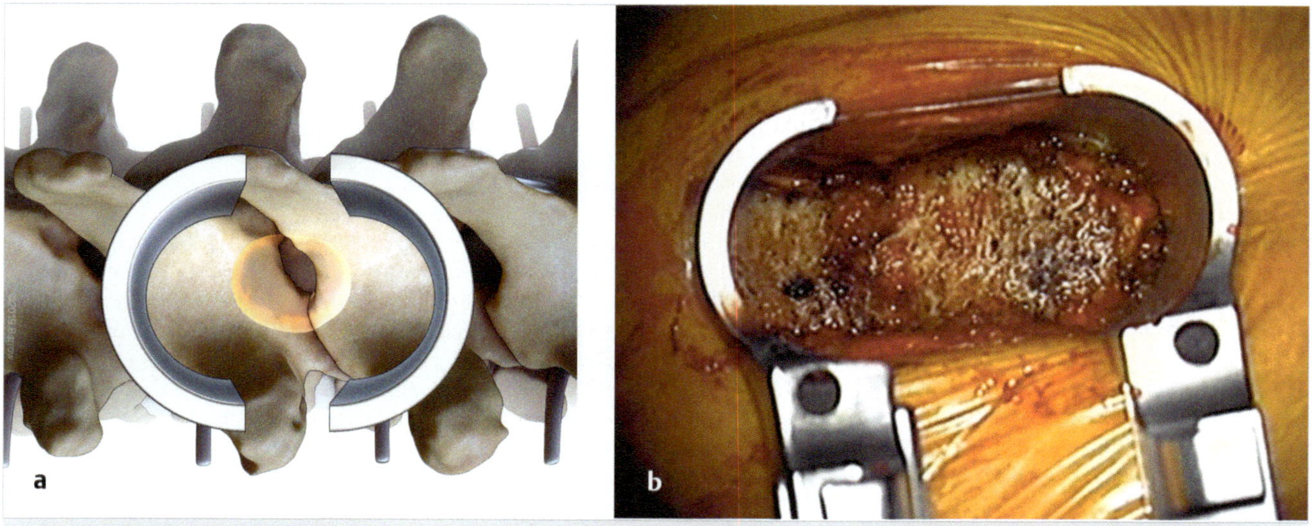

Fig. 11.17 Exposure of the spinous process, lamina, facet and transverse process for a right-sided lesion at T11. **(a)** Illustration demonstrating the exposure necessary prior to beginning the removal of the bone with the lesion ghosted in the center of the field of view. **(b)** Intraoperative photograph demonstrating 35 mm of exposure centered on the thoracic pedicle.

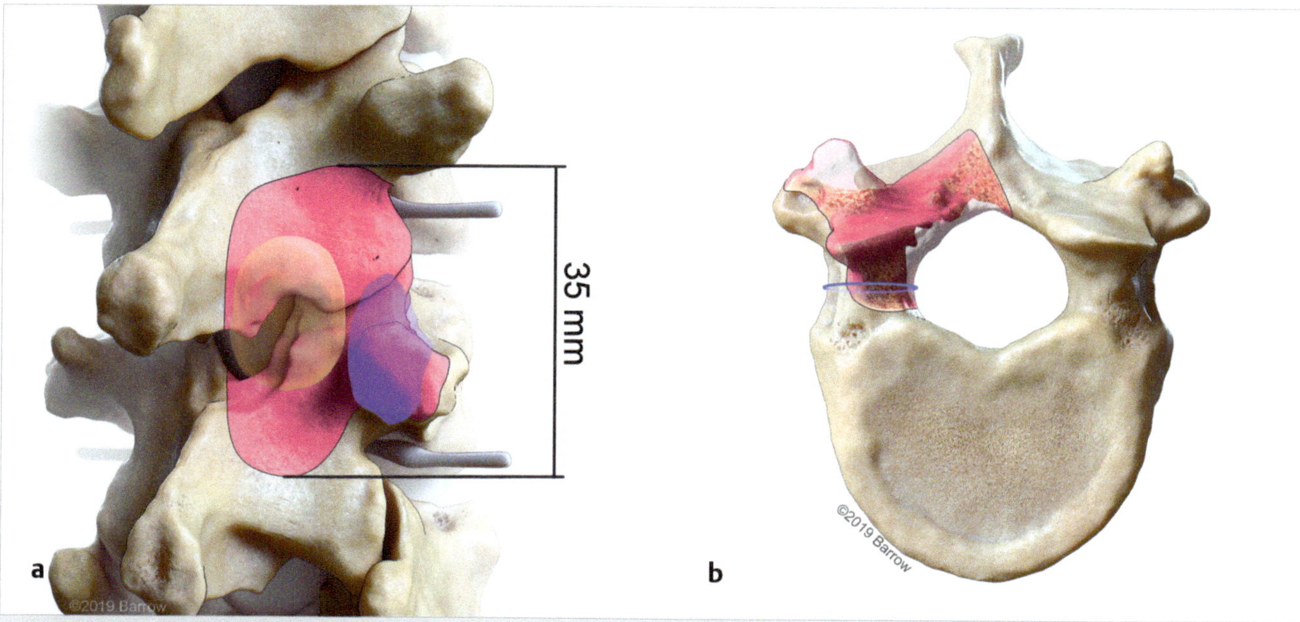

Fig. 11.18 Preliminary bone work over the top of the lesion. **(a)** The *fuchsia-shaded* area represents the preliminary bone work over the lesion. The pedicle has been highlighted in *purple*. Drilling begins on the lateral aspect of the lamina until the lateral aspect of the canal becomes evident. The medial aspect of the pedicle (*purple*) should be visible and palpable with a right-angled, ball-tipped probe before proceeding in the medial direction with the laminectomy. After identifying the medial wall of the pedicle and the lateral aspect of the canal, the objective becomes the completion of the laminectomy and undercutting the spinous process to have access to the entire canal. **(b)** Axial view demonstrating the bone work relative to the canal. The pedicle that corresponds to the lesion has been circled with a *blue ring*. Drilling the medial aspect of the pedicle enlarges the working channel for resection of the lesion.

which prevents the ideal placement of a medial–lateral retractor. By drilling down the transverse process, the lateral blade of the medial–lateral retractor may now expose the lateral aspect of the canal and prevent muscle creep, while simultaneously revealing the base of the spinous process. Hence, I drill the transverse process until it is flat. I then deepen the position of the medial–lateral retractor and angulate the blades in a medial trajectory and continue drilling (▶ Fig. 11.18).

▶ Fig. 11.19 demonstrates the first phase of the bone work to be done prior to opening the dura. The transverse process acts as a reference point for the canal and the pedicle. Once I have drilled the transverse process flat, the pedicle blush begins to reveal itself. The pedicle comes into full view as I drill in the rostral direction and approach the facet. The center of the pedicle is reliably at the midpoint of the transverse process. It is my objective to reveal the superior and inferior boundaries of

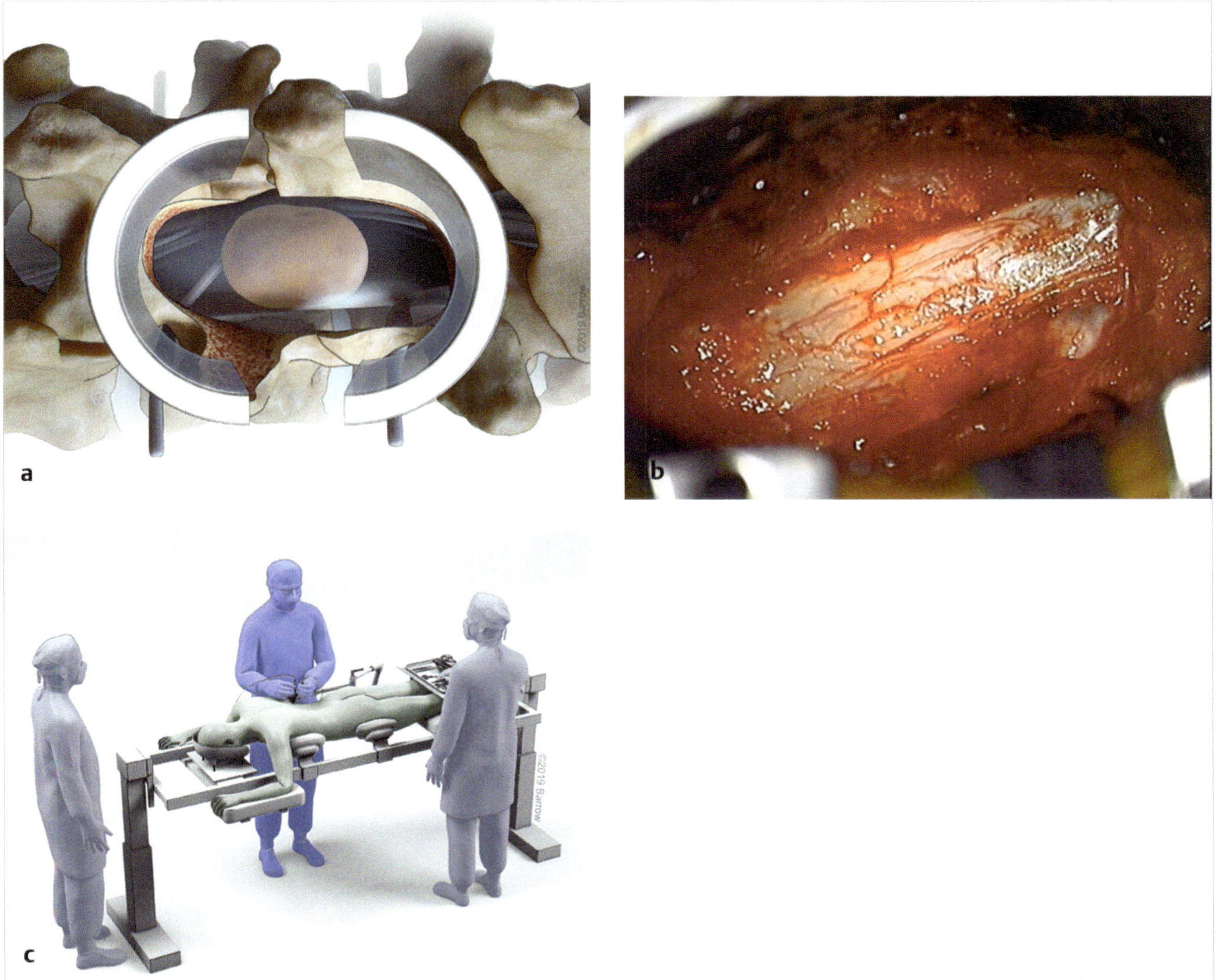

Fig. 11.19 Minimally invasive thoracic laminectomy for resection of a right-sided intradural extramedullary lesion. **(a)** Illustration of the exposure for the resection of a T12 meningioma. The entire hemilamina of T12 and the inferior half of the T11 hemilamina have been removed. A right-sided medial facetectomy at T11–12 has been completed. The transverse process of the T12 has been drilled flat, and the medial aspect of the T12 pedicle has been drilled to expand the lateral dimension of the canal. The rostral and caudal poles of the lesion may be simultaneously seen. With the bone work demonstrated in this illustration, there is an adequate working channel to close the dura in a watertight fashion. **(b)** Intraoperative photograph demonstrating the exposure of the dura prior to exposure of the lesion at T12 on the right. Note the right T11 thoracic nerve root and the lateral aspect of the thecal sac are completely exposed. **(c)** Schematic for orientation of the right-sided approach.

the pedicle. In doing so, I have provided my mind the location of the lesion. I avoid drilling into the pedicle at this point, which would cause unnecessary bleeding. Instead, I use a right-angled, ball-tipped probe to palpate the medial wall of the pedicle and take note of the superior and inferior aspects of the pedicle. Establishing the boundaries of the pedicle is valuable early in the bone removal phase, since it establishes the lateral aspect of the bone work. From the pedicle, I work to extend the medial boundary of the bone work. I drill with an oblique trajectory to undercut the spinous process and ensure an adequate midline exposure. Although the ligamentum flavum now begins to come into view, similar to the lumbar laminectomy technique, I do not resect it at this point. Instead, I complete the bone work by drilling the medial facet and the lamina of the level above the lesion down to the ligamentum flavum.

The final maneuver with the ligamentum flavum still intact is to drill down the medial aspect of the pedicle. I drill down only the medial half of the pedicle. It is essential to leave the lateral aspect of the pedicle intact where the rib head articulates with the vertebral body and pedicle for a stable articulation of the rib head into the lateral aspect of the vertebral body. I drill the medial aspect of the pedicle entirely flush with the back of the vertebral body. In doing so, I have expanded the lateral dimensions of the canal (▶ Fig. 11.20).

I make every effort to preserve the lateral half of the facet joint when completing the lateral aspect of the exposure, but at times the facet joint on the side of the lesion is removed in its entirety to access the central canal. The 5-year follow-up that I have had with the few patients with complete facetectomies have not demonstrated an untoward clinical outcome from that

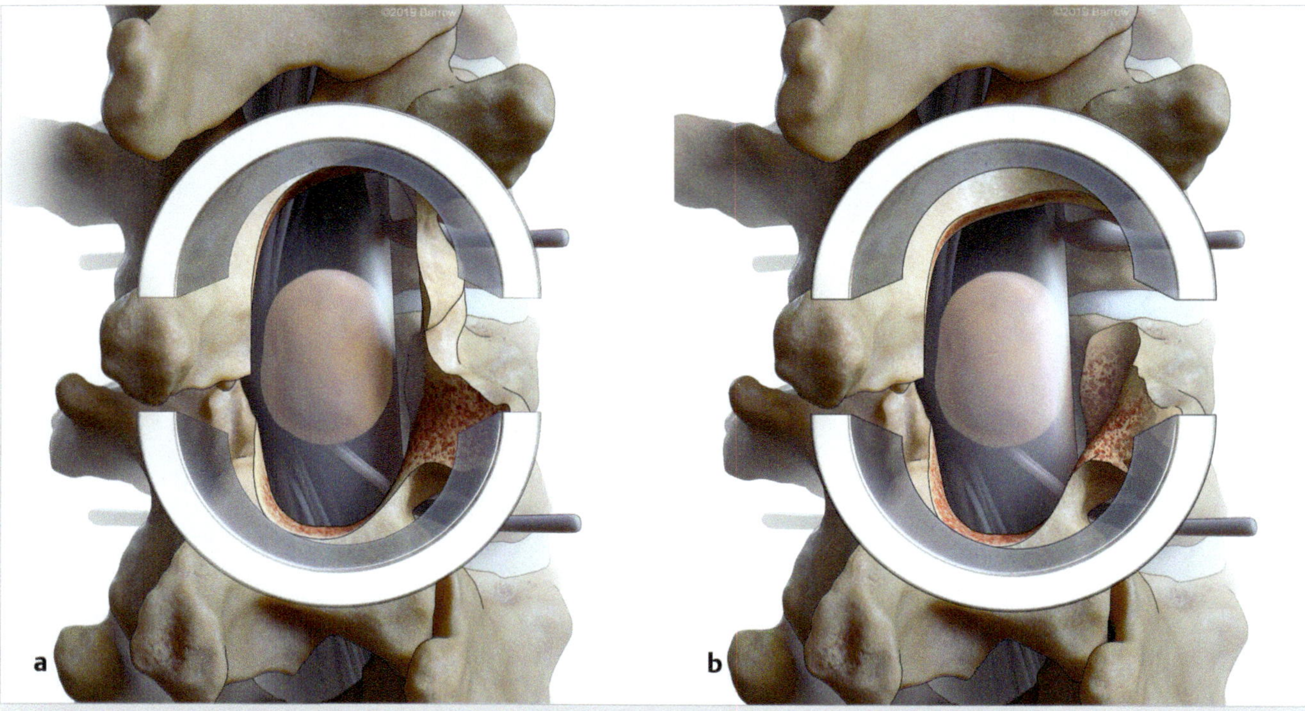

Fig. 11.20 Bone work for a thoracic meningioma. Illustration with the bone work completed. The transverse process that corresponds with the pedicle and the lesion has been drilled completely flat. The superior three-quarters of the hemilamina at the level of the lesion have been removed from the base of the spinous process to the medial aspect of the pedicle. **(a)** Every effort is made to preserve the medial facet; however, at times, **(b)** a complete facetectomy is completed to establish the lateral exposure.

bone work. From those clinical outcomes, I can only conclude that the additional support from the articulating rib, the preservation of the contralateral facet, the spinous process and posterior tension band all contribute to the stability of the segment if and when a unilateral thoracic facetectomy becomes necessary.

With the bone work complete, the entire swath of ligamentum flavum of the segment is now in view, and its en bloc resection exposes the dura of the spinal cord along with the exiting nerve root above and below the pedicle that has been drilled. It is at this time that I begin to assess whether I have enough medial exposure over the top of the dura. It is imperative to undercut the spinous process and drill the underside of the contralateral lamina to accomplish the medial bony exposure. Any additional medial removal of bone may be accomplished by increased angulation of the medial–lateral retractor. If I have met all of the above criteria, the rostrocaudal exposure should be more than adequate. I routinely measure the distance with a ruler cut precisely to 35 mm in order to confirm my exposure. For a lesion measuring 20 mm in the rostrocaudal dimension, a distance of 35 mm is more than adequate.

11.9.5 Exposure of the Lesion

As with any intradural procedure, before opening up the dura, meticulous hemostasis is imperative. Any bleeding bone should be sealed with bone wax, any visible epidural veins surrounding the dura should be cauterized and hemostatic agents should be compressed into the potential space between the lamina and the dura.

I prefer to make a paramedian opening in the dura instead of the midline for two reasons. It is straightforward to close a paramedian dural opening with a generous exposure of the dura on the ipsilateral side, where the canal has been expanded by drilling the medial aspect of the pedicle. The second and perhaps more important reason is that the lesion is off to one side, and I find it preferable to open the dura precisely over the lesion, which is also farthest from the spinal cord (▶ Fig. 11.21). Since the lesion has displaced the spinal cord laterally within the canal, a paramedian makes opening the dura in the lateral corridor the safest location to approach. A paramedian approach is certainly nothing novel. In 1983, Eggert and colleagues recommended the same approach in their series of hemilaminectomies for intradural tumors. In the summary of their article, they state, "it is emphasized that the dura should be opened only over the tumour [sic] in order to avoid protrusion of the cord."[2]

The origin of the lesion coming from a thoracic nerve root places the lesion precisely at the level of the pedicle; therefore, the dura is opened based on the midpoint of the pedicle. We know from Panjabi's anthropometric study on the thoracic pedicle that the rostrocaudal dimension of the pedicle is no more than 11 to 12 mm in the upper thoracic spine (T2–T9) and 14 to 16 mm in the lower thoracic spine (T10–T12). Therefore, opening from the caudal boundary of the pedicle and extending the opening to 7 to 8 mm above and below the pedicle provides 25 mm of a dural opening, which is then tailored, either rostrally or caudally, another 10 mm after the lesion has been identified. I keep in mind that to close the dura, 3 to 4 mm of clearance is needed from each bone edge.

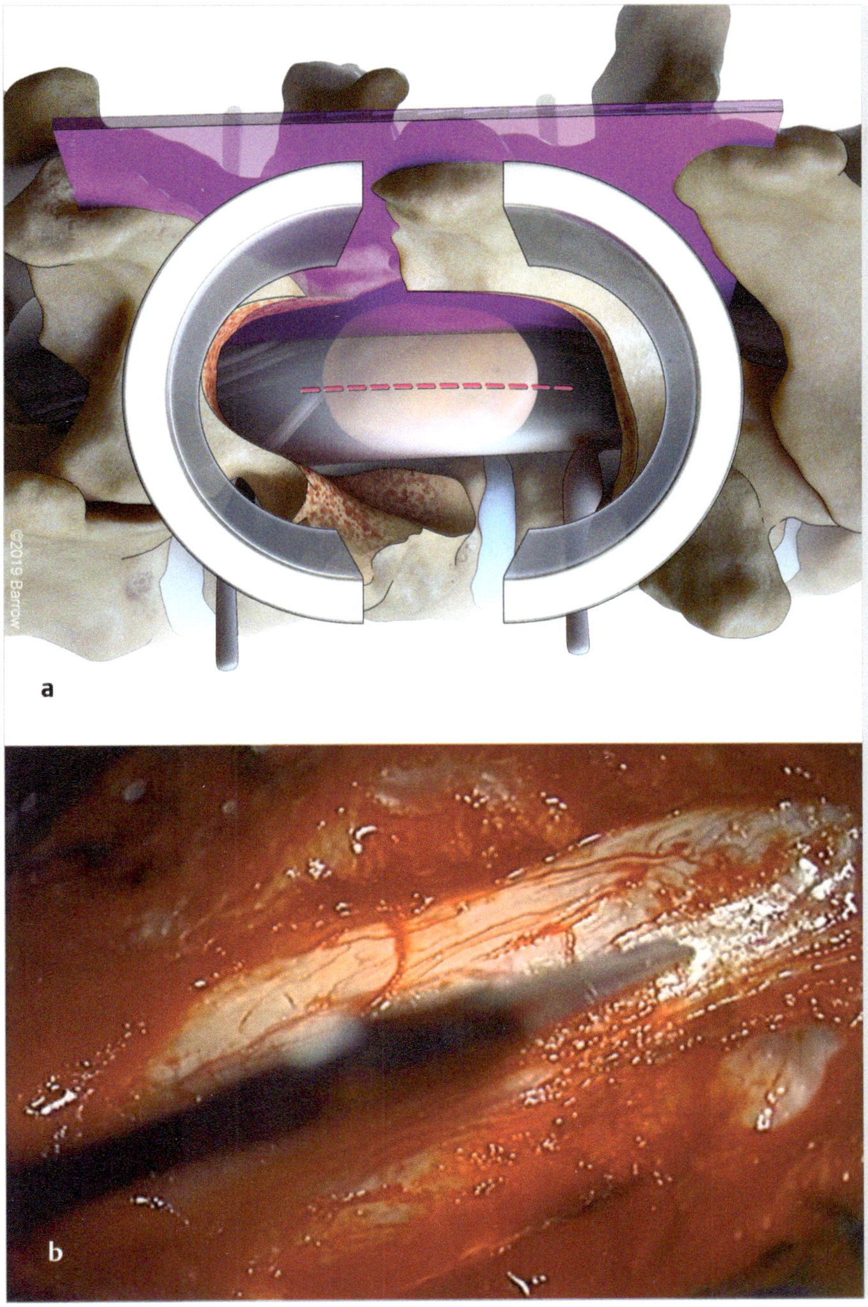

Fig. 11.21 Dural opening. **(a)** Illustration of the thoracic spine with a lesion at T12 on the right. The spine is rotated 20 degrees to demonstrate the location of the dural opening immediately over the top of the lesion (*dotted fuchsia line*). The midline is denoted by the *purple plane*. The *fuchsia* line indicates the location of the dural opening immediately above the lesion. The paramedian location of the dural opening has two main advantages. The first advantage is that it is in the center of the exposure. There is an adequate working channel on either side of the bone work to close the dura in a watertight fashion. The second advantage to a paramedian opening is that the lesion is off to that side. Therefore, the dura is being opened furthest from the spinal cord. **(b)** Intraoperative photograph showing a No. 11 blade for opening the dura above the rostral pole of the lesion.

11.9.6 Opening the Dura

I place a 6.0 polypropylene suture in the vicinity of my intended dural opening so that I may place some upward traction on the dura. I then use a No. 11 blade to open the dura beginning slightly above the lesion, as demonstrated in ▶ Fig. 11.21. An opening above the lesion places me in a place safely away from the spinal cord and allows me to identify the rostral pole of the lesion. The lesion should come into immediate view upon opening the dura. If the dura is opened to 30 mm and the lesion is not visualized, something has gone awry with the localization process. The dura is closed with one or two Nurolon sutures (Johnson & Johnson, New Brunswick, NJ), and the localization process restarted from the beginning. It is for this reason that the spinal needles are kept in position. With a meticulous and systematic approach to localization, opening the dura and not seeing the lesion should be a rare or even a never event. It has been my experience that the lesion can be seen through the dura, as the layers of the dura become diaphanous from a combination of the exposure and the microscope light. Just irrigating over the top of the dura sometimes reveals the robin's egg blue lesion below. At the minimum, there is a distinct dilatation to the dura, which leaves little doubt about what lies beneath. Once I have directly visualized the lesion, I remove the spinal needles and begin the resection of the lesion.

11.9.7 Resection of the Lesion

I open the dura until I can simultaneously visualize the rostral and caudal poles of the lesion. I tack the dural edges with a 6.0 polypropylene suture, using bayoneted Castro-Viejo needle drivers, by clamping the polypropylene strands with mosquito clamps and resting them over the minimal access port. Gravity alone maintains the opening of the dural edges (▶ Fig. 11.22). As I continue to open the dura, I use Rhoton dissectors and arachnoid knives to establish a plane between the lesion and the dura. On occasion, I have found the lesion calcified onto the dura. Such a circumstance mandates resection of the dura and sewing in a dural patch to repair the defect. However, the need for sewing a patch onto the dura is seldom the case (2 out of 26 cases), and I can typically establish a sure plane between the dura and the lesion. More often than not, I have found that the

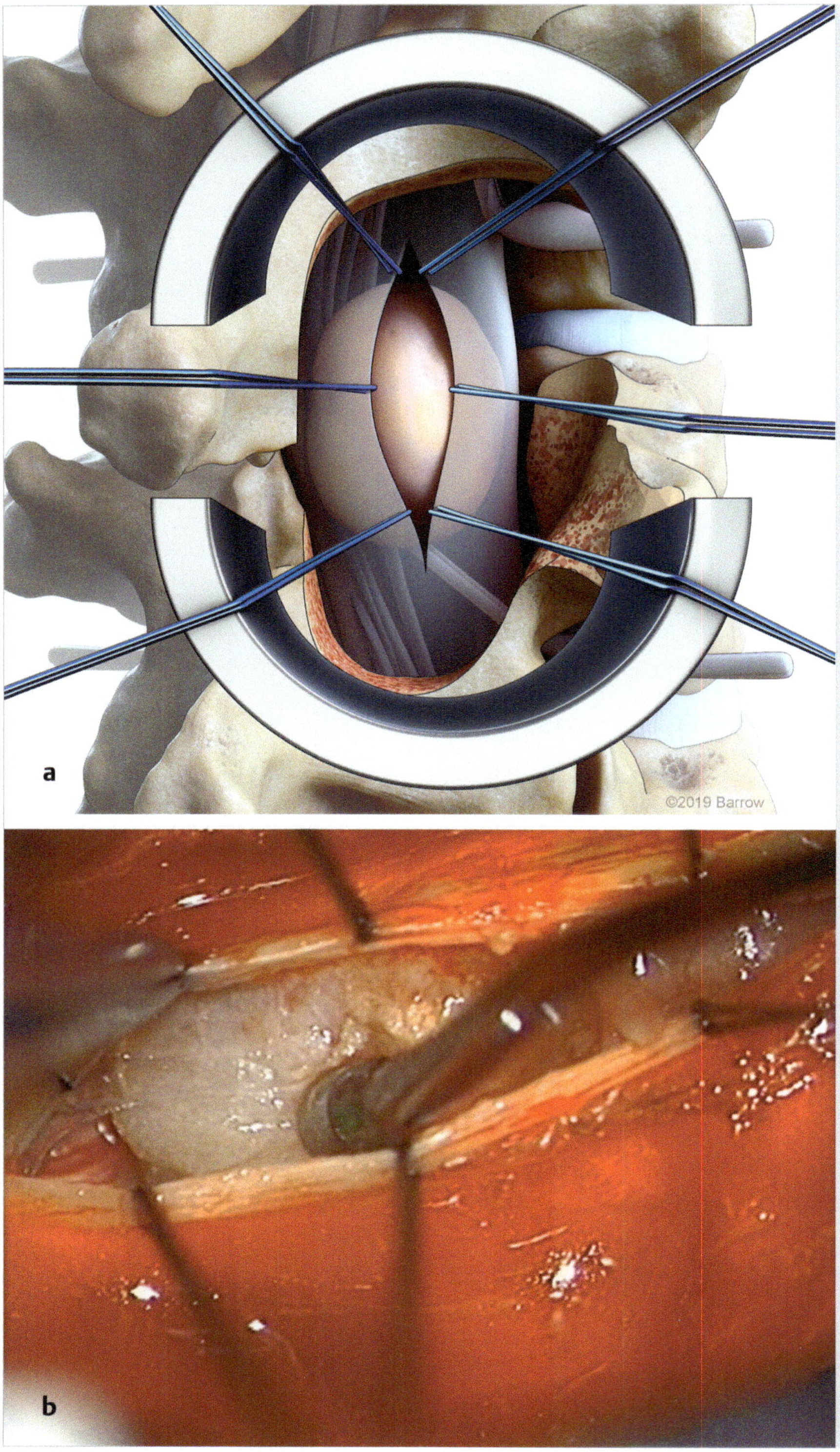

Fig. 11.22 Exposure of the lesion with dural tack up sutures. **(a)** Illustration of the dural edges tacked up with 6.0 polypropylene sutures. The dural opening should allow for exposure of the rostral and caudal poles of the lesion. The spinal cord is displaced by the lesion creating a safe corridor for resection. **(b)** Intraoperative photograph showing exposure of the lesion.

lesion has adhered to a thoracic nerve root and not the dura or the spinal cord.

With the dura tacked up, I proceed with exposure of the entire lesion. At this juncture, the operation becomes indistinguishable from its open midline counterpart. The microsurgical techniques are identical for both procedures. With the lesion in the center of the field of view, I use a No. 11 blade to incise the center of the mass, and I remove a small sample with a micropituitary rongeur for a frozen section. By peering above and below the rostral poles of the lesion, I can visualize the flattened and displaced spinal cord. It is helpful to have the knowledge of the location of the spinal cord relative to the lesion, but my priority at this point is not assessing the spinal cord. Instead, my focus is on debulking the lesion so that I can avoid any contact with the spinal cord.

I prefer to begin the resection with internally debulking the lesion. The combination of bipolar cautery, suction and Rhoton dissectors decreases the volume of the lesion and allows me to mobilize the lesion away from the spinal cord. Ultrasonic aspirators may be particularly helpful in this circumstance. In all of the cases I have performed, I have never found a single one of these lesions to be adherent to the spinal cord. Instead, I have always appreciated an arachnoid layer between the spinal cord and the lesion itself.

The main objective of internally debulking the lesion is to transform a mass that is already occupying 80 to 90% of the canal and compressing the spinal cord into an entity that I can handle and safely maneuver away from the spinal cord. I keep in mind that the spinal cord has already reached its threshold of occupancy with the lesion within the canal. There is no more room for the flattened spinal cord. In order to mitigate the risk of neurologic injury, I cannot place any downward pressure on the lesion itself, which would further compress the already flattened spinal cord. All of the vector forces need to be away from the spinal cord. Internally debulking the lesion transforms a canal-occupying mass into a more docile entity that I can deliver out of the intradural space. Intermittently alternating internal debulking with cauterizing of the outer capsule of the lesion begins to eliminate the blood flow to the mass. Over time, a gradual change in color becomes visible. Depriving the lesion of its blood flow gradually transforms an originally plump crimson lesion into a more deflated paler one. An internally debulked lesion allows me to delicately mobilize it away from the spinal cord with dissectors and finally deliver it with a micropituitary rongeur. The lesion reaches a point where the combination of depriving it of blood flow and internal debulking allows for its complete delivery out of the canal and away from the spinal cord (▶ Fig. 11.23).

With the majority of the lesion completely out of the intradural space, I can explore the canal for any residual lesion. I examine the inside of the dura to ensure I have cleared it of any residual lesion. I have found that there tends to be some extension into a thoracic nerve root, which was the likely point of origin of the lesion. Regardless, with the majority of the lesion out, I explore the lateral aspect of the dura to ensure there is no residual lesion and no lateral dural defect. I examine the thoracic nerve root under the highest magnification of the microscope and remove any residual lesion (▶ Fig. 11.24). By this time, with the canal cleared of such a space-occupying lesion, the previously displaced spinal cord begins to migrate back to midline.

I make no effort to manipulate or alter the position of the spinal cord. Instead, I take time to marvel at the resilience of the spinal cord, as I assess the resection and look for any residual tumor. I cannot help but wonder how that spinal cord was able to still conduct relatively normal neural transmission for ambulation and bowel and bladder function when it was so flattened and displaced. As the now unencumbered spinal cord slowly makes its trek back to its natural position in the canal with every pulsatile beat of the heart, I begin the closure of the dura.

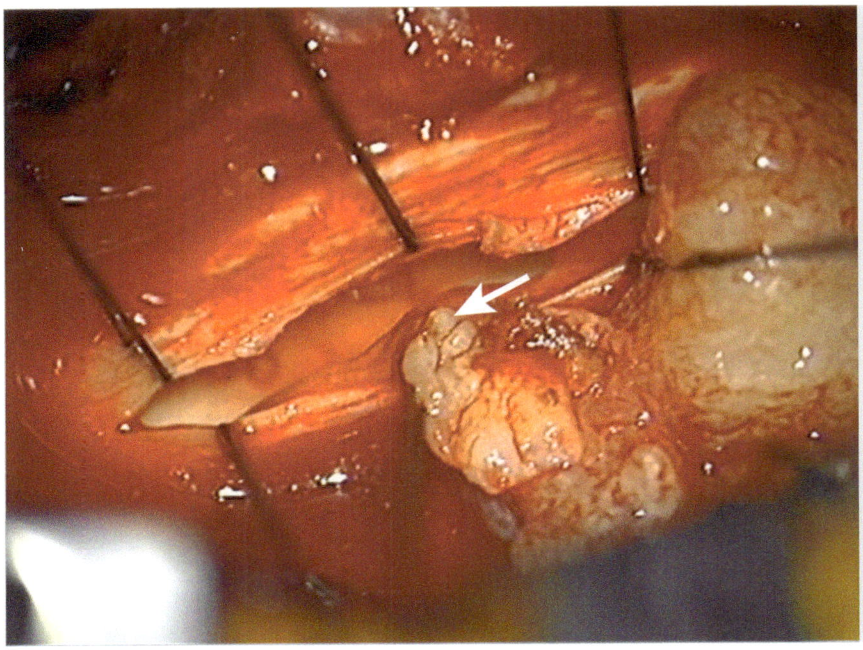

Fig. 11.23 Delivering the lesion away from the spinal cord after debulking it. Intraoperative photograph demonstrating the delivery of the lesion away from the spinal cord after a preliminary debulking of the lesion. As shown in the photograph, the lesion is adherent to the T11 thoracic nerve root (*arrow*). The spinal cord may be appreciated within the canal with the characteristic serpiginous vascularity.

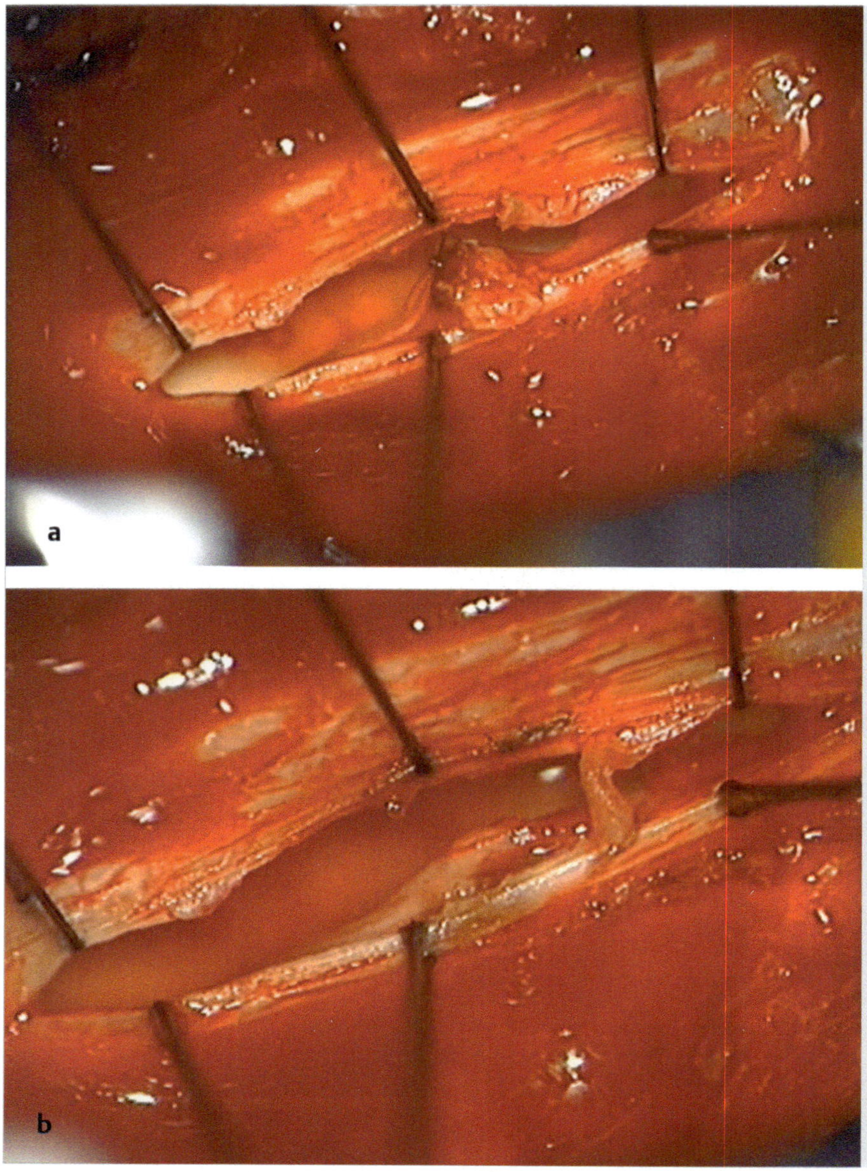

Fig. 11.24 Inspection of the thoracic nerve root for residual tumor. **(a)** Intraoperative photograph demonstrating the origin of the lesion on a thoracic nerve root identified after inspection. **(b)** The residual was removed, and the operative field was further inspected for any residual before closing the dura.

11.9.8 Dural Closure

The dura is closed with either interrupted size 4.0 Nurolon (Johnson & Johnson) sutures or a running 6.0 polypropylene suture. If I use 4.0 Nurolon, I place 8 to 10 interrupted sutures first and then proceed with tying each one. If I use 6.0 polypropylene suture, I start running the suture by anchoring it on each end of the dural opening and then tying it in the middle. Because of the narrow corridor, both passing the suture and tightening the knot are challenging. The preferred needle driver for closure in this setting is a bayoneted Castro-Viejo needle holder and long, bayoneted microforceps. After passing the suture, there is a challenge in tightening each of the six knots because of the angle of approach. The small right-angled, ball-tipped probe works proficiently as a knot pusher for this purpose. As I perform the instrument tie, the distal end of the suture is secured with the needle driver as the right-angled, ball-tipped probe, wielded by an assistant surgeon, slides the knot down. I hold the proximal end directly up, and the right-angled, ball-tipped probe tightens the knot. I repeat this process until I have securely fastened six knots. Next, I run the suture toward the center of the dural opening. Once I have completed running a suture from the rostral and caudal ends, I tie the two remaining arms of the suture in the middle (▶ Fig. 11.25). The anesthesiologist prompts the patient to perform a Valsalva maneuver to confirm a watertight repair. On occasion, an additional suture may be needed in one particular spot to complete a watertight closure. I spray a thin film of fibrin glue (or equivalent) onto the repair then collapse and remove the minimal access port. Bipolar cautery in one hand and the suction in the other allows me to obtain hemostasis, as my assistant removes the access port.

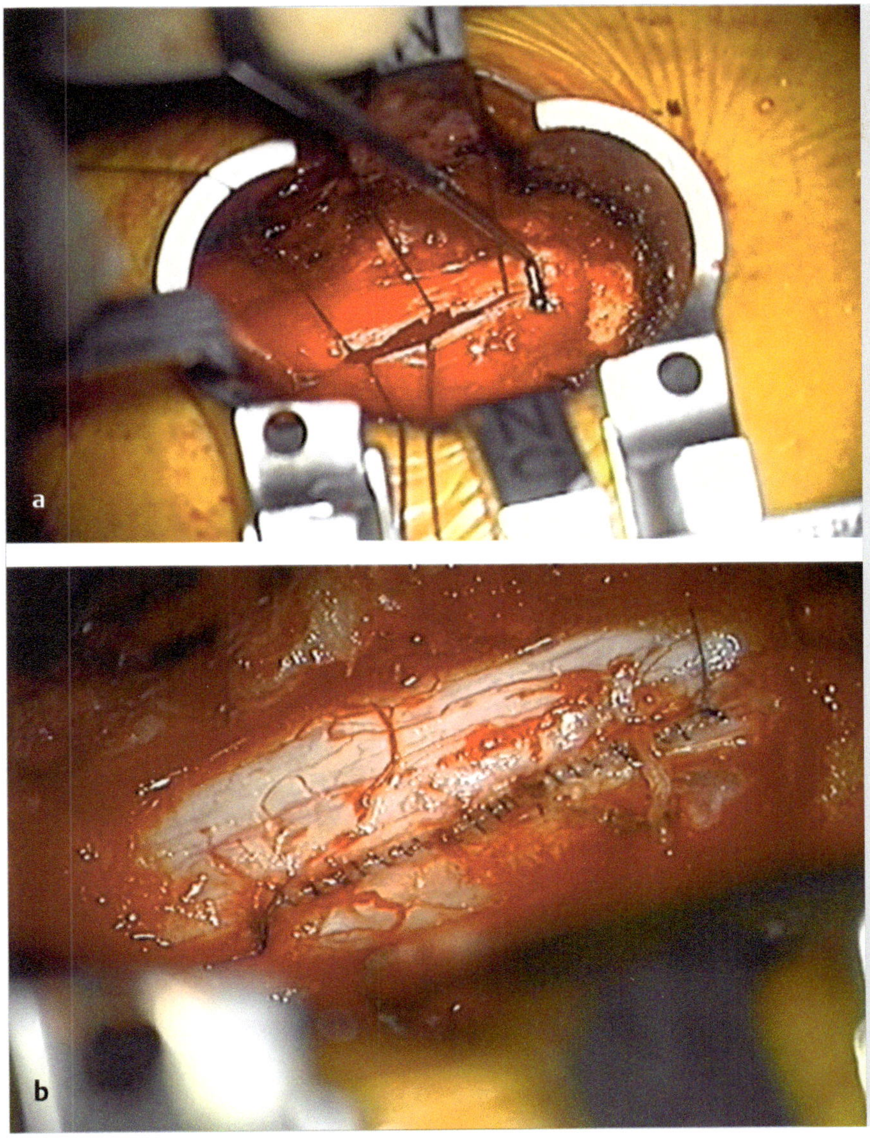

Fig. 11.25 Closure of the dura. **(a)** Intraoperative photograph demonstrating the use of a right-angled, ball-tipped probe as a knot passer to secure the knots at the rostral aspect of the dura. **(b)** Intraoperative photograph showing a running 6.0 polypropylene suture in place which has achieved a watertight dural closure.

11.9.9 Dural Patches

In the event that the lesion adhered to the dura, such as with a calcified meningioma, a large defect in the dura may result from the resection. If that is the case, the defect is repaired by sewing in a dural patch. Any suturable dural substitute matrix or bovine pericardium must be precisely trimmed to the size of the defect. I use four 6.0 polypropylene sutures to secure the dural patch to the defect in the four quadrants. Running a polypropylene suture in each direction and attempting to tie them is no small technical feat. Instead, an interrupted suture here and there around the anchoring sutures in the four quadrants is used to begin closing the gaps. I place an onlay dural graft over the repair so that the lateral aspect of the canal serves as a buttress to the repair, along with some fibrin glue.

11.9.10 Closure

After I have closed the dura and removed the minimal access port, I infiltrate the muscle and skin edges with a lidocaine–bupivacaine mixture. I bring the edges of the fascia together with interrupted size 0 polyglactin 910 sutures on a UR-6 needle. The subcutaneous layer I reapproximate with an interrupted size 2.0 polyglactin suture on an X-1 needle; finally, I bring together the skin edges with a size 3.0 polyglactin suture. Mastisol (Ferndale Laboratories, Inc., Ferndale, MI) or benzoin is applied to the skin, and Steri-Strips (3M Company, Maplewood, MN) are used to support the closure. I place a small Telfa (KPR, U.S., LLC, Dublin, OH) over the Steri-Strips and then a lidocaine patch as the final dressing.

11.10 Postoperative Care

The patient is kept in the intensive care unit overnight with an arterial line in place, and mean arterial pressure is maintained at greater than 60 mm Hg. Serial neurologic examinations are performed for the first 12 hours after surgery. The head of the bed is positioned as tolerated. I do not keep these patients flat. If the patient has demonstrated stable vital signs overnight,

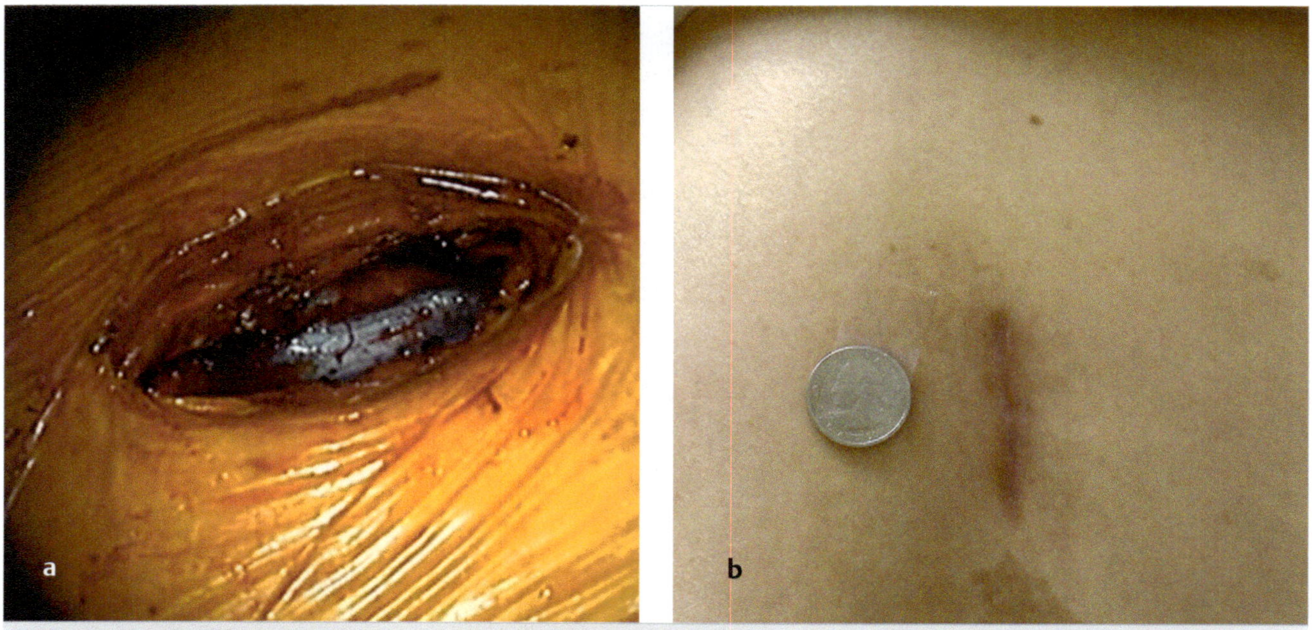

Fig. 11.26 Closure of the incision. (a) Intraoperative photograph of the incision after removal of the minimal access port. The 30-mm incision is closed in a multilayered fashion. The photograph demonstrates a favorable Caspar ratio. The incision is only a few millimeters larger than the dural exposure. Furthermore, the spinous process and contralateral lamina remain intact as does the posterior tension band. (b) Fully healed incision at 1 month.

MRI with and without gadolinium is obtained on the first postoperative day and the patient is transferred to the ward. After patients have been assessed by the neurosurgical team and the physical therapists and found to have no new deficits, nor issues with ambulation or managing their activities of daily living, they may be discharged. The mean number of hospital days in my current series of 26 patients is 2.6 days (range, 1–8 days), with the majority leaving on the second postoperative day.

Patients return 30 days after their operation for a neurologic examination and wound check (▶ Fig. 11.26). They are reevaluated again at 3 months and then annually, with surveillance MRIs to rule out recurrence.

11.11 Case Illustrations

The next section of this chapter applies the technique described above in different scenarios. The first case illustration is another example of a patient with a T11 meningioma. From there, I go on to demonstrate how applying the same standard approach allows for resection of an upper thoracic meningioma (T3). The final case exhibits how these same principles can address other intradural extramedullary pathology, specifically a midthoracic dural AV fistula.

The overarching emphasis of these case illustrations is to demonstrate how knowledge of the anatomical distances allows for standardization of the bone work. The certainty that these lesions tend to be no greater than 25 mm in any dimension not only makes such standardization possible but also proves to be the anatomical basis for a minimally invasive approach. In each of the following case illustrations, a standard pedicle-to-pedicle exposure was more than adequate to resect the intradural extramedullary lesion.

11.11.1 Case Illustration 1: T11 Meningioma

Clinical History and Neurologic Examination

A 67-year-old woman presented to her primary care physician with a 6-month history of progressive gait imbalance. After a circuitous workup, including a full metabolic workup and vitamin B12 supplementation, an MRI of the thoracic spine was ultimately obtained. On examination, the patient was independently ambulatory but incapable of a tandem walk. Strength was remarkably preserved as she demonstrated 5/5 strength through the proximal and distal muscle groups of the lower extremity. She had no issues with bowel or bladder function. The patient had a clear T11 sensory dissociation level, absent proprioception and complete loss of epicritic sensation. Reflex examination demonstrated sustained clonus at the ankle and 3 + patellar reflexes bilaterally.

Radiographic Imaging

Review of the MRI demonstrated a T11 intradural extramedullary lesion with homogeneous enhancement with gadolinium. As is typical for these lesions, it occupied almost the entire canal before the patient became symptomatic. The dimensions of the lesion are germane to the technique described in this chapter. In this circumstance, the transverse dimension was 18 mm, the AP dimension was 17 mm and, most importantly, the rostrocaudal dimension was 22 mm (▶ Fig. 11.27). Once again, the lesion was at the level of the pedicle but had grown caudally, and the majority of the lesion resided behind the vertebral body. The bone work needed to be tailored appropriately.

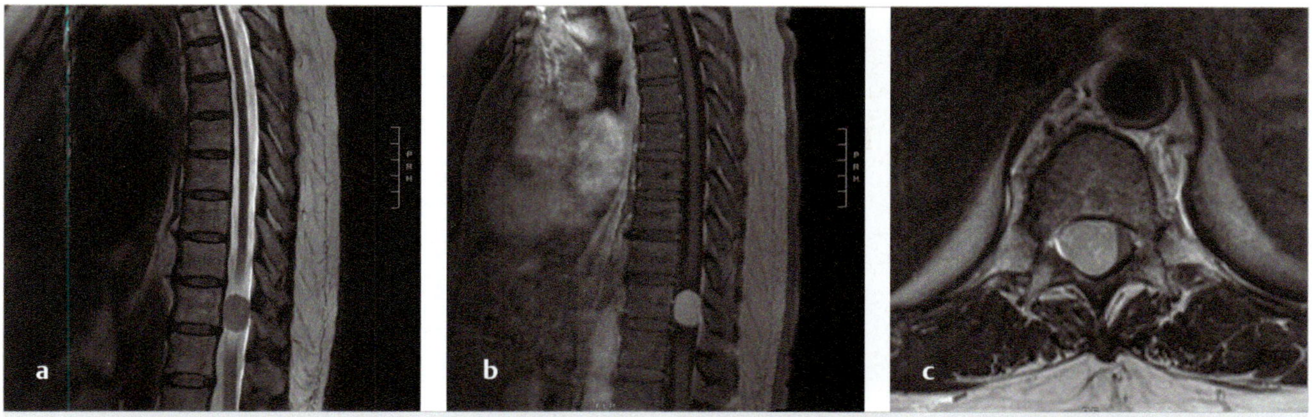

Fig. 11.27 T11 meningioma. (a) Sagittal T2-weighted magnetic resonance imaging (MRI) showing a lesion occupying the entire canal at the level of the T11 pedicle. (b) Sagittal T1-weighted MRI with gadolinium demonstrating homogeneous contrast enhancement. (c) Axial T1-weighted MRI with gadolinium showing the meningioma occupying the entire canal. The spinal cord can be seen as a crescent compressed against the pedicle on the left side of the canal.

Rationale for a Minimally Invasive Approach

In this situation, the lesion was essentially a sphere with a 20-mm diameter occupying the entire canal and displacing the spine cord off to the left. The measurements listed above would suggest that 30 mm of exposure of the dura would be more than adequate for simultaneous exposure of the rostral and caudal poles of the lesion, a criterion for resection by any technique. The geometric center of the lesion was at the T11 pedicle, which is an invaluable observation to make for surgical planning. It transforms the T11 pedicle on the right into a beacon that precisely guides you to the lesion. The knowledge that the 11th thoracic pedicle is 15 to 17 mm in height provides a sense of the dural opening needed for the lesion once the medial aspect of the pedicle has been exposed. The entire hemilamina of T11 is removed along with the medial facet. With all of these measurements in mind, a 30-mm incision was planned over the top of the T11 pedicle on the right, 25 mm lateral to the midline.

Localization

In Chapter 10, I extensively covered localization of a level in the thoracic spine. Again, I emphasize that inherent to a minimally invasive approach is precise localization. There is no room for error. As discussed in the chapter 10 case illustrations, when using fluoroscopy, confirmation on AP and lateral imaging counting up from the sacrum for a lower thoracic lesion is imperative. Although AP confirmation of the second rib-bearing vertebra may be straightforward, setting the precise trajectory in line with the pedicle on an AP projection is not. Therefore, after confirmation of the T11 level on AP and lateral, I dilate onto the spine at the T11 pedicle with lateral fluoroscopy and then take a final AP image (▶ Fig. 11.28). In this manner, I can ensure that I am precisely in line with the pedicle.

Operative Technique

With the patient positioned on a Jackson table, I prepped the entire thoracic and lumbar spine for a preliminary localization with spinal needles. AP and lateral fluoroscopy guided the placement of spinal needles into position and confirmed the level (▶ Fig. 11.28). On the basis of this preliminary localization, I planned the incision over the top of the T11 pedicle and marked each one of the spinal needle entry points so that I could repeat the process after I prepped and draped the entire operative site (▶ Fig. 11.29). Once I unequivocally confirmed the T11 level, I made a 30-mm incision centered at the T11 pedicle and divided the fascia widely with cautery to a length of 35 mm. I then palpated the T11 transverse process, and slid the first dilator just medial to it and sequentially dilated to a 22-mm diameter. With downward pressure, I secured the minimal access port in position and once again confirmed my position with AP and lateral fluoroscopic imaging (▶ Fig. 11.30). I then proceeded with the standard bone work described in the operative technique section, so that I could expose 35 mm of the dura and create a 30-mm opening for the resection (▶ Fig. 11.31, Video 11.1).

Postoperative Course

The patient tolerated the procedure well and was transferred to the intensive care unit (ICU) for postoperative monitoring of her mean arterial pressure and neurologic examination. She was transferred to the ward on the first postoperative day and home on the second. She was ambulating independently on the first postoperative day with an improvement of her gait imbalance. Postoperative MRI demonstrated a gross total resection. Surveillance MRI completed 5 years after surgery did not show any evidence of recurrence (▶ Fig. 11.32). At the time of writing, the patient continued to live a very active lifestyle well into her 70s.

11.11.2 Case Illustration 2: T3 Meningioma

Clinical History and Neurologic Examination

A 56-year-old woman presented to her primary care physician for an evaluation of left flank pain. Initially diagnosed with costochondritis, the progression of symptoms over the

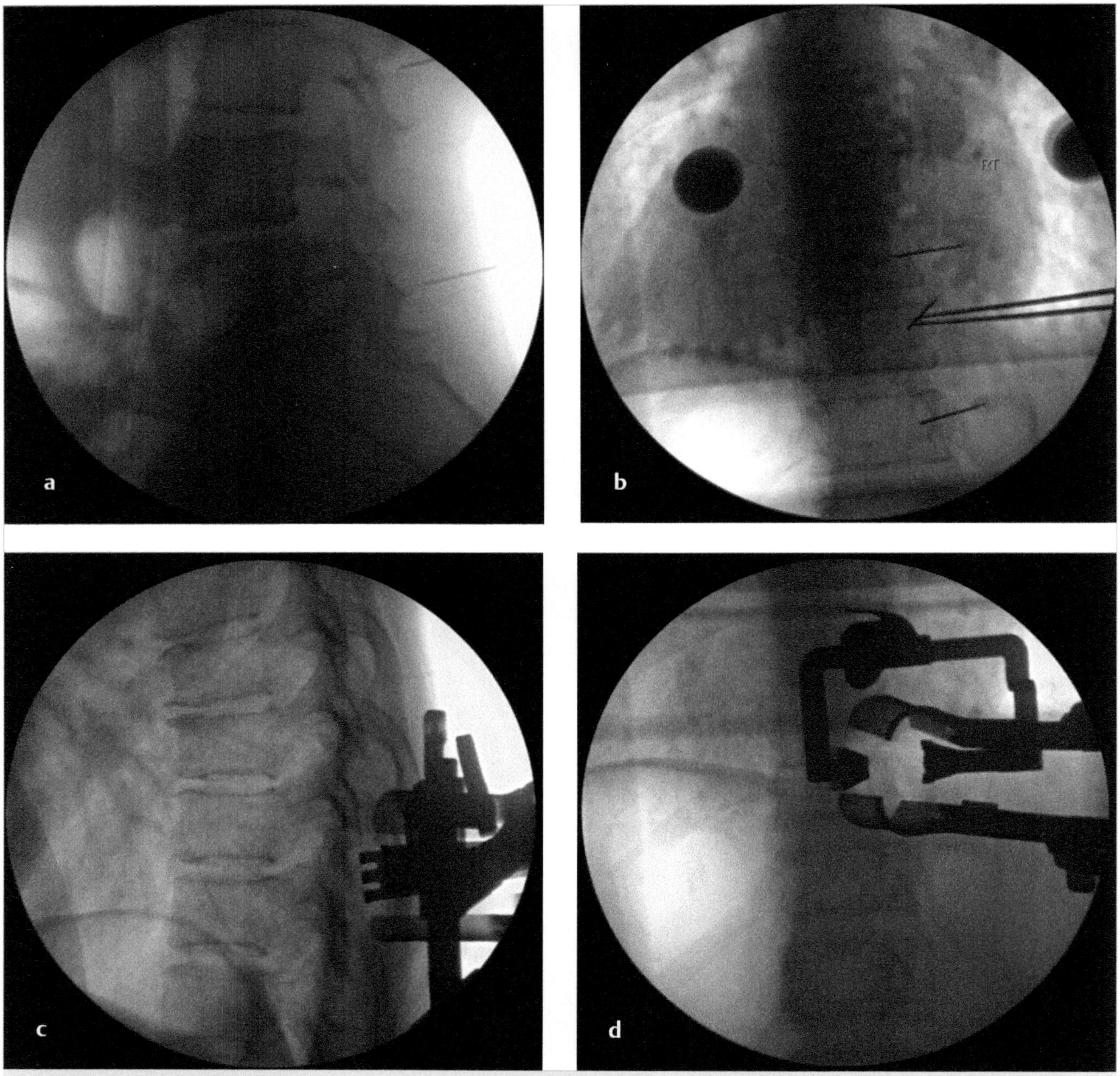

Fig. 11.28 Localization and placement of minimal access port for T11 meningioma. **(a)** Lateral fluoroscopic image demonstrating spinal needles in position counting up from the sacrum. **(b)** Anteroposterior (AP) image confirming the T11 pedicle as the second rib-bearing pedicle. **(c)** Lateral fluoroscopic image demonstrating the minimal access port secured in line with the pedicle of T11. **(d)** AP image demonstrating the preliminary exposure from the inferior aspect of T10 to the inferior aspect of T11.

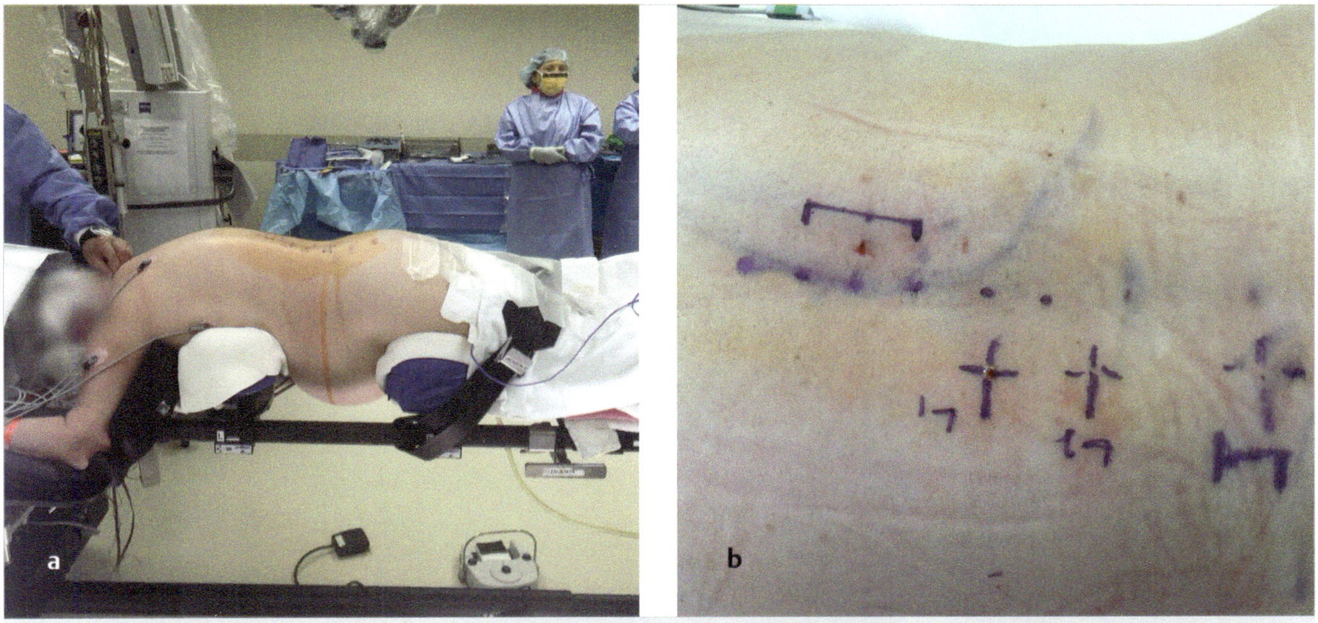

Fig. 11.29 Localization for T11 meningioma. **(a)** Intraoperative photograph showing the patient positioned on the Jackson table for a right-sided approach to a T11 meningioma. The patient has been prepped for the preliminary localization to mark the incision. After marking, the patient is prepped and draped, and the incision is confirmed a second time with spinal needles. **(b)** The spinal needle entry points are marked for the pedicles of L4, L2 and L1. The incision is planned prior to prepping and draping the patient. The same points are used to confirm the incision prior to beginning the operation.

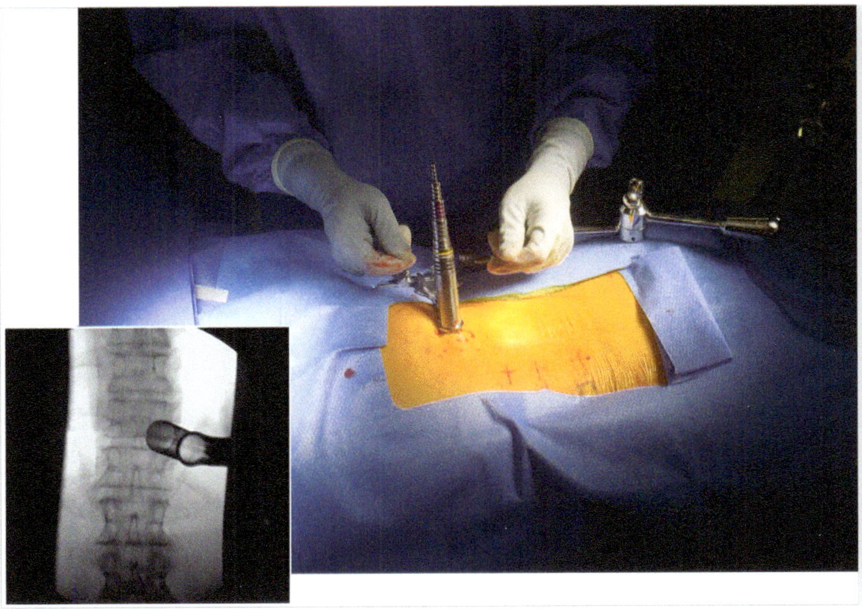

Fig. 11.30 Positioning the minimal access port for resection of a T11 meningioma. Intraoperative photograph of a minimal access port in position over the top of the T11 pedicle. The inset shows the anteroposterior fluoroscopic image of the access port just beneath the pedicle of T11, which optimizes access to the hemilamina of T11, the inferior aspect of the lamina of T10 and the superior aspect of the lamina of T12.

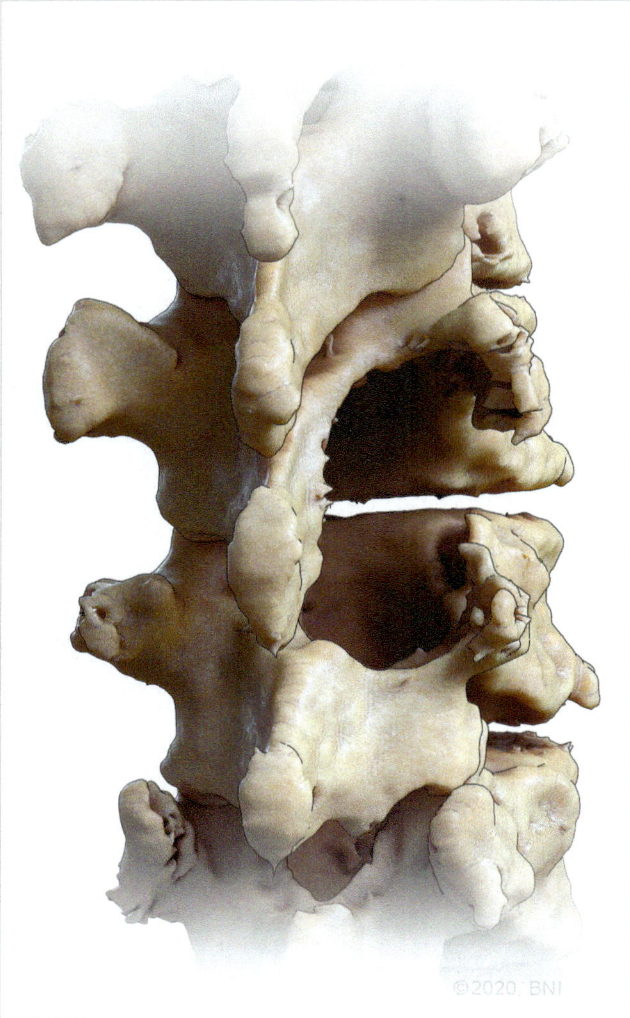

Fig. 11.31 Bone work for a T11 meningioma. Three-dimensional reconstruction of the bone work performed for resection of the lesion. In this case, the illustration was created from a postoperative computed tomographic image. A laminotomy from the pedicle of T10 to the pedicle of T11 offered an adequate working channel for resection of the lesion and closure of the dura. In this circumstance, a complete facetectomy was performed. There was no untoward clinical consequence from the unilateral facetectomy in this case. The intact spinous processes, posterior tension band and contralateral facet provide stability for the segment.

following year prompted further workup and ultimately led to MRI of the thoracic spine (▶ Fig. 11.28). Throughout the entire diagnostic workup, the patient remained fully employed and exercised two to three times a week. On examination, she ambulated without gait abnormality and denied any balance issues. The sensory examination demonstrated a left sensory dissociation level at T4. Proprioception was decreased. Her motor examination was intact, with 5/5 strength in the proximal and distal muscle groups of the lower extremities bilaterally. Babinski sign was present bilaterally. She had 3+patellar and Achilles reflexes bilaterally without clonus.

Radiographic Studies

MRI of the thoracic spine demonstrated an intradural extramedullary lesion that homogeneously enhanced with gadolinium (▶ Fig. 11.33). The axial T1-weighted MRI with gadolinium shows marked spinal cord compression, with the lesion occupying over 90% of the canal. The spinal cord had been flattened into a crescent shape in the anterior aspect of the canal.

Rationale for a Minimally Invasive Approach

Analysis of this lesion in the axial and sagittal planes revealed a lesion measuring 11 mm in the transverse dimension, 10 mm in the AP dimension and 13 mm in the rostrocaudal dimension. The lesion was eccentric to the left. Consistent with the observation made regarding the location and the growth pattern of these lesions, the geometric center of the lesion was at the T3 pedicle. A focal lesion eccentric to one side of the canal with these dimensions (in this case the left side) is readily amenable to a minimally invasive approach. The standard approach of bone work that centers on the pedicle and corresponds to the lesion provides an adequate corridor of resection.

Operative Technique

For a high thoracic lesion, I position the patient on chest rolls in a Mayfield head holder with the bed reversed, similar to the positioning for a posterior cervical foraminotomy or laminectomy (▶ Fig. 11.34). I use AP fluoroscopy to localize the T1 pedicle and adjust the fluoroscope until my view of the levels is completely parallel to the disc space (▶ Fig. 11.35).

A high thoracic lesion is one of the few circumstances where it is possible to employ only AP imaging for localization of the segment. However, definitive confirmation of the cervicothoracic junction is imperative. Positioning the fluoroscope in such a manner that the line of sight is completely parallel to the end plates of the vertebral body is an essential component of localization using AP imaging. ▶ Fig. 11.34 demonstrates marking the incision after identification of the T1 pedicle. Note the angle on the fluoroscope, which has been adjusted to have the X-ray beam parallel to the superior end plate of T2, where the rostral most aspect of the lesion resides.

The characteristic and prominent T1 transverse process is the landmark that reliably establishes the transition from the cervical to the thoracic spine. If I have any question in my ability to discern the cervicothoracic junction, I revert to lateral fluoroscopy, placing spinal needles onto the C5–6 segment (or the last cervical segment I can clearly visualize), confirm that position on lateral image and then revert to AP imaging using that reference point to establish the T1 pedicle. Confirmation of that landmark now becomes the basis for counting down into the thoracic spine.

I plan a 30-mm incision 25 mm off the midline and begin the procedure (▶ Fig. 11.35) using a No. 15 blade to make the skin incision. I use cautery to divide the fascia in an oblique trajectory onto the thoracic lamina. I palpate the third thoracic transverse process, pass the first dilator onto that prominence and then allow it to slide onto the T3 lamina. I wand a plane of dissection that spans the entire lamina of T3 and extends rostral into the lamina of T2. The subsequent dilators pass onto the lamina at a 15- to 20-degree angle. An expandable minimal

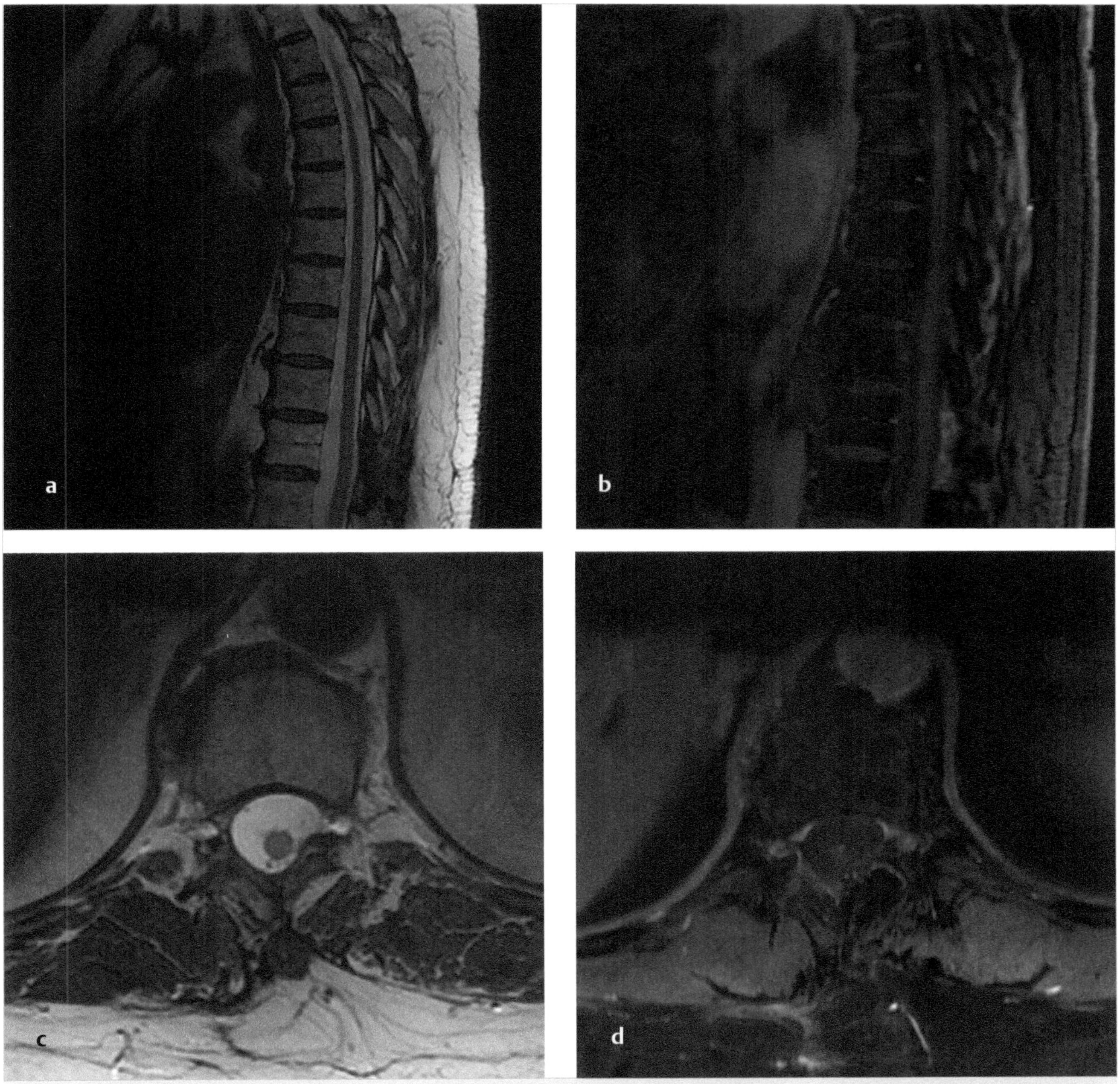

Fig. 11.32 Surveillance magnetic resonance imaging (MRI) 5 years after T11 meningioma resection. **(a)** Sagittal T2-weighted MRI. There is only a suggestion of myelomalacia within the substance of the spinal cord. **(b)** Sagittal T1-weighted MRI with gadolinium without evidence of enhancement. **(c)** Axial T2-weighted MRI showing the expansion of the central canal. **(d)** Axial T1-weighted gadolinium-enhanced MRI without evidence of enhancement.

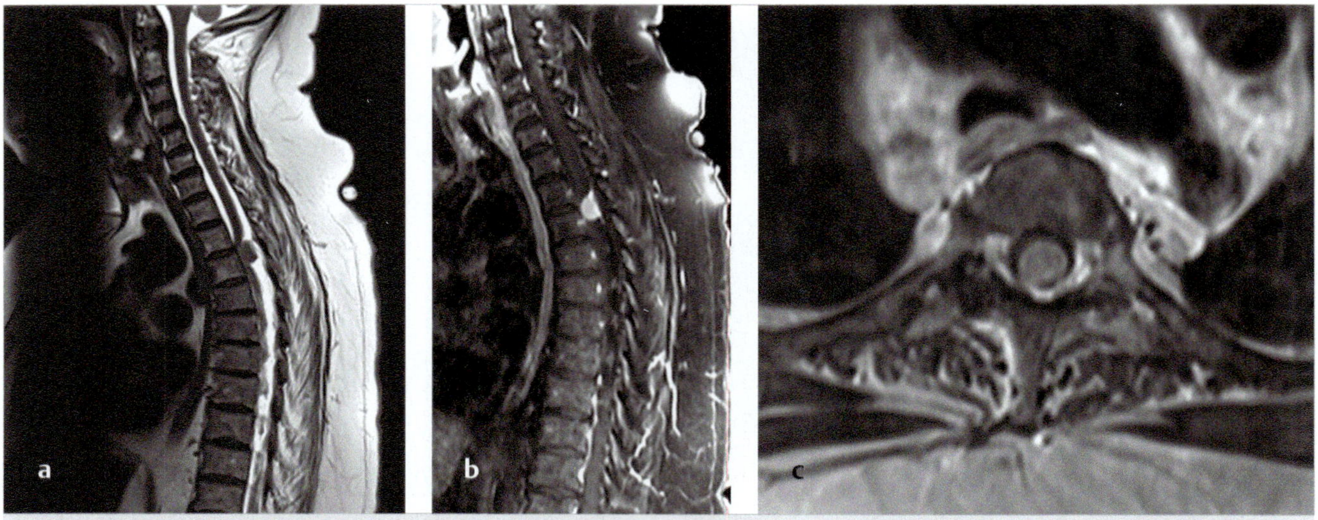

Fig. 11.33 Magnetic resonance imaging (MRI) studies of a T3 meningioma. (a) Sagittal T2-weighted MRI demonstrating an intradural extramedullary lesion at the level of the T3 vertebral body, nearly occupying the entire canal. Remarkably, there is no signal change abnormality within the substance of the spinal cord. (b) Sagittal T1-weighted MRI with gadolinium demonstrating homogeneous enhancement with a dural tail. (c) Axial T1-weighted MRI with gadolinium showing the lesion occupying nearly the entire anteroposterior and transverse dimensions of the spinal canal.

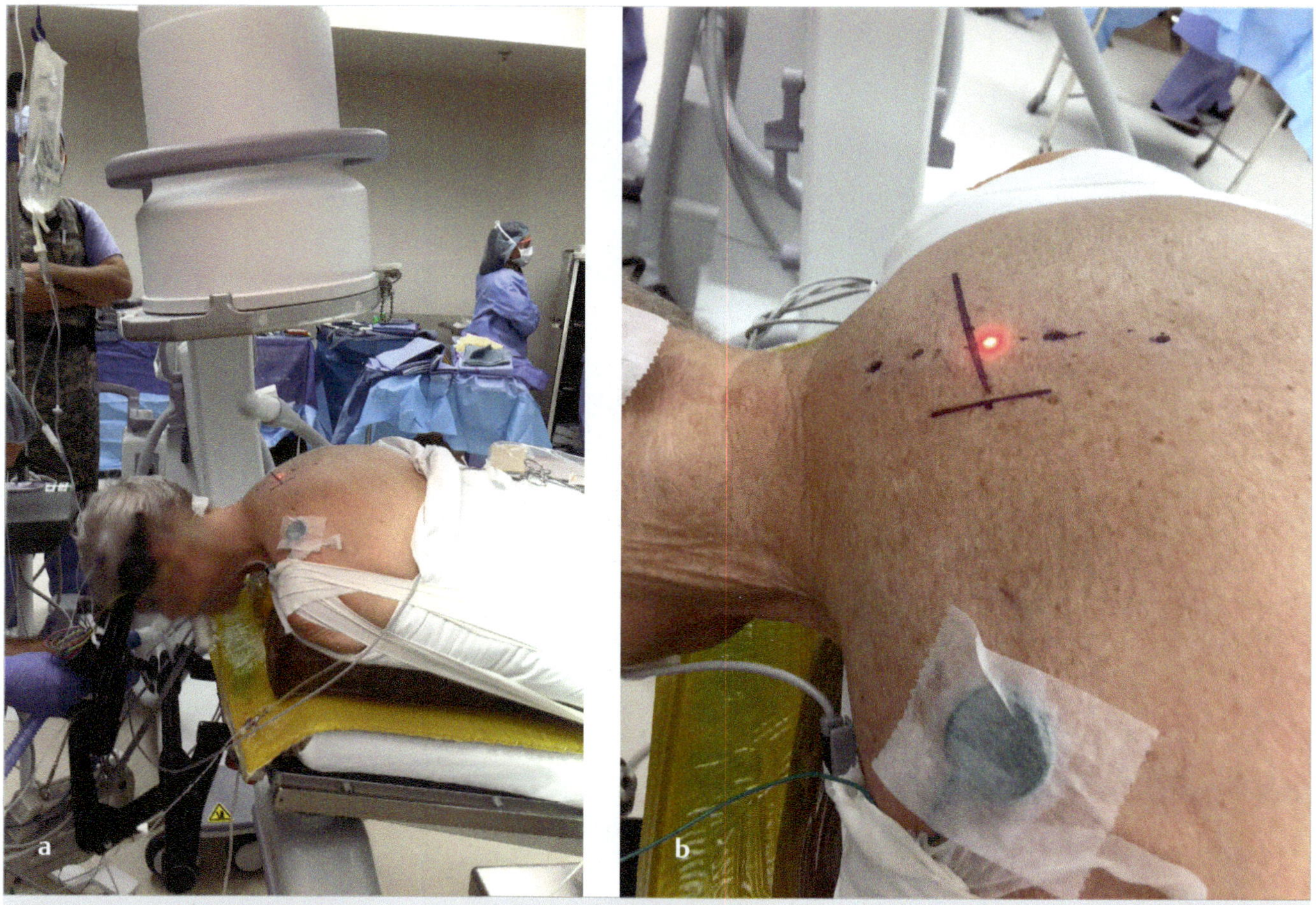

Fig. 11.34 Patient positioning for a high thoracic lesion. This particular patient had a T2 intradural intramedullary lesion. (a) The patient is positioned prone on chest rolls in a Mayfield head holder. (b) Anteroposterior fluoroscopy is used to localize the T1 pedicle and then plan the incision over the top of the T2 pedicle. An incision is planned 25 mm off the midline and 30 mm in length.

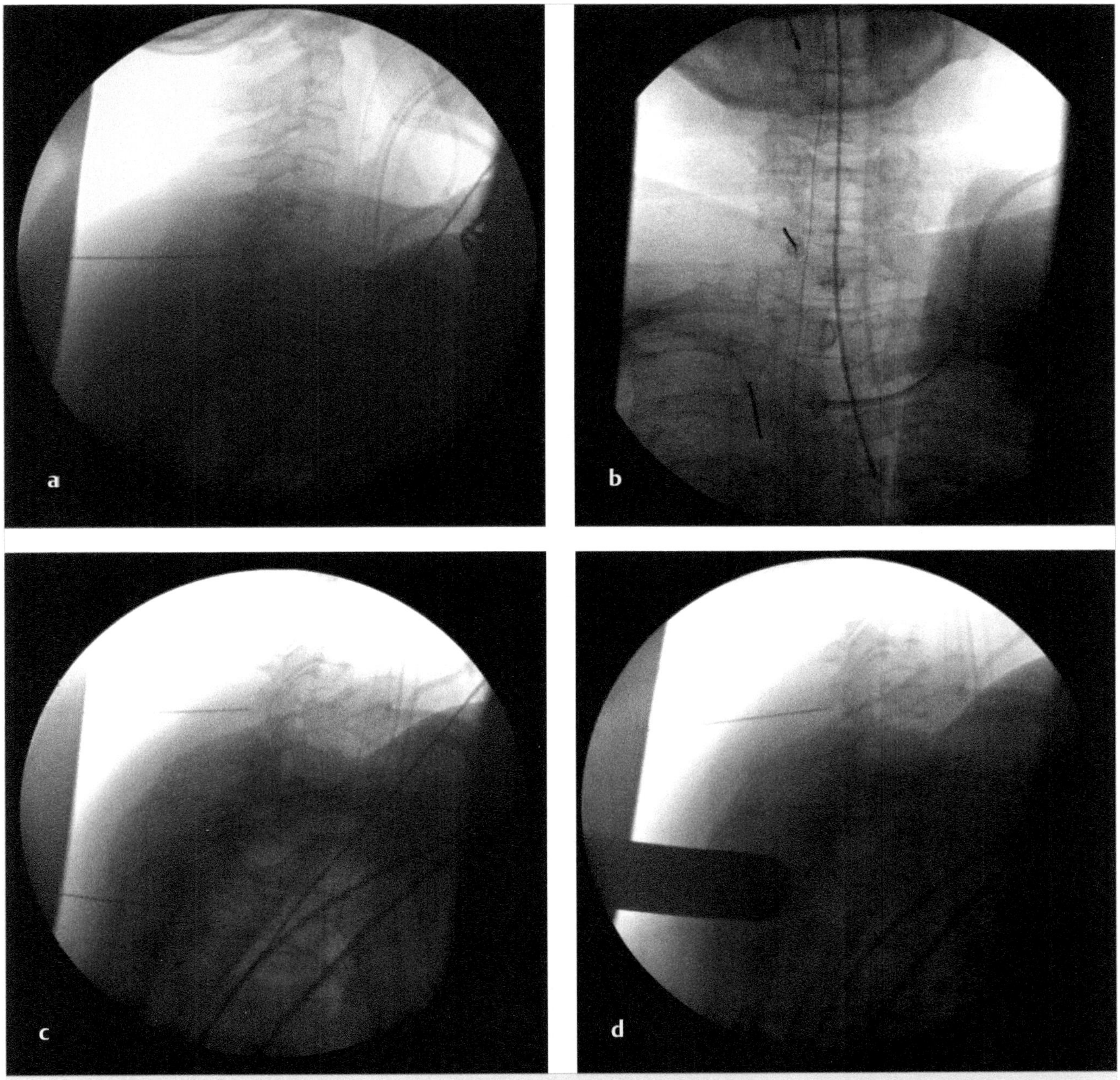

Fig. 11.35 Localization for an intradural extramedullary T3 lesion using anteroposterior (AP) and lateral fluoroscopy. **(a)** Lateral fluoroscopic image demonstrating a spinal needle pointing to the pedicle of the C6 vertebral body. **(b)** With the confirmation of the spinal needle in the lateral direction, an AP image confirms the T3 pedicle, counting down from the C6 pedicle. **(c)** Once the AP projection confirms the T3 pedicle, a lateral projection facilitates setting the trajectory. **(d)** The spinal needle at C6 remains in position and is an essential reference point for dilatation onto the spine and placement of the minimal access port.

access port encompasses the T3 transverse process and lamina when secured into position.

I continue to develop the plane of dissection as I expose the lamina to the base of the spinous process at T3. Opening the minimal access port and angling the blades facilitate placement of the medial–lateral retractors, which maintain the plane of dissection onto the lamina. Exposure of the spine continues until the landmarks of the T3 pedicle become completely evident, specifically the T2–3 facet and the T3 transverse process. Once I am convinced that I have all of the exposure of the lamina I need to expose 30 mm of the dura, I begin drilling. Like in the previous case illustration, I work in the lateral corridor and identify the canal. The medial aspect of the T3 pedicle is drilled down to enlarge the canal and consequently the working channel. From there, I extend my bone work medially to expose the entire thoracic canal from the inferior aspect of T2 to the superior aspect of T4. A ruler cut precisely to 35 mm confirms the extent of exposure before the dura is opened and the lesion removed (Video 11.2).

The frozen section, and later, the final pathology report, confirmed a meningioma. After removal of the lesion, the dura was closed with a running polypropylene suture. I removed the medial–lateral retractor, obtained hemostasis and then closed and removed the minimal access port. As previously described, the fascia is closed with interrupted size 0 polyglactin 910 sutures on a UR-6 needle; subcutaneous tissue is closed with 2.0 sutures on an X-1 needle and 3.0 polyglactin sutures for the skin edges.

Postoperative Course

After an uneventful course overnight in the ICU, the patient was transferred to the ward and discharged later on postoperative day 1. The patient had complete resolution of the left flank pain and had no new neurologic deficits. She returned to work 14 days after surgery and has had no evidence of recurrence on surveillance MRI 5 years after surgery (▶ Fig. 11.36).

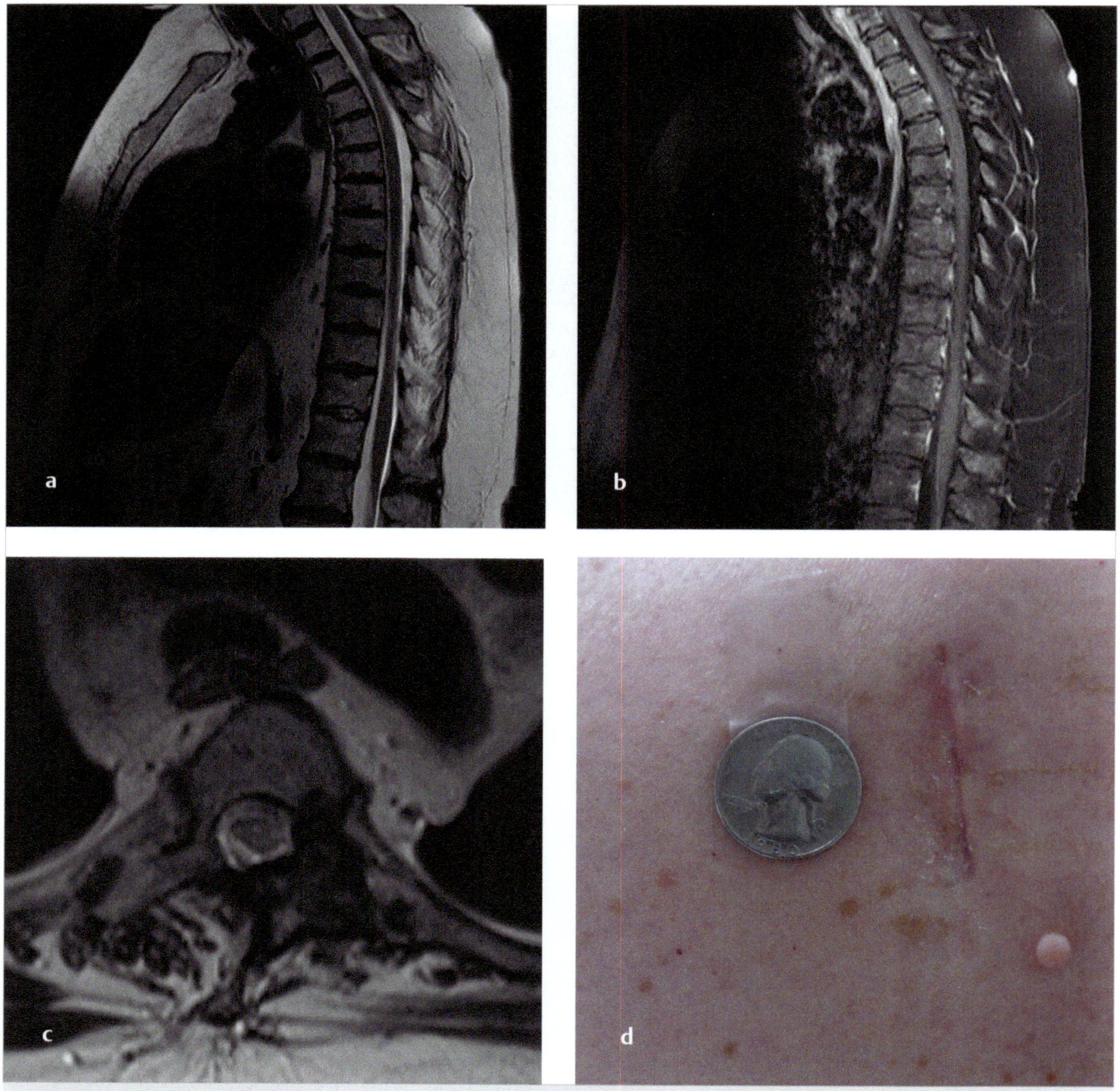

Fig. 11.36 Surveillance magnetic resonance imaging (MRI) 5 years after resection of a T3 meningioma. **(a)** Sagittal T2-weighted MRI demonstrating gross total resection of the lesion. **(b)** Sagittal T1-weighted MRI with gadolinium revealing no evidence of enhancement. **(c)** Axial T2-weighted MRI showing the spinal cord now at a normal caliber. The hypointense area of the left pedicle and lamina are indicative of the bone work that expanded the working channel. Note the preservation of the spinous process. **(d)** Photograph of the incision.

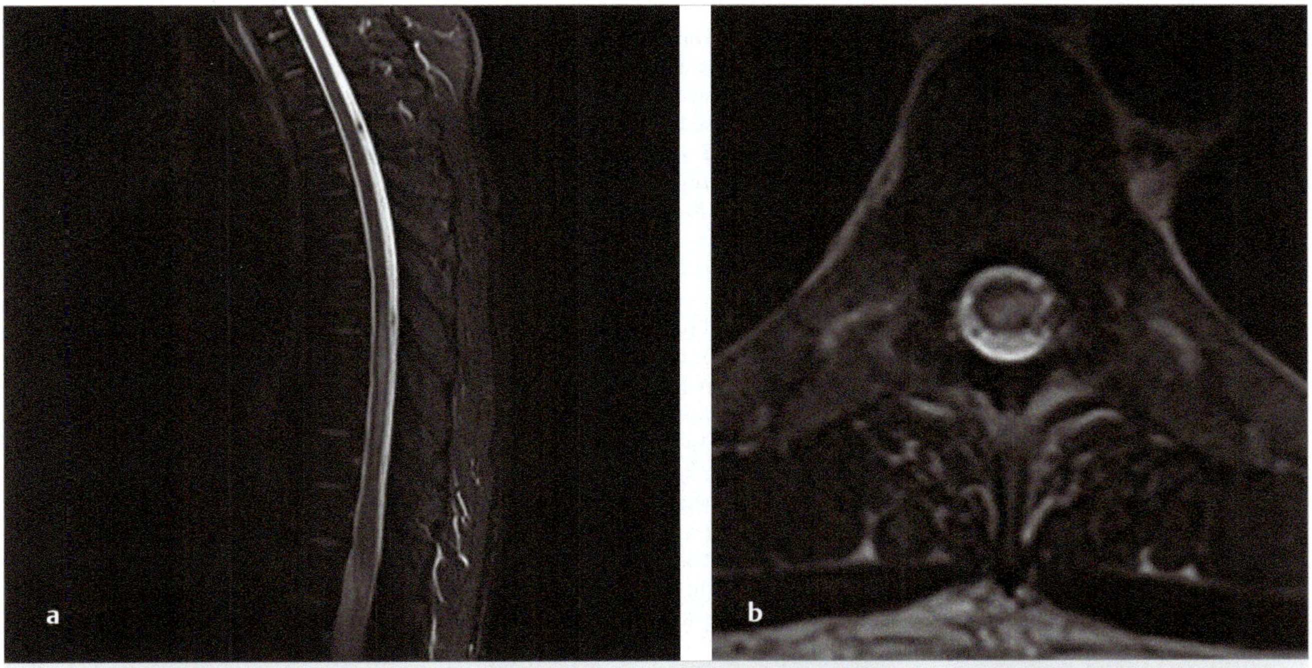

Fig. 11.37 Spinal cord type-I dural arteriovenous fistula. **(a)** Sagittal T2-weighted magnetic resonance imaging (MRI) demonstrating signal change within the spinal cord spanning T7–10. There is associated dilatation of the spinal cord in the section. **(b)** Axial T2-weighted MRI at the levels of T7–8. Spinal cord edema is most prominent on the left side. Vascularity is prominent, suggesting a potential vascular malformation.

11.11.3 Case Illustration 3: T8 Dural AV Fistula

Clinical History and Neurologic Examination

A 52-year-old man presented for evaluation of right leg numbness of 1-year duration. Initially diagnosed with lumbar radiculopathy, the patient was referred for physical therapy. Progression of the symptoms, specifically numbness extending to the abdomen and gait imbalance, prompted an MRI of the cervical and thoracic spine. On examination, the patient demonstrated intact strength in the proximal and distal muscle groups of the lower extremities. He had nondermatomal sensory loss in the right lower extremity to pinprick and light touch. Proprioception was absent in both lower extremities. He demonstrated brisk reflexes in the patellar and Achilles tendons.

Radiographic Studies

MRI of the thoracic spine demonstrated spinal cord edema extending from T7 to T10 with mild cord expansion. Spinal cord edema appeared worse on the left aspect of the cord. There was no evidence of a syrinx formation. There appeared to be prominent vascular structures along the left lateral aspect of the spinal cord near the T7–8 disc level (▶ Fig. 11.37).

There was a low level of enhancement from T7 to T10 on postcontrast images (not shown) without discrete evidence of an AV malformation. However, based on these radiographic findings, a dural AV fistula was the principal diagnosis, and conventional spinal angiography was performed demonstrating a type I dural AV fistula at T8 on the left (▶ Fig. 11.38). An embolic agent filled part of the segmental vessel, thereby marking the pedicle of T8, vastly facilitating the localization of the lesion and placement of the minimal access port.

Rationale for a Minimally Invasive Approach

The inherent limitation on the dimensions of a slow-growing neoplastic lesion within the canal was the basis for a minimally

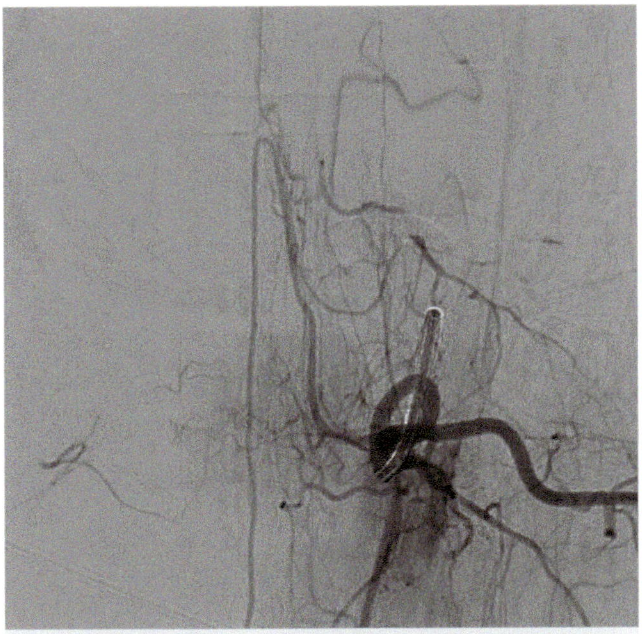

Fig. 11.38 Selective catheterization of left T8 segmental artery demonstrating a type-I dural arteriovenous fistula.

invasive approach for the previous case illustrations. In the circumstance of a dural AV fistula, the dimensions of this lesion are less important than the need to visualize the extradural and intradural components of the fistula itself. The dimension of the lesion in this circumstance is the caliber of the vessel. Furthermore, by its very nature, a dural AV fistula has laterality to it. After all, it is a segmental vessel from either the left or the right that is the root cause of the fistula. Therefore, there is no need to visualize any of the midline elements for the surgical management of this vascular lesion. The emphasis is on the lateral aspects of the spinal cord, in particular, the penetration of the segmental artery into the dura. A focal lesion with laterality meets the criteria set forth at the beginning of this chapter for a minimally invasive approach. From that standpoint, there is a compelling anatomical rationale to approach these lesions with a paramedian trajectory. Collectively, it is the limited dimensions, inherent laterality of these lesions and the need to visualize the intradural and extradural components that form the basis for a minimally invasive approach for the management of a dural AV fistula. The associations of the fistula to the thoracic nerve root make the pedicle once again the North Star of this operation. The standard 35 mm of bone work centered on the pedicle provides all of the exposure needed for safe and efficient elimination of this lesion (▶ Fig. 11.39).

Operative Technique

With the patient prone on a Jackson table, the process of localization with AP and lateral fluoroscopic images of the lumbar and thoracic spine previously covered in this chapter confirmed the T7, T8 and T9 pedicles on the left. The embolic agent marking the T8 pedicle was a useful adjunct for confirming the pedicle, but it was not used exclusively for localization. A 30-mm incision was planned 25 mm lateral to midline centered on the T8 pedicle. Cautery divided the fascia, and a plane of dissection onto the transverse process of T8 was developed. Sequential dilatation over the top of the T8 transverse process allowed for the placement of a minimally invasive expandable access port over the top of the pedicle of T8 (▶ Fig. 11.40).

Before opening the minimal access port, I continued to develop the plane of dissection onto the lamina. I began by first exposing the transverse process of T8. With the transverse process exposed, I was able to reconstruct the anatomy at depth. I visualized the pedicle and the canal in my mind. I then proceeded to expose the entire left side of the T8 lamina to the base of the spinous process. Once I was able to visualize the base of the spinous process medially, I completed the rostral and caudal exposures. It was only after complete exposure of the T8 transverse process and the entire left hemilamina of T8 that I began to open the expandable minimal access port. I extended the plane of dissection and exposure to encompass the inferior aspect of the lamina of T7 and the superior aspect of the lamina of T9. Before taking the drill to the lamina, I ensured that I had a minimum of 35 mm of the lamina exposed.

I performed a hemilaminectomy from the base of the spinous process to the medial aspect of the transverse process of T8 and then removed the inferior aspect of the lamina of T7 and the superior aspect of the lamina of T9. At T8, I ensured that I had the lateral aspect of the canal exposed by drilling down the medial aspect of the pedicle of T8. In this circumstance, there

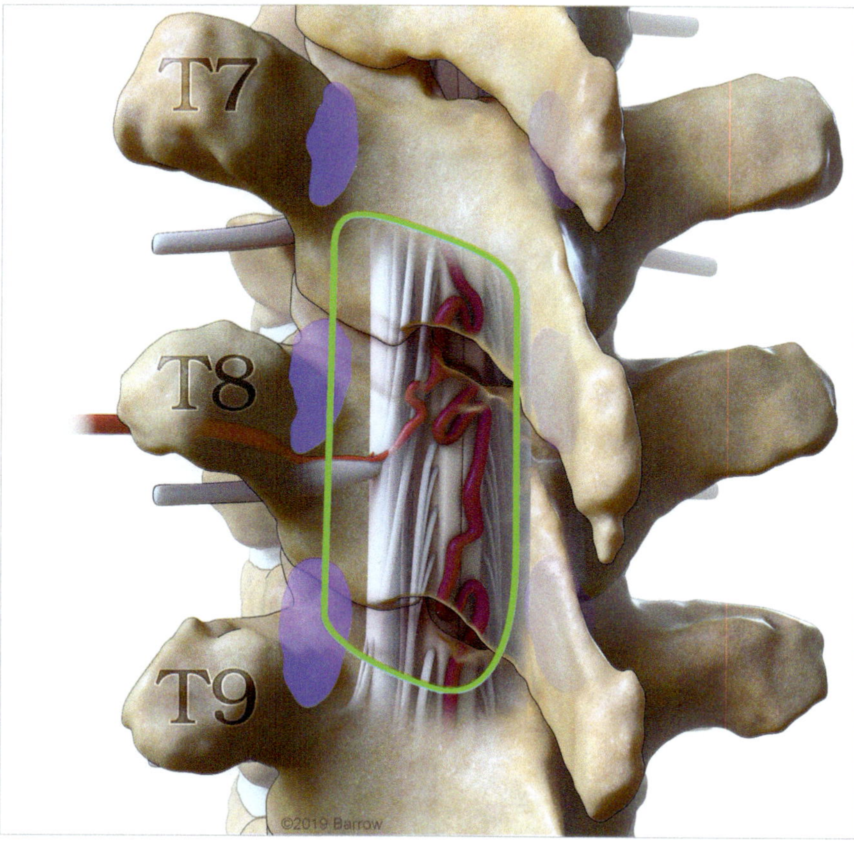

Fig. 11.39 Illustration of a Type I dural arteriovenous (AV) fistula. Since its origin is a segmental artery, laterality is inherent to a dural AV fistula. That aspect of the dural AV fistula along with its focal nature makes it an ideal target for a minimally invasive approach. In this illustration, the *green ring* outlines the bone work. The pedicles are highlighted in *purple*. The fistula is seen piercing the dura causing the arterialization of the epidural veins.

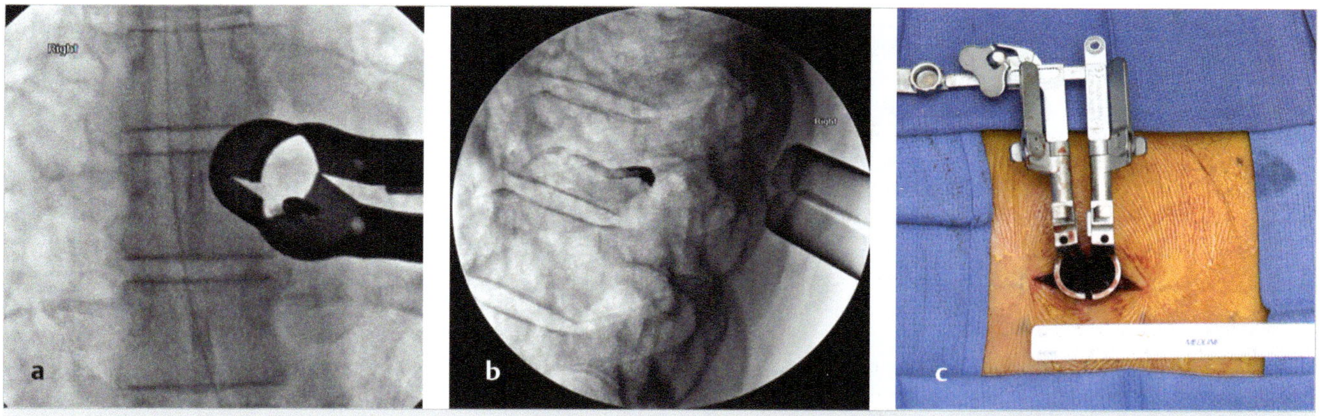

Fig. 11.40 Placement of minimal access port. (a) Anteroposterior (AP) fluoroscopic image demonstrating the placement of the minimal access port over the top of the pedicle of T8. The embolic agent marked the pedicle of T8, but confirmation with AP and lateral imaging from the sacrum to confirm T12 was still employed. (b) Lateral fluoroscopic image with the minimal access port in a trajectory in line with the pedicle of T8. (c) Intraoperative photograph of the access port in position prior to exposure of the lamina and transverse process.

was prominent vascularity from the segment penetrating the dura through the nerve root sleeve.

After I confirmed that a minimum of 30 mm of the dura was exposed, I opened the dura with a No. 11 blade and used polypropylene sutures to retract the edges of the dura. The arterialized veins of the dural AV fistula immediately came into view. At this point, careful analysis of the fistula is necessary. The use of infrared fluorescence angiography with indocyanine green is of tremendous value for identification and confirmation of the fistula. The operative video features an indocyanine green angiogram that shows the dural AV fistula (Video 11.1). A miniclip was applied to the fistula, and another injection of indocyanine green confirmed obliteration of the fistula. The tips of the bipolar then cauterized the fistula. Although the clip may be removed, leaving it in place where the fistula once resided is a useful marker for postoperative angiography.

A running 6.0 polypropylene suture is used to close the dura, and fibrin glue is employed to seal the dural repair. The blades of the minimal access port collapse and hemostasis is achieved as the port is removed. I closed the fascia, subcutaneous tissue and skin edges with a size 0 polyglactin 910 suture on a UR-6, 2.0 polyglactin on an X-1 needle and 4.0 polyglactin on an RB-1 needle, respectively. Benzoin, Steri-Strips and a lidocaine patch served as the dressing on top of the incision.

Postoperative Course

The patient maintained 5/5 strength in the proximal and distal muscle groups of the lower extremity. The nondermatomal right leg numbness demonstrated subjective improvement but persisted in the months after surgery. The patient reported immediate improvement in gait and balance. After observation in the ICU immediately after surgery, he was transferred to the ward and then home on the second postoperative day. One year after surgery, he continued to experience persistent numbness in the right lower leg, although it had improved from the preoperative condition. He denied any gait or imbalance issues.

11.12 Conclusions

This chapter represents the end of the surgical techniques that I describe in this Primer, and it is an appropriate end to this work. After all, the resection of intradural extramedullary lesions using minimally invasive techniques is the culmination of a skill set developed first with the minimally invasive microdiscectomy and further refined by the laminectomies and instrumented fusions. You will leverage every single one of these skills for safe and efficient resection of these lesions through a minimal access port. Intradural extramedullary lesions are uncommon, and so it would be unrealistic to expect that it will be the volume of these types of cases that will allow you to develop a facility managing them with minimally invasive techniques. Rather, it is taking care of the commonplace, everyday degenerative pathologies, such as lumbar stenosis and spondylolisthesis, that offers you the opportunity to develop a skill set that you can immediately translate to these intradural lesions. When the opportunity unexpectedly presents itself to apply these skills, you will be ready. Fortune favors the prepared mind.

A few closing thoughts as this chapter comes to an end. Do not take this minimally invasive skill set that you have developed for granted. When you have reached a point where you can resect an intradural extramedullary lesion with a minimally invasive approach, you have freed your mind from viewing the spine in two dimensions. You no longer must expose and see the anatomy to recognize it. Instead, you now view the spine in three dimensions with full knowledge of the anatomy at depth without having to directly see it. It has been only by peering down these minimal access ports over and over again, case after case, whether for decompressions or instrumentation or both, that you have forced your mind to reconstruct the anatomy at depth. Throughout that process, an intuitive awareness of the spine has developed. For lack of a better term, it is this sixth sense that becomes an inextricable element of the minimally invasive approach. The resection of an intradural extramedullary lesion not only requires mastery of the topography of the thoracic spine but also that valuable sixth sense that develops only as minimally invasive cases accumulate.

Intuitive awareness of the spine is difficult to describe in terms of traditional open surgery, where the anatomy lies in plain view once exposed. The perception of the spine is different in a mind prepared for the minimally invasive approach. The skill of reconstructing the anatomy at depth and viewing the pathology through smaller corridors transforms even the way that you look at an MRI or CT. You will have the capacity to see further than most in these studies. It is my prediction that, upon completion of your conversion to a minimally invasive mindset, you will find yourself looking at a study completely different from your colleague standing next to you. You will ask yourself, "why not do this minimally invasively?"

As this Primer comes to an end, one section remains. You may find it surprising that the final chapters have nothing to do with minimally invasive surgical techniques. Instead, the topic is radiation exposure and the use of the fluoroscope, which minimally invasive spine surgery requires by its very nature. Despite the development and continued advancement of computer-assisted navigation, I believe we will be walking hand in hand with fluoroscopy for the foreseeable future and perhaps for the remainder of our careers. My hope is that the final two chapters increase your understanding of how fluoroscopy works and heightens your awareness of radiation exposure. The fundamentals of fluoroscopy are topics that I feel have been missing from many a spine textbook and from the education of the next generation of spine surgeons. It is my intention, with the final section of this Primer, to fill that void.

References

[1] Chiou SM, Eggert HR, Laborde G, Seeger W. Microsurgical unilateral approaches for spinal tumour surgery: eight years' experience in 256 primary operated patients. Acta Neurochir (Wien). 1989; 100(3–4):127–133

[2] Eggert HR, Scheremet R, Seeger W, Gaitzsch J. Unilateral microsurgical approaches to extramedullary spinal tumours. Operative technique and results. Acta Neurochir (Wien). 1983; 67(3–4):245–253

[3] Yaşargil MG, Tranmer BI, Adamson TE, Roth P. Unilateral partial hemi-laminectomy for the removal of extra- and intramedullary tumours and AVMs. Adv Tech Stand Neurosurg. 1991; 18:113–132

[4] Poletti CE. Central lumbar stenosis caused by ligamentum flavum: unilateral laminotomy for bilateral ligamentectomy: preliminary report of two cases. Neurosurgery. 1995; 37(2):343–347

[5] Lin PM. Internal decompression for multiple levels of lumbar spinal stenosis: a technical note. Neurosurgery. 1982; 11(4):546–549

[6] Tredway TL, Santiago P, Hrubes MR, Song JK, Christie SD, Fessler RG. Minimally invasive resection of intradural-extramedullary spinal neoplasms. Neurosurgery. 2006; 58(1) Suppl:ONS52–ONS58, discussion ONS52–ONS58

[7] Panjabi MM, Takata K, Goel V, et al. Thoracic human vertebrae. Quantitative three-dimensional anatomy. Spine. 1991; 16(8):888–901

[8] Tumialán LM, Theodore N, Narayanan M, Marciano FF, Nakaji P. Anatomic basis for minimally invasive resection of intradural extramedullary lesions in thoracic spine. World Neurosurg. 2018; 109:e770–e777

12 Radiation and Minimally Invasive Spine Surgery

Abstract

A leading criticism of minimally invasive spine surgery is that it is associated with greater radiation exposure than open procedures. Radiation exposure also serves as a deterrent for surgeons seeking to incorporate minimally invasive techniques into their practice. The limited visualization of the anatomy in minimally invasive approaches mandates additional imaging in some form; however, there need not be a linear relationship between additional imaging and radiation exposure. Minimally invasive spine surgeons need to develop a mindset that more imaging does not necessarily equate to more radiation exposure. A thorough understanding of the fundamentals of X-ray creation and radiation exposure will enable them to begin to alter the amount of radiation they use and ultimately decrease their overall exposure to ionizing radiation during minimally invasive surgery. In this chapter, I discuss the physics of X-ray creation and then translate those basic scientific principles to the fluoroscope. My objective in this chapter is to help the reader better understand the factors that coalesce to produce an image of the spine on a screen. With an increased understanding of the fundamentals of X-ray creation and fluoroscopy, the reader will have no reason to avoid performing minimally invasive procedures with less radiation than that used with the open equivalents, if not with less radiation than ever before.

Keywords: anode, cathode, fluoroscopy, image intensifier, K-characteristic X-ray, thermionic emission, X-ray tube

To exist is to change, to change is to mature, to mature is to go on creating oneself endlessly.

Henri Bergson

12.1 Introduction

I distinctly remember walking into the operating room for my first case as a surgical intern. I was a freshly minted physician just weeks out of medical school. The case was an anterior cervical discectomy with fusion. After the patient was positioned, the cervical spine was prepped along with the anterior superior iliac spine. The attending surgeon planned and marked the incision purely on the basis of anatomical landmarks relative to the sternal notch and thyroid cartilage. The surgeon then wielded the No. 10 blade over the cervical spine as I cut a hole in the surgical drapes to reach the iliac crest, the future location of donor site pain for this patient. No fluoroscopic image or cross-table lateral radiograph held up making the incision. Once the attending surgeon exposed the presumptive level, a spinal needle found its way into the disc space as the surgeon requested a cross-table lateral radiograph.

We all wandered, like penguins, to what we perceived to be a safe distance away from the monstrous portable X-ray machine as the radiology technologist went through the elaborate process of positioning the cassette and acquiring the image. None of us was wearing protective lead. The X-ray machine hummed into a culminating high pitch, clicked and then spooled back down to a low drone.

The radiology technologist grabbed the cartridge and took it to the developing room down the hall. The portable X-ray machine was left in position just in case an additional image was needed. We stood around with our arms folded, trying not to contaminate ourselves as we awaited the verdict. We needed to know whether the spinal needle had pierced the intended target. Confirmation of the level always seemed to take an eternity. To pass time, we intermittently made awkward eye contact with one another, raised our eyebrows and looked around the room. The return of the radiograph brought a wave of excitement and anticipation to all of us in the room. We all gathered around the light box as the radiology technologist hung the film. The attending surgeon inspected the image and gruffly ordered traction on the shoulders for another image. We could not view the target level at all. After 30 minutes or so, a radiograph finally confirmed the level and we could proceed with the surgery.

My instructions were to use an oscillating saw to carve a parallel graft from the anterior superior iliac spine. Harvesting a structural graft from the hip was something I had never done before. Without asking questions, I did as I was told and handed the graft to the attending surgeon, who further shaped it to suit the segment. With a tamp and a mallet, he secured it between the vertebral bodies where the disc had been moments ago. He then placed a cervical plate in position and secured it with four screws. I remember the surgeon asking me if I thought the cervical plate was positioned straight on the cervical spine. I peered into the surgical exposure and examined the cervical plate that lay on the vertebral bodies of the cervical spine between the retractor blades. I looked back up at the surgeon and told him that I honestly could not tell. The final anteroposterior (AP) and lateral radiographs would have to wait for either closure of the incision or the postanesthesia care unit. In this manner, I completed my first case as a surgical intern at the Naval Medical Center in San Diego, California. The year was 1999.

Throughout that year, the surgeons that I worked with used very little, if any, fluoroscopy in the various spinal procedures I saw. Laminectomies, microdiscectomies and even instrumented lumbar fusions were all performed with either one or a series of cross-table lateral radiographs. I witnessed some instrumentation-related complications that, in retrospect, might have been avoided if there had been greater access to imaging. But at the time, fluoroscopy was either not readily available or not warmly embraced for spine surgery, at least at that particular institution.

I walked into neurosurgery residency in 2003 after serving several years as a deployed physician in the U.S. Navy. I had spent most of that time overseas, working in austere settings and in foreign hospitals. Upon arriving at Emory University in Atlanta, Georgia, for my first day of residency, it was obvious to me that the situation was now dramatically different. Fluoroscopy units were everywhere. At the beginning of every cervical case, the fluoroscope stood in position to help plan the incision, kept sterile in the field to efficiently confirm the level and guide the instrumentation. Similarly, all instrumented lumbar or thoracic cases had fluoroscopy from beginning to end.

Intraoperative angiography for intracranial aneurysms and arteriovenous (AV) malformations became commonplace. In contrast to what I had experienced previously, I found that having the fluoroscope readily available optimized the efficiency of the operation, improved the craftsmanship of the instrumentation and identified potential instrumentation-related complications intraoperatively, so that we could readily address them. In my estimation, expanding the availability of the fluoroscope was a step in the right direction. It was safer for the patient and more efficient for the procedure.

The rise of minimally invasive spine surgery, which coincided with the time of my residency, changed the landscape of fluoroscopy in the operating room altogether. In traditional open surgeries, fluoroscopy was helpful but not essential. To this day, some surgeons routinely perform spine operations with nothing more than a cross-table lateral radiograph to confirm a level and then proceed by anatomical landmarks or direct visualization of the pedicle and the other bony prominences. However, minimally invasive procedures mandate some form of additional image guidance. In most of these procedures, that additional image guidance takes the form of fluoroscopy. The increased availability of fluoroscopy and the expanding popularity of minimally invasive spine surgery over the past decade have combined to increase the surgeon's exposure to ionizing radiation. Couple this with interventional neuroendovascular rotations now routinely performed by neurosurgery residents and there is little doubt that the current generation of neurosurgeons in training will likely be exposed to more ionizing radiation from fluoroscopy than the preceding generations of surgeons.[1] The consequences of this increased exposure are still unknown. In fact, it will likely be another generation before the ramifications of this increased exposure are fully appreciated and understood. For several of us, it will be too late to do something about it.

At the same time, the rise of image guidance technologies has paralleled that of minimally invasive spine surgery. The use of computer-assisted navigation, combined with the technology of the various intraoperative computed tomography systems, essentially eliminates the radiation exposure for the surgeon and the operating room personnel.[2,3] The one concession we make in using this technology is the increased radiation exposure to the patient.[4] Surgeons use the rationale that it is a one-time dose to the patient, which I find to be a reasonable argument.

Analogous to the fluoroscope at the turn of the century, navigation is becoming increasingly available in our operating rooms. Few would argue its benefit over fluoroscopy in long-segment fusions or complex scoliosis cases. However, navigation remains an area ripe for debate in transpsoas approaches and in single-level or two-level transforaminal approaches where the changes in disc height cannot be captured by the navigation system with the current technology. In the coming years, navigation will undoubtedly become more accurate, more efficient and more cost-effective. I foresee navigation technologies playing an even more central role in the future of spine surgery.

However, despite the revolutionary advancements that navigation offers, it is difficult to imagine how navigation, in its current form, would supplant fluoroscopy for smaller procedures such as minimally invasive microdiscectomies, laminectomies and anterior cervical fusions. It would simply be too cumbersome for applications that have a low level of dependence on any form of image guidance but still require localization. Consequently, the role of fluoroscopy for these minimally invasive procedures remains firmly entrenched for the foreseeable future. Since we will likely continue to walk hand in hand with fluoroscopy for the remainder of our careers in spine surgery, the obvious question becomes "What can be done to minimize ionizing radiation with fluoroscopy."

The hour has arrived in the evolution of spine surgery for the pendulum to swing the other way. The next generation of minimally invasive spine surgeons needs to make every effort to decrease the amount of ionizing radiation exposure to their patients, their operating room personnel and themselves. I believe that such a paradigm shift should occur in the culture of minimally invasive spine surgery. The first step in minimizing the dose of ionizing radiation is to understand the fundamentals of fluoroscopy. Radiation physics is a topic that is often overlooked in medical schools and seldom covered in any depth in neurosurgery or orthopaedic residency training programs. I, for one, completed a residency in neurosurgery without the faintest idea about how an image of a spine appears on a screen by doing nothing more than plugging a machine into the wall and pushing a button. The second step is to harness that understanding into the application of low-dose protocols to accomplish the imaging that we need. It will be those protocols that will be the topic of the next and final chapter in this Primer.

Before proceeding with this chapter, I will leave the reader with one final anecdote, which in essence is the genesis of my interest in minimizing ionizing radiation exposure. Over the course of my military time overseas, I served intermittently aboard the *U.S.S. Buffalo*, a fast-attack nuclear submarine in the world's finest navy. Anyone serving on a nuclear-powered vessel in the U.S. Navy is assigned a dosimeter. The readings from that dosimeter become part of the permanent medical record for that service member. When I separated from the Navy to begin my residency, a final report for my radiation exposure was recorded in my medical record.

Upon completion of my residency, I returned to the Navy to the same hospital where my surgical career began as an intern a decade earlier. I was issued another dosimeter, this time for monitoring my radiation exposure in the operating room. When my Naval career ended, I was issued a final report. The juxtaposition of those two numbers was shocking. My radiation dose as an attending surgeon for 2 years performing minimally invasive spine surgery far exceeded my radiation exposure from serving on board a nuclear submarine, where I lived and breathed next to a nuclear reactor intermittently over the same period of time. I quickly did the math and extrapolated my radiation exposure over the next two decades of my life. It became evident to me that I was not on a sustainable path and had to do something. The stark contrast between the radiation exposure involved with service on a nuclear submarine and that experienced while operating next to a fluoroscopy unit heightened my awareness and set me off on a quest to understand fluoroscopy and minimize the exposure to ionizing radiation in minimally invasive spine surgeries. That mission continues to this very day.

I began this chapter with a quote from the French philosopher Henri Bergson about the need to change, mature and reinvent oneself. Over the past decade alone, spine surgery has demonstrated the capacity to do just that. We must continually reinvent our specialty for the benefit of our patients and the safety of our staff, our residents, ourselves and the generation of surgeons that follows us. The advances in minimally invasive spine surgery, transpsoas approaches, motion preservation and image guidance are perfect examples that illustrate this point. My hope is that increased radiation awareness in minimally invasive spine surgery and efforts to reduce exposure will become part of this reinvention in the years to come.

12.2 Radiology Technologists and the Minimally Invasive Surgery Ensemble

Throughout my entire residency and the first 2 years of my career, I considered fluoroscopy nothing more than a rate-limiting step to the surgery. We were either waiting for the fluoroscopy technologist to arrive with the two-part machine or waiting for the central processing unit to boot up so that we could take an image. Either way, the fluoroscope always seemed to delay the operation. Although I had plenty of time to think about it as the fluoroscope warmed up, I never considered what actually happened when someone pushed that little yellow button to generate an image.

I encourage the reader to talk to radiology technologists. You will be surprised by the knowledge that they possess once you begin to discuss radiation exposure and technique. You will quickly realize that these persons are the only ones truly qualified to acquire a fluoroscopic image. It is worthwhile to have such conversations. Over the years, I have read numerous articles and book chapters on this topic, but in the end, I learned more about radiation and fluoroscopy from the technologists I work with every day. In the introductory chapter of this Primer, I discussed the importance of the minimally invasive ensemble. Minimally invasive spine surgery is best performed by a dedicated team familiar with all aspects of minimally invasive procedures. To that end, it is important to build a good working relationship with your fluoroscopy technologists, who can anticipate, adjust and modify the position of the fluoroscope to optimize the image you need. Keep in mind that the algorithms within the central processing unit of the fluoroscope have been written with one objective in mind: image optimization. In reality, what we as spine surgeons truly need is not a perfect image every time but rather an adequate image at the lowest possible radiation dose. You can readily accomplish this goal by working closely with your fluoroscopy technologist. The first step in this endeavor is to understand the fundamentals of fluoroscopy, which is the objective of this chapter. The application of these fundamentals to reduce radiation exposure is the topic of the next and final chapter in this Primer.

12.3 Fundamentals of Fluoroscopy

In spine surgery, we plug a fluoroscope into the wall, wait for it to power up, aim it at the spine and create an image. For years I have taken that process for granted, without the slightest appreciation of what went into creating the image on the screen. In its most elemental form, that image results from converting electrical energy into electromagnetic energy. It is the electromagnetic energy that generates X-rays, which traverse the body and then interact with the image intensifier to create an image. But how does an image of the spine appear on a screen after you do nothing more than push a button? How are X-rays generated by a machine that is plugged into an electrical socket? Where does the radiation come from to generate that image? After all, there is no radioactive material in the X-ray tube. And why do we have to wait 5 minutes after turning on the fluoroscope just to generate an image?

To answer these questions, I need to take you back to your chemistry and physics courses that landed you in medical school to begin with. Kinetic energy, potential energy and Bohr's theory of the atom with orbital electrons are all familiar concepts, although perhaps distant in your memory. I will apply these theoretical principles to the fluoroscope to enable you to understand how the component parts of a cathode and an anode within an X-ray tube generate X-rays and ultimately create an image. These fundamentals are essential to understanding how a machine plugged into an electrical socket generates X-rays and creates an image on a screen that allows you to localize a level or put in a pedicle screw. I will begin with the origin of X-rays and then discuss how the component parts of the fluoroscope work together to generate these X-rays.

12.4 Origin of X-rays: A 30,000-Foot View

The transition of an electron within an atom from an outer shell to an inner shell releases energy in the form of an X-ray. In the case of fluoroscopy, the central atomic element is tungsten (▶ Fig. 12.1). The image created on the screen is therefore dependent on the transition of outer-shell electrons spinning around the tungsten nucleus to an inner electron shell. That process releases image-forming X-rays. Those X-rays penetrate the body of the patient at varying degrees and create the images that guide our surgeries.

But why would an outer electron even begin to make that transition within the tungsten atom? It does so to fill a void in an inner electron shell that is making the atom unstable. The generation of X-rays therefore depends on creating a void within an inner electron shell of the tungsten atom that must be filled by an outer electron. The ejection of an inner-shell electron makes the atom unstable, necessitating the transition of an outer electron to an inner electron shell to restore stability (▶ Fig. 12.2).

Now that we understand that the ejection of an inner-shell electron is the primary action that will produce X-rays, the next logical question becomes how to eject that inner-shell electron from the tungsten atom. The simple answer is to bombard the tungsten atom with projectiles squarely aimed at the electrons that are orbiting within their shells with the intent of knocking one of them out its shell. Conceptually, the ideal projectile to knock out an electron from a tungsten atom is something of comparable size and weight to our electron target. Collisions between billiard balls (on a subatomic scale) would be the analogous scenario. With this analogy in mind, we can see that the

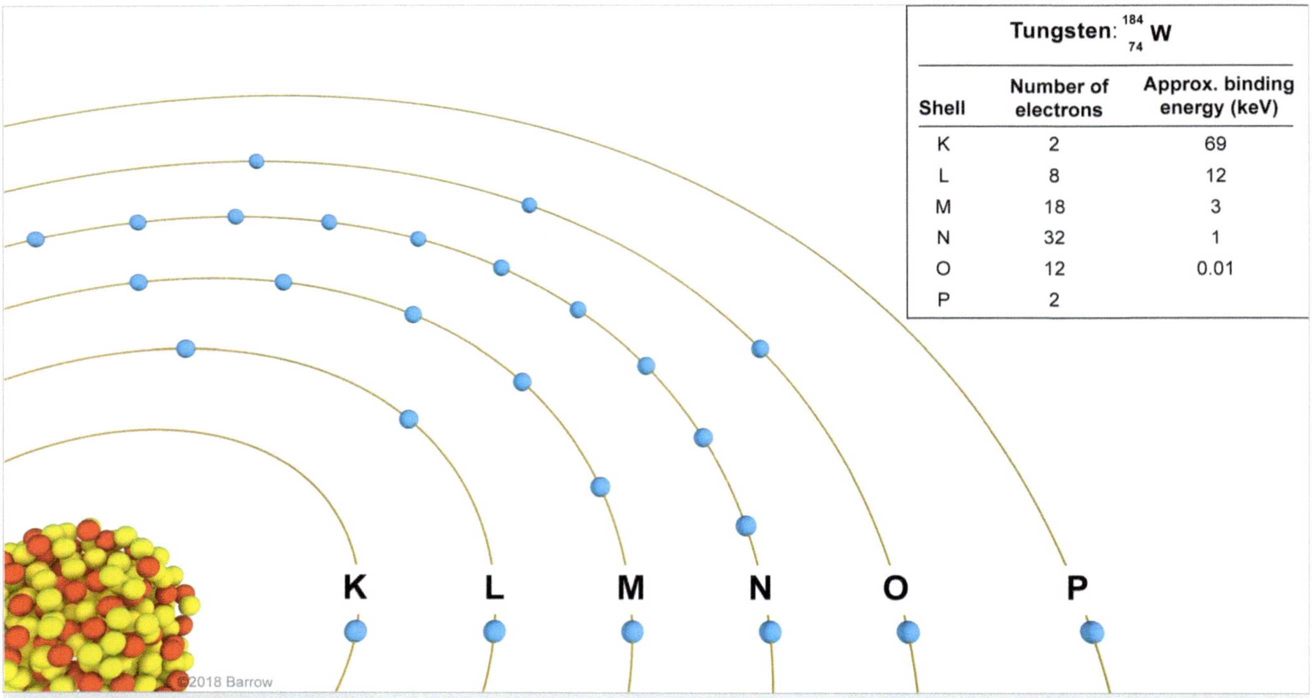

Tungsten: $^{184}_{74}W$

Shell	Number of electrons	Approx. binding energy (keV)
K	2	69
L	8	12
M	18	3
N	32	1
O	12	0.01
P	2	

Fig. 12.1 The tungsten atom has 74 electrons that orbit the nucleus. There are several electron shells (*K through P*). The closer the electron is to the nucleus, the higher the binding energy. The farther the electrons are from the nucleus, the lower the binding energy. The two electrons in the K-shell closest to the nucleus have the highest binding energy. Therefore, removing K-shell electrons from the atom requires the most energy. Removing a K-shell electron will result in an unstable atom until another electron is pulled from an outer shell to take its place. The transition of an electron from an outer shell to an inner shell is what generates radiation.

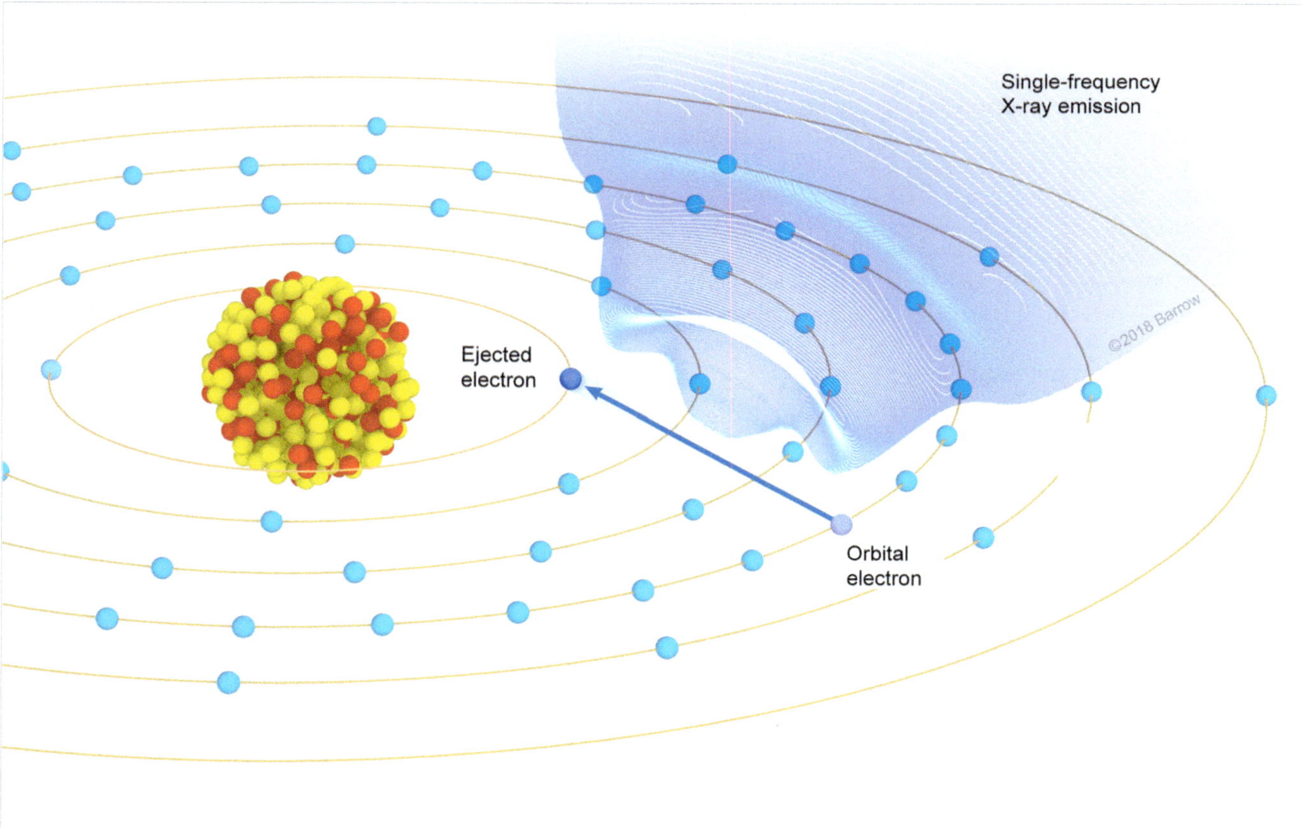

Fig. 12.2 Generation of an X-ray. The transition of an electron from an outer shell to an inner shell releases an X-ray. In this illustration, a projectile electron has ejected a K-shell electron from the tungsten atom, creating a highly unstable state. An outer-shell electron transitions into that void (*blue arrow*) and in doing so releases an X-ray. Although many X-rays will be generated with the ejection of electrons from various electron shells, only X-rays generated with transitions into the K-shell will result in X-rays with adequate energy to be useful as diagnostic X-rays. Therefore, it is the K-shell electron that is the primary focus.

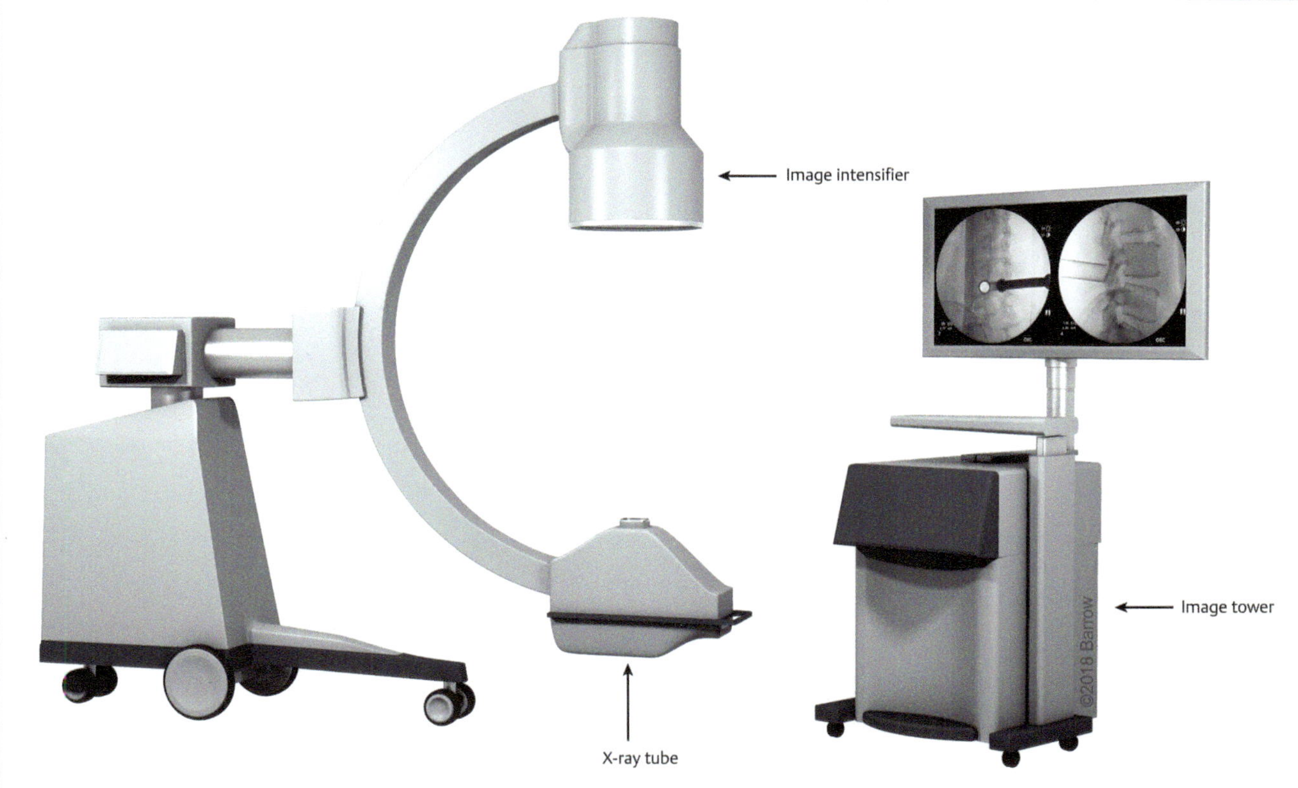

Fig. 12.3 Illustration of a fixed C-arm fluoroscope and image tower with a central processing unit. The component parts of the fluoroscope include the X-ray tube, image intensifier and image tower.

rational choice for the ideal projectile is another electron. If we could create a stream of projectile electrons aimed at the tungsten atom with enough velocity and energy to knock out an electron from the inner shell of the tungsten atom, then we could generate those precious diagnostic X-rays.

The essentials of X-ray creation, therefore, are a beam of projectile electrons and a tungsten target. With this fundamental understanding of X-ray creation, we can now discuss the components of the fluoroscope (▶ Fig. 12.3).

12.5 Components of the Fluoroscope

12.5.1 Cathode and Electron Beam

This section begins where the X-rays originate, the X-ray tube. Separating the X-ray tube from its core elements and functions will allow us to transition to the atomic level to further examine the generation of X-rays. In its most basic form, the X-ray tube is a diode with a cathode and an anode (▶ Fig. 12.4). The cathode generates the electron beam, and the beam, in turn, is directed toward the anode, which contains the target. Since the first order of business in X-ray creation is to generate a stream of projectile electrons, I will begin by focusing on the cathode component of the X-ray tube.

One way to generate this stream of electrons is to heat metal to such a high temperature that electrons will essentially boil off in a process known as thermionic emission. To accomplish this, developers of the modern-day fluoroscope used a thoriated tungsten filament in the cathode. When we turn on a fluoroscope, a current begins to warm that filament below the temperature needed for electron emission but high enough to prepare the filament for the surges of voltage that will heat the filament enough for electron emission. Warming an oven in preparation for baking is an analogous scenario.

Thermionic emission requires high voltages of electricity to surge through the thoriated tungsten filament and reach the threshold necessary to effectively boil off the outer-shell electrons of the tungsten atom. Those electrons will form the electron beam. Only a high-voltage generator allows such thresholds to be reached, and it is therefore a necessary component of the cathode. When the filament reaches a temperature high enough to make the electrons boil off, they begin to make their way to the positively charged anode (▶ Fig. 12.5).

Although forces are drawing the negatively charged electrons toward the positively charged anode, all the negatively charged electrons are trying to make their way to the same positively charged target. The electrostatic repulsion of the electrons on that journey would inevitably lead to scattering of the electron beam. Without modification, the electrons would never converge into a reliable beam capable of hitting a target. To create a beam, an even more negatively charged focusing cup electrostatically confines the electrons so that a focused beam forms and remains squarely aimed at the anode.

The combination of a high-voltage generator to produce the surge of electricity, a thoriated tungsten filament, and focusing

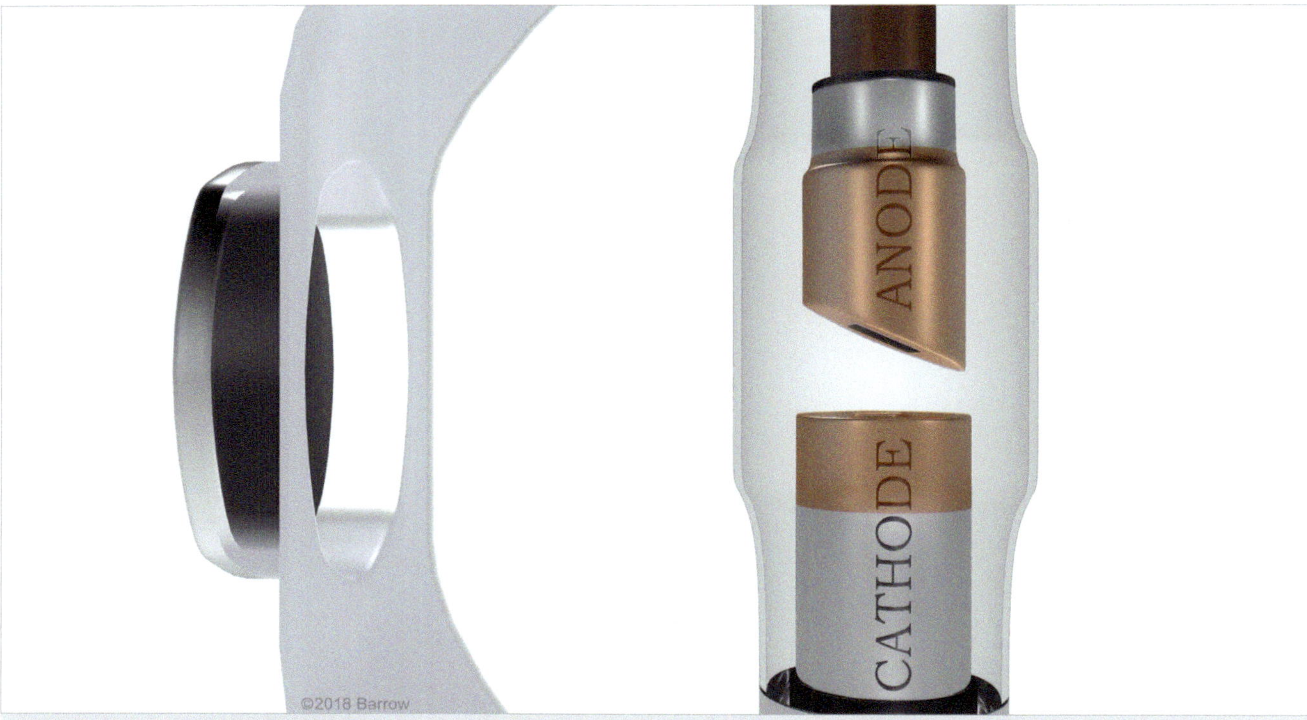

Fig. 12.4 A conceptual illustration of an X-ray tube within the housing of the fluoroscope. The X-ray tube is a diode consisting of a cathode and an anode. The cathode generates an electron beam, and the anode holds the tungsten target. The primary object of the cathode's electron beam is to collide with and then eject an inner-shell electron from the tungsten target.

cups within the cathode of the X-ray tube of the fluoroscope has addressed the creation of a stream of projectile electrons. With the formation of the electron beam, we can now turn to the target of that beam, the anode.

12.5.2 Anode

The anode is the positive side of the X-ray tube. Within the anode resides the target area for the electron beam generated by the cathode as shown in ▶ Fig. 12.5. It is the collision of this electron beam with the tungsten atoms of the anode target that has the potential to generate X-rays.

This cursory overview of X-ray generation has laid the foundation for a more granular understanding of the fundamentals of fluoroscopy that will enable you to decrease radiation exposure. A look back at Bohr's theory of the atom provides the necessary foothold for that understanding.

12.5.3 X-ray Production

As you may recall from your undergraduate studies, Bohr's theory of the atom consists of a nucleus surrounded by rings of electron shells. In the case of the tungsten atom, which is the relevant atom for diagnostic X-rays, the nucleus is made up of 74 protons, 110 neutrons and 6 electron shells (K, L, M, N, O and P) holding 74 electrons. Electron-binding energy maintains each electron in its respective shell as the electrons revolve around the atom. The closer the electron resides to the nucleus, the higher the electron-binding energy, and vice versa. It therefore follows that the two K-shell electrons will be the highest energy electrons because they are the closest to the nucleus. For diagnostic imaging, the goal is to knock out these high-energy K-shell electrons, which is the only type of electron shell that will generate a diagnostic X-ray (▶ Fig. 12.6).

Remarkably, the vast majority of the electrons generated by the cathode will do nothing more than excite—but not remove—the outer P-shell electrons in the tungsten atom on the anode target. But without the projectile electrons transferring enough energy to ionize them, no X-rays will be generated. The result is that the outer-shell electrons are temporarily raised to a higher energy level and then immediately drop back to their normal energy level. For the outer electrons, the rise and fall of their energy result in the higher emission of infrared radiation and heat. In fact, 99% of the kinetic energy from the electron beam of a cathode is converted to heat. Fluoroscopic imaging is a far from efficient process.

For the electron beam to generate an X-ray, projectile electrons must strike an inner-shell electron with enough energy to completely remove it from the atom in a process known as *ionization*. For the tungsten atom, the loss of an inner-shell electron makes it highly unstable, and the void is quickly filled by an electron from an outer shell. The transition of an outer-shell electron to fill the void in an inner shell creates an X-ray. The X-ray has energy equal to the difference in the binding energy of the orbital electron. ▶ Fig. 12.7 depicts a projectile electron ionizing a K-shell electron. The transition of an outer-shell electron into the void created by the K-shell electron creates what is known as a *K-characteristic X-ray*. If the projectile electron had ionized an M-shell electron, the transition of an outer-shell electron into the void in the M shell would have resulted in an

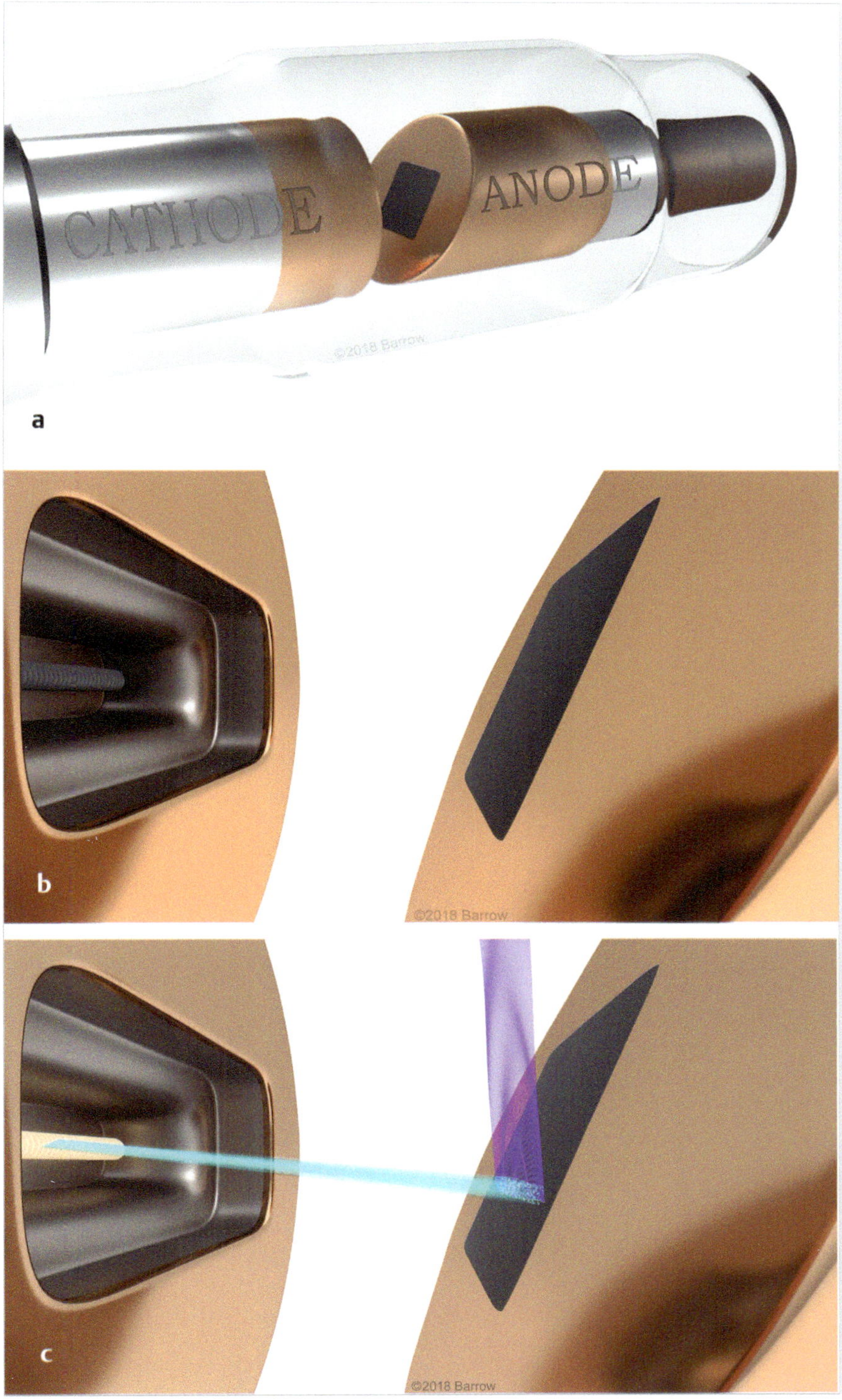

Fig. 12.5 A conceptual illustration of thermionic emission. **(a)** The X-ray tube is a diode made up of a cathode and an anode. **(b)** Close-up view of the cathode. Before the fluoroscope is turned on, the thoriated tungsten filament, in the center of the cathode, is at room temperature. When the fluoroscope is turned on, the filament heats up to prepare for the surge of electricity that will create an electron beam. **(c)** Illustration demonstrates thermionic emission. A surge of electricity has traveled through the heated thoriated tungsten filament to produce an electron beam (*turquoise*). Focusing cups (*not shown*) aim the beam toward the anode, where the tungsten target resides. The projectile electrons result in the ejection of tungsten shell electrons. When the transition of outer-shell electrons into the inner-shell voids occurs, X-rays are generated (*purple beam*).

M-characteristic X-ray, and so on. The closer the electron is to the nucleus, the higher the binding energy, which translates into higher-energy X-rays (i.e., K-characteristic X-rays rather than M-characteristic X-rays). This difference is relevant to fluoroscopic techniques in minimally invasive spine surgery because the K-characteristic X-rays of tungsten are the only useful X-rays capable of generating an image (Video 12.1).

The final type of X-rays generated in the X-ray tube results when the projectile electron misses the outer-shell and inner-shell electrons altogether and merely passes through the atom. Since the atom is mostly empty space, most of the electrons from the beam will pass freely through it. When this happens, the positively charged nucleus still attracts the negatively charged electron and alters its energy. The projectile electron approaches the atom with a certain amount of kinetic energy. As it enters electron shells and approaches the nucleus, the projectile electron is slowed by the force of the positively charged nucleus, which alters its course. The electron then exits the

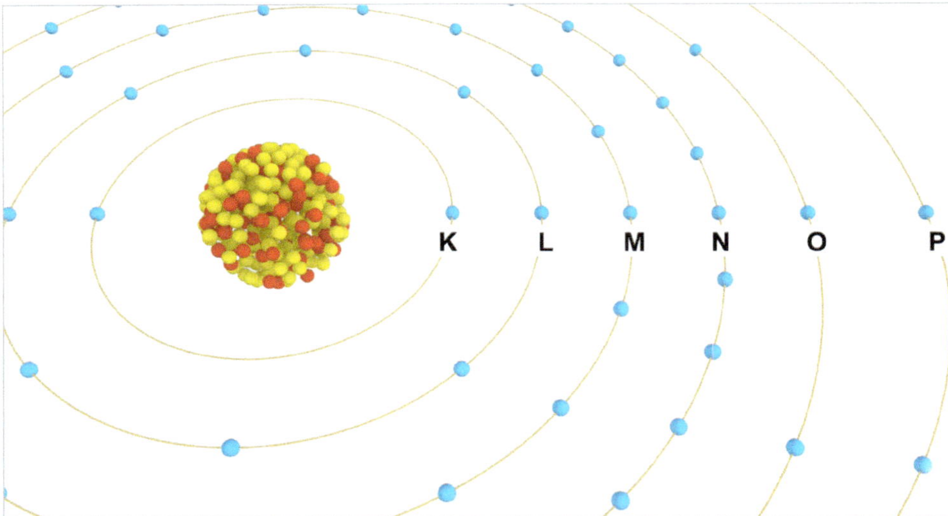

Shell	Number of electrons	Approx. binding energy (keV)
Tungsten: $^{184}_{74}W$		
K	2	69
L	8	12
M	18	3
N	32	1
O	12	0.01
P	2	

Fig. 12.6 The tungsten atom. The K-shell is the innermost shell with the highest binding energy. Although any transition of an electron from an outer shell to an inner shell will generate an X-ray, the removal of an electron from the K-shell results in the transition of an electron from an outer shell to the K-shell. This transition is what creates an X-ray with adequate energy for imaging.

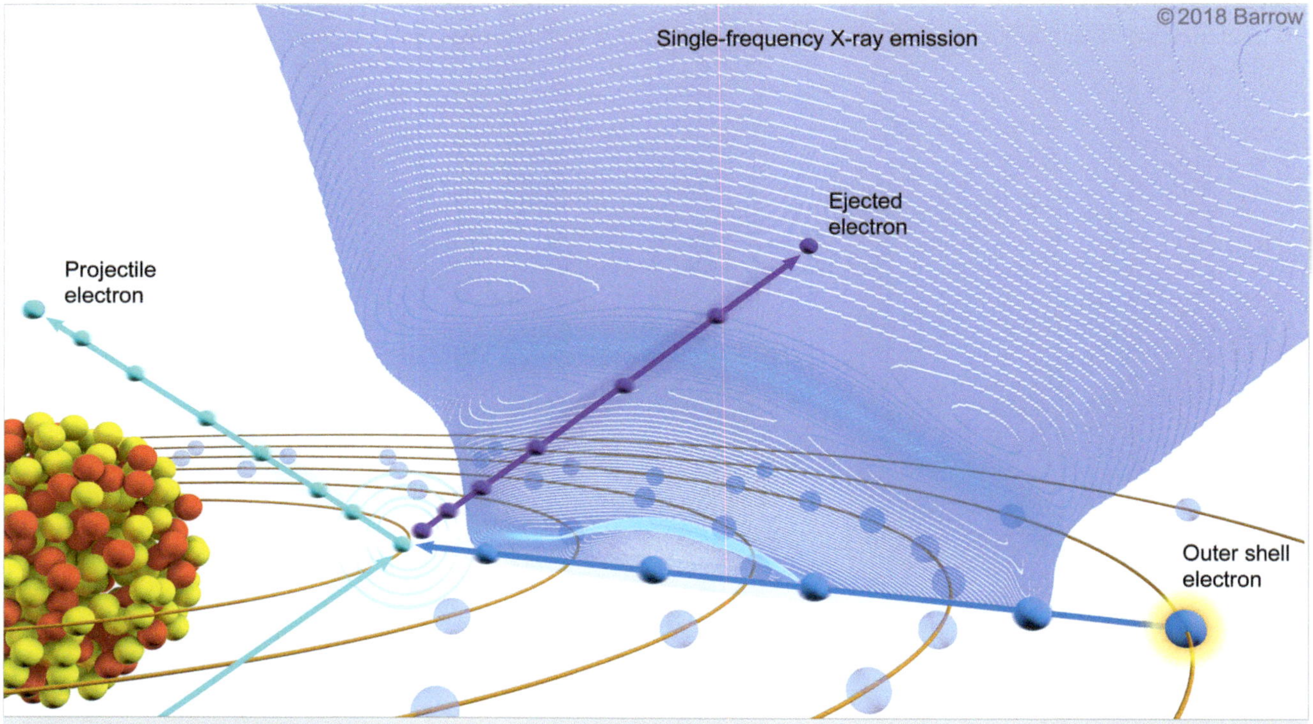

Fig. 12.7 Ionization of a K-shell electron. Illustration depicts the collision of a projectile electron with a K-shell electron, jettisoning the K-shell electron from the tungsten atom. The loss of this inner-shell electron creates an unstable state for the tungsten atom. That instability is resolved by electromagnetic forces pulling an electron from an outer shell into the void in the K-shell. The energy of this transition is released as an X-ray.

atom with a different kinetic energy. You may recall the first law of thermodynamics, also known as the law of conservation of energy. That law states that energy can neither be created nor destroyed in an isolated system. Therefore, energy is constant and can only be transferred or changed from one form to another. In the case of an electron passing through an atom, the kinetic energy is changed to radiation.

Applying the law of conservation of energy to an electron that enters an atom with one type of energy and exits with another requires a quantitative measure to account for that change in energy. That quantitative measure is the difference between the two energies. The difference is released as X-rays, known as *bremsstrahlung* radiation, from the German words *bremsen*, which means to brake, and *Strahlung*, which means radiation. Appropriately named, this type of radiation is released by the slowing (or braking) of an electron as it passes through an atom exposed to the electromagnetic forces from the protons in the nucleus. Since most of the atom is empty space, bremsstrahlung radiation makes up most of the X-rays generated in fluoroscopy. After all, projectile electrons are less likely to collide with electrons in the various shells than to pass through the mostly empty atom. Unlike the discrete energies of characteristic X-rays, bremsstrahlung radiation can encompass a wide range of energies, depending on the interaction of the nucleus with the projectile electron (▶ Fig. 12.8).

12.6 X-ray Emission Spectrum

Although the K-characteristic X-rays from the tungsten atom are the only useful X-rays for our purposes, several X-rays of several different energies are generated as the projectile electrons strike electrons in the various electron shells (L, M, N and P) of the tungsten atom. Since each X-ray generated from each electron shell has discrete energy, a plot of the various X-rays can be generated with the energy of each X-ray on the *x*-axis and the number of X-rays on the *y*-axis. A graph of the X-ray emission spectrum demonstrating the various energies would look like the image in ▶ Fig. 12.9. Because the binding energy is greatest for the K-shell electron, the K-characteristic X-rays will have the highest energy.

However, ▶ Fig. 12.9 does not show what a spectrum for tungsten would resemble with the use of fluoroscopy. For that we would have to incorporate all the events that occur within the atom. If we were to plot the various energies that resulted from all the electrons striking and ejecting inner-shell and outer-shell electrons, as well as the energy released from the electrons slowing as they pass through the atom, the graph would look like the graph in ▶ Fig. 12.10.

It is this emission spectrum that becomes the basis for understanding the effect of peak kilovoltage (kVp), milliampere (mA) and milliampere seconds (mAs), which are the parameters that we apply to the fluoroscope every time we take an image. A

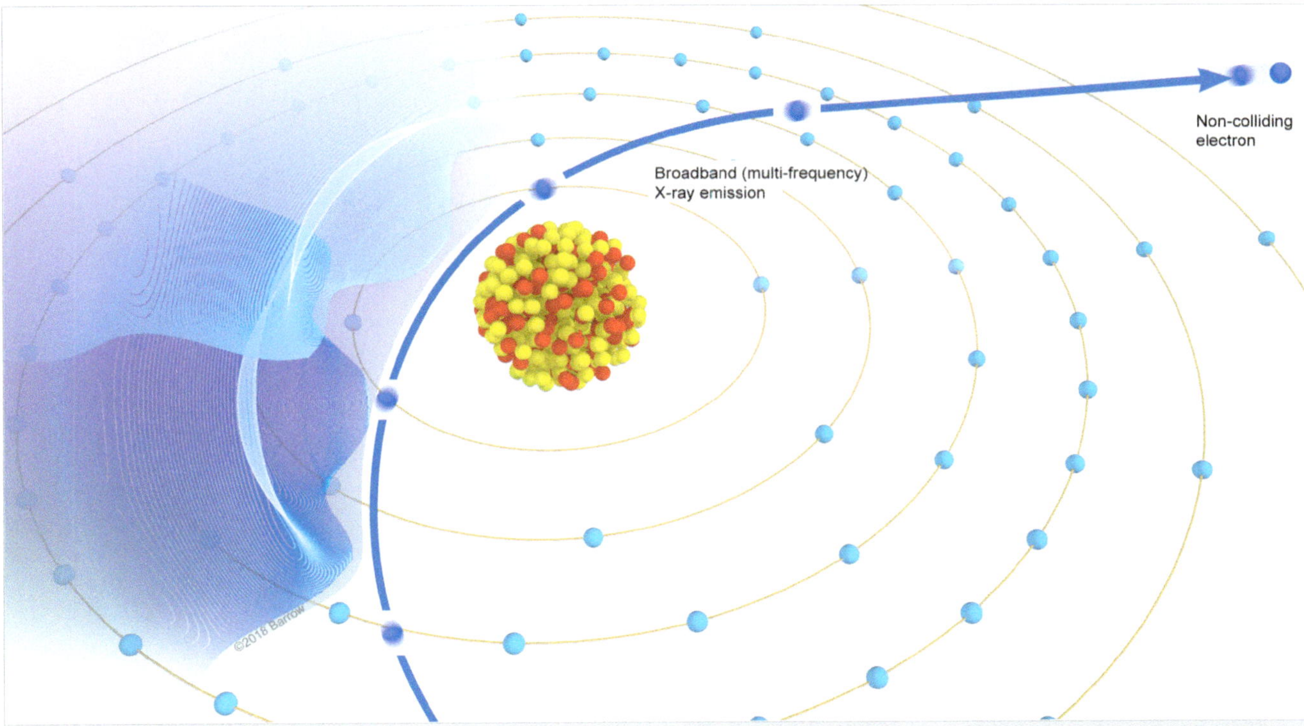

Fig. 12.8 Bremsstrahlung radiation. The vast majority of the electrons from the cathode's electron beam never strike a tungsten electron. Instead, they pass directly through the atom. The positively charged nucleus slows and alters the course of the projectile electrons, changing their energy. The difference in kinetic energy from entrance to exit is released as bremsstrahlung radiation. Unlike the change in energy produced by the ejection of an electron from a specific shell (e.g., K, L and M), this change in energy will encompass a variety of energies, depending on the electromagnetic interaction with the nucleus. The result is a broad emission spectrum.

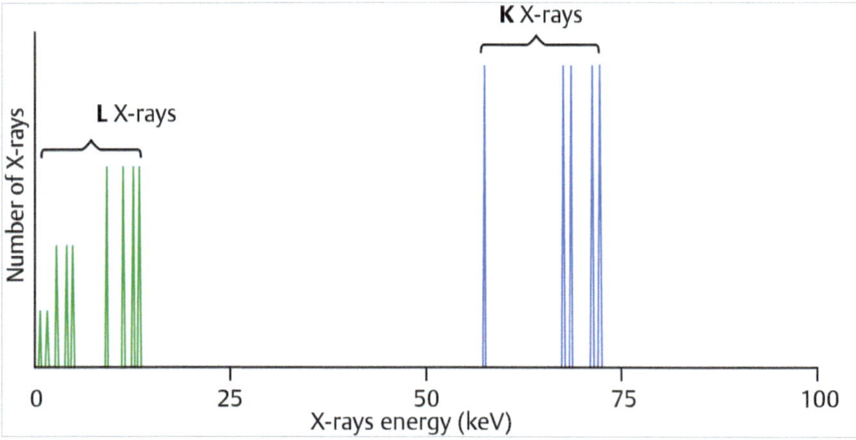

Fig. 12.9 The X-ray emission spectrum for tungsten. The spectrum has 15 different X-ray energies. The K-characteristic X-rays have the highest energy, can penetrate the body and produce a diagnostic image.

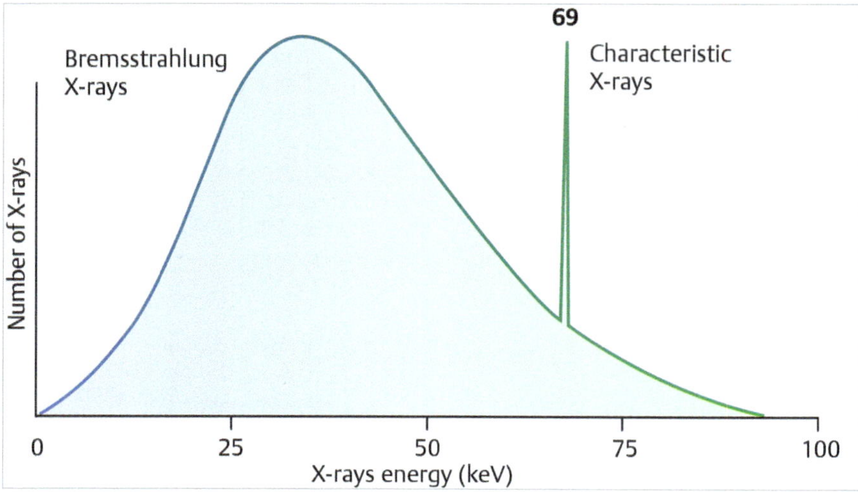

Fig. 12.10 The emission spectrum of tungsten when bremsstrahlung X-rays are included. The spike at 69 keV represents the K-characteristic X-rays.

greater understanding of those variables will serve as the basis for reducing radiation exposures, which will be discussed in the next chapter.

12.7 Impact of kVp, mA and mAs on Emission Spectrum

When we turn on the fluoroscope, three values are prominently displayed on the face of the control panel: kVp, fluoroscopy time and mA or mAs (▶ Fig. 12.11). Collectively, these values influence the radiation exposure to your patient, the operating staff and yourself. The kVp is the voltage created across the X-ray tube. The mA represents the current in the X-ray tube, also known as *tube current.* The fluoroscopy time is the cumulative time of exposure, which is hopefully always measured in seconds and never in minutes. These three values have a direct effect on the quality of image you will be looking at and on the amount of radiation exposure you will incur throughout your career. With the X-ray emission spectrum presented in ▶ Fig. 12.10 serving as a foundation, we can now leave the theoretical scenario and review real-world scenarios of the operating room we all inhabit.

12.8 Voltage

We have already established the fact that K-characteristic X-rays are the only X-rays of tungsten with sufficient energy to be of value in obtaining a meaningful image from the fluoroscope. All the other characteristic X-rays do not have enough energy to pass through the body and reach the image intensifier to create an image. Therefore, we must select a voltage for the X-ray tube to generate the valuable K-characteristic X-rays necessary to create a meaningful image. On the one hand, if we select a voltage of 25 kVp, we would find that no useful characteristic X-rays would be generated. At such a low voltage, the projectile electrons do not possess the energy to ionize enough K-shell electrons to create an image. The X-ray beam is all bremsstrahlung and outer-shell electron radiation. The result is a grainy screen. On the other hand, if we were to select a voltage of 100 kVp, sufficient energy would be transmitted into the projectile electrons to remove K-shell electrons from tungsten. The transition of outer-shell electrons can then occur and thereby generate a useful diagnostic K-characteristic X-ray beam. As mentioned previously, fluoroscopy is a highly inefficient process and K-characteristic X-rays make up only 15% of the X-ray beam, with the remaining radiation emitted as bremsstrahlung

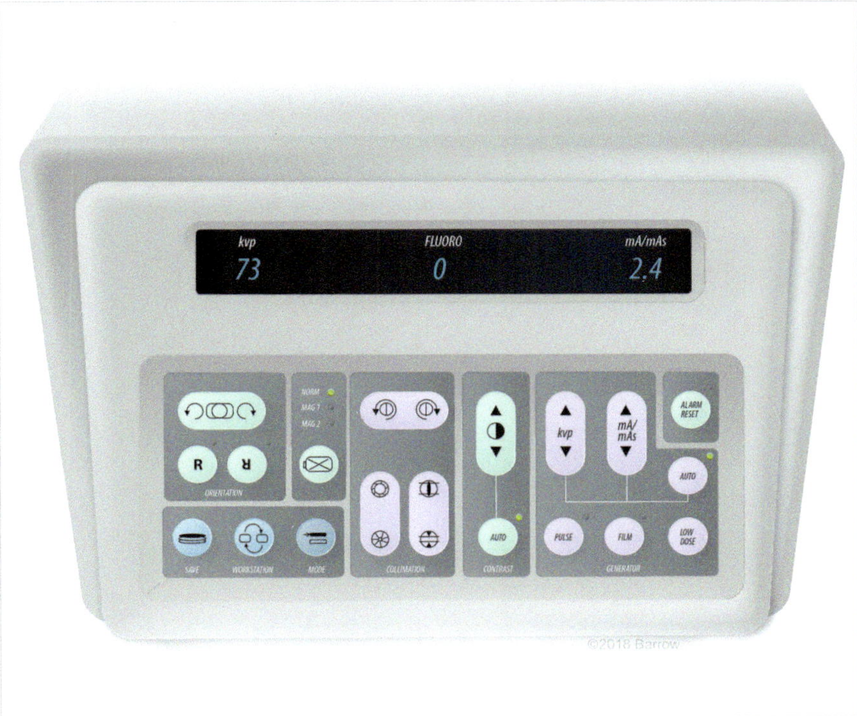

Fig. 12.11 The control panel of a GE OEC 9800 fluoroscope (General Electric Co.) displaying the three values of voltage (kVp), fluoroscopy time and current (mA/mAs). These three values will affect the quality of the image on the screen and the amount of radiation exposure.

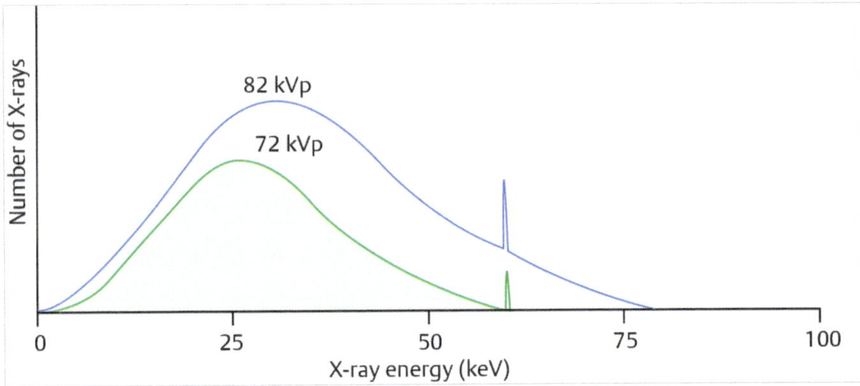

Fig. 12.12 The effect of kVp on the emission spectrum. As the kVp increases from 72 (*green area*) to 82 kVp (*blue area*), there are more K-characteristic X-rays and, consequently, a better diagnostic image. The graph demonstrates the greater amplitude of the K-characteristic energy (*blue line*). The graph also demonstrates the entire spectrum shifting to the right, which indicates that there are higher-energy X-rays. However, only the K-characteristic X-rays contribute to generating an image.

and other lower-energy characteristic X-rays (L, M, N, O and P). Nevertheless, this modest number of K-characteristic X-rays would be adequate to generate an image.

Examining the emission spectrum is another way to appreciate the effect of kVp. As kVp increases, so does the energy of the projectile electrons. The increased energy increases the likelihood of projectile electrons knocking out K-shell, M-shell or L-shell electrons and producing X-rays. The result is an increase in the relative distribution of emitted X-ray energy. As we increase kVp, we will find more K-characteristic X-rays along with other higher-energy X-rays in our spectrum. The net result is a shift of the emission spectrum to the right, where there are higher-energy X-rays. Among those X-rays are more of the sought-after K-characteristic X-rays. The result is a higher-quality image but at the cost of more radiation (▸ Fig. 12.12).

12.9 Current

The next value visible on every fluoroscope control panel is the current that runs through the X-ray filament (mA and mAs). The effect of current on the emission spectrum is distinct from the effect of voltage (kVp). For example, if the current doubles, twice as many electrons will flow from the cathode to the anode. If the kVp remains the same, doubling the current will result in twice as many X-rays at the various energy levels. Since the energy of the projectile electrons striking the anode remains the same, the emission spectrum will not shift to the right. The relevant point for the effect on imaging is that there will be twice as many K-characteristic X-rays. Again, the net effect would be a higher-quality image with more radiation (▸ Fig. 12.13).

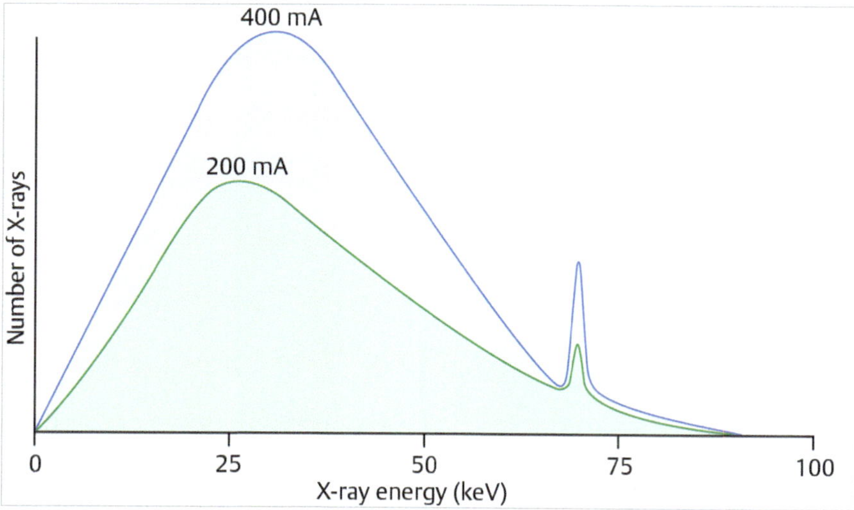

Fig. 12.13 The effect of current (mA) on the emission spectrum. Doubling the current in the X-ray tube will double the number of electrons passing from cathode to anode. The doubling of the current, in turn, doubles the number of X-rays at the various energy levels (*blue vs. green area*) without changing the distribution of X-rays at any level. With more electrons striking the anode target, there will be a greater likelihood of striking and ejecting a K-shell electron. The result is a greater number of K-characteristic X-rays. The graph demonstrates the greater magnitude of K-characteristic X-rays at 69 KeV.

12.9.1 Voltage versus Current

The goal for every fluoroscopic image should be to obtain an adequate-quality image with the least amount of radiation exposure. Understanding the fundamentals of the emission spectrum makes it evident that increasing the kVp will increase the number of higher-energy X-rays without increasing the total number of X-rays in the emission spectrum. In other words, increasing the kVp increases the energy of each projectile electron as it heads toward the anode, making it more likely that a K-shell electron will be ejected and that a K-characteristic X-ray will occur.

Another way to increase the number of K-characteristic X-rays is to increase the number of projectile electrons. But increasing the kVp does not increase the number of projectile electrons striking the anode. To increase the number of projectile electrons striking the target, one must increase the current (mA). By increasing the current, the number of K-characteristic X-rays will increase because the number of projectile electrons striking the anode will increase. Doing so results in an increased number of projectile electrons striking the target, with increased collisions and ejections of electrons from all shells occurring. Radiation-generating transitions will occur from the various outer shells to the inner shells. The result is an increased number of X-rays at all energy levels in the spectrum, including an increased number of K-characteristic X-rays.

The result of increasing the kVp and keeping mA unchanged is less absorption of the lower-energy X-rays by the patient and more X-rays that will penetrate the patient and proceed to the image intensifier to create an image. From a radiographic standpoint, just a 15% increase in kVp is equivalent to doubling the mA. The net result is a higher-quality image with less radiation exposure just by altering only one variable. I will expand upon this principle throughout the entire next chapter. Understanding kVp and mA and their effect on the emission spectrum is the foundation for minimizing ionizing radiation in fluoroscopy.

12.9.2 Image Intensifier Tube

So far in this chapter, I have covered what transpires within the X-ray tube component of the fluoroscope. I have answered the question of why we all stand around waiting after turning on the fluoroscope to generate an image. I have covered the generation of diagnostic X-rays by thermionic emission, but I have not explained how those X-rays generate an image on a screen that we can use during surgery. The final part of this equation is the image intensifier (▶ Fig. 12.14), which receives the X-rays that pass through the patient and transforms them into visible light and eventually into an image. A review of the sequence of events that occur within the image intensifier completes the process of understanding how an image appears on the screen after you hit the button to acquire an image on the fluoroscope.

The image intensifier is the bulky cylindrical part of the fluoroscope opposite the X-ray tube that is typically placed where the fellow or the resident assisting surgeon is standing. It accomplishes the task of transforming image-forming X-rays into visible light by using a series of phosphors, photocathodes and anodes to convert X-rays into photons. The X-rays that make their way through the patient strike the outer component of the unit, which is the input phosphor. The cesium iodide crystals that compose the input phosphor convert the X-rays into photons. The photocathode is bonded directly to the input phosphor. Using a process known as photoemission, the photocathode converts the photons generated by the input phosphor into electrons.

The size and shape of the image intensifier are necessary to create a potential difference between the photocathode and the anode of about 25,000 V. That potential voltage difference is something to keep in mind the next time you contort your body around this limb of the C-arm. A length of 50 cm allows the electrons to accelerate to the anode. Electrostatic lenses guide those electrons to a focal point in the anode, as shown in ▶ Fig. 12.15. Within the anode, the electrons reach the focal point and then strike the output phosphor. The electrons

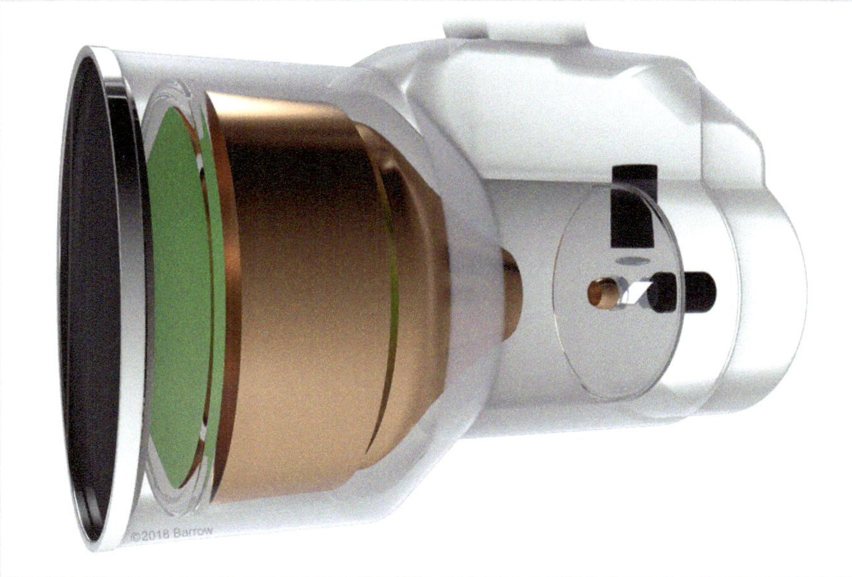

Fig. 12.14 Conceptual illustration of the image intensifier of the fluoroscope. X-rays that pass through the patient and into the image intensifier proceed through a cascade of energy transfers involving phosphors and photocathodes and eventually result in an image of the spine.

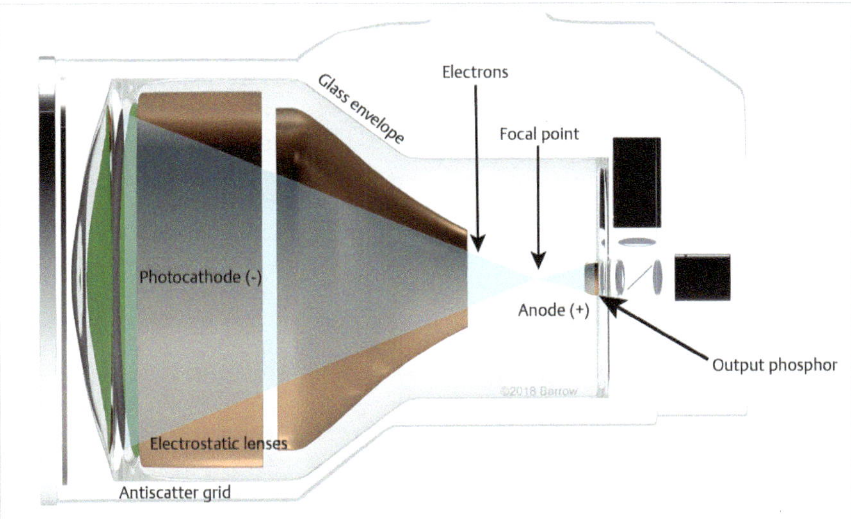

Fig. 12.15 Conceptual illustration demonstrates the schematic of the image intensifier. Note the sequence of phosphors, which are photocathodes that convert X-rays into visible light.

interact with the zinc cadmium sulfide crystals of the output phosphor, producing visible light. Finally, a specialized camera tube known as a *vidicon* transforms the photons into a video signal that appears on the screen for all of us to admire. In this manner, the cycle from when the fluoroscopy technologist hits the button to the appearance of an image on the screen is complete (▶ Fig. 12.16).

12.9.3 Putting It All Together

The goal of this chapter is to provide you with a greater understanding of what occurs in the various components of the fluoroscope the next time you request a fluoroscopic image. When you find yourself tapping your foot while waiting for the fluoroscope to become active, you will be able to visualize a low current running through that thoriated tungsten filament. Like an oven being warmed for baking, the current is slowly heating and priming the filament for the large burst of current and voltage to come that will boil off the electrons from the tungsten metal to form an electron beam. You will look at the kVp setting and know that the setting of 100 kVp will bestow enough energy on those projectile electrons leaving that tungsten filament to jettison a K-shell electron from its shell. A setting of 65 kVp will not.

The next time the fluoroscopy technologist hits the button on a fluoroscope, perhaps you will visualize the high-voltage generator within the X-ray tube surge the current and voltage within the tungsten filament of the cathode. Once the voltage and the current reach critical values, electrons begin to fire off the tip of the tungsten filament and start their voyage toward the anode. As they fly off, their negative charges repel each other, resulting in scatter until the negatively charged focusing cup in the cathode forces them into a focused beam of projectile electrons.

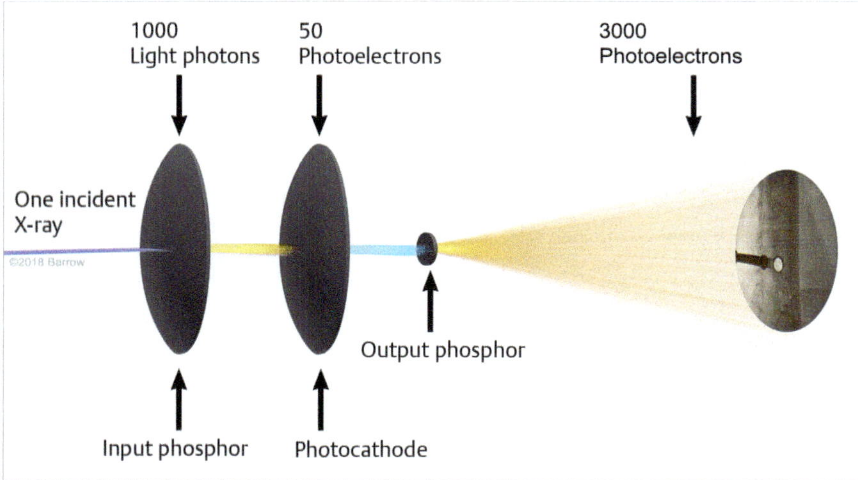

Fig. 12.16 Schematic representation of the conversion of X-rays to visible light. This illustration depicts how X-rays pass through the series of input phosphor, photocathode, anode and output phosphor. At the interface of each phosphor and photocathode, a conversion occurs from X-rays to photons, from photons to electrons, and finally from electrons to the photons that create a visible image.

As you wait for the image to appear on the screen, the electrons are making their way toward the tungsten atoms in the anode. The positively charged tungsten nuclei pull most of the projectile electrons in but do nothing more than alter their path. The affinity that the positive tungsten nucleus has for these electrons will slow them down and thus change their energy. Most of these electrons will pass right through the tungsten atoms, with the energy lost by their altered speed and course released as bremsstrahlung. You roll your eyes because you know that none of those electrons will contribute to the image you are patiently awaiting, but they still generate radiation.

What you are waiting for are those precious few projectile electrons that will find their way deep into the tungsten atom and strike one of the two K-shell electrons orbiting the nucleus. A perfect collision with either electron will overcome the binding energy holding it in orbit around the nucleus. The force of that perfect collision will jettison the electron out of the K-shell and entirely out of the tungsten nucleus, resulting in a void in the K-shell. The loss of an inner electron creates a highly unstable state, which the tungsten atom must fill. Electrons orbiting the nucleus in outer shells begin to quake as the electromagnetic force of that void begins to pull. As this is happening, projectile electrons from the beam are striking other electrons in other tungsten atoms. There are voids in electron shells in atoms all around, but the only ones that matter are the voids in the K-shells.

The stage is set for the positively charged tungsten nucleus to fill the void of the jettisoned K-shell electron. One of those orbiting electrons that began to quake moments ago now tumbles from an outer shell down into the K-shell. That transition is what you have been waiting for. A precious K-characteristic X-ray arises from the atom. That X-ray, along with other K-characteristic X-rays arising from other tungsten atoms in the anode, leaves the X-ray tube and enters your patient. You have great confidence in that X-ray because you know K-characteristic X-rays have enough energy to make it all the way through your patient.

The X-rays strike the bone and soft tissue as they pass through the patient. The bone and soft tissue, especially the bone, attenuate the X-ray beam in some areas. In other areas, the X-rays pass through unabated. All the X-rays that make it through the patient enter the bulky image intensifier, where the fellow is standing trying to find a comfortable position. Within the image intensifier, those X-rays strike the phosphors, causing photons to arise. Photons strike the photocathode and photoemission occurs, causing electrons to arise. Electrostatic lenses focus those electrons to the anode through the output phosphor, and visible light now offers the promise of an image. The vidicon takes that visible light and transforms it into a video signal. The result is the image on the screen. The image confirms the correct segment in the spine. You can now begin to operate.

12.10 Conclusion

Understanding the essentials of fluoroscopy will be an asset to you throughout your career as a minimally invasive spine surgeon. This knowledge transforms the fluoroscope from an instrument that dictates the terms of how you acquire the images you need to perform your surgeries to an instrument that you control to minimize radiation exposure. Instead of a predetermined algorithm within the fluoroscope setting radiation doses, you can determine the quality of image you need for a particular procedure. You can do so with less radiation exposure to your patient, your operating room team and yourself.

The final chapter in this Primer builds on the principles introduced in this one. But as this chapter ends, a seemingly glaring omission should be noticeable. This chapter has completely neglected one of the three values prominently displayed on the control panel: fluoroscopy time. In the realm of fluoroscopy, the time of the exposure will have the greatest impact on radiation dose. I have not omitted its discussion by accident. The goal of this chapter was to lay the foundation of fluoroscopy in a manner that will allow you to harness that understanding and apply it at the time of surgery. The goal of the next chapter is to give you the essentials to put that application to work. At the core of those essentials is time.

References

[1] Zaidi HA, Montoure A, Nakaji P, Bice A, Tumialan LMA. 5-year retrospective analysis of exposure to ionizing radiation by neurosurgery residents in the modern era. World Neurosurg. 2016; 86:220–225

[2] Abdullah KG, Bishop FS, Lubelski D, Steinmetz MP, Benzel EC, Mroz TE. Radiation exposure to the spine surgeon in lumbar and thoracolumbar fusions with the use of an intraoperative computed tomographic 3-dimensional imaging system. Spine. 2012; 37(17):E1074–E1078

[3] Van de Kelft E, Costa F, Van der Planken D, Schils F. A prospective multicenter registry on the accuracy of pedicle screw placement in the thoracic, lumbar, and sacral levels with the use of the O-arm imaging system and StealthStation Navigation. Spine. 2012; 37(25):E1580–E1587

[4] Tabaraee E, Gibson AG, Karahalios DG, Potts EA, Mobasser JP, Burch S. Intraoperative cone beam-computed tomography with navigation (O-ARM) versus conventional fluoroscopy (C-ARM): a cadaveric study comparing accuracy, efficiency, and safety for spinal instrumentation. Spine. 2013; 38(22):1953–1958

Bibliography

[1] Bushing SC. Radiologic Science for Technologist: Physics, Biology and Protection. 8th ed. St. Louis: Elsevier Mosby; 2004

[2] Halliday D, Resnick R. Fundamentals of Physics: Extended. 3rd ed. New York: John Wiley & Sons; 1988

[3] Masterton WL, Hurley CN. Chemistry: Principles and Reactions. Philadelphia: Saunders College Publishing; 1989

13 Minimizing Ionizing Radiation in Minimally Invasive Spine Surgery

Abstract
The minimally invasive spine surgeon of tomorrow will accomplish the same procedures performed today with a fraction of the radiation exposure. A sophisticated understanding of the origins of X-rays and the fundamentals of fluoroscopy will be the central tenets to achieving diminishing exposure to radiation in the coming years. The final chapter of this Primer builds upon the fundamentals introduced in the previous chapter and converts those basic science principles into practical techniques that you can apply immediately in the operating room. In this chapter, I review the principle of the inverse square law, the importance of radiation protection and different types of fluoroscopy before delving into low-dose applications of fluoroscopy in a variety of minimally invasive spine procedures. I conclude with speculation about the future of imaging for our spinal procedures. We will undoubtedly walk hand in hand with fluoroscopy for the foreseeable future, but the fluoroscope cannot remain static with the increasing amount of technology that surrounds us in our everyday lives. The coming years and decades promise changes in the imaging interface, flat panel detectors, image enhancement and navigation. Collectively, progress in each of these realms will continue to evolve to such a point that tomorrow's spine surgeons will gaze at a much higher-quality image of the spine obtained with radiation exposures so slight that we would consider them unimaginable by today's standards. The continued evolution of fluoroscopy in minimally invasive spine surgery begins with the desire to achieve the highest quality image at the lowest possible radiation exposure.

Keywords: ALARA, automatic brightness control, fluoroscopy, inverse square law, radiation exposure

Sit down before facts with an open mind. Be prepared to give up every preconceived notion. Follow humbly wherever and to whatever abyss Nature leads or you learn nothing. Don't push out figures when facts are going in the opposite direction.

Admiral Hyman G. Rickover

13.1 Introduction

All surgical procedures performed on the spine, minimally invasive or otherwise, require some form of radiographic imaging. Whether that imaging is cross-table radiography, fluoroscopy or intraoperative computed tomography (CT), radiation exposure is the inevitable consequence. Furthermore, in minimally invasive approaches, the absence of widely exposed anatomical landmarks by its very nature mandates another form of visualization. Before computer-assisted navigation, fluoroscopy assumed the role as an alternate form of visualization for spine surgery, but it rapidly took on a central role for minimally invasive spine surgery (MIS). As a result, radiation exposure was greater during minimally invasive procedures than during open procedures. At one point, greater radiation exposure seemed to be an unavoidable aspect of applying minimally invasive techniques.[1]

Perhaps the greatest detriment to the increased use of fluoroscopy that accompanied the rise of minimally invasive surgery during the early part of this century was that the increased use did not parallel a proportionate increase in knowledge about the fundamentals of fluoroscopy. There was no concerted effort to increase radiation awareness or training. As mentioned in the previous chapter, I finished a residency without the faintest idea of how a fluoroscope generated radiation or any formal training as to how to adequately protect myself from radiation. I was never issued a dosimeter. I have no idea as to the amount of radiation I was exposed to throughout my residency. Wasn't a lead gown all I needed?

Fluoroscopes are now ubiquitous both in residency training and in practice. Dosimeters are not. Although surgeons have acknowledged the greater radiation exposure with minimally invasive procedures, only recently has there been an appreciation for radiation exposure during residency training.[2] I noted my concern about the greater amount of radiation exposure associated with minimally invasive techniques at the beginning of Chapter 12. The current body of medical literature would certainly support that concern. The question now becomes what can we do about it.

My focus for this chapter is twofold. First, I want to discuss a framework in which you can decrease your exposure to radiation when you perform surgical procedures requiring a fluoroscope. Second, I would like to present alternate techniques for the fluoroscopic unit that will decrease the amount of radiation exposure. Chapter 12 provided the fundamentals of fluoroscopy that will make understanding alterations in voltage and current settings within the X-ray tube understandable. My overarching goal is for the pendulum to begin to swing in the other direction. I want surgeons to relinquish the idea that a minimally invasive technique necessitates more radiation exposure. I want the spine surgeons of tomorrow to replace that notion with the concept that they can perform minimally invasive surgical procedures with less radiation exposure than ever before.

This final chapter began with a quote from Admiral Hyman G. Rickover, the father of the nuclear navy. When the topic is radiation exposure and awareness, there may not be a better authority than Rickover. Again, it was my all-to-brief service in the nuclear navy as a diving medical officer and radiation health officer that led directly to my interest in the radiation exposure that can occur in minimally invasive approaches. Admiral Rickover transformed the diesel-powered U.S. Navy into a fleet of nuclear-propelled submarines and aircraft carriers. Perhaps his greatest legacy is the number of nuclear reactor accidents that have occurred among the 200 nuclear submarines and 23 nuclear-propelled aircraft carriers and cruisers commissioned since the birth of the nuclear navy with the launch of the *U.S.S. Nautilus* in 1954. That number is zero. Admiral Rickover created a culture of caution, awareness and precision when dealing with radiation and nuclear power. Perhaps grafting elements of Rickover's culture into MIS would be transformative. In previous chapters throughout this Primer, I examined the experience of master surgeons from decades ago to establish a basis for the various minimally invasive procedures we perform today. In a similar manner, I would like to reference Admiral Rickover's management objectives as a framework for a minimally invasive spine surgeon's work with radiation.

Rickover's management objectives:

- Require rising standards of adequacy.
- Be technically self-sufficient.
- Face facts.
- Respect even small amounts of radiation.
- Require adherence to the concept of total responsibility.
- Develop the capacity to learn from experience.

Over the years, I have often reflected on the admiral's quote that began this chapter as I listened to some of my colleagues disparage the importance of radiation awareness and summarily dismiss my efforts to minimize exposure. All the while, we are all becoming increasingly able to name spine surgeons who died too soon of cancer, including, most recently, one of my mentors from medical school who initially interested me in the study of the spine. I will readily concede that correlation does not imply causation, but it has become more and more difficult for me to dismiss the mounting evidence that there may be more to this story. The last sentence of Rickover's quotation has always lingered in my mind, "*Don't push out figures when facts are going in the opposite direction*." I saw my dosimeter readings from my time in a nuclear submarine juxtaposed with my dosimeter readings from when I performed minimally invasive spine procedures next to a fluoroscope. As much as I initially wanted to dismiss this inconvenient and pestering element of MIS, I found that I could not. I believe that when it comes to MIS and radiation exposure, we must heed the admiral's advice and follow the facts in the direction they are heading. We should respect even small amounts of radiation. We should push nothing aside, whether convenient or inconvenient to do so. We should strive to make ourselves technically self-sufficient with our understanding of fluoroscopy. Collectively, these efforts will raise the standards of adequacy regarding radiation exposure in MIS. The contents of this final chapter represent my lifelong efforts to adhere to the admiral's sage words.

13.2 As Low as Reasonably Achievable: The ALARA Principle

There is no safe dose of radiation. For this reason, the International Commission on Radiological Protection (ICRP) introduced a systematic approach to limit the radiation exposure to persons working with radiation. Our profession in MIS places us firmly in the category of radiation workers. Instead of focusing on a number or a dose, the central principle recommended by the ICRP is for each encounter with radiation to be as low as reasonably achievable (ALARA). The ALARA principle comprises three core elements: dose limitation, dose justification and dose optimization. Applying the ALARA principle in every surgery involving fluoroscopy is a central tenet for minimizing your exposure to ionizing radiation in spine surgery throughout your career.

13.3 Dose Limitation

13.3.1 The Inverse Square Law

When you strike the middle C key on a piano in an empty room, the sound waves travel outward from the source in all directions. The closer to the piano that you are standing, the louder the sound will be; the farther you are from the piano, the softer the sound. As those sound waves travel through space away from the piano, a geometric dilution occurs that results in the softer sound. If you double your distance from the piano, the intensity of the middle C note will decrease to one-fourth. If you halve the distance you are standing from the piano, the sound of that key stroke will have four times the intensity. The law that governs this phenomenon is known as the inverse square law:

$$\text{Intensity} \propto 1/r^2,$$

where r is the radius of a sphere and equal to the distance from the source.

This law of physics governs not only sound but also light and radiation. Therefore, the intensity of radiation is inversely proportional to the square of the distance from the source of the radiation. When the X-ray tube of a fluoroscope emits radiation for an image in surgery, the radiation travels through space from that point source just like the sound of the middle C key from the piano in the empty room. Geometric dilution occurs in an isotropic fashion as the radiation travels through space (▶ Fig. 13.1). The intensity of that radiation plummets as the distance from the source increases. The inverse square law is perhaps the most important principle you need to embrace when considering dose limitation. Whenever possible, always distance yourself as much as possible from the radiation source.

Radiation-Protective Apparel

At this point in the chapter, you might find it surprising to learn that the most important aspect of dose limitation is not wearing your apron or thyroid shield but wandering as far away as possible from the X-ray tube as it acquires an image. Still, the inverse square law does not supplant the importance of radiation protective apparel. Wearing radiation-protective gowns and thyroid shields is always inherent to dose limitation. Note that I have intentionally refrained from using the term *lead*, which has become the operating room vernacular for radiation-protective gowns and shields. In the interest of preserving the spines of persons who need to wear such apparel for hours at a time, manufacturers have developed lighter alternatives to leaded gowns, most of which contain no lead at all. Whether or not your radiation-protective gown contains lead, there are few better investments to make than to purchase your own radiation-protective gear, including a pair of radiation-protective glasses.

13.4 Dosimetry

I completed my residency without the faintest idea about the extent of my radiation exposure throughout my years of training. At that time, residents in my training program were not issued dosimeters. However, had it not been for the dosimeter

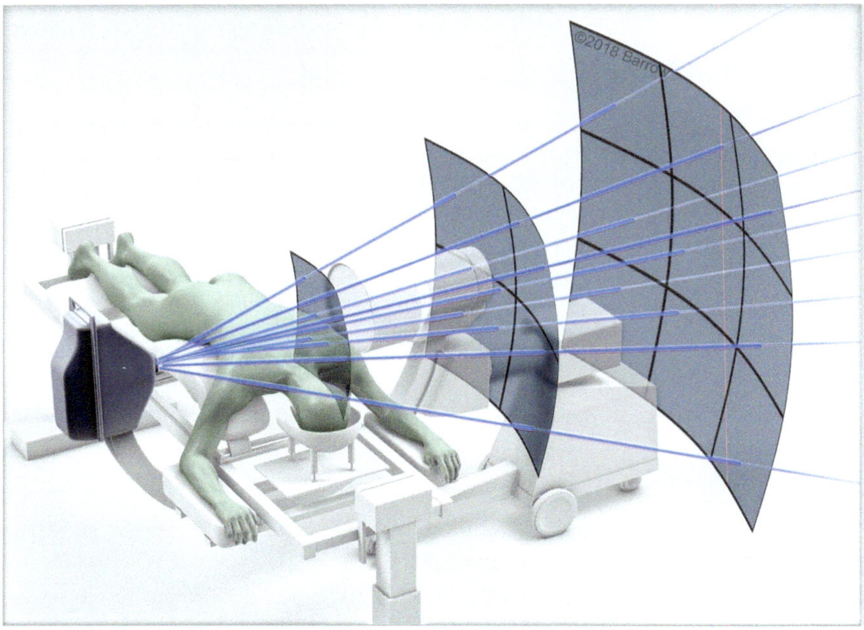

Fig. 13.1 Illustration showing the geometric dilution that occurs with radiation as the distance from the X-ray source increases. At three times the distance from the source, the dose of radiation is one-ninth of the exposure at the source. Standing on the side of the table next to the X-ray tube exposes the surgeon to a higher dose of radiation than standing on the side of the table next to the image intensifier. The inverse square law is one of the central tenets to follow to minimize your exposure to ionizing radiation throughout your career.

the Navy issued me upon my arrival at the Naval Hospital in San Diego, I would never have been able to juxtapose those dosimetry readings with my dosimetry readings aboard the *U.S.S. Buffalo*, a fast-attack nuclear submarine. Without that glaring difference in those data points, my concern about radiation exposure would never have arisen. In the absence of those data, I would never have conceived of a need to compose the final two chapters in this Primer. A dosimeter provides valuable data regarding radiation exposure. Knowledge of the data increases awareness and potentially changes behavior. Every surgeon exposed to radiation, whether in training or in practice, should have access to a dosimeter. The decision to wear and monitor that dosimeter is ultimately left to the surgeon, but the capacity to monitor exposures must be there.

The purpose of the dosimeter is to monitor exposure in the absence of a radioprotective garment. For this reason, the dosimeter should be worn outside the apron or thyroid shield. As I learned from my time in the Navy, a dosimeter is only worth the data that you can extract from it. Wearing a dosimeter does not in and of itself ward off the downstream consequences of radiation exposure. Ideally, the data from the dosimeter are collected and recorded on a quarterly basis and on an annual basis. You should strive to decrease radiation exposure year after year in your practice. Accomplishing this task would be impossible without having those values laid out before you.

13.5 Collimation

In Chapter 12, I explained how an X-ray tube generates X-rays that then make their way through the patient to the image intensifier to generate an image. What I did not explain is that those X-rays that leave the X-ray tube do not all make it across the patient. In fact, they have one of three fates: they will pass directly through the patient, they will become completely absorbed by the patient or they will interact with tissue and bone to reflect and scatter. Those X-rays that pass directly through the patient with no interaction are directly responsible for contributing to the image of the spine that appears on the screen. The appropriate title assigned to these X-rays is image-forming X-rays. Obviously, the X-rays that are completely absorbed by the patient contribute nothing to the image. The X-rays that reflect and scatter, a phenomenon known as Compton interaction, take away from the image. Scattered X-rays decrease the contrast and result in a grainy appearance to the image. Even more important is that the reflected and scattered X-rays contribute to the radiation exposure to the surgeon and operating room staff. That radiation exposure is obviously greatest for persons standing on the side of the X-ray tube where the beams reflect from the patient immediately onto the surgeon and other operating room staff; it is significantly less for persons standing on the side of the image intensifier (▶ Fig. 13.2).

In a perfect world, only the X-rays that pass through the patient with no interaction would be the ones that reach the image intensifier. But complete absorption and Compton scatter are an inevitable consequence of X-rays interacting with matter. Thus, we are faced with creating an environment wherein we optimize image-forming X-rays that contribute to the image while minimizing scattered X-rays that take away from the image. One way to optimize the image-forming X-rays and to minimize the scattered X-rays is to narrow the field of radiation. The term used to describe this is *collimation*.

Collimation is the process by which shutters within the fluoroscope narrow the field of view, analogous to an aperture on a camera limiting the light that enters the lens (▶ Fig. 13.3). The

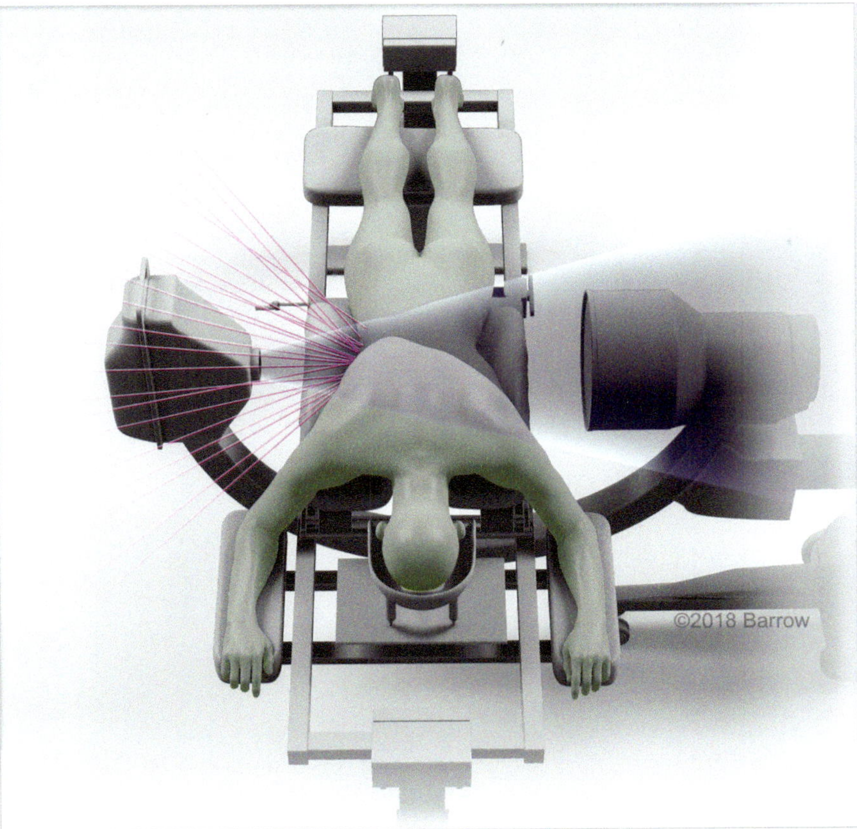

Fig. 13.2 The Compton effect. As X-rays interact with matter, they have one of three fates: (1) they pass through the patient and contribute to an image of the spine, (2) they become absorbed by the patient or (3) they strike the patient and scatter. The illustration demonstrates the Compton scatter of X-rays that can contribute to a surgeon's radiation exposure. Scattered X-rays provide no useful information on the radiograph but instead reduce the image contrast. Compton scatter is yet another reason the radiation exposure is highest on the side of the X-ray tube.

result of collimating an X-ray beam is twofold. First, a collimated X-ray beam decreases the surface area of the patient exposed to radiation, sparing unnecessary exposure to adjacent tissue. Second, the less of the patient's volume that is exposed to the X-ray beam, the less scatter there will be of X-ray incident to the detector. Reducing Compton scatter improves image contrast. The net result is less radiation exposure to the patient, less X-ray scatter to the surgeon and operating room personnel and a high proportion of image-forming X-rays. Collimating the X-ray beam will result in less radiation and a higher-quality image. As a rule, I always collimate to the smallest field of view for the segment. The capacity to collimate an image is available in almost all commercially available fluoroscopes.

13.6 Justification

Each time that you decide to acquire an image, you should be looking for information that can be provided only by a fluoroscopic image. For instance, for the placement of pedicle screws through an expandable minimal access port, the fluoroscopic image need not identify the pedicle screw entry point. Rather, it should confirm the pedicle screw entry point you have identified by your exposure of the anatomical landmarks. There is a difference. The goal is to shift your reliance away from fluoroscopy and toward direct visualization, which is the basis of my argument against percutaneous techniques. When you have direct visualization of the anatomy, the three-dimensional anatomy of the spine that you reconstruct in your mind is more valuable than any fluoroscopic image that can be acquired. After you have clearly visualized the anatomical landmarks and established the entry point, a fluoroscopic image is of value in confirming the entry point and establishing the ideal trajectory into the pedicle.

Confirmation of the operative segment is one instance in which the fluoroscopic image is the only modality that can provide the information needed to move the operation forward. However, subsequent images are of limited value. I have watched residents and fellows acquire image after image when doing nothing more than passing a dilator onto the spine at the same location for a microdiscectomy, a laminectomy or an instrumented fusion, whereas one image of the initial dilator was all that was needed until the insertion of the minimal access port. Those additional images were unnecessary because they provided no actionable information to justify taking them. I have also watched those same residents and fellows request an image with every quarter-turn of the tap. When I ask them what it is they are looking for, I have yet to hear a satisfactory answer. Once you have probed a pedicle and established a trajectory into that pedicle with a fluoroscopic image, no further imaging is necessary until the threads of the tap are buried and you would like to determine the optimal length for the pedicle screw. As noted in Chapter 4 on transforaminal lumbar interbody fusion (TLIF), after capturing an image with the instrument in the ideal position, I maintain that position relative to the blades of the minimal access port as the instrument

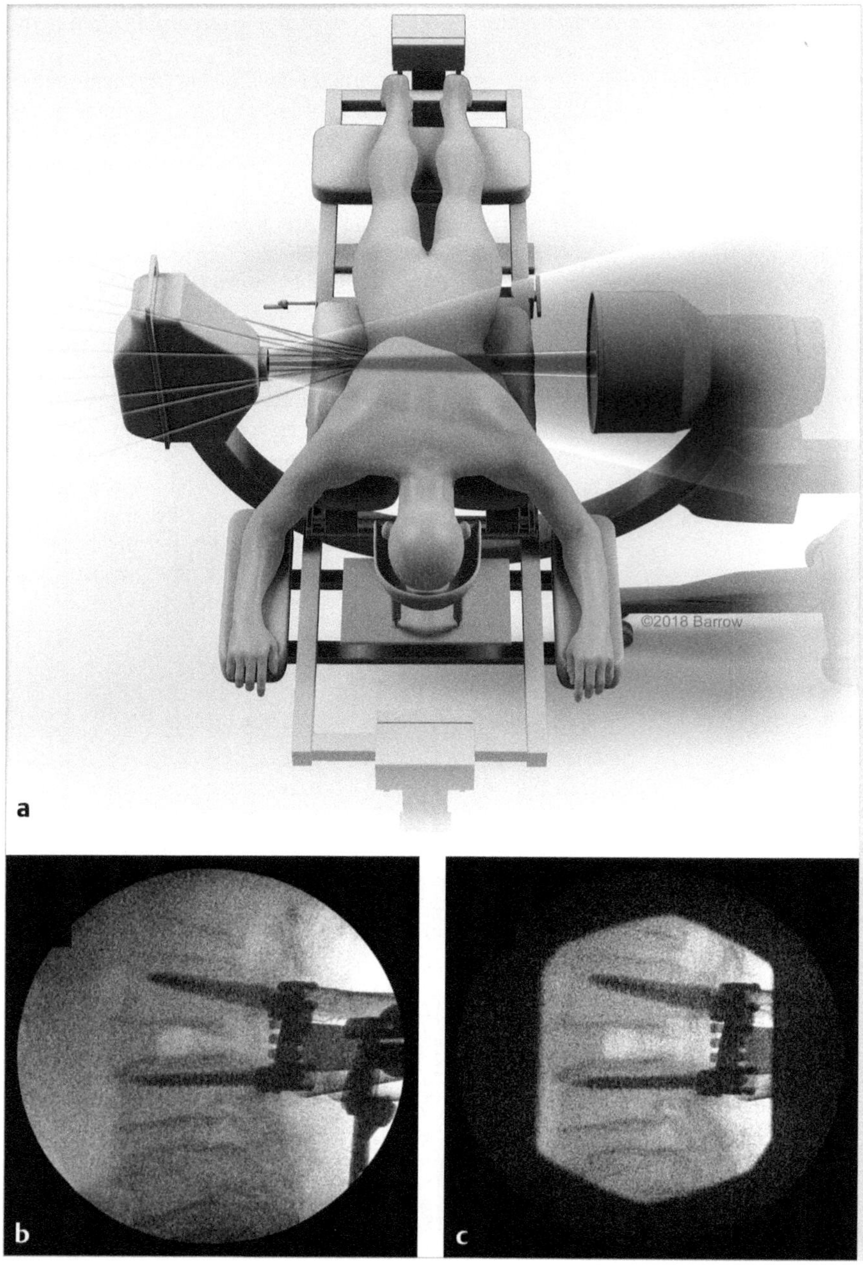

Fig. 13.3 Collimation of the useful X-ray beam. Shutters within the X-ray tube of the fluoroscope are used to decrease the exposure to adjacent tissues. **(a)** The illustration shows the decrease in Compton scatter. The reduced Compton scatter decreases radiation exposure on the side of the X-ray tube. The result is a higher-quality image at a lower radiation dose. **(b)** A lateral fluoroscopic image of a minimally invasive lumbar fusion without collimation. **(c)** The same lateral fluoroscopic image using a collimated beam. The reduction in Compton scatter sharpens and brightens the image while decreasing radiation exposure to the surgeon from the scatter off the patient. Both images were acquired at the same kVp and mA.

advances. If that position remains unaltered, subsequent images do not provide actionable information. However, an image with the threads buried will provide valuable information to help you determine the length of the pedicle screw that is needed. Images of the tap advancing along the same trajectory through the pedicle are of limited value and are not in keeping with the justification component of the ALARA principle.

It goes without saying that the safety of the patient should be your first and foremost concern. You need to acquire the imaging that is required to perform the procedure safely. I will readily acknowledge that the initial part of the minimally invasive learning curve does involve heavy reliance on fluoroscopy. Over time, however, as you develop the capacity to reconstruct the anatomy in your mind's eye, it is essential to transition to mission-essential fluoroscopy. In keeping with the theme of raising levels of adequacy, minimizing the number of fluoroscopic images for every surgical procedure (minimally invasive or otherwise) should be a central theme in your practice. The capacity to do more in surgery with less fluoroscopic guidance is a skill all its own and, as such, should be actively developed. The tactile sense of a dilator or the direct visualization of the anatomy can replace the void that a fluoroscopic image would otherwise fill. Before acquiring each image, ask yourself what information you are looking for and what you will do with that information. Justification for every image in every instance over time, and certainly over a career, is essential to reducing radiation exposure.

13.7 Percutaneous Pedicle Screws

The inability to directly visualize the anatomy while placing pedicle screws percutaneously mandates imaging at every step of the placement. When computer-assisted navigation guides the percutaneous placement of a pedicle screw, radiation exposure to the surgeon and the operating room staff becomes a moot point. However, in the absence of image guidance, radiation exposure begins to rise. The published literature documents a range of 22 to 29 seconds of fluoroscopy with a dose of up to 10.3 mREM per percutaneous screw in experienced hands.[3,4] Furthermore, the very nature of the procedure mandates the surgeon's proximity to the X-ray source, holding instruments, thereby limiting the capacity to harness the inverse square law to the surgeon's advantage. The inevitable consequence is exposure to greater amounts of radiation exposure for fluoroscopic placement of percutaneous pedicle screws compared to that for pedicle screw placement using direct visualization of anatomical landmarks with intermittent fluoroscopic guidance. Coupled with the inability to directly visualize the facets for a Smith–Petersen osteotomy or the transverse processes for a posterolateral fusion, this greater radiation exposure has made it increasingly difficult for me to use percutaneous screws for single-level and two-level fusions.

13.8 Optimization

In 1984, Wesenberg and Amundson[5] published one of the first articles detailing a low-dose protocol for the use of fluoroscopy. Their focus was the radiation exposure in children undergoing diagnostic imaging. At the root of their concern were the radiation doses and fluoroscopy times required for specific procedures (e.g., cardiac catheterization, cystourethrograms and upper gastrointestinal evaluations). Wesenberg and Amundson wanted to reduce these radiation exposures because of the inherent risk of radiation causing subsequent malignancies in growing children. Their 1984 manuscript begins with a thoughtful sentence that is still as relevant today for MIS as it was then for pediatric imaging: "the goal of diagnostic radiology is to make the most accurate diagnosis with the least amount of radiation and risk to the patient ... this is particularly applicable to pediatric radiology."[5]

Over the years, subsequent authors continued to develop techniques to minimize radiation exposure while still providing adequate diagnostic imaging for children. The pediatric cardiology literature was especially focused on this topic.[6,7] What is striking as one juxtaposes the pediatric radiology literature and the MIS literature during the same period is how diametrically opposed were the trajectories on the same topic. Pediatric radiologists kept documenting remarkably reduced exposures, whereas minimally invasive spine surgeons kept publishing reports of the exact opposite.[3,6,7,8,9] As the concern about radiation exposure in minimally invasive spinal procedures became a barrier to the application of the techniques, taking a page out of the pediatric radiology playbook was the logical step forward. In fact, when spine surgeons finally applied the well-honed fluoroscopy protocols from the pediatric radiology literature, radiation exposure and fluoroscopy times both decreased significantly without compromising the safety of the procedure.[10,11]

The remainder of this chapter focuses on exploring these low-dose protocols in the context of the final element of the ALARA principle: optimization. In the upcoming pages, I will discuss the techniques that pediatric radiology has used for decades to decrease radiation exposure with fluoroscopy. Applying these protocols will require an understanding of the types of fluoroscopy and especially the importance of acquisition time. Incorporating your understanding of peak kilovoltage (kVp) and milliampere (mA) into these protocols will serve as a background to help you harness these parameters to your advantage. You will discover that doing nothing more than altering the fluoroscopic technique or manually adjusting the kVp and mA will have a direct impact on both the radiation exposure required for each image and the quality of that image. In imaging the spine for minimally invasive spine procedures, we would do well to adopt the same attitude that Amundson and Wesenberg had more than three decades ago toward pediatric patients. Striking a balance between radiation exposure and image quality is the essence of optimization.

13.9 Types of Fluoroscopy

Let us return to the operating room, where you are waiting for the fluoroscopy technologist to turn on the fluoroscope so that you can begin a procedure. When the technologist finally plugs in the fluoroscope and turns it on, software begins to load in the central processing unit (CPU) and the thoriated tungsten filament begins to warm up, preparing for the surge of voltage coming its way. As the progress arrows populate the screen, the fluoroscopy algorithms are loaded. These are written in a manner so that when it is finally time to hit the button and obtain an image, the kVp and mA will automatically be determined such that the result will be an optimal image with ideal brightness and contrast. The type of fluoroscopy that accomplishes this ideal image is known as continuous interlaced fluoroscopy, or just continuous fluoroscopy. It is the default setting that happens simply by turning on the fluoroscope. In all likelihood, this setting is the one you have been using all along for your operations.

Continuous fluoroscopy offers a reliable image without having to manipulate any of the parameters. As the name implies, the X-ray beam is continuous. When the technologist pushes the button, that continuous X-ray beam generates 30 images per second that become interlaced to create the composite image. The kVp and the mA are initially determined by an algorithm within the CPU. The automatic brightness control (ABC) further adjusts these parameters using the patient's size through a feedback mechanism. A sensor inside the image intensifier monitors the brightness. When the brightness of the image is inadequate because of the size of the patient, the ABC algorithms increase the kVp first. The result is an increase in the number of projectile electrons striking the tungsten target, which, in turn, increases the number of diagnostic X-rays. The net increase in the number of higher-energy X-rays results in a greater proportion of X-rays that can better penetrate the body and serve as image-forming X-rays. The cervical spine has narrower dimensions than the lumbar spine, so the need for penetration is less. As a result, imaging in the cervical spine requires a lower kVp.

After the CPU establishes the kVp, the algorithm increases the mA. An increased tube current will increase the number of electrons striking the target and result in a greater total number of X-rays. The net result is a brighter image. Since these ideal images rendered by continuous fluoroscopy are contingent on the completion of the feedback loop, the result is a 1- to 3-second acquisition time per image. The first image that is obtained will typically have the longest acquisition time as the feedback loop optimizes the brightness and contrast by adjusting the kVp and mA. After the ABC has optimized the image quality, subsequent images will have shorter acquisition times, provided the fluoroscopy unit has not been moved. If you move the fluoroscope and the thickness of the patient changes, the ABC feedback loop will have to complete, which will again extend the acquisition time.

When you consider an acquisition time that ranges from 1 to 3 seconds per image, the total fluoroscopy time and exposure have the potential to quickly add up. For example, if you were to obtain 40 images throughout an instrumented lumbar fusion case using this technique, fluoroscopy times would range from 40 to 120 seconds, which is well within the reported range of fluoroscopy times for minimally invasive fusions.[4,8,12] Many authors have understandably considered that amount of radiation exposure to be a liability and, for obvious reasons, it has become one of the main criticisms of minimally invasive techniques. One approach to dealing with radiation is to use computer-assisted navigation, which can decrease radiation exposure.[3] Another approach is to use the alternative fluoroscopy technique introduced by pediatric radiologists. Fully embracing that decades-old technique alone can quickly dispel those criticisms.

13.10 Pulsed Fluoroscopy

The less time the X-ray beam is on, the less radiation exposure will occur to the patient, the surgeon and the operating room personnel. Two simple modifications to the settings on the fluoroscope will accomplish this task. The first step is to turn off the ABC. The absence of this control eliminates the feedback loop and the additional seconds of radiation exposure that are required to complete the loop. However, it also excludes the algorithm that automatically determines the ideal kVp and mA to optimize the image. Disabling the ABC is equal parts asset and liability. Every image will be acquired at the default kVp and mA settings. The drawback may be the need to manually increase or decrease these values to view an adequate image. The advantage is a substantial decrease in radiation exposure. Working closely with your radiology technologist to determine these settings will allow you to acquire an adequate image at the lowest amount of radiation exposure.

The second modification is to intermittently turn off the X-ray beam during image capture. Instead of having a continuous beam for image capture, turning the X-ray beam on and off will decrease the amount of radiation exposure. Such a setting is known as pulsed fluoroscopy (▶ Fig. 13.4). X-ray beam pulsation obviously decreases radiation exposure, but it also decreases image quality. Two key parameters guide X-ray beam pulsation: pulse width and pulse rate. The pulse width is the duration of the pulse itself, specifically how long the X-ray beam is on for image capture before turning it off. A shorter pulse width has the obvious advantage of less radiation, but it also limits the number of X-rays that contribute to image formation. The fewer the number of image-forming X-rays penetrating a patient, the lower the quality of the image and the lower the radiation exposure.

The pulse rate is the number of fluoroscopic image frames that are generated per second. For imaging a static subject, such as the spine, the pulse rate is less important. High pulse rates are necessary to study anatomy in motion, such as the assessment of diaphragmatic motion, a cardiac valve, or esophageal motility. The phenomenon known as temporal resolution is crucial for studying anatomy in motion. Since our subject matter is the motionless spine, there is little need for temporal resolution. Therefore, lowering the pulse rate will not have a significant effect on the image of a static subject. Applying the pulsed fluoroscopy setting will dramatically reduce radiation exposure for surgical procedures on the spine.[10] The combination of turning off ABC with pulsed fluoroscopy will further reduce radiation exposure by decreasing acquisition time in addition to the dose per frame. The trade-offs for these low doses and short acquisition times are the quality and the sharpness of the image. The concepts of pulse width and pulse rate are demonstrated in the accompanying video (Video 13.1).

13.11 Acquisition Time and the Digital Spot Technique

An analogous scenario to continuous fluoroscopy and even to pulsed fluoroscopy would be taking a photograph using your smartphone. Instead of the photo option, you select the video option. With activation of the video capture, the camera begins by focusing on the subject. The sensors provide feedback mechanisms within the smartphone camera to adjust the brightness and the contrast of the image before finally rendering the perfect image. Over the span of 3 seconds of video, the very last few milliseconds have perfect contrast, brightness and focus. Continuous interlaced fluoroscopy renders an image in a similar manner. The reality is that we do not use most of the footage. The final frame is all that we actually view, but the first few seconds are necessary because of the process of acquiring the image. The adjustments that occur in brightness, contrast and focus occur in the first few moments of image acquisition. For that single image, the acquisition time was quite long, and the number of frames captured for that final few milliseconds of footage was quite high. The logical question is why we would want to acquire a static image in this manner. Why would we not use the photo option with the instantaneous acquisition of a single frame?

Remarkably, the process described earlier is exactly how most of us use conventional fluoroscopy as we operate on the spine. Images created with continuous fluoroscopy default to

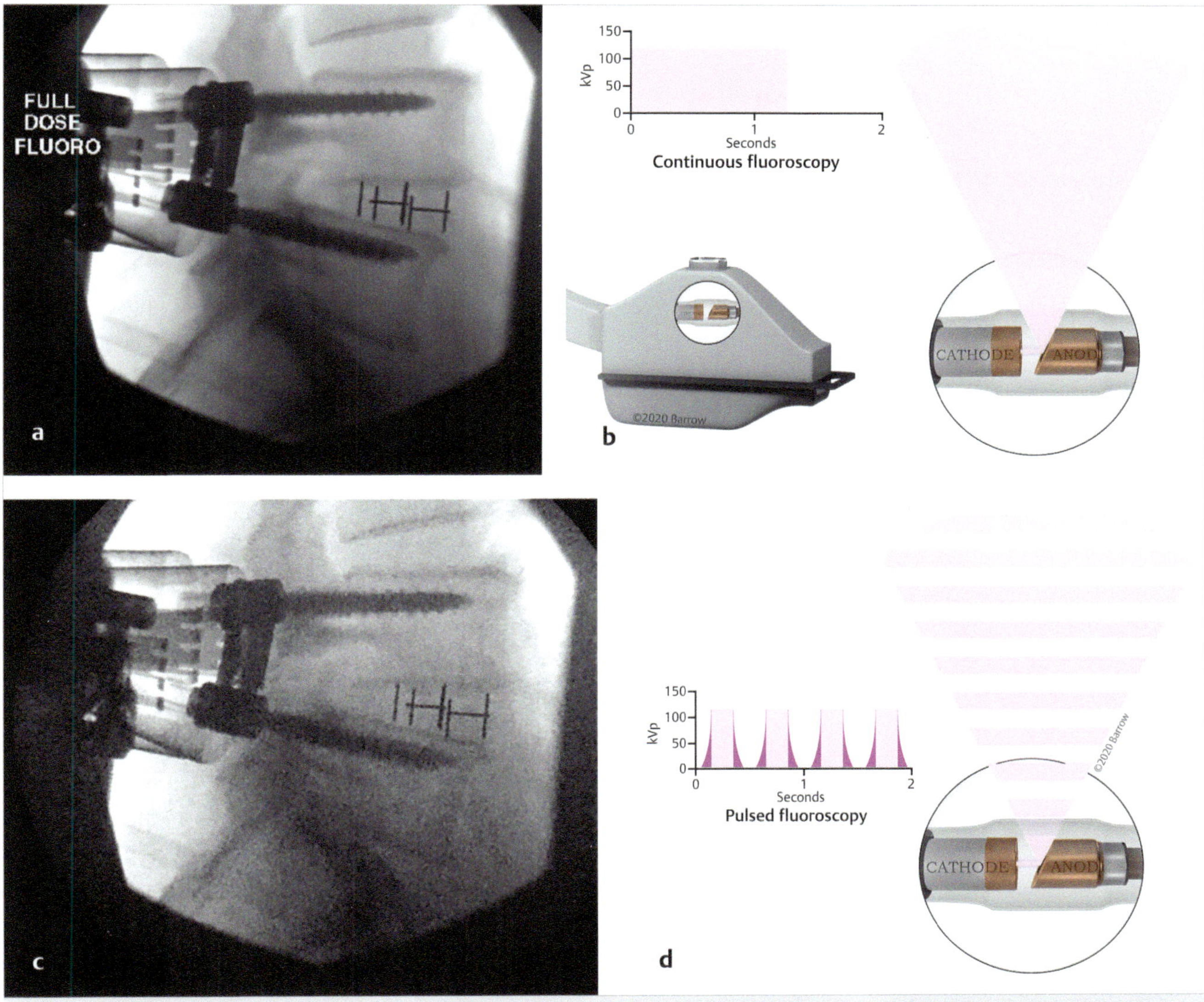

Fig. 13.4 Conventional fluoroscopy compared to pulsed fluoroscopy. **(a)** Lateral fluoroscopic image at the completion of a lumbar fusion captured at 118 kVp and 5.48 mA using conventional fluoroscopy. Conventional fluoroscopy acquires 30 frames per second to create the composite image. Acquisition time for this image was 1.2 seconds, indicating that more than 30 frames contributed to the image. **(b)** Graphical representation of radiation exposure when using conventional fluoroscopy. **(c)** A pulsed fluoroscopic image of the same region of the spine obtained at 114 kVp and 2.44 mA with a pulsed X-ray beam. Although the quality of the image is lower, the resolution of the anatomy is more than adequate for instrumentation and interbody placement. The acquisition time was 0.15 seconds. Pulsed fluoroscopy produced adequate images with less radiation in one-tenth of the time required for conventional fluoroscopy. **(d)** Graphical representation of radiation exposure when using pulsed low-dose fluoroscopy.

the "last image hold," which is the image that remains on the screen when the ray beam turns off. That image is the integration of multiple frames. The radiation exposure for that last image hold is the number of frames times the radiation exposure for the acquisition of those frames.[13] In reality, we are capturing hundreds of unnecessary frames in a video format to obtain one static composite image at the end of a feedback mechanism. Along the way, we are increasing our exposure to radiation. Instead, our goal should be to capture an image of the spine with the fewest frames and with the shortest possible acquisition time. Thus, our real goal should be to take an image of the spine with a photo setting instead of a video setting.

However, there is a reason why fluoroscopy obtains 30 frames per second to generate an image. The amount of noise in an image is inversely proportional to the square root of the number of photons used to acquire that image. As noted in Chapter 12, the number of photons that create an image is proportional to the number of diagnostic X-rays striking the image

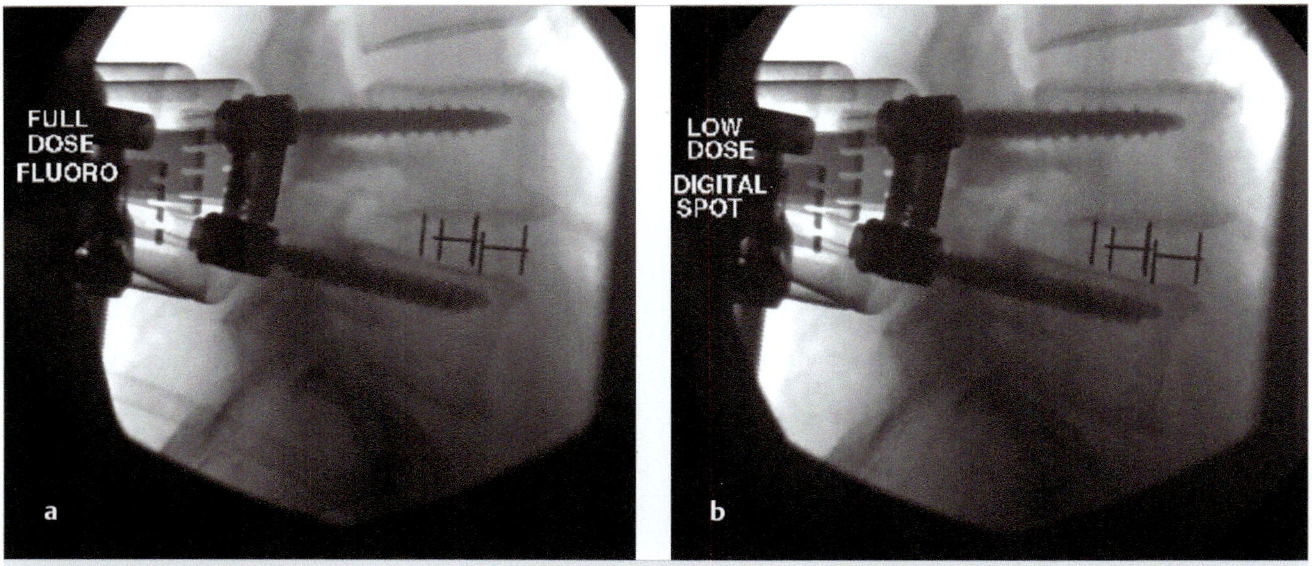

Fig. 13.5 Conventional fluoroscopy compared to digital spot fluoroscopy. **(a)** The same lateral conventional fluoroscopy image from ▶ Fig. 13.2 at the completion of a lumbar fusion captured at 118 kVp and 5.48 mA. Conventional fluoroscopy acquires 30 frames per second to create the composite image. Acquisition time for this image was 1.2 seconds, which indicates that more than 30 frames contributed to the image. **(b)** The same lateral fluoroscopic image obtained with a digital spot technique. Acquisition time was 0.15 seconds, with 120 kVp and 21.60 mA. Although the dose is significantly higher, the image is captured as a single frame. These two images are almost indistinguishable in brightness, contrast and sharpness. However, the acquisition time is significantly shorter for the digital spot technique.

intensifier. Because of the internal lag characteristics of the human eye–brain response, a real-time sequence of an image generated at 30 frames per second is perceived with much less noise than a single static fluoroscopic image. In other words, the composite image of three to five frames of fluoroscopy will appear sharper and brighter than a single frame of fluoroscopy.

Digital spot imaging solves the problem of acquisition time and the need to create a composite image (▶ Fig. 13.5). It is the equivalent of taking a photograph with the photo setting instead of the video setting. Digital spot images are immediate exposures, but the consequence of taking a single exposure is that the process requires a much higher dose of radiation than that required for a single frame of fluoroscopy. However, it is a single frame captured at a low acquisition time (typically, 0.15 seconds) with much better image quality and resolution than a pulsed fluoroscopy image. Although there is a considerable amount of radiation in a single digital spot, it must be balanced with the number of frames acquired to have an equivalent view of the anatomy with fluoroscopy. When viewed in that context, digital spot images can compare quite favorably, especially when a sharper image is needed for instrumentation.

13.12 Bringing It All Together

These fluoroscopic techniques and our newfound knowledge about radiation are meaningless if they cannot be translated to routine use in the operating room. After all, the end goal of this chapter is to provide you with the tools required to reduce your radiation exposure over the span of your entire career. The only way to create a sustainable practice that will minimize radiation is a team-based approach to fluoroscopy. The most essential element is to identify a group of radiology technologists at your hospital who will commit to working with you and will commit to learning and applying these various alternative fluoroscopic techniques to reduce radiation exposure. As with any novel technique, there will be a learning curve. However, as with the learning curve for minimally invasive techniques, it will be a worthwhile investment in time. You will no doubt be genuinely surprised at the knowledge possessed by the radiology technologists and their willingness to help you achieve lower radiation exposure. In my experience, radiology technologists self-select. Those with a true understanding of the fundamentals of fluoroscopy and an understanding of your vision will be drawn to working with you and will help you accomplish your goals. At the same time, those with little interest will make themselves less available for your cases. Without such a team, your understanding of the workings of the fluoroscope and minimizing radiation will remain trapped inside your brain and not fully put into practice. In the introductory chapter of this Primer, I emphasized the importance of the minimally invasive ensemble, in which nurses, scrub technicians and radiology technologists all work in unison with full knowledge of the procedure to move the operation forward. Minimizing the exposure of ionizing radiation to your patients, your operating room team and yourself requires a radiology technologist who can play a central role. Thus, it is essential for you to recruit a reliable cadre of radiology technologists for your spine procedures.

As you begin to incorporate these low-dose techniques, always ask yourself how much detail you truly need on an image to safely perform an operation. From this standpoint, every surgeon will have a different perspective, and the most important factor is patient safety. Surgeons should obtain images at the quality they require to confidently confirm the anatomy of the spine. Many surgeons would agree that a grainy image is more than adequate for localization of a level, but that a sharper image will perhaps be needed to confirm pedicle screw entry points or to place an interbody spacer. Adjusting the quality of the image to the appropriate phase of the operation is consistent with striking a balance between radiation dose and image quality. In reality, no surgeon requires the highest quality image at the highest dose of radiation for every component of an operation. Applying that mindset toward fluoroscopy is an essential first step to reducing your lifetime dose of radiation.

At the beginning of an operation, a digital spot fluoroscopic image or a full-dose conventional fluoroscopic image will ensure the appropriate alignment of the pedicles. The wag of the C-arm can be adjusted with these higher-quality images to ensure a perfect lateral. After the C-arm is optimally positioned, the fluoroscopic technique can be altered to use the lowest dose per image that maintains an adequate quality to visualize the anatomy (▶ Fig. 13.6 and ▶ Fig. 13.7). For these initial higher-dose images, there is no reason not to create as much distance between yourself and the X-ray source as possible. My preference is to retreat to the corner of the operating theater for these initial localizing images.

Once the fluoroscope is in the ideal position to obtain a high-quality localization image, it will begin to capture images in a pulsed low-dose technique, with the ABC turned off. Once again, the caveat to turning off the ABC is that the radiology technologist will have to manually adjust the kVp and mA to the lowest dose that provides an adequate image. Manually setting these parameters is an investment in time and exposure. Once they are set, you will be able to acquire 20 images per second of pulsed fluoroscopy without the ABC. As demonstrated in ▶ Fig. 13.4 and ▶ Fig. 13.8, a low-dose pulsed setting is more than adequate for dilating onto the facets or through the psoas muscle and then securing the minimal access port.

As the operation proceeds, higher-quality images will at times be necessary. Whether to ensure sharp end plate images for interbody placement or to confirm a pedicle screw entry point, transitioning back and forth from pulsed low-dose images to digital spot images will result in higher-quality images as needed while minimizing radiation for images not requiring precise visualization of the anatomy, such as the trajectory of a tap. ▶ Fig. 13.9a demonstrates a digital spot image with the pedicles sharply delineated by the decreased noise provided by the increased radiation exposure. After confirmation of the entry point, returning to a noisier image (▶ Fig. 13.9b) is adequate for probing, tapping and securing the pedicle screw into the pedicle.

13.13 Case Illustrations

The purpose of the following case illustrations is to review the application of low-dose fluoroscopy. In each case, I emphasize the number of images obtained for the procedure, the fluoroscope settings, the fluoroscopy time and the radiation exposure. My purpose in providing these details is to demonstrate the use of this protocol across several distinct procedures on the spine and to show the impact it has on radiation exposure.

13.14 Microdiscectomy and Laminectomy

The focus of radiation exposure among surgeons and in the literature has been on minimally invasive instrumented lumbar

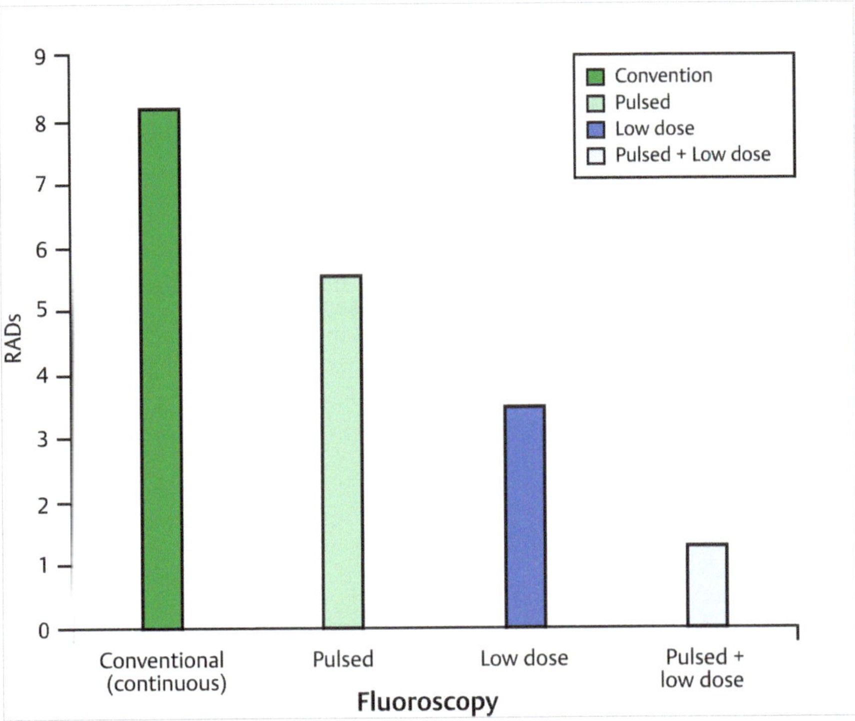

Fig. 13.6 The radiation absorbed dose for the various forms of fluoroscopy. This graph demonstrates a decreasing dose from conventional fluoroscopy to pulsed low-dose techniques per image captured. Over the span of your career, the impact on total radiation absorbed dose can be an order of magnitude less with low-dose techniques. Abbreviation: RAD, radiation absorbed dose. (Modified with permission from Vetter S, Faulkner K, Strecker EP, Busch HP. Dose reduction and image quality in pulsed fluoroscopy. Radiat Prot Dosimetry. 1998; 80(1-3):299–301.)

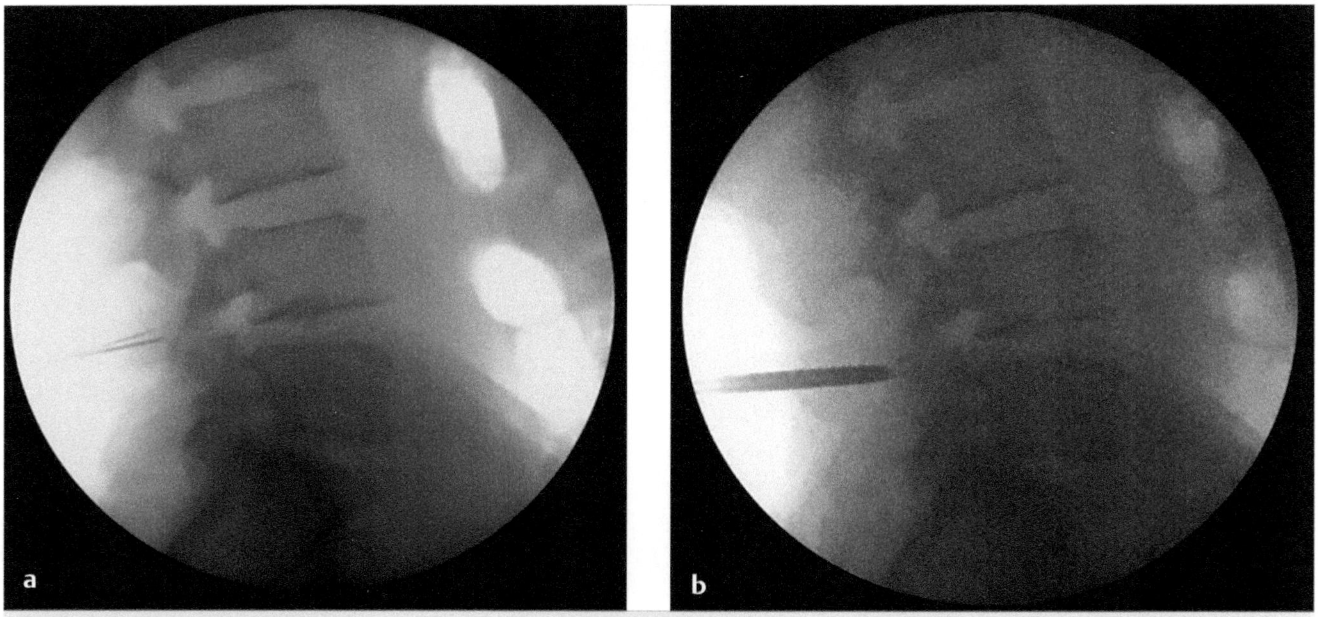

Fig. 13.7 Comparison of digital spot fluoroscopy and pulsed fluoroscopy without automatic brightness control. **(a)** Digital spot fluoroscopy was used to localize the level for an L4–5 minimally invasive transforaminal lumbar interbody fusion. Although the acquisition time for this image was low, the radiation exposure remained high. The quality of the image provides sharpness to the anatomy, which allows ideal configuration of the fluoroscopy unit, specifically for alignment of the pedicles. However, such a high-quality image is not necessary for dilating through the muscle or for securing retractors. **(b)** A pulsed fluoroscopic image with automatic brightness control turned off to decrease the acquisition time. The anatomy is clearly visible, especially with the juxtaposition of the localizing digital spot image **a** for comparison. With the quality of the pulsed fluoroscopic image, the operation can safely proceed with the next steps of dilating the paraspinal muscles and securing the retractors.

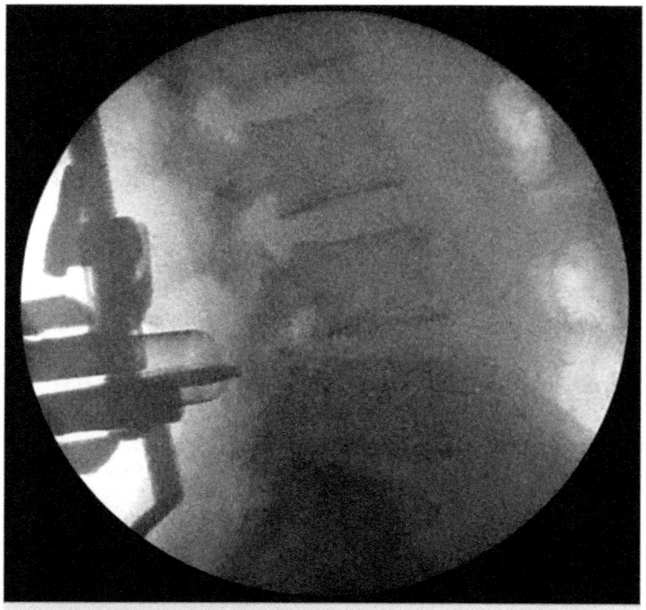

Fig. 13.8 Lateral fluoroscopic image with pulsed fluoroscopy for dilation and docking of the minimal access ports. The kVp and mA are minimized to the point that the image is degraded but remains acceptable. At such a setting, 40 images are obtained in less than 3 seconds of total fluoroscopy time and, most importantly, with less than 10 mGy of radiation for the entire case.

fusions. But the radiation exposure in a minimally invasive microdiscectomy is not inconsequential. Published reports clearly demonstrate a substantial increase in radiation exposure in minimally invasive microdiscectomies over their open equivalents.[1] The difference is understandable when you consider that securing the minimal access port with the ideal trajectory requires the surgeon to be close to the X-ray source, whereas in an open approach, the surgeon can fully embrace the inverse square law and wander as far away as possible from the source after a Penfield dissector has been placed at the segment. In my estimation, the minimally invasive microdiscectomy is not only the perfect gateway procedure into the minimally invasive arena, but it is also the ideal procedure for which to begin applying low-dose radiation protocols.

With the patient positioned for surgery, I have the fluoroscope parked in the lateral position at the level of the patient's knees. I do not obtain any preoperative images. Instead, I will palpate the intraspinous process space that corresponds with the anterior superior iliac spine and mark my incision from that presumptive L4–5 level. I drape the fluoroscope sterilely into the field and begin by passing a 20-gauge spinal needle onto the lumbar spine, always using a trajectory that diverges from the intralaminar space. When I encounter the lamina, I obtain my first fluoroscopic image. Since the needle will stay put, I can embrace the inverse square law and wander away from the X-ray source.

The fluoroscope is set to "pulsed" and "low dose." At first, I keep the ABC on so that I can determine a reasonable value for the kVp and mA. After I obtain an adequate image, I turn off the

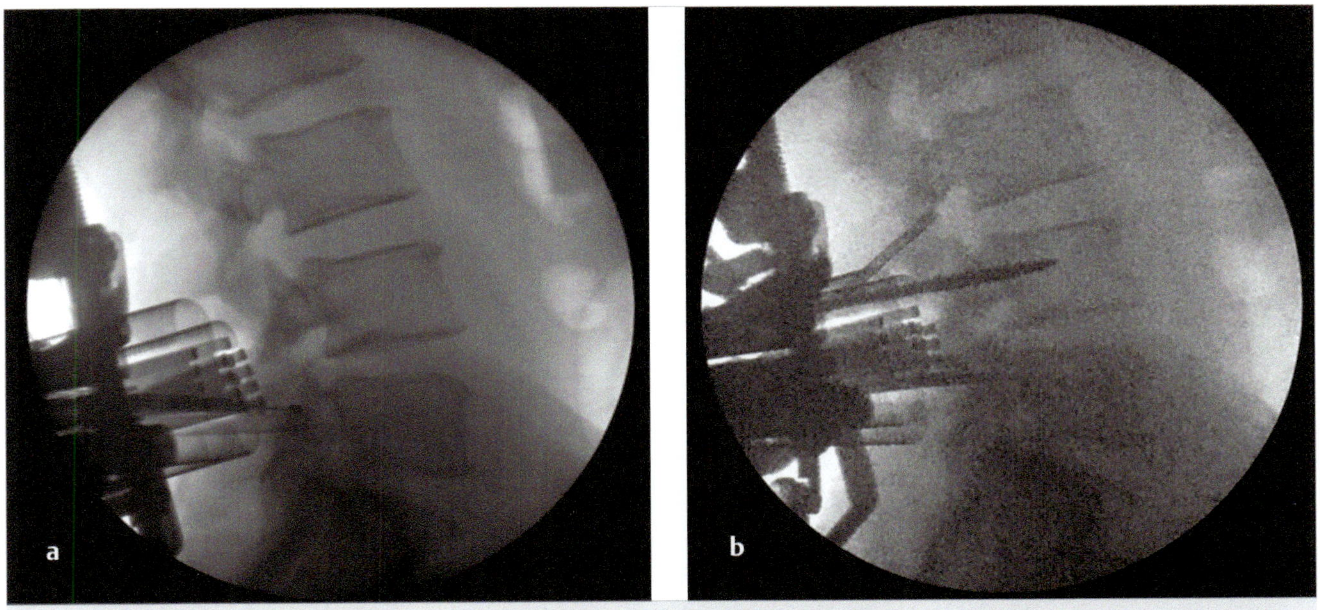

Fig. 13.9 Alternating the use of digital spot fluoroscopy and pulsed fluoroscopy. (a) A digital spot image is used to confirm an entry point identified by direct visualization of the anatomy. The higher radiation exposure decreases the noise and provides a sharp image of the pedicle. Once the entry point has been identified and confirmed, (b) a noisier image is adequate for establishing the trajectory of the probe or the tap into the pedicle.

ABC. From there, I manually adjust the kVp and mA down to achieve an adequate image at the lowest possible radiation. For example, for the microdiscectomy depicted in ▶ Fig. 13.10, the first image confirms my level and trajectory for the incision. A pulsed low-dose image at 113 kVp and 2.3 mA generates a grainy but adequate image (▶ Fig. 13.10a). These values are inherently linked with the dimensions of the patient. In this case, the patient had a body mass index (calculated as weight in kilograms divided by height in meters squared) of 32. I can now turn off the ABC and decrease my acquisition time for each subsequent fluoroscopic image. The spinal needle has a suboptimal trajectory, and I adjust it and obtain another image (▶ Fig. 13.10b). I have now adjusted my incision so that I have an ideal trajectory to the disc space. Next, I infiltrate a local anesthetic along the tract of the spinal needle and make my incision. After opening the fascia with cautery, I pass the first dilator, palpate the spine and secure the dilator firmly at the lamina facet junction. I will obtain another confirmatory image of the level before proceeding with the remaining dilators (▶ Fig. 13.10c). I will complete the dilatation process and secure the minimal access port without any additional images. The two final images are a lateral image to confirm my trajectory parallel to the disc space, and an anteroposterior image to ensure adequate convergence (▶ Fig. 13.10d, e). Since the retractor arm is securing the minimal access port for both images, I fully embrace the inverse square law once again and wander away from the X-ray source. The total fluoroscopy time for securing the minimal access port was 0.9 seconds. More importantly, the radiation dose was 1.04 mGy to obtain the five images. The sequence is identical for a minimally invasive laminectomy.

13.15 Anterior Cervical Approaches

I find the complete absence of any concern about radiation exposure in anterior cervical procedures genuinely mystifying. I have observed that the same surgeons who have demonstrated a heightened awareness of radiation exposure in minimally invasive approaches seem to have no mindfulness of their exposure in anterior cervical approaches. The surgical literature further reflects this lack of concern, as not one manuscript examining anterior approaches and radiation exposure has been published to date. It is as if the absence of a minimal access port absolves us of any hazard of radiation in an anterior cervical discectomy and fusion (ACDF). I will readily concede that the procedure is not as dependent on fluoroscopy as other minimally invasive procedures. Furthermore, radiation exposures are lower because of the nature of the anatomy of the cervical region compared to the lumbar spine. But the combination of these two elements still does not make the exposure zero. The reality of the situation in anterior cervical approaches is that spine surgeons use more fluoroscopy in the cervical spine than they realize. Collecting and analyzing my own data on radiation exposure for anterior cervical approaches was truly enlightening. I would encourage the reader of this chapter to do the same. Although these exposures may be lower than those for lumbar minimally invasive approaches, in keeping with the ALARA principle, there is no reason not to make every effort to decrease radiation exposures for this approach as much as you would for any minimally invasive lumbar approach. The following case illustration represents an effort to do just that.

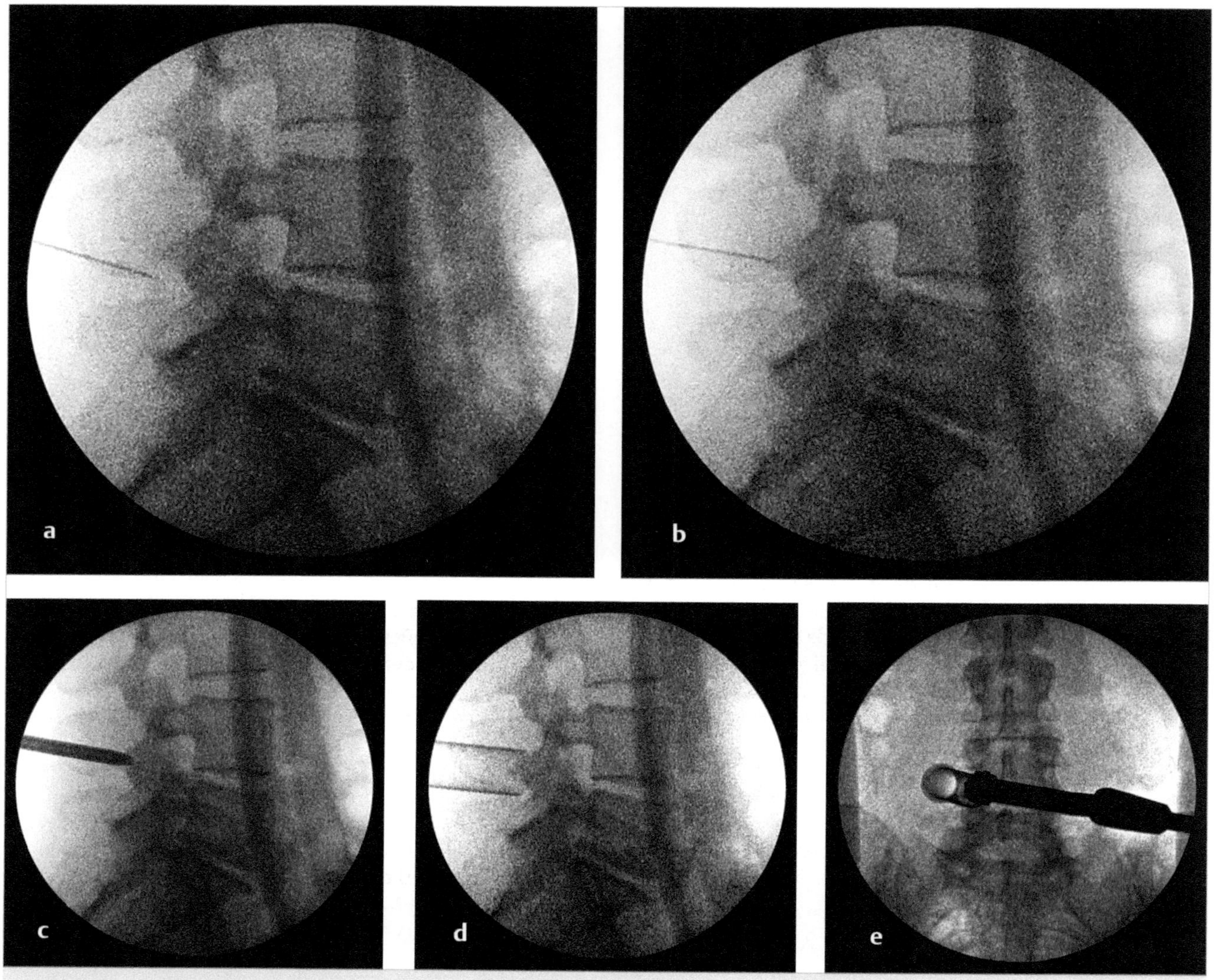

Fig. 13.10 Pulsed low-dose fluoroscopy sequence for microdiscectomy. **(a)** Lateral fluoroscopic image with a localizing spinal needle obtained with pulsed fluoroscopy at 113 kVp and 2.3 mA. Although a low-resolution image is the result, it is more than adequate for localization. With these settings established, the automatic brightness control can be turned off to decrease acquisition time. **(b)** Lateral fluoroscopic image with spinal needle repositioned to optimize the trajectory onto the lumbar spine. **(c)** Lateral fluoroscopic image of the first dilator onto the lamina facet junction. Once confirmed with imaging, the dilator remains anchored in position, precluding the need for subsequent images as the dilators traverse onto the spine. **(d)** A final lateral fluoroscopic image confirms the minimal access port in an ideal position. **(e)** Optional anteroposterior image confirms adequate convergence with kVp and mA set to lower values because an anteroposterior image has less body mass to traverse.

The first question that I have asked myself as I have tried to minimize radiation exposure in anterior cervical approaches is what images I require to perform the procedure. The list in ▶ Table 13.1 represents what I believe to be the least number of images (and the maximum) for a single-level ACDF. Note that it identifies the steps of the ACDF when imaging is required to move the operation forward.

I list the localization process as requiring two images, one image to plan the incision and the other to confirm the level after the exposure (▶ Fig. 13.11). As mentioned in Chapter 9, I do not use a spinal needle for localization, not only because reports have demonstrated accelerated degeneration in the punctured disc but also because of the highest standard of all: if it were my cervical disc, I would prefer that it not be punctured if it were not the level to be operated upon. Holding a Kittner dissector over the disc space requires me to be close to the X-ray source and therefore unable to embrace the inverse square law. In a similar manner, observing the standard of placing the Caspar posts completely perpendicular to the back wall and less than halfway up the vertebral body requires at least one image per post placement.

Confirmation of an interbody trial does not require the surgeon to be close to the X-ray source and thus provides an opportunity to embrace the inverse square law. After securing the interbody trial, wander away from the source for the image. Tapping the interbody spacer into position may require an image to ensure that it is countersunk, but not overly so. Again, there is no need for the surgeon to be near the X-ray source for this image.

Placing the shortest plate that will be a minimum of 5 mm from the disc space above and below will at times require a

Table 13.1 Mission-essential fluoroscopy for a single-level ACDF

Radiographic objective	Minimum no. of images	Maximum no. of images
Localization	2	2
Insertion of Caspar post	2	2
Interbody trial (inverse square law)	2	4
Insertion of interbody spacer	2	4
Placement of plate	0	2
Final images: AP and lateral (inverse square law)	2	2
Total	10	16

Abbreviations: ACDF, anterior cervical discectomy and fusion; AP, anteroposterior.

lateral image to confirm an appropriate variable angle and to match that same angle for the second screw. ▶ Fig. 13.12a demonstrates a variable angle drill guide in position and an image obtained to confirm an appropriate angle into the vertebral body. After I have placed that variable angle screw, I will obtain another image with the variable angle drill guide in position to match the angle (▶ Fig. 13.12b). The final anteroposterior and lateral fluoroscopic image do not require the surgeon to be near the X-ray source (▶ Fig. 13.12c).

For this case, I obtained 10 images using pulsed low-dose fluoroscopy. I captured the initial image using ABC and the subsequent image without ABC at settings of 65 kVp and 0.53 mA. All images were captured in 2.1 seconds of fluoroscopy at a dose of 0.52 mGy.

13.16 Lateral Transpsoas Interbody Lumbar Fusions

The transpsoas approach to the lumbar spine requires more images, and with the surgeon closer to the X-ray source, than any other procedure in minimally invasive spine surgery. Although computer-assisted navigation can eliminate a surgeon's radiation exposure, it cannot correct for the inevitable shift of the spine that occurs during surgery when working within the interbody space. Some of the worst-appearing interbody spacers I have secured have been done with navigation. The need to localize the level, confirm a precise location in the anteroposterior and lateral planes within the disc space, release the contralateral annulus, trial the interbody size and secure the interbody spacer are all steps that are image dependent. Radiation exposure can therefore quickly spiral out of control unless a conscious effort is made to minimize that exposure.

Deconstructing the procedure and identifying the mission-essential fluoroscopy, similar to what was done in the preceding ACDF example, will begin the systematic process of distilling those points in surgery when fluoroscopic guidance is justified to advance the operation. Having collected the number of images that I have obtained at the various phases of the operation over the past several years, I have been able to approximate a range for the number of images needed throughout the various phases of a transpsoas operation. The first column of ▶ Table 13.2 identifies those points in the procedure where I need an image to advance the procedure. The second and third columns provide a range for those radiographic objectives to be met. I fully recognize that no two cases are alike. Some single-level degenerative cases may be straightforward, whereas other complex deformity cases may be challenging. Patient safety is the most important aspect of the surgery, and thus whatever imaging is needed to perform the procedure safely is the priority. The following case illustration delineates the mission-essential images for the management of adjacent segment degeneration at L3–4, above the level of an L4–S1 fusion.

Table 13.2 Mission-essential fluoroscopy for a single-level lateral transpsoas interbody lumbar fusion

Radiographic objective	Minimum no. of images	Maximum no. of images
Preoperative AP and lateral optimization (inverse square law)	10	20
Preoperative incision planning	4	8
Traversing the psoas, placing Kirschner wire and placing minimal access port	5	10
Division of contralateral annulus	3	5
Interbody trials	5	10
Placement of interbody spacer	3	5
Final AP and lateral images (inverse square law)	2	4
Total	32	62

Abbreviation: AP, anteroposterior.

13.17 Preoperative Image Optimization and Incision Planning

In the transpsoas approach, imaging begins with the patient in the optimal position for planning the incision. Every effort should be made to position the patient perfectly lateral on the operating table and then to secure the patient firmly in that position to minimize movement. Any movement of the patient that occurs after achieving the optimal position will result in the need for additional images and adjustments in the operating table. The importance of locking in that position should be communicated both to the nursing staff and to our anesthesia colleagues, because it can only be accomplished with more tape than either of those two parties is accustomed to using. A well-secured patient will result in more efficient imaging, a more efficient surgery, and therefore less radiation exposure.

By convention, I refrain from using the terms "anteroposterior" and "lateral" throughout transpsoas cases because of the potential confusion that those terms can cause to the radiology technologist, the operating room team and me. We are all accustomed to the horizontal position of the C-arm generating a lateral image and the vertical position of the C-arm generating an anteroposterior image. The lateral position of the patient reverses the image generated by the horizontal and lateral

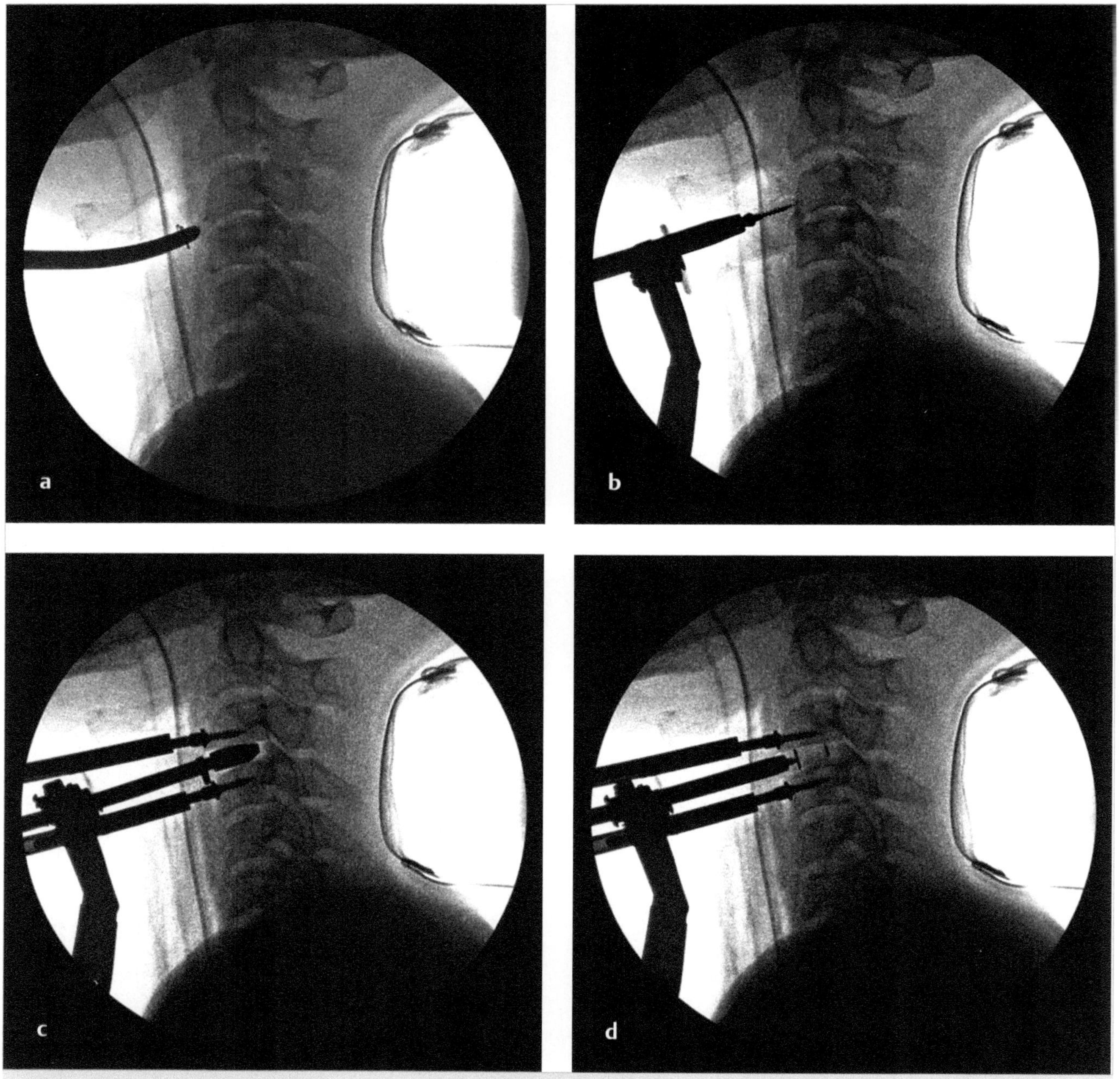

Fig. 13.11 Sequence of pulsed lateral fluoroscopic images. (a) Localization with a Kittner dissector. (b) Placement of a Caspar post. (c) Assessing an interbody trial. (d) Placement of the interbody graft. Although all these images are granular, they are more than adequate for providing the surgeon with information to continue with the procedure.

positions of the C-arm. To eliminate any potential misunderstanding by the operating room team, I use the terms "horizontal" and "vertical" when requesting images throughout the case (▶ Fig. 13.13).

It is an investment to obtain ideal horizontal (anteroposterior) and vertical (lateral) images from the outset (▶ Fig. 13.14).

It can take anywhere from 10 to 20 images to accomplish this task, depending on the degree of deformity. If I find myself having to rotate the bed too much to obtain the ideal horizontal (lateral) image, the patient is not optimally positioned on the operating table and I will release all the tape and begin repositioning the patient with the bed back in the neutral position. On a good day, I can obtain the ideal horizontal (anteroposterior) image with crisp end plates and well-aligned pedicles with minimal adjustment of the operating table and then rotate the C-arm into the horizontal position for the vertical (lateral) image, which should demonstrate the spinous process equidistant from the pedicles along with crisp end plates. Although it may require 10 to 20 images to accomplish this objective (▶ Table 13.2), there is no need to be anywhere near the X-ray source while obtaining these images. Use the inverse square law to your advantage during this phase of the operation.

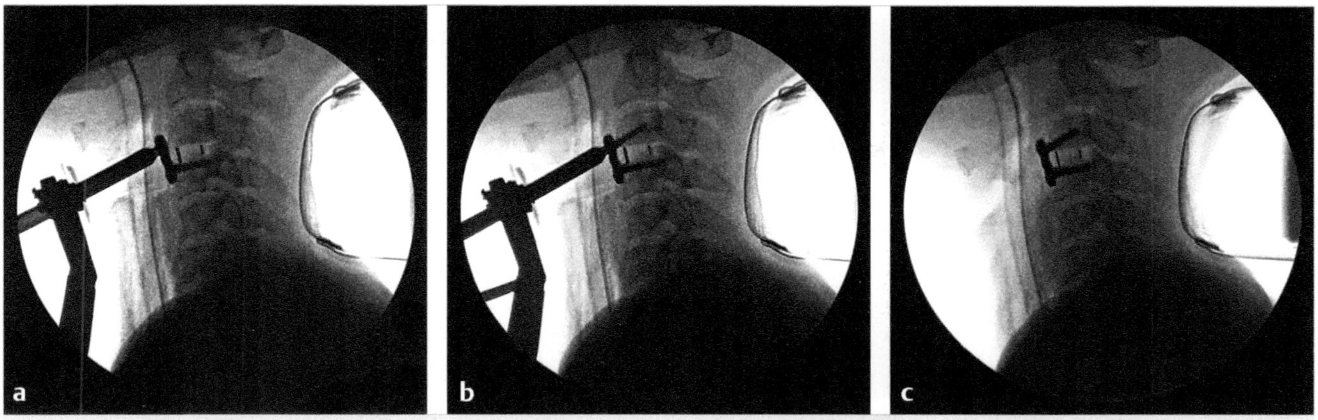

Fig. 13.12 Fluoroscopic images for securing the cervical plate. (a) Lateral pulsed low-dose fluoroscopic image used to establish the trajectory of a variable-angle screw in order to use the shortest plate. (b) The angle is matched for the other screw with the guide in position and another lateral pulsed low-dose image. (c) Final lateral pulsed low-dose image obtained while embracing the principle of the inverse square law.

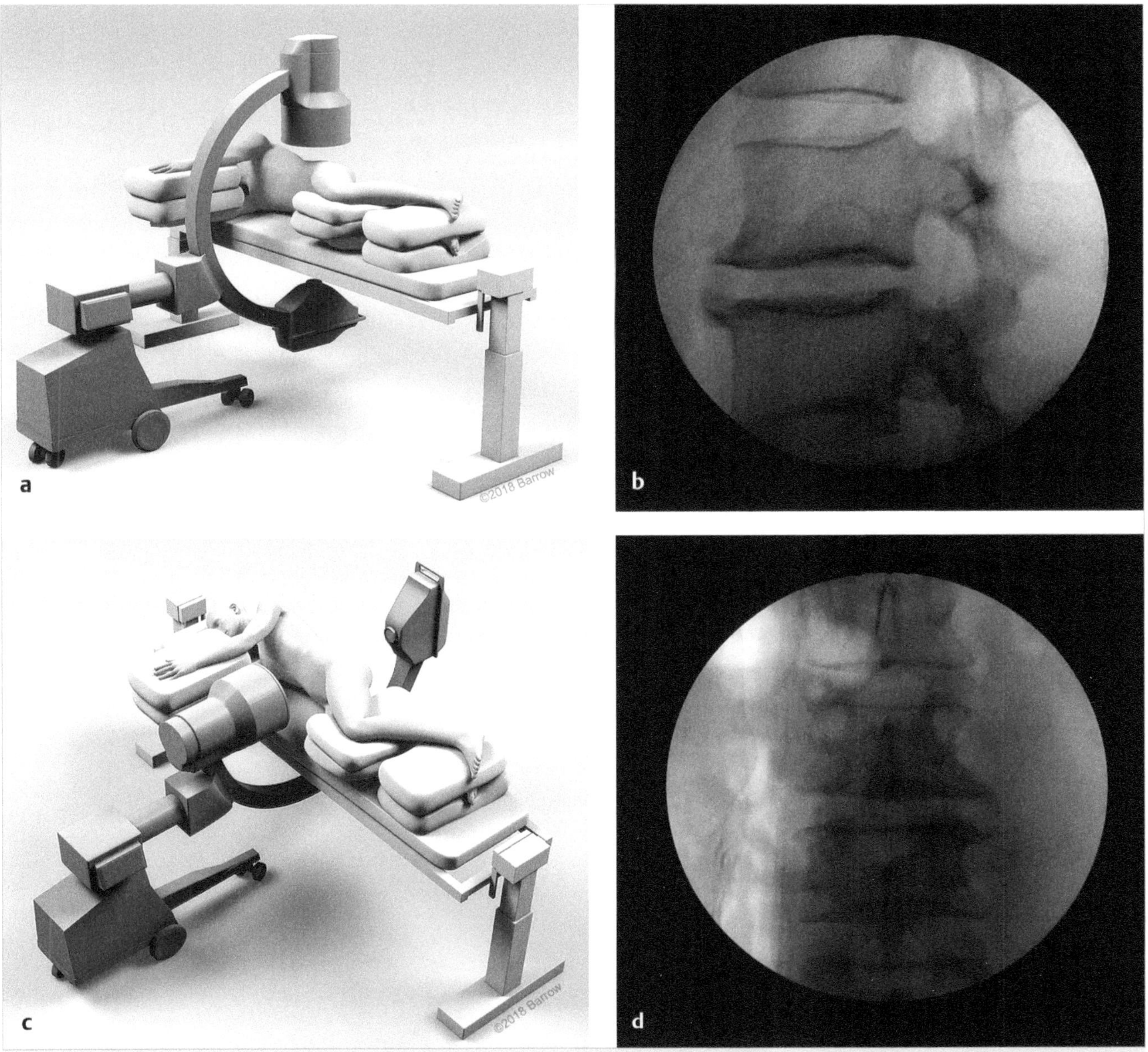

Fig. 13.13 Models illustrating the vertical and horizontal positions of the fluoroscope in transpsoas cases relative to the patient's position. (a) The vertical position of the fluoroscope provides (b) a lateral image, whereas (c) the horizontal position provides (d) an anteroposterior image. A patient who is prone with the fluoroscope in these same positions results in the opposite views.

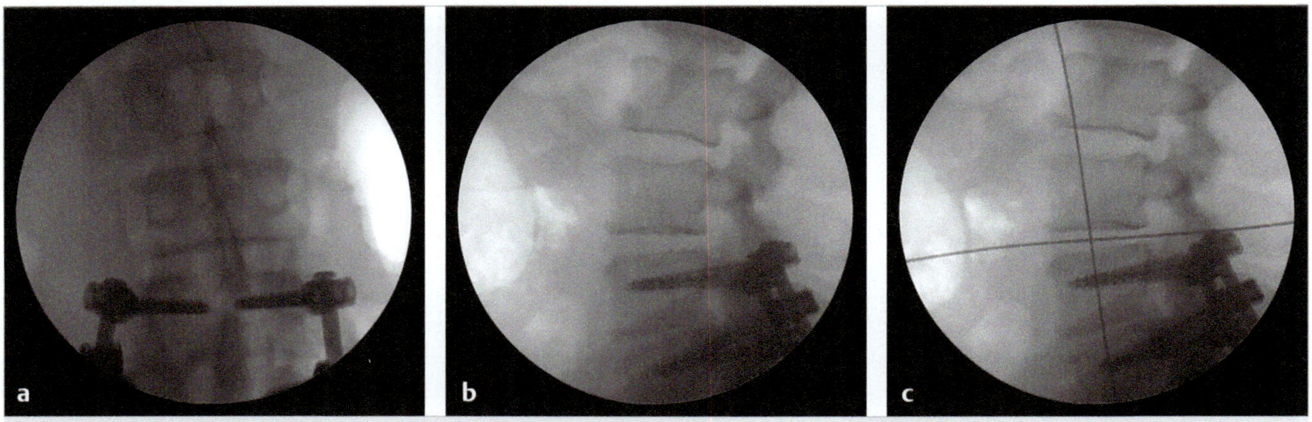

Fig. 13.14 Preoperative incision planning with fluoroscopy. **(a)** Ideal horizontal (anteroposterior) image also using pulsed low-dose fluoroscopy. **(b)** Ideal vertical (lateral) fluoroscopic image obtained with pulsed low-dose fluoroscopy. It will require several images to obtain the ideal lateral image. **(c)** The incision site is marked using a vertical (lateral) fluoroscopic image, with one Kirschner wire used to mark the L3–4 disc space and one to mark the long axis of the spine.

13.18 Traversing the Psoas and Securing the Minimal Access Port

With the patient and the fluoroscope in position for the ideal images, the surgery can proceed, with the next series of images to confirm the level, traverse the psoas and enter the disc space. This series of steps may be accomplished with as few as five images but may require as many as 10. Horizontal (anteroposterior) and vertical (lateral) imaging confirm the ideal position of the introducer, and then dilatation of the psoas may proceed along with placement of the minimal access port (▶ Fig. 13.15).

13.19 Release of the Contralateral Annulus

Once I have identified a safe corridor through the psoas, I can perform the majority of work with direct visualization and without the need for fluoroscopy. Developing the corridor with a bayoneted Penfield dissector and retracting the psoas with a nerve root retractor allow for direct exposure of the annulus, incision of the annulus, beginning the discectomy and preparation of the end plates. No additional fluoroscopic images will be needed until the release of the contralateral annulus (▶ Fig. 13.16).

The release of the contralateral annulus is primarily a tactile step, but visual confirmation with a fluoroscopic image is valuable. With the discectomy complete, a Cobb elevator may be placed up against the contralateral annulus and the release accomplished by tapping the Cobb with a mallet through the insertion. As mentioned in Chapter 6, there is an unmistakable sensation of release that occurs. Visual confirmation is valuable, which justifies an image. The superior and inferior insertions are both released, resulting in two additional images.

13.20 Trial and Placement of Interbody Spacer

The only need for fluoroscopy during these phases of the operation is to ensure the trajectory of the interbody spacer (▶ Fig. 13.17). As a result, only 5 to 10 images will be necessary, depending on the number of trials. If the appropriate trial is selected from the outset, then the number of images will be closer to five. If multiple trials are used to determine the size of the ideal interbody, then the number of images will be closer to 10. An additional one or two images at this phase is of value because where the trial goes, the interbody will follow. Ensuring a perfect trajectory into the disc space is an investment. Once the trial is in position, take advantage of yet another opportunity to embrace the inverse square law.

The placement of the interbody requires as few as three images to ensure an ideal trajectory and optimal placement across the disc space. In my experience, the range has been three to five images (▶ Fig. 13.18).

The final horizontal and vertical (anteroposterior and lateral) images may be obtained after removal of the minimal access port and before closure. I have abandoned obtaining a horizontal (anteroposterior) image with the minimal access port in position unless I believe that it has drifted far from where I secured the trial. My experience time and time again has been that wherever I secured the trial will be the final resting place of the interbody. Here is yet another opportunity to save another image or two. I will retreat as far away from the X-ray source as sterility will allow for the final two images, and with that, the fluoroscopic component of the operation is complete (▶ Fig. 13.19).

The above case illustration was completed with 4.8 seconds of fluoroscopy but, more importantly, with only 8.16 mGy at 88 kVp and 9 mA with pulse settings at 8 pulses per second. The operation was completed with 36 images, well within the range of what was predicted by ▶ Table 13.2.

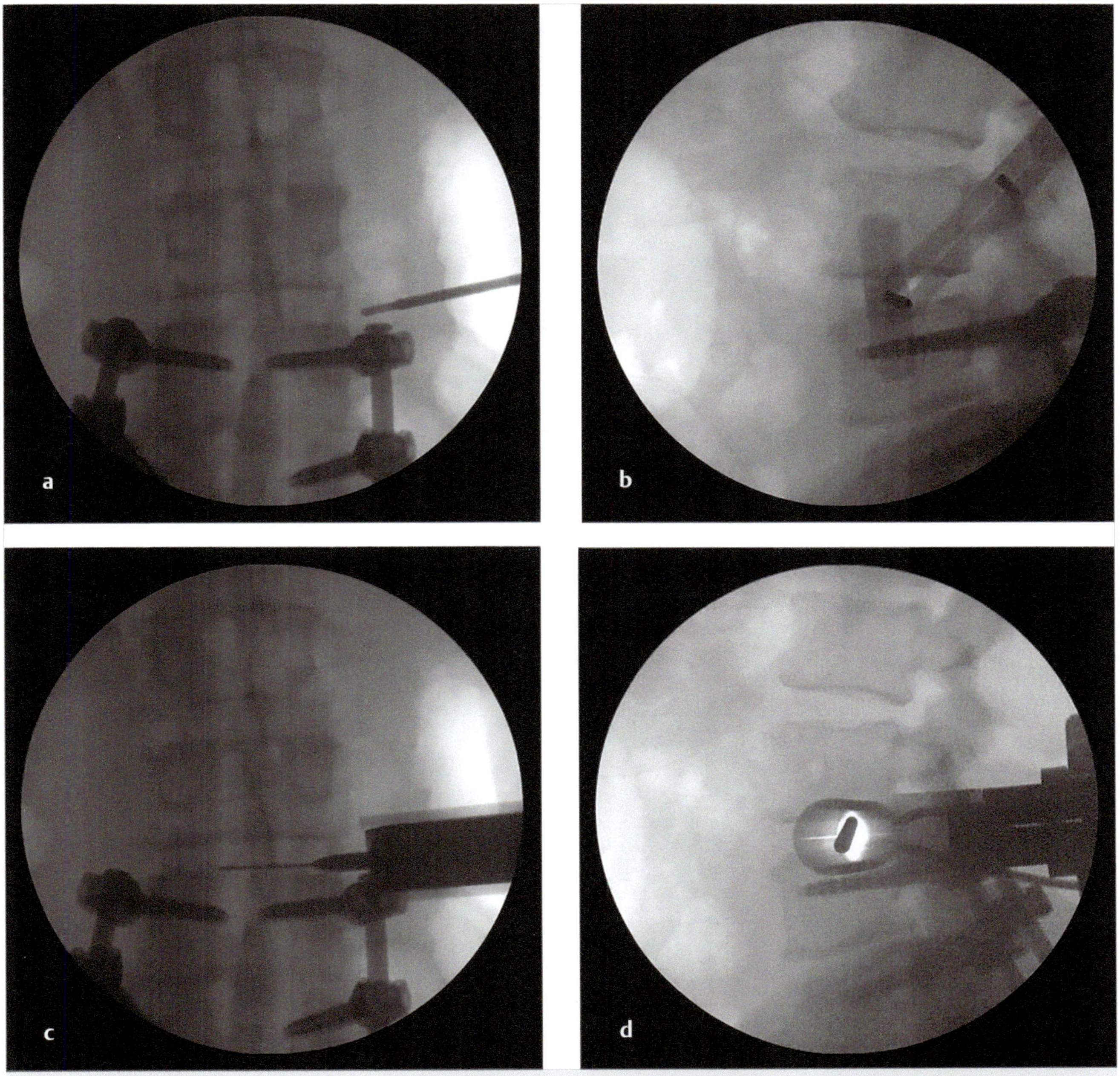

Fig. 13.15 Fluoroscopic images demonstrate localization and placement of the minimal access port for a transpsoas interbody approach. **(a)** Horizontal (anteroposterior) fluoroscopic image confirms the level as the introducer traverses the psoas. **(b)** Vertical (lateral) fluoroscopic image confirms midposition within the L3–4 disc space. **(c)** Horizontal (anteroposterior) fluoroscopic image enables positioning of the minimal access port with the dilators still in position. **(d)** Vertical (lateral) fluoroscopic image confirms ideal position of the introducer within the disc space. Once the ideal position has been confirmed, little fluoroscopy will be necessary until division of the contralateral annulus.

13.21 Minimally Invasive Transforaminal Lumbar Interbody Fusion

Few procedures have garnered more attention in the literature on radiation exposure than the MIS TLIF. The literature on radiation with this procedure far exceeds the current literature covering the transpsoas approach and radiation, which by comparison is almost absent. It was the MIS TLIF that first drew my attention to the amount of radiation I was exposed to as I explored percutaneous techniques and progressed through my learning curve. The observations that I made regarding my radiation exposure with this procedure were the impetus behind discovering these low-dose radiation protocols that I found in the pediatric literature. Thus, having the MIS TLIF as the final case illustration in this chapter could not be more appropriate. The following case illustration brings together all the material

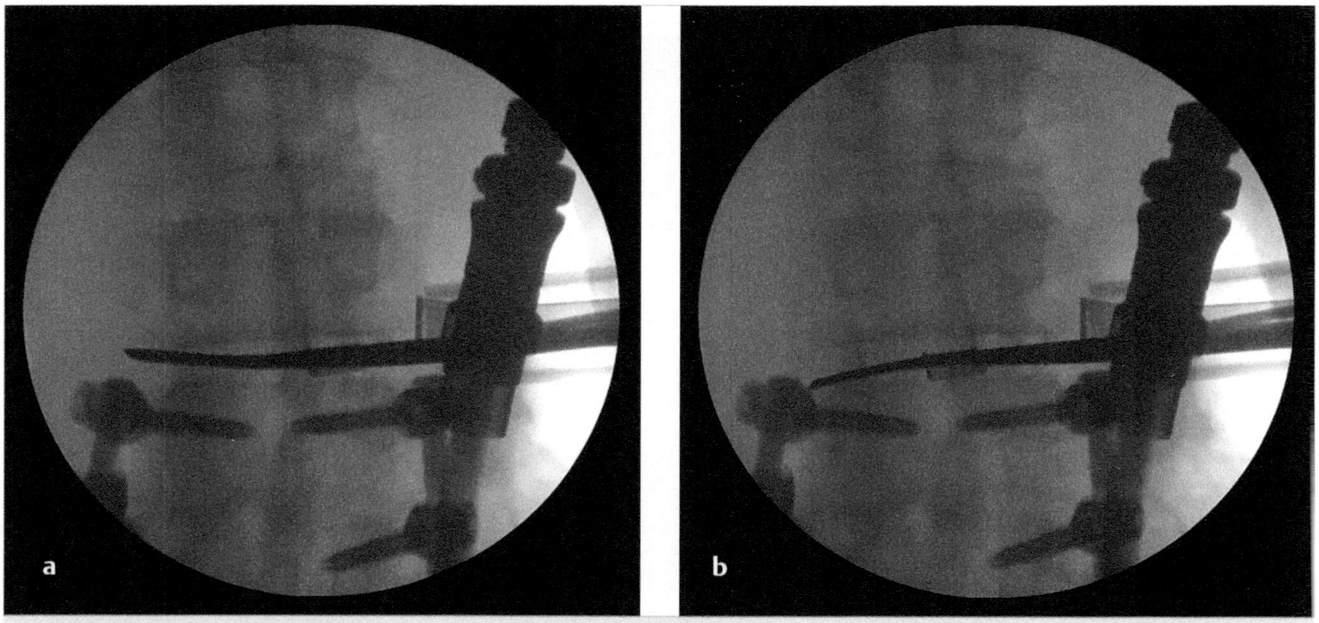

Fig. 13.16 Release of the contralateral annulus. The release of the annulus is primarily a tactile feeling of release that occurs when the Cobb gives way after tapping against it with a mallet. Visual confirmation is valuable, which justifies a fluoroscopic image to confirm release. Horizontal (anteroposterior) pulsed low-dose images obtained **(a)** for release of the contralateral annulus superior insertion and **(b)** for the inferior insertion.

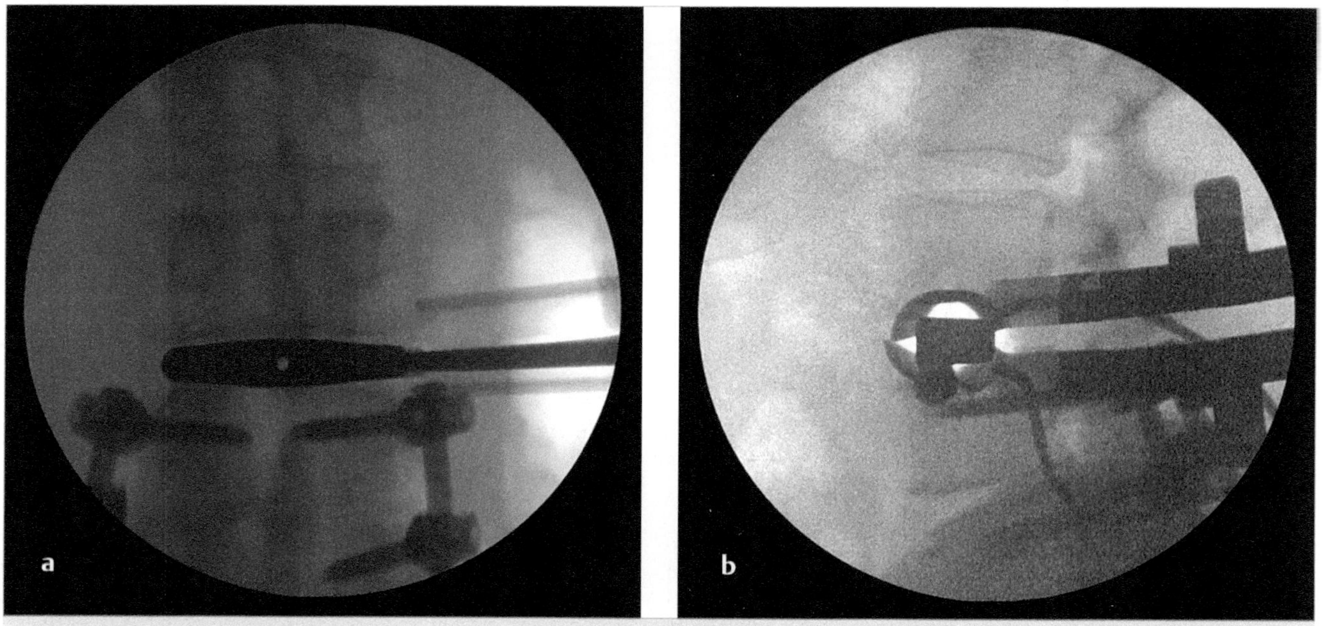

Fig. 13.17 Trial of the interbody spacer. **(a)** Horizontal (anteroposterior) pulsed low-dose image demonstrating the trial in the ideal position in the geometric center of the disc space. **(b)** Vertical (lateral) pulsed low-dose image demonstrating the interbody in the anterior one-half of the disc space.

covered in the last two chapters and lays the foundation for a systematic approach to reduce radiation exposure during the MIS TLIFs in your practice.

It should be noted that I refrained from using the digital spot technique, which offers a higher resolution image at a much higher dose of radiation, in the microdiscectomy, ACDF and transpsoas approaches. Only pulsed low-dose fluoroscopy was used in those cases. In the MIS TLIF, however, I routinely use the digital spot technique to confirm the pedicle screw entry points whenever the resolution is inadequate with pulsed fluoroscopy. ▶ Table 13.3 illustrates the various components of the MIS TLIF when fluoroscopy is needed to advance the procedure.

I have deconstructed the MIS TLIF into the various components of the operation where fluoroscopy is needed to advance

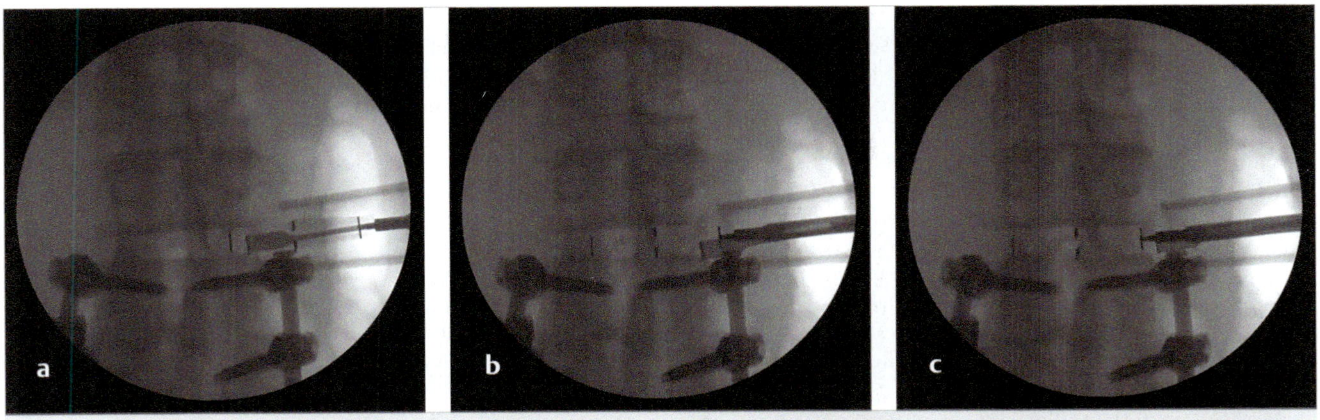

Fig. 13.18 Securing the interbody spacer into position. This series of pulsed low-dose horizontal (anteroposterior) images demonstrates the three images used to secure the interbody. **(a)** Image obtained to confirm trajectory. **(b)** Image obtained to demonstrate advancement of the interbody to the midline. **(c)** Image obtained to confirm ideal placement of the interbody.

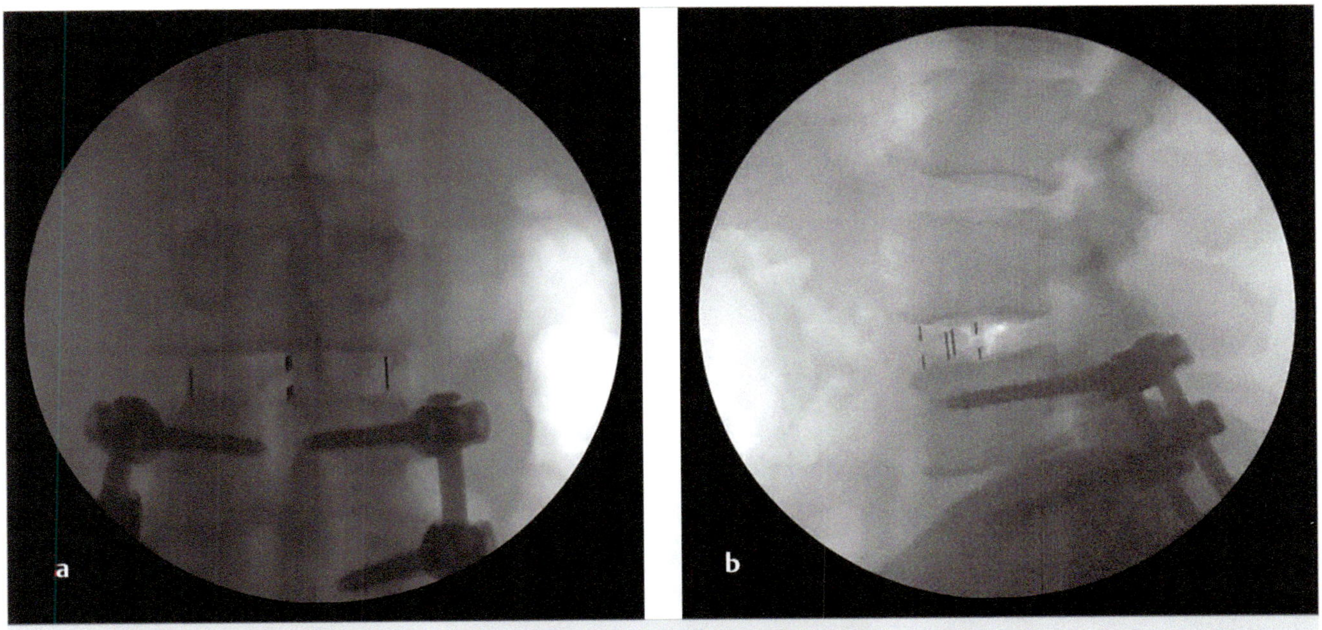

Fig. 13.19 Final horizontal (anteroposterior) and vertical (lateral) images. With the access port removed and the surgeon as far away from the X-ray source as possible, final pulsed low-dose **(a)** anteroposterior and **(b)** lateral images are obtained.

the procedure in ▶ Table 13.3. As in the previous case illustrations, I provide a range, fully cognizant that no two cases are the same. In Chapter 4, my emphasis was on describing the surgical technique, with some reference to a low-dose protocol. For this case illustration, however, fluoroscopy is the central focus.

13.22 Localization and Dilatation

Localizing and positioning the access ports require an adequate—not perfect—image that demonstrates the lumbosacral junction and allows for confirmation of the segment. An approximation of the incision at the beginning based on anatomical landmarks without any preoperative imaging saves time and decreases radiation exposure. The rationale for this approach is that any preoperative imaging will not preclude the need for imaging when it is time to make the incision. As described in Chapter 4, I will mark two 28-mm incisions 4 cm lateral to the midline and then prepare and drape the patient. Next, I will pass a 20-gauge spinal needle on one side onto the facet to confirm the level. Once an image confirms the first spinal needle is at the correct segment, I pass an 18-gauge spinal needle onto the contralateral facet. I will make the necessary adjustment to the incision to make my entry point on the skin on a trajectory completely parallel to the disc space (▶ Fig. 13.20).

13.23 Instrumentation

The next phase of the operation requires very little fluoroscopy. Instead, the focus is complete exposure of the facet joint, the pars interarticularis and the transverse processes to optimize direct visualization of the anatomy. After exposure of the junction of the pars interarticularis, transverse process and facet, one or two fluoroscopic images per pedicle is all that are needed to confirm the entry point. The key to minimizing the need for fluoroscopy at this phase of the operation is to unequivocally identify the superior and inferior aspects of the transverse process. The ideal pedicle screw entry point tends to be at the midpoint of the transverse process abutting the lateral aspect of the facet. Confirming the entry point with a single lateral fluoroscopic image may require digital spot fluoroscopy if the resolution is not adequate with a pulsed low-dose fluoroscopic image as in ▶ Fig. 13.7. In this case illustration, pulsed low-dose fluoroscopy offered adequate resolution for instrumenting the pedicles. Once I drill the entry point into the pedicle, the tip of the Lenke probe goes in search of the cancellous bone of the pedicle. The unmistakable feeling of the tip of the probe advancing into cancellous bone must be felt or else another fluoroscopic image will be required to confirm the location and trajectory of the probe. Provided the probe makes its way into the pedicle, the only role for a fluoroscopic image would be to confirm a trajectory parallel to the end plate.

Table 13.3 Mission-essential fluoroscopy for a single-level MIS TLIF

Radiographic objective	Minimum no. of images	Maximum no. of images
Localization (inverse square law)	2	4
Dilatation and securing the minimal access ports	4	8
Pedicle screw insertion × 4	16	25
Interbody trials	4	8
Placement of interbody spacer	5	10
Final AP and lateral images (inverse square law)	2	2
Total	33	57

Abbreviations: AP, anteroposterior; MIS TLIF, minimally invasive transforaminal lumbar interbody fusion.

After I remove the pedicle probe, a ball-tipped probe confirms the integrity of the pedicle and a tap prepares the way for the pedicle screw. Making note of the position of the pedicle probe relative to the minimal access port, as mentioned in Chapter 4, helps recapture the ideal trajectory into the pedicle with the tap and the pedicle screw. At this point, any additional images would be more for peace of mind than necessity. Recognizing that there is no real need for imaging at this point will help you eventually wean yourself from the need to obtain additional images. Watching the pedicle screw bottom out with direct visualization instead of with imaging is a valuable habit to develop. After all, once a pedicle screw has been tapped, the likelihood that it will take a different route is low but not absent. Taking the time to directly visualize the tip of the pedicle screw as it enters the tapped hole makes an alternate route almost impossible, whether you obtain 1 image or 10 images (▶ Fig. 13.21).

As the sole surgeon operating in this case presentation, one side was done at a time. Therefore, I repeated the sequence on the contralateral side after two pedicle screws were placed on the ipsilateral side. All four pedicle screws were secured with 16 lateral pulsed dose fluoroscopic images, after five images were required to confirm the segment and secure the minimal access ports.

13.24 Interbody Trial and Placement

After placement of the pedicle screws, no additional fluoroscopy will be necessary until I have completed the laminectomy, facetectomy, decompression and discectomy phases of the operation. In fact, the next image will not be required until it is time to try the interbody spacer. The need for imaging is low if not absent for preparation of the end plates and distraction of the disc space. A completely collapsed disc space is the one exception to that rule. The inability to access the disc space with conventional interbody instruments may require an osteo-

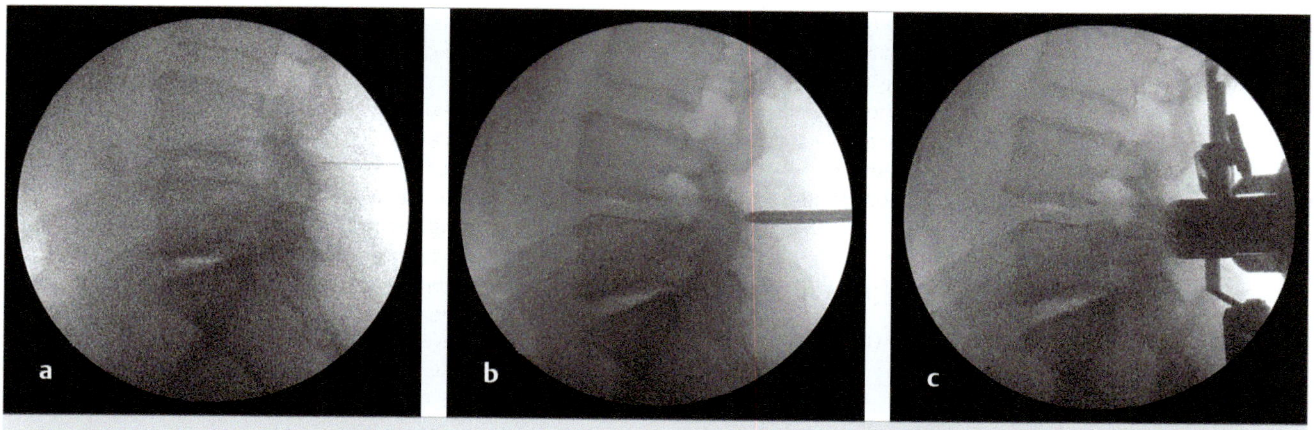

Fig. 13.20 Localization and dilatation. **(a)** Pulsed low-dose fluoroscopy with a spinal needle placed based on anatomical landmarks to confirm the operative level. The spinal needle is in an axial plane higher than the middle of the disc space. To optimize the trajectory onto the segment, the incision was slightly adjusted in the caudal direction. Although the image is not an optimal image, it is more than adequate for localization. **(b)** Pulsed low-dose fluoroscopy with slightly higher kVp to decrease the noise. Note the increased resolution over in **b** as compared to **a**. This image offers adequate resolution to secure the minimal access port. Maintaining the initial dilator in position precludes the need for subsequent images as the paraspinal muscles are dilated. **(c)** The minimal access port may be positioned and the trajectory confirmed with a lateral pulsed low-dose image before securing the access port into its final position.

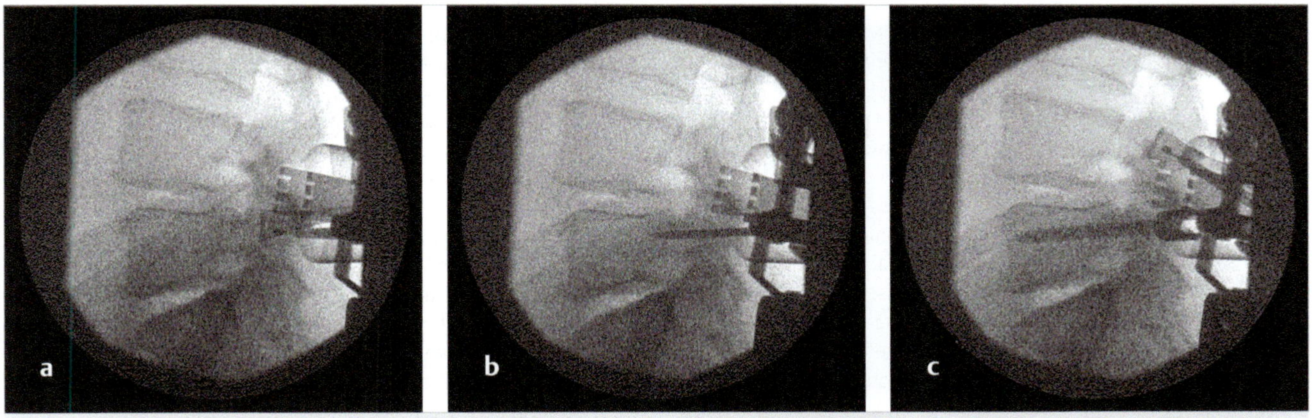

Fig. 13.21 Placement of pedicle screw with pulsed low-dose collimated fluoroscopy. **(a)** Lateral fluoroscopic image confirming pedicle screw entry point. In this case, pulsed low-dose fluoroscopy provided adequate resolution of the pedicle. **(b)** Confirmation of the trajectory of the Lenke probe parallel to the end plate. **(c)** Placement of the pedicle screw (placement of the tap not demonstrated).

tome to pry open the interbody space. Use of an osteotome requires complete alignment with the disc space to prevent the potential disruption of an end plate. Fluoroscopy is the most reliable manner to ensure that the ideal trajectory has been captured, and it is therefore needed to safely advance the operation. Fortunately, such a clinical circumstance is uncommon. Placement of the trial interbody spacer may require one or two additional images to confirm the trajectory. As the trials increase in size, an occasional additional image may be required. Placement of an interbody that rotates into position will require two or three additional images to guide the rotation of the interbody device into ideal position (▶ Fig. 13.22).

If the nested interbody technique is used, only one or two additional images are required because the second interbody tends to find its way onto the posterior aspect of the first interbody (▶ Fig. 13.23). There is little resistance to placement of a second interbody because the first interbody maintains the disc height. Furthermore, as the second interbody enters the disc space, it tends to nest into the first interbody. Thus, there is little need for additional fluoroscopy. I obtain a final anteroposterior image while I am as far away from the X-ray source as the need for sterility will allow me to be. I place the final rods and the set screws, which I torque tighten to complete the operation. In this case, the operation was completed with 3.2 seconds of fluoroscopy and 9.87 mGy of radiation exposure to the patient.

13.25 Summary of the Low-Dose Protocol in Minimally Invasive Spine Surgery

In the introduction to this Primer, I presented the concept that MIS should not necessarily equate with higher doses of radiation. Although the literature has demonstrated greater exposures with various procedures, awareness should drive radiation exposure down, not up. Minimally invasive spine surgeons must abandon the mentality that their approaches will require more imaging and thus more radiation. Instead, I suggest that we adopt the mentality that our surgical procedures should require less radiation than ever before and certainly less than the open equivalents. Adopting this mindset represents a change in culture founded upon education, awareness and the need to evolve. The theme of each of the chapters in this Primer has emphasized that MIS is part of the inevitable evolution of spine surgery. Radiation awareness, education and minimization must be part of that evolution. The continued development of image guidance, further refinements in the algorithms that govern fluoroscopy, and the use of image enhancement software will further this goal far into the future. If spine surgery adopts this thinking, the next generation of spine surgeons will be exposed to less radiation than any generation before them.

In the meantime, using the fluoroscopy techniques that our pediatric cardiology and urology colleagues developed decades ago is the surest path to accomplish that goal. ▶ Table 13.4 provides a summary of goals for radiation exposure in the common minimally invasive spinal procedures. My surgical procedures do not always fall within these parameters in every case. Some cases are more difficult than others, but I strive for these numbers with every case. Sometimes I am surprised when I have completed the operation under the stated goal. However, the most important element is not the value of milligrays at the end of the case, but the awareness of radiation exposure that comes with adopting the mindset that to safely and efficiently accomplish the goals of surgery, an adequate image at the lowest possible radiation exposure should be the one you acquire. With such a mindset, you will experience a change in culture in your operating room, one case at a time.

▶ Table 13.4 summarizes the radiation exposure goals for the common minimally invasive procedures. The most important value is that of exposure, whereas the least important is time. I would prefer 5 mGy and 10 seconds of fluoroscopy to 10 mGy and 5 seconds of fluoroscopy. The numbers of images are guidelines to help you adopt a mindset for acquiring an image only when necessary to advance the operation. The number of images required to perform an operation will decrease as you develop an aptitude to mentally reconstruct the anatomy at depth.

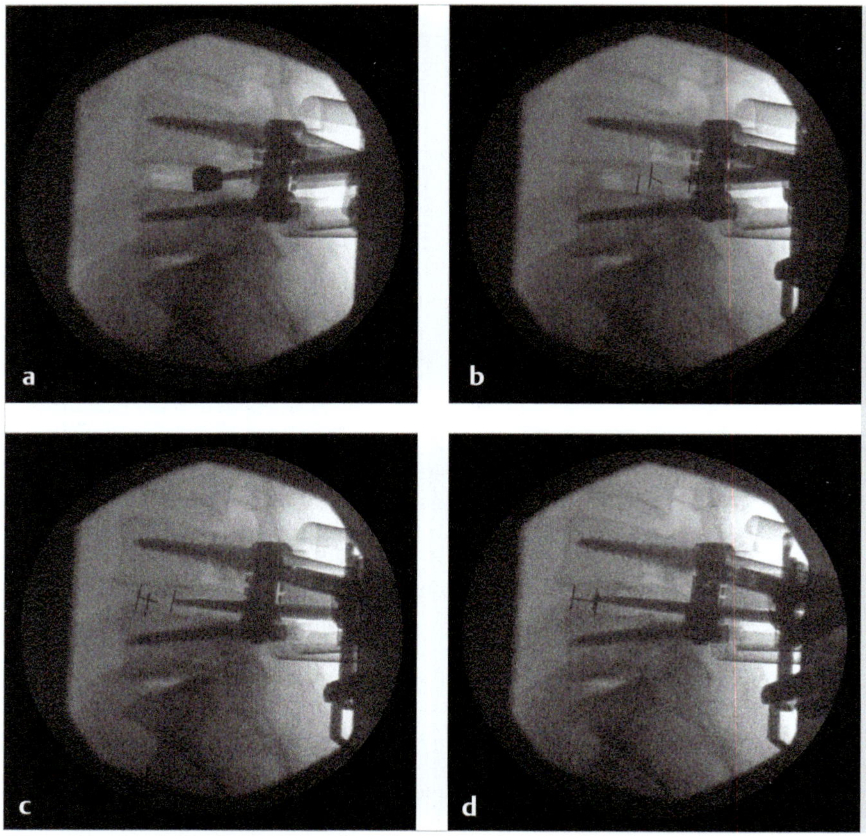

Fig. 13.22 Placement of an interbody spacer using pulsed low-dose fluoroscopic images. **(a)** A lateral fluoroscopic image confirms the trajectory of the interbody trial as it enters the disc space. **(b)** A lateral fluoroscopic image again confirms the trajectory into the disc space. **(c)** Rotation of the interbody within the disc space. **(d)** Completing the rotation into the front of the disc space.

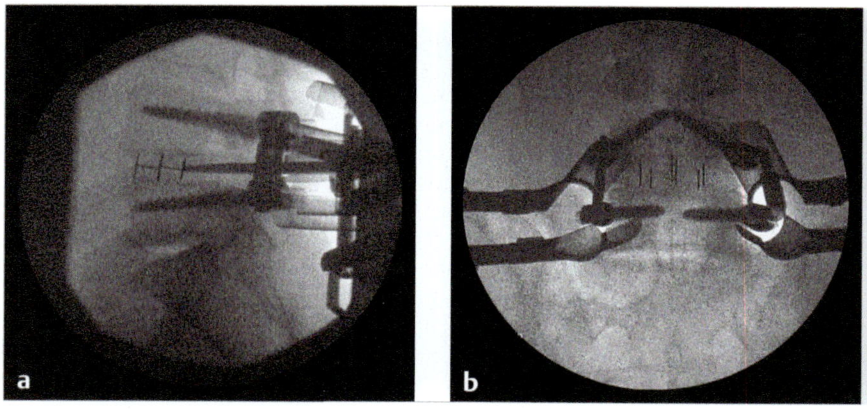

Fig. 13.23 The final **(a)** lateral and **(b)** anteroposterior (AP) images for an L4–5 minimally invasive transforaminal lumbar interbody fusion. Both images were obtained using pulsed low-dose fluoroscopy. The inverse square law can be fully embraced for the final AP image.

13.26 The Future of Imaging the Spine for Minimally Invasive Spine Surgery

It is difficult for me to end this chapter and Primer without at least some speculation about the future of imaging the spine, especially at a time when the rate of innovation only continues to increase. I will likely perform my final operation as a spine surgeon in 2038. I often wonder how different that operating room will be from the one in which I currently reside. There is little doubt that image guidance will have taken seismic leaps forward and will be seamlessly linked to the functionality of the operating room. Instead of the unwieldy process of localizing and registering as we know it today, the entire process will have receded unnoticeably into the background. Perhaps registration scans will occur as the patient rolls into the operating room and visualization of anatomy becomes linked to heads-up displays embedded within glasses or virtual reality headsets instead of monitors. Augmented reality in some form will also be present on those headsets of tomorrow.

It should not be surprising to the reader to learn that the object of most of my speculation is the fluoroscope. Will there even be one at all in the operating room in 2038? I would

Table 13.4 Goals for minimizing radiation exposure

Procedure	Total exposure (mGy)	No. of images	No. of digital spot images	Time (s)
MIS microdiscectomy	< 1	5	0	1
Single-level ACDF	< 1	10	0	2
Lateral transpsoas interbody lumbar fusion	10	50	5	10
MIS TLIF	10	35	5	5

Abbreviations: ACDF, anterior cervical discectomy and fusion; mGy, milligray; MIS, minimally invasive spine surgery; MIS TLIF, minimally invasive transforaminal lumbar interbody fusion.

venture to guess that despite all the advances in navigation technologies, the fluoroscope survives well into the future. The more pressing questions for me are what it will look like and how it will function.

The first item that I predict will disappear is the bulky vacuum tube image intensifier. Flat panel detectors, which are available today mostly in angiographic suites, will become commonplace in the operating room on the other side of the X-ray tube. The inherent design of the flat panel detector is more efficient than the image intensifier and therefore will require less radiation per image. The result will be dramatically decreased radiation exposure to patients, surgeons and operating room personnel with an increase in the quality of images.

The implementation of image-enhancement technology is my second prediction regarding the fluoroscope in the operating room of tomorrow. As of this writing, there are already various forms of image enhancement technologies based on a full-dose fluoroscopic image which can then be superimposed onto lower-quality images obtained at a much lower exposure. These technologies will continue to develop, along with other forms of image-enhancement technologies. The various images in the case illustrations in this chapter are grainy low-resolution images. Although adequate for the intended purpose, there is no reason that these images cannot be improved. The current state-of-the-art technology in image enhancement in 2020 already has the capacity to transform those images into high-resolution images. I see no reason why, by 2038, any of us will ever have to look at noisy, grainy images. Fluoroscopic images obtained with exceptionally low doses of radiation, captured by flat panel detectors and enhanced by image-editing software, will become the norm.

My final prediction is that the fluoroscope will become integrated with the operating table. Every day we conduct surgical procedures with a motionless patient on an operating table. While the table may move up and down and the fluoroscope may slide to the head or the foot of the bed, the patient remains in the same position. Despite a motionless patient, the number of wasted fluoroscopic images obtained trying to get back to that initial ideal image are too numerous to count. Our technological breakthrough for mitigating these approximating images involves the application of tape to the floor. Despite all the tape we put on the floor and all the various approximations of the operating room table height, the wasted images keep occurring. If localizing beacons could be incorporated on the fluoroscope and the operating table, as well as on the patient at the level of interest, it would not only prevent a wasted image from occurring but would ensure an ideal image every time.

Precision images guided by beacons and near-field technology will not require technologists to operate them. In fact, human involvement may be a liability. Integrated operating table–fluoroscopes will no doubt inhabit the operating room of the future. The same artificial intelligence that can scan large databases and identify a single human face from a surveillance video among the thousands of faces in that database may be employed to identify a suboptimal lateral image of a cervical spine and correct it perfectly—every time. The integration of the fluoroscope with the operating table would allow the fluoroscope to automatically rotate the bed or adjust the wag of the C-arm. It would not be an educated guess by the surgeon or the fluoroscopic technologist in one direction or another. As thoughtful and educated as our well-intended guesses may be, they reliably result in three or four additional images after the bed is moved, then the C-arm, then both. Instead, our conjecture about what to move and to what degree to move it will be replaced by a precise adjustment based on what the artificially intelligent brain of the fluoroscope knows to be a perfect lateral or anteroposterior image. All previous skeletal imaging of the patient for the relevant anatomy will have been fed into the artificially intelligent fluoroscopic brain. For instance, in a patient with scoliosis, the 36-inch standing anteroposterior and lateral X-rays will already be part of the fluoroscope's memory. Those images will have prepared the automated artificially intelligent fluoroscopic robot to precisely image the spine at the time of surgery based on thousands of images within its database.

Throughout the entire process of image optimization, the surgeon and radiology technologist would be approving preoperative images from a safe distance away, viewing the images generated by this enhanced fluoroscope from perhaps a tablet computer before approving them. At the time of surgery, the images would be acquired once again without marking the floor of the operating room with tape or pencil marks. If the fluoroscopic technologist changed because the end of a shift occurred, it would have no effect on the next image required by the surgeon. The beacons and near-field technology would guide the perfect anteroposterior and lateral view perfectly, every time. Even subtle, unnoticeable shifts in the spine from the operation would be identified, and adjustments would be made for the optimal image throughout the surgery. Requests for an image will be as they are today. However, it will be voice recognition technology that will bring the fluoroscope into the operative field to obtain the requested anteroposterior or lateral image. With such automation, the question arises as to the role of the radiology technologist. The expertise of such a technologist will still be required, but one technologist would likely be able to monitor several rooms simultaneously.

Tragically, all this technology exists today, but no bridge exists to bring these current technologies into our current operating theaters. Perhaps with increasing awareness of the importance of decreasing radiation exposure, alongside the ever-expanding and resourceful technology of today, construction of that bridge will begin. Such a bridge may span the current chasm that exists between the modern technologies outside the operating theater and may supplant the antiquated technology of yesterday that still constrains our surgical procedures today. Only time will tell how accurate these predictions will be. Perhaps a reader of this Primer will have a hand in the development of that operating room in 2038 where I will perform my final operation. After all, the mind once enlightened cannot again become dark.

The End

References

[1] Mariscalco MW, Yamashita T, Steinmetz MP, Krishnaney AA, Lieberman IH, Mroz TE. Radiation exposure to the surgeon during open lumbar microdiscectomy and minimally invasive microdiscectomy: a prospective, controlled trial. Spine. 2011; 36(3):255–260

[2] Zaidi HA, Montoure A, Nakaji P, Bice A, Tumialán LMA. A 5-year retrospective analysis of exposure to ionizing radiation by neurosurgery residents in the modern era. World Neurosurg. 2016; 86:220–225

[3] Abdullah KG, Bishop FS, Lubelski D, Steinmetz MP, Benzel EC, Mroz TE. Radiation exposure to the spine surgeon in lumbar and thoracolumbar fusions with the use of an intraoperative computed tomographic 3-dimensional imaging system. Spine. 2012; 37(17):E1074–E1078

[4] Spitz SM, Sandhu FA, Voyadzis JM. Percutaneous "K-wireless" pedicle screw fixation technique: an evaluation of the initial experience of 100 screws with assessment of accuracy, radiation exposure, and procedure time. J Neurosurg Spine. 2015; 22(4):422–431

[5] Wesenberg RL, Amundson GM. Fluoroscopy in children: low-exposure technology. Radiology. 1984; 153(1):243–247

[6] Campbell RM, Strieper MJ, Frias PA, et al. Quantifying and minimizing radiation exposure during pediatric cardiac catheterization. Pediatr Cardiol. 2005; 26(1):29–33

[7] Belanger B, Boudry J. Management of pediatric radiation dose using GE fluoroscopic equipment. Pediatr Radiol. 2006; 36 Suppl 2:204–211

[8] Bindal RK, Glaze S, Ognoskie M, Tunner V, Malone R, Ghosh S. Surgeon and patient radiation exposure in minimally invasive transforaminal lumbar interbody fusion. J Neurosurg Spine. 2008; 9(6):570–573

[9] Cohen MD. Optimizing the use of pulsed fluoroscopy to reduce radiation exposure to children. J Am Coll Radiol. 2008; 5(3):205–209

[10] Tumialán LM, Clark JC, Snyder LA, Jasmer G, Marciano FF. Prospective evaluation of a low-dose radiation fluoroscopy protocol for minimally invasive transforaminal lumbar interbody fusions. Oper Neurosurg (Hagerstown). 2015; 11(4):537–544

[11] Clark JC, Jasmer G, Marciano FF, Tumialán LM. Minimally invasive transforaminal lumbar interbody fusions and fluoroscopy: a low-dose protocol to minimize ionizing radiation. Neurosurg Focus. 2013; 35(2):E8

[12] Mroz TE, Abdullah KG, Steinmetz MP, Klineberg EO, Lieberman IH. Radiation exposure to the surgeon during percutaneous pedicle screw placement. J Spinal Disord Tech. 2011; 24(4):264–267

[13] Taylor AJ. Impact of digital spot imaging in gastrointestinal fluoroscopy. AJR Am J Roentgenol. 1999; 173(4):1065–1069

Bibliography

[1] Rockwell T. The Rickover Effect: The Inside Story of How Adm. Hyman Rickover Built the Nuclear Navy. Naval Institute Press; 1992

[2] Oliver D. Against the Tide: Rickover's Leadership Principles and the Rise of the Nuclear Navy. Naval Institute Press; 2014

Coda to the Primer

The Primer that you have before you arose more by accident than by design. As surprising as it may sound, it was never my intention to compose a book from beginning to end quite like this one. Who would voluntarily and knowingly subject themselves to such a burden? Instead, my goal was to provide inquisitive residents and fellows with some information for the rationale, anatomical basis and surgical techniques used in a few commonly performed minimally invasive spine procedures. My review of the various available minimally invasive spine texts suggested there was a need for a practical primer on the topic. I was hoping to fill a void. I initially considered addressing just three procedures: microdiscectomy, laminectomy and transforaminal lumbar interbody fusion. At the outset, I envisioned a small booklet containing a handful of pages with an image or two for good measure.

Over the years, residents and fellows asked increasingly challenging questions about how and why I do certain things in one procedure and not in others, which forced me to think long and hard to answer their questions. The research that went into answering these questions transformed the innocent but rudimentary outlines that I had scribbled down into veritable chapters that all of a sudden had the potential to be worth reading. Dr. Peter Nakaji, my friend and colleague, happened upon some of these fledgling chapters and encouraged me to present the concept to the editors at Thieme Medical Publishers. I was surprised by the warm reception the concept of the Primer received and zestfully went about the task of composing it. The year was 2015.

It goes without saying that I am indebted to those residents and fellows for their initial questions, feedback, thoughtful critiques and commentaries. Drs. Laura Snyder, Justin Clark, David Fusco and Mark Mahan were among the early residents at Barrow Neurological Institute who rotated through my service with a genuine curiosity in minimally invasive spine surgery. Their presence with me in the early years of my own learning curve not only made me a better surgeon but created the spark to begin this work. I am also appreciative of the fellows I have worked with, many of whom read various early forms of the chapters and offered me necessary feedback as to which of my analogies and metaphors were valuable for communicating a message and which fell flat. Carson Fairbanks, Ryan Godinsky, Samuel Rosenbaum, Keven Burns, Nicholas Scarcella and John McElroy all offered incredible insight, which contributed meaningfully to the chapters of this book. I am especially grateful to John McElroy, who systemically read the first draft of the entire book during the course of his fellowship. And of course, I appreciate Timothy Hiscock and Sarah Landis, the editors at Thieme, for their endless patience. They have the forbearance of Job.

It would be remiss of me not to acknowledge Georgetown University School of Medicine and the incredible culture that it fosters in the development of future physicians. In certain ways, Georgetown laid the foundation for this work. I am grateful to Ms. Donna Rae Sullivan, from the office of admissions, who saw the potential in me. I am grateful to the members of the department of orthopedics and for the time the members of that department invested in teaching medical students like myself. I will never forget the teaching rounds with Dr. John Delahay, which introduced the panoramic perspective of a person's care. Nor will I forget the late Dr. Bill Lauerman, who was the first to teach me how to assess radiographs of a lumbar spine. I would not have had the success I achieved at Georgetown had it not been for my roommates, Drs. Michael Ronald Vaughan and Derrick Joseph Fluhme. During our 4 years together, Derrick and Michael were instrumental in drilling the valuable information that lays the foundation for the practice of medicine into my rather thick head. Dr. Anthony M. Turkiewicz, my gross anatomy partner, polished my knowledge to a brilliant shine and continues to do so to this day. Thank you, Michael, Derrick and Anthony.

Had it not been for Drs. Karl Schultz and Catalino Dureza at the Balboa Naval Medical Center in San Diego, I would not have found my way into a career in neurosurgery. A fearsome thought. Both "Kip" and "Cat" fostered and encouraged my interest in neurosurgery, for which I will be eternally grateful. Along the way, Drs. Timothy Mickel and Scott Carlson bolstered me through my surgical internship and overseas operational tours. I am especially grateful to the Naval Special Warfare community, who took me in like a lost puppy and always ensured my safety in the most exotic and harrowing of places. CDR Dana DeCoster always covered my "six."

I remain convinced that the Department of Neurosurgery at Emory University provides the finest environment for a resident to seek neurosurgery training. I am indebted to that department for providing me with the opportunity to train at such an incredible institution. I was fortunate to have Drs. Bryan Barnes and Patrick Tomak as chief residents to guide a hapless junior resident transitioning from operational medicine fresh from the field through the first year of a neurosurgery residency. I was equally fortunate to have Drs. Christopher J. Farrell and Sanjay Dhall as co-residents. And no one could have a better cochief resident than Dr. Jeremy Ciporen.

At Emory, the surgical mentality espoused by Dr. Daniel Louis Barrow truly transforms the resident into a veritable neurosurgeon. The anatomical certitude orated by Dr. Nelson Oyesiku, the methodical approach of Dr. Jeffrey Olson, and the complex understanding of neuronal pathways and the surgical alteration of those pathways taught to me by Dr. Robert Gross are all fundamental building blocks that shape a neurosurgeon. The Grady Memorial Hospital experience at Emory as a chief resident is transformational. I am grateful to Dr. Sanjay K. Gupta for his willingness to take on every case I could find with me. It was at Emory that I first performed a minimally invasive transforaminal lumbar interbody fusion under the guidance of Dr. Praveen Mummaneni in 2006. The patience that Dr. Mummaneni demonstrated during those early cases was nothing short of remarkable and began my lifelong interest in minimally invasive spinal surgery. It was also at Emory, where under the mentorship of Dr. Gerald Rodts, I had the epiphany that spine surgery would be my career path. Dr. Rodts set the standard for me and countless other residents with his command of spine anatomy, surgical expertise and composed communication with patients and colleagues that I strive for even today. "Always remember that the practice of medicine is a privilege and always remember to give something back," were the words that Dr. Rodts left me with as I completed my spine rotation. Throughout the years, that adage has come frequently to mind, especially at the most difficult of times. I hope this Primer fulfills, in some small manner, part of that obligation.

Drs. Wayne Gluf, Martin Holland, Arnett Klugh and Min Park were the neurosurgeons at Balboa Naval Medical Center in San Diego when I returned to active duty in the Navy after Emory. The cross pollination that occurred in that department was transformative for me as a surgeon. It would be difficult to conceive of my career without those two years working with my shipmates in the Navy. Balboa was also where I was able to reunite and collaborate with Dr. Anthony Riccio, a fellow Georgetown classmate. I am grateful to my friend, Dr. Nicholas Theodore, for recruiting me to join him in Phoenix and thereby making this Primer a feasible project.

I made no attempt in this book to hide my genuine interest in the history of our specialty. The love of history was a gift given to me by my mother, who would regale me as a child with fascinating tale after tale of Roman battles and Greek mythology from her encyclopedic knowledge of literature and history. She would effortlessly recite entire poems from Pedro Calderón de la Barca, Rubén Darío and José Martí from memory. In doing so, she inspired a lifelong yearning for reading history and literature. My mother could always find the perfect book to put into my hands that would send me to the Battle of Lepanto or the Siege of Rhodes. And to this day, she remains incredibly adept at finding those perfect volumes to put into my grasp. Despite the concerns expressed by my editors, the fingerprints of that inclination for history and literature remain smudged all over each chapter.

I would never have found the fulfillment and satisfaction that only a career in medicine can uniquely provide were it not for my father. I have always admired the thoughtful analysis of the pathology he would provide to surgeons reviewing a case. He taught me the power of anatomical certitude. He taught me that knowledge is the true organ of sight. It was his example that guided me into this wonderful privilege that society has bestowed upon us to serve as physicians in our communities. Throughout all of my life, my sisters, Carmen and Rosa, have been a relentless cheering squad for their brother. For that, I am forever grateful.

The unwavering support that my wife Andrea has provided throughout the process of composing this Primer has always bolstered me, especially at times when I have wondered whether this book would ever see the light of day. Andrea never seemed to have a doubt. One thing is certain: without her love and support, this book would never have materialized the components parts needed to see it through to completion. Throughout my years of residency, practice and especially in the composition of this work, Andrea has been my serene Gibraltar of emotional substance. A stronger woman capable of effortlessly handling and naturally managing so many challenging aspects of family, school, community and life is difficult for me to conceive. Gratitude, awe, admiration and my unfailing love are all I can offer in return.

I am grateful for my sons, Julian Manuel, Andreas Jorge and Lucian Galen, who demonstrated exceptional patience throughout this book-writing process. These young men sat patiently waiting to start soccer drills or a baseball practice (St. Louis Cardinal baseball hats on and gloves in hand) while I finished just one more paragraph. I cherish my daughter, Alexandra Soledad, who filled the mornings with beautiful piano playing as I wrote. Her nimble little fingers deftly tapping the keys of the piano in perfect time provided me the idea for the analogy I used in Chapter 13 to describe the inverse square law that governs not only sound but radiation.

The late author Kurt Vonnegut Jr. had the revelation that most authors write to please one person that they know very, very well, even if they do not realize that they are doing so as they write. It was when I was sparring with my editors regarding some of my unconventional writing in a scientific text that I realized that Vonnegut was right. Though I did not recognize it at first, I was writing to please one particular person: my brother. I have dedicated this book to the memory of my brother Jorge. His loss so many years ago remains a wound within my heart that has been reluctant to heal despite the passage of time. Surprisingly, writing this Primer has served as a balm for that wound. My brother was a master wordsmith. His capacity to assemble a colorful argument with artful sentences had no peer. He was always my Editor-in-Chief, routinely transforming my inadequate prose into polished literary pearls. One of the last passages Jorge edited was the personal statement that I used in my application to a neurosurgery residency program. Jorge could always find that magic word or perfect phrase to hammer home a point or enlighten the mind. He could always make me smile. And so, if the reader finds a sentence here or there throughout this Primer that seems out of place but triggers a smile, you should know that it is a sentence for Jorge. For me, he lives on in this way. Amen.

Luis Manuel Tumialán
Phoenix, Arizona
December 2019

Index

Note: Page numbers set **bold** or *italic* indicate headings or figures, respectively.

D

E

F

N

O

P

U

V

W

X